THE PRINCIPLES AND PRACTICE OF MEDICINE

THE PRINCIPLES AND PRACTICE OF MEDICINE

DESIGNED FOR THE USE OF PRACTITIONERS AND STUDENTS OF MEDICINE

ORIGINALLY WRITTEN BY

THE LATE SIR WILLIAM OSLER, BT., M.D., F.R.S.

FORMERLY FELLOW OF THE ROYAL COLLEGE OF PHYSICIANS, LONDON; REGIUS PROFESSOR OF MEDICINE, OXFORD UNIVERSITY; HONORARY PROFESSOR OF MEDICINE, JOHNS HOPKINS UNIVERSITY, BALTIMORE; PROFESSOR OF THE INSTITUTE OF MEDICINE, McGILL UNIVERSITY, MONTREAL, AND PROFESSOR OF CLINICAL MEDICINE IN THE UNIVERSITY OF PENNSYLVANIA, PHILADELPHIA

TWELFTH EDITION; REVISION BY

THOMAS McCRAE, M.D.

FELLOW OF THE ROYAL COLLEGE OF PHYSICIANS, LONDON; PROFESSOR OF MEDICINE, JEFFERSON MEDICAL COLLEGE, PHILADELPHIA; PHYSICIAN TO THE JEFFERSON AND PENNSYLVANIA HOSPITALS, PHILADELPHIA; FORMERLY ASSOCIATE PROFESSOR OF MEDICINE, JOHNS HOPKINS UNIVERSITY

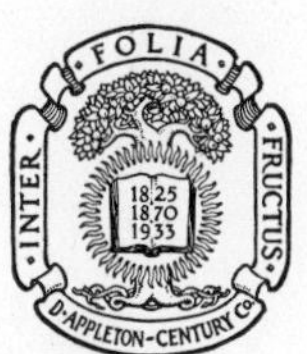

D. APPLETON-CENTURY COMPANY
INCORPORATED

NEW YORK LONDON

PRINTED IN THE UNITED STATES OF AMERICA

TO THE

Memory of Three Teachers of William Osler:

WILLIAM ARTHUR JOHNSON

PRIEST OF THE PARISH OF WESTON, ONTARIO

JAMES BOVELL

OF THE TORONTO SCHOOL OF MEDICINE, AND OF THE UNIVERSITY OF TRINITY COLLEGE, TORONTO

ROBERT PALMER HOWARD

DEAN OF THE MEDICAL FACULTY AND PROFESSOR OF MEDICINE, MCGILL UNIVERSITY, MONTREAL

PREFACE

In this edition, which is completely reset, a new type is used which permits of more words to the page and which is regarded as being more easily read. A page which gives the maximum of comfort in being read is particularly desirable in a textbook. There are certain other qualities which, in my opinion, a textbook should possess. One, that it should not be of a size and weight which make it difficult to handle and uncomfortable to hold. The contents should represent what may be regarded as sound, conservative and established knowledge; a textbook is not a year-book and should not be blown about by every wind of doctrine. It is tempting to discuss theories but the place for this is elsewhere.

In the revision of a textbook there is the constant decision to be made as to how much of what is new should displace what is older. There is no difficulty in finding material which may be added but how much of it has permanent value and represents an actual addition to knowledge is not easy to decide. It is a useful lesson to study material which was under consideration for addition to previous editions but was not included. This shows how much that appears in the literature has little or no permanent value although it may have a temporary interest. Perhaps this applies most particularly to treatment, in judging of the value of which we should pray to be delivered from hasty judgments.

In these days it is often said that the number of thoroughly trained clinicians is growing less and that internal medicine is being split up more and more into separate compartments with walls of various thickness between them. This tends to emphasize the study of one system without sufficient attention to the patient as an individual made up of many systems. Certainly we should keep before ourselves and our students the need of emphasis on the study of the patient as a whole and as a human being, and all the manifestations of disease as shown in him. Too often the idea is held that a clinician can be made over night, especially with the aid of instruments and laboratory procedures. In saying this the value of the aid from these is not made light of but time and effort and hard work must go to the acquiring of a knowledge of disease and the patient in whom it exists. We can not be Oslers but we can do our best to follow his steps. The physician and student should always make it a rule to learn everything possible about a patient by the use of his own senses and brains. For example, to have a roentgenologist make the diagnosis of fluid in a pleural cavity should cause a clinician to be thoroughly ashamed of himself. As far as possible a textbook of medicine should emphasize the clinical side of disease problems.

Diseases change in many ways and one of the interests as one grows older in his medical life is to watch these variations. New diseases, or what seem new, appear; some grow less important; others disappear. We have lost chlorosis and we do not know the reason; various forms of encephalitis have become more frequent and we have no explanation. Typhoid fever has become so infrequent in cities that our students have no proper opportunity to learn to know the disease, but in rural areas they may meet it as an unknown entity.

There are changes and additions in practically every part of the book, perhaps more especially in the discussion of diagnosis and treatment. Certain sections are new or have been materially altered. Among these are: Undulant Fever, Haverhill Fever—Erythema Arthriticum Epidemicum, Glandular Fever, Epituberculosis, Purified Protein Derivative Tuberculin, Psittacosis, Sonne Dysentery, Epidemic Diaphragmatic Pleurodynia, Lymphogranuloma Inguinale (Climatic or Tropical Bubo), Arachnidism, Manganese Poisoning, Favism, Chronic Hyperinsulinism—Hypoglycemia, von Gierke's Disease, Diabetes Mellitus (including new food tables), Uveoparotitis, Sialolithiasis, Congenital Short Esophagus—Thoracic Stomach, Para-esophageal Hernia, Cirrhosis Ventriculi—Linitis Plastica, Diseases of the Duodenum, Local Ileitis, Melanosis of the Colon, Digestive Disturbance Due to Food Allergy, Acute Fulminating Laryngo-Tracheo-Bronchitis, Silicosis, New Growths of the Bronchi, Cysts of the Lung, Cholesterol Pleurisy, Perinephritis, Tyrosinosis, Idiopathic Hypochromic Anemia, Aplastic Anemia, Achresthic Anemia, Miscellaneous Anemias, Agranulocytosis, Plummer-Vinson Syndrome, Thrombophlebitic Splenomegaly, Xanthomatoses, Hand-Schüller-Christian Disease, Subleukemic Splenic Reticulo-Endotheliosis, Pseudoxanthoma Elasticum, Vasovagal Attacks, Coronary Artery Occlusion, Congenital Heart Block, Thrombo-angiitis Obliterans—Buerger's Disease, Diseases of the Veins, Angiomatosis—Telangiectasia, Hyperparathyroidism, Simmond's Disease, Pituitary Basophilism (Cushing's Disease), Laurence-Biedl Syndrome, Acute Aseptic Meningitis, Narcolepsy, Subarachnoid Hemorrhage, Scleroedema Adultorum, Erythrocyanosis Crurum Puellarum Frigida, Panniculitis, Morquio's Disease, Hereditary Arthrodysplasia and Dystrophy of the Nails, Arachnodactyly, Hypertelorism.

Acknowledgement and thanks are due to many of my friends and associates for suggestions and advice. Of my associates, Drs. M. E. Rehfuss, H. K. Mohler, H. W. Jones, B. L. Gordon, D. W. Kramer, G. G. Duncan and A. Cantarow have given me the benefit of their knowledge on many points. Two old friends, Dr. Harvey Cushing and Dr. W. H. Witt, have aided with counsel. To physicians and students who have sent suggestions and constructive criticism, I am indebted for their interest and advice which are thoroughly appreciated.

THOMAS MCCRAE.

PREFACE TO FIRST EDITION

My thanks are due to my former first assistant, H. A. Lafleur, for much help, direct and indirect; to his successor, W. S. Thayer, for assistance in the section on Blood Diseases and for the preparation of the illustrative charts; to D. Meredith Reese, for the statistics on tuberculosis; to H. M. Thomas, for many suggestions in the section on Nervous Diseases, and particularly in the section on Topical Diagnosis; to L. P. Powell, of the Johns Hopkins University Library, for a careful revision of the manuscript; and to Miss B. O. Humpton, for valuable aid, especially in the preparation of the index.

William Osler

Johns Hopkins Hospital
Baltimore, *January 1, 1892.*

"Experience is fallacious and judgment difficult."

HIPPOCRATES: *Aphorisms, I.*

"And I said of medicine, that this is an art which considers the constitution of the patient, and has principles of action and reasons in each case."

PLATO: *Gorgias.*

CONTENTS

SECTION I

Specific Infectious Diseases

SECTION II

Diseases Due to Physical Agents

SECTION III

The Intoxications

SECTION IV

Deficiency Diseases

SECTION V

Diseases of Metabolism

SECTION VI

Diseases of the Digestive System

SECTION VII

DISEASES OF THE RESPIRATORY SYSTEM

SECTION VIII

DISEASES OF THE KIDNEYS

SECTION IX

Diseases of the Blood-Forming Organs

SECTION X

DISEASES OF THE CIRCULATORY SYSTEM

SECTION XI

Diseases of the Glands of Internal Secretion

SECTION XII

Diseases of the Nervous System

SECTION XIII

Diseases of the Locomotor System

CHARTS AND ILLUSTRATIONS

THE PRINCIPLES AND PRACTICE OF MEDICINE

THE PRINCIPLES AND PRACTICE OF MEDICINE

SECTION I

SPECIFIC INFECTIOUS DISEASES

BACTERIAL DISEASES

TYPHOID FEVER

Definition.—*A general infection caused by the typhoid bacillus* (*Eberthella typhi*), characterized anatomically by hyperplasia and ulceration of the intestinal lymph-follicles, swelling of the mesenteric glands and spleen, and parenchymatous changes in other organs. There are cases in which the local changes are slight or absent, and others with intense localization in the lungs, spleen, kidneys, or nervous system. The disease is marked by fever, roseola, abdominal tenderness, tympanites, and enlargement of the spleen; but these features are inconstant, and even the fever varies greatly.

Historical Note.—Huxham, in his Essay on Fevers, had "taken notice of the great difference there is between the *putrid malignant* and the *slow nervous fever*." In 1813 Pierre Bretonneau, of Tours, distinguished "dothiénentérite" as a separate disease; and Petit and Serres described enteromesenteric fever. In 1829 Louis' great work appeared, in which the name "typhoid" was given to the fever. At this period typhoid fever alone prevailed in Paris and many European cities, and was universally believed to be identical with the continued fever of Great Britain, where in reality typhoid and typhus coexisted. The intestinal lesion was regarded as an accidental occurrence in typhus fever. Louis' students, returning to their homes in different countries, had opportunities for studying the prevalent fevers in the thorough and systematic manner of their master. Among these were certain young American physicians, to one of whom, Gerhard, of Philadelphia, is due the honor of having first clearly laid down the differences between the two diseases. His papers in the American Journal of the Medical Sciences, 1837, are the first which give a full account of their clinical and anatomical distinctions. In 1842 Elisha Bartlett's work appeared, in which, for the first time in a systematic treatise, typhoid and typhus fever were separately considered with admirable clearness. Eberth discovered the organism in 1880.

Etiology.—General Prevalence.—Typhoid fever prevails especially in temperate climates. Widely distributed throughout the world, it presents everywhere the same essential characteristics, and is an index of the sanitary intelligence of a community. *Imperfect sewerage* and *contaminated water-supply* are two special conditions favoring the distribution of the bacilli, while from an infected person the disease may be spread by *fingers, food* and *flies.*

In *England* and *Wales* in 1931 the disease was fatal to 251 persons, a mortality of 6 per million of living persons. The rate was lower in 1931 than in any year since 1869. In the *United States* there has been a marked decrease, due largely to chlorination of the water-supplies. The death-rate per 100,000 population in the registration areas has fallen from 35.9 in 1900 to 3.7 in 1932. In 1933 the death-rate in the seventy-eight largest cities was 1.18 per 100,000. It is more prevalent in country districts than in cities, and the propagation now is largely from the country to the city.

Typhoid fever has been one of the great scourges of armies, and killed more than powder and shot. In the Spanish-American War in the national encampments among 107,973 men there were 20,738 cases of typhoid fever with 1,580 deaths. In 90 per cent of the volunteer regiments the disease broke out within eight weeks after going into camp. In the South African War the British army, 557,653 officers and men, had 57,684 cases of typhoid fever, with 8,225 deaths, while 7,582 men died of wounds received in battle. In the great European war typhoid fever did not prevail to any extent in the Western armies and the efficacy of inoculation was thoroughly demonstrated. The large proportion of paratyphoid cases was remarkable.

Season.—Almost without exception the disease is everywhere more prevalent in the autumn, hence the old popular name autumnal fever. Of 1,500 cases at the Johns Hopkins Hospital (upon the study of which this section is based), 840 were in August, September, and October.

Sex.—Males and females are equally subject to the disease, but males are more frequently admitted into hospitals, 2.4 to 1 in our series.

Age.—Typhoid fever is a disease of youth and early adult life. The greatest susceptibility is between the ages of fifteen and twenty-five. Of the 1,500 cases there were under fifteen years of age, 231; between fifteen and twenty, 253; between twenty and thirty, 680; between thirty and forty, 227; between forty and fifty, 88; between fifty and sixty, 8; above sixty, 11. Cases in advanced life are not uncommon, but as the course is often atypical the disease may not be recognized until autopsy. It is not infrequent in childhood, but infants are rarely attacked. Murchison saw a case at the sixth month.

Immunity.—Not all exposed to infection contract the disease. After recovery the immunity is apparently permanent but only against the particular infecting organism; infection with the typhoid bacillus does not protect against paratyphoid infections and *vice versa.* In 500 of our cases in which special inquiry was made as to a previous attack it was found to have occurred in 2.2 per cent. The interval varied from nine months to thirty years. Usually within a short time after recovery the immune substances disappear from the blood, yet in most cases the immunity lasts for life.

Bacillus Typhosus.—*General Characters.*—It is a rather short, thick, flagellated, motile bacillus, with round ends, about 3μ in length and 0.6μ in breadth. In cultures, filamentous forms are often found. This organism fulfills all the requirements of Koch's law—it is constantly present, and grows outside the body in a specific manner; the third requirement, the production of the disease experimentally, has been met by its conveyance to chimpanzees. The disease has resulted from the swallowing of cultures with suicidal intent.

There is more than one antigen present in the organism and **H** and **O** organisms are described. The **H** group present the flagellate forms and apparently take no part in protective immunization. The **O** antigen is divided into **OS** (smooth) which is virulent, and **OS** (rough) which is not virulent and apparently gives no protection. The **O** agglutinates both the **H** and **O** emulsion of typhoid and paratyphoid organisms. There may be difficulty in reading the agglutination results from the appearance of the suspension fluid. The **H** agglutination gives floccular and the **O** agglutination gives granular particles.

Cultures are killed within ten minutes by a temperature of 60° C. They may live for eighteen weeks at –5° C., although most die within two weeks, and all within twenty-two weeks (Park). The typhoid bacillus resists ordinary drying for months, unless in very thin layers, when it is killed in five to fifteen days. The direct rays of the sun completely destroy them in from four to ten hours' exposure. Bouillon cultures are destroyed by carbolic acid, 1 to 200, and by corrosive sublimate, 1 to 2,500.

Distribution in the Body.—The bacilli are probably in the circulating blood in the early stages of the disease in all cases. During life they may be demonstrated in the blood in a large proportion of cases. They occur in the urine in from 25 to 30 per cent of the cases (if hexamine is not given). They may be isolated from the stools in practically all cases at some stage. They are probably always present in the rose spots. They may occur in the sputum. They have been found in the milk of nursing women. At autopsy they are found widely distributed, most numerous and constant usually in the mesenteric glands, spleen, and gallbladder, but are found in almost all organs. Cultures made from the intestines at autopsy show that they are very numerous in the duodenum and jejunum, and practically constant in cultures made from the mucous membrane of the stomach. They are present in the esophagus and frequently on the tongue and tonsils. From endocardial vegetations, from meningeal and pleural exudates and from foci of suppuration, the bacilli have been isolated. They may be present in the stools of persons who show no symptoms of typhoid fever, but who have lived in close association with typhoid fever patients. This is especially true of children.

The Bacilli outside the Body.—In sterile water the bacilli retain their vitality for weeks, but under ordinary conditions, in competition with saprophytes, disappear within a few days. The question of the longevity of the typhoid bacillus in water is of great importance, and was much discussed in connection with the supposed pollution of the water of the Mississippi by the Chicago drainage canal. Whether an increase can occur in water is not settled. In sewage at room temperature, the bacilli may live from 3 to 5 weeks. Improved culture methods have made it possible to obtain positive results from water and sewage in increasing numbers.

Sedgwick and Winslow concluded that very few typhoid germs survive in ice. The Ogdensburg epidemic in 1902-'03 was apparently due to infection from ice and typhoid bacilli were grown from frozen material in it.

In *milk* the bacilli undergo rapid development without changing its appearance. They may persist for three months in sour milk, and may live for several days in butter made from infected cream.

Robertson showed that under natural conditions typhoid bacilli may live in the upper layers of the soil for eleven months. In stools which contain typhoid bacilli, at room temperature, the organisms disappear in a few days. The direct infection of exposed food-stuffs by dust may occur. The bacilli retain their vitality for many weeks; in garden earth 21 days, in filter-sand 82 days, in street dust 30 days, on linen 60 to 70 days, on wood 32 days, on thread kept under suitable conditions for a year.

Modes of Conveyance.—The essential fact is that organisms from a patient with the disease or from a carrier are taken in by a healthy individual. The methods of conveyance are many; it may be direct from the patient to an attendant; food may be infected by an attendant; flies may carry the bacilli and infect food; or a water supply may be infected by excreta. A *carrier* is always a source of danger, especially if handling food. Fingers, food and flies are the chief means of local propagation. Every patient is a possible source of infection. It is impossible for a nurse to avoid finger contamination and without scrupulous care the germs may be distributed. Even with special precautions occasional cases of infection occur in hospitals.

Infection of water is the most common source of widespread epidemics, many of which have originated in the contamination of a water supply. There are many possibilities in the infection of water supplies. One, which is due to gross carelessness, is a communication by pipes between the filtered or chlorinated water supply and polluted water, perhaps laid on for fire protection.

Typhoid Carriers.—The bacilli may persist indefinitely in the bile passages and intestines of persons in good health. They have been found in the urinary bladder and in the gallbladder, twenty and thirty years after the fever, and in cases of typhoid bone lesions the bacilli have been isolated many years after the primary attack. Many localized epidemics have been traced to carriers. Soper reported an instance in which a cook, apparently in perfect health, but in whose stools bacilli were present in large numbers, had been responsible for the occurrence of typhoid in seven households in five years. There is no limit to the length of time in which the bacilli may persist. One carrier had the attack of typhoid fever forty-seven years before. The paratyphoid bacillus may be carried in the same way.

Infection of Food.—Milk may be the source of infection. The milk may be contaminated by infected water used in cleaning the cans or by carriers or those nursing typhoid patients. The germs may be conveyed in ice, salads of various sorts, spaghetti, etc. The danger of eating celery and other uncooked vegetables, which have grown in soil on which infected material has been used as a fertilizer, must not be forgotten.

Much attention has been paid to the *oyster* as a source of infection, but it plays a small relative part. In several epidemics, as that in Middletown, reported by Conn, that in Naples by Lavis, and the outbreak at Winchester, the chain of circumstantial evidence seems complete. Mussels have been found contaminated with typhoid bacilli, and dried fish have carried the infection.

Flies.—The importance of flies in the transmission of the disease was brought out very strongly in the Spanish-American War in 1898. The report of the commission states that "flies were undoubtedly the most active agents in the spread of typhoid fever. Flies alternately visited and fed on the infected fecal matter and the food in the mess-tent. . . . Typhoid fever was much less frequent among members of the messes who had their mess-tents screened than it was among those who took no such precautions."

Contamination of the Soil.—This is important if water supplies are infected as a result. Filth, bad sewers, or cesspools can not in themselves cause typhoid fever, but they furnish the conditions suitable for the preservation of the bacillus, and possibly for its propagation. *Dust* may be an important factor, though the bacilli usually die quickly when desiccated.

Types of Infection.—We may recognize the following groups: (*a*) *Ordinary typhoid fever with marked enteric lesions.* An immense majority of all cases are of this character; and while the spleen and mesenteric glands are involved the lymphatic apparatus of the intestinal walls bears the brunt of the attack. (*b*) *Cases in which the intestinal lesions are very slight,* and may be found only after a very careful search. In reviewing the cases of "typhoid fever without intestinal lesions," Opie and Bassett call attention to the fact that in many negative cases slight lesions really did exist, while in others death occurred so late that the lesions might have healed. In some cases the disease is a general septicemia with severe intoxication, high fever and delirium. In others the main lesions may be in organs—liver, gallbladder, pleura, meninges, or even the endocardium. (*c*) *Cases in which the typhoid bacillus enters the body without causing any lesion of the intestine.* In a number of the earlier cases reported as such the demonstration of the typhoid bacillus was inconclusive. In others the intestine showed tuberculous ulcers, through which the organisms may have entered. But after excluding these, a few cases remain in which the demonstration of the typhoid bacillus was conclusive, cases in which death occurred early, and yet no intestinal lesions could be found. There were 4 cases in this series. (*d*) *Mixed infections.* It is well to distinguish between double infections, as typhoid fever with tuberculosis, diphtheria or malaria, in which two different diseases are present, and the true mixed or secondary infections, in which the conditions induced by one organism favor the growth of other pathogenic forms; thus in typhoid fever secondary infection with the colon bacillus, streptococcus, staphylococcus, or pneumococcus, may occur. (*e*) *Paratyphoid infections.* (*f*) *Local infections.* The typhoid bacillus may cause a local abscess, cystitis, or cholecystitis without evidence of a general infection. (*g*) *Terminal typhoid infections.* In rare instances the bacillus causes a fatal infection towards the end of other diseases. The subjects may, of course, be typhoid carriers. In two cases of malignant disease the bacilli were isolated from the blood, and there were no intestinal lesions.

Morbid Anatomy.—Intestines.—A catarrhal condition exists throughout the small and large bowel. Specific changes occur in the lymphoid elements, chiefly at the lower end of the ileum. The alterations which occur are most conveniently described in four stages:

Hyperplasia, which involves the glands of Peyer in the jejunum and ileum, and to a variable extent those in the large intestine.—The follicles are swollen, grayish-white, and the patches may project 3 to 5 mm. The solitary glands, which range in size from a pin's head to a pea, are usually deeply imbedded in the submucosa, but project to a variable extent. Occasionally they are very prominent, and may be almost pedunculated. Microscopic examination shows at the outset hyperemia of the follicles. There are large phagocytic cells which may be derived from the reticulo-endothelial system. The lesion is productive rather than exudative and there are few polymorphonuclear leukocytes. The lymphoid tissue is largely replaced by the mononuclear phagocytes. The necrosis is probably due to the action of toxins and blocking of the vessels by the phagocytes. The importance of the latter has been emphasized by Mallory. The infiltration, always more intense toward the lower end of the ileum, reaches its height from the eighth to the tenth day and then undergoes one of two changes, *resolution* or *necrosis.* Death rarely takes place at this stage. Resolution is accomplished by a fatty and granular change in the cells, which are destroyed and absorbed. The swollen follicles in the patch undergo resolution and shrink more rapidly than the surrounding framework, or what is more probable the follicles alone become necrotic and disintegrate, leaving the little pits. In this process superficial hemorrhages may result, and small ulcers may orginate by the fusion of these superficial losses of substance. Hemorrhage from this cause is rarely severe.

Necrosis and Sloughing.—When the hyperplasia of the lymph-follicles reaches a certain grade, resolution is no longer possible. The blood vessels become choked, there is necrosis, and sloughs form which must be separated. The process may be superficial or may extend to and involve the submucosa. The "slough" may sometimes lie upon the Peyer's patch, scarcely involving more than the epithelium (Marchand). It is always more intense toward the ileo-cecal valve, and in very severe cases the greater part of the mucosa of the last foot of the ileum may be converted into a brownish-black eschar. The necrotic area in the solitary glands forms a yellowish cap which often involves only the most prominent point of a follicle. The extent of the necrosis is exceedingly variable.

Ulceration.—The separation of the necrotic tissue—the sloughing—is gradually effected from the edges inward, and results in the formation of an ulcer, the size and extent of which are proportionate to the amount of necrosis. If this be superficial, the entire thickness of the mucosa may not be involved and the loss of substance may be small and shallow. More commonly the slough in separating exposes the submucosa and muscularis, particularly the latter, which forms the floor of a majority of typhoid ulcers. It is not common for an entire Peyer's patch to slough away, and a perfectly ovoid ulcer opposite to the mesentery is rarely seen. Irregularly oval and rounded forms are most common. A large patch may present several ulcers divided by septa of mucous membrane. The terminal 6 or 8 inches of the ileum may form a large ulcer, with here and there islands of mucosa. The edges of the ulcer are usually swollen, soft, and often undermined.

Healing.—This begins with the development of a thin granulation tissue which covers the base. Occasionally it seems as if an ulcer had healed in one place and was extending in another. The mucosa gradually extends from the edge, and a new growth of epithelium is formed. The glandular elements are re-formed; the healed ulcer is somewhat depressed and is usually pigmented. In death during relapse healing ulcers may be seen in some patches with fresh ulcers in others. In fatal cases, we seldom find evidences of cicatrization, as the majority of deaths occur before this stage. It is remarkable that no matter how extensive the ulceration has been, healing is never associated with stricture, and typhoid fever is not a cause of intestinal obstruction. Within a short time all traces of the ulcers disappear.

Large Intestine.—The cecum and colon are affected in about one-third of the cases. Sometimes the solitary glands are greatly enlarged. The ulcers are usually larger in the cecum than in the colon.

Perforation of the Bowel.—*Incidence at Autopsy.*—J. A. Scott's figures, embracing 9,713 cases, give 351 deaths from perforation among 1,037 deaths from all causes, a percentage of 33.8 of the deaths and 3.6 of the cases. The European statistics give a much lower proportion of deaths from perforation. At the Johns Hopkins Hospital among 1,500 cases of typhoid fever there were 43 with perforation. Twenty of these were operated upon, with 7 recoveries. One died of toxemia on the eighth day after operation. At the Pennsylvania Hospital there were 139 cases of perforation among 5,891 cases. The site is usually in the ileum, and as a rule, the perforation occurs within twelve inches of the ileocecal valve. There may be two or three separate perforations. Scott described two distinct varieties: first, the more common single, circular, pin-point in size, due to the extension of a necrotic process through the base of a small ulcer. The second variety, produced by a large area of tissue becoming necrotic, ranges in size from the finger-tip to 3 cm. in diameter.

Death from hemorrhage occurred in 12 of 137 deaths in our 1,500 cases. The bleeding seems to result directly from the separation of the sloughs. It is unusual to find the bleeding vessel. In one case only a single patch had sloughed, and a firm clot was adherent to it. The bleeding may come from the soft swollen edges of the patch.

The *mesenteric glands* show hyperemia and become greatly swollen. Spots of necrosis are common. In several of our cases suppuration occurred, and in one a large abscess of the mesentery was present. The rupture of a softened or suppurating mesenteric gland may cause fatal hemorrhage or peritonitis. The bunch of glands in the mesentery, at the lower end of the ileum, is especially involved. The retroperitoneal glands are also swollen.

The *spleen* is invariably enlarged in the early stages. In 11 of our series it exceeded 600 grams in weight, in one 900 grams. The tissue is soft, even diffluent. Infarction is not infrequent. Rupture may occur spontaneously, as a result of injury or from an abscess.

The *bone marrow* shows changes very similar to those in the lymphoid tissues and there may be foci of necrosis (Longcope).

The *liver* shows parenchymatous degeneration. Early in the disease it is hyperemic, and in a majority of instances it is swollen, somewhat pale, on section turbid, and microscopically the cells are granular and loaded with fat. Nodular areas (microscopic) occur in many cases, some being lymphoid, others necrotic. In 3 of our series liver abscess occurred. Pylephlebitis may follow abscess of the mesentery or perforation of the appendix.

Gallbladder. This always contains typhoid bacilli which grow readily in a medium containing bile. The gallbladder probably constantly supplies typhoid bacilli to the intestine. Acute cholecystitis may occur. In carriers the typhoid bacilli are usually in the gallbladder and may be also in its wall.

Kidneys.—Cloudy swelling with granular degeneration of the cells of the convoluted tubules, less commonly an acute nephritis, may be present. There may be numerous small areas infiltrated with round cells, which may have the appearance of lymphomata or pass on to softening and suppuration, producing the so-called *miliary abscesses,* of which there were 7 cases in this series. The typhoid bacilli have been found in these areas. The kidneys in cases of typhoid bacilluria may show no changes other than cloudy swelling. Diphtheritic inflammation of the pelvis of the kidney may occur, as in 3 of our cases. *Cystitis* is not uncommon and diphtheritic inflammation may occur.

Respiratory Organs.—Ulceration of the larynx occurs in some cases. It may be in the posterior wall, at the insertion of the cords, at the base of the epiglottis, and on the aryepiglottidean folds. The cartilages are very apt to become involved. In the later period ulcers may be present.

Edema of the glottis may require tracheotomy. Diphtheritis of the pharynx and larynx is not very uncommon. *Lobar pneumonia* may be found early (see Pneumotyphus) or may be a late event. Hypostatic congestion and the condition of the lung spoken of as splenization occur. Gangrene, abscess, and hemorrhagic infarction may occur. Pleurisy is not common. It may be fibrinous, serous or purulent.

Changes in the Circulatory System.—*Heart Lesions.*—*Endocarditis,* while not common, is probably more frequent than is generally supposed. It was present without being suspected in 3 of 105 autopsies in this series, while in 3 other cases the clinical features suggested its presence. Typhoid bacilli have been found in the vegetations. *Pericarditis* is rare. *Myocarditis* is not very infrequent. In protracted cases the muscle fibre is usually soft, flabby, and of a pale yellowish-brown color. The softening may be extreme, though rarely of the grade described by Stokes in typhus fever, in which, when held apex up by the vessels, the organ collapsed over the hand, forming a mushroom-like cap. Microscopically, the fibres may show little or no change, even when the impulse of the heart has been extremely feeble. A granular parenchymatous degeneration is common. Fatty degeneration may be present, particularly in long-standing cases with anemia. The hyaline change is not common.

Lesions of the Blood Vessels.—Changes in the arteries are not infrequent. In 21 of 52 cases in our series, in which there were notes on the state of the aorta, fresh endarteritis was present, and in 13 of 62 cases in which the condition of the coronary arteries was noted similar changes were found (Thayer). *Arteritis* of a peripheral vessel with thrombus formation occurs and bacilli have been found in the thrombi. The artery may be blocked by an embolus but in the great majority of instances they are autochthonous and due to arteritis, obliterating or partial. *Thrombosis* in the veins is very much more frequent than in the arteries, but is not as serious. It is most frequent in the femoral and in the left more often than the right.

Nervous System.—There are very few obvious changes. *Meningitis* is rare. The exudation may be serous, serofibrinous, or purulent, and typhoid bacilli have been isolated. Five cases of serous and one of purulent meningitis occurred in our series (Cole). Optic neuritis, which occurs sometimes in typhoid fever, has not been described in connection with the meningitis. The anatomical lesion of the *aphasia*—not infrequent in children—is not known; possibly it is an encephalitis. Parenchymatous changes have been found in the peripheral nerves, and appear to be not very uncommon, even when there have been no symptoms of neuritis.

The *voluntary muscles* may show the changes described by Zenker, which occur in all long-standing febrile affections, and are not peculiar to typhoid fever. The muscle substance undergoes a granular degeneration or a hyaline transformation. The abdominal muscles, the adductors of the thighs, and the pectorals are most often involved. Rupture of a rectus abdominis has been found. Hemorrhage may occur. Abscesses may develop in the muscles.

Symptoms.—General Description.—The period of incubation lasts from "eight to fourteen days, sometimes twenty-three" (Clinical Society), during which there are feelings of lassitude and malaise. The average is about ten days. The onset is rarely abrupt. In the 1,500 cases chills occurred at onset in 334, headache in 1,117, anorexia in 825, diarrhea in 516, epistaxis in 323, abdominal pain in 443, constipation in 249, and pain in the right iliac fossa in 10. The patient at last takes to bed, from which event, in a majority of cases, the definite onset may be dated. During the *first week* there is, in some cases (but by no means in all), a steady rise in the fever, the evening record rising a degree or a degree and a half higher each day, reaching 103° or 104°. The pulse is not rapid when compared with the temperature, full in volume, but of low tension and often dicrotic; the tongue is coated and white; the abdomen is slightly distended and tender. Unless the fever is high there is no delirium, but the patient complains of headache, and there may be mental confusion at night. The bowels may be constipated or there may be loose movements often due to purgation. Toward the end of the week the spleen becomes enlarged and the rash appears in the form of rose-colored spots, seen first on the skin of the abdomen. Cough and bronchitic symptoms are common at the outset.

In the *second week*, in cases of moderate severity, the symptoms become aggravated; the fever remains high and the morning remission is slight. The pulse is rapid and loses its dicrotic character. There is no longer headache, but there are mental torpor and dullness. The face looks heavy; the lips are dry; the tongue, in severe cases, becomes dry also. The abdominal symptoms, if present—diarrhea, tympanites, and tenderness—become aggravated. Death may occur during this week, with pronounced nervous symptoms, or, toward the end of it, from hemorrhage or perforation. In mild cases the temperature declines, and by the fourteenth day may be normal.

In the *third week*, in cases of moderate severity, the pulse ranges from 110 to 130; the temperature shows marked morning remissions, and there is a gradual decline in the fever. The loss of weight is more noticeable, and the weakness pronounced. Diarrhea and meteorism may occur for the first time. Unfavorable features are pulmonary complications, increasing feebleness of the heart, and pronounced delirium with muscular tremor. Special dangers are perforation and hemorrhage.

With the *fourth week*, in a majority of instances, convalescence begins. The temperature gradually reaches the normal point, the tongue cleans, and the desire for food returns. In severe cases the fourth and even the fifth week may present an aggravated picture of the third; the patient grows weaker, the pulse is more rapid and feeble, the tongue dry, and the abdomen distended. He lies in a profound stupor, with low muttering delirium and *subsultus tendinum*, and passes feces and urine involuntarily. Failure of the circulation and secondary complications are the chief dangers.

In the *fifth* and *sixth weeks* protracted cases may still show irregular fever, and convalescence may not set in until after the fortieth day. In this period we meet with relapses in the milder forms or slight recrudescence of the fever. At this time, too, occur many of the complications and sequelae.

Special Features.—*Mode of Onset.*—As a rule, this is insidious, and the patient is unable to fix definitely the time at which he began to feel ill. The most important deviations from this common course are:

Onset with Pronounced, Sometimes Sudden, Nervous Manifestations.—Headache, of a severe and intractable nature may be the initial symptom. When the patients have kept about and, as they say, fought the disease, the first manifestation may be pronounced delirium. Such patients may leave home and wander about for days. In rare cases the disease sets in with the most intense cerebrospinal symptoms, simulating meningitis—severe headache, photophobia, retraction of the head, twitching of the muscles, and even convulsions. Occasionally drowsiness, stupor, and signs of basilar meningitis may exist for days before the characteristic symptoms develop or the onset may be with maniacal and mental symptoms.

With Pulmonary Symptoms.—The initial bronchitis may be of great severity and obscure the other features. More striking are those cases in which the disease sets in with a chill, pain in the side and the features of lobar pneumonia or acute pleurisy; or tuberculosis is suspected.

With Gastro-intestinal Symptoms.—Incessant vomiting and pain may suggest acute gastro-enteritis or lead to a suspicion of poisoning, or the patient may be sent to the surgical wards for appendicitis.

With symptoms of an acute nephritis.

Ambulatory Form.—Deserving of special mention are those cases in which the patient keeps about and attempts to work, or perhaps takes a long journey to his home. He may come under observation for the first time with a temperature of 104° or 105°, and the rash well out. Many of these run a severe course, and contribute largely to the mortality. Finally, there are rare instances in which typhoid is unsuspected until perforation or a profuse hemorrhage from the bowels occurs.

Facial Aspect.—Early in the disease the cheeks are flushed and the eyes bright. Toward the end of the first week the expression becomes more listless, and when the disease is well established the patient has a dull and heavy look. There is never the rapid anemia of malarial fever, and the color of the lips and cheeks may be retained even to the third week.

Fever.—*Regular Course.*—In the stage of invasion the fever rises steadily during the first five or six days. The evening temperature is about a degree or a degree and a half higher than the morning remission, so that a temperature of 104° or 105° is not uncommon by the end of the first week. Having reached the height, the fever persists with very slight daily remissions. It may be singularly persistent and but little influenced by bathing or other measures. At the end of the second and throughout the third week the temperature becomes more distinctly remittent. The difference between the morning and evening record may be 3° or 4°, and the morning temperature may be normal. It falls by lysis as a rule.

Variations from the typical temperature curve are common. We do not always see the gradual step-like ascent in the early stage; the patients do not often come under observation at this time. When the disease sets in with a chill, or in children with a convulsion, the temperature may rise at once to 103° or 104°. Defervescence may occur at the end of the second week and the temperature fall rapidly by *crisis,* reaching normal within twelve or twenty hours. An inverse type of temperature, high in the morning and low in the evening, is occasionally seen, but has no special significance.

Sudden falls in the temperature may occur, thus, as shown in Chart I, a drop of 6.4° may follow an intestinal hemorrhage, and this may occur before blood appears in the stools. Sometimes during the anemia which follows a severe hemorrhage from the bowels there are remarkable oscillations in the temperature. Hyperpyrexia is rare. In only 58 of 1,500 cases did the fever rise above 106°. Before death the fever may rise; the highest we have known was 109.5°.

Posttyphoid Variations.—Recrudescences.—After a normal temperature of perhaps five or six days, the fever may rise suddenly to 102° or 103°, without constitutional disturbance, furring of the tongue, or abdominal symptoms. After two to four days the temperature falls. Of 1,500 cases, 92 presented these elevations, notes of which are given in the Studies on Typhoid Fever (Johns Hopkins Hospital Reports). Constipation, errors in diet, or excitement may cause them. These attacks are a frequent source of anxiety and it is not always possible to say upon what they depend. In some cases typhoid or colon bacilli are found in the blood. As a rule, if the fever is the result of a complication, such as thrombosis, there is leukocytosis. Naturally one suspects a relapse, but there is an absence of the step-like ascent, and as a rule, the fever falls after a few days.

The *Subfebrile Stage* of *Convalescence.*—In children, in nervous patients, and in cases of anemia, the evening temperature may keep up for weeks after the tongue has cleaned and the appetite has returned. This may usually be disregarded, and is often best treated by allowing the patient to get up, and by stopping the use of the thermometer. Of course, it is important not to overlook any latent complication.

Hypothermia.—Low temperatures are common, following baths, spontaneously in the third and fourth week in the periods of marked remissions and following hemorrhage. An interesting form is the persistent hypothermia of convalescence in which, particularly in protracted cases with emaciation, the temperature may be 96° or 97°. It is of no special significance.

The Fever of the Relapse.—This is a repetition in many instances of the original fever, a gradual ascent and maintenance for a few days at a certain height and then a decline. It is usually shorter than the original pyrexia, and rarely continues more than two or three weeks.

Afebrile Typhoid.—The occurrence of this is doubtful and the cases so termed are probably mild attacks with slight fever for a few days.

Chills occur: sometimes with the onset; occasionally at intervals throughout the course, and followed by sweats (so-called sudoral form); with complications, pleurisy, pneumonia, otitis media, phlebitis, etc.; with active antipyretic treatment by drugs; occasionally during defervescence without any complications, sometimes due to a septic infection; after the injection of vaccines or serum; according to Herringham, chills may result from constipation. There are cases in which throughout the latter part of the disease chills recur with great severity.

SKIN.—The characteristic rash consists of hyperemic spots, which appear from the seventh to the tenth day, usually at first upon the abdomen. They are slightly raised, flattened papules, which can be felt distinctly, of a rose-red color, disappearing on pressure, and ranging in diameter from 2 to 4 mm. They were present in 93.2 per cent of the white patients and 20.6 per cent of the colored. They come out in successive crops, and after persisting for two or three days they disappear, occasionally leaving a brownish stain. The spots may be present upon the back and not upon the abdomen. The eruption may be abundant over the whole skin of the trunk, and on the extremities. There were 81 in which they occurred on the arms, 17 on the forearms, 43 on the thighs, legs 15, face 5, hands 3. The cases with very abundant eruption are not necessarily severe. Typhoid bacilli have been found in the spots. Sometimes the spots are capped by small vesicles. A profuse miliary or sudaminal rash is not uncommon. In 38 cases in our series there were purpuric spots; 3 of the cases were true hemorrhagic typhoid fever. The rash may not appear until the relapse. In 21 cases in our series the rose spots came out after the patient was afebrile.

A branny desquamation is not rare in children and is common in adults after hydrotherapy. Occasionally the skin peels off in large flakes. A yellow color of the palms of the hands and soles of the feet is not uncommon.

Among other skin lesions the following may be mentioned:

Erythema.—It is not very uncommon in the first week of the disease to find a diffuse erythematous blush—*E. typhosum.* Sometimes the skin may have a peculiar mottled pink and white appearance. *E. exudativum, E. nodosum,* and urticaria may be present.

Herpes.—Herpes is rare in typhoid fever in comparison with its great frequency in malarial fever and in pneumonia. It was noted in 20 of our 1,500 cases, usually on the lips.

Skin Gangrene.—Areas of superficial gangrene may follow the prolonged use of an ice-bag. In children noma may occur. The nose, ears, and genitals may be attacked.

Sweats.—At the height of the fever the skin is usually dry. Profuse sweating is rare, but it is not very uncommon to see the abdomen or chest moist with perspiration. Sweats may constitute a striking feature and be associated with chilly sensations or actual chills. In this *sudoral* form there may be recurring paroxysms of chill, fever, and sweats (even several in twenty-four hours), and the case may be mistaken for malarial fever. Profuse sweats may occur with hemorrhage or perforation.

Edema of the skin occurs: (1) As the result of vascular obstruction, most commonly of a vein, as in femoral thrombosis. (2) In connection with nephritis, very rarely. (3) In association with the anemia and cachexia. The *hair* may fall out after the attack but complete baldness is rare. The nutrition of the nails suffers, and during and after convalescence transverse ridges may occur. A peculiar *odor* is exhaled from the skin in some cases and there is a very distinctive smell connected with many patients. Nathan Smith described it as of a "semi-cadaverous, musty character."

Linae atrophicae.—Lines of atrophy may appear on the skin of the abdomen, lateral aspects of the thighs and about the knees. They have been attributed to neuritis.

Bed sores are not uncommon in protracted cases with emaciation. In some cases the necroses begin in the deeper structures but, as a rule, they result from pressure and are seen upon the sacrum, more rarely the ilia, the shoulders, and the heels. These are less frequent with hydrotherapy and scrupulous care does much for their prevention, but with profound toxemia bed sores may occur with slight pressure and with astonishing rapidity.

Boils and superficial abscesses constitute a common and troublesome sequel.

CIRCULATORY SYSTEM.—The *blood* presents important changes. During the first two weeks there may be little or no change. Profuse sweats or copious diarrhea may cause the corpuscles to rise above normal. In the third week a fall usually takes place in corpuscles and hemoglobin, and the number may sink even to 1,300,000 per c.mm., gradually rising to normal during convalescence. The average maximum loss is about 1,000,000 to the c.mm.

The *hemoglobin* is always reduced, usually in a greater relative proportion than the red corpuscles, and during recovery the normal color standard is reached at a later period. *Leukopenia* is present throughout and baths increase temporarily the number of leukocytes in the peripheral circulation. The absence of leukocytosis is of value in distinguishing typhoid fever from septic fevers and inflammatory processes. The large mononuclears are relatively increased. When an acute inflammatory process occurs in typhoid fever the leukocytes show an increase in the polymorphonuclear forms, and this may be of great diagnostic moment.

The *pulse* is increased in rapidity, but not in proportion to the fever, and this is a special feature in the early stages. There is no acute disease with which a dicrotic pulse is so frequently associated. Even with high fever the pulse may not be greatly accelerated. As the disease progresses the pulse becomes more rapid, feebler and small. In 15 per cent of our cases the rate rose above 140. With extreme prostration it may reach 150 or more, and is a mere undulation—the so-called running pulse.

During convalescence the pulse gradually returns to normal, and occasionally becomes very slow. After no other acute fever do we so frequently meet with bradycardia. The pulse may be as low as 30, and instances are on record of still fewer beats to the minute. Some of these are due to temporary heart block. Tachycardia, while less common, may be a very troublesome and persistent feature of convalescence.

Blood Pressure.—There is a gradual fall during the course to about 100-110 mm. Hg. at the beginning of apyrexia. In two or three weeks later the pressure has usually returned to normal. Hemorrhage usually produces a marked fall both in the systolic and diastolic pressure. In some cases of perforation there may be a sharp rise in systolic pressure. Baths and ice sponges usually cause a rise of 10-20 mm. Hg.

The *heart sounds* may be normal throughout. In severe cases, the first sound becomes feeble and there is often heard, at the apex and along the left sternal margin, a soft systolic murmur, which was present in 22 per cent of our cases. Absence of the first sound is rare. Gallop rhythm is not uncommon. In the extreme feebleness of the graver forms, the first and second sounds become similar, and the long pause is shortened (embryocardia).

Pericarditis is rare and has been met with chiefly in children and with pneumonia. It was present in 3 of our series. *Endocarditis* was found post mortem in 3 cases, and physical signs suggested its presence in 3 other cases in the series. *Myocarditis* is more common, and is indicated by a progressive weakening of the heart sounds and feeble action.

Complications in the Arteries.—Arteritis with thrombus formation occurred in 4 cases in the series, one in the branches of the middle cerebral, two in the femoral, and one in the brachial. Gangrene usually follows. Pain, tenderness and swelling occur over the artery, with diminution or disappearance of the pulsations and coldness and blueness of the extremity. In two of the cases these symptoms gradually disappeared, and the pulsation returned. Keen refers to 46 cases of arterial gangrene, of which 8 were bilateral, 19 on the right side, and 19 on the left.

Thrombi in the veins.—In our series there were 43 instances, distributed in the following veins: femoral 23, popliteal 5, iliac 5, veins of the calf 5, internal saphenous 3, pulmonary artery and common iliac 1, axillary vein 1. *Femoral thrombosis* is the most common, and almost invariably in the left vessel, due probably to the fact that the left iliac vein is crossed by the right iliac artery, and the blood flow is not so free. The symptoms are very definite—the fever may increase or recur. Chills occurred in 11 of the cases. Pain and swelling at the site are constantly present, and the thrombotic mass can be felt, not always at first, nor is it well to feel for it. Swelling of the leg follows as a rule. In *iliac thrombosis* the pain may be severe and lead to the suspicion of perforation. Leukocytosis is usually present; in 12 cases it was above 10,000. Five of the 43 patients died, 2 only as a result of the thrombus; in the case of axillary thrombosis from pulmonary embolism, in one from embolism of the inferior cava and right auricle from the dislocation of a piece of thrombus from the left iliac vein. Thayer examined 16 of the patients at varying periods after convalescence, and found in every case more or less disability from the varices and persistent swelling. In some cases, however, the recovery is complete. Conner has emphasized the frequency of thrombosis in the small veins of the legs and feet and suggests that pulmonary embolism of slight extent is a common result.

Digestive System.—Loss of appetite is early, and, as a rule, the relish for food is not regained until convalescence. The *tongue* presents the changes inevitable in a prolonged fever. Early in the disease it is moist, swollen, and coated with a thin white fur, which, as the fever progresses, becomes denser. It may remain moist throughout. In severe cases, particularly those with delirium, the tongue becomes very dry, partly owing to the fact that such patients breathe with the mouth open. It may be covered with a brown or brownish-black fur, or with crusts between which are cracks and fissures. In these cases the teeth and lips may be covered with a dark brownish matter called *sordes*—a mixture of food, epithelial *débris,* and micro-organisms. By keeping the mouth and tongue clean from the outset, the fissures may be prevented. Acute *glossitis* is a rare complication. During convalescence the tongue gradually becomes clean. The secretion of saliva is often diminished; salivation is rare.

Parotitis occurred in 14 cases in our series; of these, 5 died. It is most frequent in the third week in very severe cases. Extensive sloughing may follow in the tissues of the neck. Usually unilateral, and in some cases going on to suppuration, it is regarded as a very fatal complication, but recovery followed in nine of our cases. It may arise from extension of inflammation along Steno's duct, probably not so serious as when it is hematogenous in origin. In four cases the submaxillary glands were involved alone, in one a cellulitis of the neck extended from the gland and proved fatal. Parotitis may occur after the fever has subsided. A remarkable localized sweating in the parotid region is an occasional sequel.

The *pharynx* may be the seat of catarrh or ulceration. Sometimes the fauces are deeply congested. Membranous pharyngitis, a serious and fatal

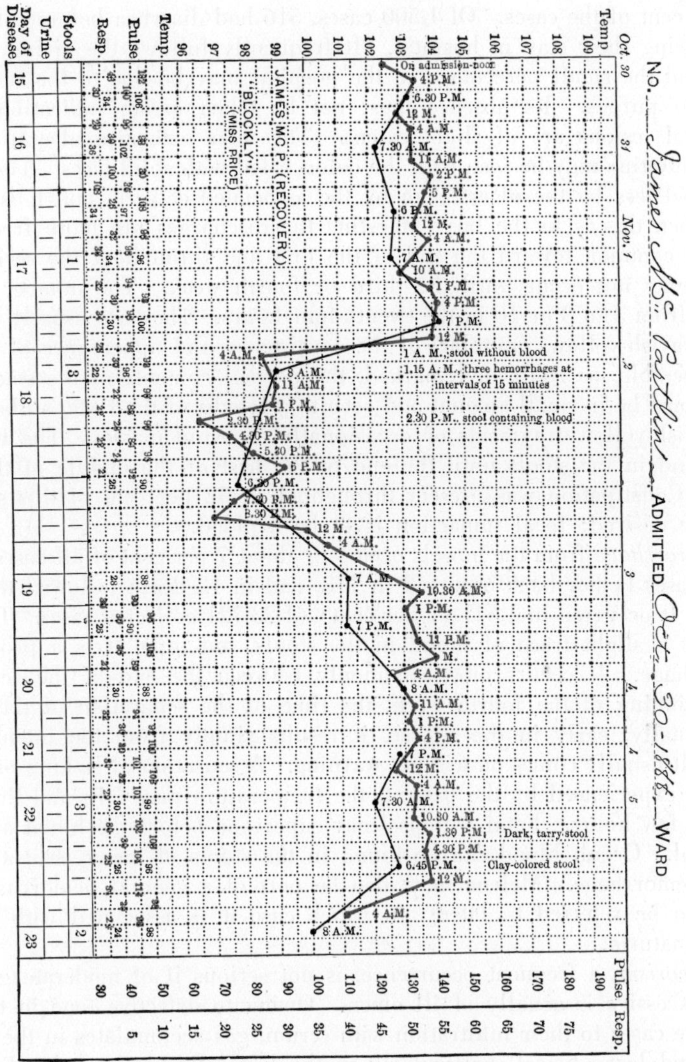

CHART I.—HEMORRHAGE FROM THE BOWEL. RAPID FALL OF TEMPERATURE.

complication, may come on in the third week. Difficulty in swallowing may result from ulcers of the esophagus, and in one of our cases stricture followed. The *thyroid* gland is often enlarged in the acute stages. Thyroiditis may occur with abscess formation years after the attack of typhoid fever. Typhoid bacilli have been found in the pus.

The *gastric symptoms* are usually few. Nausea and vomiting are not common but there are instances in which obstinate vomiting is a marked feature and may cause death from exhaustion. Vomiting does not often occur in the second and third weeks, unless associated with some complication. Ulcers have been found in the stomach. Hematemesis occurred in 4 of our cases.

Intestinal Symptoms.—Diarrhea is very variable, occurring in from 20 to 30 per cent of the cases. Of 1,500 cases, 516 had diarrhea before entering and 260 during their stay in hospital. It frequently follows the giving of purgatives and the small percentage in the hospital may be due to the fact that we used no purges. Its absence must not be taken as an indication that the intestinal lesions are of slight extent. The most extensive ulceration of the small intestine may be seen with the colon filled with solid feces. The diarrhea is caused less by the ulcers than by the associated catarrh, and it is probable that when this is in the large intestine the discharges are more frequent. It is most common toward the end of the first and throughout the second week, but it may not occur until the third or fourth week. The number of stools ranges from 3 to 8 or 10 in the twenty-four hours. They are usually abundant, thin, grayish-yellow, granular, of the consistency and appearance of pea soup, and resemble, as Addison remarked, the normal contents of the small bowel. Blood may be in small amount and occult. Sloughs of the Peyer's glands occur as grayish-yellow fragments or occasionally as ovoid masses. The bacilli are not found in the stools until the end of the first or the middle of the second week. Constipation was present throughout in 52 per cent of this series and is to be desired; fecal impaction is to be avoided.

Hemorrhage from the bowels occurs in about 7 per cent of all cases. In our 1,500 cases hemorrhage occurred in 118, and in 12 death followed the hemorrhage. It occurred in 1,641 (7 per cent) of 23,721 collected cases. There may be only a slight trace of blood in the stools, but often it is a profuse, free hemorrhage. It occurs most commonly between the end of the second and the beginning of the fourth week, the time of the separation of the sloughs. Occasionally, early in the course, it results simply from the intense hyperemia. It usually comes on without warning. A sensation of sinking or collapse may be experienced by the patient, the temperature may fall, and drop 6° or 7° in a few hours. Fatal collapse may supervene before the blood appears in the stool. Occult blood can be found in the stools of many patients without gross hemorrhage. Melena may also be part of a general hemorrhagic tendency (to be referred to later), in which case it is associated with petechiae and hematuria.

Meteorism, a frequent occurrence, is not serious if of moderate grade, but when excessive is usually of ill omen. Owing to defective tone in the walls, in severe cases to their infiltration with serum, gas accumulates in the stomach, small and large bowel, particularly in the last. Pushing up the diaphragm, it interferes with the action of the heart and lungs, and may also favor perforation. Gurgling in the right iliac fossa exists in a large proportion of cases, and indicates simply the presence of gas and fluid feces in the colon and cecum.

Abdominal pain and tenderness were present in three-fifths of a series of 500 cases studied with special reference to the point. In some it was only present at the onset. Pain occurred during the course in about one-third of the cases This is due in some instances to conditions apart from the bowel lesions, such as pleurisy, distention of the bladder, and phlebitis. It may be associated with diarrhea, severe constipation, perisplenitis, or acute abdominal complications. Pain occurs with some cases of hemorrhage, but is most constantly present with perforation. In some cases no cause could be found for the pain, and if other symptoms be associated the condition may lead to error in diagnosis. Operation for appendicitis has been performed in the early stage of typhoid fever, owing to the combination of pain in the right iliac fossa, fever, and constipation.

PERFORATION.—From one-fourth to one-third of the deaths are due to perforation. Among 34,916 collected cases perforation occurred in 3.1 per cent. While it may occur as early as the first week, in the great majority it is at the height of the disease in the third week, and much more frequently in the severe cases, particularly those associated with tympanites, diarrhea, and hemorrhage. It may occur, however, in very mild attacks and with great suddenness, when the patient is apparently progressing favorably.

Symptoms of Perforation.—By far the most important single indication is a sudden, sharp *pain* of increasing severity, often paroxysmal in character. It is rarely absent, except in patients with profound toxemia. The situation is most frequent in the hypogastric region and to the right of the middle line. Tenderness on pressure is present in the great majority of cases, usually in the hypogastric and right iliac regions, sometimes diffuse; it may only be brought out on deep pressure. When the perforation happens to be in contact with the parietal peritoneum the local features on palpation are much more marked than when the perforated ulcer is next to a coil or to the mesentery. There may be early irritability of the bladder, with frequent micturition, and pain extending toward the penis. A third important sign is muscle rigidity, increased tension, and spasm on any attempt to palpate. The temperature may rise for a few hours to fall later or may drop at once. The pulse and respiration rate are usually increased. Following these features in a few hours there is usually a reaction, and then the evidences of general peritonitis become manifest to a more or less marked degree. Among the general features, the facies shows changes; there is increased pallor, a pinched expression, and as the symptoms progress and toward the end a marked Hippocratic facies, a dusky suffusion, and the forehead bathed in a clammy perspiration. The temperature rises with the increase of the peritonitis. The pulse quickens, is running and thready, the heart's action becomes more feeble, and there is an increase in the respiration rate. Vomiting is a variable feature; it is present in a majority of the cases. Hiccough is common and may occur early, but more frequently late. In this stage there may be no complaint of pain.

The local abdominal features are often more important than the general, as it is surprising to notice how excellent the condition of a patient may be with perforative peritonitis. Limitation of the respiratory movements is usually present, perhaps confined to the hypogastric area. Increasing distention is the rule, but perforation and peritonitis may occur, it is to be remembered, with an abdomen flat or even scaphoid. Increasing pain on pressure, increasing muscle spasm and tension of the wall are important signs. Percussion may reveal a flat note in the flanks, due to exudate. A friction may be present within a few hours of the onset of the perforation. Obliteration of the liver flatness in the nipple line may be caused by excessive tympany, but rapid obliteration of liver flatness in a flat, or a not much distended abdomen, is a valuable sign. Examination of the rectum may show fullness or tenderness in the pelvis. Advance in the abdominal signs is an important point.

In some cases there is a rise in the leukocytes, which is a valuable help, but is not constant. Increase in the blood pressure is not constant.

General *peritonitis,* without perforation of the bowel, may occur by extension from an ulcer, by rupture of a softened mesenteric gland, or, as in one case in our series, from inflammation of the Fallopian tubes.

Perforation is almost invariably fatal without operation. In a few cases healing takes place spontaneously or the orifice may be closed by a tag of omentum. In some cases hemorrhage occurs with perforation and adds to the difficulty in diagnosis. In 7 of our 43 cases hemorrhage accompanied the perforation; in 3 others the hemorrhage occurred some days before.

The *diagnosis* of perforation, easy enough at times, is not without serious difficulties. The conditions for which it was mistaken in our series were: appendicitis, occurring during the course of the typhoid fever, phlebitis of the iliac vein with great pain, hemorrhage, and in one case a local peritonitis without perforation, for which no cause was found. Recovery followed the exploratory operation in all but one (hemorrhage case) of the cases. Exploration is justifiable and better than delay in suspicious cases.

ASCITES occurs in rare instances (McPhedran).

The SPLEEN is usually enlarged, and the edge was felt below the costal margin in 71.6 per cent of our cases. Percussion is uncertain, as, owing to distention of the stomach and colon, even the normal area of dulness may not be obtainable. Enlargement is often not marked in elderly patients. Rupture of the spleen occurs occasionally. Perisplenitis occurs not infrequently.

LIVER.—*Jaundice* of marked grade was present in only 8 cases of our series, but slight icterus is not uncommon. Catarrh of the ducts, toxemia, abscess, and occasionally gall stones are the usual causes.

Abscess.—Solitary abscess is exceedingly rare and occurred in but 3 cases in our series. It may occur early in the disease but most frequently is a sequel. Eberts collected 30 cases, in 9 of which the typhoid bacillus was isolated from the pus. In about half the cases the right lobe was affected. Eighteen of the patients recovered. Suppurative pylephlebitis may follow perforation of the appendix. Suppurative cholangitis has been described.

Cholecystitis occurred in 19 cases of the series. Pain in the region of the gallbladder is the most constant symptom. Tenderness, muscle spasm with rigidity, and a gallbladder tumor are present in a majority of the cases. Jaundice is inconstant. Leukocytosis usually occurs. With perforation there may be a marked drop in the fever and the signs of peritonitis. In simple cholecystitis the urgency of the symptoms may abate and recovery follow. Suppuration may occur with infection of the bile passages. Months or years later there may be cholecystitis or gall stones. Typhoid bacilli have been found in the gallbladder of patients without a history of typhoid fever.

Gall stones.—The occurrence of cholelithiasis after typhoid fever is probably associated with the presence of typhoid bacilli in the gallbladder (see under Gall Stones).

PANCREAS.—Hemorrhagic pancreatitis has occurred rarely.

RESPIRATORY SYSTEM.—*Epistaxis* occurs in the early stages of typhoid fever more often than in any other febrile affection. It is occasionally profuse and serious and may occur during the ccurse.

Laryngitis is not very common and edema, apart from ulceration, is rare. In the United States the laryngeal complications seem much less frequent than in Europe. We have twice seen severe perichondritis; both patients recovered, one after the expectoration of large portions of the thyroid cartilage. Keen and Lüning collected 221 cases of serious surgical complications of the larynx. General emphysema may follow the perforation of an ulcer. Stenosis is a serious sequence. Paralysis of the laryngeal muscles occurs; Przedborski in 100 consecutive cases found 25 with paralysis. This is nearly always due to neuritis, sometimes with affections of other nerves.

Bronchitis is one of the most frequent initial symptoms. The sputum is usually scanty. The smaller tubes may be involved, producing urgent cough and even slight cyanosis. Collapse and bronchopneumonia may also occur.

Lobar pneumonia is met with under two conditions: At the outset (*pneumotyphus*) as in three of our cases. After an indisposition of a day or so, the patient is seized with a chill, has high fever, pain in the side, with signs of consolidation and the evidences of an ordinary lobar pneumonia. The intestinal symptoms may not occur until the end of the first week or later; the pulmonary symptoms persist; crisis does not occur; the aspect of the patient changes, and by the end of the second week the picture is that of typhoid fever. Spots may then be present and the diagnosis is clear. In other instances, in the absence of a characteristic eruption, the case remains doubtful. This condition may depend upon an early localization of the typhoid bacillus in the lung.

Lobar pneumonia forms a serious complication of the second or third week —in 19 of our cases. The symptoms are usually not marked. There may be no rusty sputum, and, unless sought for, the condition is frequently overlooked. The etiological agent may vary. Typhoid bacilli have been isolated from the sputum and from the consolidated lungs at autopsy, but in such cases pneumococci may have been originally present, and the typhoid bacilli secondary invaders. In all cases of pneumonia in our series coming to autopsy, the pneumococcus was found in the consolidated lung. Infarction, abscess, and gangrene are occasional pulmonary complications.

Hypostatic congestion of the lungs and edema, due to enfeebled circulation, occur in the later periods. The physical signs are defective resonance at the bases, feeble breath sounds, and moist râles on deep inspiration. Dulness at the right base is not uncommon even early in the attack.

Hemoptysis may occur and cause death. This has resulted from hemorrhage from an eroded vessel in the edge of a laryngeal ulcer.

Pleurisy occurred in 2 per cent of our series. It may occur at the outset—*pleurotyphoid*—or during convalescence, in which case it is almost always purulent and due to the typhoid bacillus.

Pneumothorax is rare. It may be due to straining, or to the rupture of a small abscess. It may occur also during convalescence.

Nervous System.—*Cerebrospinal Form.*—The disease may set in with intense and persistent headache, or a severe neuralgia. Kernig's sign is often present without any evidence of meningeal infection. There are cases in which the effect of the disease is manifested on the nervous system early and with the greatest intensity. There are headaches, photophobia, retraction of the neck, twitchings of the muscles, rigidity, and even convulsions. The cases showing marked *meningeal features* during the course may be divided into three groups. First, those with symptoms suggestive of meningitis, but without localizing features and without the anatomical lesions of meningitis at postmortem (*meningism*). Secondly, the so-called *serous* meningitis. There is a localization of typhoid bacilli in the cerebrospinal fluid and a mild inflammatory reaction, but without suppurative meningitis. Cole in 1904 collected 13 such cases, 5 of them in our series, and Bayne-Jones collected 17 cases from the literature since 1904. Probably more frequent lumbar punctures will show that this occurs not infrequently. Thirdly, true typhoid *suppurative* meningitis due to the typhoid bacillus. Only one case occurred in our series, and Cole collected 13 from the literature. Bayne-Jones collected 18 additional cases. Meningitis in typhoid fever is occasionally due to other organisms, as the tubercle bacillus or meningococcus. Marked convulsive movements, local or general, with coma and delirium, are seen in thrombosis of the cerebral veins and sinuses.

Delirium, usually present in very severe cases, is much less frequent under rigid hydrotherapy. It may exist from the outset, but usually does not occur until the second or third week. It may be slight and only nocturnal. It is, as a rule, a quiet delirium, though there are cases in which the patient is noisy and constantly tries to get out of bed, and, unless carefully watched, may escape. The patient does not often become maniacal. In heavy drinkers the delirium may have the character of delirium tremens. Even in patients who have no positive delirium, the mental processes are usually dulled and the aspect is listless and apathetic. In severe cases the patient passes into a condition of unconsciousness. The eyes may be open, but he is oblivious to all surrounding circumstances and neither knows nor can indicate his wants. The urine and feces are passed involuntarily. In this pseudo-wakeful state, or coma vigil, the eyes are open and the patient is constantly muttering. The lips and tongue are tremulous; there are twitchings of the fingers and wrists—subsultus tendinum and carphologia. He picks at the bedclothes or grasps at invisible objects. These are serious and always indicate danger.

Convulsions are rare. There were 7 instances in our series, with 3 deaths. They occur: first, at the onset, particularly in children; secondly, as a manifestation of the toxemia; and thirdly, as a result of severe cerebral complications —thrombosis, meningitis, or acute encephalitis. Occasionally in convalescence convulsions may occur from unknown causes.

Neuritis, which is not uncommon—11 cases in the series—may be multiple or local. *Multiple neuritis* comes on usually during convalescence. The legs may be affected or the four extremities. Recovery is the rule.

Local Neuritis.—This may occur during the height of the fever or after convalescence is established. It may set in with agonizing pain and with sensitiveness of the affected nerve trunks. The local neuritis may affect the nerves of an arm or of a leg, and involve chiefly the extensors, so that there is wrist drop or foot drop. The arm or leg may be much swollen and the skin over it erythematous. A curious condition, probably a local neuritis in some but in others due to phlebitis, is that described by Handford as *tender toes.* The tips and pads of the toes, rarely the pads at their bases, become very sensitive. There is no discoloration or swelling, and the pain disappears usually within a week or ten days.

Poliomyelitis may occur with the symptoms of acute ascending paralysis and prove fatal in a few days. More frequently it is less acute, and causes either a paraplegia or a limited atrophic paralysis of one arm or leg.

Hemiplegia is a rare complication. The lesion is usually thrombosis of the arteries, less often a meningo-encephalitis. The aphasia, if present, usually disappears. *Aphasia,* apart from hemiplegia, occurs usually in children. The prognosis is good.

The superficial abdominal reflexes may disappear early in the course and not return until convalescence, but this is not constant.

True *tetany* occurs sometimes, and has been reported in certain epidemics. It may set in during the height of the disease.

Typhoid Psychoses.—There are three groups of cases: first, an initial delirium, which may be serious, and cause the patient to wander from his home, or he may become maniacal; secondly, the psychosis associated directly with the pyrexia and the toxemia; in a few cases this outlasts the disappearance of the fever for months or even years; and, lastly, the asthenic psychosis of convalescence, more common after typhoid than after any other fever. The prognosis is usually good.

There is a distressing posttyphoid *neurasthenia* which may persist for months or even for years.

Special Senses.—*Eye.*—Conjunctivitis, simple or phlyctenular, sometimes with keratitis and iritis, may develop. Panophthalmitis has occurred in association with hemorrhage (Finlay). Loss of accommodation may occur, usually in the asthenia of convalescence. Oculomotor paralysis is due probably to neuritis. Retinal hemorrhages may occur alone or with other hemorrhagic features. Double optic neuritis has been described and may be independent of meningitis. Atrophy may follow, but these complications are excessively rare. Cataract may follow inflammation of the uveal tract. Other rare complications are thrombosis of the orbital veins and orbital hemorrhage.

Ear.—Deafness is common during the course but usually is not permanent. Otitis media is not infrequent. We never found the typhoid bacillus in the discharge. Serious results are rare; only one case of mastoid disease occurred in our series. The otitis may set in with a chill and an increase of the fever but may be recognized first by the discharge.

Urinary System.—*Retention of urine* is an early symptom and may cause abdominal pain. It may recur throughout the attack. *Suppression of urine* is rare. The urine is usually diminished at first, has the ordinary febrile characters, and the pigments are increased. *Polyuria* is not very uncommon. While most common during convalescence, the increase may be sudden in the second week at the height of the fever. The amount of urine depends very much on the fluid taken.

Typhoid bacilluria occurs in about one-third of the cases if methenamine (hexamine) is not given. The urine may be turbid from their presence and in the test-tube give a peculiar shimmer. Bacilluria may occur without pyuria or any symptoms of renal or bladder trouble. The bacilli may be present for a few days, or for weeks to years after the attack.

Febrile *albuminuria* is common and of no special significance. It was present in 999 of 1,500 cases, 66 per cent. Casts were present in 568 cases, 37.8 per cent. *Hemoglobinuria* occurred in one case.

Acute nephritis at the onset or during the disease may mask the true nature of the malady. After an indisposition of a few days there may be fever, pain in the back, and the passage of bloody urine.

Nephritis during convalescence is rare, and is usually associated with anemia and edema. Chronic nephritis is a most exceptional sequel.

The lymphomatous nephritis produces, as a rule, no symptoms.

Pyuria, a not uncommon complication, may be associated with the typhoid or the colon bacillus, less often with staphylococci. It usually disappears during convalescence. It may be due to a simple catarrh of the bladder, rarely to an intense cystitis, sometimes to pyelitis. *Gangrene* of the bladder wall may occur, usually after retention. The urine is purulent and bloody, and contains fragments of bladder mucosa.

Pyelitis.—One or both kidneys may be involved, either at the height of the disease or during convalescence. There may be blood and pus at first, later pus alone, varying in amount. A severe pyelonephritis may follow. The colon bacillus is often present. *Perinephric abscess* is a rare sequel.

Generative System.—*Orchitis* is occasionally met with and may be associated with a catarrhal urethritis. Induration or atrophy may occur, and more rarely suppuration. It was present in 4 cases of our series. *Prostatitis* occurs rarely.

Acute mastitis, which may go on to suppuration, is rare and was present in 3 cases of our series during the fever and in one in convalescence.

Osseous System.—Among the most troublesome of the sequelae are the *bone lesions* which in a few cases occur at the height of the disease or even earlier. Of 237 cases collected by Keen there was periostitis in 110, necrosis in 85, and caries in 13. They are much more frequent than the figures indicate. The lesion may not appear until many years after the attack of typhoid fever. The legs are chiefly involved. In Keen's series the tibia was affected in 91 cases, the ribs in 40. The typhoid bone lesion is apt to form what the old writers called a cold abscess. Only a few of the cases are acute. Chronicity, indolence, and a remarkable tendency to recurrence are the most striking features. A bony node may be left by typhoid periostitis.

Arthritis was present in 8 cases of our series. It may be monarticular or polyarticular. One important point relating to it is the frequency with which spontaneous dislocations occur, particularly of the hip.

Typhoid Spine (Gibney).—During the disease but more often during convalescence, the patient complains of pain in the lumbar and sacral regions, perhaps after a slight jar or shock. Stiffness of the back, pain on movement, sometimes radiating, and tenderness on pressure are the chief features, but there are in addition marked nervous manifestations. There is rigidity and fixation of the spine, usually in the lower part. Kyphosis occurs in some cases. The X-ray plates may show definite bony change. There is usually spondylitis or perispondylitis. The duration is weeks or months, but the outlook is good.

The *muscles* may be the seat of degeneration but it rarely causes any symptoms. Hemorrhage occasionally occurs into the muscles, and late in protracted cases abscesses may follow. Rupture of a muscle, usually the rectus abdominis, may occur, possibly associated with acute hemorrhagic myositis. *Painful muscles* are not uncommon, particularly in the calves and painful cramps may occur. In some cases the condition is a myositis; in others the swelling and pain may be due to thrombosis in the deeper veins.

Posttyphoid Septicemia and Pyemia.—In very protracted cases after defervescence a slight fever (100°-101° F.) may recur with sweats, which is possibly septic. In other cases for two or three weeks there are recurring chills, often of great severity. They are usually of no moment in the absence of signs of a complication.

Typhoid *pyemia* is not common. Extensive furunculosis may be associated with irregular fever and leukocytosis. Following the fever there may be multiple subcutaneous "cold" abscesses, often with a dark, thin bloody pus. A crural thrombus may suppurate and cause a widespread pyemia. In rare instances suppuration of the mesenteric glands, of a splenic infarct, a sloughing parotid gland, a perinephric or perirectal abscess, acute necrosis of the bones, or a multiple suppurative arthritis may cause pyemia. In other cases following bed sores or furunculosis a general infection with pyogenic organisms occurs with fatal results.

Association of Other Diseases.—Erysipelas is a rare complication, most common during convalescence. Measles or scarlet fever may develop during the fever or in convalescence. Chickenpox and noma have been reported in children. Pseudomembranous inflammations may occur in the pharynx, larynx or genitals. Malarial and typhoid fevers may be associated, but a majority of the cases of so-called typhomalarial fever are either remittent malarial fever or true typhoid. Among 1,500 cases of typhoid fever plasmodia were found in the blood in only three.

Typhoid Fever and Tuberculosis.—The diseases may coexist. A person with chronic tuberculosis may contract the fever. Of 105 autopsies in typhoid fever, 7 presented marked tuberculous lesions. Miliary tuberculosis and typhoid fever may occur together. Cases of typhoid fever with pulmonary and pleuritic symptoms may suggest tuberculosis at the onset. There are types of tuberculosis infection which may simulate typhoid fever: the acute miliary form; the acute septicemic form; tuberculous meningitis; tuberculous peritonitis; the acute toxemia of certain local lesions; and forms of ordinary pulmonary tuberculosis. And, lastly, pulmonary tuberculosis may follow typhoid fever. In a large majority of such cases from the onset the disease has been tuberculosis.

In epilepsy and in chronic chorea the fits and movements usually cease during an attack, and in typhoid fever in a diabetic subject the sugar may be absent during the height of the disease.

Varieties.—Typhoid fever presents an extremely complex symptomatology. Many forms have been described, some of which present exaggeration of common symptoms, others modification in the course, others again greater intensity of action of the poison on certain organs. Typhoid fever has no fixed and constant course and may set in with symptoms localized in certain organs. Many of its features are extremely variable—in one epidemic uniform and textbook-like, in another slight or not present. This diversified symptomatology has led to many errors, and in the absence of the salutary lessons of morbid anatomy it is not surprising that practitioners are so often led astray. We may recognize the following varieties:

The *mild* and *abortive* forms. Much attention has been paid to the milder varieties. There is danger of neglecting these mild forms, which are often spoken of as mountain fever and malarial fever, "acclimation," "ground," and "miasmatic" fevers. There may be cases so mild that the patient does not go to bed. The onset may be sudden, particularly in children. The general symptoms are slight, the pulse rate not high, the fever rarely above 102°. Rose spots are usually present, with splenic enlargement. Diarrhea is rare. The Widal reaction is present in a majority of the patients. There may be a marked tendency to relapse. While infrequent, characteristic complications and sequelae may give the first positive clue to the diagnosis. It can not be too forcibly impressed upon the profession that it is by these mild cases, to which so little attention is paid, that the disease may be kept up in a community.

The *grave* form is usually characterized by high fever and pronounced nervous symptoms. In this category come the very severe cases, setting in with pneumonia and nephritis, and with the very intense gastro-intestinal or cerebro-spinal symptoms.

The *ambulatory* form is particularly common in hospital practice. The symptoms are usually slight, and the patient scarcely feels ill enough to go to bed. He has languor, perhaps slight diarrhea, but keeps about and may even attend to his work throughout the entire attack. In other instances delirium sets in. Hemorrhage or perforation may be the first marked sign of this ambulatory type. Sir W. Jenner called attention to the dangers of this form, and particularly to the grave prognosis in those who traveled far with the disease in progress.

Hemorrhagic Typhoid Fever.—This is excessively rare. Among Ouskow's 6,513 cases there were 4 fatal cases with general hemorrhagic features. Only three instances were present in our series. Hemorrhages may be marked from the outset, but more commonly they come on during the course. The condition is not necessarily fatal.

An *afebrile* typhoid fever is recognized by some authors, but there is usually slight fever. The patients present lassitude, headache, furred tongue, loss of appetite, slow pulse, and even the spots and enlarged spleen.

Typhoid Fever in Children.—In young children the disease is not very uncommon. The abdominal symptoms are usually mild; fatal hemorrhage and perforation are rare. Among sequelae, aphasia, noma, and bone lesions are stated to be more common in children than in adults. Two of our cases were under one year of age.

Typhoid Fever in the Aged.—After the sixtieth year the disease runs a less favorable course, and the mortality is high. The fever is less, but complications are more common, particularly pneumonia and heart failure.

Typhoid Fever in Pregnancy.—In 438 females in our series there were 6 cases. Goltdammer noted 26 pregnancies in 600 cases of typhoid fever in the female. It is more common in the first half of pregnancy. The pregnancy is interrupted in about 65 per cent of the cases, usually in the second week of the disease. There may be puerperal infection with the typhoid bacillus.

Typhoid Fever in the Fetus.—The typhoid bacillus may pass through the placenta to the child, causing a typhoid septicemia, without intestinal lesions. Infection of the fetus does not necessarily follow, but when infected the child dies, either *in utero* or shortly after birth. The agglutinating substance may filter through the placenta or be transmitted to the nursling through the milk, and cause a transient reaction.

Relapse.—Relapses vary in frequency in different epidemics, and, it would appear, in different places. The percentages of different authors range from 3 to 15 or 18 per cent. In our 1,500 cases there were 172 relapses, 11.4 per cent. Among 28,057 collected cases 8.8 per cent had a relapse. We may recognize the ordinary, the intercurrent and the spurious relapse.

The *ordinary relapse* sets in after complete defervescence. The average duration of the interval of normal temperature is five or six days but may be six weeks. As a rule, two of the three important features—steplike temperature at onset, roseola, an enlarged spleen—should be present to justify the diagnosis of a relapse. The intestinal symptoms are variable. The onset may be abrupt with a chill, or the temperature may have a typical ascent. The number of relapses ranges from 1 to 6. In one case the disease lasted for eleven months. The relapse is usually less severe, of shorter duration and the mortality is low.

The *intercurrent relapse* is common, often severe, and is responsible for many of the most protracted cases. The temperature drops and the patient improves; but after remaining between 100° and 102° for a few days, the fever again rises and the patient enters upon another attack, which may be more protracted, and of much greater intensity than the original one. The prognosis in these cases is graver than in the ordinary relapse.

Spurious relapses have been mentioned as posttyphoid elevations of temperature. They are recrudescences of the fever due to a number of causes. It is not always easy to determine whether a relapse is present, particularly in cases in which the fever persists for only five or seven days without rose spots and without enlargement of the spleen.

Undoubtedly a reinfection from within, yet of the conditions favoring the occurrence of relapse we know little. It may be due to more than one strain of the organism being present and the antibodies formed during the primary attack not giving protection against all the strains.

Diagnosis.—There are several points to note. Typhoid fever is extraordinarily variable in its manifestations; there is no such hybrid malady as typhomalarial fever; and errors in diagnosis are inevitable, even under the most favorable conditions.

General.—No single symptom or feature is characteristic. The onset is often suggestive, particularly the occurrence of epistaxis, and (if seen from the start) the ascending fever. The steadiness of the fever for a week or longer after reaching the fastigium is an important point. The irregular remittent character in the third week, and the intermittent features with chills, are common sources of errors. While there is nothing characteristic in the pulse, dicrotism is so much more common early in typhoid fever that its presence is always suggestive. The rash is the most valuable single sign and with the fever usually clinches the diagnosis. The enlarged spleen is of less importance, since it occurs in many febrile conditions, but with the fever and the rash it completes a diagnostic triad. The absence of leukocytosis is valuable. Typhoid should be suspected in every doubtful fever.

Specific.—Typhoid Bacilli from the Blood.—This is especially useful early in the disease, in doubtful cases and in the acute septic forms.

Typhoid Bacilli from the Duodenum.—Cultures from the duodenum obtained through the duodenal tube are often positive.

Typhoid Bacilli from the Stools.—Cultures from the stools are of diagnostic value at all stages.

Typhoid Bacilli from the Urine.—Positive cultures may be obtained before the Widal test is positive.

The Agglutination Test.—In 1894 Pfeiffer showed that cholera spirilla, when introduced into the peritoneum of an immunized animal, or when mixed with the serum of immunized animals, lose their motion and break up. This "Pfeiffer's phenomenon" was thoroughly studied by Durham and the specificity of the reaction demonstrated. A. S. Grünbaum and Widal made the method available in clinical work. The serum reaction is of great value and with the newer methods the reactions are of importance in inoculated and uninoculated persons.

With Dreyer's method of standard cultures of constant and known sensitiveness it is possible to follow the serum changes in typhoid or paratyphoid infection. Whatever be the infection the agglutination for that bacillus will show (*a*) a marked rise in an early stage and (*b*) a marked fall later in the infection. If the patient's serum already contains agglutinins for one or more of the bacilli (owing to inoculation), the following phenomena will be noted: (*a*) there is no change in the inoculation agglutinins or (*b*) a slight rise occurs, followed by a slight fall—an alteration which may be caused by a number of nonspecific stimuli. A well marked rise or fall of the titer is the only positive evidence of active infection that can be obtained with the agglutination test and is probably the best evidence afforded by any test except a successful blood culture.

Atropine Test (Marris).—The patient should remain as quiet as possible during the test, which should not be done until at least an hour after the last feeding. The pulse rate is counted until it is found to be steady. Atropine gr. 1/33 (0.002 gm.) is given hypodermically, and 25 minutes later the pulse is counted each minute until any rise which follows the injection has begun to pass off. The difference between the average pulse rate before the injection and the maximum after it gives the acceleration due to the atropine. The highest average count is usually about thirty minutes after the injection. If the "escape" is 14 or less, the diagnosis is probably typhoid or paratyphoid fever; if 15 or more the reaction is negative. Three negative reactions within the first fortnight of a febrile illness exclude the typhoid group. A negative reaction after the end of the second week or when the fever has fallen may be unreliable. This test is most useful from the fifth to the fourteenth day, but a series of negative reactions later than the fourteenth day is evidence against typhoid infection. A positive reaction may be obtained in those over fifty years of age, especially if arteriosclerotic. In patients with a pulse rate of 100 or over, a positive reaction has to be taken with caution; a negative reaction in patients who are very toxic is not conclusive.

Common Sources of Error in Diagnosis.—An early and intense localization of the infection in certain organs may give rise to doubt at first.

Patients with severe headache, photophobia, delirium, twitching of the muscles and retraction of the head are often regarded as having *cerebrospinal meningitis.* The lumbar puncture is a great help.

The misleading *pulmonary* symptoms have been mentioned. The bronchitis rarely causes error, though it may be intense and attract the chief attention. More difficult are the cases setting in with chill and followed rapidly by *pneumonia.* There is less danger of mistaking the pneumonia which occurs at the height of the disease. Early involvement of the pleura or the kidneys may for a time obscure the diagnosis.

Of diseases with which typhoid fever may be confounded, malaria, certain forms of pyemia, acute tuberculosis, tuberculous peritonitis, *Bacillus faecalis alkaligenes* infection, undulant fever, trichiniasis and typhus fever are the most important.

Bacillus faecalis alkaligenes infection usually has an abrupt onset and shows symptoms much like typhoid fever. The initial fever lasts for two to five days and then is normal for a few days. There may be several recrudescences. Toxemia may be marked. Blood cultures and agglutination tests are essential in diagnosis. Recovery is the rule. The treatment is symptomatic.

From *malarial fever,* typhoid is, as a rule, readily recognized. Typhoid fever and malarial fever may coexist in the same patient but this is rare. The estivo-autumnal type of malarial fever may present a striking similarity to typhoid fever and differentiation may be made only by the blood examination. There may be no chills, the remissions may be extremely slight, there is a history perhaps of *malaise,* weakness, diarrhea, and sometimes vomiting. The tongue is furred and white, the cheeks flushed, the spleen slightly enlarged, and the fever continuous, or with slight remissions. The estivo-autumnal malarial parasite may be difficult to find.

Pyemia.—The long-continued fever of obscure, deep-seated suppuration, without chills or sweats, may simulate typhoid. The more chronic cases of bacterial endocarditis may be diagnosed typhoid fever. The presence or absence of leukocytosis is an important aid. The Widal reaction and the blood cultures offer valuable help.

Acute miliary tuberculosis is not infrequently mistaken for typhoid fever. The points in differential diagnosis will be discussed under that disease. *Tuberculous peritonitis* in certain forms may simulate typhoid fever.

Undulant fever may be a source of difficulty. The absence of the positive findings in typhoid infection and the agglutination test and positive blood cultures for *Brucella militensis-abortus* are distinctive.

Trichiniasis resembles typhoid fever, but the edema, local muscular tenderness, leukocytosis and eosinophilia should make the diagnosis clear.

The early abdominal pain, etc., may lead to the diagnosis of *appendicitis.*

The mild endemic form of *typhus fever* may be regarded as typhoid fever, but the character of the rash, the absence of the agglutination reaction, negative results of blood cultures and the course are against this. The majority of cases are probably diagnosed as typhoid fever.

Prognosis.—DEATH-RATE.—The mortality is very variable, ranging in private practice from 5 to 12 and in hospital practice from 7 to 20 per cent. In some large epidemics the death-rate has been low. Hydrotherapy reduced the death-rate in a remarkable manner, even as low as 5 or 6 per cent. Of the 1,500 cases in our series, 9.1 per cent died.

SPECIAL FEATURES.—Unfavorable symptoms are high fever, toxic symptoms with delirium, meteorism, and hemorrhage. Perforation renders the outlook hopeless unless operation is done early. Fat subjects stand typhoid fever badly. The mortality in women is greater than in men. The dangers are more serious in the ambulatory form in which the patient has kept about for a time. Early involvement of the nervous system is a bad indication; and the low, muttering delirium with tremor means a close fight for life. Prognostic signs from the fever alone are deceptive. High fever may be well borne if the nervous system is not involved. The degree of bacteremia is of value; the greater this is the worse the prognosis.

Sudden Death.—It is difficult in many cases to explain this most lamentable accident. There are cases in which neither cerebral, renal, nor cardiac changes have been found. Fibrillation of the ventricle may be the cause in some cases. Sudden death occurs more frequently in men than in women. It may occur at the height of the fever or during convalescence.

Prophylaxis.—In cities the prevalence of typhoid fever is directly proportionate to the character of the drainage and the purity of the milk and water supply. With their improvement the incidence is reduced materially. In general the disease exists to a proportionately greater extent in the country than in the city. The water supply of the latter is usually better than in the country, where the privy vault is often in close proximity to the well. Chlorination of water supplies has been very largely responsible for the great decrease in typhoid fever in cities. To stamp out typhoid fever requires *the recognition of all cases, including the typhoid carriers, and, the destruction of all typhoid bacilli as they leave the patient.* It is as much a part of the physician's duty to look after these points as to take care of the patient. Mild cases of fever are to be regarded with suspicion.

In prophylaxis, the question practically narrows down to disinfection of the urine, stools, sputum (in the few cases where bacilli are present), and of objects which may be contaminated accidentally by these excretions. The nurse or attendant should regard every specimen of urine as a culture of typhoid bacilli, and exercise great care in preventing the scattering of drops of urine over the patient, bedding or floor, or over the hands of the attendant.

To disinfect the *urine* the best solutions are carbolic acid, 1-20, in an amount equal to that of the urine, or bichloride of mercury, 1-1000, in an amount one-fifth that of the fluid to be sterilized. These mixtures with the urine should stand at least two hours. Hexamine causes disappearance of the bacilli from the urine when bacilluria is present, but under no circumstances should its administration permit the disinfection of the urine to be neglected. For the *stools,* heat is the most efficient and can be employed in hospitals by special hoppers in which steam is used. Of solutions, carbolic acid or freshly prepared milk of lime is most useful. The stool should be mixed with at least thrice its volume of these solutions and allowed to stand for several hours. All *sputum* should receive the same care as in tuberculosis. It is best to collect it in paper or gauze, which may be burned.

All the *linen* from the patient's bed or person should be soaked for two hours in 1-2000 bichloride solution, and then boiled in the laundry. All dishes should be boiled before leaving the patient's room.

The nurse should wear a rubber apron when working with a typhoid patient, and this should be washed frequently with bichloride of mercury solution. She should soak her hands thoroughly in 1-1000 bichloride solution afterwards but the free use of soap and water should not be neglected.

It is impossible to deal with all the possible modes of spread of the infection. Keeping in mind that everything leaving the patient should be sterilized, a person of ordinary intelligence can carry out very satisfactory prophylaxis. Those nursing the patient should not handle food for others.

Should the typhoid fever patient be isolated? To prevent direct infection of others a moderate degree of isolation should be carried out, though this need not be absolute. The windows should have fly screens in summer. After recovery the room should be disinfected.

An important question is as to the necessity for the isolation of typhoid patients in special wards in hospitals. At present this is not generally done in the United States. When, however, we consider the cases of hospital infection the advisability of isolation of typhoid fever patients is certainly worth considering. On the other hand, in the general hospital, with students in the wards, the cases are more thoroughly studied, and in graver complications, as perforation, it is of the greatest advantage to have the early cooperation of the surgeon.

When the disease is prevalent the drinking water and the milk should be boiled. Travellers should drink mineral water rather than ordinary water or milk. Care should be taken to thoroughly cook oysters which have been fattened in streams contaminated with sewage.

During an epidemic the early recognition of all cases followed by isolation and disinfection is most important. *Preventive inoculation* should be given as generally as possible. Every effort should be made to find the source of infection with a thorough search for *carriers*, especially in local outbreaks. In the search for carriers the agglutination test is not sufficient and cultures of the contents of the duodenum, the feces and urine should be made.

Preventive Inoculation.—Introduced by Wright this has proved of inestimable value in reducing the occurrence of typhoid fever. The material used is a bouillon or agar culture of bacilli heated to a temperature of 53° to 55° C. to kill them. Lysol or tricresol may be added. Three inoculations are given at intervals of ten days. The use of a sensitized vaccine has some advantages. The smooth antigen should be employed.

A triple vaccine against typhoid and paratyphoid A and B should be used. Untoward results are rare. The inoculation fever begins in from four to six hours and may reach 101° or even 103° to 104°. Headache, chilliness, pains in the back and limbs, and vomiting may occur. In many there is only a transient indisposition. More severe symptoms may occur, such as arthritis, fugitive erythema, diarrhea, abdominal pains, septicemia, with pneumonia, pleurisy and pericarditis. In a few cases a fever resembling typhoid has followed. A light diet, avoidance of stimulants and rest lessen the possibility of serious sequels. The evidence so far points to a persistence of the protective effect for some years after inoculation. The typhoidin skin reaction is a guide to the duration of immunity. If infection results after proper inoculation it is probably due to a very large dose of typhoid bacilli. The oral administration of typhoid vaccine is advised by some and there is some evidence of its value but the hypodermic method is more reliable.

Treatment.—General Management.—Typhoid fever is not a disease to be treated mainly with drugs. Careful nursing, a proper diet, and hydrotherapy are the essentials in a majority of cases. The patient should be in a well-ventilated room, strictly confined to bed from the outset, and there remain until convalescence is well established. An intelligent nurse should be in charge. When this is impossible, the physician should write out specific instructions regarding diet and treatment of the discharges and bed linen. The common initial purge is better omitted.

Diet.—The patient should be nourished as well as possible and food given with a value of 2,500 to 3,000 calories and containing about 70 grams of protein if conditions permit. The bulk of the food should be liquid and milk or its modifications form the largest part. Milk in any form, cream, ice cream, cocoa, tea or coffee with cream, strained soups, eggs, either the white or the whole egg, raw or soft boiled, gruels and jellies may be given. The milk may be boiled or diluted, or some modification given—peptonized milk, fermented milk, malted milk, buttermilk or whey. Soft food is often permissible, such as milk toast, custard, junket, crackers and milk, bread and butter, and mashed potatoes. It is important to give carbohydrate freely to spare the body proteins, and this is aided by the addition of milk sugar to the diet. Cane sugar or dextrose can be given freely. The food should be chosen for each patient and a routine diet not followed. In case of digestive disturbance—undigested food in the stools, diarrhea, meteorism—the diet should be very simple, buttermilk, whey, peptonized milk or albumin water usually being suitable. The beef extracts, meat juices, and artificially prepared protein foods are unnecessary and sometimes harmful. *Water* should be given freely at fixed intervals. It is desirable to have the patient take at least four litres of water daily and larger amounts are an advantage. Barley water, lemonade, soda water, or iced-tea may be used. It is doubtful if alcohol is of any value except when its use enables the patient to take nourishment more freely.

Special care must be given to the mouth, which should be cleaned after each feeding. A mouth wash should be used freely (such as phenol ʒ i, 4 cc., glycerine ℥ i, 30 cc., and boric acid, saturated solution, to ℥ x, 300 cc.).

Hydrotherapy.—The use of water, inside and outside, was no new treatment in fevers at the end of the eighteenth century, when James Currie (a friend of Burns and the editor of his poems) wrote his *Medical Reports on the Effects of Water, Cold and Warm, as a Remedy in Fevers and other Diseases.* In the United States it was used with great effect and recommended strongly by Nathan Smith, of Yale. The value of bathing in fevers was especially emphasized by the late Dr. Brand of Stettin.

Hydrotherapy may be carried out in several ways, of which the most satisfactory are sponging, the wet pack, the ice-rub, and the full bath.

Sponging.—The water may be tepid or cold, according to the height of the fever. A thorough sponge-bath should take from fifteen to twenty minutes. The cold sponging and the ice-rub are not quite as formidable as the full bath, for which, when there is an insuperable objection in private practice, they are excellent alternatives.

The *wet pack* is not so generally useful in typhoid fever, but in cases with very pronounced nervous symptoms, if the tub is not available, the patient may be wrapped in a sheet wrung out of water at 60° or 65° F., and then cold water sprinkled over him with an ordinary watering-pot.

The Bath.—This has gone out of use in many city hospitals because there are so few patients with typhoid fever. When properly used it reduced the death rate by about 7 per cent. Contra-indications are peritonitis, hemorrhage, phlebitis, abdominal pain, and great prostration.

Medicinal Treatment.—There is no specific drug treatment, but it is usually advisable to give hexamine after the second week, 20 to 30 grains (1.3 to 2 gm.) daily. In private practice it may be safer, for the young practitioner especially, to order an acid or a mild fever mixture. The question of medicinal antipyretics is important: they are used far too often and too rashly. The giving of antiseptic drugs intravenously does not seem justified. The value of quinine is doubtful. In intestinal antiseptic drugs we have no faith. Most of them do no harm, except that their use too often diverts the practitioner from more rational and safer courses.

Vaccine and Serum Therapy.—The value of treatment by vaccines during the height of the disease has not been proved. Some use vaccines subcutaneously or intravenously. Doses varying from 50 to 500 million bacilli are given, usually three or four days apart. A moderate reaction should be produced. As patients react very differently, the smaller doses are safer at first, especially if given intravenously. In long-continued attacks when progress is slow, for complications due to the presence of typhoid bacilli in organs or tissues, and for carriers, vaccine therapy is helpful. No serum of proved value has been obtained.

Treatment of Special Symptoms.—For severe *toxemia* water should be given freely by mouth if possible, otherwise by the bowel or subcutaneously. Glucose may be given intravenously, 250 to 500 cc. of a 10 per cent solution. Hydrotherapy should be used actively. For headache and delirium an ice-bag or cold compresses should be kept to the head. If the patient is delirious and restless a dose of morphia hypodermically is the best treatment. Lumbar puncture is useful, the fluid being allowed to run as long as it flows under pressure. Every delirious patient should be constantly watched. It is important to secure sleep for these patients, for which morphia is most reliable. Hydrotherapy, internal and external, is our greatest aid in the treatment of the nervous conditions. The abdominal *pain* and *tympanites* are best treated with fomentations or turpentine stupes. Sir William Jenner used to lay great stress on the advantages of a turpentine stupe applied as follows: A flannel roller was placed beneath the patient, and then a double layer of thin flannel, wrung out of very hot water, with a dram of turpentine mixed with the water, was applied to the abdomen and covered with the ends of the roller. When the stomach is greatly distended the passage of a stomach tube gives relief. When the gas is in the large bowel, a rectal tube may be passed or a turpentine enema given. For tympanites, with a dry tongue, turpentine may be given, ♏ xv (1 cc.) every three hours. Whey and albumen-water should be substituted for milk. Pituitary extract or eserine 1/50 gr. (0.0013 gm.) hypodermically, may be tried. Opium should not be given.

For the *diarrhea,* if severe—that is, if there are more than three or four stools daily—a starch and opium enema may be given; or, by the mouth, a combination of bismuth, in large doses, with Dover's powder; or small doses of opium, morphia or codein. Repeated saline irrigations are sometimes helpful. The amount of food should be reduced, and whey and albumen-water in small amounts substituted for milk. An ice-bag or cold compresses relieve the soreness which sometimes accompanies diarrhea.

Constipation is present in many cases and it is well to give an ordinary enema every second day. The addition of turpentine (℥ ss, 15 cc.) is advisable if there is meteorism. Mineral oil, up to one ounce a day, may be given.

Hemorrhage.—As absolute rest is essential, the greatest care should be taken in the use of the bed-pan. Ice may be given and a light ice-bag placed on the abdomen. The amount of food should be restricted for 24 hours. If there is a tendency to collapse, stimulants should be given. Injection of salt solution beneath the skin or into a vein should only be done in case of emergency. Should opium be given? One-fifth of the cases of perforation occur with hemorrhage, and opium may obscure the features upon which the diagnosis of perforation may be made. Opium increases any tendency to tympanites and its use is not advisable. The injection of human or horse serum intramuscularly (10 to 20 cc.) is of value. Transfusion should be done in serious cases. Sodium citrate given intravenously shortens the coagulation time, reaching a maximum in one hour and returning to normal in twenty-four hours. A 30 per cent solution is used; 3 to 6 cc. being injected very slowly, taking from ten to fifteen minutes. Its use is contra-indicated in hemorrhagic blood diseases in which the platelets are decreased. Calcium lactate may be given in doses of 15 grains (1 gm.) three times a day.

Perforation and Peritonitis.—Early diagnosis and early operation mean the saving of one-third of the cases of this otherwise fatal complication. The aim should be to operate for the perforation, and not to wait until general peritonitis diminishes the chances of recovery. An incessant, intelligent watchfulness on the part of the medical attendant and the early cooperation of the surgeon are essentials. Every case of more than ordinary severity should be watched with special reference to this complication. Thorough preparation by early observation, careful notes, and knowledge of the conditions will help to prevent needless exploration. No case is too desperate; we had a recovery after three operations. In doubtful cases it is best to operate, as the patients usually stand an exploration very well.

Cholecystitis.—A majority of the cases recover, but if the symptoms are very severe and progressive, operation should be advised. For chronic cholecystitis hexamine should be given in large doses and the vaccine treatment employed; if not successful, operation should be done. Duodenal biliary drainage may be given a trial.

With signs of failure of the *circulation*, hydrotherapy should be carried on actively and strychnine given hypodermically (gr. $\frac{1}{50}$ to $\frac{1}{20}$, 0.001 to 0.003 gm.) every three hours. Saline infusions (500 cc.) are useful especially if the patient is not taking much water by mouth. Digitalis may be given as the tincture (♏ xv, 1 cc.) but if collapse or severe symptoms occur, strophanthin gr. $\frac{1}{100}$ (0.00065 gm.) intramuscularly is better. For collapse, epinephrine (♏ xv, 1 cc. of the 1–1000 solution) should be given intramuscularly. The bath treatment is the best preventive of circulatory failure. For *phlebitis* the limb should be kept absolutely at rest and wrapped in raw cotton. The application of a sedative lotion may relieve pain.

Bacilluria.—When bacilli are present, hexamine may be given in ten-grain (0.65 gm.) doses and kept up, if necessary, for several weeks. If the urine is alkaline sodium benzoate gr. x (0.6 gm.) should be added. A patient should not be discharged with bacilli in his urine. *Pyelitis* should be treated in the same way, large amounts of water being given. For *cystitis,* irrigations of bichloride of mercury (1/100,000 solution and gradually increased in strength) may be given.

For *orchitis, mastitis, parotitis,* etc., an ice-bag should be applied. Incision and drainage are advisable on the first signs of suppuration. Vaccine treatment may be helpful.

In protracted cases special care should be taken to guard against *bed sores.* Absolute cleanliness and careful drying should be enjoined. Pressure should be avoided by rubber rings. The patient should be turned from side to side and propped with pillows, and the back sponged with alcohol.

Bone Lesions.—The use of a typhoid vaccine is well worthy of trial. Typhoid periostitis does not always go on to suppuration, though, as a rule, it requires operation. This should be done very thoroughly and the diseased parts completely removed, as otherwise recurrence is inevitable. For *typhoid spine* fixation by a plaster jacket or some form of apparatus is advisable. Trauma should be guarded against. In the milder cases active counterirritation is useful. If pain is severe, large doses of sedatives are necessary.

CONVALESCENCE.—The diet can be gradually increased, but it is usually best to wait at least a week after the temperature is normal before giving ordinary meats or coarse vegetables. Solid food sometimes disagrees if it is given too early. Whether an error in diet may cause relapse is doubtful. The patient may be allowed to sit up for a short time about the end of the first week of convalescence, and the period may be prolonged with a gradual return of strength. He should move about slowly, and when the weather is favorable should be in the open air as much as possible. He should be guarded at this period against all unnecessary excitement. Emotional disturbance not infrequently is the cause of recrudescence of the fever. Constipation is not uncommon in convalescence and is best treated by mineral oil by mouth and enemata. A protracted diarrhea, usually due to ulceration in the colon, may retard recovery. In such cases the diet should be restricted to milk and the patient confined to bed; large doses of bismuth and astringent injections will prove useful. The recrudescence of the fever does not require special measures. The treatment of a relapse is that of the original attack.

Posttyphoid psychosis requires the care of an expert. The patients usually recover. The swollen leg after phlebitis is a source of great worry. A bandage or a well-fitting elastic stocking should be worn during the day. The outlook depends on the completeness with which the collateral circulation is established. In a good many cases there is permanent disability.

The *posttyphoid neuritis,* a cause of much alarm and distress, usually gets well, though it may take months, or even a couple of years, before the paralysis disappears. After the subsidence of the acute symptoms systematic massage of the paralyzed and atrophic muscles is the best treatment.

Typhoid Carriers.—Treatment of these is difficult. Hexamine should be given persistently and in large doses. Removal of the gallbladder is indicated if it is infected. The employment of an autogenous vaccine should be tried. Doses increasing from 25 to 1,000 or 1,500 million bacilli are given at intervals of 5 to 10 days. Carriers should not be allowed to handle or prepare food.

Lastly, no patient should be discharged from observation until we are certain that he can not infect others. If stool cultures continue positive, it is well to make cultures from the duodenum, after biliary drainage, to decide if biliary tract infection is responsible. The continued observation of a carrier may have to be handed over to the Board of Health.

PARATYPHOID FEVER

Definition.—An acute infection caused by the *Bacillus paratyphosus* of which there are several varieties, A, B, C and D: A and B are the most common. They are closely related to the typhoid bacillus and cause a clinical picture much like typhoid fever.

History.—In 1896 Achard and Bensaude reported a case of "typhoid fever" in which they found an organism which was not *B. typhosus* and to which they gave the name of paratyphoid. In 1898 Gwyn isolated an organism to which he gave the name of paracolon bacillus. In 1902 Buxton described the two varieties A and B.

Occurrence.—Before the World War paratyphoid A was more common in the United States and paratyphoid B in Europe. In the World War the relative proportions varied in different places, but as a rule the B form was the more common. As regards the relative incidence of typhoid and paratyphoid fever in soldiers, one army series of 4,218 cases showed 1,684 of typhoid and 2,534 of paratyphoid fever, and in another series of 5,700 cases, 93 per cent. were paratyphoid. The inoculation in the majority had been against typhoid fever only.

Etiology.—The paratyphoid organisms differ from *B. typhosus* in cultural and agglutination properties. The A form (*Salmonella paratyphi*) is nearer to the typhoid bacillus and the B (*Salmonella schottmülleri*) form closer to *B. suipestifer* and *enteritidis.* The general problems of infection are the same as those of typhoid fever with particular importance on the part played by carriers, especially in paratyphoid B. The B form at times occurs in a form suggesting meat poisoning.

Pathology.—The toxins of the paratyphoid organisms do not show the same tendency to attack lymphoid tissues as the toxin of the typhoid bacillus and appear to cause a greater variety of lesions elsewhere. As there is a bacteremia there is a possibility of any part of the body being attacked. In general the intestinal lesions are much like those of typhoid fever but show a tendency to superficial necrosis rather than to deep ulceration. In some cases the intestines are acutely inflamed without involvement of the lymphoid tissue. Some statistics suggest that the colon frequently shows ulceration. Hemorrhage and perforation are not so common as in typhoid fever. There are several forms: (1) A septicemia with little or no change in the bowels; (2) cases not distinguishable from ordinary typhoid; (3) a dysenteric form, in which the lesions are chiefly in the large bowel, and (4) cases in which the lesions are particularly in one part of the body.

Symptoms.—The average incubation period is about ten days and an acute onset is common. Headache and abdominal pain may occur at the onset, to be followed by the usual signs of an infection, malaise, chilly sensations, and general pains. Bronchitis is common early in the attack. The clinical features are variable, as in typhoid fever, and various forms have been described depending on the predominant symptoms, such as typhoid, septicemic, dysenteric, biliary, urinary, respiratory, arthritic, etc. Apathy is often marked, especially early, and severe headache is common. The striking point about the fever is its irregularity. It may be of the classical typhoid type with remissions beginning about the end of the second week, the duration of fever may be short, there may be constant remissions or the fever may be irregular throughout. The pulse rate is usually slow and with a rising temperature may be a suggestive point. The blood pressure is usually low. The *rash* is generally like the roseola of typhoid fever, but sometimes consists of large irregular spots, raised and not fading completely on pressure, leaving areas of pigmentation. It is sometimes general. Sweating is common especially in patients with a remittent type of fever. The *spleen* is usually enlarged. Intestinal disturbance may be marked, more particularly at the onset, especially in the B form. Hemorrhage is rarely profuse and perforation is rare. Relapse rarely occurs. The *course* as a rule is shorter than in typhoid fever. Some writers comment on the slow improvement after the acute features are over and emphasize mental depression in convalescence.

Complications.—These are much like those of typhoid fever with more tendency to involvement of the respiratory tract, jaundice with infection of the bile passages, nephritis, abscess formation and arthritis. The sequelae are the same as typhoid fever, even to the bone lesions.

Diagnosis.—For practical purposes typhoid and paratyphoid fever may be considered as one disease; clinically the diagnosis is based on the same findings and only a bacteriological diagnosis can be regarded as absolutely beyond doubt. The agglutination tests are fairly reliable if markedly positive.

Prognosis.—In civil life the death rate is very low, about one per cent but in the armies it was higher.

Prophylaxis.—This is the same as for typhoid fever and the use of preventive inoculation has had the same success. The triple vaccine (typhoid and both paratyphoids) should be used. The importance of carriers should be kept in mind.

Treatment.—This is the same as in typhoid fever.

COLON BACILLUS INFECTIONS

The colon bacillus, or more properly speaking the group of colon bacilli, in their biological and pathological peculiarities are closely related to the organisms of the typhoid group. Normal inhabitants of the intestines, where in all probability they serve a useful function, the *Bacillus coli* may be taken as the typical member of the group. There are great difficulties in determining the extent of the lesions caused by this organism, which varies extraordinarily in virulence. To it has been attributed a host of maladies from appendicitis to old age, but more conservative opinion limits its pathogenic scope. It is not easy to separate the effects of the *B. coli* from those of other organisms with which it is so often associated. The needful bacteriological distinction must be considered in connection with agglutination tests.

General Hemic Infections.—There are several groups of cases:

Terminal Infections.—After death the colon bacillus swarms in the body, invading the blood and contaminating all parts. In protracted illnesses, in acute intestinal and peritoneal affections it may be present in the blood some time before death and may be responsible for the terminal fever.

Cases of general infection which may be from the intestinal, biliary or urinary tract. In some instances it has followed an operative procedure. The clinical picture is not characteristic; it is that of an acute infection. The onset may be acute or gradual; chills may occur. The degree of the fever varies greatly; its average duration is usually 7 to 10 days, with termination by lysis. There is leukocytosis. Jaundice occurs relatively often and toxemia may be marked. The main complications are bronchopneumonia, infection of the lung (often septic), pyelitis, and pyelonephritis. The *diagnosis* depends on positive blood cultures. The outlook may depend on the severity of the local process rather than on the general infection.

Cases of general infection with secondary abscesses.

Secondary infection in other diseases, as for example typhoid fever.

Subinfections.—Adami suggested that a number of chronic diseases are due to a mild, continuous infection with *B. coli.*

Local Infections.—Here we are on safer ground and have definite lesions produced by the organism.

Peritonitis.—In perforation of the bowel, in strangulated hernia, in obstruction, in various types of ulcer, the peritonitis may be due to *B. coli.*

Cholecystitis and *cholangitis,* either of the simple catarrhal type or suppurative, may be caused by it.

Infection of the Urinary Tract.—The bladder and the pelvis of the kidneys are chiefly affected. There are three possible channels of infection—by the ureter, the blood stream, and the lymphatics. Hematogenous infection is the most common but lymphatic infection from the bowel plays an important rôle in many cases. Bowel troubles have been present and with slight abrasion of the mucosa of the colon the bacilli may enter the lymphatics. An interesting point is the relative frequency of involvement of the right kidney; Franke states that the cecum and ascending colon are connected by a train of lymphatics with the right kidney, an anatomical communication not present with the left. The general features may be marked, with chills, high fever, toxemia and delirium. The *fever* is variable but may continue for days, more or less constant or remittent. There is often *pain* referred to the region of the kidney, which is tender and may be found to be enlarged. There may be well-marked hematuria; the urine contains pus in varying amount and colon bacilli are present. The course varies greatly and the fever may continue for one or two weeks. Relapse is common and many cases become chronic with acute exacerbations at intervals. Some of the patients manifest general ill health and others suffer from urinary tract symptoms. The pus in the urine varies in amount from time to time. There are several groups of cases. (1) In *children,* in whom it is not uncommon, a large proportion occurring in females. (2) In connection with *pregnancy.* The cases are common and important and may occur at any time during pregnancy or follow delivery. The pelvis of the right kidney is most often attacked. (3) As a *secondary infection* in other diseases, especially typhoid fever. (4) The group in adults, in whom, without any obvious cause, and in the majority without any previous intestinal trouble, acute pyelitis or pyelocystitis comes on. The infection is obstinate and a distressing sequel is a chronic arthritis. (5) *Cystitis* and *urethritis* in newly married women are sometimes due to colon infection. Care should be taken not to regard them as gonorrheal. The colon bacillus is often present in the urethra of the female. (6) Epididymitis and orchitis.

Intestines.—To the *Bacillus coli* almost all the diseases of the bowels from ulcer of the duodenum to appendicitis have been attributed. Gastric and duodenal ulcers have been produced by feeding cultures of *B. coli* to dogs, and from the peptic ulcers of young infants Helmholz isolated the organism in pure culture. There is great difficulty in determining the precise etiological relationship of *B. coli* to the lesions of the gastro-intestinal tract.

Other local infections with which the *colon bacillus* has been associated are acute meningitis, abscess of the brain, endocarditis, and suppuration in various parts. Only in a small proportion of these cases has the association been demonstrated by cultural and biological tests.

TREATMENT.—In the cases of general infection, rest, careful diet, and large amounts of water are indicated. It is well to give a low protein diet, meat and eggs being excluded. To influence the intestinal flora, *B. acidophilus* cultures may be tried. Buttermilk in place of raw milk is useful. The bowels should be kept open and a daily enema is usually advisable. The milder laxatives are best, such as cascara and salines. In the local infections the treatment is that of the condition present, as peritonitis and cholecystitis. For infection of the urinary tract the diet should be simple and large amounts of water should be given with urinary antiseptics, especially hexamine (gr. 40 to 60 a day, 2.6 to 4 gm.) or hexylresorcinol (0.15 gm.). Local treatment by irrigations is helpful in cystitis and in some cases of pyelitis. The use of an *autogenous* vaccine is an aid in some cases and should always be tried in subacute and chronic cases. The initial dose should be small (one-half or one million organisms) and gradually increased to 250 million or even more. Vaccine treatment in intestinal infections with hemolytic varieties of the colon bacillus is worth a trial. Every effort should be made to improve the general health and special attention given to insure regularity of the bowels.

THE PYOGENIC INFECTIONS

(*Toxemia, Septicemia, Pyemia, Focal Infection, Terminal Infections*)

Definition.—A group of nonspecific diseases, induced by a number of micro-organisms, of which the pyogenic cocci are the most important, characterized by fever, chills, leukocytosis, often a profound intoxication and sometimes by foci of suppuration. A hard-and-fast line can not be drawn between an infection and an intoxication, but agents of infection alone are capable of reproduction, whereas those of intoxication are toxins, some of which are produced by bacteria, or by vegetable and animal cells. There are five chief clinical types of pyogenic infection:

LOCAL INFECTIONS WITH THE DEVELOPMENT OF TOXINS

This is the common mode of invasion of certain infectious diseases. Tetanus, diphtheria and erysipelas are diseases which have sites of local infection in which the pathogenic organisms develop; but the constitutional effects are caused by absorption of toxins. The tetanus toxin produces every feature of the disease, without the presence of the bacilli. Certain of the symptoms following the absorption of the toxins are general to all; others are special and peculiar, according to the organism which produces them. A chill, fever, general malaise, prostration, rapid pulse, restlessness, and headache are the most frequent. With but few exceptions the febrile disturbance is the most common feature. The most serious effects are upon the nervous system and the circulation, and the gravity of the changes in these systems is to some extent a measure of the intensity of the toxemia.

SEPTICEMIA

Formerly, and in a surgical sense, the term "septicemia" was used to designate the invasion of the blood and tissues of the body by the organisms of suppuration, but in the medical sense the term may be applied to any condition in which, with or without a local site of infection, there is microbic invasion of the blood and tissues, but without metastatic foci of suppuration. Owing to the development of bacteria in the blood, this condition is termed *bacteremia.* The main forms of streptococci concerned are the *S. pyogenes* or *hemolyticus* and *S. viridans.* The former usually produces general infections, often from a definite portal of entry as a wound or the uterus. The latter is often from infected teeth and tonsils and an example is subacute bacterial endocarditis.

Progressive Septicemia from Local Infection.—The common streptococcus and staphylococcus infection is, as a rule, first local, and the toxins alone pass into the blood. In other instances the cocci appear in the blood and throughout the tissues, causing a septicemia which intensifies greatly the severity of the case. The clinical features of this form are well seen in the cases of puerperal septicemia or in dissection wounds, in which the course of the infection may be traced along the lymphatics. A severe throat infection may be the source of the general invasion. The symptoms usually set in within twenty-four hours, and rarely later than the third or fourth day. There is a chill or chilliness, with moderate fever at first, which gradually rises and is marked by daily remissions and even intermissions. The pulse is small and compressible, and may reach 120 or higher. Gastro-intestinal disturbances are common, the tongue is red at the margin, and the dorsum is dry and dark. Diarrhea occurs often, especially in streptococcus infections. There may be early delirium or marked mental prostration and apathy. As the disease progresses there may be pallor of the face or a yellowish tint. Capillary hemorrhages are not uncommon. Anemia is common and leukocytosis usually occurs.

In streptococcus cases we now recognize that these infections are not always so serious as we thought. Death may occur within twenty-four hours or be delayed for several days, even for weeks, and recovery may occur. One patient showed streptococci in the blood for six weeks, but recovered (Cole). On postmortem examination there may be no gross focal lesions in the viscera, and the seat of infection may present only slight changes. The spleen is enlarged and soft, the blood may be extremely dark in color, and hemorrhages are common, particularly on the serous surfaces. Neither thrombi nor emboli are found. Certain features occur with streptococcus infection, chiefly the absence of delirium, a rather abnormal mental acuteness, and the presence of a greater degree of anemia. Staphylococcus infections more often show secondary lesions, especially in the pleura, peritoneum, bones and joints.

Many instances of septicemia are combined infections; thus in diphtheria streptococcus septicemia is a most serious event. The local disease and the symptoms produced by absorption of the toxins dominate the clinical picture; but the features are usually much aggravated by the systemic invasion. These secondary septicemias are caused most frequently by the streptococcus, but may be due to other bacteria.

Septicemia without Recognizable Local Infection.—*Cryptogenetic Septicemia.*—The subjects when attacked may be in perfect health; more commonly they are already weakened by acute or chronic illness. The pathogenic organisms are varied. *Streptococcus pyogenes* is the most common; the forms of staphylococcus more rare. Other occasional causal agents are the pneumococcus, *Bacillus proteus, Bacillus pyocyaneus* and *Bacillus influenzae.* In a period of three years, from the medical wards of the Hopkins Hospital, 21 cases of general infection came to autopsy, of which 13 were due to *Streptococcus pyogenes,* 2 to *Staphylococcus pyogenes,* and 6 to the pneumococcus. In 19 of these cases the patients were already the subjects of some other malady, which was aggravated or terminated by the septicemia. The symptoms vary somewhat with the character of the micro-organisms. In the streptococcus cases there may be chills with high, irregular fever, and a more characteristic *septic* state than in a pneumococcus infection.

These cases come correctly under the term "cryptogenetic septicemia" as employed by Leube, inasmuch as the local focus of infection is not evident during life and may not be found after death. Although most of these cases are terminal infections, yet there are instances of this form coming on in apparently healthy persons. The fever may be extremely irregular, characteristically septic, and persist for many weeks. Foci of suppuration may not develop, and may not be found at autopsy. There are cases of an intermittent pyrexia persisting for weeks, in which it is impossible to give any explanation of the phenomena, with ultimate recovery and in which tuberculosis and malaria can be excluded. These cases require to be carefully studied bacteriologically. Local symptoms may be absent, though there may be enlargement of the liver, in some due to a diffuse suppurative hepatitis. The *pyocyanic* disease, or cyanopyemia, is an interesting form of infection with *Bacillus pyocyaneus,* of which a number of cases have been reported.

SEPTICOPYEMIA

The pathogenic micro-organisms which invade the blood and tissues may settle in certain foci and there cause suppuration. When multiple abscesses are thus produced in connection with a general infection, the condition is known as pyemia or, perhaps better, septicopyemia. There are no specific organisms of suppuration, and pyemia may be produced by organisms other than streptococci and staphylococci, though these are the most common. Other forms which may cause foci of suppuration are the pneumococcus, the gonococcus, *B. coli, B. typhosus, B. proteus, B. pyocyaneus, B. influenzae.* In a large proportion of all cases of pyemia there is a focus of infection, a suppurating external wound, an osteomyelitis, a gonorrhea, an otitis media, an empyema, or an area of suppuration in a lymph-node or about the appendix. In a large majority of these cases the common pus cocci are present.

In a suppurating wound, for example, the pus organisms induce hyaline necrosis in the smaller vessels with the production of thrombi and purulent phlebitis. The entrance of pus organisms in small numbers into the blood does not necessarily produce pyemia. Commonly the transmission to various parts from the local focus takes place by the fragments of thrombi which pass as emboli to different parts, where, if the conditions are favorable, the pus organisms excite suppuration. A thrombus which is not septic or infected, when dislodged and impacted in a distant vessel, produces only a simple infarction; but, coming from an infected source and containing pyogenic organisms, an independent centre of infection is established wherever the embolus may lodge. These independent suppurative centres in pyemia, known as *embolic* or *metastatic abscesses,* have the following distribution:

In external wounds, in osteomyelitis, and in acute phlegmon of the skin, the embolic particles very frequently excite suppuration in the lungs, producing wedge-shaped pyemic infarcts; from these, or rarely by paradoxical embolism, or passage of bacteria or minute emboli through the pulmonary capillaries, metastatic foci of inflammation may occur elsewhere.

Suppurative foci in the territory of the portal system produce metastatic abscesses in the liver with or without suppurative pylephlebitis.

Endocarditis is very liable to occur in all forms of septicemia, and modifies materially the character of the clinical features. Streptococci and staphylococci are the most common organisms in the vegetations, but pneumococci, gonococci, tubercle bacilli, typhoid bacilli, and other forms have been isolated. The vegetations which grow at the site of the valve lesion become covered with thrombi, particles of which may be dislodged and carried as emboli to different parts of the body, causing multiple abscesses or infarcts.

Symptoms of Septicopyemia.—In a case of wound infection, prior to the onset of the characteristic symptoms, there may be signs of local trouble, and in the case of a discharging wound the pus may change in character. The onset of the disease is marked by a severe rigor, during which the temperature rises to 103° or 104° and is followed by a profuse sweat. These chills are repeated at intervals, either daily or every other day. In the intervals there may be slight pyrexia. The constitutional disturbance is marked and there are loss of appetite, nausea, and vomiting, and, as the disease progresses, rapid emaciation. Local symptoms usually occur. If the lungs become involved there are dyspnea and cough. The physical signs may be slight. Involvement of the pleura and pericardium is common. The anemia, often profound, causes great pallor of the skin, which later may be bile-tinged. The spleen is enlarged, and there may be intense pain in the side, pointing to perisplenitis from embolism. Usually in the rapid cases a toxic state supervenes, and the patient dies comatose.

Skin Lesions.—These are very numerous. *Erythema,* the so-called "surgical scarlet fever," may extend from the infected wound or appear on the face or chest and spread widely. *Purpura* occurs as a widespread lesion in many forms of septicemia and in the later stages as a remarkable discrete rash in various parts of the body. In the acute purpura of septicemia the skin may be completely covered within 36 hours, usually preceded by a dusky erythema. Pustules, vesicles, ecthyma, urticaria and papular rashes are occasional complications. Ordinary herpes is rare.

In chronic cases the disease may be prolonged for months; chills recur at long intervals, the fever is irregular, and the condition varies from month to month. The course is usually slow and progressively downward.

Diagnosis.—Septicemia and pyemia are frequently overlooked and often mistaken for other affections. Blood cultures are most important. Cases following a wound, an operation, or parturition are readily recognized. On the other hand, the following conditions may be overlooked:

Osteomyelitis.—Here the lesion may be limited, the constitutional symptoms severe, and the course of the disease very rapid. The cause of the trouble may be discovered only postmortem.

So, too, acute septicopyemia may follow *gonorrhea* or a *prostatic abscess.*

Cases are sometimes confounded with *typhoid fever,* particularly the more chronic instances, in which there are diarrhea, great prostration, delirium, and irregular fever. The spleen, too, is often enlarged. The marked leukocytosis is an important differential point.

In some of the instances of *ulcerative endocarditis* the diagnosis is very difficult, particularly in what is known as the typhoid, in contradistinction to the septic, type. In *acute miliary tuberculosis* the symptoms may resemble those of septicemia, more commonly those of typhoid fever.

The *postfebrile arthritides,* such as occur after scarlet fever, are really instances of mild septic infection. The joints may sometimes suppurate and pyemia develop. So, also, in *tuberculosis of the kidneys* and *calculous pyelitis* recurring rigors and sweats due to septic infection are common. In some latitudes septic and pyemic processes are too often confounded with *malaria.* In early tuberculosis, or even when signs of excavation are present in the lungs, and in cases of suppuration in various parts, particularly empyema and abscess of the liver, the diagnosis of malaria is made. The practitioner may take it as a safe rule, to which he will find very few exceptions, that *an intermittent fever which resists quinine is not malaria.*

Other conditions which may be mistaken for septicopyemia are profound anemia, infective sinus thrombosis, certain cases of Hodgkin's disease, cholecystitis, the hepatic intermittent fever associated with gall stones in the common duct, rare cases of essential fever in nervous women, perinephritic abscess, and the fever sometimes seen in rapidly growing cancer.

Treatment.—General.—Nourishment should be given liberally in the form of liquids and soft foods up to 3,000 calories with 80 grams of protein a day. Water should be forced and given by the bowel or subcutaneously if there is difficulty in taking it by mouth. The bowels should be kept open by simple laxatives. Hydrotherapy is useful. Sedatives should be given for sleep.

Surgical.—Whenever pus is accessible, free evacuation and drainage is often the only treatment required. The primary focus should be treated if possible. Unfortunately, in too many cases the focus of infection is not accessible; it then is a septicemia, and for such cases we have the treatment with serums and vaccines.

Vaccine and Serum Treatment.—By blood cultures or by cultures from the focus of infection the organism is isolated, and an autogenous vaccine prepared. The use of vaccines in acute infections is not without risk and this treatment should be employed only after careful consideration. The giving of a stock vaccine containing one or many organisms is to be condemned. Blood transfusion is indicated for severe anemia. The transfusion of blood from a donor who has been given vaccines made from cultures from the patient, in the hope of introducing antibodies, is advised by some. It is difficult to judge of its value. There is a risk of sudden death following the transfusion. In acute streptococcus cases antistreptococcus serum or a polyvalent serum may be used. Good results are sometimes obtained. In staphylococcus septicemia, encouraging results are reported from the use of serum; bacteriophage therapy may be helpful, especially in local lesions. Staphylococcus toxoid may be tried in more chronic infections.

Drugs.—There are none which control septic fever. The antipyretics and quinine are of doubtful service. The use of antiseptic drugs intravenously has not been proved to be of positive value. In the majority of cases the outcome seems to depend on the virulence of the organism (which we can not alter) and on the natural resistance of the patient. Arsenic is worthy of a trial, best in the form of sodium cacodylate (gr. i, 0.06 gm. daily) given intramuscularly or intravenously.

FOCAL INFECTION

A local focus of infection may be the source of acute septicemia, but in addition a variety of chronic infections may arise with distant and important manifestations. The resulting infection may be either local or general. The finding of focal infection gives the clue to the etiology of many obscure conditions. Foci of infection may be primary and secondary. The latter are usually the result of infection through the blood or lymph.

Etiology.—The organism most often concerned is some variety of streptococcus. The hemolytic forms are more responsible for the more acute infections; the nonhemolytic forms cause more subacute and chronic disturbances and play a large part in the etiology of subacute endocarditis. The colon bacillus is sometimes responsible. The local focus may be open to the surface or closed. An example of the former is pyorrhea alveolaris and of the latter the closed abscess at the root of a tooth. The local infection may be situated in many parts of the body but in a majority the situation is in the mouth or tonsils. Investigation has shown the frequency of deep tonsillar infection, which may show no indication on the surface, and of suppuration about the roots of teeth. Infection of the skin, nose or sinuses, bronchi, bile ducts, gall-bladder, appendix, intestine, pelvic organs and the urinary tract may be the source.

Pathology.—The lesions may be varied and situated in almost any part of the body. Perhaps the most frequent sites are in the joints and fibrous tissues. Arthritis and fibrositis are common and many of the obscure pains, termed myalgia, neuritis, "chronic and muscular rheumatism," are due to fibrositis secondary to a focal infection. Among other lesions are hyperthyroidism, endocarditis, myocarditis, gastric ulcer, cholecystitis, appendicitis and nephritis. The resulting disturbance is due to absorbed toxins or to bacteria which reach the blood stream or lymph and are carried to other parts. Systemic intoxication from absorption is not rare. The lesions produced do not show any particular characteristic. In general they are those of a chronic inflammatory process with occasional acute exacerbations, but on the whole tending to chronicity. The organisms are usually of low virulence. The disparity between the frequency of foci of infection and resulting disease is apparently largely due to natural resistance and immunity.

Symptoms.—These can not be stated in detail as so many structures may be involved. In general, there are some statements that can be made. (1) The condition is usually chronic and may vary much from time to time. Thus secondary arthritis is generally subacute or chronic, although there are cases with an acute course and more with acute exacerbations. (2) The onset of symptoms may be determined by some intercurrent disease or debilitating condition. (3) The general health is apt to be affected. (4) Active reaction as shown by marked fever is unusual, as the process is too chronic. (5) There is a tendency to anemia and disturbance of nutrition.

Diagnosis.—This can not be stated in any exact terms. The first essential is the recognition of the important part that focal infection plays. Chronic arthritis and fibrositis are not primary maladies; they are often secondary to infection somewhere. We know that if a patient has gonorrheal arthritis there is a primary local process. The primary focus has often to be searched for; it may give no symptoms. This may involve the examination of many organs. If there is no localizing indication, the teeth and tonsils may be examined first. The nose and sinuses, bronchi, gallbladder, etc., have all to be considered. Duodenal cultures are important in the recognition of biliary tract infection. Nor is it safe to conclude that a focus when found is the sole responsible one for there may be multiple foci. In some cases it seems that there is a low grade infection of many tissues.

Prognosis.—Many factors enter into this, especially the resistance of the individual and the virulence of the organism. The degree of anatomical change must be considered, thus if extensive joint changes have occurred the removal of a focus of infection can not alter these although it may prevent further damage. Naturally the earlier proper treatment is instituted the better the outlook.

Treatment.—(1) Removal of the cause, the focus of infection. This demands proper diagnosis and should not be done until this is as definite as possible. A man with mouth infection may have the real focus in his prostate. Caution should be exercised in the removal of teeth, especially in elderly persons. The mouth should be put in as clean a condition as possible and infected teeth removed at intervals. Wholesale removal of infected teeth may cause a severe reaction or be followed by a general infection. Caution should be exercised in the treatment of foci if the general symptoms are acute. (2) Vaccine therapy. In some cases this is of value and, if possible, an autogenous vaccine should be used. The use of *filtrates* seems helpful in some cases. Very small doses should be given and reaction avoided. Intradermal skin tests should be done to test the sensitivity. Toxoids may be used. (3) Injection of nonspecific protein, for example fifty millions of killed typhoid bacilli intravenously. This has proved useful but is to be employed with caution. (4) Helping the patient's powers of resistance by attention to the general health. Fresh air and sunlight, sufficient food with abundance of vitamins and proper treatment for anemia, are indicated.

TERMINAL INFECTIONS

There is truth in the paradoxical statement that persons rarely die of the disease with which they suffer. Secondary *terminal* infections carry off many patients with incurable disease. Flexner analyzed 255 cases of chronic renal and cardiac disease with bacteriological examinations at autopsy and 213 gave positive results. The infections may be local or general. The former are extremely common, and are found in a large proportion of all cases of nephritis, arteriosclerosis, heart disease, cirrhosis of the liver, and other chronic disorders. Affections of the serous membranes (acute pleurisy, pericarditis, or peritonitis), meningitis, and endocarditis are the most frequent. It is perhaps safe to say that the majority of cases of advanced arteriosclerosis and nephritis succumb to these intercurrent infections. The infective agents are very varied. The streptococcus is the most common, but the pneumococcus, staphylococcus, proteus, pyocyaneus, and gas bacillus are also found. It is surprising in how many instances of arteriosclerosis, chronic heart disease, nephritis and cirrhosis of the liver the fatal event is determined by an acute tuberculosis of the peritoneum or pleura.

The general terminal infections are somewhat less common. Of 85 cases of chronic renal disease Flexner found a general infection at autopsy in 38, and in 14 of 48 cases of chronic cardiac disease. Other diseases in which general terminal infection may occur are Hodgkin's disease, leukemia, and chronic tuberculosis. Probably of the same nature is the terminal enterocolitis so frequently found in chronic disorders.

ERYSIPELAS

Definition.—A special pyogenic infection caused by the *Streptococcus erysipelatis,* characterized by inflammation of the skin with fever and toxemia.

Etiology.—Erysipelas is a widespread affection, endemic in most communities, and at certain seasons epidemic. It is particularly prevalent in the spring and of 2,012 cases, 1,214 occurred during the first five months of the year (Anders). April had the largest number of cases. Erysipelas is both infectious and inoculable; but, except under special conditions, the infection is not very virulent and does not seem to act at any great distance. It can be conveyed by a third person. Recurrent attacks occur which may be due to bacterial allergy, there being infection in the sinuses, nose or tonsils.

The disposition to the disease is widespread, but the susceptibility is specially marked in the case of individuals with wounds or abrasions of any sort. Recently delivered women and the subjects of surgical operations are particularly prone to it. A wound, however, is not necessary, and in the so-called idiopathic form, although it may be difficult to say that there was not a slight abrasion, in very many cases there certainly is no observable external lesion. In some cases the infection spreads through the tissues from the nasal cavity to the skin. This is probably comparatively common. Erysipelas in the newborn may begin about the navel.

Chronic alcoholism, debility, and nephritis are predisposing agents. Certain persons show a special susceptibility to erysipelas, and it may recur in them repeatedly. There are instances, too, of a family predisposition.

The specific agent of the disease is a streptococcus growing in long chains, which is included under the group name *Streptococcus pyogenes,* with which *Streptococcus erysipelatis* appears to be identical. The fever and constitutional symptoms are due in great part to the toxins; the more serious visceral complications are the result of secondary metastatic infection.

Morbid Anatomy.—Erysipelas is a simple inflammation. In its uncomplicated forms there is seen, postmortem, little else than inflammatory edema.

The cocci are found chiefly in the lymph spaces and most abundantly in the zone of spreading inflammation. In the uninvolved tissue beyond the inflamed margin they are to be found in the lymph vessels. In more extensive and virulent forms there may be suppuration. Infarcts occur in the lungs, spleen, and kidneys, and there may be pyemic infection. Some cases of malignant endocarditis are secondary to erysipelas; thus, of 23 cases, 3 occurred with this disease. Septic pericarditis and pleuritis also occur. The disease may involve the meninges. Pneumonia is not a common complication. Acute nephritis is met with, often ingrafted upon an old process.

Symptoms.—The following description applies specially to erysipelas of the face and head, the form of the disease which is most common.

The *incubation* is variable, probably from three to seven days.

The stage of *invasion* is often marked by a rigor, and followed by a rapid rise in the temperature and other characteristics of an acute fever. When there is a local abrasion, the spot is slightly reddened; but if the disease is "idiopathic," there is within a few hours slight redness over the bridge of the nose and on the cheeks. The swelling and tension of the skin increase and within twenty-four hours the external symptoms are well marked. The skin is smooth, tense, and edematous. It looks red, feels hot, and the superficial layers of the epidermis may be lifted as small blebs. The patient complains of a feeling of tension in the skin; the swelling rapidly increases; and during the second day the eyes are usually closed. The first-affected parts gradually become less swollen as the disease extends at the periphery. When it reaches the forehead it progresses as an advancing ridge perfectly well defined and raised; and often, on palpation, hardened extensions can be felt beneath the skin which is not yet reddened. Even in a case of moderate severity, the face is enormously swollen, the eyes are closed, the lips greatly edematous, the ears thickened, the scalp is swollen, and the patient's features are unrecognizable. The formation of blebs is common on the eyelids, ears, and forehead. The cervical lymph nodes are swollen, but are usually masked in the edema of the neck. The temperature keeps high without marked remissions for four or five days and then defervescence takes place. Leukocytosis is present. The general condition varies much with the previous state of health. In old and debilitated persons, particularly in alcoholics, the constitutional depression may be very great. Delirium is present, the tongue becomes dry, the pulse feeble, and there is marked tendency to death from toxemia. In the majority of cases, however, even with extensive lesions, the constitutional disturbance, considering the height of the fever, is slight. The mucous membrane of the mouth and throat may be swollen and reddened. The process may extend to the larynx, but the occasional edema of this part is commonly due to the extension of the inflammation from without inward. Obstinate diarrhea is common. The general disturbance in an attack of erysipelas may be surprisingly little.

There are cases in which the inflammation extends from the face to the neck, and over the chest, and may gradually migrate or wander over the greater part of the body (*E. migrans*).

Suppuration occurs frequently in facial erysipelas. Small cutaneous abscesses are common about the cheeks, forehead and neck, and beneath the scalp large collections of pus may accumulate. Suppuration seems to occur more frequently in some epidemics than in others.

Complications.—Meningitis is rare. The cases in which death occurs with marked brain symptoms do not usually show, postmortem, meningeal affection. Pneumonia is an occasional complication. Ulcerative endocarditis and septicemia are more common. Albuminuria is almost constant, particularly in persons over fifty. Phlebitis and nephritis are occasionally seen. Severe ulceration may occur, usually about the eyes, and due to secondary staphylococcus infection. Da Costa called attention to curious irregular returns of the fever which occur during convalescence without any aggravation of the local condition.

Diagnosis.—This rarely presents any difficulty. The onset, the rapid rise in fever, and the local characters are distinctive. In *cellulitis* the swelling is more brawny and a definite edge is lacking. In old patients with chronic disease there may be areas of redness and swelling, especially on the legs, which are difficult to diagnose. If in doubt treat them as erysipelas.

Prognosis.—Healthy adults rarely die. The hospital mortality is about 7 per cent; in private practice about 4 per cent (Anders). In the newborn, when the disease attacks the navel, it is almost always fatal. In drunkards, in nephritic patients, and in the aged erysipelas is a serious affection, and death may result from a complication or from toxemia. Wandering erysipelas, with a protracted course, may cause death from exhaustion.

Treatment.—Isolation should be strictly carried out, particularly in hospitals. A practitioner in attendance upon a case of erysipelas should not attend cases of confinement.

The disease is self-limited and a large majority of the patients get well without any internal medication. The diet should be nutritious and light. Large amounts of water should be given. For the restlessness, delirium, and insomnia, chloral or the bromides may be given; or, if these fail, opium. When the fever is high the patient may be bathed or sponged, or phenacetine or acetylsalicylic acid (gr. v, 0.3 gm.) may be given.

Antitoxin.—This was introduced by Birkhaug (1926). The dose must be governed partly by the severity of the attack; 10 cc. of the concentrated serum intramuscularly is an average amount repeated daily as long as necessary. Intravenous administration should be used only if the condition is desperate. Opinions as to the value of antitoxin are divided.

Attention should be paid to any focus of infection, as in a sinus or in the tonsils. In patients with recurring attacks active immunization may be attempted by gradually increasing doses of *S. erysipelatis* vaccine.

Of *local* applications, ichthyol (as a salve, 1 to 4 of lanolin), bichloride of mercury solution (1 to 5,000), salicylic acid (1 to 500), phenol in oil (5 per cent), a saturated solution of magnesium sulphate, powdered stearate of zinc, collodion, or ichthyol in collodion (1 to 4), may be used. Painting the skin ahead of the advancing area with tincture of iodine is sometimes effectual. Perhaps as good an application as any is cold water, which was highly recommended by Hippocrates. If the disease involves the eyelids boric acid compresses should be applied and one or two drops of argyrol solution (10 per cent) instilled several times a day.

The use of X-rays over the affected area and adjoining skin, daily for three days, sometimes is of value. Ultraviolet light treatment has been used for young children, about one and a half erythema dose daily for three days. A longer period of treatment does not seem to be of advantage.

DIPHTHERIA

Definition.—A specific infectious disease, characterized by a local fibrinous exudate, usually upon the mucous membrane of the throat, and by constitutional symptoms due to toxins produced at the site of the lesion. The presence of the diphtheria bacillus is the criterion by which diphtheria is distinguished from other forms of membranous inflammation.

Cases of angina, diagnosed as diphtheria, may be due to other organisms and to these the term *diphtheroid* is applied. Though usually milder, severe constitutional disturbance, and even paralysis, may follow these forms.

History.—Known in the East for centuries, and referred to in the Babylonian Talmud, it is not until the first century A. D. that an accurate clinical account appears in the writings of Aretæus. The paralysis of the palate was recognized by Ætius (sixth century A. D.). Throat pestilences are mentioned in the Middle Ages. Severe epidemics occurred in Europe in the sixteenth and seventeenth centuries, particularly in Spain. In England in the latter part of the eighteenth century it was described by Fothergill and Huxham, and in America by Bard. Ballonius recognized the affection of the larynx and trachea in 1762; Home in Scotland described it as croup. The modern description dates from Bretonneau, of Tours (1826), who gave to it the name *diphthérite.* Throughout the nineteenth century it prevailed extensively in all known countries. After innumerable attempts, in which Klebs took a leading part, the organism was isolated by Loeffler. The toxin was determined by the work of Roux, Yersin, and others, and finally the antitoxin was discovered by Behring (1891). Schick (1913) described the intradermal test for susceptibility and immunity.

Etiology.—Everywhere endemic in large centres of population, the disease becomes at times epidemic. In England and Wales in 1931, 2,673 persons died of the disease. In the registration area in the United States the death rate per 100,000 has fallen from 43 in 1900 to 4.5 in 1932. In the tropics it is not a very serious disease. Dry seasons seem to favor the disease, which shows an autumnal prevalence.

Modes of Infection.—The disease is highly infectious. The bacilli may be transmitted (*a*) from one person to another; few diseases proved more fatal to physicians and nurses in the past. (*b*) Infected articles may convey the bacilli, which may remain alive for many months; many instances have been recorded of this mode of transmission. (*c*) Persons suffering from atypical forms of diphtheria may convey the disease; nasal catarrh, membranous rhinitis, mild tonsillitis, and otorrhea may be caused by diphtheria bacilli, and from these sources cases have been traced. (*d*) From the throats of healthy contacts—diphtheria *carriers,* persons with no signs of the disease—the bacilli have been obtained by culture. (*e*) Healthy children without any nasopharyngeal catarrh, who have not been in contact with the disease, may harbor the bacilli. Cultures from children show a varying percentage of positive results but the majority are nonvirulent forms. Only persons who harbor the virulent forms are capable of transmitting the disease. In schools the interchange of articles, such as sweets, pencils, etc., and the habit which children have of putting everything into their mouths afford endless opportunities for the transmission of the disease. (*f*) Numerous epidemics have been traced to milk. Virulent bacilli have been found in milk and virulent organisms have been found in the acquired lesions on the teats of cows. (*g*) A few instances of accidental infection from cultures and through animals are on record.

Predisposing Causes.—Age is the most important. Sucklings are not often attacked but it may occur in the newborn. Early in the second year the disposition increases rapidly, and continues at its height until the fifth year. In New York between 1891-1900 among the deaths 80.8 per cent occurred under five, 17 per cent between five and ten—figures which show the extraordinary preponderance of the disease among children. Girls are attacked in slightly larger numbers than boys. November, December, and January are the months of greatest prevalence in the United States; in London October and November. Children in the higher circles and those in small communities and in the country are more susceptible than those living in the crowded quarters of cities.

Immunity.—Individual susceptibility is a special factor; many of those exposed escape, and even those, too, in whose throats virulent bacilli lodge and grow. Probably about 80 per cent of all adults have antitoxin in the blood and so are protected. The Schick reaction is of great value in determining immunity. A negative reaction indicates the presence of antitoxin as when it is not present the toxin causes a reaction. The amount of toxin injected intradermically in the right forearm is $\frac{1}{50}$ M.L.D. in 0.2 cc. of salt solution. A control test is made on the other arm (toxin inactivated by heat). Four reactions may result: 1. *Negative.* There is no reaction on either arm. 2. *Positive.* The right arm shows an area of erythema and slight infiltration, which reaches its height in four days and persists for seven to ten days. The control test shows nothing. 3. *Negative pseudoreaction.* This is of an anaphylactic character, and is the same on both arms. It reaches its height in 24 to 36 hours and disappears about the third day. 4. *Positive combined.* This is a combination of 2 and 3. A reaction is present on both arms but in two days the left has faded and the right arm shows the usual positive test about the fourth day. In young children the reactions are usually definitely negative or positive. In older persons there may be more difficulty as to the result.

The *B. diphtheriae* (*Corynebacterium diphtheriae*) is found chiefly in the false membrane. Postmortem, the bacilli may be found in the blood and internal organs. Occasionally they are found in the blood during life. It may be the predominating or sole organism in the common bronchopneumonia. The bacillus has been found in diphtheritic conjunctivitis, in otitis media, sometimes in wound diphtheria, upon the genitals, in fibrinous rhinitis, and in ulcerative endocarditis.

Morphological Characters.—The bacillus is nonmotile, varies from 2 to 6 μ in length and from 0.3 to 0.8 μ in thickness. In appearance it is multiform, varying from short, rather sharply pointed rods to irregular bizarre forms, with one or both ends swollen, and staining more or less unevenly and intensely. Virulent and nonvirulent forms are alike. The toxicity test in the guinea-pig is necessary to distinguish them. The bacillus is Gram-positive. There are many doubtful points regarding the various forms of the bacillus. There does not seem proof that the *gravis* form is necessarily associated with severe attacks. The occurrence of epidemics in the last few years in which antitoxin did not seem to be efficient brings up the possibility of special strains.

The bacillus is very resistant, and cultures have been made from a bit of membrane preserved for five months in a dry cloth. Incorporated with dust and kept moist, the bacilli were still cultivable at the end of eight weeks; kept in a dried state they no longer grew at the end of this period (Ritter).

The Presence of the Diphtheria Bacillus in Nonmembranous Angina and in Healthy Throats.—The bacillus has been isolated from patients who show nothing more than a simple catarrhal angina of a mild type without any membrane, with diffuse redness, and perhaps huskiness and signs of catarrhal laryngitis. In other cases the picture may be that of a lacunar tonsillitis. The organisms may be present in perfectly healthy throats (diphtheria carriers), particularly in persons in the same house, or the attendants in fever hospitals. Following an attack of diphtheria the bacilli may persist in the throat or nose after the membrane has disappeared for weeks or months. Councilman called attention to the frequency with which the antrum is affected.

Toxins.—Roux and Yersin showed that a fatal result following the inoculation with the bacillus was not caused by extension of the micro-organisms within the body; and they were able to separate the toxin. The toxin killed with very much the same effects as those caused by the inoculation of the bacilli; the pseudomembrane, however, is not formed. It is suggested that in addition there is *toxone* with less affinity for antitoxin and which may be responsible for the nervous system complications.

Bacteria Associated with the Diphtheria Bacillus.—The most common is the *Streptococcus pyogenes.* Others, in addition to the organisms constantly found in the mouth, are the pneumococcus, the bacillus coli, and the staphylococcus aureus and albus. Of these, the streptococcus is the most important. The suppuration in the lymph nodes and the bronchopneumonia are usually caused by this organism.

Pseudodiphtheria Bacillus.—The Klebs-Loeffler bacillus varies very much in its virulence, and may exist in a form devoid of pathogenic properties. This organism should not be designated pseudodiphtheria bacillus. The name should be confined to bacilli, which, though resembling the diphtheria bacillus morphologically and culturally, do not produce diphtheria toxin. They may be found both in healthy and diseased throats. Another bacillus, showing certain cultural differences, has been found in the conjunctival sac in health and disease. (*B. xerosis*). *Hofmann's bacillus,* also spoken of as pseudodiphtheria bacillus, is common in the throats of healthy persons and is found also in cases of diphtheria; but how far it is responsible for pathological conditions is not settled. *Vincent's bacillus* is a fusiform organism associated with a diphtheroid angina (Vincent's angina), which occurs in two forms: a membranous and an ulcerative and destructive. The fusiform bacilli have been found in healthy throats and also with diphtheria.

Diphtheroid Inflammations.—Under the term *diphtheroid* may be grouped those membranous inflammations which are not associated with the Klebs-Loeffler bacillus. It is a more suitable designation than pseudodiphtheria or secondary diphtheria. Streptococci and pneumococci are the organisms most often found. The proportion of cases of diphtheroid inflammation varies greatly in different statistics. In a large proportion of the cases the disease develops in children, and can be differentiated from diphtheria only by the bacteriological examination. It may be simply an acute catarrhal angina with lacunar tonsillitis. Some of the cases are due to Hofmann's bacillus, a few to Vincent's fusiform bacillus. The diphtheroid inflammations are specially found with the acute fevers.

Scarlet Fever.—In a large proportion of the cases of angina in scarlet fever the Klebs-Loeffler bacillus is not present. Where diphtheria is prevalent, a large proportion of the cases of membranous throats in scarlet fever may be genuine diphtheria. Membranous angina is much less common in *measles*. *Whooping-cough* may be complicated with membranous angina. Membranous inflammations in *typhoid fever* are not very infrequent; they may occur in the throat, the pelvis of the kidney, the bladder, or the intestines. The complication may be caused by the Klebs-Loeffler bacillus, but it is frequently a streptococcus infection.

Clinical Features of the Diphtheroid Affection.—The cases, as a rule, are milder, and the mortality is low, only 2.5 per cent in the 450 cases of Park and Beebe. The diphtheroid inflammations complicating the specific fevers are often very fatal, and a general streptococcus infection is not infrequent. As in the Klebs-Loeffler angina, there may be only a simple catarrhal process. In other instances the tonsils are covered with a creamy, pultaceous exudate, without any actual membrane. Some begin as a simple lacunar tonsillitis, while in others the entire fauces and tonsils are covered by a membrane, and there is a foul sloughing angina with intense constitutional disturbance.

Are the diphtheroid cases infectious? Clinical experience shows that the membranous angina associated with the fevers is rarely communicated to other patients. Park and Beebe say that "it did not seem that the secondary cases were any less liable to occur when the primary case was isolated than when it was not."

Sequelae of the Diphtheroid Angina.—The usual mildness of the disease is in part, no doubt, due to the less frequent systemic invasion. Some of the worst forms of general streptococcus infection are, however, seen in this disease. There are no peculiarities, local or general, which are distinctive; and even the most extensive paralysis may follow an angina caused by it.

Morbid Anatomy.—Distribution of Membrane.—A definite membrane was found in 127 of 220 fatal Boston cases, distributed as follows: tonsils, 65 cases; epiglottis, 60; larynx, 75; trachea, 66; pharynx, 51; mucous membrane of nares, 43; bronchi, 42; soft palate, including uvula, 13; esophagus, 12; tongue, 9; stomach, 5; duodenum, 1; vagina, 2; vulva, 1; skin of ear, 1; conjunctiva, 1. An interesting point was the great frequency with which the accessory sinuses of the nose were infected. In the fatal cases, the exudation is very extensive, involving the uvula, the soft palate, the posterior nares, and the lateral and posterior walls of the pharynx. These parts are covered with a dense pseudomembrane, in places firmly adherent, in others beginning to separate. In extreme cases the necrosis is advanced with a gangrenous condition. The membrane is of a dirty greenish or gray color, and the tonsils and palate may show necrotic sloughing. The erosion may be deep enough to open the carotid artery, or a false aneurism may be produced in the deep tissues of the neck. The nose may be blocked by the membrane, which may extend to the conjunctivæ and through the Eustachian tubes into the middle ear. In laryngeal diphtheria the exudate in the pharynx may be extensive. In many cases it is slight upon the tonsils and fauces and abundant upon the epiglottis and larynx, which may be completely occluded. In severe cases the exudate extends into the trachea and smaller bronchi.

The membrane varies very much in consistence, depending greatly upon the stage at which death has taken place. If death occurred early, it is firm and closely adherent; if late, it is soft, shreddy, and readily detached. In the most extreme cases, with extensive necrosis, the parts look gangrenous. In fatal cases the lymphatic glands of the neck are enlarged, and there is a general infiltration of the tissues with serum; the salivary glands may be swollen. In rare instances the membrane extends to the esophagus and stomach.

The primary lesion is a necrosis and degeneration of the epithelial tissues. The organisms grow, not in the living, but in the necrotic tissues. The first step is a necrosis of the epithelium, often preceded by active proliferation of the nuclei of the cells, which become changed into refractive hyaline masses. An inflammatory exudate rich in fibrin factors is poured out, and fibrin is formed when this comes in contact with the necrotic epithelium.

The following are the important changes in the other organs:

Heart.—If death occurs in the first week the muscle is pale and there is loss of striation. Later there is edema both of the fibres and interstitial tissue. The bundle of His may show marked changes. At later periods there is interstitial myocarditis, to which some cases of fibrous myocarditis may be due. Fatty change is not marked. Pericarditis and endocarditis are rare; endocarditis was present in 7 of 220 Boston cases. The diphtheria bacilli have been found in the vegetations.

Lungs.—The *pulmonary complications* are important, and death is due to them as often as to the throat lesion. Bronchopneumonia is the most common, and was present in 131 of the 220 Boston cases; lobar pneumonia is rare. The pneumococcus is the principal agent in the lung infections but streptococci and diphtheria bacilli are frequently met with.

Kidneys.—The lesions, which are due to the action of the toxins, not to the presence of bacteria, vary from simple degeneration to an intense nephritis. There is no specific type of lesion. Interstitial and glomerular nephritis are most common in the older subjects. Degenerative changes are present in a large proportion of all the fatal cases. The liver and spleen show the degenerative lesions of acute infections.

Symptoms.—The period of incubation is "from two to seven days, oftenest two." The initial symptoms are those of an ordinary febrile attack—slight chilliness, fever, and aching pains in the back and limbs. In mild cases the symptoms are trifling, and the child may not feel ill enough to go to bed. The temperature is very variable and bears no relation to the severity of the attack; in the worst cases there may be normal or subnormal temperature. In young children there may be convulsions at the outset.

Pharyngeal Diphtheria.—In a typical case there is at first redness of the fauces, and the child complains of slight difficulty in swallowing. The membrane first appears upon the tonsils, and it may be difficult to distinguish a patchy diphtheritic pellicle from the exudate of the tonsillar crypts. The pharyngeal mucous membrane is reddened, and the tonsils themselves are swollen. By the third day the *membrane* has covered the tonsils, the pillars of the fauces, and perhaps the uvula, which is thickened and edematous, and may fill completely the space between the swollen tonsils. The membrane may extend to the posterior wall of the pharynx. At first grayish-white in color, it changes to a dirty gray, often to a yellow-white. It is firmly adherent, and when removed leaves a bleeding, slightly eroded surface, which is soon covered by fresh exudate. The glands in the neck are swollen and may be tender. The general condition of a patient in a case of moderate severity is usually good; the temperature not very high, in the absence of complications ranging from 102° to 103° F. The pulse range is from 100 to 120. The local condition of the throat is not of great severity, and the constitutional depression is slight. The symptoms gradually abate, the swelling of the neck diminishes, the membranes separate, and from the seventh to the tenth day the throat becomes clear and convalescence sets in.

Clinically atypical forms are common, and we follow Koplik's division:

(*a*) There may be no local manifestation of membrane, but a simple catarrhal inflammation associated sometimes with a croupy cough. The detection of the diphtheria bacillus can alone determine the diagnosis. Such cases are of great moment, as they may communicate the disease to other children.

(*b*) There are cases in which the tonsils are covered by a pultaceous exudate, not a consistent membrane.

(*c*) Cases presenting a punctate form of membrane, isolated, and usually on the surface of the tonsils.

(*d*) Cases which begin and often run their entire course with the local picture of a typical lacunar tonsillitis. They may be mild, and the local exudate may not extend, but in other cases there is rapid development of membrane, and extension of the disease to the pharynx and the nose, with severe septic and constitutional symptoms.

(*e*) A *hemorrhagic* form is sometimes seen with severe toxemia and hemorrhages into the skin and mucous membranes.

Systemic Infection.—The constitutional disturbance in mild diphtheria is very slight and there may be extensive local disease without grave systemic symptoms. As a rule, the general features bear a definite relation to the severity of the local disease. There are instances in which from the outset the constitutional prostration is extreme, the pulse frequent and small, the fever high, and the nervous phenomena pronounced; the patient may sink rapidly overwhelmed by the toxemia. There are cases of this sort in which the exudate in the throat may be slight, but usually the nasal symptoms are pronounced. The temperature may be very slightly raised or even subnormal. More commonly the severe systemic symptoms appear at a later date when the pharyngeal lesion is at its height. They are constantly present in extensive disease and when there is a sloughing, fetid condition. The lymphatic glands become greatly enlarged; the pallor is extreme; the face has an ashen-gray hue; the pulse is rapid and feeble, and the temperature subnormal. In the most aggravated forms there are gangrenous processes in the throat, and in rare cases, sloughing of the tissues of the neck.

A leukocytosis is present in diphtheria but does not seem to be of prognostic value, since it may be pronounced in mild cases.

Nasal Diphtheria.—In cases of pharyngeal diphtheria the Klebs-Loeffler bacillus is found on the mucous membrane of the nose and in the secretions, even when no membrane is present, but it may produce two affections similar locally but widely differing in their general features.

In *membranous* or *fibrinous rhinitis,* a remarkable affection usually in children, the nares are occupied by thick membranes, but there is an entire absence of any constitutional disturbance. Ravenel collected 77 cases, in 41 of which a bacteriological examination showed in 33 the Klebs-Loeffler bacillus. All ran a benign course, and in all but a few the membrane was limited to the nose, and the constitutional symptoms were absent or very slight. Infection of other children is extremely rare.

On the other hand, *nasal diphtheria* may present a most malignant form of the disease. The infection may be primary in the nose, and in one case there was otitis media, and the Klebs-Loeffler bacillus was separated from the discharge before the condition of nasal diphtheria was suspected. While some cases are of mild character, others are very malignant, and the constitutional symptoms most profound. The glandular inflammation is usually very intense, owing, as Jacobi pointed out, to the great richness of the nasal mucosa in lymphatics. From the nose the inflammation may extend through the tear-ducts to the conjunctivae and into the sinuses.

Laryngeal Diphtheria (*Membranous Croup*).—With a very large proportion of all the cases of membranous laryngitis the Klebs-Loeffler bacillus is associated; in a smaller number other organisms, particularly the streptococcus, are found. Of 286 cases in which the disease was confined to the larynx or bronchi, in 229 the Klebs-Loeffler bacilli were found. The streptococcus cases are more likely to be secondary to other acute diseases. Laryngeal diphtheria is rare in adults.

Symptoms.—Naturally, the clinical symptoms are almost identical in the nonspecific and specific forms of membranous laryngitis.

The affection begins like an acute laryngitis with slight hoarseness and rough cough, to which the term croupy has been applied. After these symptoms have lasted for a day or two with varying intensity, the child suddenly becomes worse, usually at night, and there are signs of impeded respiration. At first the difficulty in breathing is paroxysmal, due probably to more or less spasm of the muscles of the glottis. Soon the dyspnea becomes continuous, inspiration and expiration become difficult, particularly the latter, and with the inspiratory movement the epigastrium and lower intercostal spaces are retracted. The voice is husky and may be reduced to a whisper. The color gradually changes and cyanosis becomes marked. Restlessness comes on and the child tosses from side to side, vainly trying to get breath. Occasionally, in a severer paroxysm, portions of membrane are coughed out. The fever is rarely very high and the condition of the child may be surprisingly good. The pulse is increased in frequency and is small if cyanosis be present. In favorable cases the dyspnea is not very urgent, the color remains good, and after one or two paroxysms the child goes to sleep and wakes in the morning, perhaps without fever and feeling comfortable. The attack may recur the following night with greater severity. In unfavorable cases the dyspnea becomes more and more urgent, the cyanosis deepens, the child, after a period of intense restlessness, sinks into a semicomatose state, and death finally occurs from asphyxia or toxemia. In other cases the onset is less sudden and is preceded by a longer period of indisposition. As a rule, there is pharyngeal infection. The constitutional disturbance may be more severe, the fever higher, and there may be swelling of the glands of the neck. Inspection of the fauces may show the presence of false membrane on the pillars or tonsils. Bacteriological examination alone can determine whether these are due to the diphtheria bacillus or a streptococcus. Ware, of Boston, whose essay on croup is one of the most solid contributions to the subject, reported the presence of exudate in the fauces in 74 out of 75 cases of croup. Pulmonary signs may be caused by laryngeal obstruction, blocking of the bronchi by membrane, collapse and bronchopneumonia. During the paroxysm the vesicular murmur is scarcely audible, but the laryngeal stridor may be loudly communicated.

Diphtheria of Other Parts.—Primary diphtheria occurs occasionally in the *conjunctiva.* It follows in some instances the affection of the nasal mucous membrane. Some of the cases are severe and serious, but it has been shown that the diphtheria bacilli may be present in a conjunctivitis catarrhal in character, or associated with only slight membraneous deposits.

Diphtheria of the *external auditory meatus* is seen when a diphtheritic otitis media has extended through the tympanic membrane.

Diphtheria of the *skin* is most frequently seen in the severer forms of pharyngeal diphtheria, in which the membrane extends to the mouth and lips, and invades the adjacent portions of the skin of the face. The skin about the anus and genitals may also be attacked. Pseudomembranous inflammation is not uncommon on ulcerated surfaces and wounds. In very many of these cases it is a streptococcus infection, but in a majority, perhaps, in which the patient is suffering with diphtheria, the Klebs-Loeffler bacillus will be found in the fibrinous exudate. As proposed by Welch, the term "wound diphtheria" should be limited to infection of a wound by the Klebs-Loeffler bacillus. Paralysis may follow wound diphtheria. The fibrinous membrane so common in the neighborhood of the tracheotomy wound in diphtheria is rarely associated with the Klebs-Loeffler bacillus. Diphtheria of the *genitals* is occasionally seen in both sexes.

Complications and Sequelae.—Hemorrhage from the nose or throat may occur in the severe ulcerative cases. Skin rashes are not infrequent, particularly diffuse *erythema.* Occasionally there is urticaria and in the severe cases purpura. Local gangrene may occur. Fatal cases almost invariably show *bronchopneumonia* and large patches of collapse, or septic particles may reach the bronchi and excite gangrenous processes which may lead to severe and fatal hemorrhage. Jaundice is rarely of serious import.

Albuminuria, present in all severe cases, is alarming only when the albumin is in considerable quantity and associated with epithelial or blood casts. *Nephritis* may appear early, setting in occasionally with complete suppression of urine. In comparison with scarlet fever the renal changes lead less frequently to chronic nephritis. In rare instances there may be coma, and even convulsions, without albumin in the urine or edema.

Of the sequelae, *paralysis* due to toxic neuritis is by far the most important. It can be experimentally produced in animals by the toxin. The proportion of the cases in which it occurs ranges from 10 to 15 and even to 20 per cent. It usually comes on in the second or third week of convalescence. It may follow very mild cases; indeed, the local lesion may be so trifling that the paralysis calls attention to the true diagnosis. It is proportionately less frequent in children than in adults. J. D. Rolleston's study indicates that the early use of antitoxin diminishes the liability to paralysis. In 494 cases collected by Woodhead, the palate was involved in 155, the ocular muscles in 197, in 10 other muscles. Ninety-one of the patients died.

Of the local paralyses the most common is that which affects the *palate.* This gives a nasal character to the voice, and, owing to a return of liquids through the nose, causes a difficulty in swallowing. The palate is relaxed and motionless, and sensation in it is much impaired. The affection may extend to the constrictors of the pharynx, and deglutition become embarrassed. Within two or three weeks or even a shorter time the paralysis disappears. In many cases the palate affection is part of a general neuritis. Of other local forms perhaps the most common are paralyses of the *eye muscles,* intrinsic and extrinsic. There may be strabismus, ptosis, and loss of power of accommodation. Facial paralysis is rare. The neuritis may be confined to the nerves of one limb, though more commonly the legs or the arms are affected together. Very often with the palatal paralysis is associated a weakness of the legs without definite palsy but with loss of the knee jerk. J. D. Rolleston found the Babinski sign present in 172 of 877 cases in the acute stage and most often in severe forms. In *diaphragmatic paralysis,* from involvement of the phrenic nerve, the breathing is intercostal, the diaphragm is high in position and the abdomen scaphoid. It usually occurs about the sixth week and is almost always fatal. An *ataxic* paralysis sometimes occurs with incoordination of movements and loss of muscle sense. It may be mistaken for tabes dorsalis.

The *multiple* form of neuritis may begin with the palatal affection, or with loss of power of accommodation and loss of the tendon reflexes. This last is an important sign, which may occur early, but is not necessarily followed by other signs of neuritis. There is paraplegia, which may be complete or involve only the extensors of the feet. The paralysis may extend and involve the arms and face and render the patient entirely helpless. The muscles of respiration may be spared. Sensory is less common than motor disturbance.

Heart.—Myocardial changes are common and may be serious. The blood pressure often falls markedly. An increase in the heart rate is common early in the attack. Irregularity is common, also sinus arrhythmia, sino-auricular block and premature contractions. *Heart block* of high grade may occur not infrequently and its possibility should always be in mind. The murmurs, so common in children with fever, as a rule are not important. Tachycardia which is persistent, especially with gallop rhythm and a feeble first sound, is of serious omen. A rapid drop in rate to 40, 30 or 20 (heart block) is always ominous, especially if accompanied by vomiting without evident cause. Attacks of acute circulatory failure occur with marked change in the pulse, precordial pain, rapid respiration and cyanosis. Death may occur very suddenly. Experimental evidence is against the vasomotor centre being involved. Possibly in some cases there is degeneration of the vagus, supported by the frequency of paralysis of the palate with vomiting, epigastric pain and tenderness.

Diagnosis.—The presence of the diphtheria bacillus is regarded as the sole criterion of true diphtheria, and as this organism may be associated with all grades of throat affections, from a simple catarrh to a sloughing, gangrenous process, it is evident that in many instances there will be a striking discrepancy between the clinical and the bacteriological diagnosis.

The bacteriological diagnosis is simple as a rule. In cases which are suspicious clinically a single negative result should not be regarded as conclusive;

further cultures should be made. In carriers, it may be necessary to determine if the organisms are virulent by animal test. An immediate diagnosis may be possible by making a smear preparation of the exudate. The Klebs-Loeffler bacilli may be present in sufficient numbers and may be characteristic enough to make the diagnosis reasonably certain.

Where a bacteriological examination can not be made, the practitioner must regard as suspicious all forms of throat affections in children, and carry out measures of isolation and treatment. In this way alone can serious errors be avoided. It is not, of course, in the severer forms of infection that mistake is likely to occur, but in the milder forms. *Acute tonsillitis* is usually bilateral and the exudate is rarely marked. The temperature is generally higher than in diphtheria. *Vincent's angina* may resemble diphtheria closely, having a membrane which may extend to the soft palate. A form of tonsillitis due to *mycotic* infection, most common in the tropics, simulates diphtheria as the membrane may extend to the palate, pharynx and larynx. In all these the smears and cultures usually give the diagnosis. *Syphilis* with marked throat involvement has caused difficulty, especially if the tonsils are swollen and show patches. The findings elsewhere, negative cultures and a positive Wassermann reaction are important.

A large proportion of the cases of *diphtheroid* inflammation of the throat are due to streptococci. They are usually milder, and the liability to general infection is less intense; still many virulent cases of throat disease, with intense systemic infection, are caused by this organism. The diagnosis between scarlet fever and diphtheria is discussed in the section on scarlet fever.

Laryngeal diphtheria offers many difficulties, and signs of laryngitis in a child should always suggest its possibility. If membrane can be seen in the pharynx or on the epiglottis or diphtheria bacilli obtained by a swab the diagnosis is clear. Any sputum should be examined for portions of membrane. Direct examination of the larynx is of great help if it can be done. Laryngitis due to various causes and laryngismus stridulus may cause doubt and it may be impossible to be sure until longer observation and cultures give aid. In such cases antitoxin should be given at once if there is any doubt. Edema of the larynx, a foreign body in the larynx or trachea and retropharyngeal abscess are possible causes of difficulty.

Prognosis.—The outlook depends greatly on the promptness and thoroughness with which antitoxin treatment is carried out. In hospital practice the mortality was formerly from 30 to 50 per cent. In the Boston City Hospital the death-rate between 1888 and 1894 was only once below 40 per cent, and in 1892 and 1893 rose to nearly 50 per cent. Following the introduction of antitoxin from 1895 to 1912 the death rate was not once above 15 per cent, and in 6,080 cases was 7.8 per cent (McCollom). In cases of ordinary severity the outlook is usually good. Extensive membrane, a marked septic state, laryngeal involvement, bronchopneumonia, evidence of serious myocarditis, nervous system complications, especially bulbar, vomiting, absence of fever and hemorrhagic features are of serious significance. In children below the age of five years the outlook is more serious as 80 per cent of the deaths from diphtheria occur in this period. Much depends on the day on which antitoxin is given. If this is on the first or second day the mortality is very low; it increases with each day of delay.

Prophylaxis.—Isolation of the sick, disinfection of everything that has come in contact with the patient, careful scrutiny of the milder cases of throat disorder, and more stringent surveillance in the period of convalescence are important in prevention. Suspected cases should be at once isolated or removed to an infections hospital. When a death has occurred from diphtheria, the body should be wrapped in a sheet soaked in corrosive sublimate solution (1 to 2,000), and placed in a sealed coffin. The funeral should always be private. It is important to insist on these precautions.

In cases of well-marked diphtheria these precautions are usually carried out, but the chief danger is from the milder cases, particularly the ambulatory form, in which the disease has perhaps not been suspected. But from such patients mingling with susceptible children the disease is often conveyed. The healthy children in a family in which diphtheria exists may carry the disease. Removal of the patients to isolation hospitals is an important factor in controlling the disease.

A very important matter relates to the period of convalescence as after all the membrane has cleared away, virulent bacilli may persist in the throat for weeks to months. The disease may be communicated by these *carriers* and they should be isolated and treated, but some are very resistant to all forms of treatment. Antitoxin may be applied locally to the throat and spraying the throat and nose with a culture of lactic acid bacilli is sometimes efficient. The application of iodized phenol (phenol 60, iodine crystals 20, glycerine 20) every second day is sometimes effectual. Removal of the tonsils and adenoids is usually the most efficient measure in those with bacilli in the throat. For carriers with bacilli in the nose mild alkaline douches are useful. The possibility of sinus infection should be considered.

The important elements in the prophylaxis of diphtheria are the rigid scrutiny of the milder types of throat affection, the thorough isolation and disinfection of individual patients and *immunization* of those who are susceptible to the disease. During an epidemic there should be repeated examinations of all those exposed to infection to detect carriers. Efforts should be made to educate the public to give early attention to throat and laryngeal symptoms and to realize the value of immunization.

Careful attention should be given to the throats and mouths of children, particularly to the teeth and tonsils. Diseased tonsils should be removed. Cats and dogs may carry infection and should be excluded from contact with patients. Physicians and nurses should wear gowns and caps. Everyone in contact with patients should be proved to be immune to the disease.

IMMUNIZATION.—The giving of *antitoxin* as a preventive measure (passive immunity) has an important place. The usual dose for adults is 1,000 units, for older children 750 units, and for children under two years of age 500 units. The immunity lasts about three weeks. The same precautions should be taken as in giving antitoxin to those with the disease. The giving of *antitoxin* as a preventive measure is indicated when there has been exposure to infection or in case of a sudden epidemic. It is only necessary for those who are not known to be immune. However, in case of any doubt it is wiser to give a prophylactic dose.

The value of *toxin-antitoxin* and *toxoid* immunization (active immunity) is thoroughly proved. The ideal would be to immunize all children between the ages of six months and two years as the majority of children are susceptible at the age of one year. At birth about 85 per cent of infants are immune (derived from the mother), but this immunity usually disappears at the age of six to nine months. Three injections of the *toxin-antitoxin* mixture are given, one to two weeks apart. The immunity develops slowly (six weeks to three months) and therefore antitoxin should be given in case of exposure to the disease. The immunity persists for at least five years in 98 per cent of cases (Park) and probably is permanent in many cases. Immunization should not be done in infants below the age of six months. *Toxoid* (anatoxin), diphtheria toxin treated with formaldehyde or alum, is coming into more extensive use to produce immunity. To determine those who are liable to severe reactions the Maloney test is used. A minute amount of toxoid is injected intracutaneously and a positive reaction indicates susceptibility.

Treatment.—Hygienic Measures.—The patient should be in a room from which the carpets, curtains, and superfluous furniture have been removed. The temperature should be about 68°, and thorough ventilation should be secured. The air may be kept moist by a kettle or a steam-atomizer. The physician should wear a gown and cap, and on leaving the room he should thoroughly wash his hands and face in corrosive sublimate solution. The strictest quarantine should be employed.

Rest.—This should be absolute and for a period of two to four weeks in the average attack. It is specially important in patients who have circulatory disturbance, paralysis, respiratory difficulty or vomiting. When the patient is allowed to sit up, the effect on the pulse should be noted and if irregularity or marked change in rate appears further rest is indicated. Special emphasis should be placed on the need of prolonged rest if there is circulatory disturbance. Sudden death may follow slight exertion. Small children may require constant watching.

Local Treatment.—In this especial care should be taken to avoid mechanical injury to the tissues. Since the introduction of antitoxin, local treatment is much less important and many patients do perfectly well with little or none. As a rule there is no advantage in struggling with a child to carry out local treatment. If it is employed the frequency should be determined by the results. In some patients it gives comfort.

Boric acid solutions, peroxide of hydrogen, Dobell's solution, and bichloride of mercury (1-2000) may be employed in the form of sprays, but in many cases the use of irrigations is the most satisfactory. This should always be done very gently with the patient lying on the side. Either a saline solution or a 2 per cent boric acid solution is satisfactory.

In nasal diphtheria salt solution, saturated boric acid or bichloride of mercury (1-5000) may be used. To be effectual the injection must be properly given. The nozzle of the syringe should be passed horizontally, not vertically; otherwise the fluid will return through the same nostril.

When the larynx is involved, a steam tent may be arranged, so that the child may breathe an atmosphere saturated with moisture. When the signs of obstruction are marked there should be no delay in the performance of intubation or tracheotomy. The choice between these must depend on the circumstances in each case. *Intubation* may be regarded as the operation of choice in the majority of cases. *Tracheotomy* is preferable in adults and may be the operation of necessity. The patient requires more skilful care after intubation than after tracheotomy. When the membrane is loose, suction with direct laryngoscopy may be used. This should be done only by one skilled in direct laryngoscopy. This procedure may have to be repeated and there should be no hesitation in doing it.

Hot applications to the neck are useful, particularly in young children, though in older children and adults the ice bag is to be preferred.

General Measures.—Every effort should be made to nourish the patient. The food should be liquid—milk, beef juices, barley water, ice cream, albumen water, and soups. If there is difficulty in swallowing, these should be given by a tube. The patient should be encouraged to drink water freely. If there is difficulty in taking it by mouth, it should be given by the bowel or subcutaneously. The bowels should be freely opened, for which a calomel and saline purge is usually best. When the pharyngeal involvement is very great and swallowing painful, a 5 per cent glucose solution can be given by the bowel. In toxic cases, in addition to the giving of antitoxin freely, dextrose-insulin therapy is useful. This is based on the effect of diphtheria toxin on carbohydrate metabolism which in severe cases causes increased glycogenesis and hyperglycemia. Later glycogen disappears from the liver and there may be hypoglycemia. If the toxin damages the pancreas, the insulin supply is less. The blood sugar curve may be like that in diabetes. Dextrose should be given freely by mouth or 20 grams in a 25 per cent solution intravenously, followed one to two hours later by insulin (10 to 20 units). Dextrose up to 100 grams may be given in twenty-four hours.

For the circulation the early giving of antitoxin is the best preventive of trouble. When symptoms arise, stimulants, such as caffeine and epinephrine are indicated. Absolute rest is most important and morphia hypodermically in proper dosage for the age is useful in myocardial conditions. Digitalis should not be given if there is any indication of heart block. Dextrose should be given intravenously, 25 cc. of a 25 per cent solution, and 15 units of insulin. This may be repeated every twelve hours if indicated.

Antitoxin Treatment.—As the years go on experience has shown that, thoroughly carried out, this is both safe and efficacious. It should be given as early as possible in the course of the disease as every hour's delay adds to the danger of the attack. The antitoxin unit is the amount of antitoxin which, injected into a guinea-pig of 250 grams in weight, neutralizes 100 times the minimum fatal dose of toxin of standard strength.

Dosage.—The ideal dose is one sufficiently large so that a second is not required. If there is any doubt as to what dose should be given choose the larger. The danger is of giving too small and not too large a dose, as the object is to neutralize the free toxin as quickly as possible. The antitoxin persists in the blood for a number of days and hence the value of a sufficient single dose. An insufficient dose at first cannot be entirely made up for by subsequent administration. In case of doubt as to the diagnosis it is wise to give antitoxin at once rather than wait for the result of cultures. The amount given should be decided by the severity of the attack, whether early or late in the course and by the seat of the local disease. When seen early and the attack is mild the smaller doses are proper. If late in the course, with severe features or in nasal or laryngeal involvement large doses should be given. In a general way the following dosage is a guide: for children up to the age of two years 2,000 to 10,000 units, from two to twelve years 3,000 to 20,000 units, and above twelve years 5,000 to 50,000 units. If a sufficient amount has been given, a second dose will not be required, but repeated doses should be given if indicated by lack of improvement or advance in the symptoms.

Administration.—Antitoxin should be given intramuscularly or intravenously. An intramuscular injection is absorbed about three times as rapidly as a subcutaneous one, and when given intravenously the whole amount is immediately available. The last is advisable in severe cases. The serum should be strongly potent, not show turbidity, warmed to body temperature and given at the rate of 1 cc. per minute. The usual care should be taken with the needle and skin.

Favorable effects are seen in the improvement in both the local and general condition. The swelling of the fauces subsides, the membrane begins to disappear, the temperature falls, and the pulse becomes slower.

Untoward Effects.—"Serum Disease."—This may appear in any normal individual and is due to the serum and not to the antitoxin. Following the injection after an interval, which varies from one to eighteen days, but is usually between seven and ten days, a local reaction appears which may be accompanied by general symptoms. The site of injection shows edema, urticaria or erythema, which may become more or less general. Malaise, vomiting, fever, adenitis, albuminuria, arthralgia and arthritis may occur. The symptoms are usually not severe and disappear in three or four days. Calcium lactate (gr. xv, 1 gm. three times a day) may be given as a prophylactic or when the symptoms have appeared. Epinephrine, 10 μ (0.6 cc.) of the 1-1000 solution hypodermically may relieve the urticaria. There is another reaction which is much more serious. In individuals who have been given antitoxin previously, even at a long interval —who have been sensitized—in some who have had asthma and in some of those who are affected by the proximity of horses, an acute dangerous condition may be caused by the injection of serum—*anaphylaxis.* This comes on very suddenly and with acute symptoms, among which are extreme distress, dyspnea, cyanosis, edema, collapse, respiratory failure and convulsions; death may follow rapidly. Fortunately this occurs rarely, but its possibility should be kept in mind, and before giving antitoxin the patient should be asked as to a history of asthma, an idiosyncrasy to horses and previous administration of antitoxin. This must be kept in mind in the case of patients who have a relapse, as if seven days have elapsed since the first dose the patient may be sensitized. If there is any reason to suspect the possibility of allergy, the patient should be tested for hypersensitiveness. The scratch test on the skin is done with serum diluted 100 times with salt solution. If he is susceptible a reaction usually occurs in an hour, but it is safer to wait three hours. The intradermic injection of 0.2 cc. of horse serum (1 to 10 dilution) or 0.2 cc. of antitoxin solution in a strength of 1 to 100 of salt solution produces a local reaction in a few minutes in a sensitive individual. If the patients are sensitive and the need of antitoxin is great, small doses (0.1 to 0.2 cc. intramuscularly) should be given every 15 or 20 minutes. In the absence of reaction it is safe to give the usual dose, for a sensitized individual, after receiving a small dose, is refractory to larger doses some hours later. Children seem to be much less liable to sensitization than adults. If anaphylaxis should occur, morphia (gr.

¼, 0.016 gm.) and atropine (gr. $\frac{1}{100}$, 0.0006 gm.) hypodermically should be given at once followed by epinephrine (1 cc. of a 1-1000 solution). Artificial respiration should be done if there is respiratory failure.

Results.—Of 183,256 cases treated in 150 cities previous to the serum period, the mortality was 38.4 per cent. In 88 cities in the United States (37 million population) the death rate in 1933 was 2.32 per 100,000; in 1923 it was 13.13 per 100,000.

Convalescence.—If there are signs of cardiac disturbance, the patient should be kept absolutely at rest. Nourishment should be given freely, strychnine administered in full doses, and iron with arsenic if there is anemia. With the postdiphtheritic paralysis the patients should be kept in bed, fed liberally and given strychnine hypodermically. Antitoxin may be given. In chronic forms with muscular wasting, electricity and massage should be used. The patient should not be discharged from quarantine until two successive cultures from the throat and nose, two days apart, have been negative.

SCARLET FEVER

Definition.—An infectious disease, the infection being local in the nasopharynx, caused by certain specific strains of hemolytic streptococci. A soluble toxin is produced which is absorbed, causing the general and special features of the disease. There may be a secondary systemic streptococcal infection. The organism is the *Streptococcus scarlatinae.*

History.—In the sixteenth century Ingrassias of Naples and Coyttarus of Poitiers recognized the disease; but Sydenham in 1675 gave a full account of it under the name febris scarlatina. The isolation of the strains of streptococci, the production of scarlet fever experimentally in human subjects and the preparation of an antitoxin (by injection of the toxin into the horse) by G. F. and G. H. Dick are outstanding achievements. Dochez and his co-workers did important work in the study of the strains of organisms. They produced an antitoxin by immunizing the horse with the organisms. Variation in the severity of the disease is a striking feature in its history.

Etiology.—No acute infection varies so greatly in the intensity of the outbreaks, a point to which both Sydenham and Bretonneau called attention. In some years it is mild; in others, with equally widespread epidemics, it is fearfully malignant. It is widespread, occurring in nearly all parts of the globe and attacking all races. Sporadic cases occur from time to time. The epidemics are most intense in the autumn and winter. There is an extraordinary variability in the severity of the outbreaks, which on the whole appear to be lessening in severity. In England and Wales the disease is declining. In 1883 there were over 12,000 deaths; in 1903, 4,158; and in 1931, 540 deaths. Newsholme attributes this in part to the general improvement in sanitation, to hospital isolation, and in part to the decline in the severity of the disease. In the United States registration areas the mortality in 1900 was 10.2 and in 1932 2.1 per 100,000.

Seibert's studies in New York show that the disease increases steadily from week to week until the middle of May; the frequency diminishes gradually until the end of June, and increases through October, November, and December.

He associates the drop in July, August, and September with the closure of the schools and less daily congregation of children in small areas.

Age is the most important predisposing factor; 90 per cent of the fatal cases are under the tenth year. Sucklings are rarely attacked. The general liability to the disease is less widespread than in measles. Many escape in childhood; others escape until adult life; some never take it.

Family susceptibility may be illustrated by the death in rapid succession of four or five members. An attack as a rule confers subsequent immunity. In rare instances there have been one or even two recurrences.

Immunity.—Most newborn children are immune, this being acquired from the mother, as in diphtheria. Many children lose this immunity and become susceptible. This may be determined by the intracutaneous injection of 0.1 cc. of a 1-1000 dilution of the toxin—*Dick test.* With a positive reaction, signs appear in six hours, reaching a maximum in from eighteen to thirty-six hours. An area of erythema measuring 10 mm. in diameter is regarded as positive. The local reaction rapidly subsides and rarely persists more than forty-eight hours. In patients who are convalescent from scarlet fever the reaction is negative or only slightly positive. The production of active immunity is possible by the injection of the toxin in proper amounts. The serum from a convalescent patient and the antitoxin produce a passive immunity.

Infectivity.—The source of infection is often not discovered in a given case. The organisms are given off with the secretions of the nose and throat and in the discharge from an otitis media. *Carriers* are important, especially those with nasal or ear discharges. The mild angina of ambulatory cases may convey the disease, and in this way it is spread in schools, and the "return cases" may find in this way their explanation. The intractable character of the nasal discharge after scarlet fever is well recognized and this secretion is highly infectious. Direct contact is probably important but the organism can persist for a long time in garments, etc.

The disease may be conveyed by *milk.* Of 99 epidemics studied by Kober the disease prevailed in 68 either at the dairy or the milk farm. There appear to be two groups of cases: first, genuine scarlet fever, in which the infection is conveyed through the milk having come in contact with infected persons; and, secondly, outbreaks of an infection resembling scarlet fever, associated with disease of the udder of the cows and due to streptococci.

By *surgical scarlatina,* first brought to attention by Sir James Paget in 1864, is understood an erythematous eruption following an operation or occurring during septic infection. It differs from scarlet fever in the large number of adults attacked, the shorter incubation, the mildness of the throat symptoms, the starting of the eruption at the wound, and the precocious desquamation. Alice Hamilton, after analyzing 174 reported cases, concludes that the eruption is most frequently due to septic infection and in cases in which the disease was undoubtedly scarlet fever it is probable that the relation between the wound and the scarlet fever was coincidence. Allergy may be a factor, the sensitization occurring early in life.

Organism.—The association of hemolytic streptococci with scarlet fever has long been recognized but the etiological relationship was in doubt. Dochez and his coworkers isolated this streptococcus from a wound and an infected burn in scarlet fever, from the lochial discharge in puerperal scarlet fever and from both the patients and infected milk in a milk-borne epidemic. G. F. and G. H. Dick produced scarlet fever experimentally in human subjects by two types of hemolytic streptococci which do and do not ferment mannite. Does the organism represent a specific type? There is not general agreement on this and some hold that there is no definite serological distinction between it and other hemolytic streptococci.

Morbid Anatomy.—Except in the hemorrhagic form, the skin after death shows no traces of the rash. There are no specific lesions. Those in the internal organs are due partly to the fever and partly to infection with pus organisms. The anatomical changes in the throat are those of simple inflammation, follicular tonsillitis, and, in extreme grades, of diphtheroid angina. In severe cases there are intense lymphadenitis and inflammatory edema of the tissues of the neck, which may go on to suppuration, or even to gangrene. The lymph nodes and the lymphoid tissue may show hyperplasia and the spleen, liver, and other organs may be the seat of widespread focal necroses. Endocarditis and pericarditis are infrequent. Myocardial changes are not common. The renal changes will be considered with the diseases of the kidney. Affections of the respiratory organs are not frequent. When death results from the pseudomembranous angina, bronchopneumonia is not uncommon. Cerebrospinal changes are rare but meningeal hemorrhage has been found.

Symptoms.—Incubation.—"From one to seven days, oftenest two to four." McCollom considered the usual period to be ten to fourteen days.

Invasion.—The onset is as a rule sudden. It may be preceded by a slight, scarcely noticeable, indisposition. An actual chill is rare. Vomiting is one of the most constant initial symptoms; convulsions are common. The fever is intense; rising rapidly, it may on the first day reach 104° or even 105°. The pulse rate is usually high. The skin is unusually dry and to the touch gives a sensation of very pungent heat. The tongue is furred, cough and catarrhal symptoms are uncommon. The face is often flushed and the patient has the objective features of an acute fever. There is frequently marked dryness and pain in the throat with redness of the pharynx and soft palate. The uvula may be red and edematous. The injection of the fauces and tonsils may be very intense and exudate may form. The lymph nodes at the angles of the jaws may be enlarged and tender.

Eruption.—Usually on the second day, in some instances within the first twenty-four hours, the rash appears in the form of scattered red points on a deep subcuticular flush; at first on the neck and chest, and spreading so rapidly that by the evening of the second day it may have invaded the entire skin. After persisting for two or three days it gradually fades. At its height the rash has a vivid scarlet hue, quite distinctive and unlike that seen in any other eruptive disease. It is an intense hyperemia, and the anemia produced by pressure instantly disappears. There may be fine punctiform hemorrhages, which do not disappear on pressure. The relative prominence of the punctate and erythematous elements gives different appearances. In some cases the rash does not become uniform but remains patchy, and intervals of normal skin separate large hyperemic areas. Tiny papular elevations may sometimes be seen, but they are not so common as in measles. With each day the rash becomes of a darker color, and there may be in parts even a bluish-red shade. Smooth at the beginning, the skin gradually becomes rougher, and to the touch feels like "goose skin." At the height of the eruption sudaminal vesicles may develop, the fluid of which may become turbid. The entire skin may at the same time be covered with small yellow vesicles on a deep red background—*scarlatina miliaris.* McCollom laid stress upon a punctate eruption in the armpits, groins, and on the roof of the mouth. There is special involvement of the flexor surfaces of the joints. Marked transverse lines at the bend of the elbow may occur early. Apart from the virulent hemorrhagic form there are other occurrences of a hemorrhagic character. There may be a widespread purpuric eruption early or purpura may appear about the third week. Ecchymoses may appear, often about the sacrum or buttocks. Hemorrhagic bullae may occur and necrosis may follow. In some cases the purpura takes the Henoch form. Two factors may be responsible, injury to the capillaries by the toxin and deficiency of the blood platelets. The former seems the more probable. The subject was discussed by Box (1933). Small skin hemorrhages

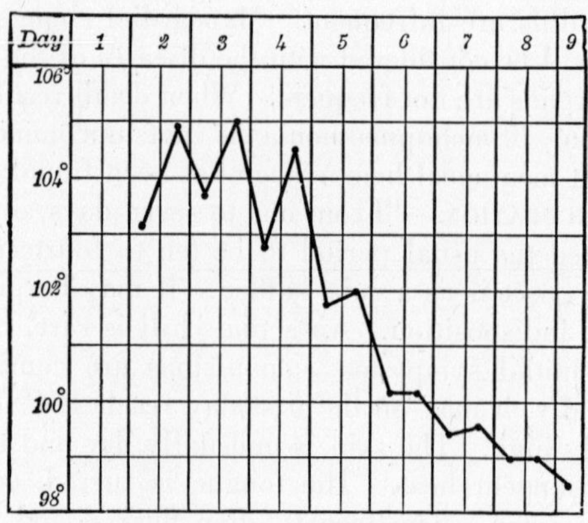

Chart II.—Scarlet Fever.

may occur into the skin at the elbow after constriction of the upper arm (Leeds-Rumpel phenomenon).

The eruption does not always appear upon the face. Circumoral pallor is often marked. There may be a good deal of swelling of the skin, which feels uncomfortable and tense. The itching is variable; not as a rule intense at the height of the eruption. The rash may be transitory, lasting only a few hours, and rarely persists longer than a week. The tongue at first is red at the tip and edges, furred in the centre; and through the white fur are often seen the swollen red papillae, which give the so-called "strawberry" appearance to the tongue, particularly if the child puts out the tip of the tongue between the lips. In a few days the "fur" desquamates and leaves the surface red and rough, and it is this condition which some writers call the "strawberry," or, better, the "raspberry" tongue. The breath often has a heavy, sweet odor. Enlargement of the papillae is a very constant sign.

The pharyngeal features are: (1) Redness, which may be marked, with swelling of the pillars of the fauces and of the tonsils. (2) A more intense grade of swelling and infiltration of these parts with a follicular tonsillitis. (3) Diphtheroid angina with intense inflammation of all the pharyngeal structures, swelling of the glands below the jaw, and in very severe cases a thick brawny induration of all the tissues of the neck.

The *fever*, which sets in with such suddenness and intensity, may reach 105° or even 106° F. It persists with slight morning remissions, gradually declining with the disappearance of the rash. In mild cases the temperature may not reach 103° F.; on the other hand, in very severe cases there may be hyperpyrexia, 108° F., or before death even 109° F.

The *pulse* ranges from 120 to 150; in severe cases with very high fever from 190 to 200. The respirations show an increase proportionate to the intensity of the fever. A polymorphonuclear *leukocytosis* (15,000-30,000) is usually present and inclusion bodies may be seen in the leukocytes. The gastro-intestinal symptoms are not marked after the initial vomiting, and food is usually well taken. In some instances there are abdominal pains. The edge of the spleen may be palpable. The liver is not often enlarged. The cervical, axillary and inguinal lymph nodes are usually enlarged. With the initial fever nervous symptoms are present in a majority of the cases; but as the rash comes out the headache and the slight delirium disappear. The urine has the ordinary febrile characters, being scanty and high colored. Slight albuminuria is common during the stage of eruption. Careful examination of the urine should be made every day. There is no cause for alarm in the trace of albumin which is so often present, not even if associated with a few casts.

DESQUAMATION.—With the disappearance of the rash and the fever the skin looks somewhat stained, is dry, a little rough, and gradually the upper layer of the cuticle begins to separate. The process usually begins about the neck and chest, and flakes are gradually detached. Desquamation often begins over the papillae and spreads in a ring shape. Peeling along the edges of the nails is characteristic and of value in late diagnosis. The degree and character of the desquamation bear some relation to the intensity of the eruption. When the latter has been very vivid and of long standing large flakes may be thrown off. In rare instances the hair and even the nails have been shed. There are cases in which the desquamation is prolonged to the seventh or eighth week. The average time is from ten to fifteen or even twenty days.

Varieties of Scarlet Fever.—MILD AND ABORTIVE FORMS.—In cases of exceptional mildness the rash may be scarcely perceptible. Desquamation, however, may follow, and in these very mild forms nephritis may occur. During epidemics, when several children of a household are affected, one child may have a sore throat and the "strawberry tongue," but the rash does not appear. In such cases desquamation may follow.

MALIGNANT SCARLET FEVER.—With all the characteristics of an acute intoxication, the patient is overwhelmed by the intense toxemia and may die in 24 or 36 hours. The disease sets in with great severity—high fever, extreme restlessness, headache, and delirium. The temperature may rise to 107° or even higher. Convulsions may occur and the initial delirium rapidly gives place to coma. The dyspnea may be urgent; the pulse is rapid and feeble.

HEMORRHAGIC FORM.—Hemorrhages occur into the skin, and there are hematuria and epistaxis. Scattered petechiae appear, which gradually become more extensive, and ultimately the skin may be universally involved. Death may take place on the second or third day. While this form is more common in feeble children, it may attack adults apparently in full health.

SEPTIC FORM.—The throat symptoms appear early and progress rapidly; the fauces and tonsils swell and are covered with a thick membranous exudate, which may extend to the posterior wall of the pharynx, forward into the mouth, and upward into the nostrils. The glands of the neck rapidly enlarge. Necrosis occurs in the tissues of the throat, the fetor is extreme, the constitutional disturbance profound, and the child dies with the clinical picture of a malignant diphtheria. Occasionally the membrane extends into the trachea and the bronchi. The Eustachian tubes and the middle ear are usually involved. When death does not take place rapidly from toxemia there may be extensive abscess formation in the tissues of the neck with sloughing.

SEPTICEMIC FORM.—In this there is a marked secondary infection and death occurs in the second or third week from severe toxemia.

Complications and Sequelae.—ALBUMINURIA.—At the height of the fever there is often a slight trace of albumin in the urine, which is not of special significance. In a majority of cases the kidneys escape without greater damage than occurs in other acute febrile affections.

NEPHRITIS is most common in the second or third week and may follow a very mild attack. It may be delayed until the third or fourth week. As a rule, the earlier it occurs the more severe the attack. It occurs in from 10 to 20 per cent of the cases. Watch should be kept for decrease in the amount of urine and the presence of blood and albumin. Three grades of severity may be recognized:

Acute hemorrhagic nephritis. There may be suppression of urine or only a small quantity of bloody fluid laden with albumin and tube casts. Vomiting is constant, there are convulsions, and the child may die with the symptoms of acute uremia. In severe epidemics an acute, rapidly fatal, nephritis due to scarlet fever may occur without an exanthem.

Less severe cases without serious acute symptoms. There is edema of the eyelids, with slight edema of the feet; the urine is diminished in quantity, smoky, and contains albumin and casts. The kidney symptoms then dominate the entire case, the dropsy persists, and there may be effusion into the serous sacs. The condition may become chronic, or the patient succumbs to uremia. Fortunately, in a majority of the cases recovery takes place.

Cases so mild that they can scarcely be termed nephritis. The urine contains albumin and a few casts, but rarely blood. The edema is slight or transient, and the convalescence is scarcely interrupted. Occasionally serious symptoms supervene. Edema of the glottis may prove rapidly fatal, and in one case the child died of acute effusion into the pleural sacs.

In other cases the edema disappears and the child improves, though he remains pale, and a slight amount of albumin persists in the urine for months or even for years. Recovery may take place or a *chronic nephritis* may follow. Occasionally edema occurs without albuminuria or signs of nephritis. Possibly it may be due to the anemia; but there are instances in which marked changes have been found in the kidney after death, when the urine did not show the features characteristic of nephritis.

ARTHRITIS.—There are two forms: first, a severe pyemia, with suppuration of one or more joints—part of a widespread streptococcus infection. This is an extremely serious and fatal form. Secondly, scarlatinal arthritis, analogous to that in other infections. It occurs in the second or third week; many joints are attacked, particularly the small joints of the hands. The heart may be involved. Chorea, subcutaneous nodules, purpura, and pleurisy may be complications. The outlook is usually good.

Cardiac Complications.—In the severe septic cases a malignant endocarditis, sometimes with purulent pericarditis, closes the scene. Simple endocarditis may occur. It may not be easy to say whether an apex systolic murmur signifies a valvular lesion. The persistence after convalescence, with enlargement of the heart, may alone decide that the murmur indicated an organic change. As is the rule, such cases give no symptoms. There may be a severe toxic myocarditis, sometimes leading to acute dilatation and sudden death. The cardiac complications are often latent. Changes in the electrocardiograms are common, especially from the second to the fifth weeks. Changes in conduction may persist for some months.

Acute Bronchitis and Bronchopneumonia.—These are not common. *Empyema* is an insidious and serious complication.

Ear Complications.—Common and serious, due to extension of the inflammation from the throat through the Eustachian tubes, they rank among the most frequent causes of deafness in children. The severe forms of membranous angina are almost always associated with otitis, which goes on to suppuration and perforation of the drum. The process may extend to the labyrinth and rapidly produce deafness. In other instances there is mastoiditis. Williams (1933) in 14,733 cases found 10.8 per cent of otitis media and 1.1 per cent of mastoiditis. In the necrosis which follows the middle-ear disease the facial nerve may be involved and paralysis follow. Later, still more serious complications may follow, such as thrombosis of the lateral sinus, meningitis, or abscess of the brain. *Sinusitis* is not infrequent.

Adenitis.—In comparatively mild cases the submaxillary lymph nodes may be swollen. In severer cases the swelling of the neck becomes extreme and extends beyond the limits of the glands. Acute phlegmonous inflammations may lead to widespread destruction, in which vessels may be eroded and fatal hemorrhage ensue. The suppurative processes may also involve the retropharyngeal tissues. The swelling of the lymph nodes usually subsides, and within a few weeks even the most extensive enlargement gradually disappears. There are rare cases in which the lymphadenitis becomes chronic, and the neck remains with a glandular collar which almost obliterates its outline and proves intractable to all treatment.

Peritonitis.—Primary peritonitis, without any demonstrable focus in the peritoneal cavity, is rare. It is not clear whether the infection is from the blood stream, lymphatics or by direct extension. There is a thick fibrinopurulent exudate which simulates a pseudomembrane. The amount of fluid is usually not large. Diarrhea is sometimes marked. In treatment, laparotomy with drainage should be done. The majority of the few cases of recovery have occurred after operation.

Nervous Complications.—Chorea occasionally complicates the arthritis and endocarditis. Sudden convulsions followed by hemiplegia may occur. In 7 of a series of 120 cases of infantile hemiplegia the onset was during scarlet fever. Progressive paralysis of the limbs with wasting may present the features of a subacute ascending spinal paralysis. Thrombosis of the cerebral veins may occur. Mental symptoms, mania, and melancholia have been described.

Encephalitis is rare and also meningitis which may develop late. Vagotonia may be marked in convalescence.

Other complications and sequelae are edema of the eyelids, without nephritis, symmetrical gangrene, enteritis, noma, and perforation of the soft palate. Rhinitis is comparatively common. Paronychia may occur.

The fever may persist for several weeks after the disappearance of the rash, and the child may remain in a septic state. This is usually the result of some chronic suppurative process about the throat or the nose, occasionally the result of a chronic adenitis, but in a few cases nothing whatever can be found to account for the fever.

RELAPSE was noted in 7 per cent of 12,000 (Caiger), in 1 per cent of 1,520 (Newsholme), and in 3 per cent of 5,000 cases (McCollom).

COEXISTENCE OF OTHER DISEASES.—Of 48,366 cases of scarlet fever in the Metropolitan Asylum Board Hospitals complicated by some other disease, in 1,094 cases the secondary infection was diphtheria, in 899 cases chickenpox, in 703 measles, in 404 whooping-cough, in 55 erysipelas, in 11 typhoid fever, and in 1 typhus fever (F. F. Caiger).

Diagnosis.—This is not difficult in typical attacks when the patient is seen early but in mild cases with a transitory rash or after the acute features are over, it may be very difficult. The following are the most common conditions with which scarlet fever may be confounded:

ACUTE EXFOLIATING DERMATITIS.—This simulates scarlet fever very closely. It has a sudden onset, with fever. The eruption spreads rapidly, is uniform, and after persisting for five or six days begins to fade. Even before it has entirely gone desquamation usually begins, sometimes leaving erythematous skin. Some cases cannot be distinguished from scarlet fever in the stage of eruption. The throat symptoms are usually absent, and the tongue rarely shows the changes so marked in scarlet fever. In the desquamation of this affection the hair and nails are commonly affected. It is, too, a disease liable to recur. Some of the instances of second and third attacks of scarlet fever have been cases of this form of dermatitis.

MEASLES is distinguished by the longer period of invasion, the characteristic prodromes, and the later appearance of the rash. The greater intensity of the measly rash upon the face, the more papular character and the irregular crescentic distribution are distinguishing features. Other points are the absence in measles of the sore throat, the peculiar character of the desquamation, the absence of leukocytosis, and the presence of Koplik's sign.

RUBELLA.—The rash is sometimes strikingly like that of scarlet fever. In cases of doubt the mild general symptoms are our best guide. The catarrhal symptoms and adenitis are helpful.

SEPTICEMIA.—The so-called puerperal or surgical scarlatina shows an eruption which may be identical in appearance with that of scarlet fever.

DIPHTHERIA.—The practitioner may be in doubt whether he is dealing with scarlet fever with intense membranous angina, a true diphtheria with an erythematous rash, or coexisting scarlet fever and diphtheria. A rash in diphtheria is, after all, not common, is limited usually to the trunk, is not so persistent, and is generally darker than the scarlatinal rash. Cultures are important in doubtful cases. Scarlet fever and diphtheria may coexist, but in a case presenting widespread erythema and extensive membrane with diphtheria bacilli, only the specific skin reaction may determine if scarlet fever is present. The streptococcus angina is not so apt to extend to the larynx, nor are recurrences so common; but general infection may occur, the membrane may spread downward with great rapidity, and all the nervous sequelae of diphtheria may follow a streptococcus infection.

FOOD, SERUM AND DRUG RASHES.—The history and general features are important, while the rashes are partial, and seldom more than a transient hyperemia. Occasionally they are diffuse and intense, and in such cases very deceptive. They are not associated with the characteristic symptoms of invasion and there is no fever. They are most apt to follow the use of belladonna, quinine, phenobarbital and iodide. The antitoxin erythema may cause doubt, particularly in hospitals for infectious diseases.

Specific Reaction.—The intracutaneous injection of serum from a person immune to or convalescent from scarlet fever or 0.1 cc. of scarlet fever antitoxin into a patient with scarlet fever produces a local area of blanching which persists until the rash has faded. These phenomena suggest the neutralization of a toxin in the tissues. A positive reaction with the Dick test early in convalescence from a doubtful attack is against scarlet fever as also a negative reaction early in the illness.

How Long Is a Child Infective?—Usually in six weeks the danger is thought to be over, but the occurrence of so-called "return cases" shows that patients may remain infective even at this stage. With 15,000 cases submitted to an average period of isolation of 49 days or under, the percentage of return cases was 1.86; with an average period of 50 to 56 days the percentage was 1.12; where the isolation extended to between 57 and 65 days the percentage of return cases was 1 (Neech). Special care should be taken of patients with rhinorrhea, otorrhea and throat trouble, as the secretions from these parts are often infective.

Prognosis.—The death rate has been falling of late years. Epidemics differ remarkably in severity and the mortality is extremely variable. Among the better classes the death-rate is much lower than in hospital practice. There is a curious variability in the local mortality from this disease. In England, for example, in some years, certain counties enjoy almost immunity from fatal scarlet fever. The younger the child the greater the danger. In infants under one year the death rate is very high. The great proportion of fatal cases occurs in children under six years of age. Serious features are high fever, severe toxemia, bronchopneumonia, the occurrence of hemorrhages (cutaneous or visceral), intense throat infection, cervical cellulitis, and laryngeal obstruction. Nephritis is always serious, and setting in with suppression of urine may quickly prove fatal; a large majority of the patients recover.

Prophylaxis.—A rigid system of school inspection, and general recognition of the importance of latent cases and the persistence of infection in the secretions of the nose and throat will aid. The attendant in a case of scarlet fever should take the most careful precautions against the conveyance of the disease. The duration of quarantine varies with the attack: six to eight weeks is the average period. Patients with discharge from the ear or nose require longer isolation. The quarantine period for contacts is 10 days.

Passive immunity may be secured by the intramuscular injection of 10 to 20 cc. of convalescent serum or 5 to 10 cc. of scarlet fever antitoxin. This is useful in epidemics; the immunity is temporary and for a few weeks. *Active immunity* is secured by the use of the specific toxin, given subcutaneously, in increasing doses from 500 to 80,000 skin-test-doses, once a week for three or four weeks. The Dick test should be done to determine if the individual is susceptible. The immunity lasts for two or three years and may be permanent. The reaction may be fairly severe. All those who come in contact with the disease should be immunized, if susceptible.

Treatment.—The patient may be treated at home or sent to an isolation hospital. The difficulty in *home treatment* is in securing complete isolation. The risks are well illustrated by the studies of Chapin, of Providence, who found that 26.1 per cent of 4,412 persons under twenty-one years of age in infected families took the disease. When practicable, it is better to send the other children out of the house. Chapin's experience is interesting. In seventeen years, from 652 families infected with scarlet fever, 1,051 children, none of whom had had the disease, were removed. Only 5 per cent were attacked while away from home; 19 who had been sent away from the infected houses were attacked on their return.

The patient should be isolated, in charge of a competent nurse and be kept in bed for three weeks at least. The temperature of the room should be constant and the ventilation thorough. The child should wear a light flannel nightgown, and the bedclothing should not be too heavy. The mouth should be kept clean and rinsed freely with a mild antiseptic solution. The diet should consist of milk, buttermilk, whey, and ice cream; water and fruit juices should be freely given. Cream and lactose may be added to the milk. With the fall of the temperature the diet may be increased very slowly, farinaceous food being added first, later the child may gradually return to ordinary fare. An occasional warm bath may be given. At any time during the attack the skin may be sponged with warm water. In convalescence great care should be exercised to prevent exposure to cold. The renal complications are very apt to occur during convalescence, and after all danger is apparently past. Ordinary cases may be given a simple fever mixture. The bowels should be carefully regulated but drastic purgation avoided.

When the fever is above 103° F. tepid sponges may be given. In severe cases, with the temperature rapidly rising, this will not suffice, and more thorough measures of hydrotherapy should be practised. With pronounced delirium and nervous symptoms the wet pack should be used. When the fever is rising rapidly but the child is not delirious, he should be placed in a warm bath, the temperature of which can be gradually lowered. In giving the pack a rubber sheet and a thick layer of blankets should be spread upon a sofa or a bed, and over them a sheet wrung out of water. The naked child is laid upon it and wrapped in blankets. An intense glow of heat quickly follows the preliminary chilling, and from time to time the blankets may be unfolded and the child sprinkled with water. The good effects are often striking, particularly in allaying the delirium and jactitation, and procuring quiet sleep. The child may be removed from the warm bath, placed upon a sheet wrung out of tolerably cold water, and then folded in blankets. The ice-cap is useful and may be kept constantly applied when there is a high fever. Medicinal antipyretics are not of much service in comparison with cold water. If the child is restless or sleepless, hydrotherapy is usually effectual. If not, moderate doses of bromide may be given. With *hemorrhagic* features blood transfusion should be done, preferably from a patient convalescent from scarlet fever. The administration of liver extract has been advised.

The *throat* symptoms, if mild, do not require much treatment. If severe, the local measures mentioned under diphtheria should be used. The nose should be kept clean, for which a simple alkaline douche, given gently, is best. Cold applications to the neck are to be preferred to hot, though it is sometimes difficult to get a child to submit to them. If cervical adenitis occurs, an ice bag should be applied, and with the first signs of suppuration an incision made. The *ears* should be specially watched and careful disinfection of the mouth and fauces by suitable antiseptic solutions should be practised. When the inflammation extends through the tubes to the middle ear, the practitioner should examine daily the condition of the drum, or, when available, a specialist called in to assist. An early puncture when required may save the hearing. The operation may be repeated at intervals if the pain and distention return. Watch should be kept for mastoiditis.

The nephritis should be dealt with as in ordinary cases; indications for treatment will be found under the appropriate section. Many insist upon the great value of milk diet in scarlet fever as a preventive of nephritis.

Among other indications for treatment is cardiac weakness, for which digitalis, or if urgent strophanthin intramuscularly, may be given.

Serum Treatment.—Antitoxin should be given as early as possible in doses of 10-20 cc. intramuscularly. If given intravenously care should be taken to determine if hypersensitiveness exists. It may be given daily for 3 or 4 days if necessary. There is difference of opinion as to its value in preventing complications. It is not likely to be of value if given on the fifth day or later.

THE PNEUMONIAS AND PNEUMOCOCCIC INFECTIONS

A variety of diseases are caused by the pneumococcus, among which lobar and bronchopneumonia are the most important. Various inflammatory affections of the lungs may be caused by other organisms, but the pneumococcus plays the important rôle in the common lobar pneumonia and in the ordinary bronchopneumonia. It may set up also many local affections and is the cause of many terminal infections in chronic diseases.

LOBAR PNEUMONIA

(*Croupous or Fibrinous Pneumonia, Lung Fever*)

Definition.—An infection usually caused by the pneumococcus, characterized by inflammation of the lungs, a toxemia of varying intensity and a fever which terminates by crisis in about 50 per cent of the cases.

History.—The disease was known to Hippocrates and the old Greek physicians, by whom it was confounded with pleurisy. Among the ancients, Aretæus gave a remarkable description. "Ruddy in countenance, but especially the cheeks; the white of the eyes very bright and fatty; the point of the nose flat; the veins in the temples and neck distended; loss of appetite; pulse, at first, large, empty, very frequent, as if forcibly accelerated; heat indeed, externally, feeble, and more humid than natural, but, internally, dry and very hot, by means of which the breath is hot; there is thirst, dryness of the tongue, desire of cold air, aberration of mind; cough mostly dry, but if anything be brought up it is a frothy phlegm, or slightly tinged with bile, or with a very florid tinge of blood. The blood-stained is of all others the worst." At the end of the seventeenth and the beginning of the eighteenth century Morgagni and Valsalva made many accurate clinical and anatomical observations on the disease. Our modern knowledge dates from Laënnec (1819), whose masterly description of the physical signs and morbid anatomy left little for subsequent observers to add or modify.

Incidence.—One of the most widespread of acute diseases, pneumonia has become the "Captain of the Men of Death," among acute infections, to use the phrase applied by John Bunyan to consumption. In England and Wales in 1931 there were 23,573 deaths from this cause. In the United States in the registration area in 1930 there were 98,657 deaths; of these 53,810 were due to lobar pneumonia, 40,663 to bronchopneumonia, and 4,184 were unclassified.

Etiology.—AGE.—To the sixth year the predisposition to pneumonia is marked; it diminishes to the fifteenth year, but then for each subsequent decade it increases. For children Holt's statistics of 500 cases give: First year, 15 per cent; from the second to the sixth year, 62 per cent; from the seventh to the eleventh year, 21 per cent; from the twelfth to the fourteenth year, 2 per cent. Lobar pneumonia has been met with in the new-born. The relation to age is well shown in the U. S. Census Report for 1900. The death-rate in persons from fifteen to forty-five years was 100.05 per 100,000 of population; from forty-five to sixty-five years it was 263.12; and in persons sixty-five years of age and over it was 733.77. Pneumonia may well be called the friend of the aged. Taken off by it in an acute, short, not often painful illness, the old escape those "cold gradations of decay" that may make the last stage of all so distressing.

SEX.—Males are more frequently affected than females; of 12,098 collected cases 73 per cent were in males and 27 per cent in females.

RACE.—In the United States pneumonia is more fatal in negroes than among the whites.

SOCIAL CONDITION.—The disease is more common in the cities. Overcrowding probably is a factor. Individuals who are much exposed to hardship and cold are particularly liable to the disease. Newcomers and immigrants are stated to be less susceptible than native inhabitants.

PERSONAL CONDITION.—Debilitating causes of all sorts render individuals more susceptible. Alcoholism is perhaps the most potent predisposing factor. Robust, healthy men are, however, often attacked.

PREVIOUS ATTACK.—No other acute disease recurs in the same individual with such frequency. Instances are on record of individuals who have had ten or more attacks. The percentage of recurrences has been placed as high as 50. Netter gives it as 31, and in collected statistics found 27 per cent. In the recurrent attacks the prognosis is usually good.

TRAUMA.—*Contusion Pneumonia.*—Pneumonia may follow directly upon injury, particularly of the chest, without necessarily any lesion of the lung. Collapse of the lung may be mistaken for it. Stern describes three clinical varieties: first, the ordinary lobar pneumonia following a contusion of the chest wall; secondly, atypical cases, with slight fever and not very characteristic physical signs; thirdly, cases with the physical signs and features of broncho-pneumonia. The last two varieties have a favorable prognosis.

COLD has been regarded as an important etiological factor. The frequent occurrence of an initial chill has been one reason for this widespread belief. As to the close association of pneumonia with exposure there can be no question. We see the disease occur promptly after a wetting or a chilling due to some unusual exposure, or come on after an upper respiratory tract infection of a few days' duration. Cold is regarded simply as a factor in lowering the resistance of the bronchial and pulmonary tissues.

CLIMATE AND SEASON.—Climate does not appear to have very much influence, as pneumonia prevails in hot and cold countries. It is stated to be more prevalent in the southern than in the northern states, but the Census Reports show little difference in the various state groups. The disease is less prevalent in England than in the United States, where the dry, overheated air of the houses favors catarrhal processes in the air passages. More important is the influence of *season.* Statistics are almost unanimous in placing the highest incidence in the winter and spring months. In many localities the highest percentage is in January, February and March.

Bacteriology.—PNEUMOCOCCUS OR DIPLOCOCCUS PNEUMONIAE.—In September, 1880, Sternberg inoculated rabbits with his own saliva and isolated a micrococcus. The publication was not made until April, 1881. Pasteur discovered the same organism in the saliva of a child dead of hydrophobia in December, 1880, and the priority of the discovery belongs to him, as his publication is dated January, 1881. There was no suspicion that this organism was concerned in the etiology of lobar pneumonia, and it was not really until 1884, that Fraenkel determined that the organism found by Sternberg and Pasteur in the saliva was the most frequent germ in pneumonia.

The organism is a somewhat elliptical, lance-shaped coccus, usually occurring in pairs; hence the term diplococcus. There are a number of groups based upon well defined immunological differences. Types I and II each comprise about one-third of the cases with a mortality of 25-30 per cent. Type III comprises 10-15 per cent with a mortality about 40 per cent and Group IV, the remainder with a mortality about 12 per cent. A large number of strains (29) are included in Group IV. The relative figures vary in different years. Young persons seem especially susceptible to Type I and the elderly to Type III infections. Organisms of Group IV are the commonest forms in the mouths of healthy individuals.

Distribution in the Body.—In the bronchial secretions and in the affected lung the pneumococcus is readily demonstrated in smears, and in the latter in sections. It is possible to isolate the pneumococcus from the blood in about one-third of all cases of lobar pneumonia.

In the Mouth.—The pneumococcus is present in the mouths of a large proportion of healthy individuals (Type III and Group IV), various observers giving 80 to 90 per cent. Types I and II are not often found in the mouths of healthy individuals and infection due to these is acquired from without. The virulence is not always uniform and may increase during the winter months. Some persons always harbor a virulent variety. It seems proved that normal individuals—*i.e.*, persons in whose mouths virulent pneumococci were proved to be absent—acquired the organisms by association with cases of pneumonia, or with healthy persons in whom these pneumococci were present.

Outside the Body.—The viability of the pneumococcus is not great. It has been found in the dust and sweepings of rooms, but Wood has shown (New York Commission Report) that the germs exposed to sunlight die in a very short time—an hour and a half being the limit. In moist sputum kept in a dark room the germs lived ten days, and in a badly ventilated room in which a person with pneumonia coughed, the germs suspended in the air retained their vitality for several hours.

PNEUMOBACILLUS OF FRIEDLÄNDER.—This is a larger organism than the pneumococcus, and appears in the form of plump, short rods. It shows a capsule but presents marked differences from the pneumococcus. The exudate caused by this bacillus is usually more viscid and poorer in fibrin than that in pneumococcus pneumonia. It may be the primary organism or a secondary invader. It is not a common cause: Cecil found 9 cases in 2,000 cases of pneumonia in which it was apparently the primary cause and 9 cases in which it occurred with the pneumococcus. The process may be lobar or lobular, the latter usually becoming confluent.

OTHER ORGANISMS.—Various bacteria may be associated with the pneumococcus in lobar pneumonia, the most common of these being streptococci and staphylococci. The pneumonias caused by *B. typhosus*, *B. diphtheriæ*, and the influenza bacillus are not to be identified with true lobar pneumonia.

Clinically, the *infectious nature* of pneumonia was recognized long before we knew of the pneumococcus. It may occur in epidemic form, in certain houses, barracks, jails, and schools. As many as ten occupants of one house have been attacked. Several members of a family may be attacked consecutively with a most malignant form. In the Middlesborough epidemic, studied by Ballard, 682 persons were attacked, with a mortality of 21 per cent. Direct infection is suggested by the fact that a patient in the next bed to one with pneumonia may take the disease, or 2 or 3 cases may follow in rapid succession in a ward. It is very exceptional, however, for nurses or doctors to be attacked.

Infection and Immunity.—Under ordinary conditions practically everyone harbors some type of pneumococcus and for periods one may have predominantly one fixed type. There are carriers of pathogenic varieties of the pneumococcus who do not have pneumonia but who distribute the organisms. It is probable that pneumonia results when infection with a pathogenic strain of the pneumococcus coincides with lowered resistance in the individual. It is usually impossible to trace the source of infection.

There are three phases in the infection—a period of incubation and onset, the clinical manifestations, and the immunization characterized by the crisis. The attack is usually attributed to lowered general resistance, but there is basis for the view that local conditions in the lung, such as catarrhal processes, favor the development of pneumococci. Changes leading to lobar consolidation may be regarded as local defensive reactions. The explosive onset bears a certain resemblance to the anaphylactic reaction. The attack begins abruptly in about 50 per cent of the cases; in the other 50 per cent it is secondary to a preceding respiratory tract infection. The process apparently begins about the hilus in many cases.

The clinical features are a toxemia, plus disturbances of respiratory and circulatory functions. The intoxication bears no proportion to the local lesion. There are profound general infections with little or no pulmonary involvement. Some of the most toxic cases, particularly in the aged, have very slight lesions, while a lung may be solid and the patient show no signs of toxemia. The nature of the toxemia is unknown or, possibly due to absorption of the products of the local exudate, which does not seem likely, as the symptoms abate after crisis when this absorption is most active. To regard the symptoms as due to absorption of an endotoxin is natural. Studies on the oxygen and carbon dioxide contents of the blood by Peabody showed no change in the reaction of the body tissues beyond the mild grade of acidosis common in all fevers.

The explanation of the crisis is obscure. Immune bodies are not constantly increased after it, or they may not appear for several days. Upon what the neutralization of the toxins depends is doubtful.

Anoxemia.—Oxygen deficiency is an important factor and the amount in the arterial blood may be reduced from the normal 95 per cent to 75 per cent. This increases the dyspnea and the heart rate and causes serious disturbance in the nervous system. It is not possible to separate accurately the features caused by anoxemia from those due to toxemia.

Morbid Anatomy.—Since the time of Laënnec, three stages have been recognized: engorgement, red hepatization and gray hepatization.

In the stage of *engorgement* the lung tissue is deep red in color, firmer and more solid, and on section the surface is bathed with blood and serum. It still crepitates, though not so distinctly as healthy lung, and excised portions float. The air cells can be dilated by insufflation from the bronchus. The capillary vessels are greatly distended, the alveolar epithelium swollen, and the air cells occupied by a variable number of blood corpuscles and detached alveolar cells. In the stage of *red hepatization* the lung tissue is solid, firm, and airless. If the entire lobe is involved it looks voluminous, and shows indentations of the ribs. On section, the surface is dry, reddish-brown in color, and has lost the deeply congested appearance of the first stage. One of the most remarkable features is the friability; in striking contrast to the healthy lung, which is torn with difficulty. The surface has a granular appearance due to the fibrinous plugs filling the air cells. The distinctness of this appearance varies greatly with the size of the alveoli, which are about 0.10 mm. in diameter in the infant, 0.15 or 0.16 in the adult, and from 0.20 to 0.25 in old age. On scraping the surface a reddish viscid serum is removed, containing small granular masses. The smaller bronchi often contain fibrinous plugs. If the lung has been removed before the heart, it is not uncommon to find solid moulds of clot filling the blood-vessels. Microscopically, the air cells are occupied by coagulated fibrin in the meshes of which are red blood corpuscles, leukocytes, and alveolar epithelium. The alveolar walls are infiltrated and leukocytes are seen in the interlobular tissues. Cover-glass preparations from the exudate, and thin sections show, as a rule, the diplococci, many of which are contained within cells. In the stage of *gray hepatization* the tissue has changed from a reddish-brown to a grayish-white color. The surface is moister, the exudate is more turbid, the granules in the acini are less distinct, and the lung tissue is still more friable. The air cells are densely filled with leukocytes, the fibrin network and the red blood corpuscles have largely disappeared. A more advanced condition of gray hepatization is that known as *purulent infiltration*, in which the lung tissue is softer and bathed with a purulent fluid. Small abscess cavities may form, and by their fusion larger ones, though this is rare in ordinary pneumonia.

Resolution.—The changes in the exudate which lead to resolution are due to an autolytic digestion by proteolytic enzymes, which are present more abundantly in gray hepatization than in the preceding stage. The dissolved exudate is for the most part excreted by the kidneys. By following the nitrogen excess in the urine the progress of resolution may be followed and even an estimate formed of the amount of the exudate thus eliminated.

General Details of the Morbid Anatomy.—In 100 autopsies at the General Hospital, Montreal, in 51 cases the right lung was affected, in 32 the left, in 17 both organs. In 27 cases the entire lung, with the exception, perhaps, of a narrow margin at the apex and anterior border, was consolidated. In 34 cases, the lower lobe alone was involved; in 13 cases, the upper lobe alone. When double, the lower lobes were usually affected together, but in three instances the lower lobe of one and the upper lobe of the other were attacked. In 3 cases both upper lobes were affected. Occasionally the disease involves the greater part of both lungs. In a third of the cases, red and gray hepatization existed together. In 22 instances there was gray hepatization. As a rule the unaffected portion of the lung is congested or edematous. When the greater portion of a lobe is attacked, the uninvolved part may be in a state of almost gelatinous edema. The unaffected lung is usually congested, particularly at the posterior part. This may be largely due to postmortem subsidence. The uninflamed portions are not always congested and edematous. The upper lobe may be dry and bloodless when the lower lobe is consolidated. The average weight of a normal lung is about 600 grams, while that of a pneumonic lung may be 1,500 or even 2,500 grams.

The bronchi contain, as a rule, at the time of death a frothy serous fluid, rarely the tenacious mucus so characteristic of pneumonic sputum. The mucous membrane is usually reddened, rarely swollen. In the affected areas the smaller bronchi often contain fibrinous plugs, which may extend into the larger tubes, forming perfect casts. The bronchial glands are swollen and may be soft and pulpy. The *pleural* surface of the inflamed lung is invariably involved when the process becomes superficial. Commonly, there is only a thin sheeting of exudate. The pleura was not involved in only 2 of the 100 cases. In some cases the fibrinous exudate may form a creamy layer an inch in thickness. A serous exudation of variable amount is not uncommon.

Lesions in Other Organs.—The *heart,* particularly its right chamber, is distended with firm, tenacious coagula, which can be withdrawn from the vessels as dendritic moulds. In no other acute disease do we meet with coagula of such solidity. The spleen is often enlarged, though in only 35 of the 100 cases was the weight above 200 grams. The *kidneys* show parenchymatous swelling, turbidity of the cortex, and, in a very considerable proportion of the cases—25 per cent—chronic interstitial changes.

Pericarditis was present in 35 of 658 cases in our series (Chatard). *Endocarditis* occurred in 16 of the 100 postmortems; in 5 of these it was of the simple character; in 11 the lesions were ulcerative. Of 209 cases of malignant endocarditis collected from the literature, 54 occurred in pneumonia. Of 517 fatal cases of acute endocarditis, 22.3 per cent were in pneumonia (E. F. Wells). It is more common on the left than on the right side of the heart. Among 658 cases of pneumonia in the Johns Hopkins Hospital endocarditis occurred in 15 (Marshall). *Myocarditis* and fatty degeneration of the heart may be present in protracted cases.

Meningitis, which is not infrequent, may be associated with malignant endocarditis. It was present in 8 of the 100 autopsies. Of 20 cases of meningitis in ulcerative endocarditis 15 occurred in pneumonia. Changes are found in the cells of the *medullary centres* and *pons.* It is suggested that the cells of the respiratory and vasomotor centres show the most marked change.

Croupous or diphtheritic inflammation may occur in other parts. A *croupous colitis* is not very uncommon. It is usually a thin, flaky exudation, most marked on the tops of the folds of the mucous membrane. The liver shows parenchymatous changes, and often extreme engorgement of the hepatic veins. Degeneration of the muscle fibres of the diaphragm is common, probably due to anoxemia.

Symptoms.—COURSE IN TYPICAL CASES.—We know but little of the incubation period, but it is probably very short. There may have been a previous respiratory tract infection. As a rule, the disease sets in abruptly with a severe *chill,* which lasts from fifteen to thirty minutes or longer. In no acute disease is an initial chill so constant or so severe. The patient may be taken abruptly in the midst of his work or awaken out of sleep in a rigor. The temperature during the chill shows that the fever has already begun. If seen shortly after the onset, the patient usually has features of an acute fever and complains of headache and general pains. Within a few hours there is pain in the side, often agonizing; a short, dry, painful cough begins, and the respirations are increased in frequency. When seen on the second or third day, the picture in typical pneumonia is more distinctive than in any other acute disease. The patient lies often on the affected side; the face is flushed, particularly one or both cheeks; the breathing is hurried, accompanied often with a short expiratory grunt; the alæ nasi dilate with each inspiration; herpes is usually present on the lips or nose; the eyes are bright, the pupils are often unequal, the expression is anxious, and there is a frequent short cough which makes the patient wince and hold his side. The expectoration may be blood-tinged and extremely tenacious. The temperature may be 104° or 105°. The pulse is full and bounding and the pulse-respiration ratio much disturbed. Examination of the lungs shows the physical signs of consolidation with blowing breathing and fine râles. After persisting for seven to ten days if a crisis occurs, with the fall in temperature the patient passes from a condition of extreme distress and anxiety to one of comparative comfort.

SPECIAL FEATURES.—The *fever* rises rapidly, and may be 104° or 105° within twelve hours. Having reached the fastigium, it is remarkably constant. Often the two-hour temperature chart will not show more than a degree of variation for several days. In children and in patients without chill the rise is more gradual. In old persons and in drunkards the fever is lower than in children and healthy individuals; one occasionally sees an afebrile pneumonia. The degree of fever is no guide to the severity of the infection.

Pain.—There is early a sharp, agonizing pain, generally referred to the region of the nipple or lower axilla of the affected side, and much aggravated by deep inspiration and coughing. It is associated, as Aretæus remarks, with involvement of the pleura. It is absent in central pneumonia, and much less frequent in apex pneumonia. The pain may be severe enough to require morphia. With involvement of a lower lobe, especially in children, the pain may be altogether abdominal, suggesting some acute condition. Operation for appendicitis or cholecystitis has been performed.

Dyspnea is almost constant and even early the respirations may be 30 in the minute, and on the second or third day between 40 and 50. In children the respirations may be 80 or even 100. The movements are shallow, evidently restrained, and if the patient is asked to draw a deep breath he cries out with the pain. Expiration is frequently interrupted by an audible grunt. At first with the increased respiration there may be no sensation of distress. Later this may be present in a marked degree. Many factors combine to produce the shortness of breath—pain, toxemia, fever, anoxemia, acidosis possibly, and loss of function in a considerable area of the lung. There is more pulmonary work required and less lung to do it. Sometimes there appear to be nervous factors at work. That it does not depend upon the consolidation is shown by the fact that after the crisis, without any change in the lung, the respirations may drop to normal. *Cyanosis* of some degree is usually present and if severe it means a serious condition of anoxemia.

Cough.—This usually comes on with the pain, and at first is dry, hard, and without any expectoration. Later it becomes very characteristic—frequent, short, restrained, and associated with great pain in the side. In old persons, in drunkards, in terminal pneumonias, and sometimes in young children, there may be no cough. After the crisis the cough usually becomes much easier and the expectoration more easily expelled. The cough is sometimes persistent, continuous, and by far the most aggravated and distressing symptom of the disease. Paroxysms of coughing of great intensity after the crisis suggest a pleural exudate.

Sputum.—A brisk *hemoptysis* may be the initial symptom. At first the sputum may be mucoid, but usually after twenty-four hours it becomes blood-tinged, viscid, and very tenacious. At first quite red from the unchanged blood, it gradually becomes rusty or of an orange yellow. The tenacious viscidity of the sputum is remarkable; it often has to be wiped from the lips of the patient. When jaundice is present it may be green or yellow. In low types of the disease the sputum may be fluid and of a dark brown color, resembling prune juice. The amount is very variable, ranging from 100 to 300 cc. in the twenty-four hours. In 100 cases studied by Emerson, in 16 there was little or no sputum; in 32 it was typically rusty; in 33 blood-streaked; in 3 cases the sputum was very bloody. In children and old people there may be no sputum whatever. After the crisis the quantity is variable, abundant in some cases, absent in others. This does not seem to have any bearing on the rapidity of resolution.

Microscopically, the sputum consists of leukocytes, mucus corpuscles, red blood corpuscles in all stages of degeneration, and bronchial and alveolar epithelium. Hematoidin crystals are occasionally met with. The pneumococcus is usually present, and sometimes other organisms. Very interesting constituents are small cell moulds of the alveoli and fibrinous casts of the bronchioles; the latter may be plainly visible to the naked eye and sometimes may form good-sized dendritic casts. Chemically, the expectoration is particularly rich in calcium chloride.

PHYSICAL SIGNS.—*Inspection.*—The position of the patient is not constant.

He usually rests more comfortably on the affected side, or he is propped up with the spine curved toward it. Orthopnea is rare.

In a small lesion no difference may be noted between the sides; as a rule, movement is much less on the affected side, which may look larger. With involvement of a lower lobe, the apex on the same side may show greater movement. The compensatory increased movement on the sound side is sometimes very noticeable. The intercostal spaces are not usually obliterated. When the cardiac lappet of the left upper lobe is involved there may be a marked increase in the area of visible cardiac pulsation. Pulsation of the affected lung may cause a marked movement of the chest wall (Graves). Other points to be noticed are the frequency of respiration, the action of the accessory muscles, and the dilatation of the nostrils with each inspiration. Asynchronous contractions of the respiratory muscles occur in some cases. When fully developed the diaphragm and thoracic respiratory muscles contract alternately (Coleman). This is of grave significance.

Mensuration may show a definite increase in the volume of the side affected, rarely more, however, than 1 or 1½ cm.

Palpation.—The lack of expansion on the affected side is sometimes more readily perceived by touch than by sight. The pleural friction may be felt. The voice fremitus is greatly increased. It is to be noted that if the bronchi are filled with thick secretion, or if, in what is known as massive pneumonia, they are filled with fibrinous exudate, the tactile fremitus may be diminished. It is always well to ask the patient to cough before testing the fremitus.

Percussion.—In the stage of engorgement the note is higher pitched and may have a tympanitic quality. This can often be obtained over the lung tissue just above a consolidated area. L. A. Conner calls attention to a point which all observers must have noticed, that, when the patient is lying on his side, the percussion at the dependent base is "deeper and more resonant than that of the upper side," which by contrast may seem abnormal, and there may even be a faint tubular element added to the vesicular breathing on the compressed side. When the lung is hepatized, the percussion note is dull, the quality varying from a note which has a certain tympanitic quality to one of absolute flatness. There is not the wooden flatness of effusion and the sense of resistance is not so great. There are many different combinations of dulness and tympany. The student must not expect to find typical physical signs in all cases; they may show great variation. During resolution the tympanitic quality of the percussion note usually returns. For weeks or months after convalescence there may be a higher-pitched note on the affected side. Wintrich's change in the percussion note when the mouth is open may be present in pneumonia of the upper lobe. Occasionally there is an almost metallic quality over the consolidated area, and when this exists with a pronounced amphoric quality in the breathing the presence of a cavity may be suggested. In deep-seated pneumonias there may be no change in the percussion note for several days. *Tympany* is common in lobar pneumonia. It occurs with beginning and clearing consolidation, with consolidation over a bronchus, where air-containing lung is over consolidated lung and sometimes over an area close to consolidation.

Auscultation.—Quiet, suppressed breathing in the affected part is often a marked feature in the early stage, and is always suggestive. Only in a few cases is the breathing harsh or puerile. Very early there is heard at the end of inspiration the fine crepitant râle, a series of minute cracklings heard close to the ear, and perhaps not audible until a full breath is drawn. Sometimes this may be a fine pleural crepitus, as Leaming maintained; it is usually believed to be produced in the air-cells and finer bronchi by the separation of the sticky exudate. In the stage of red hepatization and when dulness is well defined, the respiration is tubular. It is heard first with expiration (a point noted by James Jackson, Jr.), and is soft and of low pitch. Gradually it becomes more intense, and finally presents an intensity unknown in any other pulmonary affection—of high pitch, perfectly dry, and of equal length with inspiration and expiration. It is simply the propagation of the laryngeal and tracheal sounds through the bronchi and consolidated lung tissue. The permeability of the bronchi is essential to its production. Tubular breathing is absent in the rare cases of massive pneumonia in which the larger bronchi are completely filled with exudation. When resolution begins mucous râles of all sizes can be heard. At first they are small and have been called the *redux-crepitus.* The voice-sounds and the expiratory grunt are transmitted through the consolidated lung with great intensity and may have a curious nasal quality. There are cases in which the consolidation is deeply seated—so-called central pneumonia, in which the physical signs are slight, yet the cough, rusty expectoration, and general features make the diagnosis certain.

Circulatory Symptoms.—During the chill the *pulse* is small, but in the succeeding fever it becomes full and bounding. In cases of moderate severity it ranges from 100 to 120. It is not often dicrotic. In strong, healthy individuals and in children there may be no sign of failing pulse throughout the attack. With extensive consolidation the left ventricle may receive a diminished amount of blood and the pulse in consequence may be small. In the old and feeble it may be small and rapid from the outset. The pulse may be full, soft, very deceptive, and of no value whatever in prognosis from its character but an increased rate is always important.

Heart.—The *heart* sounds are usually loud and clear. During the intensity of the fever, particularly in children, murmurs are not uncommon both in the mitral and pulmonic areas. The second sound over the pulmonary artery is accentuated. Attention to this sign gives a valuable indication as to the condition of the lesser circulation. With distention of the right chambers and failure of the right ventricle to empty itself completely, the pulmonary second sound becomes much less distinct. When the right heart is engorged there may be an increase in the dulness to the right of the sternum. With circulatory failure diastole is greatly shortened and the sounds approach each other in tone (embryocardia). Disturbances of rhythm, especially extra systoles, occur in about 10 per cent of cases and disturbance of conduction in about the same number. Auricular fibrillation may occur, often for short periods and is not necessarily of serious omen.

There may be a sudden collapse of the circulation with a very feeble, rapid pulse and increasing cyanosis. This may happen on the third day. Even when these symptoms are very serious recovery may take place. In other instances without any special warning death may occur in robust, healthy men. Some of these cases are due to heart block. The soft, easily compressed pulse, the gray facies, cold hands and feet, clammy perspiration, and the progressive prostration tell of a toxic action on the circulation.

Blood Pressure.—During the first few days there is usually no change. The extent of involvement seems to have no effect upon the blood pressure. In the toxic cases the pressure may begin to fall early; a drop of 15-20 mm. Hg is perfectly safe, but a progressive fall indicates the need of stimulation. A sudden drop is rarely seen except just before death. The crisis has no effect on the blood pressure. The opinion commonly held, that when the blood pressure as expressed in millimeters of Hg does not fall below the pulse rate expressed

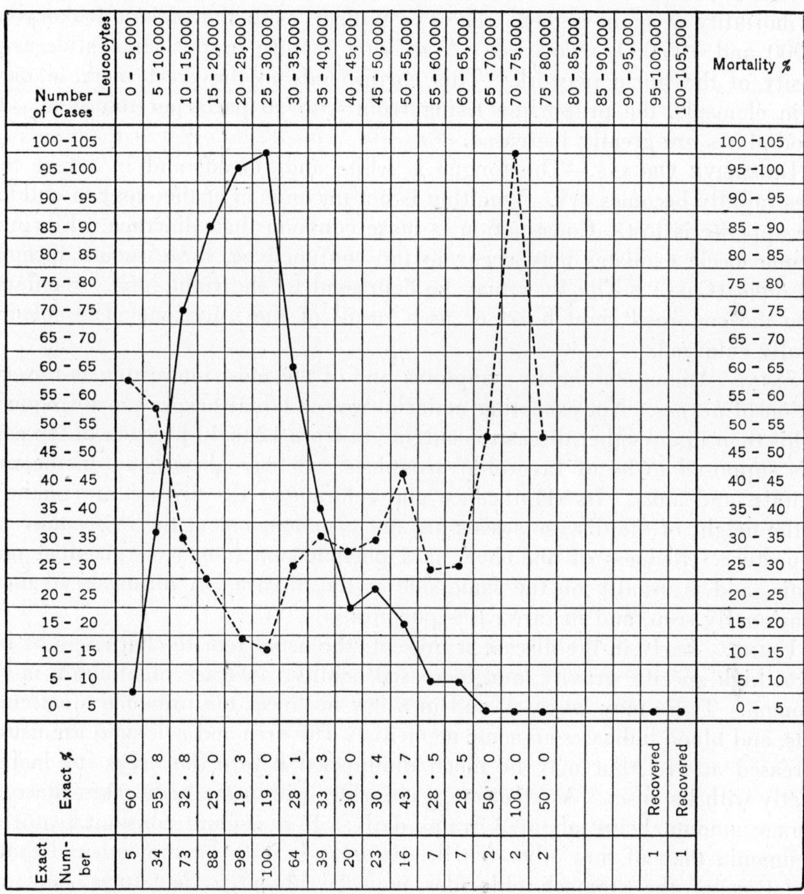

Chart III.—Blood Count in Pneumonia and Comparative Mortality. Continuous Line Represents Number of Cases of Pneumonia. Broken Line Represents Mortality Percentage of Same.

in beats per minute, the outlook is good, and *vice versa,* is by no means always correct.

Blood.—Pneumococci are present in the blood in about 30 per cent of all cases. Anemia is rare. A decrease in the red cells may occur at the time of the crisis. There is in most cases a leukocytosis, which appears early, persists, and disappears with the crisis. Absence of leukocytosis or leukopenia is an ominous sign. The leukocytes may number from 12,000 to 40,000 or even 100,000 per

c. mm. The fall in the leukocytes is often slower than the drop in the fever, particularly when resolution is delayed or complications are present. The annexed chart gives a study by Chatard of the leukocytes in 582 cases at the Johns Hopkins Hospital. More than half of the patients, about 350, had a leukocytosis between 15,000 and 35,000, and one-third (198) between 20,000 and 30,000. The broken line represents the mortality which is high when the leukocytes are below 10,000, but steadily decreases and is lowest when they are between 20,000 and 30,000. With the leukocytes between 30,000 and 60,000 the mortality is again higher. The two patients with the highest leukocytosis, 95,000 and 105,000, recovered. A striking feature in the blood-slide is the density of the fibrin network. This corresponds to the great increase in the fibrin elements, the proportion rising from 4 to 10 parts per thousand. The blood-plates are greatly increased.

Digestive Organs.—The tongue is white and furred, and in severe toxic cases rapidly becomes dry. Vomiting is not uncommon at the onset in children. The appetite is lost. Constipation is more common than diarrhea. Fibrinous, pneumococcic exudates may occur in the conjunctivae, nose, mouth, prepuce, and anus (Cary). The liver may be depressed by the right lung, or enlarged from the engorged right heart or as a result of the infection. The spleen is usually enlarged.

Skin.—Among *cutaneous* symptoms one of the most interesting is the association of *herpes*. Not excepting malaria, we see labial herpes more frequently in this than in any other disease, occurring in from 12 to 40 per cent of the cases. It is supposed to be of favorable prognosis. It may also occur on the nose, genitals, and anus. Its significance and relation to the disease are unknown. At the height of the disease sweats are not common, but at the crisis they may be profuse. Redness of one cheek is a phenomenon long recognized in pneumonia, and is usually on the same side as the disease. A diffuse erythema is occasionally seen, and in rare cases purpura.

Urine.—Early in the disease it presents the usual febrile characters of high color, high specific gravity, and increased acidity. A trace of albumin is very common. There may be casts, and in a few instances the presence of albumin, casts, and blood indicates an acute nephritis. The urea and uric acid are usually increased at first, but may be much diminished before the crisis, to increase greatly with its onset. A retention of chlorides within the body takes place, the average amount being about 2 grams daily. It is a more constant feature of pneumonia than of any other febrile disease. It is to be remembered that in dilatation of the stomach chlorides may be absent. Hematuria is a rare complication.

Cerebral Symptoms.—Headache is common. In children vomiting or convulsions may occur at the outset. Apart from meningitis, considered separately, one may group the cases with marked cerebral features into:

First, the so-called cerebral pneumonias of children, in which the disease sets in with a convulsion, and there are high fever, headache, delirium, great irritability, muscular tremor, and perhaps retraction of the head and neck with Kernig's sign and an extensor plantar reflex. The diagnosis of meningitis may be made, and the local affection overlooked.

Secondly, the cases with maniacal symptoms. These may occur at the very outset, with no suspicion that the disease is pneumonia.

Thirdly, alcoholic cases with the features of delirium tremens. It should be an invariable rule, even if fever be not present, to examine the lungs in a case of *mania à potu.*

Fourthly, cases with toxic features, rather resembling those of uremia. Without a chill and without a cough or pain in the side, a patient may have fever, a little shortness of breath, and then gradually grow dull mentally, and within three days be in profound toxemia with low, muttering delirium.

It is stated that apex pneumonia is more often accompanied with severe delirium. Occasionally the cerebral symptoms occur after the crisis. Mental disturbance may persist during and after convalescence, and in a few instances delusional insanity follows, the outlook in which is favorable.

Hemiplegia may be due to thrombosis, embolism, abscess or edema. Withington called attention to a form associated with *encephalitis.* It may be transient and recovery complete. Transient *aphasia,* with or without hemiplegia, may occur and there are cases in which no gross lesions have been found, so that it has been suggested that it is due to edema or to a relative ischemia. Inequality of the pupils is not uncommon but has no special significance.

The Crisis.—After the fever has persisted for from five to nine or ten days there may be an abrupt drop, known as the *crisis,* which is a most characteristic feature. The day of the crisis is variable. It is very uncommon before the third day, and rare after the twelfth. We have seen it as early as the third day. From the time of Hippocrates it has been thought to be more frequent on the uneven days, particularly the fifth and seventh; the latter has the largest number of cases (Musser and Norris). A *precritical rise* of a degree or two may occur. In one case the temperature rose from 105° to nearly 107°, and then in a few hours fell to normal. The usual time is from five to twelve hours, but often in an hour there may occur a fall of six or eight degrees. The temperature may be subnormal after the crisis, as low as 96° or 97°. Usually there is an abundant sweat, and the patient sinks into a comfortable sleep. The day after the crisis there may be a slight postcritical rise. A *pseudocrisis* is not very uncommon, in which on the fifth or sixth day the temperature drops from 104° or 105° to 100° or to normal and then rises again. When the fall takes place gradually within twenty-four hours it is called a protracted crisis. If the fever persists beyond the twelfth day, the fall is likely to be by *lysis.* Occasionally in debilitated individuals the temperature drops rapidly just before death; more frequently there is an antemortem elevation. In delayed resolution the fever may persist for six or eight weeks. The crisis appears to represent the stage of active immunity to the toxin of the pneumococcus. The fever, dyspnea and general symptoms disappear when the immunity reaches a certain stage. With the fall in the fever the respirations become reduced almost to normal, the pulse slows, and the patient passes from a state of hazard and distress to one of safety and comfort, and yet, so far as the physical examination indicates, there is no special change in the condition of the lung. Crisis occurs most often in Type I and least often in Type III infections.

Complications.—Compared with typhoid fever, pneumonia has but few complications and still fewer sequelae. The most important are:

Pleurisy is an inevitable event when the inflammation reaches the surface of the lung, and can scarcely be termed a complication. But there are cases in which the pleuritic features take the first place. The exudation may be serofibrinous with copious effusion, differing from that of an ordinary acute pleurisy in the greater richness of the fibrin, which may form thick, tenacious, curdy layers. An extensive *serous effusion* may form very rapidly and cause extreme dyspnea which may be regarded as due to the pneumonia. The error is serious as removal of the fluid may be necessary to save the patient's life. Pneumonia on one side with extensive pleurisy on the other is sometimes a puzzling complication to diagnose, and an aspirating needle may be required to settle the question.

Empyema is a common complication occurring in 2.2 per cent of 13,550 cases (Musser and Norris) and in 3.6 per cent of the Johns Hopkins Hospital series. The pneumococcus is usually present; in some the streptococcus, in which case the prognosis is not so good. Some cases may be due to extension from or rupture of a small lung abscess. It can not be emphasized too strongly that empyema in lobar pneumonia is almost always a *complication—not a sequel.* It is present before the crisis or lysis in the great majority of cases. The temperature does not reach normal as a rule and if it does, only for a short time, rarely more than one day. The persistence of fever, perhaps with sweating, the persistence of leukocytosis and continued cough, especially in paroxysms, are suspicious. The effusion is usually small at first and must be looked for. There may be no great change in the percussion note but the resistance is increased. The breath sounds become distant or are absent, and the voice sounds have a nasal quality different from that over consolidated lung. Râles may be heard despite the presence of fluid. The signs are often found over a limited area and a difference in signs over areas not more than an inch or two apart is very suggestive. Such a condition may be closely simulated by a layer of fibrinous exudate or a thickened pleura. Exploratory aspiration may settle the question and should not be delayed. There are obscure cases in which the pus has been found only at operation, as the collection may be very small or interlobar. The X-rays rarely give aid in the *early* diagnosis. The clinician has no right to expect the roentgenologist to make the diagnosis for him.

Abscess.—This occurred in 4 of the 100 autopsies. Usually the lung breaks down in limited areas and the abscesses are not large, but they may fuse and involve a considerable portion of a lobe. The condition is recognized by the sputum, which is usually abundant and contains pus and elastic tissue, sometimes cholesterin crystals and hematoidin crystals. The cough is often paroxysmal and of great severity; usually the fever is remittent, or in protracted cases intermittent. When a case is seen for the first time it may be difficult to determine whether it is one of abscess of the lung or empyema which has perforated the lung. The X-ray study is of aid in the diagnosis.

Gangrene.—This is most common in old debilitated persons. It was present in 3 of the 100 autopsies. It very often occurs with abscess. The gangrene is associated with the growth of saprophytic bacteria on a soil made favorable by the presence of the pneumococcus or the streptococcus. Gangrene is rendered very evident by the horribly fetid odor of the expectoration and its characteristic features. In some instances gangrene is found postmortem when clinically there has been no evidence of its existence.

Edema of the Lungs.—This is always serious and it is important to recognize the early signs. Increased dyspnea and cyanosis, more marked signs of circulatory disturbance and increase in the heart rate suggest it. On auscultation showers of fine to medium râles with a mucous character and later coarser bubbling râles are heard. Portions of lung which are not involved by pneumonia show them more markedly than over the consolidated area.

Pericarditis, one of the most serious complications, was present in 35 of 658 patients in the Hopkins Hospital (Chatard). It is often terminal and overlooked. It may not be possible to hear the friction rub owing to the noisy respiration. The mortality is very high; 21 of the 35 patients died. It was most frequently associated with pneumonia of the right lung. In only 3 cases was the amount of fluid above 500 cc. Pleurisy is an almost constant accompaniment, not infrequently being purulent.

Endocarditis.—The valves on the left side are more commonly attacked, and particularly if the seat of arteriosclerosis or old valvular disease. There may be no symptoms even in very severe cases. It may, however, be suspected in cases (1) in which the fever is protracted and irregular; (2) when signs of septic mischief arise, such as chills and sweats; (3) when embolic phenomena appear. The frequent complication of meningitis with the endocarditis of pneumonia gives prominence to the cerebral symptoms in these cases. The physical signs may be deceptive and in some cases no cardiac murmurs have been heard. In others the occurrence under observation of a loud, rough murmur, particularly if diastolic, is extremely suggestive.

Antemortem clotting in the heart, upon which the old writers laid great stress, is very rare. *Thrombosis* in the peripheral veins is also uncommon. In 35 of 44 cases which were fully reported, the thrombosis occurred during convalescence. It is almost always in the femoral veins. A rare complication is *embolism* of one of the larger arteries. In one instance embolism of the femoral artery at the height of pneumonia necessitated amputation at the thigh. The patient recovered.

Meningitis varies at different times and in different regions. The Montreal series is rather exceptional, as 8 per cent of the fatal cases had this complication. In twenty years at the Johns Hopkins Hospital there were 25 cases of pneumococcus meningitis, in 18 of which pneumonia was present. Endocarditis was present in 7 of the 18 cases. The percentage of meningitis in the pneumonia cases was 2.4, which is lower than the figures of Musser and Norris of 3.5 per cent in 4,883 autopsies. It usually comes on at the height of the fever, and in the majority of the cases is not recognized unless the base is involved, which is not common. Occurring later in the disease, it is more easily disagnosed. The prognosis is bad and few instances of recovery are on record. *Peripheral neuritis* is a rare complication.

Gastric complications are rare. Fussell drew attention to the occurrence of acute *dilatation of the stomach.* Persistent vomiting, sudden abdominal distention and collapse are the most common features. A croupous gastritis has been mentioned. The *croupous colitis* may induce severe diarrhea. It is by no means uncommon to have early *pain,* in the region of the umbilicus or in the right iliac fossa, and a suspicion of appendicitis is aroused; indeed, a catarrhal form of this disease may occur with pneumonia. In other instances so localized may the pain be in the region of the pancreas, associated with meteorism and high fever, that the diagnosis of acute pancreatitis is made. *Peritonitis* is a rare complication, sometimes in the upper peritoneum, due to direct extension through the diaphragm. It is usually in the severer cases and not easy to recognize. In one case in which there was a friction along the costal border, which was thought to indicate a peritonitis, it was communicated from the diaphragmatic pleura. *Meteorism* is common and usually occurs with severe toxemia. In some cases it may be due to a defect in the action of the diaphragm, in others to an acute septic catarrh of the bowels, or to a toxic paresis of the walls, occasionally to peritonitis. *Jaundice* occurs with curious irregularity in different years. It seems to be more common among the negro patients. It sets in early and is rarely very intense but there are cases in which it assumes a serious form. The mode of production is not well ascertained. It may be due to hemolysis which occurs in the pulmonary exudate. It is not unfavorable; in fact it often seems that jaundiced patients do well.

Parotitis occasionally occurs, commonly in association with endocarditis. In children, middle-ear disease is not an infrequent complication.

Nephritis does not often follow pneumonia.

Arthritis occurred in 5 of 658 cases at the Johns Hopkins Hospital (Howard). It may precede the onset, and the pneumonia, possibly with endocarditis and pleurisy, may occur as a complication. In other instances at the height of the pneumonia one or two joints become involved or after the crisis has occurred pain and swelling may come on in the joints. It is a serious complication as recovery is often slow and a stiff joint may result.

Relapse.—There are cases in which the fever subsides, and after the temperature has been normal for a day or two a rise occurs and fever may persist for ten days or two weeks. Though this might be termed a relapse, it is more correct to regard it as an anomalous course or delayed resolution. When it does occur, the attack is usually abortive and mild. In one patient the crisis occurred on the seventh day, and after a normal temperature for thirteen days he was discharged. That night he had a shaking chill, followed by fever with reappearance of the pneumonia. In a second case the crisis occurred on the third day, and there was recurrence of pneumonia on the thirteenth day.

Recurrence is more common in pneumonia than in any other acute disease. Rush gives an instance in which there were 28 attacks. Other authorities narrate cases of 8, 10, and even more attacks.

Convalescence is usually rapid, and sequelae are rare. After the crisis, sudden death has occurred when the patient has got up too soon.

Delayed Resolution.—The lung is restored to its normal state by the liquefaction and absorption of the exudate. There are cases in which resolution takes place rapidly without any increase in (or, indeed, without any) expectoration; on the other hand, during resolution it is not uncommon to find in the sputum little plugs of fibrin and leukocytes which have been loosened from the air cells and expelled by coughing. A variable time is required for resolution. Sometimes within a week or ten days the dulness is greatly diminished, the breath sounds become clear, and, so far as physical signs are any guide, the lung seems perfectly restored. Delayed resolution occurs in from 3 to 4 per cent of cases. Of 40 cases at the Johns Hopkins Hospital, 33 were males and 7 females; 23 of the patients were negroes, a very high incidence. The lower lobe is most frequently involved, 37 cases in this series, usually the right one and as a rule only one lobe. The duration was to the fourth week 5 cases, fifth week 10 cases, sixth week 4 cases, ninth week 3 cases, tenth, eleventh and twelfth weeks each one case. In one patient the left lung remained solid for eleven weeks and then cleared perfectly. Syphilis is possibly a contributing factor in some cases.

Clinically, there are several groups of cases: First, those in which the crisis occurs naturally, the temperature falls and remains normal; but the local features persist—well-marked flatness with tubular breathing and râles. Resolution may occur very slowly and gradually, taking several weeks. In a second group the temperature falls by lysis, and with the persistence of the local signs there is slight fever, sometimes sweats and rapid pulse. The condition may persist for three or four weeks and during all this time there may be little or no sputum. The practitioner naturally dreads tuberculosis. In a third group the crisis occurs or the fever falls by lysis; but consolidation persists, and there may be intense bronchial breathing, with few or no râles, or the fever may recur and the patient may die exhausted.

Termination in Fibrosis.—The exudate may organize and the alveolar walls thicken with the gradual production of a chronic interstitial or fibroid "pneumonia." In a patient aged 58, dead on the thirty-second day from the initial chill, the right lung was solid and the cut surface grayish in color with a smooth, translucent appearance. This is most frequent as a sequence of delayed resolution in debilitated subjects. Milne found 10 instances of organization of the exudate among 150 fatal cases. The shortest duration in the series was twenty-three days.

Ordinary lobar pneumonia never terminates in tuberculosis. The instances of caseous pneumonia and softening which have followed an acute pneumonic process have been tuberculous from the outset.

Clinical Varieties.—Local variations are responsible for some deviations from the usual type. *Apex pneumonia* is said to be more often associated with adynamic features and marked cerebral symptoms. The expectoration and cough may be slight. *Migratory* or *creeping pneumonia* successively involves one lobe after the other. *Double pneumonia* has no peculiarities other than the greater danger connected with it. *Massive pneumonia* is a rare form, in which not alone the air cells but the bronchi of an entire lobe or even of a lung are filled with the fibrinous exudate. The auscultatory signs are absent; there is neither fremitus nor tubular breathing, and on percussion the lung is absolutely flat. It closely resembles pleurisy with effusion. The moulds of the bronchi may be expectorated in violent fits of coughing. *Streptococcus infection* occasionally follows the pneumonia and may not occur until some days after it is over. The onset is usually sudden, the course is rapid and the outlook very serious.

Central Pneumonia.—The inflammation may be deep-seated at the root of the lung or centrally placed in a lobe, and for several days the diagnosis may be in doubt. It may not be until the third or fourth day that a pleural friction is detected, or that dulness or blowing breathing and râles are recognized. Sometimes the diagnosis has to be made from the general features or by an X-ray study.

Pneumonia in Infants.—It is sometimes seen in the newborn. In infants it often sets in with a convulsion. The apex of the lung seems more frequently involved than in adults, and the cerebral symptoms are more marked. The torpor and coma, particularly if they follow convulsions, and the preliminary stage of excitement, may lead to the diagnosis of meninigitis. Pneumonic sputum is rarely seen in children.

Pneumonia in the Aged.—The disease may be latent and set in without a chill; the cough and expectoration are slight, the physical signs ill-defined and changeable, and the constitutional symptoms out of all proportion to the extent of the local lesion.

Pneumonia in Alcoholic Subjects.—The onset is insidious, the symptoms masked, the fever slight, and the clinical picture usually that of delirium tremens. The thermometer alone may indicate the presence of an acute disease. Often the local condition is overlooked, as the patient makes no complaint, and there may be very little dyspnea, no cough, and no sputum.

Terminal Pneumonia.—The wards and the postmortem room show a very striking contrast in their pneumonia statistics, owing to the occurrence of terminal pneumonia. Patients with arteriosclerosis, heart disease, nephritis, etc., are not infrequently carried off by a pneumonia which may give few or no signs. There may be slight fever, with increase in the respirations, but the patient is near the end and perhaps not in a condition in which a thorough physical examination can be made. There is often no leukocytosis. In diabetic patients the disease may run a rapid course, and end in abscess or gangrene.

Secondary Pneumonia.—This is met with chiefly in the fevers as diphtheria, typhoid fever, typhus and the plague. Anatomically, it rarely presents the typical form of red or gray hepatization. The surface is smoother, not so dry, and it is often a pseudolobar condition, a consolidation caused by closely set areas of lobular involvement. It shows in many instances a more cellular, less fibrinous exudate, which may also infiltrate the alveolar walls. The pneumococcus may be the dominant organism; but Friedländer's bacillus, streptococci, staphylococci, the influenza and colon bacillus have been found. The pneumonia due to the Friedländer bacillus is usually very severe and fatal in a few days. However, there are cases (perhaps in which it is a secondary invader) in which it is chronic with signs suggestive of delayed resolution.

The symptoms of the secondary pneumonias often lack the striking definiteness of primary lobar pneumonia. The pulmonary features may be latent or masked altogether. There may be no cough and only a slight increase in the number of respirations. The lower lobe of one lung is most commonly involved, and the physical signs are obscure and rarely amount to more than impaired resonance, feeble breathing, and a few crackling râles.

Epidemic Pneumonia is, as a rule, more fatal, and often displays minor complications which vary in different outbreaks.

Larval Pneumonia.—Mild, abortive types are seen, particularly in institutions when pneumonia is prevailing extensively. A patient may have the initial symptoms of the disease, a slight chill, moderate fever, a few indefinite local signs, and herpes. The whole process may only last for two or three days; some authors recognize even a one-day pneumonia.

Asthenic, Toxic or Typhoid Pneumonia.—The toxic features dominate; the local lesions may be slight and subjective phenomena absent. The nervous symptoms usually predominate. Very frequently there is jaundice. Gastrointestinal symptoms may be present, particularly diarrhea and meteorism. In such a case, seen about the end of the first week, it may be difficult to say whether the condition is asthenic pneumonia or typhoid fever with early localization in the lung. The Widal reaction and blood cultures are important aids. Possibly, too, there is a mixed infection, and a streptococcus may be in large part responsible for the toxic features.

Association of Pneumonia with Other Diseases.—*With Malaria.*—A malarial pneumonia is described. Pneumonia is not uncommon in the tropics and may attack the subjects of malaria. The prognosis is bad in the estivo-autumnal infections. Is there a special form of pneumonia due to the malarial parasite? There are cases reported by Craig and others in which in an acute malarial infection the features suggest pneumonia at the onset, but parasites are found in the blood, and under the use of quinine the fever drops rapidly and the pneumonia signs clear. In some instances a chill in the course of a pneumonia is associated with malarial infection.

Pneumonia and Tuberculosis.—Subjects of chronic pulmonary tuberculosis may die of acute lobar pneumonia, but often it is surprising how well they do even with a severe attack. A point to be specially borne in mind is the fact that acute tuberculous pneumonia may set in with all the features and physical signs of lobar pneumonia.

POSTOPERATION PNEUMONIA.—Before the days of anesthesia, pneumonia was a well-recognized cause of death after surgical injuries and operations. Norman Cheevers, in an early number of the Guy's Hospital Reports, called attention to it as a frequent cause of death after surgical procedures. In the statistics collected by Homans the mortality due to lung complications after laparotomies ranged from 0.56 to 12.5 per cent. Operations on the stomach are peculiarly liable to be followed by pneumonia. The cases may be divided into three groups: (1) Inhalation or anesthesia pneumonia which may be lobar or bronchopneumonia. (2) Hypostatic pneumonia due to enfeebled circulation. (3) Embolic cases with sudden onset which may simulate pneumonia very closely. It must be emphasized that some cases regarded as postoperative or posttraumatic pneumonia are really instances of *collapse* of the lung as shown by W. Pasteur. Careful examination and an X-ray study should give the diagnosis.

ANESTHESIA PNEUMONIA.—The anesthetic may have a damaging influence on the bronchial and alveolar epithelium, but a more important influence is the aspiration of mucus and saliva into the air passages during the anesthesia. Thorough disinfection of the mouth and throat before operation is a useful preventive measure. The pneumonia may be lobar or patchy and as a rule the signs are well marked within the first two days after operation. *Collapse* may involve both lower lobes or one lobe or one lung, and may simulate pneumonia very closely. When unilateral, the mediastinum and heart are drawn towards the affected side. It may come on with great suddenness and prove fatal. Pneumonia may follow collapse of the lung.

Prognosis.—Pneumonia is one of the most fatal of all acute diseases. In America the mortality appears to be increasing. It varies greatly in different years.

The statistics of the Johns Hopkins Hospital from 1889 to 1905 were analyzed by Chatard. There were 658 cases with 200 deaths, a mortality of 30.4 per cent. Excluding 35 cases of terminal pneumonia, the percentage is 26.4 The death-rate among 245 negroes was very little above that of the whites. Greenwood and Candy in a study of the pneumonia statistics at the London

Hospital from 1854-1903, a total of 5,097 cases, conclude that the mortality has not appreciably changed in this period. In comparing the figures from various hospitals, there is an extraordinary uniformity in the mortality rate. Between the ages of 21-30 the mortality is about 20 per cent; between the ages of 31-40, 30 per cent; and then after each decade it rises, until above the age of 60 more than one-half die.

Age.—As Sturges remarks, the old are likely to die, the young to recover. Under one year it is more fatal than between two and five. Of 50 cases under 10 years of age, 4 died; of 119 cases under 20, 16 died (Chatard). Above sixty the death rate is very high, amounting to 60 or 80 per cent; 33 of 44 cases in our series. From the reports of its fatality in some places, one may say that to die of pneumonia is almost the natural end of old people.

Previous habits of life and the condition of health at the time of the attack are important factors. In a series of fatal cases one is very much impressed by the number in which the organs show signs of degeneration. This applies particularly to the kidneys. In 25 of the 100 autopsies at the Montreal General Hospital the kidneys showed extensive interstitial changes. Individuals debilitated from sickness or poor food, hard drinkers, and that class of hospital patients, composed of robust laborers between the ages of forty-five and sixty, whose organs show signs of wear and tear, and who have used alcohol to excess fall an easy prey. *Obesity* as a rule adds to the danger. Patients with valvular cardiac disease and good compensation as a rule do surprisingly well. In every attack there is always an element of uncertainty.

Bacteremia.—The presence of pneumococci in the blood adds to the gravity of the prognosis. In the Bellevue Hospital series the mortality was almost seven times greater in the patients with bacteremia than in those with negative blood cultures (Cecil). A high degree of blood infection as shown by cultures is a bad omen.

Certain *complications* and *terminations* are particularly serious. The meningitis of pneumonia is almost always fatal. Endocarditis is extremely grave, more so than pericarditis. Much stress has been laid upon the factor of *leukocytosis* as an element in the prognosis. A very slight or complete absence of leukocytosis or leukopenia is very unfavorable.

Toxemia is an important prognostic feature, to which in a majority of the cases the degree of pyrexia and the extent of consolidation are entirely subsidiary. Marked nervous symptoms, dilatation of the heart, a pulse rate persistently above 125, low blood pressure, marked cyanosis, edema of the lungs, meteorism, scanty secretion of urine and severe exhaustion are unfavorable signs. With multilobar involvement the mortality is about double that when only one lobe is involved.

The determination of the *type* of organism is of assistance. The death-rate in Types I and II is from 25 to 30 per cent; in Type III about 40 per cent, and in Type IV 15 per cent. These figures may show considerable variation in different years.

Death is rarely due to direct interference with the function of respiration, even in double pneumonia. Sometimes it is caused by the extensive involvement with edema of the other parts of the lung, usually with progressive weakness of the right heart. But death is most frequently due to the action of the toxin on the circulation, with circulatory failure.

Diagnosis.—No disease is more readily recognized in a large majority of the cases. The general characters, the sputum, and the physical signs combine to make one of the clearest of clinical pictures. The ordinary lobar pneumonia of adults is rarely overlooked. Errors are particularly likely to occur in the intercurrent pneumonias, in those complicating chronic affections, and in the disease in children, the aged, and drunkards. Acute pneumonic tuberculosis is easily confounded with pneumonia. Pleurisy with effusion is not often mistaken except in children.

In nephritis, chronic heart disease, cancer, etc., an acute pneumonia often ends the scene, and is frequently overlooked. In these cases the temperature is perhaps the best index, and should, more particularly if cough occurs, lead to a careful examination of the lungs. The absence of expectoration and of pulmonary symptoms may make the diagnosis very difficult.

In children there are two special sources of error: the disease may be entirely masked by the cerebral symptoms and the case mistaken for one of *meningitis*. It is remarkable how few indications there may be of pulmonary trouble. Lumbar puncture is of great aid in such cases. The other condition is *pleurisy with effusion*, which may have deceptive physical signs. The breathing may be intensely tubular and tactile fremitus may be present. The exploratory needle is sometimes required to decide the question. In the old and debilitated a knowledge that the onset of pneumonia is insidious, and that the symptoms are ill-defined and latent, should put the practitioner on his guard and make him very careful in the examination of the lungs in doubtful cases. In chronic alcoholism the cerebral symptoms may completely mask the local process. The disease may assume the form of violent mania, but more commonly the symptoms are those of delirium tremens. In any case, rapid pulse, rapid respiration, and fever are symptoms which should invariably excite suspicion of pneumonia. The acute signs due to a *foreign body* in a bronchus are often mistaken for those of pneumonia.

Pneumonia is rarely confounded with pulmonary tuberculosis, but to differentiate *acute pneumonic tuberculosis* is often difficult. The attack may set in with a chill. It may be impossible to determine which condition is present until softening occurs and elastic tissue and tubercle bacilli appear in the sputum. With *typhoid fever*, pneumonia may be confounded. There are instances of pneumonia with the local signs well marked in which the patient rapidly sinks into what is known as the typhoid state, with dry tongue, rapid pulse, and diarrhea. The diagnosis from *bronchopneumonia* is discussed under that disease. *Infarct* of the lung should be considered in patients with cardiac disease. The sputum is usually more bloody and the signs in the lung not as marked. *Collapse* of the lung may suggest pneumonia but the marked displacement of the heart to the affected side is important evidence. The X-ray study is decisive. The occurrence of *abdominal pain* with involvement of a lower lobe may lead to a diagnosis of appendicitis, especially in children. A proper examination should prevent this error.

In addition an exact etiological diagnosis should be made as rapidly as possible. If due to the pneumococcus the type should be determined from the sputum if obtainable, otherwise by puncture of the lung or blood culture.

Prophylaxis.—We do not know in how many cases pneumonia is an auto-infection, the lowered resistance due to exposure or to alcohol, or a trauma furnishing conditions which favor the spread and growth of an organism already present. Individuals who have had pneumonia should be careful to keep the teeth in good condition, and the mouth and throat in as healthy a state as possible. Antiseptic mouth washes may be used.

The evidence suggests that there is value in vaccines as a preventive, but the immunity produced is of short duration. When done it should be regarded as an experiment and careful records kept.

We know practically nothing of the conditions under which the pneumococcus lives outside the body, or how it gains entrance in healthy individuals. Patients should be isolated more carefully than is the ordinary custom, especially in institutions. The sputum should be sterilized, and gauze or paper napkins used to receive it should be burned. Gauze should be held before the mouth of the patient during coughing.

Treatment.—Pneumonia is a self-limited disease and even under the most unfavorable circumstances it may terminate abruptly and naturally. So also, under the favoring circumstances of good nursing and care, the experience of many physicians in different lands has shown that pneumonia runs its course in a definite time, terminating sometimes on the third or fifth day, or continuing until the tenth or twelfth. It is an advantage to have the patient in a hospital as early in the course as is possible. Later in the course with a patient seriously ill, the danger of moving him should always be kept in mind. Good judgment is required in the decision.

General Management.—The same careful hygiene of the bed and sickroom should be carried out as in typhoid fever. Everything should be done to make the patient comfortable, save him exertion and secure sufficient sleep. Needless disturbance of the patient is to be avoided, for unnecessary examinations are tiring and may do harm. To secure sleep, the use of morphia hypodermically is the most efficient measure but common sense must be exercised as to abolish the cough reflex may be harmful. Whenever possible the patient should be in the open air if this adds to his comfort or improves his condition. It does both in the majority of cases. In cold weather he should have sufficient covering to keep him warm, but should not be overburdened by a heavy weight of clothes. A blanket and rubber sheet, under the mattress, which can be folded up over the bed prevent chilling from below. A hot-water bag should be kept at the feet. The patient is brought indoors when necessary for treatment. If the patient is indoors the room should be thoroughly ventilated. The clothing should be as light as possible; there is no advantage in a "pneumonia jacket." The patient should be carefully sponged with tepid water. This should be done with as little disturbance as possible. Special care should be taken to keep the mouth and nose clean. The giving of an alkali, such as potassium citrate (gr. xv, 1 gm. four times a day) is advisable. Alcohol should be given to chronic alcoholics.

Diet.—Plain water, a pleasant table water, or lemonade should be given freely. The water should be given at fixed intervals and by the bowel or subcutaneously if it is not taken by mouth. Tea and coffee are sometimes taken better than water. The food should be liquid and semisolid consisting of milk and its modifications, ice cream, broths, custard, milk toast, cereals and eggs. Carbohydrate, as milk sugar or dextrose, can be added to each feeding of milk, and as cane sugar to lemonade.

Bowels.—These can be kept open by simple laxatives, salines or enemata. Drastic purgation is not advisable. It is important to prevent *meteorism,* if possible, by care in the diet, giving water freely and preventing constipation. If present, measures for relief should be begun at once. Turpentine stupes, turpentine (℥ ss, 15 cc.) added to an enema, an asafetida enema and the use of the rectal tube, are helpful. Strychnine and pituitary extract hypodermically are also useful. If the stomach is distended a stomach tube should be passed.

Bleeding.—The reproach of Van Helmont, that "a bloody Moloch presides in the chairs of medicine," can not be brought against this generation. Before Louis' iconoclastic paper on bleeding in pneumonia it would have been regarded as almost criminal to treat a patient without venesection. We employ it more often late in the disease than early. To bleed at the onset in robust, healthy individuals in whom the disease sets in with great intensity and high fever is good practice. Late in the course marked dilatation of the right heart is the usual indication. The quantity removed must be decided by the effect; small amounts are often sufficient.

Specific Treatment.—The value of the antipneumococcic serum is established for Type I if begun in the first three days. The serum for Type II is less efficient but may be of value. The serum should be given intravenously as soon as possible in doses of 50-100 cc. diluted one half with freshly prepared salt solution. This is repeated twice or thrice daily, four or five doses usually being necessary. A rise in temperature indicates further dosage. Immune bodies are found in the blood after the first injection and remain if the treatment is continued. It is well to give 0.5 cc. of serum subcutaneously a few hours before the first intravenous injection to desensitize. The first injection should be given very slowly. There are polyvalent serums and if typing can not be done there is justification for their use. There is no proof that the use of vaccines is of value in treatment.

Pneumothorax.—This has been successful in some cases; it should only be used if the pneumonia is unilateral. It should be done by one who is experienced in pneumothorax treatment.

Hydrotherapy.—This—internal and external—is our principal means of combating toxemia and circulatory failure. Cold sponging is usually the best measure, done every three hours and with the least possible disturbance of the patient. A large flat ice bag may be kept to the side or back constantly, unless it causes distress. Probably the best effect of hydrotherapy is on the vasomotor and nervous systems.

Symptomatic Treatment.—*To Relieve Pain.*—The stitch in the side at onset, which is sometimes so agonizing, is best relieved by a hypodermic injection of morphia (gr. 1/4, 0.016 gm.). When the pain is less intense and diffuse a hot water bag or mustard poultice may be applied but the ice bag is usually more efficacious. When the disease is fairly established the pain is not, as a rule, distressing, except when the patient coughs, and for this codein (gr. 1/2, 0.03 gm.), heroin (gr. 1/12, 0.005 gm.), may be used or morphia hypodermically (gr. 1/6 0.01 gm.), according to the patient's needs.

To Combat Toxemia.—Abundance of water should be given to promote the flow of urine, and fluid given by bowel or subcutaneously if necessary but care must be taken not to give too large an amount subcutaneously if the circulation is failing; 500 cc. is usually sufficient. In toxic patients the administration of glucose solution intravenously (250-300 cc. of a 10 per cent solution) two or three times a day may be helpful. External hydrotherapy should be kept up actively.

An all-important indication is *to support the circulation.* Hydrotherapy and keeping the patient out of doors are of great value for this. Mechanical disturbance, as from meteorism, should be prevented if possible. Drugs should not be given in any routine way and not until they are required. Strychnine is useful (also for its effects on the respiratory centre). It should be given hypodermically and in full doses (gr. $\frac{1}{20}$, 0.003 gm., and even gr. $\frac{1}{10}$, 0.006 gm., for short periods) every two or three hours. Atropine is useful, especially when there is excessive secretion or pulmonary edema, and should be given in full doses hypodermically. In severe cases it is well to begin the use of digitalis early in the form of the tincture (♏ x, 0.6 cc.) three times a day. With signs of weakness of the circulation, intramuscular injections of one of the digitalis preparations are advisable. In severe conditions the use of strophanthin is often more efficient (gr. $\frac{1}{100}$, 0.0006 gm.) intramuscularly or intravenously. This may be repeated once in twelve or twenty-four hours. For severe circulatory failure caffeine (sodio-benzoate) gr. v. (0.3 gm.), or epinephrine solution (♏ xv, 1 cc.) may be given hypodermically. Pituitary extract (posterior lobe) has been warmly recommended. An injection of hot saline solution given in the bowel or saline subcutaneously is helpful.

Respiratory Tract.—The most comfortable position, avoidance of exertion, and abundance of fresh air are important aids in preventing dyspnea. Pain should be relieved as much as possible. Expectorant drugs are not indicated and often upset the stomach. When the cough is severe it is well to give sedatives, of which codein and heroin are the best. Morphia in small doses may be required but should be given only when necessary. For *edema* of the lungs digitalis or strophanthin should be given intramuscularly and atropine (gr. $\frac{1}{50}$, 0.0012 gm.) and caffeine hypodermically. Venesection is advisable if the right heart be dilated. The dosage of atropine should be governed by the degree of edema and the results. There should be no hesitation in giving large doses when required.

Oxygen.—The occurrence of cyanosis is an indication for its use. The oxygen chamber is rarely available. Tents and masks are useful if the patient is not disturbed by them. A nasal tube may be the only method possible; about 2 litres of oxygen per minute should be given.

Nervous System.—The patient with delirium should be constantly watched. An ice bag to the head and frequent sponges are useful. *Sleep* is important for every patient and the need for this is often forgotten. While such drugs as the bromides, chloral hydrate and barbital may be effectual, it is wiser, as a rule, to give morphia hypodermically in a sufficient dose (gr. $\frac{1}{4}$, 0.016 gm.) to secure rest and sleep.

Crisis.—As this approaches constant watch should be kept for signs of collapse. If sweating is profuse and the patient feeble, atropine (gr. $\frac{1}{50}$, 0.0013 gm.) should be given hypodermically with epinephrine and repeated as necessary.

TREATMENT OF COMPLICATIONS.—As empyema usually is a complication care should be taken to recognize it early. If present, aspiration should be done at once as by this some cases clear promptly. If aspiration is not effectual drainage is necessary and should be done early in cases due to the pneumococcus. In streptococcus cases delay is uually advisable, aspiration being done in the interval. The occasional serous effusion should be aspirated promptly. In a complicating pericarditis with a large effusion aspiration may be necessary. Delayed resolution is a difficult condition to treat. The use of the X-rays is perhaps the most effective treatment but tuberculosis should be excluded. Vaccine treatment has been useful in some cases.

CONVALESCENCE.—The diet should be increased as rapidly as possible, the patient kept out of doors and after an ordinary attack allowed up in about a week. If the heart has suffered rest should be more prolonged.

BRONCHOPNEUMONIA

(*Lobular Pneumonia, Capillary Bronchitis*)

Definition.—A bacterial infection of the finer bronchi and their related lobules. The process begins with inflammation of the bronchioles and smaller bronchi, a capillary bronchitis, which extends to the alveoli, and the whole lobule or a group of lobules becomes filled with exudate, cellular and hemorrhagic but distinctly less fibrinous than in lobar pneumonia.

Etiology.—Bronchopneumonia occurs either as a primary or as a secondary affection. The relative frequency in 443 cases is thus given by Holt: Primary, without previous bronchitis, 154; secondary to bronchitis of the larger tubes, 41; to measles, 89; to whooping cough, 66; to diphtheria, 47; to scarlet fever, 7; to influenza, 6; to varicella, 2; to erysipelas, 2; and to acute ileocolitis, 19. The proportion of primary to secondary forms as shown in this list is probably too low.

PRIMARY ACUTE BRONCHOPNEUMONIA attacks those of any age and is not uncommon in adults. The etiological factors are very much those of lobar pneumonia, and probably the pneumococcus is often associated with it.

SECONDARY BRONCHOPNEUMONIA occurs: As a sequence of the infectious fevers—measles, diphtheria, whooping cough, scarlet fever, etc. In children it forms the most serious complications of these diseases, and in reality causes more deaths than are due directly to the fevers. Following, as it does, the infectious diseases which principally affect children, a large majority of cases occur during early life and it is most fatal during the first two years of life. The number of cases increases or decreases with the prevalence of measles, scarlet fever, and diphtheria. It is most prevalent in the winter and spring months. In the febrile affections of adults bronchopneumonia is not very common. Thus in typhoid fever it is not so frequent as lobar pneumonia, though isolated areas of consolidation at the bases are by no means rare in protracted cases. In old people it may follow debilitating causes of any sort, and is met with in chronic nephritis and various acute and chronic maladies.

In the second division are embraced the cases of so-called *aspiration* or *deglutition* pneumonia. Whenever the sensitiveness of the larynx is benumbed, as in the coma of apoplexy or uremia, minute particles of food or drink may enter the trachea, and, reaching the smaller tubes, excite an intense inflammation. Cases occur after operations about the mouth and nose, after tracheotomy, and in cancer of the larynx and esophagus. In some cases suppuration or gangrene supervenes. The ether pneumonia may be lobular in type.

An aspiration bronchopneumonia may follow hemoptysis, the aspiration of material from a bronchiectatic cavity, and occasionally the material from an empyema which has ruptured into the lung. A common and fatal form of bronchopneumonia is that excited by the tubercle bacillus.

Terminal Bronchopneumonia. This is common in patients with chronic disease of many kinds.

Among general predisposing causes may be mentioned *age.* It is prone to attack infants, and a majority of cases of pneumonia in children under five years of age are of this form. At the opposite extreme of life it is common with influenza and with various debilitating circumstances and chronic diseases. In children, rickets and diarrhea are marked predisposing causes, and bronchopneumonia is a frequent postmortem lesion in infants' homes and foundling asylums. The disease prevails most extensively among the poorer classes.

Morbid Anatomy.—On the pleural surfaces, particularly toward the base, are seen depressed bluish or blue-brown areas of collapse, between which the lung tissue is of a lighter color. Here and there are projecting portions over which the pleura may be slightly turbid or granular. The lung is fuller and firmer than normal, and, though in great part crepitant, solid, nodular bodies can be felt in places throughout the substance. The dark depressed areas may be isolated or a large section of one lobe may be in the condition of collapse. Inflation by a blow-pipe in the bronchus will distend a great majority of these collapsed areas. On section, the general surface has a dark reddish color and usually drips blood. Projecting above the level of the section are lighter red or reddish-gray areas representing the patches of bronchopneumonia. These may be isolated and separated from each other by tracts of uninflamed tissue or they may be in groups; or the greater part of a lobe may be involved. Study of a favorable section of an isolated patch shows: (*a*) A dilated central bronchiole full of tenacious purulent mucus. A fortunate section parallel to the long axis may show a racemose arrangement—the alveolar passages full of mucopus. (*b*) Surrounding the bronchus for from 3 to 5 mm. or even more, an area of grayish-red consolidation, usually elevated above the surface and firm to the touch. It may present a perfectly smooth surface, though in some instances it is distinctly granular. In a late stage small grayish-white points may be seen, which on pressure may be squeezed out as purulent droplets. A section in the axis of the lobule may present a somewhat grape-like arrangement, the stalks and stems representing the bronchioles and alveolar passages filled with a yellowish or grayish-white pus, while surrounding them is a reddish-brown hepatized tissue. (*c*) In the immediate neighborhood of this peribronchial inflammation the tissue is dark in color, smooth, airless, at a lower level than the hepatized portion, and differs distinctly in color and appearance from the other portions of the lung.

There are three groups of cases: (1) Those in which the bronchitis and bronchiolitis are most marked, and in which there may be no definite consolidation, and yet on microscopic examination many of the alveolar passages and adjacent air-cells appear filled with inflammatory products. (2) The disseminated bronchopneumonia, in which there are scattered areas of peribronchial hepatization with patches of collapse, while a considerable proportion of the lobe is still crepitant. This is by far the most common condition. (3) The pseudolobar form, in which the greater portion of the lobe is consolidated, but not uniformly, for intervening strands of dark congested lung tissue separate the groups of hepatized lobules.

Microscopically, the centre of the bronchus is seen filled with a plug of exudation, consisting of leukocytes and swollen epithelium. Section in the long axis may show irregular dilatations of the tube. The bronchial wall is swollen and infiltrated with cells. The air cells next the bronchus are mostly densely filled, while toward the periphery the alveolar exudation becomes less. The contents of the air cells are made up of leukocytes and swollen epithelial cells in varying proportions. Red corpuscles are not often present and a fibrin network is rarely seen, though it may be present in some alveoli. In the swollen walls are seen distended capillaries and numerous leukocytes. The *interstitial* inflammation is the special feature of bronchopneumonia.

The histological changes in the aspiration or deglutition bronchopneumonia differ from the ordinary post-febrile form in a more intense infiltration of the air cells with leukocytes, producing suppuration and foci of softening; even gangrene may be present.

Bacteriology.—The organisms most commonly found are the pneumococcus, *Streptococcus pyogenes* (alone or with the pneumococcus), *Staphylococcus aureus et albus,* Friedländer's bacillus, and the influenza bacillus. The Klebs-Loeffler bacillus is not infrequent in the secondary lesions of diphtheria. Except the pneumococcus these organisms are rarely found in pure cultures. In the lobular type the streptococcus is the most constant organism, in the pseudolobar the pneumococcus. Mixed infections are almost the rule in bronchopneumonia.

Terminations of Bronchopneumonia.—(*a*) In *resolution,* which when it once begins goes on more rapidly than in fibrinous pneumonia. Bronchopneumonia of the apices, in a child, persisting for three or more weeks, particularly if it follow measles or diphtheria, is often tuberculous. In these instances, when resolution is supposed to be delayed, caseation has in reality taken place. (*b*) In *suppuration,* which is rarely seen apart from the aspiration and deglutition forms, in which it is common. (*c*) In *gangrene,* which occurs under the same conditions. (*d*) In *fibroid changes*—a rare termination in the simple, a common sequence of the tuberculous, disease. When due to Friedländer's bacillus the consolidation may resolve very slowly, almost be chronic, and simulate pulmonary tuberculosis.

Symptoms.—The *primary* form sets in abruptly with a chill or a convulsion. The patient has not had a previous illness, but there may have been slight exposure. The temperature rises rapidly and is more constant; the physical signs are more local and there is not the widespread diffuse catarrh of the smaller tubes. Many cases are mistaken for lobar pneumonia. In others the pulmonary features are in the background or are overlooked in the intensity of the general or cerebral symptoms. The termination is often by crisis, and the recovery is prompt. The mortality of this form is slight. It is important to recognize the frequency of these primary cases and their resemblance to lobar pneumonia. The primary form is not uncommon in adults and as a rule the attack is not severe.

The *secondary* form begins usually as a bronchitis of the smaller tubes. Much confusion has arisen from the description of capillary bronchitis as a separate affection, whereas it is only a part, though a primary and important one, of bronchopneumonia. It may be said that if in convalescence from measles or whooping cough a child has an accession of fever with cough, rapid pulse, and rapid breathing, and if, on auscultation, fine râles are heard at the bases, or widely spread throughout the lungs, even though neither consolidation nor blowing breathing can be detected, the diagnosis of bronchopneumonia may safely be made. The onset is rarely sudden or with a distinct chill; but after a day or so of indisposition the child has fever and begins to cough and be short of breath. The fever is variable; a range of from 102° to 104° is common. The skin is very dry and hot. The cough is hard, distressing, and may be painful. Dyspnea gradually becomes a prominent feature. Expiration may be jerky and grunting. The respirations may rise as high as 60 or even 80 per minute. Within the first forty-eight hours the percussion resonance is not impaired; the note, indeed, may be very full at the anterior borders of the lungs. Percussion yields varying notes; tympany may be adjacent to dulness which depends on areas of consolidation or collapse near the surface. On auscultation, many râles are heard, chiefly the fine subcrepitant variety, with sibilant rhonchi. There may be no signs indicating that the parenchyma of the lung is involved, but even at this early stage, within forty-eight hours of the onset of pulmonary symptoms, scattered nodules of lobular hepatization may be found. *Collapse* of small areas of lung tissue is probably common and explains some of the sudden changes in signs over a given area. The dyspnea is constant and progressive and cyanosis is marked in severe cases. The face becomes a little suffused and the finger-tips bluish. The patient has an anxious expression and gradually enters upon the most distressing stage of asphyxia. At first the urgency of the symptoms is marked, but soon the influence of the toxins is seen and there are no longer strenuous efforts to breathe. The cough subsides, and, with a gradual increase in lividity and a drowsy restlessness, the right ventricle becomes more and more distended, the bronchial râles become more liquid as the tubes fill with mucus, and death follows. These are symptoms of a severe case of bronchopneumonia, or what the older writers called *suffocative catarrh.*

The PHYSICAL SIGNS may at first be those of capillary bronchitis, as indicated by the absence of dulness and the presence of fine subcrepitant and whistling râles. In many cases death takes place before any definite pneumonic signs are detected. When these exist they are much more frequent at the bases, where there may be areas of impaired resonance or of positive dulness. When numerous foci involve the greater part of a lobe the breathing may become tubular, but in the scattered patches of ordinary bronchopneumonia, following the fevers, the breathing is more commonly harsh than blowing. In grave cases there is retraction of the lower sternum and of the lower costal cartilages during inspiration, pointing to deficient lung expansion. The duration is usually longer than in lobar pneumonia or in the primary form. The termination is by lysis and convalescence is prolonged. There is a group in which an area of consolidation at the base may persist for some time, weeks or months.

Complications are not common. Empyema may occur, sometimes of small extent and the area may be walled off, making diagnosis difficult. Abscess and gangrene occur most often in the aspiration cases and in debilitated persons. Endocarditis, pericarditis, meningitis, otitis media, etc., are occasional complications. Of *sequels* the most important is fibrosis which may be local. Associated with or due to it are some cases of bronchiectasis.

Diagnosis.—The clinical picture is so variable that no exact rules can be given. In some cases the diagnosis is made from the symptoms and general condition rather than from the physical signs. The most frequent error is to miss a bronchopneumonia rather than to confuse it with some other disease. A *suspicion* of bronchopneumonia is usually justified. In the primary form there is rarely much difficulty in recognizing pneumonia but the distinction from the lobar form may not be easy. Bronchopneumonia is bilateral; even with large areas of consolidation this rarely involves the whole of a lobe; it tends to involve the lower lobes, and its physical signs are rarely so definite. The consolidation of bronchopneumonia may be variable from day to day (probably due to varying grades of collapse) and is usually patchy. The breath sounds show change if small areas are carefully observed with comparison of the adjacent lung, and the whispered voice may be unusually clear and nasal in quality. In the secondary form, the increase in fever with cough, the rise in the respiration rate, cyanosis, toxemia and signs usually most marked in the lower lobes, suggest the diagnosis.

For the student the distinction from *acute bronchitis* perhaps gives the greatest difficulty. Bronchitis alone is not a serious disease, the temperature is not high, dyspnea is slight or absent, there is rarely cyanosis, and the only sign is the occurrence of medium or coarse râles. The presence of fine crackling râles, especially in the lower lobes, should always suggest pneumonia. A severe "bronchitis" with marked general features is usually bronchopneumonia. If the student remembers that the areas involved vary from multiple minute "dots" to consolidation of a lobe, with every gradation between, the variation in the physical signs will cause less difficulty. In children the signs caused by a foreign body, especially a nut, in a bronchus may be mistaken for those of bronchopneumonia.

In many instances the decision whether a bronchopneumonia is simple or *tuberculous* cannot be made, as the onset and physical signs may be identical. There are cases of bronchopneumonia which time alone enables us to distinguish from tuberculosis. The existence of extensive disease at the apices or central regions is suggestive and signs of softening may be detected.

Terminal Bronchopneumonia.—Fever, or an increase if it is already present, dyspnea, cyanosis and increasing toxemia are the general features. The signs in the lungs may not be distinctive especially if myocardial failure is already present.

Some forms show special features, as the bronchopneumonia of *influenza.* In that due to the hemolytic streptococcus the features are severe with marked toxemia, dyspnea and cyanosis, bloody sputum and a remarkable frequency of empyema which may come on very rapidly. The picture is that of a severe septic infection. In the form due to *staphylococci* there are chills, a remittent fever curve, thick purulent sputum containing many of the organisms and severe toxemia. Abscess of the lung is fairly common. The mortality is high.

Cerebral symptoms may mask the true nature of the disease, as in lobar pneumonia, and lead to the diagnosis of *meningitis.* Lumbar puncture or autopsy may be necessary to determine whether the child had tuberculous meningitis or a cerebral complication of an acute pulmonary affection.

Prognosis.—In the *primary* form the outlook is good. In children enfeebled by constitutional disease and prolonged fevers bronchopneumonia is terribly fatal, but in cases with whooping cough or after measles recovery may take place in the most desperate cases. It is in this disease that the truth of the old maxim is shown—"Never despair of a sick child." The death rate in children under five has been variously estimated at from 30 to 50 per cent. After diphtheria and measles thin, wiry children seem to stand bronchopneumonia much better than fat, flabby ones. In adults the aspiration or deglutition pneumonia is very fatal.

Prophylaxis.—Much can be done to reduce the probability of attack after febrile affections. Thus, in the convalescence from measles and whooping-cough, it is very important that the child should not be exposed to cold, particularly at night, when the temperature of the room naturally falls. The use of light flannel "combinations" obviates this nocturnal chill, which is an important factor in the pulmonary affections of young children. Catarrhal troubles of the nose and throat should be carefully attended to, and during fevers the mouth should be kept clean with an antiseptic solution. For old persons in bed with infections frequent change of position is advisable.

Treatment.—The frequency and the seriousness of bronchopneumonia render it a disease which taxes to the utmost the resources of the practitioner. There is no acute pulmonary affection over which he at times so greatly despairs. On the other hand, there is not one in which he will be more gratified in saving patients who have seemed past all succor. The general measures are much as in lobar pneumonia. The patient should be in the open air if a trial shows that he is more comfortable than inside; if indoors, the windows should be open with the patient protected from drafts. Some patients are relieved by a moist atmosphere. In cases due to the pneumococcus Type I, serum may be given as in lobar pneumonia.

Diet.—As much food as possible should be given. Milk and its modifications, ice cream, eggs, broths, cocoa, and gruels are suitable. Water should be given freely by mouth and if this is not possible by the bowel or subcutaneously. The *bowels* should be opened by castor oil or calomel and care taken to secure a daily movement by simple laxatives or enema. Severe purgation should be avoided.

Hydrotherapy.—This may be given by various methods to be chosen for each patient, depending on the condition and results. Sponges may be given to any patient. Packs are useful, hot if there is much restlessness or cold if the temperature is high, or baths may be given to children for short periods, using water at 95° F. and gradually reducing to 75° or 80° F. Compresses, made out of linen covered by flannel or of flannel alone, wrung out of water 60° to 70°, are often useful. They should not be covered by oiled silk. A mustard bath is of value for children, especially early in the attack. Hydrotherapy is especially indicated for patients with high fever, delirium or stupor, severe toxemia, or circulatory failure.

Local Applications.—Poultices have gone out of fashion but are sometimes of value. They should be light and are best kept in place by being slipped in pockets in a flannel jacket so that the poultice can be replaced without disturbing the patient. The use of dry cups is often advised; they should be applied frequently. The ice bag should be used if it gives comfort.

Medicinal.—The indications must be carefully studied and drugs which may disturb the stomach given with care. If cough is distressing the use of the compound tincture of benzoin in an inhalation should be tried. The expectorant drugs may aid and of these ammonium chloride (gr. ii to v, 0.13 to 0.3 gm.) and the wine of ipecacuanha (♏ x to xx, 0.6 to 1.3 cc.) are the most useful. To these a sedative, such as paregoric (ʒ i, 4 cc.), codein (gr. ¼, 0.016 gm.) or heroin (gr. 1-20, 0.0032 gm.) should be added if the cough is very distressing. Strychnine hypodermically in the proper dose for the age is an aid to the respiratory centre. For circulatory failure the treatment is the same as described under lobar pneumonia. Inhalations of oxygen are advisable if they give relief to the dyspnea and lessen cyanosis.

In old persons early stimulation is usually advisable and every effort should be made to persuade them to take nourishment. Cold applications must be used with caution and the use of heat is generally better. At all ages frequent change in position is advisable and in young children this may be done by taking them out of bed and holding them in the arms.

OTHER PNEUMOCOCCIC INFECTIONS

The organism causes a number of affections other than pulmonary:

Acute Septicemia.—Without any recognized local lesion there may be a general infection with the pneumococcus. The features are those of an acute general infection and death may result in a short time. The diagnosis can only be made by blood culture. If due to Type I or II, the serum should be administered as in lobar pneumonia.

Local Affections.—The local affections caused by the pneumococcus are numerous and described under the appropriate sections. In the *mouth*, erosions, gingivitis and glossitis; in the *pharynx*, inflammation and tonsillitis; in the *ear*, acute and chronic suppuration; in the accessory sinuses, of which it is a common habitant, inflammation and suppuration; it is a common cause of *meningitis;* in the *bronchi* it has been found associated with acute and chronic bronchitis, and bronchiectasis; in the *lungs*, in addition to pneumonia, it may cause acute edema and is associated with tuberculosis and many chronic affections. It has been found in acute *pleurisy* and it is one of the common causes of *empyema;* acute arthritis, primary and secondary forms; acute peritonitis, particularly in children; appendicitis; endocarditis; pyelitis and local abscesses in various parts may be caused by it.

CEREBROSPINAL FEVER

Definition.—An infectious disease, occurring sporadically and in epidemics, caused by the *meningococcus*, characterized by inflammation of the cerebrospinal meninges, a general infection in some cases, and a clinical course of great irregularity. It is also designated meningococcus meningitis, spotted fever and epidemic cerebrospinal meningitis.

History.—Vieusseux first described a small outbreak in Geneva in 1805. In 1806 L. Danielson and E. Mann (Medical and Agricultural Register, Boston) gave an account of "a singular and very mortal disease which lately made its appearance in Medfield, Mass." The Massachusetts Medical Society, in 1809, appointed James Jackson, Thomas Welch, and J. C. Warren to investigate it. Elisha North's book (1811) gives a full account of the early epidemics. Stillé's monograph (1867) and the elaborate section in vol. i of Joseph Jones' works contain details of the later American outbreaks. In his Geographical Pathology, Hirsch divides the outbreaks into four periods: From 1805 to 1830, when the disease was most prevalent throughout the United States; a second period, from 1837 to 1850, when the disease prevailed extensively in France, and there were a few outbreaks in the United States; a third period, from 1854 to 1874, when there were outbreaks in Europe and several extensive epidemics in America. During the Civil War there were comparatively few cases. In the fourth period, from 1875 to the present, the disease has broken out in a great many regions. In the United States, during 1898-1899, it prevailed in mild form in 27 states and since 1899 there have been extensive outbreaks. In New York in 1904-'05 there were were 6,755 cases and 3,455 deaths. In Glasgow in 1907 there were nearly 1,000 cases with 595 deaths (Chalmers). There were 1,974 deaths in England and Wales in 1915, the average for the five years before being 153, and 1,440 deaths in 1931. In the winter of 1914-'15 the disease was carried by Canadian troops to England. It broke out in many home camps and, spreading to the civil population, for the first time the disease prevailed widely in England.

Etiology.—Cerebrospinal fever occurs in epidemic and in sporadic forms. The *epidemics* are localized and are rarely very widespread. Only in the tropics have there been extensive killing pandemics. As a rule, country districts have been more afflicted than cities. Mining districts and seaports have suffered severely. The outbreaks have occurred most frequently in the winter and spring. The concentration of individuals, as of troops in barracks, is a special factor; recruits and young soldiers are specially liable. In civil life children and young adults are most susceptible. Overexertion, depressing mental and bodily surroundings, and the misery and crowding of the tenement houses in cities are predisposing causes. The disease is not highly infectious. It is very rare to have more than one or two cases in a house, and in a city epidemic the distribution of the cases is very irregular. The organism enters and leaves the body by the nasopharyngeal mucous membrane, and hence infection may be by contact or by coughing and sneezing. Meningitis *carriers* play an important rôle in transmitting the disease. They are found also when the disease is not epidemic.

Sporadic Cerebrospinal Fever.—The disease lingers indefinitely after an outbreak, and cases occur in all large cities. The posterior basic meningitis of Gee and Barlow has been shown to be due to the meningococcus.

Bacteriology.—In 1877 Weichselbaum described the *meningococcus.* In the tissues the organism is almost constantly within the polynuclear leukocytes. Some hold that there are four fixed types, and perhaps others, distinguishable from one another by immune reactions. Types I and II are said to be more likely to involve the meninges and III and IV to cause septicemia and metastases. The mortality at different stages of epidemics suggests a marked difference in the susceptibility of the hosts or in the virulence of the organism. It has not been possible to identify any one strain with a high mortality. The type of organism in the cerebrospinal fluid is the same as in the nasopharynx and apparently if one variety infects the mucous membrane it is not likely that another will be superimposed on it. The use of agglutination tests has been of great value in identifying the organism. The presence of the organism in the nasopharynx both in patients and in healthy contacts (carriers) is an important point. The meningococcus may be in the blood without meningitis resulting (meningococcus septicemia, which may be chronic). The blood infection is probably present in many cases before meningitis occurs.

Morbid Anatomy.—In malignant cases there may be no characteristic changes, the brain and spinal cord showing only extreme congestion, which was the lesion described by Vieusseux. In a majority of the acutely fatal cases death occurs within the first week. There is intense injection of the pia-arachnoid. The exudate is usually fibrinopurulent, most marked at the base of the brain, where the meninges may be greatly thickened and plastered over with it. On the cortex there may be much lymph along the larger fissures and in the sulci; sometimes the entire cortex is covered with a thick, purulent exudate. It deserves to be recorded that Danielson and Mann made five autopsies and were the first to describe "a fluid resembling pus between the dura and pia mater." The cord is always involved with the brain. The exudate is more abundant on the posterior surface, and involves, as a rule, the dorsal and lumbar regions more than the cervical portion.

In the more chronic cases there is general thickening of the meninges and scattered yellow patches mark where the exudate has been. The ventricles in the acute cases are dilated and contain a turbid fluid, or in the posterior cornua pure pus. In the chronic cases the dilatation may be very great. The brain substance is usually a little softer than normal and has a pinkish tinge; foci of hemorrhage and of encephalitis may be found. The cranial nerves are usually involved, particularly the second, fifth, seventh, and eighth. The spinal nerve roots are also found imbedded in the exudate.

Microscopically, the exudate consists largely of polynuclear leukocytes closely packed in a fibrinous material. In some instances there are foci of purulent infiltration and hemorrhage. The neuroglia cells are swollen, with large, clear, and vesicular nuclei. The ganglion cells show less marked changes. Meningococci are found in variable numbers in the exudate, being more numerous in the brain than in the cord.

The sphenoidal sinuses may be full of pus and the surrounding bone inflamed. The frequency of catarrhal and other changes in the nasopharynx and sinuses suggests that the infection reaches the meninges through this route. Pneumonia, pleurisy, empyema, congestion with edema, intracranial abscess, endocarditis (sometimes without meningitis), pericarditis and peritonitis have occurred.

The *spleen* varies a good deal in size. *Acute nephritis* may be present. The intestines may show swelling of the follicles.

Symptoms.—Cases differ remarkably in character and many different forms are described. These are perhaps best grouped into three classes:

Malignant Form.—This fulminant type is found with variable frequency in epidemics and may occur sporadically. The onset is sudden, usually with violent chills, headache, somnolence, spasms in the muscles, great depression, moderate elevation of temperature, and feeble pulse, which may fall to 50 or 60. Usually a purpuric rash develops. In a Philadelphia case, a young girl, apparently quite well, died within twenty hours of this form. There are cases in which death has occurred within a shorter time.

Ordinary Form.—The stage of incubation is probably four or five days. The disease usually sets in suddenly. There may be premonitory symptoms: headache, pains in the back, and loss of appetite. More commonly, the onset is with headache, severe chill, and vomiting. The temperature rises to 101° or 102°. The pulse is full and strong. An early and important symptom is a painful stiffness of the muscles of the neck. The headache increases and there are photophobia and great sensitiveness to noises. Children become very irritable and restless. In severe cases the contraction of the muscles of the neck sets in early, the head is drawn back, and when the muscles of the back are also involved, there is orthotonos, which is more common than opisthotonos. The pains in the back and in the limbs may be very severe. The motor symptoms are most characteristic. Tremor of the muscles may be present with tonic or clonic spasms in the arms or legs. Rigidity of the muscles of the back or neck is very common, and the patient lies with the body stiff and the head drawn so far back that the occiput may be between the shoulder-blades. Except in early childhood convulsions are not common. Strabismus is a frequent and important sign. Spasm or paralysis of the muscles of the face may occur. Cases have been described with such general rigidity and stiffness that the body could be moved like a statue.

The *onset* may be with local infection of the nose and throat with coryza, pharyngitis and tonsillitis, or conjunctivitis may occur. If there is a period of septicemia before meningitis occurs, the patient is dull and disturbed by handling and complains of headache and general malaise with hyperesthesia. Arthralgia or arthritis may be present.

Of *sensory* symptoms, headache is the most dominant and persists from the outset. It is chiefly in the back of the head, and the pain extends into the neck and back. There may be great sensitiveness along the spine, and in many cases there is general hyperesthesia.

The *psychical* symptoms are pronounced. Delirium occurs at the onset, occasionally of a furious and maniacal kind. The patient may display marked erotic symptoms at the onset. The delirium gives place in a few days to stupor, which, as the effusion increases, deepens to coma.

The *temperature* is irregular and variable. Remissions occur frequently, and there is no uniform or typical curve. In some instances there is little or no fever, or the temperature may reach 105° or 106° or, before death, 108°. The pulse may be very rapid in children; in adults it is at first usually full and strong. In some cases it is remarkably slow. Sighing respirations and Cheyne-Stokes breathing occur in some instances. Unless there is pneumonia the respirations are not often increased in frequency.

The *cutaneous* features are important. *Herpes* occurs with a frequency almost equal to that in pneumonia. The *petechial rash,* which gave the name "spotted fever" to the disease, is very variable. It appears to have been more frequent in the epidemics in America than in Europe. The petechiae may be numerous and cover the entire skin. An erythema or dusky mottling may be present. In some instances there are rose-colored hyperemic spots like the typhoid rash. Urticaria or erythema nodosum, ecthyma, pemphigus, and in rare instances gangrene of the skin have been noted.

Leukocytosis is an early and constant feature, and ranges from 25,000 to 40,000. It persists even in the protracted cases. The meningococcus may be present in the blood and has been demonstrated in the leukocytes.

Vomiting may be a special feature at the onset; as a rule, it subsides but in some instances it persists and becomes a most serious and distressing symptom. Diarrhea is not common, the bowels being usually constipated. The abdomen is not tender. In the acute form the spleen is usually enlarged. The urine is sometimes albuminous and the quantity may be increased. Glycosuria has been noted, and hematuria in the malignant types.

The *duration* is extremely variable. Hirsch states that it may range from a few hours to several months. More than half of the deaths occur within the first five days. In favorable cases, after five or six days, improvement is indicated by a lessening of the spasm, reduction of the fever, and a return of the intelligence. A sudden fall in the temperature is of bad omen. Convalescence is extremely tedious, and may be interrupted by a relapse or recrudescence, complications and sequelae.

ANOMALOUS FORMS.—*Abortive Type.*—The attack sets in with great severity, but in a day or two the symptoms subside and convalescence is rapid. Strümpell distinguished between this abortive variety, which begins with such intensity, and the mild ambulant cases. In the mild cases, as distinguished from the abortive, the patients complain of headache, nausea, sensations of discomfort in the back and limbs, and stiffness in the neck. There is little or no fever, and only moderate vomiting. These cases could be recognized only during an epidemic and are easily regarded as influenza.

An *intermittent* type was recognized by von Ziemssen and Stillé. It is characterized by exacerbations of fever, which may recur daily or every second day, or follow a curve of an intermittent or remittent character. The pyrexia resembles that of pyemia rather than malaria. These are probably instances of the chronic septicemic form.

Chronic Form.—An attack may be protracted for from two to five or even six months, and may cause the most intense marasmus. It is characterized by a series of recurrences of the fever, and may present the most complex symptomatology. These patients show extreme emaciation, bed sores form, rigidity is marked, blindness and deafness are common, so that death comes as a welcome release. It is probable that in these protracted cases chronic hydrocephalus or abscess of the brain is present.

Posterior Basic Form.—This occurs in young children and the early stages may show nothing peculiar. Retraction of the head is marked. Vomiting is persistent and emaciation is rapid. The course is chronic, the child lying without motion for hours, often with marked arching of the back. Lumbar puncture may give the usual findings early, but later the meningococcus disappears and it may be impossible to obtain any fluid by lumbar puncture due to the closure of the foramen. Internal hydrocephalus is marked. Death usually results in some weeks.

Chronic Septicemic Form.—This may begin as an acute upper respiratory tract infection followed by headache, fever which may be very variable, skin rashes and arthralgia or arthritis. The fever may be intermittent with afebrile periods of several days. Chills may occur. The rashes appear after the first week; erythema, roseola, herpes and various forms of hemorrhagic rash may be present. Joint pains are common with or without arthritis. The spleen may be enlarged. A moderate leukocytosis is common. Pneumonia may occur and also endocarditis with features much like those of *Streptococcus viridans* cases (Gwyn, 1931). Meningitis may occur, usually late. The *diagnosis* may be difficult and depends on positive blood cultures and agglutination tests. The *duration* may be for months.

Complications.—Pleurisy, pericarditis, and parotitis are not uncommon. The last has been associated with thyroiditis and orchitis.

Pneumonia is described as frequent in certain outbreaks. Councilman suggested that it is not the true lobar form, but due to the meningococcus. This was found in eight of the Boston cases, and in one was so extensive that it could have been mistaken for ordinary lobar pneumonia. Cerebrospinal fever sometimes prevails extensively with ordinary pneumonia. *Arthritis* has been the most frequent complication in certain epidemics. Many joints are affected simultaneously with swelling, pain, and exudation, sometimes serous, sometimes purulent. This was first observed by James Jackson, Sr., in the epidemic which he described. *Spondylitis* occurs rarely. *Enteritis* is rare. *Epididymitis* is common in some epidemics.

Hydrocephalus occurs in two forms. In the *generalized* form there is an increased amount of cerebrospinal fluid present without obstruction of the foramina. The patient has headache, stupor of some degree, vomiting and dilated pupils. Lumbar puncture should be done repeatedly and marked results support the diagnosis. In *internal* hydrocephalus the foramina are closed and the symptoms are usually more marked than in the generalized form. In young children the fontanelles may bulge. Persistent vomiting, convulsions, increasing stupor, tremors, incontinence of urine and feces, and a negative lumbar puncture are suggestive. On percussion of the skull behind the junction of the frontal, parietal and temporal bones there is a tympanitic quality to the note (Macewen). In these cases puncture of the lateral ventricles is indicated. Mental feebleness and aphasia have been noted. Paralysis of individual cranial nerves or of the lower extremities may persist for some time. In some of these cases there may be peripheral neuritis. Headache may persist for months or years after an attack.

Special Senses.—*Eye.*—Optic neuritis may follow involvement of the nerve in the exudation at the base. The inflammation may extend directly into the eye along the pia-arachnoid of the optic nerve, causing purulent choroido-iritis or even keratitis. A neuritis of the fifth nerve may be followed by keratitis and purulent conjunctivitis.

Ear.—Deafness often occurs early and is bilateral and permanent. It may follow inflammation of the labyrinth. Otitis media, with mastoiditis, may occur from direct extension. Of 64 patients with meningitis who recovered, Moos found that 55 per cent were deaf. He suggests that the abortive form of the disease may be responsible for many cases of early acquired deafness. In children this not infrequently leads to deafmutism.

Nose.—Coryza is not infrequent early in the disease, probably associated with the presence of the organism on the nasal mucous membrane. In carriers the organism may persist for weeks; in some for months.

Diagnosis.—General Features.—The fever, headache, delirium, retraction of the neck, tremor, and rigidity of the muscles are most important signs.

In the meningitis of cerebrospinal fever the spinal symptoms are very much more marked than in other forms. One has to bear in mind that certain cases of typhoid fever and pneumonia closely simulate meningitis. Lumbar puncture is of great aid in recognizing the cases of *meningism.* Mild cases of meningitis are often mistaken for influenza.

Among the SPECIAL DIAGNOSTIC FEATURES may be mentioned:

Kernig's Sign.—When the thigh is flexed at right angles to the abdomen, the leg can be extended upon the thigh nearly in a straight line. If *meningeal irritation* be present, strong contractures of the flexors prevent the full extension of the leg on the thigh.

Brudzinski's Sign.—Flexing the head on the chest causes flexion of the legs at the hip and knee joints, and flexing one leg on the trunk produces the same movement in the other leg.

Lumbar Puncture.—This can usually be done without general anesthesia. The fluid runs, as a rule, with increased pressure which may reach 250-300 mm., the normal being about 120 mm., and when meningitis is present it is usually turbid, sometimes purulent, occasionally bloody. Meningitis may be present with a clear fluid. There is absence of sugar in the spinal fluid. The cytology is important. At an early stage there is an increase in the lymphocytes but usually when puncture is done the polymorphonuclear leukocytes are in great excess. In the late stages and in the posterior basic form the formula may be reversed. In the majority of cases extra- and intracellular meningococci are found in smears. Cultures should always be made. There is rarely great difficulty in distinguishing between the pneumococcus and the meningococcus. If there is any doubt as to the organism the agglutination test should be done or the meningococcus searched for in the nasopharynx. Meningitis due to the pyogenic organisms is usually easily recognized by a careful study of the cerebrospinal fluid. A thorough search will usually show tubercle bacilli in cases of tuberculous meningitis, cultures may be made, or a guinea-pig inoculated.

Prognosis.—The mortality before the use of serum was about 75 per cent; now it is about 25 per cent. In children below the age of two years the death-rate is high. A severe onset, marked coma or delirium, convulsions, high fever and hydrocephalus are of grave omen. The earlier the serum is given the better the outlook.

Prophylaxis.—The patient should be strictly isolated. Cultures from the nasopharynx of those in immediate contact should be taken and *carriers* should be isolated until proved to be free of infection. The use of chloramin (1 per cent) and zinc sulphate (1.5 per cent) solution has been helpful in some cases. These may be applied directly to the mucous membrane or the chloramin used in an oil spray after thorough cleansing with saline solution. A 1 per cent solution of peroxide of hydrogen or a solution of iodine (1 per cent) and glycerine may be used as a spray. Some carriers prove very resistant; in others the germs disappear after a few days. Hexamine, 30 to 50 grains daily, may be given. Protective vaccination was tried extensively in the last English epidemic.

Treatment.—The patient should be kept as quiet as possible, handled gently and all causes of irritation removed. Special attention should be given to the care of the skin, owing to the danger of bed sores. The hair should be clipped close and an ice-bag applied to the head. The diet should be liquid, as concentrated as possible, and given at short intervals. If swallowing is difficult the patient can be fed through a tube. Water should be given freely. The bowels are to be opened by a calomel and saline purge, and laxatives or enemata used later if necessary. For severe headache, general pains or vomiting, morphia hypodermically is usually best. The administration of hexamine, sixty grains (4 gm.) a day, is worthy of a trial.

Serum Therapy.—To Flexner we owe the specific serum which has reversed the mortality and recovery rates—one of the most striking advances in modern therapy. The serum should be given as early as possible and also in doubtful cases. It should be given intravenously in severe cases with signs of septicemia (rash or arthritis) in doses of 100 cc. every eight hours, first desensitizing by giving 1 cc. subcutaneously. As bacteremia, if it occurs, is early and transient, later intravenous administration is not necessary. Whenever the fluid obtained by lumbar puncture is purulent the serum should be given intraspinally, but repeated only if the meningococcus is found. Before giving the serum as much cerebrospinal fluid as possible should be withdrawn. If this has been large in amount (over 40 cc.) and in severe cases, 45 cc. of serum should be introduced slowly through the needle and by gravity. In ordinary cases 30 cc. of the serum should be given. In all cases with abnormal resistance to the injection of serum after an amount equal to the fluid removed has been injected, it is well to stop. If the symptoms are very severe or increasing, the injection should be repeated in twelve hours. Otherwise the usual dose (30 cc.) should be given daily for four days. It is well to continue to give serum until two successive spinal fluids are free of organisms. The return of sugar is of more value than the cell count. If meningococci are found after this, daily injections should be continued. Continuance or exacerbation of the symptoms demands further injections. If the condition remains stationary after four days' interval, the four daily injections should be given again and this repeated until the organisms disappear and the symptoms abate. Injection by cisternal puncture is sometimes more effectual. If there is a block the serum should be given into the ventricle, if the fontanelle is still open, or by cisternal puncture. An average dosage of serum is 400-600 cc. intravenously and 100 cc. intraspinally. The failure of the serum is sometimes due to its preparation from a different strain from the one infecting the patient and the need of a polyvalent serum is evident. In the chronic forms serum should be given if organisms are present and in the posterior basic form in the hope of benefit. In the chronic septicemic form, a polyvalent serum should be given intravenously.

Vaccine Therapy.—This may be useful in subacute and chronic cases, for conditions such as arthritis, in nervous system and eye complications and in cases not responding to the usual treatment. In acute cases in early stages it is of no value. The first dose may be 5 to 10 millions; every third day the dose is doubled until 600 millions are given. In young children about one-quarter of these doses may be given.

Hydrotherapy.—This may give relief to the symptoms. Hot baths or hot packs may be given for fifteen minutes every three hours.

Lumbar Puncture.—Done for injection of the serum it is often of value in itself. Severe headache and marked cerebral features are indications. As much fluid as possible should be removed and if under high pressure early repetition is advisable. Lumbar or cisternal puncture should be done early and frequently with signs of accumulation of fluid in the ventricles.

Complications.—Conditions due to extension to the cranial nerves are not influenced by treatment. *Otitis* requires early incision and *arthritis* rest, local applications and incision if suppuration occurs. With signs of generalized hydrocephalus, repeated drainage with injection of serum may be tried. With *internal hydrocephalus* the ventricle should be punctured, fluid withdrawn and serum injected. This is readily done through the anterior fontanelle, if it is still open, the ventricle being reached at a depth of about 3 cm. In older patients a flap of bone has to be removed. In the chronic cases every effort should be made to nourish the patient well and especial precautions taken against bed sores. For the pain and stiffness sometimes occurring on convalescence, hot baths and massage are useful.

INFLUENZA (LA GRIPPE)

Definition.—An acute infectious disease, which is pandemic, epidemic and endemic. The pandemics occur irregularly about three to a century and are characterized by a remarkable rapidity of extension and the large number attacked. Following the pandemic there are, as a rule, for several years endemic, epidemic, or sporadic outbreaks in different regions. Clinically, the disease has protean aspects, but a special tendency to attack the respiratory mucous membranes. The term "influenza" is often used loosely and applied to acute upper respiratory tract infections, acute febrile illnesses of various kinds and even to digestive tract disturbances. It is often used as a term to fit an illness without any proof of its correctness.

History.—Great pandemics have been recognized since the sixteenth century. There were four with their succeeding epidemics during the last century —1830-'33, 1836-'37, 1847-'48, and 1889-'90. The last seems to have begun, as many others, in the Far East. The pandemic of 1918 far exceeded any of its predecessors in its intensity. It is unusual to have the culmination in the summer months as was the case in some countries. A special feature was the high mortality in young adults, the very young and the old being comparatively immune. The accompanying pneumonia was very virulent. Pregnant women seemed particularly susceptible.

The duration of an epidemic in a locality is from six to eight weeks. With the exception, perhaps, of dengue, there is no disease which attacks indiscriminately so large a portion of the inhabitants, about 40 per cent, as a rule. Fortunately, the rate of mortality is low if all cases are included.

Etiology.—What relation has epidemic influenza to the ordinary cold or catarrhal fever (commonly called the *grippe*), which is constantly present in the community? Leichtenstern answered this question by making the following divisions: (*a*) Epidemic *influenza vera;* (*b*) endemic-epidemic *influenza vera,* which often occurs for several years in succession after a pandemic; (*c*) endemic *influenza nostras,* pseudo-influenza or catarrhal fever, commonly called the *grippe,* is caused by various organisms, alone or in combination.

Since the pandemic of 1889-'90 we have not been free from local outbreaks in some part of the world. In some places the disease seems to have been continually present. We do not know what determines the sudden increase in virulence which characterizes the pandemics. During the pandemics and the subsequent epidemic outbreaks the disease assumes a severity quite different from that of the inter-epidemic disease. The outstanding features are not the same in the pandemics; in that of 1889-'90 the nervous system was specially attacked, in 1918 the respiratory tract. The student must remember that descriptions of the severe epidemic cases do not apply to the usual endemic form.

The disease is highly infectious; it spreads with remarkable rapidity, which, however, is not greater than modern methods of conveyance. In the great pandemics some institutions escaped entirely. The outbreak of epidemics is independent of all seasonal and meteorological conditions. One attack does not necessarily protect from a subsequent one.

Bacteriology.—In 1892 Pfeiffer isolated a bacillus, a small nonmotile organism, which stains well in Loeffler's methylene blue, or in a dilute solution of carbolfuchsin in water. It has been found in the blood in a number of cases. There are various strains. The bacilli are present in enormous numbers in the nasal and bronchial secretions. They persist often after the severe symptoms have subsided. Is it the responsible organism or a secondary invader? The influenza bacillus (*Haemophilus influenzae*) has a close association with the disease, whether as a primary or secondary agent. There is considerable evidence that a virus is the cause. It may be that both organisms are required to produce the disease and are associated. A variety of other organisms may be found as secondary invaders. The influenza bacillus is actively pathogenic as seen in meningitis due to it. By using the virus, Smith, Andrewes and Laidlaw (1933) transmitted the disease to ferrets. Mice are also susceptible. Convalescent serum is protective against the virus. There seems to be a relation between the virus and canine distemper.

Pathology.—As death results usually from bronchopneumonia this is the usual finding at autopsy. The lesions vary with the predominating organism, thus in 1918 in the United States many cases of pneumonia were associated with the *Streptococcus haemolyticus*. When the influenza bacillus predominates there may be acute peribronchial infiltration with marked hemorrhage and edema. There is primarily injury of and desquamation of the epithelium with distention of the alveoli and rupture with hemorrhage into the air spaces. A hyaline membrane is formed with hyaline degeneration in the terminal bronchioles. There is a severe tracheitis and bronchitis, often hemorrhagic. Hemorrhage, edema and acute emphysema were marked features in the 1918 epidemic.

Symptoms.—The incubation period is from one to four days and has an average of two days. The onset is usually abrupt, with fever and its associated phenomena, headache, general pains, prostration and sometimes sore throat and an irritating cough. The manifestations are so many that it is best to describe them under various headings.

Respiratory Form.—The mucous membrane of the respiratory tract from the nose to the air cells of the lungs may be regarded as the seat of election of the infection. In the simple forms the disease sets in with coryza, and presents the features of an acute catarrhal fever, with perhaps rather more prostration and debility than is usual. In other cases after catarrhal symptoms tracheitis and bronchitis occur, the fever increases, there is delirium and much prostration with severe toxemia. The cough is usually very severe and persistent. Edema of the larynx was not uncommon in the 1918 epidemic. The graver respiratory conditions are bronchitis, pleurisy, and pneumonia. The *bronchitis* has really no special peculiarities but the sputum is supposed by many to be distinctive. Sometimes it is in extraordinary amounts, very thin, and containing purulent masses. Some regard sputum of a greenish-yellow color and in coin-like lumps as almost characteristic of influenza. In other cases there may be a bright or dark red, bloody sputum. The process tends to go on to bronchopneumonia.

Influenza *pneumonia* is one of the most serious manifestations, and may depend upon Pfeiffer's bacillus itself or a secondary infection. The true influenza pneumonia is lobular and probably never lobar. It was a special feature of the 1918 pandemic and responsible for most of the deaths. It may be present from the onset or develop after some days of general infection. The signs were often atypical for several days and suppression of breath sounds and fine crackling râles were the common early signs. Severe cough with bloody sputum or hemoptysis is common. Cyanosis is usually marked. There is a special tendency to the secretion of fluid so that the lungs are "water-logged." Resolution may be slow and signs persist for some time. Abscess or gangrene follows not infrequently. The toxemia is often extreme but the circulation shows remarkably little change in many cases. The blood pressure is usually low. *Subcutaneous emphysema* was common in the 1918 epidemic, usually over the neck and upper thorax but sometimes very widespread. In many of these cases there was extreme emphysema of the lungs. Probably the air escaped, after rupture of a surface bleb, into the mediastinum and then reached the tissues of the neck.

Influenza *pleurisy* is more rare, but cases of primary involvement of the pleura are reported. It is very apt to lead to empyema. Pulmonary tuberculosis is usually aggravated by an attack of influenza.

Nervous Form.—Without any catarrhal symptoms there are severe headache, pain in the back and joints, with profound prostration. Among the more serious complications may be mentioned meningitis and encephalitis, the latter leading to hemiplegia or monoplegia. Abscess of the brain has followed. Myelitis, with symptoms like acute Landry's paralysis, has occurred, and spastic paraplegia or a pseudotabes may follow an attack. In the 1918 epidemic there were cases of widespread hemorrhage into the spinal thecae. All forms of *neuritis* are not uncommon, and in some cases are characterized by marked disturbance of motion and sensation. Judging from the literature, almost every form of disease of the nervous system may follow influenza. Among the sequelae are depression, melancholia, and in some cases dementia.

Gastro-intestinal Form.—With the onset of the fever there may be nausea and vomiting, or the attack may set in with abdominal pain, profuse diarrhea, and collapse. In some epidemics jaundice has been a common symptom. In a considerable number of the cases there is enlargement of the spleen, depending chiefly upon the intensity of the attack.

Febrile Form.—The fever in influenza is very variable, but it is important to recognize that it may be the only manifestation of the disease. It is sometimes markedly remittent, with chills; or in rare cases there is a protracted, continued fever of several weeks' duration, which simulates typhoid closely. Sometimes the fever resembles that of a tertian malaria.

Blood.—*Leukopenia* is the rule, sometimes with an increase in the lymphocytes and decrease or absence of the eosinophiles. Complications may cause a leukocytosis but in the 1918 epidemic leukopenia often persisted through a bronchopneumonia.

Complications.—*Pericarditis* is apt to be latent. Of *endocarditis,* cases have been reported in which micro-organisms morphologically like influenza bacilli have been isolated from the vegetations. The malignant form may occur. *Myocarditis* may occur and has been a cause of sudden death. Functional disturbances are common, palpitation, bradycardia, tachycardia, and angina-like attacks. *Phlebitis* and *thrombosis* of various vessels have been described. Influenzal *meningitis* occurs most often in infancy and early childhood. It was found in 111 of 2,727 cases of meningitis (Neal *et al.*). It may be primary or secondary. The early features are fever, irritability and digestive disturbance. Leukocytosis is usually marked with a high proportion of polymorphonuclear cells. The spinal fluid is cloudy or purulent and the bacilli can be demonstrated in it by smear or culture. A positive culture is necessary for diagnosis. The bacilli from meningitis cases tend to belong to one group (Neal *et al.,* 1934). Bronchopneumonia is common and endocarditis occurs occasionally. The duration is often from 10 to 20 days, but may be 60 days. The mortality is high, over 90 per cent. *Peritonitis* is rare. *Cholelithiasis* may follow an attack.

Various renal affections have been noted, but *nephritis* was rare in the 1918 pandemic. *Orchitis* has been seen. *Herpes* is common. A diffuse erythema sometimes occurs, occasionally purpura. *Catarrhal conjunctivitis* is a frequent event. *Iritis,* and in rare instances *optic neuritis,* have been met with. *Acute otitis media* is a common complication and sinus infection is not rare. Severe and persistent *vertigo* may follow influenza, probably from involvement of the labyrinth. *Bronchiectasis* is a common sequel and the sputum may contain influenza bacilli in large numbers.

After epidemics it has been the fashion to date various chronic ailments from influenza. In many cases this is correct. It is astonishing how many people are crippled in health after an attack, particularly with bronchial, nervous or circulatory disturbances.

Diagnosis.—During a pandemic the cases offer but slight difficulty. The profoundness of the prostration, out of all proportion to the intensity of the disease, is one of the most characteristic features. The leukopenia is important. The diagnosis of gastro-intestinal influenza should be made with caution, except in pandemics. "Intestinal influenza" is usually a cover for ignorance. The more chronic pulmonary infections are sometimes mistaken for tuberculosis. The diagnosis of influenza is often made carelessly in various forms of coryza and respiratory tract infection.

Prognosis.—In epidemics the outlook depends largely on the existence of bronchopneumonia. At other times age is important; in the very young and the aged, especially if debilitated, the danger is greater.

Treatment.—Isolation should be practised when possible, and old people should be guarded against all possible sources of infection. There is no conclusive proof that vaccines have a preventive effect or that they are useful in treatment. The secretions, nasal and bronchial, should be thoroughly disinfected. In every case the disease should be regarded as serious, and the patient confined to bed at once and for some days after the fever has disappeared, as relapse is common. In this way serious complications may be avoided. From the outset the treatment should be supporting, and the patient carefully fed and well nursed. Water should be given freely. The bowels should be opened by a dose of calomel or a saline draught. At night 10 grains (0.65 gm.) of Dover's powder may be given. At the onset a warm bath is sometimes grateful in relieving the pain in the back and limbs, but great care should be taken to have the bed well warmed, and the patient should be given a hot drink after it. The patient should be sponged several times a day and an ice-bag applied to the head. If the fever is high or there is much discomfort, acetylsalicylic acid (gr. x, 0.6 gm.) may be given. The medicinal antipyretics should be used with caution, as profound prostration sometimes occurs after their employment. An alkali, such as potassium citrate (gr. xv, 1 gm.) four times a day, should be given. Too much stress should not be laid upon the mental features. Delirium may be marked even with slight fever. In the cases with cardiac weakness stimulants should be given freely, and during convalescence strychnia in full doses. In *meningitis* frequent lumbar puncture should be done. The serum should be used both intravenously and intraspinally.

The intense bronchitis, pneumonia, and other complications should receive their appropriate treatment. The convalescence requires careful management, and it may be weeks or months before the patient is restored to full health. A good nutritious diet, change of air, and pleasant surroundings are essential. The depression following this disease is one of its most unpleasant and obstinate features.

WHOOPING COUGH

Definition.—A specific affection due to the *B. pertussis* (*Haemophilus pertussis*), characterized by catarrh of the respiratory passages and a series of convulsive coughs which end in a long-drawn inspiration or "whoop."

History.—Ballonius, in his *Ephemerides*, describes the disease as it appeared in 1578. Glisson and Sydenham in the following century gave brief accounts. Willis (Pharmaceutice Rationalis, second part, 1674) gave a much better description and called it an "epidemical disorder."

Etiology.—The disease occurs in epidemic form, but sporadic cases appear in a community from time to time. It is directly infectious from person to person; but rooms, houses, school-rooms, and other localities may be infected by a sick child. It is, however, in this way less infectious than other diseases, and is probably most often conveyed by direct contact. Epidemics prevail for some months, usually during the winter and spring, and have a curious relation to other diseases, often preceding or following epidemics of measles, less frequently of scarlet fever.

Children from one to ten years of age are most liable to be attacked. Sucklings are not exempt, and severe attacks may occur in infants under six weeks. It is stated that girls are more subject to the disease than boys. Adults and old people are sometimes attacked, and in the aged it may be a very serious affection. It is most infectious in the catarrhal period. A natural immunity has been mentioned, but it must be remembered that a child may have the disease in a very mild form and as a rule, one attack protects. The disease is more than twice as fatal in the negro race as in others. There were 2,512 deaths from it in 1931 in England and Wales and 5,707 in the U. S. registration areas in 1930.

The *B. pertussis* is found in early stages of the disease (in 75 per cent during the catarrhal stage) but not often after the third week of the paroxysmal stage. In convalescents the deviation of complement reaction is present and the serum agglutinates the organism. The complement fixation test is not given early and so is not of great value in diagnosis. Apes have been successfully inoculated. Some regard a filterable virus as the causal agent.

Morbid Anatomy.—Whooping cough itself has no special pathological changes. In fatal cases pulmonary complications, particularly bronchopneumonia, are usually present. Collapse and compensatory emphysema, vesicular and interstitial, are found, and the tracheal and bronchial glands are enlarged. There is a constant lesion of the trachea with the presence of bacilli between the columnar cells.

Symptoms.—The incubation period is difficult to give exactly and extremes of four to twenty days are given; probably ten days is a fair average. Catarrhal and paroxysmal stages can be recognized. In the *catarrhal stage* the child has the symptoms of an ordinary cold, which may begin with slight fever, running at the nose, injection of the eyes, and a bronchial cough, usually dry, and sometimes with a spasmodic character. Trousseau called attention to the *incessant* character of the early cough. The fever is usually not high and the symptoms may be thought to be those of a simple cold. After a week or ten days, instead of subsiding, the cough becomes worse and more convulsive. Paroxysmal sneezing may take the place of the cough.

The *paroxysmal stage,* marked by the characteristic cough, dates from the first appearance of the "whoop." The fit begins with a series of from fifteen to twenty forcible short coughs of increasing intensity, between which no inspiratory effort is made. The child gets blue in the face, and then with a deep inspiration the air is drawn into the lungs, making the "whoop," which may be heard at a distance, and from which the disease takes its name. A deep inspiration may precede the series of spasmodic expiratory efforts. Several coughing fits may succeed each other until a tenacious mucus is ejected, usually small in amount, but after a series of coughing spells a considerable quantity may be expectorated. *Vomiting* often takes place at the end of a paroxysm, and may recur so frequently that the child does not get enough food and becomes emaciated. There may be only four or five attacks in the day; an average is twenty attacks daily. They may be more frequent and severe at night. In severe and fatal cases the paroxysms may exceed one hundred daily. During the paroxysm the thorax is strongly compressed by the powerful expiratory efforts, and, as very little air passes in, there are signs of defective aëration of the blood; the face becomes swollen and congested, the veins are prominent, the eyeballs protrude, and the conjunctivae become deeply engorged. Suffocation indeed seems imminent, when with a deep, crowing inspiration air enters the lungs and the color is quickly restored. The child knows for a few moments when the attack is coming on, and tries in every way to check it, but failing to do so, runs terrified to the nurse or mother to be supported, or clutches anything near by. Few diseases are more painful to witness. In severe paroxysms the sphincters may be opened. An ulcer may form under the tongue from rubbing on the teeth (Riga's disease). Among circumstances which precipitate a paroxysm are emotion, such as crying, and any irritation in the throat. Even the act of swallowing sometimes seems sufficient. In a close dusty atmosphere the coughing fits are more frequent. After lasting for three or four weeks the attacks become lighter and finally cease. In cases of ordinary severity the course of the disease is rarely under six weeks.

During the attack, if the chest be examined, the resonance is defective in the expiratory stage, full and clear during the deep, crowing inspiration; but on auscultation during the latter there may be no vesicular murmur heard, owing to the slowness with which the air passes the narrowed glottis. Bronchial râles are occasionally heard.

Blood.—There is usually a marked leukocytosis (15,000-25,000) which may appear early. There is generally a marked increase in the lymphocytes and myelocytes may be found.

Complications and Sequelae.—During the extensive venous congestion hemorrhages are very apt to occur in the form of petechiae, particularly about the forehead, ecchymosis of the conjunctivae, and even tears of blood (Trousseau) from the rupture of the vessels, epistaxis, bleeding from the ears, and occasionally hemoptysis. Hemorrhage from the bowels is rare. Glycosuria occurs occasionally. Death has occurred from spasm of the glottis. Convulsions are not very uncommon, vascular lesions, including venous stasis, meningo-encephalitis and angiospasm are possible causes. Sudden death has been caused by extensive subdural hemorrhage. Choked disk, relieved by decompression, has occurred. Paralysis is a rare event. It was associated with 3 in a series of 120 cases, but in none did the hemiplegia come on during the paroxysm, as in a case reported by S. West. A spastic paraplegia may follow. Acute polyneuritis is a rare sequel. Arthritis occurs occasionally. Otitis media is not uncommon.

The *pulmonary* complications are extremely serious. During the severe coughing spells interstitial emphysema may be induced, more rarely pneumothorax. Occasionally the air reaches the subcutaneous tissues of the neck, and the condition may become general. Capillary bronchitis and bronchopneumonia are the dangerous complications, responsible for nine out of ten deaths in the disease. In some cases the process is tuberculous. Pleurisy is sometimes met with and occasionally lobar pneumonia. Enlargement of the bronchial glands is very common in whooping cough. During the spasm the radial pulse is small, the right heart engorged, and during and after the attack the cardiac action is disturbed. It is doubtful if serious damage results, or if valvular disease in children can be attributed to whooping cough. Rupture of the omentum has occurred. Serious renal complications are very uncommon, but albumin sometimes and sugar frequently are found in the urine. A distressing sequel in adults is asthma, which may recur at intervals for a year or more. Bronchiectasis is an occasional sequel. A paroxysmal cough may persist for months after an attack, especially in adults.

Diagnosis.—A persistent paroxysmal cough, without sufficient signs to explain it, should excite suspicion. When the "whoop" occurs the diagnosis is easy; but there are doubtful cases, particularly during epidemics, in which a series of expiratory coughs occurs without any "whoop." The spasmodic cough due to enlarged bronchial glands may cause difficulty. In adults a diagnosis of acute tracheitis and bronchitis may be made in the early stages but the paroxysmal character of the cough should excite suspicion. The earlier that cultures are made, the more likely are positive results. This is best done by the "cough-plate" method—a Petri dish with special media into which the patient coughs is held four inches from the mouth.

Prognosis.—If we include its complications, whooping cough is a very fatal affection, ranking high among the acute infections as a cause of death in children under five years of age and especially in the first year.

Prophylaxis.—The patient should be isolated and the sputum collected and disinfected. As the organism usually disappears within four weeks from the appearance of the whoop there seems little danger of infection in the later stages. A prophylactic vaccine has been used, three injections of 500 million, 2 and 3 billion, being given every third day. There is no agreement as to its value.

Treatment.—The gravity of the disease is scarcely appreciated by the public. Children with the disease should not be sent to school or exposed in public in any way. There is more reprehensible neglect in connection with this than with any other acute infectious disease. The patient should be in bed if the paroxysms are severe or there is fever. Fresh air, night and day, is important, but in cities in the winter this is not easy to manage. Stock vaccine has been used for treatment early in the attack; some patients seem to benefit. The average initial dose is 500 million for children over one year. With two-day intervals doses of 1 and 2 billion are given. Convalescent serum has been employed. Treatment by X-ray exposures is sometimes successful. Treatments are given every second day to a total of three; a second similar course is given after seven days in severe cases. Ephedrine hydrochloride may be useful in doses of gr. $\frac{1}{12}$ (gm. 0.005) for children under one year and gr. $\frac{1}{6}$ (gm. 0.01) for older children, given in the evening or two or three times a day. Belladonna or atropine may be given. The use of benzoin and eucalyptus inhalations is often helpful. Sedatives are by far the most trustworthy drugs in severe cases, and paregoric may be given freely, particularly to give rest at night. Codein and heroin in doses proper for the age often give much relief. Antipyrin and chloral hydrate may be tried. Chloretone may be used in doses of gr. 1 (0.065 gm.) four times a day for a young child. Painting the throat with a 2 per cent solution of silver nitrate is sometimes useful. Children can often be taught to inhibit an attack. The wearing of a tight abdominal binder is sometimes of value. If vomiting is severe it is well to give food in small amounts immediately after the paroxysm.

After convalescence has begun, the child should be watched with the greatest care. It is at this period that bronchopneumonia is apt to develop. The cough sometimes persists for months and the child remains weak and delicate. Change of air should be tried. Such a patient should be fed with care and given tonics and codliver oil.

GONOCOCCUS INFECTION

Definition.—An acute infection with a primary lesion, usually urethritis, and secondary and systemic manifestations, of which prostatitis and epididymitis, salpingitis, arthritis, synovitis and endocarditis are the most important. The gonococcus (*Neisseria gonorrhoeae*) was described by Neisser, in 1879. Gonorrheal conjunctivitis is an important local lesion.

Gonorrhea, a widespread and serious disease, presents many features for consideration. It is not a killing disease but as a cause of ill health and disability the gonococcus occupies a position of the very first rank among its fellows. While the local lesion is too often thought to be trifling, in its singular obstinacy, in the possibilities of permanent sexual damage to the individual himself and still more in the "grisly troop" which may follow in its train, gonorrhea does not fall very far short of syphilis in importance.

Etiology.—The organism is a biscuit-shaped micrococcus, occurring in pairs, usually within the leukocytes, and is present in the primary and systemic lesions. Gonococcus strains represent a number of distinct types serologically. It may be that certain cases of infant forms of infection are due to a different strain from those causing the disease in adults. The disease has been reproduced by inoculation of the pure culture.

The disease occurs as a result of impure sexual intercourse, by accidental infection, and in the newborn from vaginal contamination. Ophthalmia neonatorum is one of the great causes of blindness, but an active campaign of education has reduced the number of cases. The gonococcus vaginitis and ophthalmia are very serious diseases in children's hospitals and infants' homes. The story of the gonococcus infection in the Babies' Hospital, New York, for eleven years, as told by Holt, illustrates its singular obstinacy. In eleven years, there were 273 cases of vaginitis, only 6 with ophthalmia and 26 with arthritis. Other institutions have had equally sad experiences. Constant vigilance is required to prevent the disease gaining entrance. Isolation and prolonged quarantine are the only measures to combat the disease successfully.

The effects of the gonococcus may be considered under:

I. The primary infection.
II. The spread in the genito-urinary organs by direct continuity.
III. Systemic gonococcus infection.

The primary lesion we need not here consider, but we may call attention to the frequency of the local complications, as periurethral abscess, gonorrheal prostatitis and seminal vesiculitis in the male, and vaginitis, endocervicitis, salpingitis and inflammation of the glands of Bartholin in the female. An acute salpingitis may cause difficulty in diagnosis in the female and in the male involvement of the seminal vesicles and prostate may give a variety of symptoms, especially referred pain.

Serious sequels result from the *spread* by continuity. Gonococcus salpingitis is not infrequent. Metritis and ovaritis are also met with, and peritonitis. The gonococcus has been found in pure culture in acute general peritonitis. Gonococcal *peritonitis* in children may result in a curious condition in which there are a remarkable number of adhesions, which may be general or most marked in the upper abdomen. Equally important is the cystitis, which is probably more frequently the result of a mixed infection than due to the gonococcus itself. There is some danger of extension to the kidneys. The pyelitis, like the cystitis, is usually a mixed infection.

In *gonococcal stomatitis* the gums are swollen and inflamed. The soft palate, pillars of the fauces, and parts of the tongue may show whitish patches with inflammation around them. Potassium permanganate solution (1-5000) as a mouth wash and silver preparations applied locally are helpful.

Systemic Gonococcal Infection.—GONOCOCCUS SEPTICEMIA AND PYEMIA.—Thayer and Blumer first cultivated gonococci from the blood of a patient in Osler's wards. Of 29 cases in which septicemia was demonstrated by positive blood cultures, 12 died. Cole divided the cases into four groups: (1) Those with *endocarditis,* 11 of the 29 cases collected by him. The clinical features are those of malignant endocarditis; two recovered. In gonococcus *endocarditis* the aortic valve is frequently attacked and the right heart is involved more often than in endocarditis due to other organisms. Embolic phenomena may occur. (2) Cases with *local suppuration* and the general features of a *pyemia* —of the six cases three died. The septicemia associated with a small focus of suppuration may be very intense. A man ten days after the onset of urethritis had chills and high fever; he became profoundly toxemic and died on the morning of the fourth day from the chill. There was a small prostatic abscess. (3) Cases *with no metastatic local affections* or perhaps only slight arthritis. In a case at the Johns Hopkins Hospital, three months after an acute gonorrhea the patient had a fever resembling typhoid, which lasted seven weeks. Gonococci were cultivated from the blood. (4) Cases of *gonorrheal puerperal septicemia.* The *treatment* is that of a severe general infection. Chemotherapy seems of little value.

GONOCOCCAL ARTHRITIS.—In many respects this is the most damaging and disabling of all the complications, occurring in from 2 to 5 per cent of the cases. Lees (1931) found 338 cases in 13,000 patients with gonorrhea. It occurs more frequently in males than in females. It occurs, as a rule, during an acute attack of gonorrhea but it may occur as the attack subsides or even when it has become chronic. A severe gonorrheal arthritis may occur in a newly married woman infected by an old gleet in her husband. In women it is not always easy to find evidence of local infection; the cervix should be carefully examined. As a rule, many joints are affected at the onset but usually the process persists in one or two.

The *anatomical changes* are variable. The inflammation is often peri-articular, and involves especially the sheaths of the tendons. Effusion of varying amount is common. In other cases the joint shows a diffuse brawny swelling and is very tender. This form is usually more severe than that with effusion. When effusion occurs it rarely becomes purulent. It has more commonly the characters of a synovitis. About the wrist and hand suppuration sometimes occurs in the sheaths. The gonococcus may be present in the inflamed joint or in the peri-arthritic exudate, and obtained in pure culture. Mixed infection is very rare.

Clinical Course.—Variability and obstinacy are the two most distinguishing features. The following are the most important clinical forms:

Arthralgic, in which there are pains about the joints, without redness or swelling. These may persist for a long time.

Polyarthritic.—The fever is usually slight; the local inflammation may fix itself in one joint, but less commonly several become swollen and tender. In other cases one joint is especially involved, the others subsiding rapidly. The knee joint is most often involved—64 per cent of Lees' series. The pain is severe, the swelling extensive, due chiefly to peri-articular edema, and synovitis is often marked. The fever is not at all proportionate to the intensity of the local signs. The exudate usually resolves, though suppuration occasionally supervenes. Ankylosis may occur.

Chronic Hydrarthrosis.—This is usually mono-articular, and is particularly apt to involve the knee. It may come on without pain, redness, or swelling. Formation of pus is rare.

Bursal and Synovial Form.—This attacks chiefly the tendons and their sheaths and the bursae and the periosteum. The articulations may not be affected. The bursae of the patella, the olecranon, and the tendo Achillis are most apt to be involved.

Spondylitis.—This may be due to gonococcus infection and is usually in the lower spine. It presents no special peculiarities.

Painful Heel.—This is due to local periosteal thickening and exostosis on the os calcis, causing pain and great disability. Baer demonstrated the gonococcus in the periosteal lesion.

Complications.—Iritis is not infrequent and may recur with successive attacks. Meningitis, myelitis and true neuritis occur rarely. Endocarditis, pericarditis, phlebitis and pleurisy occur. *Sciatica* is fairly common, usually secondary to spondylitis or prostatitis, although a toxic factor has been suggested. Myositis and a variety of skin conditions occur, especially hyperkeratosis of the palms and soles.

Diagnosis.—The thought of the possibility of gonococcus infection and a search for the primary lesion are the best safeguards. The usual error is to mistake an acute gonococcus polyarthritis for rheumatic fever. The persistence, usually in one or two joints, and the occurrence of changes in the joints should make the diagnosis clear. The swelling often extends more above and below the joint than in other forms of arthritis. Gonococci may be found in fluid from the joint or peri-articular tissues. The complement fixation and the intradermal skin tests are sometimes of value.

Prognosis.—Much depends on the time at which proper treatment is begun. In early acute cases the outlook is good unless there is a purulent arthritis in which case some disability will probably remain. If damage of the articular surfaces has occurred, complete restoration is not to be expected. Many cases are protracted.

Treatment.—The primary infection—usually urethritis—should be actively treated. Of special measures, the use of foreign protein injection and vaccine treatment are worthy of trial; either helps some cases, both fail in many. Good food, fresh air, and open bowels are important. Drugs are of little value, but the syrup of ferrous iodide (ʒ i, 4 cc.) is sometimes useful. Phenacetine or acetylsalicylic acid may be given for the pain.

The local treatment is very important. In acute cases, fixation of the joints for a short period is beneficial (but care should be taken to avoid ankylosis), and in the chronic forms, massage and passive motion. Counter-irritation by the cautery or blisters and active hyperemia are useful. Diathermy may be useful. A distended joint may be tapped and then tightly bandaged or air introduced. The surgical treatment is more satisfactory in severe cases and good results usually follow incision and irrigation.

The use of fever therapy, including diathermy and the employment of short waves, seems to be of value in various forms of gonococcal infection.

BACILLARY DYSENTERY

Definition.—A form of intestinal infection, usually acute, occurring sporadically and in epidemics, characterized by pain, frequent passages of blood and mucus, and due to a specific bacillus, of which there are various strains. It may attack individuals of any age.

Etiology.—Owing to improved sanitation, dysentery has become less frequent. In temperate climates sporadic cases occur from time to time, and at intervals epidemics prevail. Records of widespread epidemics were collected by Woodward. The most serious was that which prevailed from 1847 to 1856. In institutions, particularly if overcrowded, dysentery is common. In the tropics "dysentery is a destructive giant compared to which strong drink is a mere phantom" (Macgregor). Dysentery is one of the great camp diseases, and has been more destructive to armies than powder and shot. In the Federal service during the Civil War, according to Woodward,[1] there were 259,071 cases of acute and 28,451 cases of chronic dysentery. A fatal form of dysentery has prevailed in Japan, with a mortality about 26 per cent. Severe epidemics of acute dysentery are usually of the bacillary type. It is a mistake to regard bacillary dysentery as a tropical disease only; it is not uncommon in temperate zones.

Bacillus Dysenteriae.—There are various strains of dysentery bacilli. The first was discovered by Shiga in 1898 in Japan and the second by Flexner in Manila. The organisms belonging to the first group are identical, but there are several varieties of the Flexner group which react more or less to a serum prepared from any one. This immune serum has little effect on the Shiga group and vice versa. In general, infection with the Shiga group is more severe than with the other forms. The Shiga bacilli form two toxins, exotoxin and endotoxin; the Flexner bacilli endotoxin only. The organism appears to be constantly present in the acute dysentery of the tropics. Certain forms of summer diarrheas of infants are due to infection with *B. dysenteriae.*

The strains of the bacillus most frequently found in the United States are the "Flexner-Y" group. The lesions produced by the different strains are identical. The organism agglutinates with the blood serum of cases with acute dysentery as well as with the serum of immunized animals. It is rarely found in the blood.

Infection takes place by the mouth. The organisms are widely distributed by the feces of persons suffering with the disease and also by dysentery "carriers." In institutions food and drink readily become contaminated. Possibly, too, the germs are distributed by flies and dust.

Morbid Anatomy.—In acute cases, the mucous membrane of the large intestine is swollen, of a deep-red color, and presents elevated, coarse corrugations and folds. In addition to the intense hyperemia there are hemorrhagic areas. Over the surface there is usually a superficial necrotic layer, which may be in patches, or uniform over large areas. Following the necrosis there is superficial ulceration but the edges are not undermined as in amebic dysen-

---

[1] Medical and Surgical History of the War of the Rebellion, Medical, vol. ii. The most exhaustive treatise extant on intestinal fluxes—an enduring monument to the industry and ability of the author.

tery. In cases of great intensity the colon may be stiff and thick and the mucous membrane enormously increased in thickness, grayish black, extensively necrotic, and, in places, gangrenous. The serous surface is often deeply injected. The ileum may be involved, having a deeply hemorrhagic mucosa, with a superficial necrosis.

Symptoms.—According to Strong and Musgrave, the period of incubation is not more than forty-eight hours. The onset, which is usually sudden, is characterized by slight fever, pain in the abdomen, and frequent stools. At first mucus is passed, but within twenty-four hours blood appears with it, or there is pure blood. There is a constant desire to go to stool, with great straining and tenesmus; every hour or half hour there may be a small amount of blood and mucus passed. The temperature rises and may reach 103° or 104°. The pulse increases in frequency, and in the severer cases becomes very small. The tongue is coated with a white fur, and there is excessive thirst. Vomiting may occur. In the very acute cases the patient becomes seriously ill within forty-eight hours, the movements increase in frequency, the pain is of great intensity, the patient becomes toxic and delirious, and death may occur on the third or fourth day. In cases of moderate severity the urgency of the symptoms abates, the stools lessen, the temperature falls, and within two or three weeks the patient is convalescent. The mortality in the severe forms is high. There is a subacute form which lasts for many weeks or months. The patients become greatly emaciated, having from three to five stools in the twenty-four hours. The *B. dysenteriae* is found in the stools, and it agglutinates readily with the blood serum.

The foregoing account describes the essential features of bacillary dysentery as seen in the tropics. The clinical features of bacillary dysentery in adults in temperate climates differ in no essential manner from those described. Although the evidence hardly warrants the statement that all nonamebic cases of dysentery are bacillary in origin yet probably this is the case. What is known as acute catarrhal dysentery is probably a sporadic form due to the *B. dysenteriae*. Diphtheritic dysentery is a type of the bacillary form with great necrosis and infiltration of the mucosa. There may be rapid gangrene and a fatal termination within twenty-four hours. A secondary dysentery is a common terminal event in many acute and chronic diseases. In young children the disease is usually serious. There may be high fever with vomiting and rapid loss of weight. Dehydration and toxemia are usually marked. The persistent occurrence of stools containing blood or pus, or both, in infants suggests bacillary dysentery. The *Sonne variety* is relatively slightly toxic. It is usually recognized in children and is often from contact infection. The symptoms may be very slight and the patient may not feel ill. Severe forms have fever and the usual features of dysentery; they are often regarded as food poisoning. The course is usually short.

Chronic Form.—The acute form may gradually pass into this or the patient may have recovered apparently and relapses occur with a transition to the chronic form. There may be four to eight stools a day with blood and mucus. The general health suffers and emaciation is marked, but some patients live for many years and have a fair measure of health. The mucous membrane is inflamed and edematous with shallow ulcers. Before a diagnosis of chronic dysentery is made care should be taken to exclude chronic poisoning and syphilis or carcinoma of the rectum. The same methods are indicated as in the diagnosis of acute dysentery.

Complications and Sequelae.—*Peritonitis* is rare, due either to extension through the wall of the bowel or to perforation. When this occurs about the cecal region, perityphlitis results; when low down in the rectum, periproctitis. In 108 autopsies collected by Woodward perforation occurred in 11. Abscess of the liver, so common in the amebic form, is very rare. It is interesting to note, as illustrating the probable type of the disease, how comparatively rare abscess of the liver was during the American Civil War. Very few cases occurred in the South African War (Rolleston). Hemorrhage from the bowel sometimes occurs and is occasionally profuse. In the tropics malaria and acute dysentery often coexist.

Sydenham noted that dysentery was sometimes associated with arthritic pains, and in certain epidemics *arthritis* has occurred. In severe cases there may be parotitis, pleurisy, thrombosis, pericarditis, endocarditis, epididymitis, and occasionally pyemic manifestations, among which is pylephlebitis and abscess of the spleen. Chronic nephritis is an occasional sequel. In protracted cases there may be an anemic edema. An interesting sequel is paralysis of which Woodward reported 8 cases. Weir Mitchell mentioned it as not uncommon, occurring chiefly in the form of paraplegia. As in other acute fevers, this is due probably to a neuritis. Intestinal stricture is a rare sequence—so rare that no case was reported during the Civil War. It appears to be not uncommon in the East.

Diagnosis.—The recognition of dysentery itself is rarely difficult. Some cases of ulcerative colitis may cause confusion, but local examination by the sigmoidoscope and the results of cultures should make the diagnosis clear. Metallic poisoning, especially bichloride of mercury, may be mistaken for dysentery in the absence of a complete history, but chemical examination of the stools, the renal involvement and stomatitis should prevent error. Syphilis and carcinoma of the bowel should be excluded. The recognition of the *form* of dysentery is important, particularly for treatment. The amebic, Bilharzial, and flagellate forms can generally be recognized by careful examination of fresh stools or the material obtained by a rectal tube or on direct examination. The dysentery bacillus may be obtained on culture from the stools. The agglutination test is usually positive. Houghwout emphasizes the value of a study of the cellular exudate as shown in the stools. In bacillary dysentery there is a rich purulent exudate, consisting mainly of polymorphonuclear leukocytes (about 90 per cent) and phagocytic endothelial macrophages. The cells show marked degeneration. In amebic dysentery the exudate is scanty and without the inflammatory character of the bacillary form.

Prognosis.—Flint showed that sporadic dysentery is, in its slighter grades at least, a self-limited disease, which runs its course in eight or nine days. In epidemics the death rate averages 10 to 40 per cent. The outlook is serious in young children and in debilitated persons.

Treatment.—PROPHYLACTIC.—The same precautions should be followed as in typhoid fever. Flexner and Gay have shown that animals can be protected from infection by a previous treatment with immune serum. Protective and curative serums have been prepared. Vaccines, in doses of three billion have been given by mouth daily for three days, at least an hour before food.

Acute Dysentery.—The patient should be absolutely at rest in bed. He should be kept warm and have a flannel abdominal binder applied. The diet should be very simple—whey, egg albumen, barley or rice water, and strained gruels. Milk and lactose may be added later. Enough water should be given to relieve thirst. If vomiting occurs, nothing should be given by mouth for some hours, and if the patient requires fluid this can be given subcutaneously. Hot applications to the abdomen are useful. If the patient is seen early in the attack, free purgation is advisable, for which sodium sulphate and Rochelle salts are best. Either may be given in doses of two drams (8 gm.) for two doses an hour apart and later half the amount every three hours until the bowels have moved freely. By this treatment the course is sometimes cut short. If the attack is well established, the use of purgatives must be determined by the conditions present. If solid fecal matter is being passed, a purgative is indicated, castor oil being the best (ʒ vi, 25 cc.). Until the bowels have been thoroughly cleared, purgation is indicated.

Medicinal.—Bismuth in large doses often has a beneficial effect. Thirty to sixty grains (2 to 4 gm.) should be given every hour. For the relief of pain and to quiet the bowel, morphia is most useful and to be preferred to opium by mouth. It should be given hypodermically (gr. 1/4 to 1/3, 0.016 to 0.022 gm.), and repeated according to the needs. If tenesmus is not marked, opium can be given as the starch and laudanum enema, with 30 minims (2 cc.) of laudanum. In severe cases salt solution may be given subcutaneously or 10 per cent dextrose solution intravenously (up to 300 cc.).

Local Treatment.—During the acute stages this may be out of the question, but should be employed whenever possible. Normal saline or sodium bicarbonate (1 per cent) solution at the body temperature can be used as an irrigation. This should be given very gently and with the hips elevated. If there is a rectal irritation, a cocaine or morphia suppository should be given beforehand. As the symptoms lessen, the quantity of fluid can be increased and other solutions used, such as boric acid (5 per cent) or alum (1 to 200).

With convalescence the diet should be increased very gradually and only simple foods allowed. The patient should be kept quiet until all danger of a relapse is over. This is most important to prevent chronic dysentery.

Specific Therapy.—Good results have been reported from the use of polyvalent serums, which should be given in doses of 50 to 100 cc. Bacteriophage has been used and seems to be of value in some cases.

Chronic Dysentery.—The patient should be at rest in bed and on simple diet, milk, boiled, peptonized or fermented, whey, beef juice, and eggs. In some cases milk may have to be given well diluted or in small amounts, but it usually agrees well. It is well to give an occasional purge (castor oil, ℥ ss, 15 cc.) to empty the bowels. Drugs by mouth are not of great value. Bismuth, if used, should be in large doses (ʒ i, 4 gm.) every three hours while the patient is awake. Opium should not be given as a routine as there is great danger of forming a habit; it is best given in the starch and laudanum enema. The serum is of little value; vaccine therapy is more promising.

Local Treatment.—This should be carried out thoroughly. If the rectum is irritable, a cocaine or morphine suppository can be given previously. The irrigation, at the body temperature, should be given very gently, the patient encouraged to retain it as long as possible, and the amount gradually increased up to two litres if possible. One irrigation a day is usually enough. Silver nitrate solution is probably the best (1 to 5,000 at first and increased to 1 to 500). Boric acid (5 per cent), salicylic acid (2 per cent), alum, or tannic acid (3 per cent) may be used. With any of these an occasional irrigation of saline solution is useful. With improvement the frequency of the irrigations is reduced. To ulcers in the bowel which can be reached silver nitrate solution (25 per cent) should be applied. In obstinate cases an appendicostomy or cecostomy may be done and the bowel irrigated through the opening.

UNDULANT FEVER: BRUCELLOSIS

Definition.—A specific fever caused by organisms of the *Brucella melitensis-abortus* group characterized by fever, sweating, arthritis and an enlarged spleen. The organisms fall into closely related serological types. The *melitensis* is caprine and the *abortus* bovine and porcine. Both may infect man.

Distribution.—The disease as first recognized was derived from goat's milk and prevailed extensively in the Mediterranean littoral. Wherever goats were infected and the milk was drunk the disease occurred. From its prevalence in Malta arose the designation Malta fever. Bruce in 1886 isolated the organism *Brucella melitensis.* Subsequently it was shown that the organism which causes abortion in cattle (Bang in 1897 described it as *Bacillus abortus*) has close relations with *Brucella melitensis.* They are regarded as distinct serological types of the same species. Wherever infection of animals with *B. abortus* occurs, and that is wherever there are cattle, the disease, undulant fever, may be conveyed to man.

Etiology.—The detection of the cause of undulant fever in Malta as due to *B. melitensis* conveyed in infected goat's milk was a brilliant piece of work, due largely to Marston, Bruce and Hughes. The recognition of the close relationship between the organisms was due to A. E. Evans (1918). Later proof of the occurrence of infection due to *B. abortus* in man was found (Keefer, 1924; Carpenter *et al.,* 1926). The recognition of this infection has been rapid and cases have been reported from many countries. Infection is usually due to the use of raw dairy products as by drinking infected milk from goats or cows. The organisms may enter through abrasions or wounds of the skin and those handling infected animals, or infected meat or pork, may so contract the disease. Infection has occurred in laboratory workers.

In the United States the bovine and porcine forms are the most important. The caprine form is found in the southwestern parts of the country. The porcine and caprine infections are the most severe.

Age.—Children seem to be relatively immune. Males predominate (70 to 80 per cent), due to exposure in handling animals and meats.

The organism is pathogenic for man, animals and fowls. It is small (0.3 to 0.5 by 1.5 microns) and grows slowly. It is pleomorphic, bacillary forms usually being found on media and coccoid forms in tissues. In cattle the infection is chronic, the main result being the occurrence of abortion. Herds have shown the infection for long periods. The organisms are in the uterus and male genitalia. They may be excreted in the milk. In goats the organisms are in the milk and urine.

Pathology.—There is often a bacteremia and the organisms may be found in many organs. They have been found in the bile obtained by duodenal biliary drainage and in the stools and urine. The gallbladder may be a source of infection in a carrier. There are no specific lesions. The spleen is enlarged and cloudy swelling occurs in the liver and kidneys. In the intestine there may be areas of congestion with swelling of the mucosa; ulceration occasionally results and intestinal hemorrhage has been reported. Endocarditis, acute nephritis and endophlebitis may occur.

Clinical picture.—This is so varied that it is difficult to give a description which covers all forms. As a general rule in North America the disease hardly deserves the term "Undulant Fever," as this form of fever curve is exceptional. The *incubation* period varies from ten to twenty days. The *onset* is usually gradual but may be acute with a chill or chilly sensation. There may be headache, backache, weakness, general malaise, and anorexia. The occurrence of fever may not be noted and the patients go about for weeks before the disease is recognized. In some instances the weakness is marked and in others a single symptom or sign may predominate. With the progress of the disease, fatigue, irritability, general malaise, anorexia, constipation and chills, or chilly sensations, become more marked. The fever may be absent in the morning and only present towards evening. Profuse *sweating* is common, and chills with fever and sweating may occur in the latter part of the day. The pulse rate is not greatly altered.

Fever.—In some the fever is very slight. In others, perhaps the more common form, it may last for weeks or months, usually in a remittent or intermittent form, and varying in height. Temperature of 98°-100° in the morning and 101°-102° in the evening may be regarded as an average range. In the undulant form there may be waves of fever which recur a number of times but this is less marked in the American cases.

Certain features are usually present; weakness is common, and may be very marked. Anorexia, nausea and vomiting may occur, and constipation is frequent. Some patients have abdominal pain with tenderness. Irritability and insomnia may be rather striking, but many of the patients do not suggest serious illness and are remarkably well considering the fever and duration of the disease. Arthralgia is common and arthritis may occur. Intermittent hydrarthrosis has been described, the organism being found in the joint fluid.

There is marked *leukopenia* and often a considerable increase in the mononuclear cells. Secondary anemia is common. The agglutinins are present in the blood usually in the second week. The titer reaches usually 100-160, or higher, in the third or fourth week.

Complications.—Bronchitis may occur; bronchopneumonia is rare. Pleurisy with effusion has occurred. In males orchitis, prostatitis and epididymitis may occur. In pregnant women abortion may result and mastitis sometimes. Various bone lesions may be present, as osteomyelitis, spondylitis, disease of the hip joint with the formation of a sterile abscess, psoas abscess probably from caries of the lumbar vertebrae (the organisms have been found in the pus) and arthritis. Meningitis has occurred rarely.

Certain *sequels* may be striking. There may be marked weakness and disability for a time. In some patients stiffness of the joints persists. Cholecystitis may persist with the organisms present in the gallbladder.

The *duration* of the disease may be from a few weeks to a year or longer. There is a remarkable tendency to recurrences. The mortality is low and averages 2 or 3 per cent.

Diagnosis.—This disease has to be considered as a possibility in all doubtful cases of fever and the assistance of thorough laboratory work is important. Blood cultures should be made as early as possible. The agglutination test is of great value and should be done in all suspicious cases. Agglutination in a dilution of 1-80 should be demanded; in a dilution of 1-40, suspicion should be aroused and further studies made. A dermal reaction, using diluted vaccine, has been used. Animal inoculation tests may be done. In these guinea-pigs are inoculated intraperitoneally with blood from the patient. When positive the animals show loss of weight with orchitis, and at autopsy the organism may be obtained. Particularly important are small areas of necrosis in the liver. The frequency of ambulatory cases and the slight grade of fever in some instances, especially in those with digestive disturbance or weakness as the main symptom, suggest the wisdom of agglutination tests and a consideration of this disease in what may seem to be slight febrile ailments.

Prophylaxis.—In localities where goats' milk is drunk, its use should be abandoned or the milk thoroughly boiled. The *abortus* form is due to drinking raw milk or cream. Pasteurization should be done or the milk boiled. Particular care should be taken in the country in districts where abortion in cattle occurs. The organisms may be in large numbers in the vaginal discharges of infected animals and infect those working with them.

The difficulty of *prophylaxis* in country districts is evident as probably 20 per cent of the cattle are infected. Milk should be boiled on farms where the cows are infected. Special care should be taken, especially by dairymen and those working in packing houses or with pork, to avoid infection by the hands.

Treatment.—Thus far we have no specific serum therapy and vaccine treatment does not seem to have proved its value. The treatment is that of a general infection. The patient should be given as much nourishment as possible. In patients who have shown the bacillus in the stools the administration of thyolin and methylene violet in pills coated with phenyl salicylate in dosage of 25-200 mgm. per day apparently has been of value. The same drugs may be given in the form of an enema 300 cc. of a 1:100,000 to 1:25,000 strength to be retained for some time. Foreign protein therapy may be tried, using typhoid and paratyphoid vaccine, with an initial dose of 50 millions, increasing this gradually and giving a dose every five days. Brucellin and filtrates have been used with apparent benefit. A change of climate seems to aid convalescence.

TULAREMIA

This is a specfic infectious disease due to *Bacterium tularense,* transmitted from rodents to man by insects (fly and tick) or acquired by handling infected animals.

History.—In 1910, R. A. Pearse of Brigham City, Utah, reported cases of infection due to the bite of a fly and described the symptoms. McCoy and Chapin in 1912 discovered *Bacterium tularense* as the cause of a disease in rodents resembling plague. The first human case with proved bacteriological findings was in Cincinnati in 1913 (Wherry and Lamb), the cultures being made from conjunctival ulcers. Subsequently the organism was obtained from patients in Utah. There have been a number of cases in laboratory workers contracted while working with the organism. The name tularemia was suggested by Francis in 1921 (from Tulare county, California).

Etiology.—The disease in animals affects rabbits particularly but many other wild animals and some game birds suffer from it. Sheep have been infected; there is doubt regarding cattle. The disease has not been conveyed from the human patient to a healthy individual. It is widely distributed in the United States.

Clinical Features.—The incubation period may be from one to ten days with an average of three or four days. The onset is sudden with headache, malaise, fever, chills and prostration. The disease takes various forms, about 90 per cent being ulceroglandular. Fever occurs and lasts from two to three weeks. There is usually a leukocytosis of 15,000 to 20,000. Various skin eruptions may occur, macular to pustular. Peritonitis and ascites have occurred with the organisms in the fluid. Lobar or bronchopneumonia may occur; pleurisy and pericarditis with effusion have been noted. The mortality is about 5 per cent. Various forms of the disease have been described.

Ulceroglandular Form.—This is by far the most common. The situation of the lesion will depend on the site of the area of infection. It is on the hand if contracted from skinning infected animals; on an exposed surface if contracted from the bite of a fly; under the clothing or in the hair if from a tick bite. The patient complains of pain in the lymph nodes which drain the area of infection; the nodes are tender and enlarged in the local areas only. About a day later the site of infection becomes inflamed, showing a painful papule which breaks down; there is a necrotic area which leaves an ulcer about 1 cm. in diameter. There is redness of the skin over the inflamed lymph nodes which suppurate in about half the cases. In the others the glands are hard and tender for several months. Suppuration of lymph nodes may occur many months after the acute features are over. Subcutaneous nodules have occurred on the arms; they may suppurate.

Oculoglandular Form.—In this the primary involvement is in the conjunctiva (60 cases reported up to 1932). There is irritation of the eye with swelling of the lids, edema of the ocular conjunctiva and often a papule on the conjunctiva of the lower lid. Various lymph nodes in the surrounding areas may be involved, sometimes even the axillary glands. Ulcers appear on the conjunctival surface of both lids. Purulent dacrocystitis may occur. Blindness may follow.

Glandular Forms.—In these there is no evident primary lesion and the epitrochlear and axillary glands are especially involved.

Typhoid Form.—In this there are the features of a general infection without any local lesion. The laboratory infections in man (30 up to 1932) have been of this form.

Diagnosis.—The local lesions are suggestive. The organism has been obtained from guinea-pigs inoculated from the patient's blood or from the pus from the suppurating glands. Complement fixation and agglutination tests are positive. As some patients show no glandular features and others very slight general disturbances mild cases are easily overlooked. The specific agglutinins do not appear until the second week but remain for many years. Some serums agglutinate *Brucella abortus-melitensis*.

Prevention.—Rubber gloves should be worn by those who dress wild rabbits and hares. Special precautions should be taken by laboratory workers in handling infected material or cultures. The meat of infected animals is safe to eat if thoroughly cooked. The liver and spleen of an infected rabbit are studded with small spots which suggest the diagnosis.

Treatment.—The use of a *serum* prepared from goats by Foshay has given encouraging results. Two doses of 15 cc. are given intravenously on successive days; larger doses are used for patients seriously ill. Exposure of the primary lesions to X-rays has been advised. The general treatment is that of an acute infection.

CHOLERA ASIATICA

Definition.—A specific, infectious disease, caused by the "comma bacillus" of Koch, and characterized clinically by violent purging and rapid collapse.

Historical Summary.—Cholera has been endemic in India from a remote period, but only within the last century did it make inroads into Europe and America. An extensive epidemic occurred in 1832, in which year it was brought in immigrant ships from Great Britain to Quebec. It travelled along the lines of traffic up the Great Lakes, and finally reached as far west as the military posts of the upper Mississippi. In the same year it entered the United States by way of New York. There were recurrences of the disease in 1835-36. In 1848 it entered the country through New Orleans, and spread widely up the Mississippi Valley and across the continent to California. In 1849 it again appeared. In 1854 it was introduced by immigrant ships into New York and prevailed widely throughout the country. In 1866 and in 1867 there were less serious epidemics. In 1873 it again appeared in the United States, but did not prevail widely. Although occasional cases have been brought by ship to the quarantine stations of Great Britain and the United States, the disease has not gained a foothold in either country since 1873. It has prevailed extensively in the Philippines and in the Near and Far East. In 1911 cholera prevailed in Italy, North Africa and Madeira. There were outbreaks in Asia Minor, Arabia and Turkey, and the usual prevalence in India.

Etiology.—In 1884 Koch announced the discovery of the specific organism (*Vibrio cholerae*). It has the form of a slightly bent rod, which is thicker, but not more than about half the length of the tubercle bacillus, and sometimes occurs in corkscrew-like or S forms. The organisms grow upon a great variety of media and display characteristic appearances. Koch found them in the water tanks in India, and they were isolated from the Elbe water during the Hamburg epidemic of 1892. The bacilli are found in the intestine, in the stools from the earliest period of the disease, and very abundantly in the rice-water evacuations, in which they are in almost pure culture. They very rarely occur in the vomitus. Postmortem, they are found in enormous numbers in the intestine also in the gallbladder and biliary tract, urine, lungs and spleen in some cases. In acutely fatal cases they do not seem to invade the intestinal wall, but with a more protracted course they are found in the glands and deeper tissues. Varieties of paracholera organisms are described.

IMMUNITY.—Animals may be immunized by repeated injections of non-fatal doses of the dead and later of the living organisms. The serum of an immunized animal has agglutinative and other antibacterial properties. The blood serum of convalescent patients also possesses these properties.

Modes of Infection.—As in other diseases, individual peculiarities count for much, and during epidemics virulent cholera bacilli have been isolated from the stools of healthy men. Cholera cultures have been swallowed with impunity. The disease is not highly infectious; those in close contact with patients are not often affected. On the other hand, washerwomen and those who handle the linen of the cholera patients, or their stools, are prone to contract the disease. There have been instances of "laboratory cholera," in which students have been accidentally infected while working with the cultures. Vegetables which have been washed in infected water may convey the disease. Milk may also be contaminated. The bacilli live on fresh bread, butter, and meat, for from six to eight days. The possibility of the infection of food by flies should be borne in mind, since the bacilli may live for at least three days in their intestines.

The disease is propagated chiefly by contaminated *water* and the virulence of an epidemic in any region is in direct proportion to the imperfection of its water-supply. In India the demonstration of the connection between drinking-water and cholera infection is complete. The Hamburg epidemic is a remarkable illustration. The unfiltered water of the Elbe was the chief supply, although taken from the river in such a situation that it was directly contaminated by sewage. In August, 1892, there was a sudden explosive epidemic, and within three months nearly 18,000 persons were attacked, with a mortality of 42.3 per cent. The neighboring city of Altona, which also took its water from the Elbe, but which had an efficient filtration system, had in the same period only 516 cases.

Two main types of epidemics are recognized: the first, in which many individuals are attacked simultaneously, as in the Hamburg outbreak, and in which there is widespread contamination of the drinking-water. In the other the cases occur in groups, so-called cholera nests; individuals are not attacked simultaneously, but successively. A direct connection between the cases may be very difficult to trace. Both these types may be combined, and in an epidemic which has started in a widespread infection through water, there may be other outbreaks, examples of the second type. The disease follows the lines of human travel. In India it has, in many notable cases, been spread by pilgrims. Cholera *carriers* have an important influence. In Manila nearly 8 per cent of 376 healthy persons harbored the bacilli.

The disease affects persons of all ages. It is particularly prone to attack the intemperate and those debilitated by want of food and by bad surroundings. Depressing emotions, such as fear, may have an influence. It is doubtful whether an attack furnishes immunity against a second one.

Morbid Anatomy.—A postmortem diagnosis can be made by any competent bacteriologist, as the organism is distinctive. The body has the appearances associated with profound collapse. There is often marked postmortem elevation of temperature. The *rigor mortis* sets in early and may produce displacement of the limbs. The lower jaw has been seen to move, the eyes to rotate and movements of the arms and legs have been noted. The blood is thick and dark, and there is a remarkable diminution in the amount of its water and salts. The peritoneum is sticky, and the coils of intestines are congested and look thin and shrunken. The small intestine usually contains a turbid serum, similar to that passed in the stools. The mucosa is, as a rule, swollen, and in acute cases slightly hyperemic; later the congestion is more marked, especially about the Peyer's patches. The bacilli are found in the contents of the intestine and in the mucous membrane. The spleen is usually small. The liver and kidneys show cloudy swelling, and the latter extensive coagulation-necrosis and destruction of the epithelial cells.

Symptoms.—A period of incubation of uncertain length, probably not more than from two to five days, precedes the onset of the symptoms.

Three stages may be recognized in the attack: the preliminary diarrhea, the collapse stage, and the period of reaction.

THE PRELIMINARY DIARRHEA may set in abruptly without any previous indications. More commonly there are, for one or two days, colicky pains in the abdomen, with looseness of the bowels, perhaps vomiting, with headache and depression of spirits. There may be no fever.

COLLAPSE STAGE.—The diarrhea increases, or without any of the preliminary symptoms, sets in with the greatest intensity, and profuse liquid evacuations succeed each other rapidly. There are in some instances griping pains and tenesmus. More commonly there are exhaustion and collapse. The thirst becomes extreme, the tongue is white; cramps of great severity occur in the legs and feet. Within a few hours vomiting sets in and becomes incessant. The patient sinks into a condition of collapse, the features are shrunken, the skin has an ashy-gray hue, the eyeballs sink in the socket, the nose is pinched, the cheeks are hollow, the voice becomes husky, the extremities are cyanosed, and the skin is shriveled, wrinkled, and covered with perspiration. The temperature sinks and in the axilla or mouth may be subnormal, but in the rectum it may be 103° or 104°. The blood pressure falls greatly and is often below 70 mm. Hg. The pulse becomes extremely feeble and the patient passes into coma, though consciousness is often retained until near the end. Uremia with acidosis is common.

The stools are at first yellowish in color but soon become grayish-white and look like turbid whey or rice-water; whence the term "rice-water stools." Numerous small flakes of mucus and granular matter, and at times blood are found in them. The reaction is usually alkaline. The fluid contains albumin and the chief mineral ingredient is chloride of sodium. Microscopically, mucus and epithelial cells and innumerable bacteria are seen.

The condition of the patient is largely the result of toxemia with concentration of the blood consequent upon the loss of serum in the stools. Acidosis has some influence. The specific gravity of the blood rises to 1.060 to 1.072. There is almost complete arrest of secretion of saliva and urine, but the sweat glands increase in activity, and in nursing women it has been stated that the lacteal flow is unaffected. This stage sometimes lasts not more than two or three hours, but more commonly from twelve to twenty-four.

REACTION STAGE.—When the patient survives the collapse, the cyanosis gradually disappears and warmth returns to the skin, which may have for a time a mottled color or present a definite erythematous rash. The heart's action becomes stronger, the urine increases, the irritability of the stomach disappears, the stools are at longer intervals, and there is no abdominal pain. In the reaction the temperature may not rise above normal. This may be interrupted by a recurrence of diarrhea and the patient dies in a relapse. Others pass into what has been called *cholera-typhoid,* in which the patient is delirious, the pulse rapid and feeble, and the tongue dry. Death finally occurs with coma. These symptoms have been attributed to uremia and acidosis.

During epidemics attacks are found of all grades of severity. There are cases of diarrhea with griping pains, liquid stools, vomiting, and cramps, with slight collapse. They resemble the cases of *cholera nostras.* At the opposite end of the series are the instances of *cholera sicca,* in which death may occur in a few hours after the onset, without diarrhea.

Complications and Sequelae.—The consecutive nephritis rarely induces dropsy. Diphtheritic colitis has been described. There is a special tendency to diphtheritic inflammation of the mucous membranes, particularly of the throat and genitals. Pneumonia and pleurisy may follow, and destructive abscesses may occur in different parts. Suppurative parotitis is not very uncommon. In rare instances local gangrene may occur. A troublesome symptom of convalescence is cramps in the muscles of the arms and legs.

Diagnosis.—Difficulty may occur from *cholera nostras,* the severe choleraic diarrhea which occurs during the summer months in temperate climates. The clinical picture of the two affections is identical. The extreme collapse, vomiting, and rice-water stools, the cramps, the cyanosed appearance, are all seen in the worst forms of cholera nostras. In enfeebled persons death may occur within twelve hours. The diagnosis has to be made by bacteriological methods. Attacks similar to Asiatic cholera are produced in poisoning by arsenic, corrosive sublimate and certain fungi; but a difficulty in diagnosis could scarcely arise.

The *prognosis* is always uncertain, as the mortality ranges in different epidemics from 30 to 80 per cent. Intemperance, debility, and old age are unfavorable conditions. The more rapidly the collapse sets in, the greater is the danger, and as Andral truly says of the malignant form, "It begins where other diseases end—in death." Patients with marked cyanosis and very low temperature rarely recover.

Prophylaxis.—Efficient quarantine has prevented the disease entering England or the United States since 1873. During epidemics the greatest care should be exercised in the disinfection of the stools and linen of the patients. When an epidemic prevails, persons should not drink water unless previously boiled. The milk should be boiled and all food and drinks carefully protected from flies. Uncooked vegetables and salads should not be eaten. As the disease is not more infectious than typhoid fever, the chance of passing safely through an epidemic depends very much upon how far one is able to carry out prophylactic measures thoroughly. Digestive disturbances are to be treated promptly, particularly diarrhea, which so often is a preliminary symptom. For this, opium and large doses of bismuth should be given. Protective inoculation by vaccines has been carried out with success. In epidemics it is important to search for cholera "carriers" and isolate them. The stools from patients should be thoroughly disinfected and protected from flies.

Treatment.—The patient should be at rest in bed, kept warm, and given boiled milk, whey and egg albumen. Water may be given freely. If vomiting occurs food should be withheld and the stomach washed with an alkaline solution. Hot applications to the abdomen should be used and hot baths given if they prove helpful. Favorable results have been reported from the use of cholera bacteriophage. It is best not to attempt to give remedies by the mouth, as they disturb the stomach, but kaolin (a suspension in water given *ad lib.*) appears to be useful if given early. In the collapse stage, writers speak strongly against the use of opium. Undoubtedly it must be given with caution, but, judging from its effects in cholera nostras, it would seem that collapse *per se* is not a contra-indication. Potassium permanganate (gr. ii, 0.13 gm. in keratin coated pills) is given every 15 minutes for two to four hours and then every half hour until the color of the stools is green or yellow. For collapse pituitary extract and caffeine are useful.

Owing to the profuse serous discharges the blood becomes concentrated and to meet this, intravenous injections were introduced by Latta, of Leith, in the epidemic of 1832. Bovell first practised the intravenous injections of milk in Toronto, in the epidemic of 1854. Saline injections, intravenous and into the bowel, have been much used and with great success by the method introduced by Leonard Rogers. The hypertonic solution is composed of sodium chloride, grains 120; potassium chloride, grains 6; calcium chloride, grains 4; water, 1 pint. If the blood pressure is below 70 or the specific gravity of the blood 1.060 or over the hypertonic solution is given intravenously (1500-3000 cc.) and repeated as often as required to keep the blood pressure above 70 and the specific gravity below 1.060. Normal saline solution (500 cc.) with glucose (5 per cent) is given by the bowel every two hours and at longer intervals if the urine increases. If there is suppression of urine with the danger of uremia, sodium chloride 4 gm. and sodium bicarbonate 10 gm. in 500 cc. of water are given intravenously. This treatment has markedly reduced the mortality.

In the stage of reaction sponges should be given if the fever is high and pituitary extract intramuscularly if the blood pressure is low. If diarrhea returns potassium permanganate and kaolin may be given by mouth. The amount of urinary secretion should be watched and if it becomes small in amount, alkaline solutions should be given intravenously or subcutaneously. In convalescence the diet should be simple and a long period of rest advised.

THE PLAGUE

Definition.—A specific, infectious disease, caused by *Bacillus pestis*, and occurring in two chief forms: a bubonic, involving the lymphatic glands, and a pneumonic, causing an acute and rapidly fatal inflammation of the lungs.

History and Geographical Distribution.—The disease was probably not known to the classical Greek writers. The earliest positive account dates from the second century of our era. The plague of Athens and the pestilence of the reign of Marcus Aurelius were apparently not this disease (Payne). From the great plague in the days of Justinian (sixth century) to the middle of the seventeenth century epidemics of varying severity occurred in Europe. Among the most disastrous was the famous "black death" of the fourteenth century, which overran Europe and destroyed a fourth of the population. In the seventeenth century it raged virulently, and during the great plague of London, in 1665, about 70,000 people died. During the eighteenth and nineteenth centuries the ravages of the disease lessened. Throughout the nineteenth century it waned progressively, outbreaks of some extent occurring in Turkey, Asia Minor and Astrakhan; but we had begun to place it among the diseases of the past. We knew that it slumbered in parts of China, and in northwest India, but the outbreak in 1894 at Hongkong showed that the "black death" was still virulent. Since then it has spread over many parts of the world. In Europe, cases have been carried to Marseilles and other Mediterranean ports and to Hamburg and Glasgow. There have been small outbreaks in the United States at intervals from 1907 with infection of rats and ground squirrels.

The distribution in India is chiefly in the Punjab, Bombay, and the United Provinces, which have a combined population of about 100 millions. In these three provinces between 1896 and the middle of 1911, about five and a half million deaths occurred from plague. In the remaining provinces of India, with a population of some 200 millions, only about two millions of plague deaths occurred. The Manchurian outbreak of pneumonic plague in the winter of 1910-11 was one of the most virulent on record, carrying off more than 45,000 persons in a few months.

Etiology.—The specific organism is a bacillus discovered by Kitasato (*Pasteurella pestis*). It resembles somewhat the bacillus of chicken cholera, and grows in a characteristic manner. It occurs in the blood, in the organs of the body and in the sputum, and has also been found in the dust and in the soil of houses in which the patients have lived, but outside the body the life of the bacillus is thought to be short. Bedbugs may harbor it.

The disease prevails most frequently in hot seasons, though an outbreak may occur during the coldest weather. Persons of all ages are attacked. It spreads chiefly among the poor, in the slums of the great cities.

The following conclusions of the Plague Commission (1908) relate to bubonic plague: (*a*) Contagion occurs in less than 3 per cent of the cases, playing a very small part in the general spread of the disease. (*b*) Bubonic plague in man is entirely dependent on the disease in the rat. (*c*) The infection is conveyed from rat to rat and from rat to man solely by means of fleas. (*d*) A case in man is not in itself infectious. (*e*) A large majority of cases occur singly in houses. When more than one case occurs in a house, the attacks are generally nearly simultaneous. (*f*) Plague is usually conveyed from place to place by imported fleas, which are carried by people on their persons or in their baggage. The human agent may himself escape infection. (*g*) Insanitary conditions have no relation to the occurrence of plague, except in so far as they favor infestation by rats. (*h*) The nonepidemic season is bridged over by acute plague in the rat, accompanied by a few cases among human beings.

In the pneumonic form direct infection from one person to another is the common way, as the bacilli are sprayed into the air by coughing. The possibility of the human flea as a carrier must be considered.

Clinical Forms.—PESTIS MINOR.—In this variety, also known as the ambulant, the patient has a few days of fever, with swelling of the glands of the groin, and possibly suppuration. He may not be ill enough to seek medical relief. These cases, often found at the beginning and end of an epidemic, are a very serious danger, as the urine and feces contain bacilli.

Bubonic Plague.—This constitutes the common variety with a usual incubation period of three or four days. The stage of invasion is characterized by headache, backache, stiffness of the limbs, a feeling of anxiety and restlessness, and great depression of spirits. There is a steady rise in the fever until the third or fourth day, when there is a drop of two or three degrees. There is then a secondary fever, in which the temperature reaches a still higher point. The tongue becomes brown, collapse symptoms are apt to supervene, and in very severe infections the patient may die at this stage. In at least two-thirds of all cases there are glandular swellings or buboes. The inguinal and femoral glands, the axillary glands and the submaxillary and cervical glands are involved in that order as regards frequency. The swelling appears usually from the third to the fifth day. Resolution may occur, or suppuration, or in rare cases gangrene. Suppuration is a favorable feature, as noted by De Foe in his graphic account of the London plague. There is a high leukocytosis.

Petechiae are common and may be extensive. These have been called the "plague spots," or the "tokens of the disease," and gave to it in the middle ages the name of the Black Death. Hemorrhages from the mucous membranes may also occur; in some epidemics hemoptysis has been especially frequent. The hemorrhagic features are due to toxic injury of the endothelial lining.

Septicemic Plague.—In this, the most rapid form, the patient succumbs in three or four days with a virulent infection before the buboes appear. Hemorrhages are common. The bacilli can be obtained from the blood.

Pneumonic Plague.—In the ordinary bubonic type, pneumonia is not uncommon, but the true pneumonic plague begins abruptly with fever, shortness of breath, cough, and sometimes pain in the chest. The fever increases, the signs of the involvement of the lung occur early; there may be impaired resonance at both bases with harsh and tubular breathing; the sputum becomes bloody and is more fluid than in ordinary pneumonia. Cyanosis is an early feature; the pulse is small and rapid; the spleen enlarges rapidly, as early as the second day, and a fatal result follows in from two to four days. Recovery is very rare.

In other varieties the chief manifestations may be in the skin and subcutaneous tissues, or in the intestines, causing diarrhea and sometimes the features of typhoid fever.

Diagnosis.—At the early stage of an outbreak plague cases are easily overlooked, but if the suspicious cases are studied by a competent bacteriologist, there is no disease which can be more positively identified. The San Francisco epidemic illustrates this. The nature of the cases was recognized by Kellog and by Kinyoun, but with an amazing stupidity (which was shared by not a few physicians, who should have known better) the Governor of the State refused to recognize the presence of plague, and the United States Government had to intervene and send a board of experts to settle the question. The finding of marked lymph node swelling may suggest the diagnosis, but a definite conclusion must depend on the bacteriological study. Acute, rapidly fatal pneumonia or septicemia should arouse suspicion.

Prophylaxis.—A careful watch should be kept on the mortality of rats. Epidemics in rats precede human epidemics. When found infected, energetic measures should be taken to destroy them. Three things are necessary—the cleansing of premises, particularly stables and outhouses, so that rats cannot find nesting places or food; systematic rat destruction; and making buildings rat proof. Certain measures prevent the access of plague to healthy ports; fumigation of ships to destroy the rats, careful inspection of passengers and crew, and detention over a period which covers the incubation of the disease.

When a centre becomes infected, the sanitary organization should carry out the segregation of the sick in hospitals, the disinfection of infected rooms, destruction of infected bedding, and thorough cleansing of the entire district; old, badly infected buildings should be destroyed.

Preventive Inoculation.—Haffkine's vaccine has given satisfactory results both in prevention of the disease and in reducing the mortality if the disease should develop after inoculation. The protection lasts for six to twelve months.

Treatment.—In a disease the mortality of which may reach as high as 80 or 90 per cent the question of treatment resolves itself into making the patient as comfortable as possible, and following out certain general principles. Cantlie recommends purgation and stimulation from the outset, and the use of morphia for the pain. The local treatment of the buboes is important. Hot applications are made to them; incision should be done if suppuration occurs. The pyrexia is best treated by hydrotherapy. A plague serum, chiefly the Lustig and the Yersin-Roux, has been used. Doses of 100-200 cc. are necessary. Plague bacteriophage has been used but its value is not established.

TETANUS (LOCKJAW)

Definition.—An infectious disease characterized by tonic spasms of the muscles with marked exacerbations. The tetanus bacillus occurs in earth, in putrefying fluids, and manure, and is a normal inhabitant of the intestines of many animals.

Etiology.—In the United States, according to Anders and Morgan, it is most frequent in the Hudson valley, in Long Island and in the Atlantic States. In 1930 there were 1,287 deaths from tetanus in the U. S. registration area, of which 136 were in children under one year. A large number of cases followed the accidents of the July 4th celebrations, but the propaganda of the Journal of the American Medical Association succeeded in reducing these fatalities in a remarkable way. In England the disease is not very common. There were 121 deaths in 1931. It is more prevalent in certain districts, *e.g.*, the Thames valley. It is more common in the summer months and males are more frequently attacked than females.

In the tropics tetanus is a much more severe disease especially in infants. For years the island of St. Kilda, one of the Western Hebrides, was scourged by the "eight days sickness" among the new born. Of 125 children, 84 died within fourteen days of birth. Since the introduction of proper methods of treating the umbilical cord the disease has practically disappeared.

The tetanus bacillus has contaminated vaccines, and its presence in commercial gelatine is a danger. Outbreaks have occurred in hospitals from infected catgut. The disease has occurred after use of a hypodermic needle and has followed the use of gelatine as a hemostatic.

The disease usually follows an injury and particularly lacerated wounds of the hands which have been contaminated by dirt and splinters. It may occur without any recognizable wound, so-called idiopathic tetanus.

THE TETANUS BACILLUS.—The organism is widely diffused in earth, in garden mould, in and about stables and farmyards, and is a normal inhabitant of the intestines of many herbivora. Living bacilli occur in the intestines of 5 per cent of healthy men and up to 20 per cent of hostlers and dairymen. It is a slender motile bacillus, one end of which is swollen and occupied by a spore. It is anaërobic and grows at ordinary temperatures. The spores are the most resistant known. From two steel nibs dipped in a tetanus culture in 1891 a growth of virulent bacilli was obtained from one in 1902 and from the other in 1909 (Semple). The spores may remain in the tissues for months. The toxin is very virulent. Whereas the fatal dose of strychnine for a man weighing 70 kilos is from 30 to 100 mgm. that of the tetanus toxin is estimated at 0.23 mgm. Every feature of the disease can be produced by it experimentally without the presence of the bacilli. Abel holds that the toxin is carried by the blood and not by the nerves or lymphatics; it may be excreted in the urine of patients. A high degree of antitoxic immunity can be conferred on animals, which then yield a protective serum. It is stated that the blood serum of persons with the bacilli in the intestines contains antitoxin which must give some degree of immunity.

Morbid Anatomy.—No characteristic lesions have been found in the cord or in the brain. Congestions occur in different parts, and perivascular exudations and granular changes in the nerve cells have been found. The condition of the wound is variable. The nerves are often found injured, reddened, and swollen. In tetanus neonatorum the umbilicus may be inflamed.

Symptoms.—The incubation period is from one to twenty days. Of 1,092 cases (E. W. Hill) in 17.49 per cent it was from one to five days and in 55.06 per cent from five to ten days. In only 8 cases was the incubation as long as twenty days. If the disease develops after antitoxin has been given for prevention, the incubation period may be greatly prolonged. The patient complains at first of slight stiffness in the neck, or a feeling of tightness in the jaws, or difficulty in mastication. Occasionally chilly feelings or actual rigors may precede these symptoms. Sometimes the muscles near the wound show spasticity and increased excitability early. Gradually a tonic spasm of the muscles of these parts produces the condition of trismus or lockjaw. The eyebrows may be raised and the angles of the mouth drawn out, causing the so-called sardonic grin—*risus sardonicus.* In children the spasm may be confined to these parts. Sometimes the attack is associated with paralysis of the facial muscles and difficulty in swallowing, which has most commonly followed injuries in the neighborhood of the fifth nerve. Gradually the process extends and involves the muscles of the body. Those of the back are most affected, so that during the spasm the victim may rest upon the head and heels—*opisthotonos.* The rectus abdominis muscle has been torn across in the spasm. The entire trunk and limbs may be perfectly rigid—*orthotonos.* Flexion to one side is less common—*pleurothotonos;* while spasm of the muscles of the abdomen may cause the body to be bent forward—*emprosthotonos.* In very violent attacks the thorax is compressed, the respirations are rapid, and spasm of the glottis may occur, causing asphyxia. The paroxysms are momentary or last for several seconds but even in the intervals *the relaxation is not complete.* The slightest irritation is sufficient to cause a spasm. The paroxysms are associated with agonizing pain, and the patient may be held as in a vice, unable to utter a word. Usually he is bathed in a profuse sweat. The temperature may remain normal or show only a slight elevation toward the close. In other cases fever is marked from the outset; the temperature reaches 105° or 106°, and before death 109° or 110°. The leukocytes are increased. The spinal fluid usually shows increased pressure with a normal cell count and negative globulin test. The course is sometimes very rapid, with fever and general spasms; death may take place on the third day. Death occurs during the paroxysm from heart failure or asphyxia, or is due to exhaustion.

In those who have been given antitoxin as a preventive there may be anomalous forms. The onset of symptoms may be delayed for weeks or months and may be determined by a secondary operation. *Local tetanus* may be limited to muscles near the wound or to an extremity. In *chronic tetanus* the symptoms appear late, are not severe and may persist for a long time. *Cephalic tetanus* originates usually from a wound of the head, and is characterized by stiffness of the muscles of the jaw and paralysis of the facial muscles on the same side as the wound, with difficulty in swallowing. There may be no other symptoms. The progress is good in the chronic cases, which may show slight symptoms only.

Tetanus neonatorum occurs particularly in hot climates and in districts where the tetanus bacillus is very prevalent. The infection follows imperfect treatment of the navel. The symptoms may come on in a few days or be delayed for ten days. Trismus and difficulty in crying and taking food are the earliest symptoms, followed in a few days by more general spasms. It is very fatal. A form known as *visceral tetanus* is described by the French in which the disease originates in the intestines, and the possibility of this must be considered, as the organism may be present in the human intestine. *Post-operative tetanus* occurs particularly after peritoneal operations in a large proportion of which catgut has been used. It is very fatal with a short incubation and rapid course. Operation on an individual who has recently recovered from tetanus may cause a relapse.

Diagnosis.—Well-marked cases following a trauma could not be mistaken for any other disease. The spasms are not unlike those of *strychnia poisoning,* and in the celebrated Palmer murder trial this was the plea for the defence. The jaw-muscles, however, are never involved early, if at all, and between the paroxysms in strychnia poisoning there is no rigidity. In *tetany* the distribution of the spasm at the extremities, the peculiar position, the greater involvement of the hands, and the condition under which it occurs make the diagnosis clear. In doubtful cases cultures should be made from the pus of the wound. In rabies there is the history of a bite, there is no continuous rigidity and the spasms are particularly of the muscles of respiration and deglutition. In meningitis and hysteria a careful examination should prevent error. A mild trismus may occur with throat and mouth infection and should not be mistaken for head tetanus.

Escherich described in children a form of generalized tonic contractures of the muscles of the jaw, neck, back, and limbs, usually a sequel of some acute infection, occasionally occurring as an independent malady. The contractures may be intermittent or persistent. The condition may last from a week to a couple of months. The patients as a rule recover.

Prognosis.—Two of the Hippocratic aphorisms express tersely the general prognosis: "The spasm supervening on a wound is fatal," and "such persons as are seized with tetanus die within four days, or if they pass these they recover." Of 1,264 cases (E. W. Hill) only 414 recovered. If the disease lasts beyond the tenth day the patient has an even chance, and from this time the prognosis improves. The mortality is greatest in children. Favorable indications are: late onset of the attack, localization to the muscles of the neck and jaw, an absence of fever, anomalous forms and a prompt administration of antitoxin after the injury.

Prophylaxis.—Suspicious wounds should be freely opened and thoroughly disinfected by hydrogen peroxide and iodine. In districts where the disease prevails, special precautions should be taken with all injuries, and a prophylactic dose of antitetanic serum (500 to 1,500 units) administered. It should be carried out promptly in all street and infected injuries. As the serum is expensive, Boards of Health should arrange, if necessary, to provide it. The experience of the Great War showed the value of antitoxin as a preventive. In the U. S. Civil War the incidence was one case of tetanus among 487 wounded; in the U. S. troops in the Great War it was one among 6,224 wounded. Tetanus *toxoid* can be used to secure active immunity in those exposed to the possibility of wounds which may be infected with tetanus. This causes the production of tetanus antitoxin in the blood and the immunity (produced in 3 to 6 months) lasts probably for several years. Two doses of 1 cc. are given 2 or 3 months apart.

Treatment.—The patient should be kept in a darkened room, absolutely quiet, and attended by only one person. All possible sources of irritation should be avoided. Veterinarians appreciate the importance of this complete seclusion in treating horses.

When the lockjaw is extreme the patient may not be able to take food by the mouth and it is best to feed by a catheter passed through the nose. The spasms should be controlled by chloroform, which may be repeatedly used. It is well to keep the patient thoroughly under the influence of morphia given hypodermically. Chloral hydrate, chloretone, and bromide of potassium may be helpful. Phenobarbital (luminal) may be effectual, 3-5 grains (0.2-0.3 gm.) being given by mouth or rectum every few hours. Avertin may be used as for anesthesia or sodium amytal given intravenously. Intraspinal injections of a solution of magnesium sulphate (25 per cent) have been used (Meltzer); 1 cc. is injected for every 25 pounds weight of the patient. *Tetanus antitoxin* should be given promptly and in sufficient dosage, the object being to saturate the patient as quickly as possible. The wound should be cleaned, if necessary, and left open with a dry sterile dressing; 5,000 units of antitoxin should be injected about the wound. The antitoxin should be given intravenously (20,000 to 50,000 units) with the usual precaution of a preliminary skin test; the serum is given slowly, diluted with an equal volume of salt solution. Lumbar or cisternal puncture is done—for which an anesthetic is generally advisable—and if possible 10,000 units are given intraspinally. The same dosage, intravenously and intraspinally, is given on the two following days. Intramuscular injections of 10,000 units are given daily. Improvement may suggest a decrease in the dosage on the second or third day but it must be remembered that the failure of antitoxin in *treatment* has often been due to insufficient dosage. Some suggest much larger doses especially intravenously. Smaller doses can be given to young children. Sometimes after a period of improvement severe symptoms recur. In this event the serum should be given again intravenously and intraspinally.

GLANDERS

(*Farcy*)

Definition.—An infectious disease of the horse and ass, caused by *Bacillus mallei,* communicated occasionally to man, characterized by the formation of nodules, chiefly in the nares (glanders) and beneath the skin (farcy).

Etiology.—The disease belongs to the infective granulomata. The specific germ is a short, nonmotile bacillus, not unlike that of tubercle, but it exhibits different staining reactions. It grows readily on the ordinary culture media. For the full recognition of glanders in man we are indebted to Rayer, whose monograph remains one of the best descriptions of the disease. Man becomes infected by contact with diseased animals, and usually by inoculation on an abraded surface. In a Montreal case a man was probably infected by the material expelled from the nostril of his horse, which was not suspected of having the disease. It is a rare disease. Only 5 deaths were registered in England and Wales from 1921 to 1931 inclusive, and 1 death in the U. S. registration area for 1930. Among laboratory workers the *Bacillus mallei* has caused a number of deaths and in working with it the greatest precautions should be taken.

Morbid Anatomy.—The disease may be localized in the nose (glanders) or beneath the skin (farcy). The essential lesion is the granulomatous tumor, with numerous lymphoid and epithelioid cells, among and in which are the glanders bacilli. These nodular masses tend to break down rapidly, and on the mucous membrane result in ulcers, while beneath the skin they form abscesses. The nodules may occur in the internal organs.

Symptoms.—An acute and a chronic form of glanders may be recognized in man, and an acute and a chronic form of farcy.

Acute Glanders.—The period of incubation is rarely more than three or four days. There are signs of general febrile disturbance. At the site of infection there are swelling, redness, and lymphangitis. Within two or three days there is involvement of the mucous membrane of the nose, the nodules break down rapidly to ulcers, and there is a mucopurulent discharge. An eruption of bullae or papules, which rapidly become pustules, breaks out over the face and about the joints. It has been mistaken for variola. There may be areas in the subcutaneous tissue which break down; gangrene may follow. There is a great swelling of the nose. There may be an eruption like erysipelas. The ulceration may go on to necrosis, in which case the discharge is very offensive. The lymph glands of the neck are usually much enlarged. This form runs its course in about eight or ten days, and is invariably fatal. *Glanders pneumonia* may appear after subcutaneous infection (one case from infection with a hypodermic syringe stuck into the thumb). Grossly the lung appeared like a caseous pneumonia.

CHRONIC GLANDERS is rare and is usually mistaken for a chronic coryza. There are ulcers in the nose and often laryngeal symptoms. It may last for months and recovery sometimes takes place. Tedeschi described a case of chronic osteomyelitis, due to the *B. mallei,* which was followed by a fatal glanders meningitis. The diagnosis may be extremely difficult. In such cases a suspension of the secretion, or of cultures upon agar-agar made from the secretion, should be injected into the peritoneal cavity of a male guinea-pig. At the end of two days, in positive cases, the testicles are swollen and the skin of the scrotum reddened. The testicles continue to increase in size and finally suppurate. Death takes place after two or three weeks, and generalized glanders nodules are found in the viscera. The use of *mallein* for diagnostic purposes is highly recommended.

ACUTE FARCY in man results usually from an inoculation into the skin. There is an intense local reaction with a phlegmonous inflammation. The lymphatics are early affected, and along their course there are nodular subcutaneous enlargements, the so-called *farcy buds,* which may rapidly go on to suppuration. There are pains and swelling in the joints, and abscesses may form in the muscles. The symptoms are those of an acute infection, almost like an acute septicemia. The nose is not involved and the superficial skin eruption is not common. The bacilli have been found in the urine in acute cases in man and animals. The disease is fatal in a large proportion of the cases, usually in from twelve to fifteen days.

CHRONIC FARCY is characterized by the presence of localized tumors which break down into abscesses, and sometimes form deep ulcers, without much inflammatory reaction and without special involvement of the lymphatics. The disease may last for months or years. Death results from pyemia or acute glanders develops. The French veterinarian Bouley had it and recovered.

Diagnosis.—The occupation is very important. The acute forms may be mistaken for smallpox or septicopyemia and the chronic forms for syphilis or tuberculosis. In cases of doubt the inoculation should be made in animals or the complement fixation test used. In the acute cases there is very little hope. In the chronic cases recovery is possible, though often tedious.

Treatment.—If seen early, the site of inoculation should be excised or destroyed by caustics and an antiseptic dressing applied. The farcy buds should be opened early. Antiseptic solutions such as potassium permanganate and hydrogen peroxide should be used. Vaccine treatment may be tried cautiously with doses from 10 to 100 millions every two to four days in chronic cases. Increase in dosage must be governed by the reaction. Those handling the patient should take great care to avoid infection.

Melioidosis, a disease of the Far East, is caused by *Bacillus whitmori,* closely related to *B. mallei.* It occurs in rodents and man is infected from them. The lesion is a caseous nodule which breaks down or coalesces into large caseous masses, especially in the lungs. In acute cases there are vomiting, diarrhea and collapse with death in a few days. In less acute forms there are fever, multiple abscesses and caseation, and toxemia. Recovery is rare. The *diagnosis* depends on finding the organism in the blood, urine, sputum or abscesses. The *treatment* is symptomatic.

ANTHRAX

(*Splenic Fever; Charbon; Wool-sorter's Disease*)

Definition.—An acute infectious disease caused by *Bacillus anthracis*, occurring in three forms, cutaneous, pulmonary and intestinal. In animals, particularly sheep and cattle, the disease has the character of an acute septicemia with enlargement of the spleen—hence the name *splenic* fever. In man it occurs sporadically or as a result of accidental inoculation.

Etiology.—*Baccilus anthracis* is a nonmotile, rod-shaped organism with a length of from 2 to 25 μ; the rods are often united. The bacilli themselves are readily destroyed, but the spores are very resistant, and survive after prolonged immersion in a 5 per cent solution of phenol, or withstand for some minutes a temperature of 212°. They are capable of resisting gastric digestion. Outside the body the spores are very durable.

In Animals.—Geographically and zoölogically the disease is widespread and is much more prevalent in Europe and Asia than in America. Its ravages among the herds of cattle in Russia and Siberia, and among sheep in parts of Europe, are not equalled by any other animal plague. In the United States anthrax is not very prevalent. In France from 6 to 10 per cent of the sheep and about 5 per cent of the cattle formerly died of it.

The disease is conveyed sometimes by direct inoculation, as by the bites and stings of insects, by feeding on carcasses of animals which have died of the disease, but more commonly by grazing in pastures contaminated by the germs. Pasteur thought that the earthworm played an important part in bringing to the surface the bacilli from the buried carcass of an infected animal. Certain fields may thus be infected for an indefinite period. It seems probable that, if the carcass is not opened or the blood spilt, spores are not formed in the buried animal and the bacilli quickly die.

In man the disease results from an infection through the skin, intestines or lungs. Workers in wool and hair, and persons whose occupations bring them into contact with animals or animal products, as stablemen, shepherds, tanners, and butchers, are specially liable to the disease. In the United States the disease is usually found in the workers in hides, in butchers, and in veterinarians. Cases have resulted from the use of infected shaving brushes. It is rare in general hospital work. In the United States there was an average of 33 deaths a year from 1911 to 1920 in the registration area and in 1930, 15 deaths; in England and Wales from 1921-1931 inclusive there were 98 deaths. Ponder states that 40 per cent of the cases of anthrax in British leather workers are due to handling Chinese or East Indian goods; 80 per cent of the cases are due to skin infection while handling hides at the docks or in tanneries.

Various forms of the disease have been described, and two chief groups may be recognized: the external anthrax and the internal anthrax, of which there are pulmonary and intestinal forms.

Symptoms.—External Anthrax.—The incubation period is one to three days. At the site of inoculation, usually on an unprotected exposed surface—the hands, arms, neck, or face—there are, within a few hours, itching and uneasiness, and the gradual formation of a small papule, which soon becomes vesicular. Inflammatory induration extends around this, and within thirty-six hours at the site of inoculation there is a dark brownish eschar, at a little distance from which there may be a series of small vesicles. There is usually some pus below the scab. The brawny induration may be extreme. The edema produces very great swelling of the parts. The inflammation extends along the lymphatics, and the neighboring lymph glands are swollen and sore. The fever at first rises rapidly, and the concomitant phenomena are marked. Subsequently the temperature falls, and in many cases becomes subnormal. Death may take place in from three to five days. In patients who recover the constitutional symptoms are slighter, the eschar gradually sloughs out and the wound heals. The cases vary much in severity. In the mildest form there may be only slight swelling. At the site of inoculation a papule is formed, which rapidly becomes vesicular and dries into a scab, which separates in the course of a few days.

A form in which edema is marked occurs in the eyelid, and also in the head, hand, and arm, and is characterized by the absence of the papule and vesicle forms, and by the most extensive *edema,* which is associated with the presence of anthracomucin. The edema reaches such a grade of intensity that gangrene results, and may involve a considerable area. The constitutional symptoms are extremely grave and the cases usually prove fatal. The progress in this form may be very rapid.

The greatest fatality is seen with inoculation about the head and face, when the mortality, according to Nasarow, is 26 per cent; the least in infection of the lower extremities, when it is 5 per cent.

In a case at the Johns Hopkins Hospital in 1895, in a hair-picker, there were most extensive enteritis, peritonitis, and endocarditis, which last lesion has been described by Eppinger. Meningitis has also occurred.

A feature in both these forms is the absence of feelings of distress or anxiety on the part of the patient, whose mental condition may be perfectly clear. He may be without any apprehension, even though the condition be most critical. In some cases there is no fever.

The *diagnosis* in most instances is readily made from the character of the lesion and the occupation of the patient. There is a remarkable freedom from pain which distinguishes anthrax from furuncle, carbuncle and cellulitis. When in doubt, the examination of the fluid from the pustule or beneath the scab may show anthrax bacilli. Cultures should be made, or a mouse or guinea-pig inoculated from the local lesion. The blood may not show the bacilli in numbers until shortly before death.

INTERNAL ANTHRAX.—*Intestinal Form.*—In these cases the infection results from eating the flesh or drinking the milk of diseased animals; it may, however, follow an external infection if the germs are carried to the mouth. Butler and Huber described an epidemic in which twenty-five persons were attacked after eating the flesh of an animal which had had anthrax. Six died in from forty-eight hours to seven days. The symptoms are those of intense poisoning. The disease may set in with a chill, followed by vomiting, diarrhea, moderate fever, and pains in the legs and back. It may be mistaken for intestinal obstruction. In acute cases there are dyspnea, cyanosis, great anxiety and restlessness, and toward the end convulsions or spasms of the muscles. Hemorrhage may occur from the mucous membranes. Occasionally there are small phlegmonous areas or petechiae on the skin. The spleen is enlarged.

The blood is dark and remains fluid for a long time after death. Late in the course the bacilli may be found in the blood.

Wool-sorter's Disease, Pulmonary Anthrax.—This form occurs in establishments in which wool or hair is sorted and cleansed. The hair and wool imported from Russia and South America appear to have induced the largest number of cases. Many of these show no external lesion. The infective material has been swallowed or inhaled with the dust. There are rarely premonitory symptoms. The patient is seized with a chill, becomes faint and prostrated, has pains in the back and legs, and the temperature rises to 102° or 103°. The breathing is rapid, and he complains of much pain in the chest. There may be a cough and signs of bronchitis. The pulse is feeble and very rapid. There may be vomiting, and death may occur within twenty-four hours with profound collapse. Other cases are more protracted, and there may be diarrhea, delirium, and unconsciousness. The cerebral symptoms may be intense; in at least four cases the brain seems to have been chiefly affected and its capillaries stuffed with bacilli (Merkel). The recognition of wool-sorter's disease as a form of anthrax is due to J. H. Bell, of Bradford.

In certain instances the symptoms of internal anthrax are associated with the external lesions of malignant pustule. Meningitis may occur with anthrax bacilli in the spinal fluid.

The *rag-picker's disease* was studied by Eppinger who showed that it is a local anthrax of the lungs and pleura, with general infection.

Prognosis.—The disease is always serious and recovery is rare in the internal forms. Cutaneous lesions about the face are more serious than elsewhere; the mortality was high in the cases due to infected shaving brushes. Marked toxemia and the occurrence of bacilli in the blood are ominous. Meddlesome treatment of the local lesion renders the outlook more serious. The average case of external anthrax usually does well.

Prophylaxis.—This is important, and should be carried out by rigid disinfection of hair, and rags before they are placed in the hands of workmen. Those handling infected material should have the arms and neck covered and wear gloves. Wounds in such workers should be promptly disinfected. Animals may be immunized against the disease and Pasteur's method of vaccination has been employed in France with good results. The immunity is lost within a year in nearly 50 per cent of the animals.

Treatment.—In the cutaneous form, the local lesion should be left alone, as surgical treatment may spread the infection. The part should be kept absolutely at rest, without any dressing and exposed to the air. The anti-anthrax serum should be injected around the area in amounts of 10 to 15 cc. every four hours. The serum has given good results and should be given except in mild cases. An initial dose of 100 to 150 cc. is given intravenously with the usual precautions and repeated each 24 hours for one or two days depending on the condition. The general treatment is that of an acute infection. In malignant forms, particularly the intestinal cases, little can be done. Active purgatives may be given at the outset, so as to remove the infecting material. The use of normal bovine serum (20-30 cc. heated twice for half an hour to 56° C.) intravenously appears to give good results. Benefit is reported from bacteriophage. Neoarsphenamine has been used (0.9 gram intravenously, given daily for two or three doses).

HAVERHILL FEVER: ERYTHEMA ARTHRITICUM EPIDEMICUM

Definition.—An infectious disease characterized by fever, rash and arthritis.

History.—In 1926, Place, Sutton and Willner described the occurrence of this disease in Haverhill, Mass., and studied 45 cases. The organism obtained was studied by Parker and Hudson. Beach and Hazard (1932) report a case which was thoroughly studied.

Etiology.—The source of infection is not known but conveyance by milk has been suspected. The organism, *Haverillia multiformis,* shows marked polymorphism influenced greatly by the medium on which it is grown. An average size is 2 to 5 microns in length and 0.1 to 0.4 microns in width. It is gram negative. The organism agglutinates with the patient's serum.

Clinical Features.—The onset is sudden, sometimes with a chill, followed by malaise, severe headache, fever, vomiting in some cases, and prostration. Sore throat occurs in some cases. The temperature may reach 105° soon after the onset and usually subsides by the third or fourth day. The *rash* appears early, increases for two or three days and persists for three to seven days. It consists of dull red maculopapular lesions of 2 to 4 mm. in diameter, mostly on the extensor surfaces of the arms and legs, and about the joints, occasionally on the trunk and face. The rash is sometimes hemorrhagic. Desquamation follows in some cases. The *arthritis* appears in the first few days and varies from slight involvement to severe swelling with effusion. Both large and small joints are involved. The arthritic manifestations may persist for a few days or as long as two weeks. There may be a leukocytosis but this is not constant.

Diagnosis.—The association of clinical features should suggest the diagnosis. A positive blood culture and agglutination test are necessary for definite proof.

Treatment.—This is largely symptomatic, acetylsalicylic acid for the pain, hydrotherapy for the fever, and local applications to the affected joints.

LEPROSY

Definition.—A chronic infectious disease caused by *Bacillus leprae,* characterized by the presence of tubercular nodules in the skin and mucous membranes (tubercular leprosy) or by changes in the nerves (anesthetic leprosy). At first these forms may be separate, but ultimately are combined, and in the characteristic tubercular form there are disturbances of sensation.

History.—The disease appears to have prevailed in Egypt as far back as three or four thousand years B. C. The Hebrew writers refer to it, but, as is evident from the description in Leviticus, different forms of skin disease were embraced under the term leprosy. Both in India and China the affection was known before the Christian era. The old Greek and Roman physicians were familiar with its manifestations. Evidence of a pre-Columbian existence of leprosy in America has been sought in the Peruvian pottery representing deformities suggestive of this disease. Throughout the Middle Ages leprosy prevailed extensively in Europe, largely spread by the crusades, and the number of leper asylums has been estimated as at least 20,000. During the sixteenth century it gradually declined.

Geographical Distribution.—In Europe leprosy prevails in Iceland, Norway and Sweden, parts of Russia, particularly about Dorpat, Riga, and the Caucasus, and in certain provinces of Spain and Portugal. In Great Britain there are about 500 recognized cases. In Canada there are a few lepers in New Brunswick and British Columbia (nearly all Chinese). The number has gradually lessened. The disease appears to have been imported from Normandy about the end of the eighteenth century.

Leprosy is endemic in the West India Islands and also occurs in Mexico and Brazil. In the Sandwich Islands it spread rapidly after 1860, and strenuous attempts have been made to stamp it out by segregating all lepers on the island of Molokai. In British India there are a large number of lepers. In China leprosy prevails extensively and in Africa it has increased rapidly. In Australia, New Zealand, and the Australasian islands it also prevails, chiefly among the Chinese. It occurs both in Central and South America. It is estimated that there are about 3,000,000 lepers in the world.

Etiology.—*Bacillus leprae* (*Mycobacterium leprae*) discovered by Hansen, of Bergen, is recognized as the cause of the disease. It has many points of resemblance to the tubercle bacillus, but can be readily differentiated. The organism has been grown by special methods.

MODES OF INFECTION.—*Inoculation.*—While it is highly probable that leprosy may be contracted by accidental inoculation, the experimental evidence is inconclusive. With one possible exception, negative results have followed the attempts to reproduce the disease in man. The Hawaiian convict, under sentence of death, who was inoculated on September 30, 1884, by Arning, four weeks later had rheumatoid pains and gradual painful swelling of the ulnar and median nerves. The neuritis gradually subsided, but a small lepra tubercle developed at the site of the inoculation. In 1887 the disease was manifest, and the man died of it six years after inoculation. The case is not regarded as conclusive, as he had leprous relatives and lived in a leprous country. Insects may take up the bacilli.

Heredity.—For years it was thought that the disease was transmitted from parent to child, but opinion is now against this view. The possibility of its transmission cannot be denied, and in this respect leprosy and tuberculosis occupy very much the same position, though men with very wide experience have never seen a newborn leper. The youngest cases are rarely under two years of age.

By Infection.—The bacilli are given off from the open sores; they are found in the saliva and expectoration of patients with leprous lesions in the mouth and throat, and occur in large numbers in the nasal secretion. Sticker found in 153 lepers, subjects of both forms of the disease, bacilli in the nasal secretion in 128, and herein, he thinks, lies the chief source of danger. Schaffer collected lepra bacilli on clean slides placed on tables and floors near to lepers whom he had caused to read aloud. The bacilli have also been isolated from the urine and the milk of patients. It seems probable that they may enter the body through the mucous membranes and by abrasions of the skin. Sticker believes that the initial lesion is in an ulcer above the cartilaginous part of the nasal septum. One of the most striking examples of the infectiousness of leprosy is the following: "In 1860, a girl who had hitherto lived at Holstfershof, where no leprosy existed, married and went to live at Tarwast with her mother-in-law, who was a leper. She remained healthy, but her three children (1, 2, 3) became leprous, as also her younger sister (4), who came on a visit to Tarwast and slept with the children. The younger sister developed leprosy after returning to Holstfershof. At the latter place a man (5), fifty-two years old, who married one of the 'younger sister's' children, acquired leprosy; also a relative (6), thirty-six years old, a tailor by occupation, who frequented the house, and his wife (7), who came from a place where no leprosy existed." There is evidence that the disease may be spread by infected clothing.

CONDITIONS INFLUENCING INFECTION.—The disease attacks persons of all ages but infection is rare after the age of thirty. Evidently intimate contact is essential. The doctors, nurses and Sisters of Charity who care for the patients are very rarely attacked. In the lazaretto at Tracadie not one of the Sisters who have so faithfully nursed the lepers contracted the disease. Father Damien, in the Sandwich Islands, and Father Boblioli, in New Orleans, both fell victims in the discharge of their priestly duties.

Morbid Anatomy.—The leprosy tubercles consist of granulomatous tissue made up of cells of various sizes in a connective tissue matrix. The bacilli in extraordinary numbers lie partly between and partly in the cells. The process gradually involves the skin, giving rise to tuberous outgrowths with intervening areas of ulceration or cicatrization, which in the face may gradually produce the so-called *facies leontina.* The mucous membranes, particularly the conjunctiva, the cornea, and the larynx, may gradually be involved. In many cases deep ulcers form which result in extensive loss of substance or loss of fingers or toes, the so-called *lepra mutilans.* In anesthetic leprosy there is a peripheral *neuritis* due to the development of the bacilli in the nerve-fibres. Indeed, this involvement of the nerves plays a primary part in the etiology of many of the important features, particularly the trophic changes in the skin and the disturbances of sensation.

Clinical Forms.—TUBERCULAR LEPROSY.—Prior to the appearance of the nodules there are areas of cutaneous erythema which may be sharply defined and often hyperesthetic. This is sometimes known as *macular* leprosy. The affected spots in time become pigmented. In some instances this superficial change continues without the development of nodules, the areas become anesthetic, the pigment gradually disappears, and the skin gets perfectly white—the *lepra alba.* In the early stage there may be a patchy erythema with slight swelling of the skin. The nodules or tubercles appear, sometimes after recurrences of the rash, and may be fairly general. They may gradually disappear but often break down and form ulcers which may involve large areas. There are recurring attacks of irregular fever. The eyelashes and eyebrows and the hairs on the face fall out. The mucous membranes finally become involved, particularly in the mouth, throat, and larynx; the voice becomes harsh and finally aphonic. Death may result from the laryngeal complications and pneumonia, but usually from cachexia after an average period of ten years. The conjunctivae are frequently attacked, and the sight is lost by a leprous keratitis.

ANESTHETIC LEPROSY.—This form has, in characteristic cases, no external resemblance to the other variety. It usually begins with pains in the limbs and areas of hyperesthesia or numbness. Maculae appear upon the trunk and extremities, and after persisting for a variable time gradually disappear, leaving areas of anesthesia, but the loss of sensation may come on independently of the outbreak of maculae. Trophic changes may appear very early. The nerve trunks, where superficial, may be felt to be large and nodular. The trophic disturbances are usually marked. Pemphigus-like bullae break and leave ulcers which may be very destructive. The fingers and toes are liable to contractures and to necrosis, so that in chronic cases the phalanges are lost. The course of this form is very chronic and it may persist for years without much deformity. We knew a prominent clergyman who had anesthetic leprosy for over thirty years, which did not seriously interfere with his usefulness, and not in the slightest with his career.

Prognosis.—The outlook for recovery is improved by modern treatment. Lepers usually die of tuberculosis, nephritis or sepsis, rarely of leprosy alone. With involvement of the larynx and generally in the nodular form, the prognosis is more serious.

Diagnosis.—Even in the early stage the dusky erythematous maculae with hyperesthesia or areas of anesthesia are very characteristic. In an advanced grade neither the tubercular nor anesthetic form is likely to be mistaken. Lupus and syphilis may cause difficulty in the nodular form, and syringomyelia, neuritis and Raynaud's disease in the anesthetic form. The finding of lepra bacilli in the nasal secretion and the study of a nodule are definite.

Prevention.—Segregation of the patient should be carried out in as humane a manner as possible. Contacts should be examined every few months for several years.

Treatment.—The general treatment should be much as in tuberculosis with every effort to improve the condition of the patient as much as possible. Chaulmoogra oil has been extensively used. Heiser advises chaulmoogra oil 60 cc., camphorated oil 60 cc., and resorcin 4 gm.; this is sterilized and 1 cc. given subcutaneously once a week. The dose is gradually increased to 3 cc. Rogers advises the intravenous injection of gynocardate of soda (prepared from the fatty acids of chaulmoogra oil) gr. $\frac{1}{10}$ to $\frac{4}{5}$ (0.006 to 0.05 gm.), in a 2 per cent saline solution and 0.5 per cent phenol. Ethyl chaulmoograte and sodium hydnocarpate are also employed. Ultraviolet light treatment is useful for nerve pains and is given over areas of necrosis and induration. The use of epinephrine by injection or ephedrine by mouth is said to relieve the nerve pains.

TUBERCULOSIS

GENERAL ETIOLOGY AND MORBID ANATOMY

Definition.—An infection caused by *Bacillus tuberculosis* (*Mycobacterium tuberculosis hominis*) the lesions of which are characterized by nodular bodies, tubercles, and diffuse infiltrations, which either undergo caseation, necrosis, and ulceration, or heal with sclerosis and calcification.

The very varied clinical features depend upon the organ involved, the intensity of the infection, and the degree of resistance offered by the body.

History.—The Greek physicians made many observations upon the clinical features of pulmonary tuberculosis, and our description of the symptoms and of the consumptive form dates from Hippocrates. Galen recognized its infectious nature. In the seventeenth century F. Sylvius indicated the connection between the tuberculous nodule and phthisis, and Richard Morton, a friend of Sydenham, wrote (1689) the first modern treatise in which the clinical side of the disease was well considered. He regarded it as contagious. Pierre Desault, William Stark, and Matthew Baillie laid the foundation of our knowledge of the coarse characters of tubercle as the anatomical basis of tuberculosis. Our real knowledge is a nineteenth century contribution, beginning with the work of Bayle on the structure of the tubercle and its identity in the widely distributed lesions. With the Traité d'Auscultation Médiate (1819) Laennec laid the foundation not only of our modern knowledge of tuberculosis, but of modern clinical medicine. This work (easily to be had in an English translation) should be read from cover to cover by every young doctor, and, when possible, by every senior student. The unity of the forms of the tubercle—the miliary granule, the infiltration and the caseous mass—was recognized, and for the first time physical signs and anatomical features were correlated, and the course of the disease carefully studied. Virchow led a battle against the unity of tuberculous lesions, and held that the products of any simple inflammation might become caseous, and that the ordinary so-called catarrhal pneumonia might terminate in tuberculosis.

The infectiousness of the disease, a belief in which had long been held by individuals, and was widely spread in certain countries—as in Italy—was emphasized and confirmed by the brilliant work of Villemin, who first placed the infective nature of the disease on a solid experimental basis. There is nothing more masterly in the literature of experimental medicine than his work. Then came the demonstration by Robert Koch (in 1882) of the *Bacillus tuberculosis*. The preliminary article in the Berliner klin. Wochenschrift (1882) and the more complete work (Mitteilungen a. d. k. Gesundheitsamte, Bd. 2) should be studied by all who wish to appreciate the value of scientific methods. The thoroughness of Koch's work is manifested by the fact that, in the years that have elapsed, the innumerable workers have amplified and extended, but in no way essentially modified his original position. The account of this discovery should be read by every medical student.

Distribution.—The disease is widely spread zoölogically.

In Animals.—Of animals the cold-blooded are rarely affected. In birds the disease is not uncommon, particularly in fowls, but there are minor differences between the avian and mammalian forms. In the domestic animals tuberculosis is a common disease, particularly in cattle. In sheep, goats, and horses it is rare. In pigs it is not uncommon in certain parts of Europe. Cats and dogs are not prone to the disease. In monkeys in confinement it is very common. The most important single fact in the distribution of the disease in animals is its widespread prevalence in bovines, from which nearly all the milk and a large proportion of our meat are derived.

In Man.—Tuberculosis is his most universal scourge, well deserving the epithet bestowed upon it by Bunyan: "Captain of the Men of Death." Probably about one-eighth of all deaths are due to it. In England and Wales there were 35,818 deaths from all forms of tuberculosis in 1931. In the

United States it is responsible for about 8 per cent of all deaths. The rate in the registration areas was 201.9 per 100,000 in 1900 and 71.5 in 1930.

Practically everywhere in the civilized world, there has been a reduction in the death rate—the most encouraging feature of modern sanitation. To what is this to be attributed? (1) To the improved social condition of the people, better housing, better food, better habits and better working conditions. The falling death rate began before the present campaign against the disease. (2) The education of the people, which has made great strides, and a large proportion are striving to lead hygienic lives. There are less drunkenness, less overcrowding, better air, and better food. The habit of spitting in public has been checked and the seeds of the disease are not spread so broadcast. Child welfare work with its education of parents and children in matters of health and the attention given to under-nourished children have had a good influence. (3) Segregation has done much to protect the healthy from the sick and a larger number of advanced cases are in hospitals. (4) The patients are seen earlier and the condition is recognized before it is hopeless. In a larger number of persons with pulmonary disease the diagnosis is made at a stage when complete healing is possible. (5) The search for contact cases and the careful study of those exposed to infection with more attention to the children in tuberculous families. (6) The use of artificial pneumothorax resulting in the closing or collapse of many cavities. (7) The better education of the patient himself. The important elements then are, fewer seeds, more stony soil.

The economic loss from tuberculosis is enormous. It is estimated that in many communities, about 1 per cent of the population has active tuberculosis and 1 per cent has arrested disease. There are approximately 9 active cases for each death per annum. The cost of death and sickness from tuberculosis each year is hundreds of millions of dollars!

Etiology: Bacillus tuberculosis.—The Seed.—The tubercle bacillus is a minute rod-shaped organism slightly bent or curved, with an average length of from 3 to 4 μ. When stained it may present a beaded appearance. Aberrant forms are not uncommon, *i.e.*, long filaments or branched forms. It stains in a characteristic way with aniline dyes, is "acid fast," and in cultures the growth is distinctive. The bacillus apparently multiplies by more complex processes than was formerly thought and it may undergo changes ("dissociation") so that different forms may grow from one colony. "Branching" tubercle bacilli are usually found in chronic and not very active cases; of greater significance may be the fact that they are usually present in the individual throughout the course. There is some question as to differences in the virulence of the strains of the human bacillus; in animal studies, the local and general reactions are essentially the same. It seems more a matter of dosage and individual resistance; large doses, especially the first, are more harmful than small repeated doses (other conditions being equal).

Specific varieties are recognized. The *avian* form has well-marked peculiarities, but the great point of discussion has been the relation of the bacillus causing human to that which causes *bovine* tuberculosis. Differences in the character of the tubercles of these two classes had long been recognized, and Theobald Smith pointed out special differences between human and bovine bacilli. The matter was brought to a focus in 1901 by Koch's statement that the bacilli of bovine tuberculosis did not cause human tuberculosis, and *vice versa.* The question has been submitted to the test and it is recognized that there are differences between the two forms. The bovine organism is capable of producing the disease in man, in whom it may often be recognized as a special form.

In the Body.—The bacilli are found in all tuberculous lesions, particularly in those actively growing, but in the chronic disease of the lymph nodes and joints they are scanty. In all caseous foci they are few in number. In the sputum in pulmonary tuberculosis they may be present in countless myriads. They are sometimes found in the blood, particularly in cases of miliary tuberculosis, but this is not common in open cases of pulmonary tuberculosis.

Outside the Body.—Tubercle bacilli are widely scattered and found in varying numbers wherever human beings are crowded together. There are two chief sources—the expectoration of persons with advanced disease of the lungs and the milk of tuberculous cows.

From a patient in the Johns Hopkins Hospital, with moderately advanced disease, Nuttall estimated that from 1½ to 4 billions of bacilli were thrown off each twenty-four hours. Allowed to dry, the sputum becomes dust and is distributed far and wide; they may live in dried sputum for three years. Experiments have shown the presence of the bacilli in dust samples from hospital wards, from public buildings, streets, railway carriages and various localities. So widely spread are the bacilli that in cities few individuals pass a week without affording opportunity for their lodgment, usually in the throat or air passages, inhaled with dust. The young child, especially at the crawling stage, is close to the floor and so runs extra risk of infection. They may readily contaminate food. The hands of tuberculous subjects are almost always contaminated. From the street, tuberculous sputum may be brought into the house on shoes, on long skirts, on the hair of dogs, etc. In some of the places most frequented by tuberculous subjects, *e.g.*, sanatoria, the dust may be free from bacilli.

Bovine bacilli are distributed by the milk, rarely by the flesh, and still more rarely by contact with the animals. A proportion of all cases of infection in childhood are with this variety. Bovine tuberculosis is practically negligible in adults but in young children may cause about 10 per cent of the deaths from tuberculosis when cattle are not inspected or the milk pasteurized. It is much more prevalent in Great Britain than in North America. A certain number of cases of pulmonary infection are bovine.

So widely spread everywhere is the seed, that the soil, the conditions suitable for its growth, is practically of equal moment.

THE SOIL.—Many years ago the senior author drew the parallel between infection in tuberculosis and the parable of the sower, which though now somewhat hackneyed illustrates in an effective way the importance of the nature of the ground upon which the seed falls. "*Some seeds fell by the wayside and the fowls of the air came and devoured them up.*" These are the bacilli scattered broadcast outside the body, an immense majority of which die. "*Some fell upon stony places.*" These are the bacilli that find lodgment in many of us, perhaps, with the production of a small focus, but nothing comes of it; they wither away "because they have no root." "*Some fell among thorns, and the thorns sprang up and choked them.*" This represents the cases of tuberculosis, latent or active, in which the seed finds the soil suitable and grows, but the conditions are not favorable, as the thorns, representing the protecting force of the body, get the better in the struggle. "*But others fell on good ground and sprang up and bare fruit an hundredfold.*" Of this fourth group were the 84,741 who died of the disease in 1930 in the United States—the soil suitable, the protecting forces feeble.

What makes a good soil? Fortunately the human body is not a very good culture medium for the tubercle bacillus. About one-eighth of the human race dies of tuberculosis, but a large proportion of all individuals become infected before reaching adult life. The studies of Naegli, Burkhardt, and others show that in 90 per cent of the bodies of city dwellers who have died of disease other than tuberculosis small tuberculous lesions are present. This is probably too high an estimate for England or the United States. The proportion of young adults who give a positive tuberculin reaction varies with locality but is always large. This means, of course, that in a small proportion of those upon whom the seed falls is the soil suitable for active growth—only a natural immunity keeps the race alive.

What this suitable soil is has been the subject of much discussion. From the time of Hippocrates the profession has recognized a tuberculous habitus, variously described as disposition, diathesis, dyscrasia, temperament, constitution, or by the German word "Anlage." These terms are not always interchangeable, but here Ribbert's definition suffices, that a disposition is "that peculiarity in the organism which allows of the effective working of the exciting causes of a disease." Manifestly, such a disposition or constitution may be inherited or acquired. Pearson concludes that "the diathesis of pulmonary tuberculosis is certainly inherited, and the intensity of the inheritance is sensibly the same as that of any normal physical character yet investigated in man. Infection probably plays a necessary part, but in the artisan classes of the urban population of England it is doubtful if their members can escape the risks of infection, except by the absence of diathesis—*i.e.*, the inheritance of what amounts to a counter-disposition."

Hippocrates defined the *habitus phthisicus* in the following words: "The form of body peculiar to subjects of phthisical complaints was the smooth, the whitish, that resembled the lentil; the reddish, the blue-eyed, the leukophlegmatic, and that with the scapulae having the appearance of wings." The so-called scrofulous type has broad coarse features, opaque skin, large thick bones, and heavy figure.

Acquired disposition may arise through a lowering of the resistance of the body forces. Dwellers in cities in the dark, close alleys, and tenement houses, workers in cellars and ill-ventilated rooms, persons addicted to drink, are much more prone to the disease. The influence of environment was demonstrated in the experiment of Trudeau, who found that rabbits inoculated with tuberculosis if confined in a dark, damp place, without sunlight and fresh air, rapidly succumbed, while others treated in the same way, but allowed to run wild, recovered or showed very slight lesions. The occupants of prisons, asylums, and poorhouses, too often, indeed, in barracks and workshops, are in the position of Trudeau's rabbits in the cellar, and under conditions most favorable to foster the development of the bacilli which have lodged in their tissues. But the disease will not develop from the influence of surroundings; the danger is from persons with open lesions.

No *age* is exempt. The disease is met with in the suckling and in the octogenarian, but fatal tuberculosis is, as Hippocrates pointed out, more common between the eighteenth and thirty-fifth year. The influence of *race* is important. It is a fatal disease in negroes, particularly in the United States, and in the North American Indians. This is often due to massive dosage and crowded living conditions; under proper circumstances negroes seem to do about as well as whites. The Irish, both at home and in the United States, are more prone to the disease than other European races. The Hebrews everywhere have a low mortality from tuberculosis but not necessarily a low incidence of the disease. They seem to have a strong resistance to it.

Occupation has an influence, in so far as insanitary surroundings, exposure to dust, close confinement, long hours and low wages favor the prevalence of the disease. Economic factors are important and the social and home conditions should be considered in estimating the influence of occupation. Certain local conditions influence the soil very greatly. Catarrh of the respiratory passages appears to lower the resistance and favor the conditions which enable the bacilli to enter. It is doubtful whether the specific fevers predispose to tuberculosis; although any lowering disease may do so, but in such cases it is often not a fresh infection, but the blazing of a smouldering fire. The soil of diabetes is favorable to the tubercle bacillus. Many chronic affections lower resistance and very often the fatal event in arteriosclerosis, cirrhosis of the liver, etc., is a terminal acute tuberculosis. There is no evidence that being gassed in war favors tuberculous infection.

Trauma, as for example a blow on the chest, injury to the knee, a blow upon the head, may be followed by local tuberculosis. The injured part for a time is a *locus minoris resistentiae,* and the bacilli already present grow in the favorable conditions caused by the injury.

Specific Reactions of the Bacilli.—In its growth the bacillus so far as we know does not form soluble toxins, at least not in the cultures. It causes (1) a local tissue reaction which results in the formation of a new growth, the tubercle; (2) changes in the immunity reactions of the body fluids. The local tissue reactions will be considered later; here we may speak of the phenomena grouped under the term immunity.

Tuberculin Reaction.—An animal inoculated subcutaneously with tubercle bacilli, or with dead cultures, has a local reaction associated with the formation of a tubercle; the neighboring lymph glands become involved, and in susceptible animals the disease generalizes and causes death if living organisms were inoculated. Koch found that if to a guinea-pig with a subcutaneous focus of tuberculosis so caused a second injection of the bacillus was given, healing occurred in the primary nodule, and the animal did not die. Upon these facts his tuberculin treatment was based. The first tuberculin was the sterilized filtered concentrate of glycerine bouillon cultures of the tubercle bacillus ("old" tuberculin, O.T.). If into a healthy person .025 cc. of original tuberculin is injected, there is a slight fever with malaise which passes off in from twelve to twenty-four hours. If into an individual with tuberculosis doses of .015 cc. of tuberculin are injected subcutaneously, there is an active *focal* reaction about the tuberculous lesion and a *constitutional* reaction (fever, general pains, etc.). This "tuberculin reaction," is not used now for diagnosis. The reaction may be local, focal or constitutional. The *skin reactions* are the safest because the reaction is local. The chief methods are the intracutaneous of Mantoux and the cutaneous of Pirquet.

Intracutaneous Test.—The new preparation—*purified protein derivative*—should be used. This is obtained from the filtrate of cultures of strains of the human type grown on synthetic medium. It does not sensitize or cause antibody formation. For single tests, or for small numbers, there are tablets of two sizes, containing 0.0002 mgm. of the material to be used in the first test and 0.05 mgm. for the second test. There is also a vial of sterile salt solution. The stoppers of the bottles are cleaned with alcohol and allowed to dry. Then 1 cc. of the diluent is passed through the stopper of the vial containing the tablet by a sterile tuberculin syringe and needle. The vial is shaken to dissolve the tablet. The skin of the forearm is cleaned with alcohol or acetone. For the first dose 0.1 cc. of the dissolved protein derivative (first strength test tablet) is injected into the skin. This represents 0.000,02 mgm. of the derivative. If no reaction occurs in 48 hours, 0.1 cc. of the solution of the second strength test tablet, prepared in the same way, is used. This contains 0.005 mgm. of the derivative and is injected into the skin of the other arm. Only freshly prepared solutions should be used. A positive reaction consists of a swelling from 5 to 20 mm. in diameter with hyperemia and edema. It reaches a maximum in one or two days and disappears in about six days. A doubtful reaction is characterized by swelling measuring 5 mm. or less in diameter.

In the *cutaneous* test of Pirquet a small abrasion is made on the inner surface of the forearm and a drop of tuberculin placed on it. A positive reaction appears within 48 hours, a papule surrounded by hyperemia.

Immunity Changes.—In an infected person certain changes occur in the blood serum, depending upon the development of so-called antibodies, the presence of which may be demonstrated by complement fixation; and the serum also contains agglutinins. Either directly themselves or through the toxic products there are brought into play certain cellular and humoral reactions which are capable of destroying the infecting agents or of neutralizing their effects or of limiting their activities. Experimentally in animals, according to the virulence of the organism and the dose, all gradations may be produced, from the slightest local reaction to the profoundest septicemia with high fever and death. In a local tuberculous infection, such as happens to the great majority of us at some time in our lives, happily the protective mechanism suffices to localize and limit the invaders. It may amount only to a skirmish, such as is constantly going on at the frontiers of a great empire, but if the local infection is more virulent, or becomes wider spread, the products of the growth of the bacilli or the bacilli themselves enter the circulation, an auto-inoculation, in which case the general metabolism is disturbed, fever is produced, and antibodies are formed.

Allergy.—With the first infection a condition of allergy is produced which is permanent, so that the individual reacts in a different way to further infection. This hypersensitiveness renders subsequent infection more dangerous. There has been much controversy as to the relations between allergy and immunity. They are apparently distinct processes; allergy does not mean immunity. Much depends on the degree of infection; it may be so severe that it kills quickly, as is seen in very young children, or so slight that it heals or remains quiescent without symptoms. The tissue response is largely noninflammatory and the bacilli usually survive at the point of entrance and in the regional lymph nodes. With this changes occur and substances are liberated which pass into the body fluids and render the body cells sensitive to the tubercle bacillus and its protein. Any further infection occurs in a sensitized individual. Focal allergic reactions occur whenever bacilli spread to new tissue and vary from hyperemia to marked exudation. There may be caseation, necrosis, resolutions or fibrosis as a result. Reinfections find allergic tissues and the reaction may be marked. It is evident that reinfections may be from outside or from foci in the patient's body. Such infections probably increase the resistance unless they are too severe to be overcome.

We speak of *productive* or *proliferative* and *exudative* lesions but the terms are not always used with the same meaning in the literature. In the productive lesion new tissue is formed, as in the tubercle. In the exudative lesion there is an exudate which infiltrates the normal tissue but does not replace it. If it caseates, the exudate and the elements of the involved tissues are involved. Lesions may be both proliferative and exudative. In the tubercle it is the new formed granulation tissue which breaks down. The two lesions may coexist but one is superimposed on the other. Much of the inflammation in tuberculosis is exudative which may clear by resolution. The shadows seen in lungs after hemorrhage probably are caused by an exudation.

Koch observed a marked difference in the reaction of healthy and tuberculous animals to cutaneous inoculation with tubercle bacilli. In healthy animals the wound closes and for a few days seems to heal, but in from ten to fourteen days a hard nodule appears, which soon breaks down. General infection occurs and the ulcer remains open to the time of the death of the animal. In tuberculous animals an acute inflammatory ulceration occurs on the second or third day after inoculation, but the ulcer heals quickly and permanently, without even the neighboring lymph glands becoming infected.

Modes of Infection.—*Hereditary Transmission.*—In order that the disease be transmitted by the sperm it would be necessary that tubercle bacilli should lodge in the individual spermatozoön which fecundates an ovum. The chances that this could occur are extremely small, from a numerical point of view, although we know that bacilli are occasionally present in the semen; they become still smaller when we consider that the spermatozoön is made up of nuclear material, which the tubercle bacillus is never known to attack. The possibility of transmission by the ovum must be accepted. Baumgarten in one instance found the tubercle bacillus in the ovum of a female rabbit which had been artificially fecundated with tuberculous semen.

Congenital.—The almost constant method of transmission in congenital tuberculosis is through the blood current, the tubercle bacilli penetrating by the placenta which is usually the seat of tuberculosis. But there are undoubted instances in which, with an apparently sound placenta, both the placental blood and the fetal organs contained tubercle bacilli, although the organs appeared normal. The number of cases of congenital tuberculosis in man is very small; it is more common in cattle.

Latency of the Tubercle Germs.—Baumgarten and his followers assume that tubercle bacilli, present in the newborn child, lie latent in the tissues and subsequently develop when, for some reason or other, the individual resistance is lowered. The small number of congenital cases is against this view. The more modern view is that adult infection is not necessarily derived from childhood infection but may be endogenous or exogenous.

Inoculation.—Cutaneous.—The infective nature of tuberculosis was first demonstrated by Villemin, who showed in 1865 that it could be transmitted to animals by inoculation. The experiments of Cohnheim and Salomonsen, who produced tuberculosis in the eyes of guinea-pigs and rabbits by inoculating fresh tubercle into the anterior chamber, confirmed and extended Villemin's observations and paved the way for Koch's announcement. This mode of infection is seen in persons whose occupation brings them in contact with dead bodies or animal products. Demonstrators of morbid anatomy, butchers and handlers of hides are subject to a local tubercle of the skin, which forms a reddened mass of granulation tissue, usually on the dorsal surface of the hand or a finger. This is the so-called postmortem wart, the *verruca necrogenica* of Wilks. The proof of its nature is shown by the presence of tubercle bacilli and by inoculation experiments in animals.

In the performance of circumcision children have been accidentally inoculated. Infection in these cases is probably always associated with disease in the operator and occurs with the habit of cleansing the wound by suction. Other means of inoculation are described: as the wearing of earrings, washing the clothes of tuberculous patients, the bite of a tuberculous subject, or a cut by a broken sputum cup of a consumptive; Czerny reported two cases of infection by transplantation of skin.

It has been urged by the opponents of vaccination that tuberculosis may be thus conveyed, but of this there is no evidence. Lupus has originated at the site of vaccination in a few cases (C. Fox, Graham Little). Inoculation in man plays a trifling rôle in the transmission of tuberculosis.

Mucous membrane inoculation is probably important in childhood through abrasions of the lips, tongue or gums, though a primary focus is not often seen. The open door in the mouth and throat is more often by loss of the protective epithelium due to catarrhal and ulcerative processes.

Infection in Childhood.—The special points favoring this are: (*a*) The intimate contact between children and parents and other adults in households where tuberculosis exists. (*b*) The habit of playing about the floor and putting objects in the mouth. (*c*) The influence of certain infections, but such cases are probably rare. (*d*) The large place which milk takes in the diet. (*e*) The close contact with other children in school. The result may be: (i) Acute tuberculosis and death. (ii) An infection of short duration with slight symptoms and recovery. (iii) A more chronic condition. (iv) Latency of the disease until adult life, when, as the result of lowered resistance by many factors, the infection becomes active.

Infection by Inhalation.—A belief in the infectiousness of pulmonary tuberculosis originated with the early Greek physicians and persisted among the Latin races. The investigations of Cornet afford conclusive proof that the dust of a room or other locality frequented by patients with pulmonary tuberculosis is infective. The bacilli attached to fine particles of dust are inhaled and gain entrance through the respiratory tract.

Flügge denied that the bacillus-containing dust is the dangerous element in infection. Experimentally he only succeeded in producing the disease when there is some lesion in the respiratory tract. He regarded the danger of infection by dry sputum as slight and held that the infection is chiefly conveyed by the finely divided particles of sputum produced in coughing.

It is well remarked by Cornet, "The consumptive in himself is almost harmless, and only becomes harmful through bad habits." It has been fully shown that the expired air of consumptives is not infective. The bacilli are in the sputum, which when dry is widely disseminated and constitutes the great medium for the transmission of the disease. Among the points in favor of the inhalation view are:

Primary tuberculous lesions are in many cases connected with the respiratory system. The frequency with which foci are found in the lungs and bronchial glands is extraordinary, and a considerable proportion of all persons dying of accident or by suicide present evidences of the disease in these parts. The post-mortem statistics show the widespread prevalence of infection through the air passages. In 125 autopsies at the Foundling Hospital, New York, the bronchial glands were tuberculous in every case.

The greater prevalence of tuberculosis in institutions in which the residents are confined and restricted in the matter of fresh air and a free open life—conditions which favor the presence of the bacilli in the atmosphere and lower the resistance of the individual. The investigations of Cornet upon the death rate among certain religious orders give some striking facts. In a review of 38 cloisters, with an average number of 4,028 residents, among 2,099 deaths in twenty-five years, 1,320 (62.88 per cent) were from tuberculosis. In some cloisters more than three-fourths of the deaths are from this disease, and the mortality in the residents, up to the fortieth year, is greatly above the average, the increase being due entirely to tuberculosis. The more perfect the hygienic arrangements of an institution, the lower the death rate from tuberculosis. The mortality in prisons is sometimes four times as great as outside. The death rate from tuberculosis in prisons constitutes in some countries over 60 per cent of the total mortality. Flick studied the distribution of the deaths from tuberculosis in a single city ward in Philadelphia for twenty-five years. His researches go far to show that it is a *house* disease. About 33 per cent of infected houses had more than one case.

Marital Infection.—Opie and McPhedran (1932) conclude from a study of 533 married couples that husbands and wives in contact with tuberculosis in the other partner are infected from five to nine times as often as those with no known contact with the disease. In such studies a distinction must be made between infection with the tubercle bacillus and the disease tuberculosis.

Infection by Ingestion.—There are two other channels, the tonsils and the intestines, both of great importance.

Tonsillar Infection.—The bacilli pass to the glands of the neck and mediastinum, and reach the circulation through the lymph channels. Or an infected bronchial gland becomes adherent to a branch of the pulmonary artery; if a large number of bacilli escape, miliary tuberculosis follows; if only a small number, they reach the lungs. Through this tonsillar-cervical route bacilli may gain entrance without causing local disease at the portal of entry. In a study of nearly 9,000 cases by Weller *active* tuberculosis of the tonsils was found in 2.35 per cent. The age varied from 2 to 59 years. Many of the individuals with tuberculous tonsils seemed in good health. There is nothing characteristic in the appearance of the tonsil. There are several forms: (1) Infection of the crypts with submucous tubercles; this is the most common and is probably primary. (2) Ulcerative lesions which may follow the first form; (3) A diffuse miliary form, probably hematogenous; (4) Mixed cases. Involvement of the glands was not always present.

Intestinal Infection.—Behring announced in 1903 that pulmonary tuberculosis could be induced through intestinal infection, and further maintained that milk fed to infants was the chief cause of tuberculosis in adults, the infection remaining latent. Behring's first contention was supported by Ravenel and others, who produced pulmonary tuberculosis in animals by feeding experiments, and it was demonstrated that the intestinal surface itself might remain intact. This does away with the objection raised by Koch that, if infection through the milk of tuberculous cattle is common, primary intestinal tuberculosis should be more frequent, whereas among 3,104 cases of tuberculosis in children there were only 16 of primary bowel infection. Experiments have shown how the lungs act as filters for particles absorbed from the intestines. Vansteenberghe and Grysez produced anthracosis of the lungs by introducing china-ink emulsion directly into the stomach. They found a remarkable difference in young and adult guinea-pigs; in the former the carbon particles were filtered out by the mesenteric glands, while the lungs remained free; in the latter the glands were unaffected, but the lungs were carbonized. Calmette and Guérin showed how easily the lungs may be infected through the intestinal route without leaving the slightest trace of disease of the bowel. The truth is that this ubiquitous bacillus is not particular, and gains entrance through either portal. The important matter for the individual is the nature of the soil on which it falls and the severity of the infection.

Milk is a common source of infection. The commercial pasteurization kills tubercle bacilli and is responsible for the great decrease in tuberculous adenitis and bone lesions, in places where its use is general. The flesh of tuberculous animals is rarely dangerous.

Re-infection.—This is not uncommon in adult life but its frequency is difficult to state. Repeated slight infections may be important.

Primary Infection.—"Childhood Form." While this usually occurs in early life, it may be in the adult. In the lungs the lesion may be in any part and there is secondary involvement of the lymph nodes to which the lymph flow from the involved area goes. In early infancy the disease is usually severe and fatal. Deaths in childhood begin in the first months of life and increase to the end of the first year, falling during the next two years. The fatal results are due to acute miliary disease or tuberculous meningitis. From the age of five years to puberty, the number infected steadily increases as shown by the growing percentage of those who react to tuberculin and show signs of involvement of the lungs. Healed lesions in the lungs and lymph nodes are found in increasing numbers in those who die of other diseases.

The *clinical features* in many with the primary infection are slight and the diagnosis may be possible only by the X-ray study or tuberculin test. Much depends on the dosage of the infection and how much further infection occurs. With healing, the lesion in the lung, usually at the periphery, becomes fibrosed and may be calcified (tubercle of Parrot or Ghon). The lymph nodes at the hilus are enlarged and may be calcified. Probably if the first infection occurs in adult life the process is the same. With this there may be extensive parenchymatous infiltration. This may give little in the way of physical signs but is evident in the X-ray plates. In the lung, both with a primary infection and reinfection, spread of the disease may occur by the bronchi. In the pulmonary disease of adults, this spread by the bronchi is probably the important method of progress.

Much has been learned by the discovery of infection (by the tuberculin test and X-ray study) which does not give symptoms or signs sufficient for a clinical diagnosis. Opie reports that 86 per cent of children exposed to a parent with open tuberculosis reacted to tuberculin and 53 per cent had lesions shown in X-ray plates. In children with no contact with tuberculosis in the family, 44 per cent reacted to tuberculin and 21 per cent showed lesions by the X-ray study. It is evident that many of the lesions can not be found in the X-ray films. What is the subsequent course of these cases of primary infection? In some there is complete recovery, but probably in the majority the apt illustration used by J. A. Myers applies: "The first infection may be compared to a bomb which is placed in the body without any knowledge as to the time when it will explode." There may never be any explosion or it may be determined by various factors, such as a lowering of resistance.

Reinfection.—When this occurs the body reacts in a different way from the primary infection as there is hypersensitiveness to the tubercle bacillus. Reinfection may be from the lesions of the first infection (perhaps influenced by lowering of resistance, etc.) or from without. The evidence points to the fact that reinfection is a much more serious matter and it operates in a different fashion. There has been much discussion as to the relative importance of endogenous and exogenous infection. It is evident that it may be very difficult to decide which has occurred in a given patient.

Morbid Anatomy.—DISTRIBUTION OF THE TUBERCLES IN THE BODY.—Clinically in adults, the lungs may be regarded as the seat of election; in children, the lymph nodes, bones, and joints. In 1,000 autopsies there were 275 cases with tuberculous lesions. With but two or three exceptions the lungs were affected. The distribution in the other organs was as follows: Pericardium, 7; peritoneum, 36; brain, 31; spleen, 23; liver, 12; kidneys, 32; intestines, 65; heart, 4; and generative organs, 8. Among 1,287 tuberculous surgical patients at the Würzburg clinic, the distribution of lesions was: Bones and joints, 1,037; lymph nodes, 196; skin and connective tissues, 77; mucous membranes, 10; genito-urinary organs, 20.

THE CHANGES PRODUCED BY THE TUBERCLE BACILLI.—*The Nodular Tubercle.*—A "tubercle" *presents in its early formation nothing distinctive or peculiar, either in its components or in their arrangement.* Identical structures are produced by other parasites, such as actinomyces.

The following changes occur in the evolution of a tubercle:

The tubercle bacilli multiply and disseminate in the surrounding tissues, partly by growth, partly in the lymph currents.

The fixed cells, especially those of connective tissue and the endothelium of the capillaries, multiply and form rounded, cuboidal, or polygonal bodies with vesicular nuclei—the *epithelioid cells*—inside some of which the bacilli are soon seen.

Leukocytes, chiefly polynuclear, migrate in numbers and accumulate about the focus of infection. They do not survive. Many undergo rapid destruction.

Later, as the tubercle grows, the leukocytes are chiefly mononuclear, which do not undergo the rapid degeneration of the polynuclear forms.

A reticulum of fibres is formed by the fibrillation and rarefaction of the connective-tissue matrix. This is most apparent, as a rule, at the margin.

In some, but not all, tubercles *giant cells* are formed by an increase in the protoplasm and in the nuclei of an individual cell, or possibly by the fusion of several cells. The giant cells seem to be in inverse ratio to the number and virulence of the bacilli.

The Degeneration of Tubercle.—*Caseation.*—At the central part of the growth, owing to the direct action of the bacilli or their products, a process of coagulation necrosis goes on in the cells, which lose their outline, become irregular, no longer take stains, and are finally converted into a homogeneous, structureless substance. This may be due to the blood supply being cut off or to the toxins of the tubercle bacillus. Proceeding from the centre outward, the tubercle may be gradually converted into a yellowish-gray body, in which the bacilli are still abundant. No blood vessels are found in them. Aggregated together these form cheesy masses which may undergo softening, fibroid limitation (encapsulation) or calcification.

Sclerosis.—With the necrosis of the cell elements at the centre of the tubercle, hyaline transformation proceeds, together with great increase in the fibroid elements; so that the tubercle is converted into a firm, hard structure. Often the change is rather of a fibrocaseous nature; but the sclerosis predominates. In some situations, as in the peritoneum, this seems to be the natural transformation and it is by no means rare in the lungs.

In all tubercles two processes go on: the one—*caseation*—destructive and dangerous; and the other—*sclerosis*—conservative and healing. The ultimate result in a given case depends upon the capabilities of the body to fight the invaders. There are tissue soils in which the bacilli are, in all probability, killed at once. There are others in which a lodgment is gained and more or less damage done, but finally the day is with the protecting forces. Thirdly, there are tissue soils in which the bacilli grow luxuriantly, caseation and softening, not limitation and sclerosis, prevail, and the day is with the invaders.

The action of the bacilli injected directly into the blood vessels illustrates many points in the histology and pathology of tuberculosis. If into the vein of a rabbit a pure culture of the bacilli is injected, they accumulate chiefly in the liver and spleen. The animal dies usually within two weeks, and the organs apparently show no trace of tubercles. Microscopically, in both spleen and liver the young tubercles in process of formation are very numerous, and karyokinesis is going on in the liver cells. After an injection of a more dilute culture, or one of less virulence, instead of dying within a fortnight the animal survives for five or six weeks, by which time the tubercles are apparent in the spleen and liver, and often in the other organs.

The Diffuse Exudative Lesion.—This is most frequent in the lungs and results from the fusion of many small foci, so small that they may not be visible to the naked eye, but which histologically are composed of scattered centres, surrounded by areas in which the air cells are filled with the products of exudation and the proliferation of the alveolar epithelium. Caseation takes place, usually in small groups of lobules, occasionally in an entire lobe, or even the greater part of a lung. This inflammatory response is the result of fresh infection in sensitized tissues. In the early stage the tissue has a gray gelatinous appearance, the *gray infiltration* of Laennec. These cells accumulate and undergo coagulation necrosis, forming areas of caseation, the scrofulous or cheesy pneumonia of later writers. There may also be a diffuse infiltration and caseation without any special foci, a widespread tuberculous pneumonia induced by the bacilli.

The essential feature of the allergic reaction is *exudation,* appearing as inflammation in tissues and effusion in serous spaces. The process may develop rapidly. Tubercles present at the time of reinfection may also show an acute inflammatory reaction and a stimulation of fibrosis.

Secondary Inflammatory Processes.—The irritation caused by the bacilli produces an inflammation which may be limited to exudation of leukocytes and serum, but may also be much more extensive and vary with changing conditions. We find, for example, about the smaller tubercles in the lungs, pneumonia—either catarrhal or fibrinous—proliferation of the connective-tissue elements in the septa (which also become infiltrated with round cells), and changes in the blood and lymph vessels.

In processes of minor intensity the inflammation is of the slow reactive nature, which results in the production of a cicatricial connective tissue which limits and restricts the development of the tubercles and is the essential conservative element. In chronic pulmonary tuberculosis much of the fibroid tissue is not in any way associated with the action of the bacilli. Persistent infection from the upper respiratory tract, as from sinusitis, may be responsible for fibroid changes in the same way as in the nontuberculous.

Suppuration.—Do the bacilli themselves induce suppuration? In so-called cold tuberculous abscess the material is not histologically pus, but a *débris* consisting of broken-down cells and cheesy material. It is moreover sterile—that is, does not contain the usual pus organisms. The products of the tubercle bacilli are probably able to induce suppuration, as in the joint and bone tuberculosis pus is frequently produced, although this may be due to a mixed infection. Tuberculin is one of the best agents for the production of experimental suppuration. In tuberculosis of the lungs the suppuration is largely the result of infection with pus organisms.

ACUTE MILIARY TUBERCULOSIS

The modern knowledge of this remarkable form dates from the statement of Buhl (1856), that miliary tuberculosis is a specific infection dependent on the presence in the body of an unencapsulated yellow tubercle or a tuberculous cavity in the lung; and that it bears the same relation to the primary lesion as pyemia does to a focus of suppuration.

Carl Weigert established the truth of this brilliant conception by demonstrating the association of miliary tuberculosis with tuberculosis of the blood vessels. There are two groups of *vessel tubercle*—the tuberculous *periangitis* in which there is invasion of the adventitia, and the *endangitis* in which the tubercles start in the intima. The parts most frequently affected are the pulmonary veins and the thoracic duct, less often the jugular vein and the vena cava superior, and the sinuses of the dura mater, the aorta and the endocardium. To the branches of the pulmonary veins caseous glands may be adherent, penetrating the walls and showing a growth of miliary tubercles in the intima. A special interest belongs to tuberculosis of the thoracic duct, first accurately described by Sir Astley Cooper. Benda in cases of vessel tuberculosis found in many instances an enormous number of bacilli, particularly in the caseous tubercles of the thoracic duct.

The bacilli do not increase in the blood, but settle in the different organs, producing a generalized tuberculosis, of which Weigert recognized three types or grades: I. The acute general miliary tuberculosis, in which the various organs of the body are stuffed with miliary and submiliary nodules. II. A second form characterized by a small number of tubercles in one or many organs. III. The occurrence of numerous tuberculous foci widely spread throughout the body, but in a more chronic form; the tubercles are larger and many are caseous. It is the chronic generalized tuberculosis of children. Transitional forms between these groups occur. In the first variety, which we are here considering, there is an eruption into the circulation of an enormous number of bacilli. Benda suggests in explanation of the profound toxemia seen in certain cases (the typhoid form) that in addition the blood is surcharged with toxins from a large caseous focus which has eroded a vessel.

Clinical Forms

The cases may be grouped into those with the symptoms of an *acute general infection*—the typhoid form; cases in which *pulmonary* symptoms predominate; and cases in which the *cerebral* or *cerebrospinal* symptoms are marked—tuberculous meningitis. Other forms have been recognized, but this division covers a large majority of the cases. Taking any series of cases it will be found that the meningeal form of acute tuberculosis exceeds in numbers the cases with general or marked pulmonary symptoms.

General or Typhoid Form.—The patient presents the symptoms of a profound infection which simulates and may be mistaken for typhoid fever. After a period of failing health, with loss of appetite, he becomes feverish and weak. Occasionally the disease sets in more abruptly, but in many instances the anamnesis closely resembles that of typhoid fever. Nose-bleeding, however, is rare. The temperature increases, the pulse becomes rapid and feeble, the tongue dry; delirium becomes marked and the cheeks are flushed. The pulmonary symptoms may be slight; usually bronchitis exists, but is not more severe than is common in typhoid fever. The pulse is seldom dicrotic, but is rapid in proportion to the pyrexia. Perhaps the most striking feature of the fever is the irregularity; and if seen from the outset there is not the steady ascent noted in typhoid fever. There is usually an evening rise to 103° F., sometimes 104° F., and a morning remission of from two to three degrees. Sometimes the fever is intermittent, and the temperature may be below normal during the early morning hours. The inverse type of temperature, in which the rise takes place in the morning, is held by some to be more frequent in general tuberculosis than in other diseases. In rare instances there may be little or no fever. On four occasions we had a patient admitted with profound debility and a history of illness of from three to four weeks' duration, with rapid pulse, flushed cheeks, dry tongue, and very slight fever in whom (postmortem) the condition proved to be general tuberculosis. Reinhold called attention to these afebrile forms of acute tuberculosis. In 9 of 52 cases there was no fever, or only a transient rise.

In some cases the respirations are increased in frequency, particularly in the early stage, and there may be diffuse bronchitis and slight cyanosis. Cheyne-Stokes breathing occurs toward the close. Active delirium is rare. More commonly there are torpor and dullness, gradually deepening into coma, in which the patient dies. In some cases the pulmonary symptoms become more marked; in others meningeal or cerebral features occur. The duration is usually from four to six weeks. Practically all the patients die.

Diagnosis.—The diagnosis from typhoid fever may be difficult. A point of importance is the irregularity of the fever curve. The greater frequency of the respirations and the tendency to slight cyanosis are much more common in tuberculosis. There are cases, however, of typhoid fever in which the initial bronchitis is severe with dyspnea and cyanosis. The cough may be slight or absent. Diarrhea is rare in tuberculosis; the bowels are usually constipated; but diarrhea may occur and persist for days. In certain cases the diagnosis is complicated still further by the occurrence of blood in the stools. Enlargement of the spleen occurs in general tuberculosis, but is neither so early nor so marked as in typhoid fever. In children the enlargement may be considerable. The urine may show albumin and contain tubercle bacilli in a considerable number of cases. The absence of the characteristic roseola is important. Occasionally in acute tuberculosis reddish spots may occur and cause difficulty, but they do not come out in crops, and rarely have the characters of the true typhoid eruption. Herpes is perhaps more common in tuberculosis. Toward the close, petechiae may appear on the skin, particularly about the wrists. A rare event is jaundice, due possibly to tubercles in the liver. The lesions of acute tuberculosis and of typhoid fever have been found in the same body.

A negative Widal test and blood-culture may be of decisive importance in these doubtful cases. In rare instances tubercle bacilli have been found in the blood. Leukocytosis is more common in miliary tuberculosis than in typhoid fever, in which leukopenia is the rule. Careful examination of the eyes may show choroidal tubercles, though we have never known a diagnosis made on their presence alone. In the spinal fluid the tubercle bacilli may be abundant, even when there is no active meningitis.

Pulmonary Form.—From the outset the pulmonary symptoms are marked. The patient may have had a cough for months or years without much impairment of health, or he may be known to have chronic pulmonary tuberculosis. In other instances, particularly in children, the affection follows measles or whooping cough, and is of a bronchopneumonic type. The disease begins with the symptoms of diffuse bronchitis. The cough is marked, the expectoration mucopurulent, occasionally rusty. Hemoptysis has been noted in some instances. From the outset *dyspnea* is a striking feature and may be out of proportion to the physical signs. There is *cyanosis* and apart from emphysema and severe pneumonia, there is no other pulmonary condition in which the cyanosis is so marked. The physical signs are those of bronchitis. In children there may be defective resonance at the bases, from scattered areas of bronchopneumonia; or, what is equally suggestive, areas of hyperresonance. Indeed, the percussion note, particularly in the front of the chest, in some cases of miliary tuberculosis, is full and clear, and it will be noted (postmortem) that the lungs are unusually voluminous. This is probably the result of more or less widespread acute emphysema. On auscultation, the râles are sibilant and sonorous or small, fine, and crepitant. There may be fine crepitation from tubercles on the pleura (Jürgensen). In children there may be high-pitched tubular breathing at the bases or toward the root of the lung. Toward the close the râles may be larger and more mucous. The temperature rises to 102° or 103° F., and may present the inverse type. The pulse is rapid and feeble. In very acute cases the spleen is always enlarged. The disease may prove fatal in ten or twelve days, or be protracted for weeks or even months. *Chronic* cases are described, in which the diagnosis is based largely on the X-ray findings, also used to estimate the progress.

Diagnosis.—The diagnosis of this form offers less difficulty and is more frequently made. There is often a history of previous cough or the patient is known to be the subject of tuberculosis. In children these symptoms following measles or whooping cough indicate in the majority of cases acute miliary tuberculosis, with or without bronchopneumonia. Occasionally the sputum contains tubercle bacilli. The choroidal tubercle occurs in a limited number of cases. More important is the combination of dyspnea with cyanosis and a diffuse bronchitis. In some instances the cerebral symptoms give a clew to the diagnosis. The X-ray examination may be of great aid. Of late years diagnoses of acute miliary tuberculosis have been made more frequently by some roentgenologists when the clinical features were not very severe and recovery followed. It may be difficult to prove the nature of the lesions but if they represent miliary tuberculosis we have to modify our views as to its outcome.

Meningeal Form (*Tuberculous Meningitis*).—This is essentially an acute tuberculosis in which the membranes of the brain, sometimes of the cord, bear the brunt of the attack. Our first accurate knowledge of it dates from the publication of Robert Whytt's Observations on the Dropsy of the Brain, Edinburgh, 1768. He studied 20 cases and divided the disease into three stages, according to the condition of the pulse.

Though Guersant had as early as 1827 used the name *granular meningitis* for this form of inflammation of the meninges, it was not until 1830 that Papavoine demonstrated the nature of the granules and noted their occurrence with tubercles in other parts. In 1832 and 1833, W. W. Gerhard, of Philadelphia, made a very careful study of the disease in the Children's Hospital at Paris, and his publications, more than those of any other author, served to place the disease on a firm anatomical and clinical basis.

There are several special *etiological* factors in this form. It is much more common in young children than in adults. In a majority of the cases a focus of old tuberculous disease will be found, commonly in the bronchial or mesenteric glands. In a few instances the affection seems to be primary in the meninges. It is very difficult, however, in an ordinary postmortem to make an exhaustive search, and the lesion may be in the bones, in the middle ear, or in the genito-urinary organs. There is doubt as to how often the infection is hematogenous and how often from a caseous nodule of the brain or a caseous focus in the meninges. In some series in Great Britain about 25 per cent showed the bovine bacillus.

Morbid Anatomy.—The meninges at the base are most involved, hence the term basilar meningitis. There may be only slight turbidity and matting of the membranes, and a certain stickiness with serous infiltration; but more commonly there is a turbid exudate which covers the structures at the base, surrounds the nerves, extends into the Sylvian fissures, and appears on the lateral, rarely on the upper, surfaces of the hemispheres. The tubercles may be very apparent, particularly in the Sylvian fissures, appearing as small, whitish nodules. They vary much in number and size, and may be difficult to find. The amount of exudate bears no definite relation to the abundance of tubercles. The arteries of the anterior and posterior perforated spaces should be carefully withdrawn and searched, as upon them nodular tubercles may be found when not present elsewhere. In doubtful cases the middle cerebral arteries should be carefully removed, spread on a glass plate with a black background, and examined with a lens. The tubercles are seen as nodular enlargements on the smaller arteries. The lateral ventricles are dilated (acute hydrocephalus) and contain a turbid fluid; the ependyma may be softened, and the septum lucidum and fornix are usually broken down. The convolutions are often flattened and the sulci obliterated owing to the increased pressure. The meninges are not alone involved, but the contiguous cerebral substance is more or less edematous and infiltrated with leukocytes, in reality a *meningo-encephalitis.*

There are instances in which the acute process is associated with chronic meningeal tuberculosis, which may for months present the clinical picture of brain tumor. Although in a majority of instances the process is cerebral, the spinal meninges may also be involved, particularly those of the cervical cord. There are cases in which the symptoms are chiefly spinal.

Clinical Features.—Tuberculous meningitis presents an extremely complex clinical picture. *Prodromal* symptoms are common. The child may have been in failing health for some weeks, or may be convalescent from measles or whooping cough. In many instances there is a history of a fall. The child gets thin, is restless, peevish, irritable, loses its appetite, and the disposition may completely change. Suggestive symptoms may then set in, either suddenly with a convulsion, or more commonly with headache, vomiting and fever, three essential features of the onset which are rarely absent. The pain may be intense and agonizing. The child puts its hand to the head and occasionally gives a short, sudden cry, the so-called hydrocephalic cry. Sometimes the child screams continuously until exhausted. The vomiting is without apparent cause and independent of taking of food. Constipation is usually present. The fever is slight, but gradually rises to 102° to 103° F. The pulse is at first rapid, subsequently irregular and slow. The respirations are rarely altered. During sleep the child is restless and disturbed. There may be twitchings of the muscles or sudden startings; or the child may wake up from sleep in great terror. In this early stage the pupils are usually contracted. These are the chief symptoms of the initial stage, or the *stage of irritation.*

In the second period these irritative symptoms subside; vomiting is no longer marked, the abdomen becomes retracted, boat-shaped or *carinated.* The bowels are obstinately constipated, the child no longer complains of headache, but is dull and apathetic, and when roused is more or less delirious. The head is often retracted and the child utters an occasional cry. The pupils are dilated or irregular, and a squint may develop. Sighing respiration is common. Convulsions may occur, or rigidity of the muscles of one side or of one limb. The temperature is variable, ranging from 100° to 102.5° F. A blotchy erythema is not uncommon.

In the final period, or stage of *paralysis,* the coma increases and the child can not be roused. Convulsions are not infrequent, and there are spasmodic contractions of the muscles of the back and neck. Spasms may occur in the limbs of one side. Optic neuritis and paralysis of the ocular muscles may be present. The pupils become dilated, the eyelids are only partially closed, and the eyeballs are rolled up. Diarrhea may occur, the pulse becomes rapid, and the child may sink into a toxic state with dry tongue, low delirium and involuntary passages of urine and feces. The temperature often becomes subnormal, sinking in rare instances to 93° or 94° F. In some cases there is an antemortem elevation to 106° F. The duration is from a fortnight to several weeks. A leukocytosis is not infrequently present throughout.

The clinical picture may be very varied, especially in adults, and some cases pursue a rapid course. They set in with great violence, often in persons apparently in good health, and may prove fatal within a few days. In these instances, more common in adults, the convex surface of the brain is usually involved. There are instances which are essentially chronic with symptoms of a limited meningitis, sometimes with pronounced psychical features or those of cerebral tumor. The symptoms may vary from time to time; some are probably due to toxemia rather than to a local lesion.

There are certain features which call for special comment. The irregularity and slowness of the *pulse* in the early and middle stages of the disease are points upon which all authors agree. Toward the close, as the heart's action becomes weaker, the pulse is more frequent. The temperature is usually elevated but there are instances in which it does not rise much above 100° F. It may be extremely irregular and the oscillations are often as much as three or four degrees in the day. The *ocular* symptoms are of special importance. In the early stages narrowing of the pupils is the rule. Toward the close, with increase in the intracranial pressure, the pupils dilate and are irregular. There may be conjugate deviation of the eyes. The third nerve is most frequently involved, sometimes with paralysis of the face, limbs, and hypoglossal nerve on the opposite side (syndrome of Weber). In some cases when the head is flexed on the chest strabismus occurs in one or both eyes, lasting as long as the head is held flexed. The retinal changes are important. *Neuritis* is the most common. According to Gowers, the disk at first becomes full colored and has hazy outlines, and the veins are dilated. Swelling and striation become pronounced, but the neuritis is rarely intense. Tubercles in the choroid are less frequently seen during life than post-mortem figures indicate.

Among the motor symptoms *convulsions* are most common, but there are other changes which deserve mention. A tetanic contraction of one limb may persist for several days, or a cataleptic condition. Tremor and athetoid movements are sometimes seen. The paralyses are either hemiplegias or monoplegias. Hemiplegia may result from disturbance in the cortical branches of the middle cerebral artery, occasionally from softening in the internal capsule, due to involvement of the central branches. Of monoplegias, that of the face is perhaps most common, and if on the right side it may occur with aphasia. Brachial monoplegia may be associated with it. In the more chronic cases the symptoms persist for months, and there may be a characteristic Jacksonian epilepsy. Kernig's sign may be present, but is not constant. The Babinski sign is sometimes found. The motor phenomena occur more often in adults and the usual signs of meningitis may be few. Unexplained constant severe headache may be the first symptom.

The DIAGNOSIS is rarely difficult. The sudden onset of persistent severe headache in tuberculous adults should excite suspicion, especially if there is any cranial nerve paralysis. Points upon which special stress is to be laid are a tuberculous focus in the body, the mode of onset and the symptoms, and the evidence obtained on *lumbar puncture*. The cerebrospinal fluid is usually clear or slightly turbid, and after standing for 12 to 24 hours, a feathery clot of fibrin forms down the centre of the fluid. In this clot the tubercle bacilli are usually found. By centrifugalization, careful staining and long search, tubercle bacilli can be found in a large proportion of cases—in 135 of 137 in one series (Hemenway). The cells are usually much increased in number; over 90 per cent are small lymphocytes, though occasionally an excess of polymorphonuclear leukocytes is found. Tubercle bacilli may be grown in culture.

The PROGNOSIS is always most serious. We have seen neither a case proved to be tuberculous recover, nor postmortem evidence of past disease of this nature but cases of recovery have been reported by reliable authorities. In some of these there may have been a local area in some part of the meninges from which tubercle bacilli entered the cerebrospinal fluid.

TREATMENT.—In a disease which is practically always fatal this does not offer much. The patients should be nourished as well as possible and given sedatives to control restlessness or pain. In the meningeal form, lumbar puncture should be done frequently. There should be no hesitation in using sedatives freely when required. Treatment by X-rays has been employed, three or four applications being given.

TUBERCULOSIS OF THE LYMPHATIC SYSTEM

Tuberculosis of the Lymph Nodes (Scrofula)

Scrofula is tubercle and the bacillus of Koch is the essential element. In a considerable number of cases the bovine organism is responsible. The observations of Lingard are important as showing a variation in the virulence of the tubercle bacillus. Guinea-pigs inoculated with ordinary tubercle showed lymphatic infection within the first week and died within three months; infected with material from tuberculous glands, the lymphatic enlargement did not appear until the second or third week, and the animals survived for six or seven months. The proportion of cases of bovine infection is highest in children but it is not very rare in adults. The cases of bovine infection in cervical gland tuberculosis vary greatly in different countries.

Tuberculous *adenitis*, met with at all ages, is more common in children than in adults, and may occur in old age. A special predisposing factor in lymphatic tuberculosis is catarrh of the mucous membranes, which excites slight adenitis of the neighboring glands. In a child with constantly recurring nasopharyngeal catarrh, the bacilli which lodge on the mucous membranes find in all probability the gateways less strictly guarded and are taken up by the lymphatics and passed to the nearest glands. The importance of the *tonsils* as an infection-atrium has been urged. In good health the local resistance is active enough to deal with the invaders, but the irritation of a chronic infection weakens the resistance and the bacilli are enabled to grow and change a simple into a tuberculous adenitis. The association of tubercle in the mesenteric glands with intestinal catarrh is thus explained. There has been a great decrease in tuberculous adenitis in the cities of the United States, probably due to pasteurization of milk.

The following are some of the features of interest in tuberculous adenitis:

The *local* character. The glands of the neck, or at the bifurcation of the bronchi or those of the mesentery, may be alone involved. But there is usually a pulmonary lesion with involvement of the tracheobronchial nodes.

The tendency to *spontaneous healing*. In a large proportion of the cases the battle between the bacilli and the protective forces is long; but the latter are finally successful, and we find in the calcified remnants in the bronchial and mesenteric lymph nodes evidences of healing. Too often in the bronchial glands a truce only is declared and hostilities break out afresh in the form of an acute tuberculosis.

The tendency of tuberculous adenitis to pass on to *suppuration*. The frequency with which, particularly in the glands of the neck, the tuberculous process is associated with suppuration is a special feature. In nearly all instances the pus is sterile. Whether the suppuration is excited by the bacilli or by their products, or whether it is the result of a mixed infection with pus organisms, which are subsequently destroyed, is not settled.

An *unhealed* tuberculous adenitis is a constant menace and in a large proportion of the instances of acute tuberculosis the infection is from this source. On the other hand, there is evidence that tuberculous adenitis in childhood gives some immunity in adult life. Only a small number of adults with pulmonary tuberculosis show scars from adenitis—3.2 per cent of one series of 2,000 patients. Certain autopsy studies suggest that in adults with mesenteric gland tuberculosis, pulmonary tuberculosis is less frequent.

Generalized Tuberculous Lymphadenitis.—In exceptional instances we find diffuse tuberculosis of nearly all the lymph nodes of the body with little or no involvement of other parts. The most extreme cases which we have seen have been in negro patients. Two well-marked cases occurred at the Philadelphia Hospital. In a woman, the chart from April, 1888, until March, 1889, showed persistent fever, from 101° to 103°, occasionally rising to 104° F. On December 16th the glands on the right side of the neck were removed. She died on March 5th. The lungs presented only one or two puckered spots at the apices. The bronchial, retroperitoneal and mesenteric glands were greatly enlarged and caseous. There was no intestinal, uterine or bone disease. The continuous fever depended apparently upon the tuberculous adenitis. In these instances the enlargement is most marked in the retroperitoneal, bronchial and mesenteric glands, but may be also present in the external glands. Occurring acutely, it presents a picture resembling Hodgkin's disease. In infants and children there is a form of general tuberculous adenitis in which the various groups of glands are successively, more rarely simultaneously, involved, and in which death is caused either by cachexia or by an acute miliary process.

Local Tuberculous Adenitis.—CERVICAL.—This is the most common form in children, and is seen particularly among the poor and those who live among unsanitary conditions. Children in foundling hospitals and asylums are specially prone to the disease. In the United States it is most common in the negro race. It often occurs with catarrh of the nose and throat, or chronic tonsillitis.

The involvement is usually greater on one side than on the other. As they increase in size, the individual tumors can be felt; the surface is smooth and the consistence firm. They may remain isolated, but more commonly they form large, knotted masses, over which the skin is, as a rule, freely movable. In many cases the skin ultimately becomes adherent, and inflammation and suppuration occur. An abscess points and, unless opened, bursts, leaving a sinus which heals slowly. The disease is frequently associated with coryza, with eczema of the scalp, ear, or lips, and with conjunctivitis or keratitis. When the glands are large and growing actively there is fever. The subjects are usually anemic, particularly if suppuration has occurred. The progress of this form is slow and tedious. Death, however, rarely follows, and many severe cases in children do well. Not only the submaxillary group, but the glands above the clavicle and in the posterior cervical triangle may be involved. In other instances the cervical and axillary glands are involved together, forming a continuous chain which extends beneath the clavicle and the pectoral muscle. The bronchial glands may also be enlarged and caseous. The enlargement of the supraclavicular and axillary glands may precede a tuberculous pleurisy or pulmonary tuberculosis.

TRACHEOBRONCHIAL.—The mediastinal lymph nodes constitute filters in which lodge the various foreign particles which escape the normal phagocytes of bronchi and lungs. Among these foreign particles, and probably attached to them, tubercle bacilli are not uncommon, and we find tubercles and caseous matter with great frequency in this group. Northrup found them involved in every one of 125 cases of tuberculosis at the New York Foundling Hospital. The tuberculosis adenitis may, in the bronchial glands, attain the dimensions of a tumor of large size. In children the bronchial adenitis is apt to be associated with suppuration. The glands at the bifurcation of the trachea are first involved and chiefly on the right side—74 per cent of Wollstein's cases. Irregular fever, failure of nutrition, loss of appetite, and lassitude may be found; pain is rare, though it is complained of sometimes in the mammary region. The cough is paroxysmal, often brassy, so that it has been mistaken for whooping cough. Stridor, when present, is more often expiratory. The *physical signs* are not very definite. Dilated veins over the anterior aspect of the thorax or in the axilla, absence of descent of the larynx during inspiration, and pain on pressure over the upper dorsal vertebrae are mentioned. Extension of the normal dulness over the upper four thoracic vertebrae to the fifth and sixth is of importance, and there may be paravertebral dulness on delicate percussion. Some writers lay stress upon whispered bronchophony over the upper thoracic vertebrae, and a venous hum may be heard over the manubrium. The X-ray pictures are usually distinctive but do not tell whether the process is tuberculous or not, unless a nodule is found in the lung.

Some of the uncommon effects are: Compression of the superior cava, of the pulmonary artery and of the azygos vein. The trachea and bronchi, though often flattened, are rarely seriously compressed. The vagus nerve may be involved, particularly the recurrent laryngeal branch. More important are perforations of the softened glands into the bronchi or trachea, or a sort of secondary cyst may be formed between the lung and trachea. Asphyxia has been caused by blocking of the larynx by a caseous gland which ulcerated through the bronchus (Voelcker), and Ogle reported a case in which the ulcerated gland practically occluded both bronchi. Perforations of the *vessels* are much less common, but the pulmonary artery and the aorta have been opened. Perforation of the esophagus has been described. One serious effect is infection of the lung or pleura by caseous glands situated deep along the bronchi. This may be by direct contact, and it may be difficult to determine where the caseous bronchial gland terminates and the pulmonary tissue begins. In other instances it takes place along the root of the lung and is subpleural. Among other sequences are mentioned diverticulum of the esophagus following adhesion of an enlarged gland and subsequent retraction; and from the anterior mediastinal and aortic groups, the production of pericarditis by contact or rupture of a softened gland into the sac. A serious danger is systemic infection, which takes place through the vessels.

MESENTERIC; TABES MESENTERICA.—In this affection, the glands of the mesentery and retroperitoneum become enlarged and caseate; more rarely they suppurate or calcify. A slight tuberculous adenitis is extremely common in children, and is often accidentally found (postmortem) when they have died of other diseases. It may be a primary lesion or secondary to tuberculous disease of the intestines.

The statistics of abdominal tuberculosis show a great variation in different localities. The small percentage in North America contrasts with the high figures given for Scotland by John Thomson. "Scotland enjoys the unenviable distinction of having more abdominal tuberculosis than any other civilized country—twice as much at least as England generally, and more than ten times as much as Europe and North America." The involvement of the glands interferes seriously with nutrition, and the patients are puny, wasted and anemic. The abdomen is enlarged and tympanitic; diarrhea is a constant feature; the stools are thin and offensive. There is moderate fever, but the general wasting and debility are the most characteristic features. The enlarged glands can not often be felt, owing to the distended abdomen. These cases are often spoken of as "consumption of the bowels," but in a majority the intestines do not present tuberculous lesions. In a considerable number of the cases of tabes mesenterica the peritoneum is also involved, and in such the abdomen is large and hard, and nodules may be felt.

In *adults* tuberculous disease of the mesenteric glands may occur as a primary affection, or in association with pulmonary disease. It may exist without tuberculous disease in the intestines or in any other part. The tumor mass is usually a little to the right of the umbilicus, freely movable. The general symptoms are loss of weight and slight fever; locally there is pain, sometimes diarrhea and appendicitis is often suspected.

The condition is now so rare in the United States that an incorrect diagnosis may be made because it is not considered. In some cases the correct diagnosis is made only by abdominal section. Calcified mesenteric lymph nodes are easily recognized by an X-ray study.

Tuberculosis of the Serous Membranes

General Serous Membrane Tuberculosis (*Polyorrhomenitis.*—The serous membranes may be chiefly involved, simultaneously or consecutively, presenting a distinctive form of tuberculosis. There are three groups of cases. First, those in which an acute tuberculosis of the peritoneum and pleuræ occurs rapidly, caused by disease of the tubes in women, or of the mediastinal or bronchial lymph nodes. Secondly, more chronic cases with exudation into peritoneum and pleurae, the formation of cheesy masses, and the occurrence of ulcerative and suppurative processes. Thirdly, there are cases in which the pleuroperitoneal affection is still more chronic, the tubercles hard and fibroid, the membranes thickened, and with little or no exudate. In any of these forms the pericardium may be involved with the pleurae and peritoneum. It is important to bear in mind that there may be no visceral tuberculosis in these cases.

Tuberculosis of the Pleura.—*Acute Tuberculous Pleurisy.*—It is difficult to estimate the proportion of instances of acute pleurisy due to tuberculosis (see Acute Pleurisy). The cases are rarely fatal. There are three groups: (1) Acute tuberculous pleurisy with subsequent chronic course. (2) Secondary and terminal forms of acute pleurisy (these are not uncommon in hospital practice). And (3) acute tuberculous suppurative pleurisy. A considerable number of the purulent pleurisies, designated as latent and chronic, are caused by tubercle bacilli, but it is not so widely recognized that there is an acute, ulcerative and suppurative disease which may run a very rapid course. The pleurisy sets in abruptly, with pain in the side, fever, cough, and sometimes with a chill. There may be nothing to suggest tuberculosis, and the subject may have a fine physique and come of healthy stock.

Subacute and chronic tuberculous pleurisies are more common. The largest group comprises those with serofibrinous effusion. The onset is insidious, the true character is frequently overlooked, and almost always there are tuberculous foci in the lungs and bronchial glands. These are cases in which the termination is often in pulmonary tuberculosis or general miliary tuberculosis. In a few cases the exudate becomes purulent.

Lastly, there is a *chronic adhesive pleurisy*, a primary proliferative form which is of long standing, and may lead to very great thickening of the membrane, and sometimes to invasion of the lung.

Secondary tuberculous pleurisy is very common. The visceral layer is usually involved in pulmonary tuberculosis. Adhesions form and a chronic pleurisy results, which may be simple, but usually tubercles are scattered through the adhesions. An acute tuberculous pleurisy may result from direct extension. The fluid may be serofibrinous or hemorrhagic, or may become purulent. And, lastly, in pulmonary tuberculosis, a superficial spot of softening may perforate with the production of *pyopneumothorax*.

The general symptomatology of these forms will be considered under disease of the pleura.

Tuberculosis of the Pericardium.—Miliary tubercles may occur as a part of a general infection, but the term is properly limited to those cases in which, either as a primary or secondary process, there is extensive disease of the membrane. Tuberculosis is not so common in the pericardium as in the pleura and peritoneum, but it is more common than the literature indicates. George Norris found 82 instances among 1,780 postmortems in tuberculous subjects. The onset of symptoms may be insidious and without any evident cause. Some fever is common. The features of myocardial insufficiency may increase steadily with little or no response to treatment. There are no characteristic symptoms.

We may recognize four groups of cases: First, those in which the condition is entirely latent, and the disease is discovered accidentally in individuals who have died of other affections or of chronic pulmonary tuberculosis.

A second group, in which the symptoms are those of cardiac insufficiency following dilatation and hypertrophy with chronic adhesive pericarditis. The symptoms are those of cardiac insufficiency, and suggest idiopathic hypertrophy and dilatation, or, if there is a loud blowing systolic murmur at the apex, mitral valve disease. The adherent pericardium is usually overlooked.

In a third group the clinical picture is that of an acute tuberculosis, either general or with cerebrospinal manifestations, which has had its origin from the tuberculous pericardium or tuberculous mediastinal lymph glands.

A fourth group, with symptoms of acute pericarditis, includes cases in which the affection is acute and accompanied with more or less exudation of a serofibrinous, hemorrhagic or purulent character. There may be no suspicion whatever of the tuberculous nature of the trouble.

The *diagnosis* may be suggested by tuberculosis elsewhere and the absence of any history of other causes of pericarditis, such as rheumatic fever. In case of effusion, tubercle bacilli may be found in the fluid. In chronic cases calcification may be made out by X-ray study. In *treatment* the general measures for tuberculosis should be carried out. If effusion is causing difficulty, tapping should be done. The usual measures for myocardial insufficiency have little effect.

Tuberculosis of the Peritoneum.—In connection with miliary and chronic pulmonary tuberculosis it is not uncommon to find the peritoneum studded with small gray granulations. They are constantly present on the serous surface of tuberculous ulcers of the intestines. Apart from these conditions the membrane is often the seat of extensive tuberculous disease, which occurs, in the following forms:

Acute miliary tuberculosis with serofibrinous or bloody exudation.

Chronic tuberculosis, with larger growths, which tend to caseate and ulcerate. The exudate is purulent or seropurulent, and often sacculated.

Chronic fibroid tuberculosis, which may be subacute from the onset, or which may represent the final stage of an acute miliary eruption. The tubercles are hard and pigmented. There is little or no exudation, and the serous surfaces are matted together by adhesions.

The process may be primary and local, which was the case in 5 of 17 postmortems. In children the infection appears to pass from the intestines, and in adults this is the source in the cases associated with chronic tuberculosis. In women the disease extends commonly from the fallopian tubes. In at least 30 or 40 per cent of the instances of laparotomy in this affection the infection was from them. The prostate or the seminal vesicles may be the starting point. In many cases the peritoneum is involved with the pleura and pericardium, particularly with the former membrane.

Certain conditions of the abdominal organs predispose to the disease; thus patients with cirrhosis of the liver often die of an acute tuberculous peritonitis. The frequency with which the condition is met with in operations upon ovarian tumors has been noted by gynecologists. Many cases have followed trauma of the abdomen. An interesting feature is the not uncommon occurrence of tuberculosis in hernial sacs. In a majority of the instances it is discovered accidentally during the operation for radical cure or strangulation. In some instances the sac alone is involved.

It is generally stated that males are attacked oftener than females, but in the collected statistics the cases are twice as numerous in females as in males. Tuberculous peritonitis occurs at all ages, but is most frequent between the ages of 20 and 40. It may occur in advanced life; one patient was 82 years of age. It is common in children with intestinal and mesenteric disease. Of 357 cases from the literature, there were under ten years, 27; between ten and twenty, 75; from twenty to thirty, 87; between thirty and forty, 71; from forty to fifty, 61; from fifty to sixty, 19; from sixty to seventy, 4; above seventy, 2. In America it is more common in the negro than in the white race.

Clinical Features.—In certain special features the tuberculous varies considerably from other forms of peritonitis. It presents a symptom-complex of extraordinary diversity.

The process may be *latent* and met with accidentally in an operation for hernia or ovarian tumor. An *acute* onset is not uncommon. Four cases in our records were diagnosed appendicitis, two acute cholecystitis, and six had symptoms of intestinal obstruction, in two of these coming on with great abruptness (Hamman). The cases have been mistaken for strangulated hernia. Other cases set in acutely with fever, abdominal tenderness and the symptoms of acute peritonitis. Cases with a slow onset, abdominal tenderness, tympanites, and continuous fever may be mistaken for *typhoid fever*.

Ascites is frequent, but the effusion is rarely large. It is sometimes hemorrhagic. In this form the diagnosis may rest between acute malignant disease, cirrhosis of the liver, and a chronic simple peritonitis—conditions which usually offer no special difficulties in differentiation. A most important point is the simultaneous presence of a pleurisy. The tuberculin test may be used. *Tympanites* may be present in very acute cases, when it is due to loss of tone in the intestines owing to inflammatory infiltration; or it may occur in old, long-standing cases when universal adhesion has taken place between the parietal and visceral layers. *Fever* is marked in the acute cases, and the temperature may reach 103° or 104° F. In many cases the fever is slight. In the more chronic cases subnormal temperatures are common, and for days the temperature may not rise above 97°. An occasional sign is pigmentation of the skin, which has led to the diagnosis of Addison's disease. A striking peculiarity of tuberculous peritonitis is the frequency with which it simulates or is associated with *tumor*. This may be:

Omental, due to puckering and rolling of this membrane until it forms an elongated firm mass, attached to the transverse colon and lying athwart the upper part of the abdomen. This cord-like structure is found also with cancerous peritonitis, but is much more common in tuberculosis. Gairdner called special attention to this tumor and in children saw it undergo gradual resolution. A resonant percussion note may sometimes be elicited above the mass.

Though usually near the umbilicus, the omental mass may form a prominent tumor in the right iliac region.

Sacculated exudation, in which the effusion is limited and confined by adhesions between the coils, the parietal peritoneum, the mesentery, and the abdominal or pelvic organs. This encysted exudate is most common in the middle zone, and may be mistaken for ovarian tumor. It may occupy the entire anterior portion of the peritoneum, or there may be a more limited saccular exudate on one side or the other. Within the pelvis it is associated with disease of the fallopian tubes. Eighteen cases in the gynecological wards (J. H. H.) were operated upon for pyosalpinx (Hamman).

In rare cases the tumor formations may be due to great retraction or thickening of the *intestinal coils.* The small intestine is shortened, enormously thickened, and the entire coil may form a firm knot close against the spine, suggesting a solid mass. The entire bowel from the duodenum to the rectum has been found forming such a hard nodular tumor.

Mesenteric glands may form large, tumor-like masses, more common in children than in adults. This may be confined to the abdominal glands. Ascites may coexist. The condition must be distinguished from that in children, in which, with ascites or tympanites—sometimes both—there can be felt irregular nodular masses, due to large caseous formations between the intestinal coils. No doubt in a considerable number of cases of tabes mesenterica, particularly with enlargement and hardness of the abdomen—which the French call *carreau*—there is involvement also of the peritoneum.

The *diagnosis* of these peritoneal tumors is sometimes very difficult. The omental mass is a less frequent source of error than any other; but a similar condition may occur in cancer. The most important problem is the diagnosis of the saccular exudation from ovarian tumor. In fully one-third of the recorded cases of laparotomy in tuberculous peritonitis the diagnosis of ovarian disease has been made. The most suggestive points for consideration are the history and the evidence of old tuberculous lesions. The physical condition is not of much help, as in many instances the patients are robust and well nourished. Irregular febrile attacks, gastro-intestinal disturbance, and pains are more common in tuberculous disease. Unless inflamed there is usually not much fever with ovarian cysts. The local signs are very deceptive, and may conform in every particular to those of cystic disease. The outlines in saccular exudation are rarely so well defined. The position and form may be variable, owing to alterations in the size of the coils of which in parts the walls are composed. Nodular cheesy masses may sometimes be felt at the periphery. Depression of the vaginal wall is mentioned as occurring in encysted peritonitis; but it is also found in ovarian tumor. The condition of the fallopian tubes, of the lungs and the pleurae, should be thoroughly examined. The association of salpingitis with an ill-defined anomalous mass in the abdomen should arouse suspicion, as should also involvement of the pleura, the lung, or an epididymis or seminal vesicle in the male.

Treatment.—General measures should be carried out as in pulmonary tuberculosis. Direct exposure of the abdomen to heliotherapy and to the X-rays has proved useful in some cases. Surgical treatment is most helpful in cases with ascites, but when there are tuberculous tumors and many adhesions the results are not satisfactory. In some cases the removal of a focus of infection, such as tuberculous mesenteric glands, a diseased appendix or a tuberculous fallopian tube, has been of benefit.

PULMONARY TUBERCULOSIS

Three clinical groups may be recognized: *acute pneumonic tuberculosis; chronic tuberculosis;* and *fibroid tuberculosis.*

According to the mode of infection there are two distinct types of lesions: (*a*) When the bacilli reach the lungs through the blood vessels or lymphatics the primary lesion is usually in the tissues of the alveolar walls, in the capillary vessels, the epithelium of the air cells, and in the connective-tissue framework of the septa. Small, gray, miliary nodules are formed, involving several alveoli and consisting largely of round, cuboidal, epithelioid cells. Depending upon the number of bacilli which reach the lung in this way, a localized or a general tuberculosis is excited. The tubercles may be scattered through both lungs and form part of a general miliary tuberculosis, or be confined to the lungs, or even in great part to one lung. The further stages may be: (1) Arrest of the process of cell division, gradual sclerosis of the tubercle, and ultimately complete fibroid transformation. (2) Caseation of the centre of the tubercle, extension at the periphery by proliferation of the epithelioid and lymphoid cells, so that the individual tubercles or small groups become confluent and form diffuse areas which undergo caseation and softening. (3) Occasionally as a result of intense infection of a localized region through the blood vessels the tubercles are thickly set. The intervening tissue is acutely inflamed, the air cells are filled with the products of a desquamative pneumonia, and many lobules are involved.

(*b*) When the bacilli reach the lung through the bronchi—inhalation or aspiration tuberculosis—the picture differs. The smaller bronchi and bronchioles are more extensively affected; the process is not confined to single groups of alveoli, but has a more lobular arrangement, and the tuberculous masses from the onset are larger, more diffuse, and may in some cases involve an entire lobe or the greater part of a lung. It is in this mode of infection that we see the characteristic peribronchial granulations and the areas of the so-called nodular bronchopneumonia. These bronchopneumonic areas, with on the one hand caseation, ulceration, and cavity formation, and on the other sclerosis and limitation, make up the essential elements in the anatomical picture of pulmonary tuberculosis.

Acute Pneumonic Tuberculosis

This form, known also as *galloping consumption,* occurs both in children and adults. The cases may be mistaken for simple pneumonia.

Two types may be recognized, the *pneumonic* and *bronchopneumonic.*

Pneumonic Form.—In this one lobe may be involved, or in some instances an entire lung. The organ is heavy, the affected portion airless; the pleura is usually covered with a thin exudate, and on section the picture resembles closely that of ordinary hepatization. The following is an extract from the report of a case in which death occurred twenty-nine days after the onset with the characters of an acute pneumonia: "Left lung weighs 1,500 grams (double the weight of the other organ) and is heavy and airless, crepitant only at the anterior margins. Section shows a small cavity the size of a walnut at the apex, about which are scattered tubercles in a consolidated tissue. The greater part of the lung presents a grayish-white appearance due to the aggregation of tubercles which in some places have a continuous, uniform appearance, in others are surrounded by injected and consolidated lung-tissue. Toward the margins of the lower lobe strands of this firm reddish tissue separate anemic, dry areas. There are in the right lung four small groups of tubercles but no caseous masses. The bronchial glands are not tuberculous." Here the intense local infection was due to the small focus at the apex, probably an aspiration process.

Only the most careful inspection may reveal the miliary tubercles, or the attention may be arrested by tubercles in the other lung or in the bronchial glands. The process may involve only one lobe. There may be older areas which are of a yellowish-white color and distinctly caseous. A remarkable picture is presented by cases in which the disease lasts for some months. A lobe or an entire lung may be enlarged, firm, airless throughout, and converted into a dry, yellowish-white, cheesy substance. In some cases the entire lung is in this condition, with perhaps only a narrow area of air-containing tissue on the margin. More commonly, if the disease has lasted for two or three months, rapid softening has taken place at the apex with extensive cavity formation.

Males are much more frequently attacked than females. Of a series of 15 cases, 11 were males. The onset was acute in 13, with a chill in 9. Bacilli were found in the sputum in one case as early as the fourth day.

Clinical Features.—The attack sets in abruptly with a chill, usually in a healthy individual, although in many cases the onset has been preceded by exposure to cold, or there have been debilitating circumstances. The temperature rises rapidly after the chill, there are pain in the side and cough, with at first mucoid, subsequently rusty expectoration which may contain tubercle bacilli. The dyspnea may become extreme and the patient may have suffocative attacks. The examination shows involvement of one lobe or of one lung, with dulness, increased fremitus, at first feeble or suppressed breath sounds, and subsequently well-marked bronchial breathing.

At this time, as a rule, the practitioner has no suspicion that the case is anything but one of frank lobar pneumonia. Occasionally there may be suspicious circumstances in the history but, as a rule, no stress is laid upon them in view of the characteristic mode of onset. Between the eighth and tenth day, instead of the expected crisis, the condition becomes aggravated, the temperature is irregular, and the pulse more rapid. There may be sweating, and the expectoration becomes mucopurulent and greenish in color—a point of special importance, to which Traube called attention. Even in the second or third week, with the persistence of these symptoms, the physician tries to console himself with the idea that the case is one of unresolved pneumonia, and that all will yet be well. Gradually, the severity of the symptoms, the presence of physical signs indicating softening, the existence of elastic tissue and tubercle bacilli in the sputum present the mournful proofs that the case is one of acute pneumonic tuberculosis. Death may occur on the sixth day. The earliest death in our series was on the thirteenth day. A majority of the cases drag on and death does not occur until the third month. In a few cases, even after a stormy onset and active course, the symptoms subside and the patient passes into a chronic stage.

Diagnosis.—Waters, of Liverpool, called attention to the difficulty in distinguishing these cases from ordinary pneumonia. Certainly the mode of onset affords no criterion whatever. A healthy young Irishman, a cab-driver, who had been kept waiting on a cold, blustering night until three in the morning, was seized the next afternoon with a violent chill, and the following day was admitted to the University Hospital, Philadelphia. He was the subject of a clinical lecture on the fifth day, when there was absent no single feature in history, symptoms or physical signs of acute lobar pneumonia of the right upper lobe. It was not until ten days later, when bacilli were found in the sputum, that we realized the true nature of the case. There is no criterion by which cases of this kind can be distinguished in the early stage. A point to which Traube called attention is the absence of breath sounds in the consolidated region; but this does not hold good in all cases. The tubular breathing may be intense and marked as early as the fourth day; and how common it is to have, as one of the earliest and most suggestive of signs of lobar pneumonia, suppression or enfeeblement of the breath sounds. In many cases, however, there are suspicious circumstances in the onset: the patient has been in bad health, may have had previous pulmonary trouble, or there are recurring chills. Careful examination of the sputum and a study of the physical signs from day to day can alone determine the true nature. A point of some moment is the fever, which in true pneumonia is more continuous, particularly in severe cases, whereas in this form of tuberculosis remissions are not infrequent. When lobar pneumonia occurs in a patient with chronic pulmonary tuberculosis, time alone can determine whether it is pneumococcal or tuberculous.

Acute Tuberculous Bronchopneumonia.—This is more common, particularly in children, and forms a majority of the cases of *phthisis florida*, or "galloping consumption." In the early stages the areas have a grayish red, later an opaque white, caseous appearance. By the fusion of contiguous masses an entire lobe may be rendered nearly solid, but crepitant areas can usually be found. This is not uncommon in the acute tuberculosis of adults but is more frequent in children. The following is from the postmortem report of a case on a child aged four months, who died in the sixth week of illness: "On section, the right upper lobe is occupied with caseous masses from 5 to 12 mm. in diameter, separated from each other by an intervening tissue of a deep red color. The bronchi are filled with cheesy substance. The middle and lower lobes are studded with tubercles, many of which are becoming caseous. Toward the diaphragmatic surface of the lower lobe there is a small cavity the size of a marble. The left lung is more crepitant and uniformly studded with tubercles of all sizes, some as large as peas. The bronchial glands are very large, and one contains a tuberculous abscess."

There is a form of tuberculous *aspiration* pneumonia, to which Bäumler called attention, occurring as a sequence of hemoptysis, and due to the aspiration of blood and the contents of pulmonary cavities into the finer tubes. There are fever, dyspnea, and signs of a diffuse bronchopneumonia. Some of these cases run a very rapid course. This accident may occur early in the disease or follow hemorrhage in a well-marked pulmonary tuberculosis.

In children the enlarged bronchial glands usually surround the root of the lung, and even pass deeply into the substance; the lobules may be involved by direct contact. In other cases the caseous bronchopneumonia involves groups of alveoli or lobules in different portions of the lungs, more commonly at both apices, forming areas from 1 to 3 cm. in diameter. The size of the mass depends largely upon that of the bronchus involved. There are cases which probably come in this category, in which, with an acute illness of from four to eight weeks, the lungs are extensively studded with large gray tubercles, ranging in size from 5 to 10 mm. In some instances there are cheesy masses the size of a cherry. All of these are grayish-white, distinctly cheesy, and between the adjacent ones, particularly in the lower lobe, there may be recent pneumonia or splenization. In such a case at the Philadelphia Hospital death took place about the eighth week from the abrupt onset with hemorrhage. There were no extensive areas of consolidation, but the cheesy nodules were uniformly scattered throughout both lungs. No softening had taken place.

Secondary infections are not uncommon; but Prudden was able to show that the tubercle bacillus could produce not only distinct tubercle nodules, but also the various kinds of exudative pneumonia, the exudates varying in appearance in different cases, which phenomena occurred absolutely without other organisms. These exudative phenomena represent the result of reinfection in tissues sensitized by previous infection.

Symptoms.—The symptoms of acute bronchopneumonic tuberculosis are very variable. In adults the disease may attack persons in good health, but over-worked or "run down." Hemorrhage initiates the attack in a few cases. There may be repeated chills; the temperature is high, the pulse rapid, and the respirations increased. The loss of flesh and strength is striking.

The physical *signs* may at first be uncertain and indefinite, but finally there are areas of dulness, usually at the apices; the breath sounds are harsh and tubular, with numerous râles. The sputum may early show elastic tissue and tubercle bacilli. In the acute cases, within three weeks, the patient may be in a marked toxic state, with delirium, dry tongue and high fever. Death may occur within three weeks. In other cases the onset is severe, with high fever, rapid loss of flesh and strength, and signs of extensive unilateral or bilateral disease. Softening takes place and there are sweats, chills and progressive emaciation. Six or eight weeks later the patient may begin to improve, the fever lessens, the general symptoms abate, and a case which looked as if it would terminate fatally drags on and becomes chronic.

In *children* the disease most commonly follows the infectious diseases, particularly measles and whooping cough. At least *three groups* of these tuberculous bronchopneumonias may be recognized. In the *first* the child is taken ill suddenly while teething or during convalescence from fever; the temperature rises rapidly, the cough is severe, and there may be signs of consolidation at one or both apices with râles. Death may occur within a few days, and the lung shows areas of bronchopneumonia, with perhaps here and there scattered opaque grayish-yellow nodules. Macroscopically the affection does not look tuberculous, but histologically miliary granulations and bacilli may be found. Tubercles are usually present in the bronchial glands, but the appearance of the bronchopneumonia may be exceedingly deceptive, and it may require careful examination to determine its tuberculous character. The *second* group is represented by the case of the child previously quoted, who died in the sixth week with the ordinary symptoms of severe bronchopneumonia. The *third group* is that in which, during the convalescence from an infectious disease, the child is taken ill with fever, cough and dyspnea. The severity of the symptoms abates within the first fortnight; but there is loss of flesh, the general condition is bad, and examination shows scattered râles throughout the lungs, and areas of defective resonance. The child has sweats, the fever becomes irregular, and in many cases the picture gradually passes into that of chronic pulmonary tuberculosis.

Treatment.—In tuberculous pneumonia, we have no specific treatment and general measures for comfort and nutrition are indicated. With the process confined to one lung collapse therapy might be tried.

Chronic Tuberculosis of the Lungs

Under this heading may be grouped the great majority of cases of pulmonary tuberculosis.

Morbid Anatomy.—The lungs show a remarkable variety of lesions, nodular tubercles, diffuse tuberculous infiltration, caseous masses, pneumonic areas and cavities with changes in the pleura, bronchi and bronchial glands.

Distribution of the Lesions.—As a rule the most advanced lesions are in the upper lobes, and the disease progresses downward, usually more rapidly in one of the lungs. This general statement, accepted ever since the description of Laënnec, was elaborated by Kingston Fowler, who found that the disease in its onward progress through the lungs follows, in a majority of the cases, distinct routes. In the upper lobe the primary lesion of the adult form is not, as a rule, at the extreme apex, but from an inch to an inch and a half below it, and nearer to the posterior and external borders. The lesion here tends to spread downward, probably from inhalation and this accounts for the frequent circumstance that examination behind, in the supraspinous fossa, may give indications of disease before any evidences exist at the apex in front. Anteriorly this initial focus corresponds to a spot below the centre of the clavicle, and the direction of extension in front is along the anterior aspect of the upper lobe, along a line running about an inch and a half from the inner ends of the first, second, and third interspaces. A second less common site of the primary lesion in the apex "corresponds on the chest wall with the first and second interspaces below the outer third of the clavicle." The extension is downward, so that the outer part of the upper lobe is chiefly involved.

In the middle lobe of the right lung the affection usually follows disease of the upper lobe on the same side. In the involvement of the lower lobe the first secondary infiltration is about an inch to an inch and a half below the posterior extremity of its apex, and corresponds on the chest wall to a spot opposite the fifth dorsal spine. This involvement is of great importance clinically, as "in the great majority of cases, when the physical signs of the disease at the apex are sufficiently definite to allow of the diagnosis of phthisis being made, the lower lobe is already affected." Examination, therefore, should be made carefully of this area in all suspicious cases. In this situation the lesion spreads downward and laterally along the line of the interlobular septa, a line marked by the vertebral border of the scapula, when the hand is placed on the opposite scapula and the elbow raised above the level of the shoulder.

Once present, the disease usually extends in time to the opposite upper lobe; but not, as a rule, until the lower lobe of the lung first affected has been attacked.

Lesions of the base may be primary, though this is rare. The proportion of basal to apical tuberculosis has been given as 1 to 500 but this is probably too low. In the Jefferson Hospital we have proved a number of cases of basal involvement to be tuberculous only by finding tubercle bacilli in material obtained by the bronchoscope. Other findings were inconclusive. In very chronic cases there may be arrested lesions at the apex and more recent lesions at the base.

The Lesions in Pulmonary Tuberculosis.—*Miliary Tubercles.*—They have one of two distributions: (1) A dissemination due to aspiration of tuberculous material, the tubercles being situated in the air cells or the walls of the smaller bronchi; (2) the distribution due to dissemination of tubercle bacilli by the lymph current, the tubercles being scattered about the old foci in a radial manner—the secondary crop of Laënnec. Much more rarely there is a scattered dissemination from infection here and there of the smaller vessels, the tubercles being situated in the vessel walls. Sometimes, with cavity formation at the apex, the greater part of the lower lobes presents many groups of sclerotic, miliary tubercles, which may form the distinguishing anatomical feature—a chronic miliary tuberculosis.

Tuberculous Bronchopneumonia.—In a large proportion of cases of chronic tuberculosis the terminal bronchiole is the point of origin of the process, so that we find the smaller bronchi and their territories blocked with the products of inflammation in all stages of *caseation.* At an early period a cross-section of an area of tuberculous bronchopneumonia gives a characteristic appearance. The central bronchiole is seen as a small orifice or is plugged with cheesy contents, while surrounding it is a caseous nodule, the peribronchial tubercle. The picture depends much upon the slowness or rapidity with which the process advanced. The following changes may occur:

Ulceration.—When the caseation takes place rapidly or ulceration occurs in the bronchial wall, the mass may break down and form a small cavity.

Sclerosis.—In other instances the process is more chronic and fibroid changes gradually produce a sclerosis. This may be confined to the margin, forming a limiting capsule, within which is a uniform, firm, cheesy substance, in which lime salts are often deposited. This represents the healing of these areas of caseous bronchopneumonia. It is only, however, when complete fibroid transformation or calcification has occurred that we can really speak of healing. In many instances the colonies of miliary tubercles about these areas show that the process is still active. Subsequently, in ulcerative process, these calcareous bodies—lung-stones—may be expectorated.

Pneumonia.—An important though secondary place is occupied by inflammation of the alveoli surrounding the tubercles, which become filled with epithelioid cells. The consolidation may extend for some distance about the tuberculous foci and unite them into areas of uniform consolidation. Although in some instances this inflammatory process may be simple, in others it is undoubtedly specific and is excited by the tubercle bacilli. It may present a very varied appearance; in some instances resembling ordinary red hepatization, in others being more homogeneous and infiltrated. In other cases the contents of the alveoli undergo fatty degeneration, and appear on the cut surface as opaque white or yellowish-white bodies. In early tuberculosis much of the consolidation is due to this infiltration.

Cavities.—A cavity is produced by necrosis and ulceration. The process usually begins in the wall of the bronchus in a tuberculous area. Dilatation is produced by retained secretion, and necrosis and ulceration of the wall occur with gradual destruction of the contiguous tissues. By extension of the necrosis and ulceration the cavity increases, contiguous ones unite, and there may be a series of small excavations communicating with a bronchus. In nearly all instances the process extends from the bronchi, though necrosis and softening may take place in the centre of a caseous area without primary involvement of the bronchial wall. Three forms may be recognized.

The *fresh ulcerative*, seen in acute cases, in which there is no limiting membrane, but the walls are made up of softened, necrotic, and caseous masses. A small cavity of this sort, just beneath the pleura, may rupture and cause pneumothorax. In acute pneumonic tuberculosis they may be large, occupying the greater portion of the upper lobe. In the chronic ulcerative form, cavities of this sort are invariably present in those portions of the lung in which the disease is advancing. At the apex there may be a large old cavity with well-defined walls, while at the interior margin of the upper lobes, or in the apices of the lower lobes, there are recent ulcerating cavities communicating with the bronchi.

Cavities with Well-defined Walls.—A majority of the cavities in the chronic cases have a well-defined limiting membrane, the inner surface of which constantly produces pus. The walls are crossed by trabeculae which represent remnants of bronchi and blood vessels. Even the cavities with well-defined walls extend gradually by a slow necrosis and destruction of contiguous lung tissue. The contents are usually purulent. Not infrequently the membrane is vascular or it may be hemorrhagic. Occasionally, when gangrene has occurred, the contents are horribly fetid. These cavities may occupy the greater portion of the apex, forming an irregular series which communicate with each other and with the bronchi, or the entire upper lobe except the anterior margin may be excavated, forming a thin-walled cavity. In rare instances there is total excavation of the lung, not a remnant of which remains, except perhaps a narrow strip at the anterior margin. In a case of this kind, the cavity held 40 fluid ounces, in another 42 ounces.

Quiescent Cavities.—When quite small and surrounded by dense cicatricial tissue communicating with the bronchi they form the *cicatrices fistuleuses* of Laënnec. Occasionally one apex may be represented by a series of these small cavities, surrounded by dense fibrous tissue. The lining membrane of these old cavities may be quite smooth, almost like a mucous membrane.

In the formation of cavities the blood vessels gradually become closed by obliterating inflammation. They are the last structures to yield and may be completely exposed in a cavity, even with the circulation going on in them. The erosion of a large vessel which has not been obliterated is not infrequent and causes profuse hemorrhage. Another event is the formation of aneurisms on the arteries in the walls of cavities. These may be small or form sacs the size of a walnut or larger. They are important with regard to hemoptysis.

And finally, about cavities of all sorts, the connective tissue grows, tending to limit their extent. The thickening is particularly marked beneath the pleura, and in chronic cases an entire apex may be converted into a mass of fibrous tissue, inclosing a few small cavities.

Pleura.—Practically, in all cases of chronic tuberculosis the pleura is involved. Adhesions take place which may be thin or dense and firm, uniting layers of 2 to 5 mm. in thickness. This pleurisy may be simple, but in many cases it is tuberculous, and miliary tubercles or caseous masses may occur in the thickened membrane. Effusion is not infrequent: serous, purulent or hemorrhagic. Pneumothorax is a common accident.

Smaller Bronchi.—Changes in the *smaller bronchi* control the situation in the early stages of pulmonary tuberculosis, and play an important rôle throughout. The process very often begins in the walls of the smaller tubes and leads to caseation, distention with products of inflammation, and bronchopneumonia. In many cases the implication of the bronchus is an extension upward of a process which began in the smallest bronchiole. This involvement weakens the wall, leading to bronchiectasis, not an uncommon event. The mucous membrane of the larger bronchi is more or less swollen, and in some instances ulcerated. Besides these specific lesions, they may be the seat, especially in children, of inflammation due to secondary invasion, most frequently by the *pneumococcus* with the production of a bronchopneumonia.

The bronchial glands.—In the more acute cases these are swollen and edematous. Miliary tubercles and caseous foci are usually present. In cases of chronic tuberculosis the caseous areas are common, calcification may occur, and not infrequently purulent softening.

Changes in the Other Organs.—Tuberculosis is the most common. In 275 autopsies the brain presented tuberculous lesions in 31, the spleen in 33, liver in 12, kidneys in 32, intestines in 65, and the pericardium in 7. Other groups of glands besides the bronchial may be affected.

Amyloid change may occur in the liver, spleen, kidneys, and mucous membrane of the intestines. The *liver* is often the seat of extensive fatty infiltration, which may cause marked enlargement. *Intestinal tuberculosis* occurs in advanced cases and is responsible in great part for the diarrhea.

Endocarditis was present in 12 of 275 postmortems and in 27 of Kidd's 500 cases. Tubercle bacilli may be found in the vegetations. Tubercles may be present on the endocardium, particularly of the right ventricle.

The *larynx* may be involved, and ulceration of the vocal cords and destruction of the epiglottis are not at all uncommon.

Modes of Onset.—We have already seen that tuberculosis of the lungs may occur as the chief part of a general infection, or may set in with symptoms which closely simulate acute pneumonia. In the ordinary type of pulmonary tuberculosis the invasion is gradual and less striking, but presents an extraordinarily diverse picture. As has been noted in the primary infection (or childhood form) the manifestations are surprisingly few unless miliary or pneumonic disease occurs. We are here specially concerned with the adult form, representing reinfection (endogenous or exogenous). The great variations must be remembered as the progress represents a series of remissions and exacerbations. New areas of involvement will vary with the character of the infection and the reaction of the patient. We should think of irregularity rather than a fixed course as characteristic. This applies with equal force to the modes of onset among which are the following:

Latent Types.—Many cases are found in routine examinations and it is probable that many slight, ill-defined ailments are due to unrecognized tuberculosis. In the history of patients with tuberculosis such attacks are not infrequently mentioned. The disease may make considerable progress before serious symptoms arouse the attention of the patient and may advance to excavation of an apex before he seeks advice. It is remarkable how slight the lung symptoms may have been. They may be masked by serious disease elsewhere as in the peritoneum, intestines or bones.

With Symptoms of Dyspepsia and Anemia.—The gastric mode of onset is very common, and the early manifestation may be irritability of the stomach with vomiting or acid dyspepsia with eructations. In young girls and children with this dyspepsia there is frequently a pronounced anemia, and the patient complains of palpitation of the heart, increasing weakness, slight afternoon fever and amenorrhea.

Malarial Symptoms.—In some cases the onset is with symptoms which suggest malarial fever. The patient has repeated paroxysms of chills, fevers, and sweats, which may recur with regularity.

With Pleurisy.—The first symptoms may be from a dry pleurisy over an apex, with a persistent friction murmur. In other instances the pulmonary symptoms follow an attack of pleurisy with effusion. The exudate gradually disappears, but cough persists, the patient becomes feverish, and signs of disease gradually become manifest. About one-third of all cases of pleurisy with effusion subsequently have pulmonary tuberculosis.

With Laryngeal Symptoms.—The. primary localizations may be in the larynx, though in a majority of the instances in which huskiness and laryngeal symptoms are the first noticeable features there are foci already in the lung. The group in which throat and larynx symptoms precede the manifestations of pulmonary tuberculosis is a very important one.

With Hemoptysis.—The first indication may be a brisk hemorrhage, following which the pulmonary symptoms may come on with great rapidity. In other cases the hemoptysis recurs, and it may be months before the symptoms become well established. There should be no glib explanation of hemoptysis as due to bleeding from the throat. In a majority of these cases the local tuberculous lesion exists at the date of the hemoptysis. Blood-streaked sputum may have the same significance.

With Tuberculosis of the Cervico-axillary Glands.—Preceding the onset of pulmonary disease for months, or even years, the lymph nodes of the neck or of the neck and axilla of one side may be enlarged. These cases are of importance because of the latency of the pulmonary lesions and in such patients the corresponding apex of the lung may be extensively involved.

With General Symptoms.—Malaise, fatigue and indefinite nervous disturbances with loss of weight may be the marked features and suggest neurasthenia or hyperthyroidism. Special attention should be given to fatigue for which there is no evident cause.

With Bronchial Symptoms.—In by far the largest number the onset is with a *bronchitis* or "a cold." There has been, perhaps, a liability to catch cold easily or the patient has been subject to nasopharyngeal catarrh; then a cough begins, which may be frequent and irritating. The examination of the lungs may reveal fine râles at one apex and perhaps wheezing bronchitic râles in other parts. In a few cases the early symptoms are suggestive of asthma with wheezing and piping râles.

Miscellaneous Group.—(1) Following acute infections, such as influenza. (2) With or after pregnancy. (3) After an operation in which ether anesthesia was used. (4) In association with ischiorectal abscess and fistula-in-ano. In all of these an inactive process may be rendered active.

Clinical Features.—Anatomical stages can not be satisfactorily correlated with corresponding clinical periods, and a patient with a well-marked cavity may be in a better condition and with greater prospects of recovery than a patient with diffuse consolidation. It is a mistake to try and classify all patients into various stages. Each patient is a distinct problem.

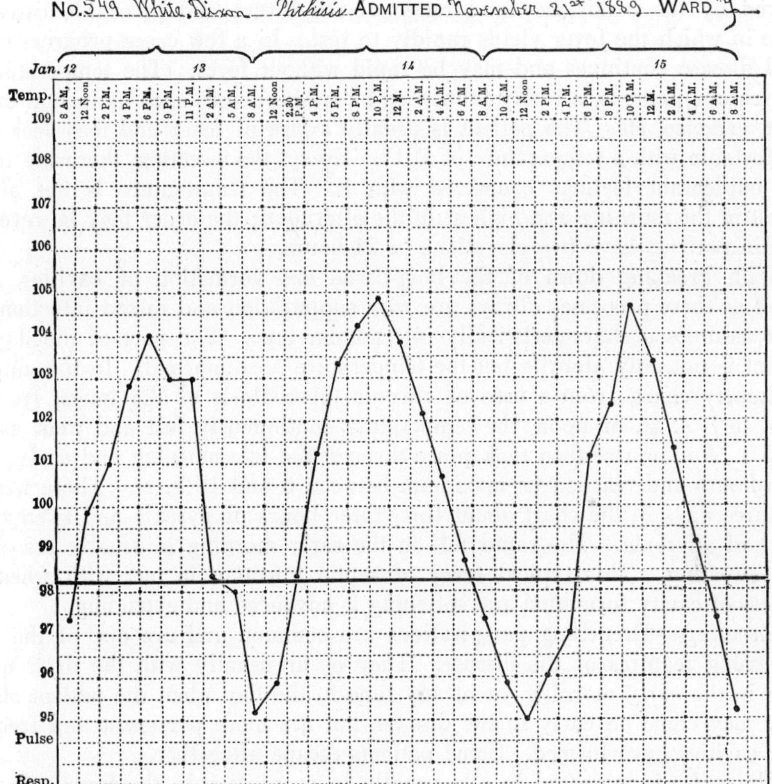

Chart IV.—Temperature Record. Chronic Tuberculosis.

Fever.—The temperature varies in normal individuals, and the afternoon range may be 99° F. The difference between the mouth and rectal temperature may be a degree, and in full-blooded persons, in the nervous, and after exercise the normal rectal temperature may be 100.5° or even 101° F. To get a correct idea of the temperature range it is necessary to make observations every two hours at first. The usual morning and evening record may be deceptive, giving neither the minimum nor maximum. The former usually occurs between 2 and 6 A. M., and the latter between 2 and 6 P. M. but this may be reversed. In a tuberculous female there is often an increase of fever at the time of menstruation.

Fever, one of the earliest and most important signs, is due to the effect of the toxins or materials absorbed from the tuberculous focus. Later the hectic fever is caused in part by other organisms. It is an auto-inoculation comparable with the fever produced by an injection of tuberculin. Anything that stimulates the local lymph and blood flow favors the discharge of the toxins and causes fever. A patient at rest may be afebrile; after exercise the temperature may be 102.5°. In acute cases the fever is more or less continuous, resembling that of typhoid fever or pneumonia, with slight morning remissions. It may set in with a chill and be followed by sweats, and there are cases with a marked intermittent pyrexia from the onset. As a rule, the degree of activity may be gauged by the persistency and range of the fever; and favorable cases are those in which the fever yields rapidly to rest. In a few cases progress of the local disease continues and may be rapid without fever. The temperature of tuberculous patients is easily influenced by trivial causes such as mental excitement, exercise, etc. The patient is usually aware of fever and may feel more comfortable with a temperature of 101°. Except the sweating, there are rarely any unpleasant feelings connected with it. The temperature is not always lowest in the morning and highest in the afternoon; the order may be reversed. Certain patients have two elevations in 24 hours.

With breaking down of the lung-tissue and formation of cavities, associated as these processes always are with suppuration and mixed infection, the fever assumes a characteristically intermittent type. For part of the day the patient is not only afebrile but the temperature is subnormal. In the annexed two-hourly chart, from a case of chronic tuberculosis of the lungs, from 10 P. M. to 8 A. M. or noon, the temperature continuously fell and went as low as 95°. A slow rise then took place through the late morning and early afternoon hours and reached its maximum between 6 and 10 P. M. There were in the three days in the chart about forty-three hours of pyrexia and twenty-nine hours of apyrexia. The rapid fall in the early morning is usually associated with sweating. This typical fever of septic infection is met with when the process of cavity formation and softening is advanced and extending.

Sweating.—Drenching perspirations are common and are one of the most distressing features of the disease. They occur usually with the drop in the fever in the early morning, or at any time in the day when the patient sleeps. They may come on early in the disease, but are more persistent and frequent after cavities have formed. Some patients escape altogether.

The *pulse* is increased in rate usually in proportion to the fever. Even at rest and afebrile the pulse may be rapid, but the excitement of counting it may increase the rate 20 to 30 beats. The pulse is often full, soft and compressible; even after recovery it may remain rapid. Pulsation may sometimes be seen in the capillaries and in the veins on the back of the hand.

Emaciation is a pronounced feature, from which the two common names of the disease have been derived. The loss of weight is gradual and, if the disease is extending, progressive. The scales give one of the best indications of the progress. It is most rapid early in the disease, when the loss may be five or six pounds a week; and usually is in direct relation to the intensity and duration of the fever. With arrest of the progress and fall in temperature the patient usually begins to regain weight. The average gain in weight of 901 patients at the Adirondack Sanatorium was fourteen pounds (L. Brown). A gain of two pounds a week is satisfactory. Loss of strength may be out of proportion to and quite independent of loss of weight.

Pain in the chest may be early and troublesome or absent throughout. It is usually associated with pleurisy, and may be sharp and stabbing, and either constant or felt only during coughing. Perhaps the commonest situation is in the lower thorax, though in some cases it is beneath the scapula or referred to the apex. The attacks may recur at long intervals.

Cough is one of the earliest symptoms, and is present in the majority of cases from beginning to end. There is nothing peculiar or distinctive about it. At first dry and hacking, and perhaps scarcely exciting the attention of the patient, it subsequently becomes looser, more constant and associated with a glairy, mucopurulent expectoration. In the early stages the cough is bronchial in its origin. When cavities have formed it becomes more paroxysmal, and is most marked in the morning or after a sleep. Cough is not a constant symptom, however, and a patient may have well-marked excavation at one apex with little or no cough. So, too, there may be well-marked physical signs without expectoration or cough. In well-established cases the nocturnal paroxysms are distressing and prevent sleep. The cough may be so persistent and severe as to cause vomiting, and the patient becomes emaciated from loss of food—Morton's cough (Phthisiologia, 1689, p. 101). The laryngeal complications give a peculiar husky quality to the cough, and when erosion and ulceration have proceeded far in the vocal cords the cough is much less effective.

Sputum.—This varies greatly in amount and character with the different stages. There are patients with well-marked signs at one apex, with slight cough and moderately high fever, without sputum. So, also, there are patients with extensive consolidation but without enough expectoration to enable an examination for bacilli to be made. In the early stage of pulmonary tuberculosis the sputum is chiefly catarrhal and has a glairy, sago-like appearance, due to alveolar cells which have undergone myeline degeneration. There is nothing distinctive or peculiar in this expectoration, which may persist for months without indicating serious trouble. The earliest trace of characteristic sputum may show small grayish or greenish-gray purulent masses. These are always suggestive and should be picked out for microscopic examination. As softening comes on, the expectoration becomes more profuse and purulent, but may still contain a quantity of alveolar epithelium. Finally, when cavities exist, the sputum assumes the nummular form; each mass is isolated, flattened, greenish-gray in color, quite airless, and, when spat into water, sinks to the bottom.

By the microscopic examination of the sputum we determine whether the process is tuberculous, and whether softening has occurred. The bacilli in stained preparations are seen as elongated, slightly curved, red rods, sometimes presenting a beaded appearance. Only one or two may be found on a slide, or they are so abundant that the entire field is occupied. Repeated examinations may be necessary. In *basal tuberculosis* the sputum may be negative for long periods.

The continued presence of tubercle bacilli in the sputum is an infallible indication of tuberculosis. One or two may possibly be due to accidental inhalation. In nummular sputa the bacilli are very abundant.

Elastic tissue may be derived from the bronchi, the alveoli, or from the arterial coats; and its appearance will vary with the locality from which it comes. In the examination for this it is not necessary to boil the sputum with caustic potash. In almost all instances if the sputum is spread in a sufficiently thin layer the fragments of elastic tissue can be seen with the naked eye. The thick, purulent portions are placed upon a glass plate 15 x 15 cm. and flattened into a thin layer by a second glass plate 10 x 10 cm. In the layer between the glass plates any fragments of elastic tissue show on a black background as grayish-yellow spots; the uppermost piece of glass is slid along until the fragment is exposed, when it is picked out and placed upon an ordinary slide. Fragments of bread, etc., may present an opaque white appearance, but can readily be recognized. Fragments of epithelium from the tongue, infiltrated with micrococci, are more deceptive.

The bronchial elastic tissue forms an elongated network, or two or three long, narrow fibres are found close together. From the blood vessels a somewhat similar form may be seen and occasionally a distinct sheeting is found as if it had come from a good-sized artery. The elastic tissue of the alveolar wall is distinctive, the fibres are branched and often show the outline of the arrangement of the air cells. The elastic tissue from bronchi or alveoli indicates extensive erosion of a tube and softening of the lung tissue.

Another occasional constituent is blood, which may be the chief characteristic of the sputum in hemoptysis or may simply tinge the sputum. In cases with large cavities, in addition to bacteria, various fungi may be found, of which the aspergillus is the most important. Sarcinae may occur.

Albumin Reaction.—Albumin is found in the sputum in a majority of cases and its continued absence is evidence against tuberculosis. It occurs in other destructive conditions.

Calcareous Fragments.—The size varies from a small pea to a large cherry. As a rule, a single one is ejected; sometimes large numbers are coughed up in the course of the disease. They are formed in the lung by the calcification of caseous masses, and it is said also occasionally in obstructed bronchi. They may come from the bronchial glands by ulceration into the bronchi, and there is a case of record of suffocation in a child from this cause.

The daily *amount* of expectoration varies. In rapidly advancing cases, with much cough, it may reach as high as 500 cc. in the day. In cases with large cavities the chief amount is brought up in the morning. The expectoration of tuberculous patients usually has a heavy, sweetish odor, and occasionally it is fetid, owing to decomposition in the cavities.

Hemoptysis.—One famous Hippocratic axiom says, "From a spitting of blood there is a spitting of pus." The older writers thought that the "phthisis" was directly due to the inflammatory or putrefactive changes caused by the hemorrhage into the lung. Morton, however, in his section, *Phithisis ab Haemopeöe*, rather doubted this sequence. Laënnec and Louis, and later Traube, regarded the hemoptysis as an evidence of existing disease of the lung. From the accurate views of Laënnec and Louis the profession was led away by Graves, and particularly by Niemeyer, who held that the blood in the air cells set up an inflammatory process, a common termination of which was caseation. We have learned that many cases in which the physical examination is negative show, either during the period of hemorrhage or immediately after it, tubercle bacilli in the sputum and we regard hemoptysis as an indication of existing disease. In young, apparently healthy, persons cases of hemoptysis may be divided into three groups. In the first the bleeding has come on without pneumonia, without overexertion or injury, and there is no family history of tuberculosis. The physical examination is negative, and the sputum at the time of the hemorrhage and subsequently shows no tubercle bacilli although the X-ray study may show disease. Some of these individuals retain good health and have no further trouble. Of 386 cases of hemoptysis noted by Ware in private practice 62 recovered, and pulmonary disease did not subsequently occur.

In a second group individuals apparently in perfect health are suddenly attacked, perhaps after a slight exertion or during some athletic exercises. The physical examination is negative, but tubercle bacilli may be found in the bloody sputum, more frequently a few days later, and the X-ray study shows a lesion.

In a third set of cases the individuals have been in failing health for a month or two, but the symptoms have not been urgent and perhaps not noticed. Physical examination shows well-marked tuberculous disease, and there are both tubercle bacilli and elastic tissue in the sputum.

An interesting study of hemoptysis was made in the Prussian army by Stricker. During 1890-'95 there were 900 cases admitted to the hospitals; in 480 the hemorrhage came on without recognizable cause. Of these, 417 cases, 86 per cent, were certainly or probably tuberculous but in only 221 was the evidence conclusive. In a second group of 213 cases the hemorrhage came on during military exercise, and of these 75 were shown to be tuberculous. In 118 cases the hemorrhage followed special exercises, as in the gymnasium or riding or swimming. In 24 cases it occurred during the exercise of the voice as in singing or in the use of wind instruments. In 24 cases the hemorrhage followed trauma, a fall or a blow upon the thorax. In 7 of these tuberculosis was positively present, and in 6 other cases there was a strong probability of its existence.

Hemoptysis occurs in from 60 to 80 per cent of all cases of pulmonary tuberculosis and as an early symptom in about 10 per cent. In a majority of cases the bleeding recurs. Sometimes it is a special feature so that a hemorrhagic form has been recognized. The amount of blood varies from a couple of drams to a pint or more. In 69 per cent of 4,125 cases of hemoptysis at the Brompton Hospital the amount was under half an ounce.

A distinction may be drawn between hemoptysis early in the disease and that which occurs in the later periods. In the former the bleeding is usually slight, is apt to recur, and fatal hemorrhage is very rare. In these cases the bleeding is usually from small areas of softening or from erosions in the bronchial mucosa. In the later periods, after cavities have formed, the bleeding is, as a rule, more profuse and is more apt to be fatal. Single large hemorrhages, proving quickly fatal, are very rare, except in advanced stages when the bleeding comes from an erosion of a good-sized vessel in the wall of a cavity or from the rupture of an aneurism of a pulmonary vessel.

Hemoptysis, as a rule, sets in suddenly. Without warning the patient may notice a warm salt taste and the mouth fills with blood. It may come up with a slight cough. The total amount may not be more than a few drams, and for a day or two the patient may spit up small quantities. When a large vessel is eroded or an aneurism bursts, the amount of blood is large, and in a short time a pint or two may be expectorated. Fatal hemorrhage may occur into a very large cavity without any blood being coughed up. The character of the blood is, as a rule, distinctive. It is frothy, mixed with mucus, generally bright red, except when large amounts are expectorated, and then it may be dark. The sputum may be blood-tinged for some days, or shows brownish-black streaks, or friable nodules consisting of blood corpuscles may be coughed up. Blood moulds of the smaller bronchi are sometimes expectorated.

The microscopic examination of the sputum in hemorrhage cases is most important. If spread out, there may be noted, even in an apparently pure hemorrhagic mass, little portions of mucus from which bacilli or elastic tissue may be obtained. Flick and others called attention to the frequency with which hemoptysis is associated with intercurrent infections.

Dyspnea is not common in ordinary tuberculosis. The greater part of one lung may be diseased and local trouble exist at the other apex without any shortness of breath. Even with high fever the respirations may not be much increased. Dyspnea occurs with the rapid extension in both lungs of broncho-pneumonia; with miliary tuberculosis; with pneumothorax; in old cases with much emphysema and fibrosis and it may be associated with cyanosis; in cases with marked adhesions to the diaphragm and the flat diaphragm often found with emphysema; in long-standing cases, with contracted apices or great thickening of the pleura, the right heart is enlarged, and the dyspnea may be cardiac; and with acute pleurisy or large effusion.

Physical Signs.—The presence of definite physical signs means that a relatively considerable degree of change has occurred. In the earliest stage the most careful examination may not show any sign of disease. The aid of the X-ray study is essential but we must remember that in this the man is all important. He is drawing conclusions from plates and shadows and much depends on his skill in interpretation. The whole burden of diagnosis should not be put on the roentgenologist. There are cases in which the X-ray study shows nothing and yet there are tubercle bacilli in the sputum. We have no right to decide that a patient is free of pulmonary tuberculosis from the absence of physical signs and of bacilli in the sputum; there must be a negative X-ray study also.

Inspection.—The shape of the chest is often suggestive, though the disease may be found in chests of any build. Practically, in a considerable proportion of cases the thorax is long and narrow, with wide intercostal spaces, the ribs more vertical in direction, and the costal angle narrow. The scapulae are "winged," a point noted by Hippocrates. Another common type of chest is that which is flattened in the anteroposterior diameter. The costal cartilages may be prominent and the sternum depressed. The shoulder, the nipple or the scapula on the affected side may be lower. Asymmetry of the scapulae is often seen. Inspection of the back is always important. There may be muscular atrophy, especially of the trapezius. Special examination should be made of the clavicular regions to see if one clavicle or if the spaces above or below it are more marked. Defective *expansion* at one apex is an early and important sign. the precordia should be noted, as a wide area of impulse, particularly in the second to fourth interspaces, often results from disease of the left apex. From behind the patient, looking over the shoulders, one can often better estimate the relative expansion of the apices. Atrophy of the muscles of the shoulder-girdle on the affected side is common, and slight scoliosis may be present. Movement may be restricted on the affected side, particularly at the apex. Pleurisy with adhesions or with effusion, fibrosis, and pneumonic consolidation may limit the movement of one side. The Litten phenomenon (seen best on the right side) may be restricted or absent. The chest expansion may be much reduced.

Palpation.—Deficiency in expansion can be gauged by placing the hands in the subclavicular spaces and then in the lateral regions of the chest and asking the patient to draw a full breath slowly. Standing behind the patient and placing the thumbs in the supraclavicular and the fingers in the infraclavicular spaces one can judge as to the relative mobility. There may be tenderness above the clavicle and in the suprascapular region. The tactile fremitus is increased wherever there is local growth of tubercle or extensive caseation. In comparing the apices it is important to bear in mind that normally the fremitus is stronger over the right than the left. In the later stages, when cavities form, the fremitus is usually much exaggerated over them. When the pleura is greatly thickened the fremitus may be diminished. The use of the ulnar side of the hand is useful in comparisons.

Percussion.—Tubercles, inflammatory products, fibroid changes, and cavities produce changes in the pulmonary resonance. There may be localized disease, even of some extent, without much alteration, as when the tubercles are scattered there is air-containing tissue between them. If there is local emphysema the note may be hyperresonant. In early stages percussion may be negative as it requires a fair-sized area of infiltration to cause a change in the percussion note. An early and valuable sign is defective resonance upon and above a clavicle. In a considerable proportion of cases the dulness is first noted in these regions. The comparison between the two sides should be made also when the breath is held after a full inspiration, as the defective resonance may then be more clearly marked. In early stages the percussion note is usually higher in pitch, and it may require an experienced ear to detect the difference. In recent consolidation from caseous pneumonia the percussion note often has a tympanitic quality. Confusing and varying signs may be due to areas of collapse or a small pneumothorax. A wooden dulness is rarely heard except in old cases with extensive fibroid change. Over large, thin-walled cavities at the apex the cracked-pot sound may be obtained. Percussion should be carefully done in the supraspinous fossae and the interscapular space, as they correspond to important areas involved early. By light percussion along the border of the trapezius and in the supraclavicular and supraspinous fossae, areas of apical resonance may be mapped out (Kronig's apical resonance zones). Consolidation or retraction of an apex causes narrowing of the zone on the affected side. The procedure gives valuable information in the early stage of infiltration. In cases with numerous isolated cavities at the apex, without much fibroid tissue or thickening of the pleura, the percussion note may show little change, and the contrast between the signs on auscultation and percussion is most marked. In direct percussion, particularly in thin patients over the pectorals, one frequently sees the phenomenon known as myoidema, a local contraction of the muscle causing bulging, which persists for a variable period and gradually subsides.

Auscultation.—Feeble breath sounds are among the most characteristic early signs and it is well to compare carefully the corresponding points on the two sides of the chest without asking the patient to draw a deep breath or cough. With early apical disease the inspiration on quiet breathing may be scarcely audible. Expiration is usually prolonged. On the other hand, there are cases in which the earliest sign is a harsh, rude, respiratory murmur. On deep breathing it is frequently noted that inspiration is jerking or wavy, the so-called "cog-wheel" rhythm; which, however, is by no means confined to tuberculosis. With extension of the disease the inspiratory murmur is harsh, and, when consolidation occurs, whiffing and bronchial. With these changes in the breath sounds there are râles. The patient should first breathe quietly, then take a full breath, and then cough. When heard with quiet breathing, if they persist and are present in one area only, they are of great importance. The fine rustling crepitus heard when the patient first takes a deep breath is of no moment. It may also be present at the bases. Râles at the end of a deep inspiration which disappear on repeated breathing may be suspicious but are not positive. Râles which are brought out by coughing (most useful during expiration), which persist, and are repeatedly heard at the same spot are of the greatest importance. It is of equal import when moist, clicking râles are present with change in the percussion note. We should hesitate to make a diagnosis of pulmonary tuberculosis on auscultatory signs alone.

When softening occurs the râles are louder and have a bubbling, sometimes a characteristic clicking quality. These "moist sounds" when associated with change in the percussion note are extremely suggestive. When cavities form the râles are louder, more gurgling, and resonant in quality. When there is consolidation of any extent the breath sounds are tubular, and in the large excavations loud and cavernous, or have an amphoric quality. In the unaffected portions of the lobe and in the opposite lung the breath sounds may be harsh. The vocal resonance is usually increased in all stages and bronchophony and pectoriloquy are met with in the regions of consolidation and over cavities. Pleuritic friction may be present at any stage and sometimes occurs very early. In some cases it is a marked feature throughout. When the lung over the heart is involved there may be a pleuropericardial friction, and when this area is consolidated there may be curious clicking râles synchronous with the heart beat, due to the compression by the heart of this portion with expulsion of air from it. In thin-chested persons, nervous patients, and often in early pulmonary tuberculosis the so-called cardiorespiratory murmur may be heard. It is best heard during inspiration and in the anterolateral regions of the chest.

A systolic murmur is frequently heard in the subclavian artery on either side, the pulsation of which may be very visible. The murmur is probably due to pressure on the vessels by the thickened pleura.

The signs of *cavity* may be briefly enumerated, always remembering that there may be no distinctive signs over small cavities, the presence of which may be proved only by the X-ray study.

(1) When there is not much thickening of the pleura or infiltration of the surrounding lung tissue, the percussion sound may be full and clear, resembling the normal note. More commonly there is dulness or a tympanitic quality which may be purely amphoric. The pitch of the percussion note changes over a cavity when the mouth is opened or closed (Wintrich's sign),

or it may be brought out more clearly on change of position. The cracked-pot sound is obtainable over large cavities with thin walls or when one cavity is above another. It is best elicited by a firm, quick stroke, the patient having the mouth open. (2) On auscultation there are various grades of modified breathing—blowing or tubular, cavernous or amphoric. There may be a curiously sharp hissing sound, as if air was passing from a narrow opening into a wide space. In large cavities both inspiration and expiration may be typically amphoric. There are coarse bubbling râles which have a resonant quality, and on coughing may have a metallic or ringing character or be loud and gurgling. In large thin-walled cavities, and more rarely in medium-sized cavities, surrounded by recent consolidation, the râles may have a distinctly amphoric echo, simulating those of pneumothorax. There are dry cavities in which no râles are heard. The vocal resonance is greatly intensified, and the whispered voice is clearly heard. In large apical cavities the heart-sounds are well heard, and occasionally there may be an intense systolic murmur, probably always transmitted to and not produced in the cavity itself. In large excavations of the left apex the heart impulse may cause gurgling sounds or clicks synchronous with systole which may be heard at a distance from the chest wall. A large cavity with smooth walls and thin fluid contents may give a succussion sound and even the coin sound may be obtained. *Pseudocavernous* signs may be given by an area of consolidation near a large bronchus and the condition may be most deceptive.

Epituberculosis.—This term has been applied to various conditions and the meaning is not always clear. It occurs in young children and as a rule the child is not seriously ill; slight fever may be present and generally an unproductive cough. If sputum can be obtained, tubercle bacilli are not found. The tuberculin test as a rule is positive. In the thorax there is dulness, usually over the upper lobe with rough breath sounds; râles may or may not be present. The X-ray picture shows a very definite shadow which reaches from the hilus to the periphery. The lower border has a clean cut margin with a slight concavity. The upper border extends to the apex. These signs may remain for weeks or months and gradually disappear. Apparently recovery always follows.

As to the mechanism, it is suggested that it may be: (1) *collapse* which may be due to pressure on the bronchus by a tuberculous gland. In some instances the area has cleared rapidly following bronchoscopy. (2) It may represent an *allergic phenomenon,* a nonspecific infiltration of the lung in the vicinity of a tuberculous focus. (3) That it represents a *tuberculous* process. In some cases tubercle bacilli have been obtained by passing a needle into the involved portion of the lung. Possibly various factors may be causal. Bronchoscopy would seem advisable when possible.

Fibroid Tuberculosis

In their monograph on Fibroid Diseases of the Lung, Clark, Hadley, and Chaplin make the following classification: 1. Pure fibroid—in which there is no tubercle. 2. Tuberculofibroid disease—primarily tuberculous but which has run a fibroid course. 3. Fibrotuberculous disease—primarily fibroid but which has become tuberculous. The *tuberculofibroid* form may come on gradually as a sequence of a chronic tuberculous bronchopneumonia or follow a chronic tuberculous pleurisy. In other instances the process supervenes upon ordinary pulmonary tuberculosis. The disease becomes limited to one apex, the cavity is surrounded by dense fibrous tissue, the pleura is thickened, and the lower lobe is gradually invaded by the sclerotic change. Ultimately the picture differs little from fibrosis of the lungs. It may be difficult to say that the process is tuberculous, but in advanced cases the bacilli are usually present in the walls of the cavity at the apex, or old, encapsulated caseous areas are present, or there may be tubercles at the apex of the other lung and in the bronchial glands. Dilatation of the bronchi is present; the right ventricle, or the entire heart, is hypertrophied.

The disease is chronic, lasting from ten to twenty or more years, and the patient may have fair health. The chief *symptoms* are cough, often paroxysmal and most marked in the morning, and dyspnea on exertion. The expectoration is purulent, and in some instances, when the bronchiectasis is extensive, fetid. There is rarely any fever.

The physical *signs* are very characteristic. The chest is sunken and the shoulder lower on the affected side; the heart is often displaced. If the left lung is involved there may be a large area of cardiac pulsation. Heart murmurs are common. There are dulness and deficient tactile fremitus over the affected side, except over cavities where fremitus is increased. At the apex there may be well-marked cavernous sounds; at the base, distant bronchial breathing. In some cases the other lung becomes involved, or the patient has repeated attacks of hemoptysis. Amyloid degeneration may take place; dropsy frequently supervenes from failure of the right heart.

Complications of Pulmonary Tuberculosis

In the Respiratory System.—The larynx is often involved. The first sign may be huskiness of the voice. There are pain, particularly in swallowing, and cough which is often wheezing and in the later stages very ineffectual. Aphonia and dysphagia are distressing features of laryngeal involvement. When the epiglottis is seriously diseased and the ulceration extends to the lateral wall of the pharynx, the pain in swallowing may be intense; there may be coughing spells and regurgitation of food through the nose. Bronchitis and tracheitis are almost invariable accompaniments.

Pneumonia is an occasional complication of pulmonary tuberculosis. It usually runs a perfectly normal course, but resolution may be delayed, and one is in doubt as to the presence of a simple or a tuberculous pneumonia. In some cases pneumonia is a terminal complication.

Emphysema of the uninvolved portions of the lung is common, rarely producing any special symptoms. There are cases of chronic tuberculosis in which emphysema dominates the picture, coming on slowly during a period of many years. General subcutaneous emphysema is due to perforation of the trachea or the rupture of a cavity adherent to the chest wall.

Collapse of the lung may occur with hemoptysis or pneumothorax. Varying grades of distress, acute dyspnea, cyanosis and tachycardia may result.

Gangrene of the lung is an occasional event, due in almost all instances to sphacelus in the walls of the cavity, rarely in the lung tissue itself.

Complications in the Pleura.—A *dry* pleurisy is common in the early stages of tuberculosis. It is always a conservative, useful process. In some cases it is extensive, and friction murmurs may be heard over the sides and back sometimes without pain. The cases with dry pleurisy and adhesions are much less liable to pneumothorax. Pleurisy with *effusion* more commonly precedes than occurs with pulmonary tuberculosis. Still, there are cases in which a serofibrinous effusion arises in the course of the chronic disease. In some it is a special feature and seems to favor chronicity. A patient may for years have signs of local disease at one apex with recurring effusion on the same side. Owing to adhesions, the effusion may be encapsulated. *Hemorrhagic* effusions, not uncommon with tuberculous pleurisy, are comparatively rare in pulmonary tuberculosis. Chyliform or milky exudates are sometimes found. Purulent effusions are not frequent apart from pneumothorax. An empyema may occur in the course of the disease or as a sequence of a serofibrinous exudate.

Pneumothorax is a common complication. Of 49 cases at the Johns Hopkins Hospital, 23 were tuberculous (Emerson). It may prove fatal in twenty-four hours. A pyopneumothorax may follow and the patient linger for weeks or months. In some patients it seems to have a beneficial effect.

Small Pneumothorax.—Barlow and Thompson have drawn attention to its frequency and to the importance of its recognition in the interpretation of puzzling physical signs. The pneumothorax may be superficial, interlobar or mediastinal. The symptoms are very variable. The onset may be sudden with pain, dyspnea and bloody sputum. The signs depend on the size of the pneumothorax, the amount of collapse of the lung, and the extent of pleural exudate. Previous signs of lung involvement may disappear and suggest improvement. There may be deviation of the trachea to the affected side (the opposite of large pneumothorax). The percussion note shows combinations of tympany and dulness, depending on the amount of air, the pleural exudate and the extent of collapse. A superficial pneumothorax gives decreased breath sounds and exudate cuts them off. A friction rub may be heard in adjoining areas. The whispered voice is often high pitched and amphoric and near the area there may be bronchophony. There are usually fine râles over the area of collapse. The X-ray diagnosis requires special methods and training. The interpretation of "ring-shaped" areas (annular shadows) may be difficult; they may represent cavities or areas of pneumothorax.

Changes in Other Organs.—*Cardiovascular.*—The retraction of the left upper lobe exposes a large area of the heart and in thin-chested subjects there may be marked visible pulsation. Sometimes with much retraction of the left upper lobe the heart is drawn up. A systolic murmur over the pulmonary area and in the subclavian arteries is common in all stages. Apical murmurs are not infrequent and may be rough and harsh without endocarditis. The association of heart disease with tuberculosis is not very uncommon. There were 12 instances of endocarditis in 216 autopsies. The arterial tension is usually low and the pulse is often full and soft even in the later stages. *Phlebitis* may occur early, usually in the legs and more often in the saphenous than in the femoral vein. It is usually gradual in onset, does not cause severe pain, and edema is slight unless the femoral vein is involved.

Blood.—Anemia is often more apparent than real and severe anemia is rare. The blood-plates are, as a rule, increased and are seen as the so-called

Schultze's granule masses. Without any significance, they are of interest chiefly from the fact that every few years some tyro announces their discovery as a new diagnostic sign of tuberculosis. The leukocytes are increased, particularly in the later stages. The percentage of lymphocytes is higher in the milder and more chronic cases. The Arneth index is of some value. With progress of the disease there is a shift to the left with an increase of the younger cells; with improvement there is a shift to the right. The same applies to the Schilling hemogram. *Sedimentation test.* Sedimentation is usually more rapid than normal with active disease and may suggest activity when other signs are lacking.

Gastro-intestinal System.—The tongue is usually furred, but may be clean and red. Small aphthous ulcers are sometimes distressing. A red line on the gums may be found. Extensive tuberculous disease of the pharynx, with a similar affection of the larynx, may interfere seriously with deglutition and prove very distressing and intractable.

Tuberculosis of the *stomach* is rare. Ulceration may occur as an accidental complication and multiple catarrhal ulcers are not uncommon. Interstitial and parenchymatous changes in the mucosa are common (possibly associated with venous stasis) and lead to atrophy, but these can not always be connected with the symptoms, and may be found when not expected. On the other hand, when the gastric symptoms have been severe the mucosa may show little change. It is impossible always to refer the anorexia, nausea and vomiting to local conditions. Fever and neurotic influences may play an important rôle. There is interference with both the secretory and motor functions early in the course. Hyperacidity is rare (Mohler and Funk).

Anorexia is often marked at the onset; there may be positive loathing for food, and even small quantities cause nausea. Sometimes, without any nausea or distress, the feeding of the patient is a daily battle. When practicable, forced alimentation is of great benefit in such cases. Nausea and vomiting, though occasionally troublesome early, are more marked in the later stages. The latter may be caused by severe attacks of coughing. S. H. Habershon refers to four causes of vomiting: Central, as from tuberculous meningitis; pressure on the vagi by caseous glands; stimulation from the peripheral branches of the vagus, either pulmonary, pharyngeal, or gastric; and mechanical causes.

Of *intestinal* symptoms diarrhea is the most serious. It may come on early, but more usually in the later stages, and associated with ulceration, particularly of the large bowel. Extensive ulceration of the ileum may exist without any diarrhea. The associated catarrhal condition may account in part for it, and in some amyloid degeneration of the mucous membrane. Perforation occurred in 13 of 475 autopsies in pulmonary tuberculosis.

Nervous System.—(1) *Focal lesions* are due to coarse tubercles and areas of tuberculous meningo-encephalitis. Aphasia may result from the growth of meningeal tubercles in the fissure of Sylvius, or hemiplegia may occur. The solitary tubercles are more common in the chronic tuberculosis of children. (2) *Basilar meningitis* is an occasional complication. It may be confined to the brain, though more commonly it is a (3) *cerebrospinal meningitis,* which may come on in persons without well-marked signs in the chest so that the pulmonary disease is not discovered until the postmortem. (4) *Peripheral neuritis,* which is not common, may cause an extensor paralysis of the arm or leg, more commonly the latter, with footdrop. It is usually a late manifestation. (5) The *brachial plexus,* close to the pleuropulmonary apex, is sometimes involved, either by adhesion to tuberculous glands or in the thickening of the tissues about the pleura itself. There may be pains in the arm, trophic disturbances and occasionally paralysis, particularly in the distribution of the lower cord in the plexus. (6) *Mental* symptoms. Many consumptives have a peculiarly hopeful temperament, and the *spes phthisica* forms a curious characteristic. Frequently, however, this is assumed to conceal depression. Apart from tuberculosis of the brain, there is sometimes in chronic tuberculosis a form of *psychosis* not unlike that in the convalescence from acute affections.

Eyes.—The conjunctiva is rarely involved. Iritis may occur and not always tuberculous. Keratitis, choroiditis, scleritis and episcleritis occur. The pupils are often dilated. With apical pleurisy, irregularity of the pupils may be present. Myosis with narrowing of the palpebral fissure and retraction of the eye or mydriasis with associated vasomotor features may occur with small lesions of the apex and pleural involvement.

Hypertrophy of the mammary gland may occur in pulmonary tuberculosis, most commonly in males. It may be only on the affected side. It is a chronic interstitial, nontuberculous mammitis (Allot). Mastitis adolescentium is not necessarily suggestive of pulmonary tuberculosis.

Genito-urinary System.—The urine presents no special peculiarities but fever has a marked influence upon it. Albuminuria is frequent and may be associated with the fever or is the result of definite renal changes. Tubercle bacilli may be present in the urine without disease of the kidney. Amyloid disease of the kidneys occurs.

Pus in the urine may be due to disease of the bladder or of the pelves of the kidneys. In some instances the entire urinary tract is involved. In pulmonary tuberculosis extensive tuberculous disease is rarely found in the urinary organs. *Hematuria* is not common and occurs occasionally as a result of congestion of the kidneys. In other instances it results from disease of the pelvis or of the bladder, associated with early tuberculosis or more commonly with ulceration. In a medical clinic the routine inspection of the epididymis for tubercle will save two or three mistakes a year. *Amenorrhea* is common in women. Bartholin's gland may show tuberculous infection.

Cutaneous System.—The skin is often dry and harsh. Local tubercles occasionally occur on the hands. There may be pigmentary staining, the *chloasma phthisicorum,* which is more common when the peritoneum is involved. Upon the chest and the back the brown stains of *pityriasis versicolor* are frequent. The hair may become dry. The terminal phalanges, in chronic cases, become clubbed and the nails incurvated—the Hippocratic fingers. Landouzy called attention to a curious bending, usually of the ring and little fingers, which permits flexion, but not extension—which he calls camptodactaly. An unusual complication is general emphysema, which may result from ulceration of an adherent lung or perforation of the larynx or trachea.

Diagnosis of Pulmonary Tuberculosis

The *early diagnosis* of pulmonary tuberculosis may be said to mean the recognition of lesions which do not give positive signs. Suspicion is an important factor in the early diagnosis with a determination to leave nothing undone to decide whether or not tuberculosis is present. But the diagnosis should not rest with the answer that tuberculosis is present in the patient. Two other questions should be answered. From whom did he contract the disease? Has he infected any other individual? Until this is done the diagnosis should not be regarded as complete.

With fever, well-marked physical signs and bacilli in the sputum, no disease is more easily diagnosed. Successful treatment depends largely upon early diagnosis, and special attention must be paid to the obscure, variable, and uncertain symptoms and signs of the initial stage. The active crusade against the disease has made both the public and the profession more alert, but some have, as so often happens, gone to an extreme, and are apt to see early tuberculosis in trivial complaints. The following are of importance in the diagnosis of early cases:

History.—Tuberculosis in the family, "Phthisical habitus," exposure to infection, special debilitating circumstances, as worry, dissipation, or a chronic illness, pleurisy, "bronchitis" which persists, and blood-tinged sputum. There may be a history suggestive of previous infection.

Symptoms.—Loss of weight, loss of strength, marked nervous and physical exhaustion and anemia, if progressive and not otherwise accounted for, are of first importance. *Fever* is both trustworthy and fallacious. The thermometer has needlessly condemned many patients to a sanatorium. Regard should be had to the points already mentioned in speaking of the fever. In nervous persons, particularly in flabby young girls, a temperature from 99.5° to 100° may mean nothing, and the rectal temperature is often deceptive: if taken after exercise or excitement it may be a degree and a half above normal. In a suspicious case a two-hour temperature record should be taken during the day for ten days and the influence of exercise upon it carefully estimated. Fever, otherwise unexplained, is always suggestive of tuberculosis but other causes should be excluded; focal infection, syphilis and genito-urinary tract infection may be overlooked.

A *cough* is always suspicious in the young, more in the winter than in the summer, and more in the morning than at other times. Throat and sinus conditions should be carefully excluded, particularly the irritation from cigarette smoking. The spitting of blood has been considered and its importance in the diagnosis of tuberculosis is universally recognized. An early hemoptysis is often helpful, not only for the positive information it gives but for its useful moral effect on the patient. The greater the care with which the bloody sputum is examined the more likely it is that bacilli are found. A short dry cough, especially on exertion, is suspicious.

Sputum.—The patient should be instructed to collect what is expectorated, particularly early in the morning, and everything brought up should be sent. The difficulty is that it requires a long series of examinations to exclude positively the presence of tubercle bacilli. Time and again with suspicious cases the clinical clerk has been asked day by day "Any bacilli yet?" and in one instance none was found until the twentieth examination! It is well to bear in mind that one or two negative examinations are not sufficient. Various methods of digesting the sputum and examining the centrifugalized sediment are important when few bacilli are present. The antiformin method often reveals tubercle bacilli missed by an ordinary examination. In children it may be impossible to secure any sputum. The examination of swabs from the throat, of the stomach contents or of the feces may show tubercle bacilli. The study of material obtained through the bronchoscope may give the diagnosis in a doubtful case.

Physical Signs.—These raise the difficulty. The position resembles that of years ago in respect to the heart, when any murmur was regarded as serious. Of the physical signs, change in the breath sounds and the presence of râles are the two most important, as dulness is rarely present in early cases. Altogether too much stress has been laid upon roughened or impure inspiration associated with a few râles. Only upon repeated examinations should a decision be reached.

In regard to the extent of disease in the lung, caution is advisable in patients seen for the first time with fever and acute symptoms. Signs may be found over a large area, but these may be due to an acute intercurrent infection and lessen materially in a few days or to an allergic lesion which may be absorbed rapidly.

Certain conditions may be *wrongly diagnosed as tuberculous.* Foreign bodies in the bronchi may be a cause of error. In patients with infection of the mouth or throat, tonsillitis, sinusitis, and adenoids, there may be a persistent cough with bronchitis and fever. Recognition and proper treatment of the cause may result in the prompt disappearance of the pulmonary signs. In some cases these nontuberculous infections cause definite fibroid change. There may be enlargement of the glands about the hilus and considerable peribronchial thickening. Too often an X-ray study by one not sufficiently trained supports an erroneous diagnosis of tuberculosis. There are certain nontuberculous chronic bronchial and pulmonary diseases which may be mistaken for tuberculosis. Mycotic infections, spirochetal bronchitis, abscess, neoplasm, syphilis, chronic bronchitis, fibrosis and bronchiectasis are in this group. It is a good rule that with signs of advanced chronic disease in the lungs and no tubercle bacilli in the sputum, the condition is not likely to be tuberculous. A diagnosis of tuberculosis based on *marked* lung changes without finding tubercle bacilli in the sputum is often wrong. Atypical forms of pneumonia, disease of the pleura, especially apical, an azygos lobe and aneurism may lead one astray. *Pneumoconiosis,* especially *silicosis,* plus tuberculosis may give difficulty. *Hemorrhage* with bronchiectasis or from an ulcer in a bronchus may cause confusion but bronchoscopy is of great aid in the recognition of such cases. Signs in the lungs secondary to *cardiac* disease not infrequently cause error; râles due to circulatory disturbance may be apical as well as basal. Mitral stenosis is the lesion most likely to mislead; the persistence of the lung signs, the occurrence of hemoptysis and the occasional presence of dulness above the third rib on the left side (Goodman) all contribute to the mistake. *Basal lesions* are not uncommon. The symptoms may be mild and the diagnosis difficult as sputum is often scanty and negative for tubercle bacilli. The use of the bronchoscope to obtain material which may contain tubercle bacilli is important. The X-ray study may not be definite and if a cavity is present, the walls are often thinner than usual.

Postinfluenzal changes and conditions in soldiers who were gassed often cause difficulty. There may be complaint of general ill health, weakness, cough and pain or discomfort in the chest. Wheezing and shortness of breath with rapid heart action on exertion occur in some. The signs are varied and usually most marked on auscultation, harsh breath sounds, râles of different kinds, usually coarse and on both sides. The X-ray may show much diffuse thickening but no definite local lesion. Fibrosis and emphysema seem to be the important factors in many cases.

Specific Reaction.—*Tuberculin Test.*—The cutaneous or intradermal test is used. A positive reaction signifies the presence of a tuberculous lesion but does not prove that the patient has active tuberculous disease, in the ordinary sense of the term disease. As a large proportion of adults (60 to 80 per cent) show tuberculin hypersensitiveness, a positive test has little value in diagnosis. It is more useful in young children but in them it must be interpreted with caution. In the absence of acute or advanced disease a negative test is strong evidence against tuberculosis and therefore of decided value. The conjunctival test is no longer used and the subcutaneous method is rarely employed; it has practically been discarded.

Complement Fixation Test.—This has not proved of much value in doubtful cases. It may be of help in deciding as to the arrest of the disease.

Cultures.—The improvement in cultural methods has made this much more useful in diagnosis. The results are often very satisfactory.

X-ray Diagnosis.—In skilful hands the study with the Roentgen rays is of great value. In diseased conditions changes are seen in the hilum, shadows due to enlarged or calcified glands and to the increase in the fibrous and lymphatic tissues in the mediastinum. The pulmonary vessels with their contained blood play an important part in the production of the shadow. The X-rays undoubtedly show very early changes in the lungs, but they can not always determine the etiological factor. Much depends on the roentgenologist who examines the plates; with a skilled man the results are of great value. The estimation of the meaning of changes in an X-ray plate needs skill, knowledge and good judgment as much as does the estimation of the clinical features. The physician and roentgenologist should examine the plates together. In some cases with signs and positive sputum results the X-ray examination is negative. More than any others, *some* roentgenologists need the salutary lessons of the dead house to correct their visionary interpretations of shadows.

Concurrent Infections.—Many cases of pulmonary tuberculosis are combined infections; streptococci and pneumococci may be found in the sputum, and the former have been isolated from the blood. The pneumonia complicating tuberculosis may be due to the tubercle bacillus or follow secondary infection with other germs. An infection by other organisms may be followed by increased fever and an aggravation of the general symptoms. It is probable that the effect of infection with the pus organisms is important in hastening necrosis and softening, and in the chronic cases they doubtless produce some of the toxins which are responsible for many of the symptoms.

Diseases Associated with Pulmonary Tuberculosis.—*Lobar pneumonia* is not a common cause of death. It may occur as a terminal event or occur early and be difficult to distinguish from an acute caseous pneumonia. The sputum in the latter is rarely rusty, while the fever in the former is more continuous and higher, but often it is impossible to differentiate them.

The association of tuberculosis and *typhoid fever* has been discussed.

Erysipelas not infrequently attacks old *poitrinaires* in almshouses. There are instances in which the attack seems to be beneficial, as the cough lessens and the symptoms ameliorate. It may prove fatal.

Erythema Nodosum.—Some regard it as a symptom of the disease, a "tuberculide" as the French call it. Tubercle bacilli have been found in the lesions and a number of patients with erythema nodosum later develop frank tuberculosis.

The *eruptive fevers,* particularly measles, sometimes precede but rarely occur in the course of pulmonary tuberculosis. In the revaccination of a tuberculous subject the vesicles run a normal course.

Fistula in ano, so often associated with pulmonary tuberculosis, in a majority of such cases is a tuberculous process. The general affection may progress rapidly after an operation.

Heart Disease.—Cardiac hypoplasia seems uncommon in tuberculosis, though it was much referred to by the older writers. It was present in only 3 cases in 1,764 autopsies on tuberculous patients (Norris). All forms of congenital heart disease predispose to tuberculosis, particularly pulmonary stenosis. Mitral stenosis, on the other hand, has a distinctly inhibitory influence and the two conditions are rarely associated. Endocarditis has been mentioned. A terminal acute tuberculosis, particularly of the serous membranes, is not uncommon in cardiovascular disease.

In chronic and arrested tuberculosis *arteriosclerosis* and *phlebosclerosis* are not uncommon. Chronic renal disease is not uncommon.

Diabetes mellitus.—Among 31,834 cases of tuberculosis there were 151 with glycosuria. The lesions often spread in a fan shape from the hilus. There may be marked exudation without much fibrosis. The association means an unfavorable prognosis. In treatment the diabetes should be handled in the usual way.

Cancer.—Not often associated with active tuberculosis, many persons dying of cancer show foci of old tuberculosis. There does not seem to be any active antagonism between the diseases.

Peculiarities of Pulmonary Tuberculosis at the Extremes of Life

Old Age.—It is remarkable how common tuberculosis is in the aged, particularly in institutions. Laënnec met with a case in a person over ninety-nine years of age. At the Philadelphia Hospital, in the bodies of aged persons from the almshouse, it was extremely common to find either old or recent tuberculosis. One patient died at the age of eighty-two with extensive peritoneal tuberculosis. Pulmonary tuberculosis in the aged is usually *latent* and runs a slow course. The physical signs are often masked by emphysema and chronic bronchitis. The diagnosis may depend entirely upon the discovery of bacilli and elastic tissue. Tuberculosis is by no means uncommon with senile emphysema. Some cases of tuberculosis in the aged are instances of quiescent disease which may have dated from an early period.

Infancy.—The occurrence of acute tuberculosis in children has been mentioned, and also that the disease is occasionally congenital. Chronic ulcerative tuberculosis of the lungs is much more rare than in adults. The form in children (primary infection) has special features. Much depends on the infection; if severe the course is rapid, especially if miliary tuberculosis results, as occurs, for example, if a caseous lymph node discharges into a blood vessel. In many cases the infection is not severe and recovery follows.

Modes of Death in Pulmonary Tuberculosis

By asthenia, a gradual failure of the strength. The end is usually peaceable and quiet, occasionally disturbed by paroxysms of cough. Consciousness is often retained until near the close.

By asphyxia, as in some cases of acute miliary and acute pneumonic tuberculosis. In chronic pulmonary tuberculosis it is rarely seen, even when pneumothorax develops.

By syncope. This may happen in patients who insist upon going about when in the advanced stages. Syncope may follow hemorrhage or be due to pulmonary thrombosis, embolism or pneumothorax.

From hemorrhage. The fatal bleeding in chronic tuberculosis is due to erosion of a large vessel or rupture of an aneurism in a cavity, most commonly the latter. Of 35 cases collected by Kidd, aneurism was present in 30. In a case at the Philadelphia Hospital, the bleeding proved fatal before hemoptysis occurred, as the vessel opened into a large cavity.

With cerebral symptoms. Coma may be due to meningitis, less often to uremia. Death in convulsions is rare. Hemorrhagic pachymeningitis occasionally causes loss of consciousness, but is rarely a direct cause of death. In one case death resulted from thrombosis of the cerebral sinuses with symptoms of meningitis.

TUBERCULOSIS OF THE ALIMENTARY CANAL

Lips.—Tuberculosis of the lip is very rare. It occurs occasionally as a solid tuberculoma or in the form of an ulcer, either alone or more commonly with laryngeal or pulmonary disease. The ulcer is usually very sensitive and may be mistaken for a chancre or an epithelioma. The diagnosis may be made by culture, inoculation or the examination of a portion for tubercle bacilli. The cheeks, gums and floor of the mouth are very rarely involved. Lupus occasionally extends to the mouth from the skin.

Tongue.—The disease begins by an aggregation of small granular bodies on the edge or dorsum. Ulceration proceeds, leaving an irregular sore with a distinct but uneven margin, and a rough, often caseous base. The disease extends slowly and may form an indolent ulcer of considerable size. It may be mistaken for epithelioma and the tongue excised. It is rare except when other organs are involved. The glands at the angle of the jaw are not enlarged and the sore does not yield to iodide, which are points of distinction between the tuberculous and syphilitic ulcer. In doubtful cases a portion should be excised for examination.

Salivary Glands.—These seem to possess a relative immunity; very few cases have been reported. The *parotid gland* shows two forms; (1) an acute inflammatory process with swelling and perhaps fluctuation, in which case incision is required and (2) a chronic fibroid encapsulated process. This may be mistaken for syphilis or a mixed tumor.

Palate.—Tubercles of the palate usually follow extension from neighboring parts. The lesions are usually multiple and ulcerated.

Tonsils.—This is mentioned previously. Some claim that the majority of cases of tuberculous cervical glands result from infection with tubercle bacilli which gain admission by the tonsil. There may be infection of the crypts, superficial ulceration or an infiltration with miliary tubercles, that produces hypertrophy which it is impossible to distinguish from ordinary enlargement of the tonsil without microscopic examination.

Pharynx.—In extensive laryngeal tuberculosis an eruption of miliary granules on the posterior wall of the pharynx is not very uncommon. In chronic tuberculosis an ulcerative pharyngitis, due to extension of the disease from the epiglottis and larynx, renders deglutition acutely painful. Adenoids of the nasopharynx may be tuberculous.

Esophagus.—A few instances occur in the literature of tuberculosis of the esophagus. The condition is a pathological curiosity, except in the slight extension from the larynx, which is not infrequent; but in a case described by Flexner, the ulcer perforated and caused purulent pleurisy.

Stomach.—Many cases are reported which are doubtful. In 2,000 autopsies at the Brompton Hospital, a tuberculous ulcer was found twice (Fenwick). In 2,051 gastric operations at the Mayo Clinic in four years only one instance was found. Ulcer is the most common lesion and occurs in about 80 per cent of the cases. Miliary tubercles, pyloric stenosis and the occurrence of a nodule are the other lesions. Perforation of the stomach occurred in 6 of 12 cases collected by Marfan.

Intestines.—The tubercles may be (1) primary in the mucous membrane, or more commonly (2) secondary to disease of the lungs, or in rare cases the affection may (3) pass from the peritoneum.

Primary intestinal tuberculosis is most frequent in children, in whom it may be associated with enlargement and caseation of the mesenteric glands, or with peritonitis. There is great discrepancy in the statistics on this point. Biedert gives 16 cases in 3,104 instances of tuberculosis in children. In adults primary intestinal tuberculosis is rare, occurring in but 1 instance in 1,000 autopsies upon tuberculous adults at the Munich Pathological Institute; but cases occur in which the disease sets in with irregular diarrhea, moderate fever, and colicky pains. In a few cases hemorrhage has been the initial sign. Regarded at first as a chronic catarrh, it is not until emaciation becomes marked or signs of disease appear in the lungs that the true nature is apparent. Still more deceptive are the cases in which the tuberculosis begins in the *cecum* and there are symptoms of appendicitis—tenderness in the right iliac fossa, constipation, or an irregular diarrhea and fever. These signs may gradually disappear, to recur in a few weeks and further complicate the diagnosis. Fatal hemorrhage has occurred. Perforation into the peritoneum may take place, a pericecal abscess may form, or in very rare instances there is partial healing with great thickening of the walls and narrowing of the lumen. Tuberculosis of the *appendix* is found in about one per cent, but often can only be diagnosed microscopically. The symptoms are those of a suppurative appendicitis.

Secondary involvement of the bowels is very common in chronic pulmonary tuberculosis, *e.g.*, in 566 of the 1,000 Munich autopsies in tuberculosis. In only three of these cases were the lungs not involved. The *clinical* features are loss of appetite, nervous disturbances, such as depression, dyspepsia, abdominal pain more or less persistent, constipation if the small bowel and diarrhea if the colon is involved. The patient may fail to gain or lose ground without evident cause. The lesions are chiefly in the ileum, cecum, and colon. Tuberculosis of the duodenum is rare; Matthews (1932) found 123 cases. The lesions may be ulcerative, caseous or hyperplastic (very rare). In the colon the recognition of an overactive portion of the bowel is important. Ulceration is usually in the ileocecal region. It is difficult to recognize in the small bowel. The caseation and necrosis lead to ulceration, which may be extensive. In the ileum the Peyer's patches are chiefly involved and the ulcers may be ovoid, but in the jejunum and colon they are usually round or transverse to the long axis. The tuberculous *ulcer* has the following characters: (*a*) It is irregular, rarely ovoid or in the long axis, more frequently girdling the bowel; (*b*) the edges and base are infiltrated, often caseous; (*c*) the submucosa and muscularis are usually involved; and (*d*) on the serosa may be seen colonies of young tubercles or a tuberculous lymphangitis. Perforation and peritonitis are not uncommon in the secondary ulceration. Stenosis of the bowel from cicatrization may occur; the strictures may be multiple.

Localized chronic tuberculosis of the *ileocecal region* is of great importance. The cecum may present a chronic hyperplastic tuberculosis, which not uncommonly extends into the appendix and a definite tumor-like mass is formed in the right iliac fossa. This varies in size, is usually elongated in a vertical direction, hard, slightly movable, or bound down by adhesions and very sensitive to pressure. The tumor simulates more or less closely a neoplasm. There are gradual constriction of the bowel, periodic attacks of severe pain, and alternating diarrhea and constipation. The extremely localized character of the disease warrants an exploratory operation, as the results of operation are favorable. In a second form, less frequent, there is no definite tumor mass, but a general induration and thickening in the right iliac fossa similar to the local changes produced by a recurring appenditicis. In this variety a fistula discharging fecal matter occasionally results. Both forms may be distinguished from the diseases they simulate by finding tubercle bacilli in the stools or in the discharge from the fistula when such exists.

Tuberculosis of the *rectum* has a special interest in connection with *fistula in ano,* which occurs in about 3.5 per cent of cases of pulmonary disease. In many instances the lesion is tuberculous. It is very rarely primary, but if the tissue on removal contains bacilli and is infective the lungs are almost invariably involved. It is a common opinion that the pulmonary symptoms progress rapidly after the fistula is cut. This may have some basis if the operation consists in laying the tract open, and not in a free excision.

Extension from the peritoneum may excite tuberculous disease in the bowels. The affection may be primary in the peritoneum or extend from the tubes in women or the mesenteric glands in children. The coils of intestines become matted together, caseous and suppurating foci develop between the folds, and perforation may take place between the coils.

The *diagnosis* of intestinal tuberculosis should be made early, in which the general digestive disturbances, especially anorexia, are important. The X-ray study is of considerable aid. In *treatment,* the general measures, open air, careful diet, etc., are important. The use of light therapy, either by sunlight or artificial light, is often successful. X-ray exposures help some patients. Operation is indicated when the process is localized. Advanced disease of the lung or small bowel is a contra-indication.

TUBERCULOSIS OF THE LIVER

This organ is very constantly involved in (*a*) *miliary tuberculosis.* This is seen in the general form, though the granules may be small and have to be looked for carefully. In chronic tuberculosis miliary tubercles are not uncommon in the liver. (*b*) *Solitary tubercle.* Occasionally tuberculous masses are found, sometimes with perihepatitis or tuberculous peritonitis, and in children with tuberculous adenitis. In a few cases the masses are large, though only in exceptional cases can the tumor be felt through the abdominal wall. The organ may be enlarged by numerous caseous masses and present the clinical picture of an enlarged rough tender liver with jaundice. The solitary tubercles may be infected with pus organisms, soften and form an abscess. (*c*) *Tuberculosis of the bile ducts.* This is the most characterisic tuberculous change in the organ, and is not uncommon. It was well described by Bristowe in 1858. The liver is enlarged, and section shows numerous small cavities, which look at first like multiple abscesses in suppurative pylephlebitis, but the pus is bile-stained and the process is a local tuberculous cholangitis. (*d*) *Tuberculous cirrhosis.* With the eruption of miliary tubercles there may be slight increase in the connective tissue, overshadowed by the fatty change. In all the chronic forms of tubercle in this organ there may be fibrous overgrowth. Hanot states that the condition may be primary. Practically it is very rare, except with chronic tuberculous peritonitis and perihepatitis, when the organ may be much deformed by a sclerosis involving the portal canals and the capsule, which may be involved in a polyserositis.

Jaundice is not common. It is usually due to some form of tuberculosis of the liver, either solitary tubercles or larger nodules. It is important to note its frequency in acute general miliary tuberculosis.

TUBERCULOSIS OF THE BRAIN AND CORD

Tuberculosis of the *brain* occurs as (*a*) an *acute miliary infection* causing meningitis and acute hydrocephalus; (*b*) as a *chronic meningo-encephalitis,* usually localized, and containing small nodular tubercles; and (*c*) as the so-called *solitary tubercle.* Between the last two forms there are all gradations, and it is rare to see the meninges uninvolved. The acute variety has already been considered. The *chronic* form, which comes on slowly and has the clinical characters of a tumor, is more common in children. Of 148 cases collected by Pribram 118 were under fifteen years of age. Other organs are usually involved, particularly the lungs, bronchial glands, or bones. In rare instances no tubercles are found elsewhere. They occur most frequently in the cerebellum; next in the cerebrum, and then in the pons. The growths are often multiple and range in size from a pea to a walnut; large tumors occasionally occur, and sometimes an entire lobe of the cerebellum is affected. On section the tubercle presents a grayish-yellow, caseous appearance, usually firm and hard, and encircled by a translucent, softer tissue. The centre of the growth may be semidiffluent. As in other localities the tubercle may calcify. The tumors are as a rule attached to the meninges, often to the pia at the bottom of a sulcus so that they look imbedded in the brain-substance. About the longitudinal fissure there may be an aggregation of the growths, with compression of the sinus, and the formation of a thrombus. The tuberculous tumor not infrequently excites *acute meningitis.* In localized meningo-encephalitis the pia is thickened, tubercles are adherent to the under surface and grow about the arteries. It is often combined with cerebral softening from interference with the circulation. In the *spinal cord* the same forms are found. The acute tuberculous meningitis is almost always cerebrospinal. The solitary tubercle of the cord is rare and usually secondary. The symptoms are those of spinal tumor or meningitis.

TUBERCULOSIS OF THE GENITO-URINARY SYSTEM

Any part of the genito-urinary system may be invaded. The disease may be limited for a long time to the urinary or to the genital tract. As a rule only in the later stages does involvement of both systems occur. The successive involvement of the organs may be so rapid that unless the patient is seen early it may be impossible to state with any certainty which has been the primary seat. There may be simultaneous involvement of various portions of the tract. In tuberculosis of the genito-urinary system one always has to bear in mind the possibility of latent disease elsewhere. There may be a tuberculous process of extremely slow development elsewhere without any symptoms. From this point bacilli may enter the blood stream, lodge in the epididymis, and produce nodules which are readily discovered. Such a case might be easily regarded as primary genital tuberculosis, whereas the primary tuberculous focus is far distant.

Infection of the genito-urinary tract occurs in various ways:

CONGENITAL.—It has been met with in the fetus. The comparative frequency of tuberculosis of the testicle in young children suggests that the urogenital organs may be involved as a result of direct transmission.

BY INFECTION FROM OTHER AREAS OF TUBERCULOSIS.—*Hematogenous.*—In many cases of urogenital tuberculosis it appears most probable that infection has been by the blood. Jani's observations, published by Weigert after the author's death, strongly support this theory. In sections of the organs of patients who died of pulmonary tuberculosis, he found tubercle bacilli in 5 out of 8 cases in the testicle, and in 4 out of 6 cases in the prostate, without microscopic evidences of tubercles in these organs. The bacilli in the testis were partly within and partly close beside the cellular and granular contents of the seminal tubules, while in the prostate they were always situated in the neighborhood of the glandular epithelium.

From the Peritoneum.—This source of infection is much more frequent than is commonly supposed. The intimate relationship between the peritoneum and bladder in both sexes, and with the vesiculae seminales and vasa deferentia in the male, allows a ready way of invasion by direct extension. The peritoneum is a frequent source of genital tuberculosis in the female. No doubt many cases of tuberculosis of the Fallopian tubes originate from this source. The fact that the fimbriated extremity of the tube is often most seriously involved points in this direction, although this might be taken as a point in favor of blood infection, favored by its greater vascularity. The action of the cilia lining the lumina of the Fallopian tubes apparently tends to attract particles introduced into the peritoneal cavity. Jani's observation showed the possibility of tubercle bacilli entering the tubes from the peritoneal cavity without there being any tuberculous peritonitis. He found typical tubercle bacilli in the lumen, in sections of a normal Fallopian tube, in a woman who died of pulmonary and intestinal tuberculosis. The explanation was that the bacilli made their way through the thin peritoneal coat from an intestinal ulcer to the peritoneal cavity, and thence were attracted into the Fallopian tube by the action of the cilia. The tubes are affected in from 30 to 40 per cent of cases of tuberculous peritonitis in females.

Direct Extension.—The occurrence of direct extension from the peritoneum has been mentioned. In tuberculous ulceration of the intestine adhesions to the bladder or to the uterus and vagina in the female may occur, with resulting fistulae and a direct extension of the disease. Perirectal tuberculous abscesses may lead to secondary involvement of some portion of the genito-urinary tract. Tuberculosis of the vertebrae may be followed by tuberculosis of the kidney as a result of direct extension.

FROM WITHOUT.—Whether urogenital tuberculosis may occur as a result of the entrance of tubercle bacilli into the urethra or vagina is a disputed question. That bacilli gain admission to these passages during coitus with a person the subject of urogenital tuberculosis, or by the use of foul instruments, seems quite probable. The possibility of genital tuberculosis in the female as a result of coitus with a male the subject of tuberculosis in the genito-urinary system was suggested by Cohnheim, who stated, however, that it rarely, if ever, occurred. In a patient with intestinal tuberculosis the tubercle bacilli might reach the urethra or vagina from the rectum.

Urogenital tuberculosis is commonest between the ages of twenty and forty years—that is, during the period of greatest sexual activity. Males are affected much more frequently than females, the proportion being 3 to 1. This great difference is no doubt partly due to the more intimate relationship between the urinary and genital systems in the former than in the latter.

Once the urogenital tract has been invaded the disease is likely to spread rapidly, and the method of extension is important. Frequently this is direct, as when the bladder is involved secondarily to the kidney or when the tuberculous process extends along the vas deferens to the vesiculae seminales. No doubt surface inoculation occurs in some instances, and to this may be attributed a certain percentage of cases of vesical and prostatic disease following tuberculosis of the kidney. Although this probability is acknowledged, there is doubt as to the possibility of the kidney becoming affected secondarily to the bladder or prostate by the passage of the bacilli up the lumen of one ureter; for in such a case we have to suppose that a nonmotile bacillus ascends against a current of urine flowing in the opposite direction. The lymphatics may afford a means for the spreading of the disease, but in the majority of cases the infection is *hematogenous.* Cystoscopic examinations of the bladder not infrequently show the presence of tubercles beneath the mucous membrane before there is any evidence of superficial ulceration—a fact suggesting strongly a blood infection.

The discovery of tubercle bacilli in the urine or semen and the production of tuberculous lesions in animals by inoculation with the urinary sediment afford positive evidence of genito-urinary tuberculosis. Tubercle bacilli have been found in the semen of men with tuberculosis of the testicle or vesiculae seminales. As the smegma bacillus has the same staining reaction as the tubercle bacillus and resembles it morphologically, the greatest care must be used to eliminate all chances of error.

Kidneys.—In general tuberculosis the kidneys frequently present scattered miliary tubercles. In pulmonary tuberculosis it is common to find a few nodules in the organ or there may be pyelitis. In 17,000 admissions to the medical wards of the Johns Hopkins Hospital there were 1,085 cases of tuberculous infection. In 17 of these a clinical diagnosis of renal tuberculosis was made. Walker analyzed the first 1,369 autopsies in the same hospital and found that 784 had tuberculosis in some part of the body. In all there were 61 cases of renal tuberculosis. Of 482 cases of pulmonary tuberculosis showing symptoms during life, one or both kidneys were involved in 23. There were 36 cases of acute general miliary tuberculosis, and in every instance the kidney was affected. Primary tuberculosis of the kidneys is rare, and in no instance in the above series did Walker demonstrate a primary infection in the kidney. In a majority of the cases the process involves the pelvis and the ureter, sometimes the bladder and prostate. It may be difficult to say in advanced cases whether the disease began in the bladder, prostate, or vesicles, or whether it started in the kidneys and proceeded downward. Walker thinks that a hematogenous infection takes place in 90 per cent of the cases, and that this is the channel of infection in the majority of instances where renal follows vesical tuberculosis rather than along the ureter. One kidney alone may be involved, and the disease creeps down the ureter and may only extend a few millimetres on the vesical mucosa.

In a series of 386 cases collected by Walker, 182 of the patients were males and 204 females. In the earliest stage, which may be met with accidentally, the disease is seen to begin in the pyramids and calyces. Necrosis and caseation proceed rapidly, and the colonies of tubercles start throughout the pyramids and extend upon the mucous membrane of the pelvis. As a rule, from the outset it is a tuberculous pyonephritis. It may be confined to one kidney or progress more extensively in one than in the other. At autopsy both organs are usually found enlarged. In only 3 of 61 autopsies was the disease unilateral. One kidney may be completely destroyed and converted into a series of cysts containing cheesy substance. In the contents of these cysts lime salts may be deposited. In other instances the walls of the pelvis are thickened and cheesy, the pyramids eroded, and caseous nodules are scattered through the organ, even to the capsule, which may be thickened and adherent. The other organ is usually less affected, and shows only pyelitis or a superficial necrosis of one or two pyramids. The ureters are usually thickened and the mucous membrane ulcerated and caseous. Involvement of the bladder, vesiculae seminales and testes is not uncommon in males.

The SYMPTOMS are those of pyelitis. The urine may be purulent for years, and there may be little or no distress. *Pain* occurs in a number at an early stage but is more common later. Urination may be painful. Even before the bladder becomes involved micturition is frequent, and many instances are mistaken for cystitis. The *frequent micturition* is in part due to an initial polyuria, in part to reflex irritation, but chiefly to a nontuberculous inflammation over the trigone of the bladder. It is usually the earliest and most constant symptom. *Hematuria,* of a mild grade, occurs at some time in the majority of cases. Dull, aching pain in the lumbar region is frequently complained of and may be the first symptom. The condition is for many years compatible with fair health. The curability is shown by the accidental discovery of a kidney converted into cysts containing a putty-like substance. In cases in which the disease becomes advanced and both organs are affected constitutional symptoms are more marked. There is irregular fever, with chills and loss of weight and strength. General tuberculosis is common and the lungs are usually involved. In a case at the Montreal General Hospital a cyst perforated and caused fatal peritonitis.

Examination may detect tenderness on one side, or the kidney may be palpable in front on deep pressure; but tuberculous pyonephritis seldom causes a large tumor. Occasionally the pelvis becomes enormously distended; but this is rare in comparison with its frequency in calculous pyelitis. The urine shows pus cells, epithelium, often red blood cells and occasionally definite caseous masses. It is nearly always acid. Albumin is present but casts are rare. Tubercle bacilli may be demonstrated and should be searched for when there are any unusual sensations. There may be "showers" of bacilli at these times. The renal function is sometimes diminished.

Diagnosis.—To distinguish the condition from calculous pyelitis is often difficult. Hemorrhage may be present in both, though not nearly so frequently in the tuberculous disease. The appearance of the ureteral orifices on cystoscopic examination is often characteristic. The diagnosis rests on: (1) The detection of some focus of tuberculosis, as in the epididymis; (2) the presence of tubercle bacilli in the sediment; (3) the use of tuberculin; and (4) cystoscopic examination and catheterization of the ureters. (5) Pyelography may aid by showing an irregular outline.

Treatment.—With only one kidney involved, immediate removal is indicated. If there is marked pulmonary disease or extensive involvement elsewhere, the decision is difficult but disease of the bladder often improves after removal of a tuberculous kidney. The usual general treatment should be given and tuberculin is sometimes useful.

Tuberculosis of the adrenal glands is considered under Addison's Disease.

Ureter and Bladder.—This is rarely primary but nearly always secondary to involvement of other parts, particularly the kidney. Protracted cystitis without apparent cause is always suggestive of tuberculosis. The renal regions, the testes, the seminal vesicles and the prostate should be examined with care. It may follow a pyonephritis or be associated with primary disease of the prostate or vesiculae seminales. Primary tuberculosis of the posterior wall of the bladder may simulate stone.

Prostate and Vesiculae seminales.—The prostate is frequently involved in urogenital tuberculosis. Barney collected 1,862 cases of genito-urinary tuberculosis, the majority of the genital tract alone. Of 821 cases the epididymis showed tuberculosis in 617 (75 per cent); of 1,675 cases the prostate and vesicles were involved in 1,169 (70 per cent); disease of the testicle was found in 58 per cent of 739 cases. The prostatic lobes contain nodules varying in size from a pea to a bean. There is great irritability of the bladder and agonizing pain on catheterization. The seminal vesicles may be involved primarily or secondarily. They become thickened, enlarged and tender, sometimes nodular, and tubercle bacilli may be found in the fluid expressed by massage. An extremely rare lesion is primary urethral tuberculosis, which may simulate stricture. Pelouze states that lymphocystic urethral lesions are suggestive of active systemic tuberculosis. Chronic hyperplastic tuberculosis of the corpus cavernosum of the penis is described.

Testes and Epididymes.—This may be primary but, more frequently, is secondary to tuberculous disease elsewhere. Cases occur before the second year, and it is stated to have been found in the fetus. In infants it is serious and usually associated with tuberculous disease in other parts. In 20 cases (Jullien) 6 were under one year, and 6 between one and two years old. In 5 of the cases both testicles were affected. Koplik held that most of these cases are congenital, in Baumgarten's sense. In young children the testis proper may be involved first, but in adults the epididymis is first affected. Trauma and previous inflammation are predisposing factors. Extension to the testicle and other parts of the genital tract occurs later. The initial *symptoms* may be acute, resembling acute epididymitis, followed by a chronic condition. More often the onset is insidious and painless enlargement is found. Pain may occur later, frequently dull with sharp paroxysms. The cord may be thickened. Sexual desire may be unchanged but azoospermia is frequent. The semen may contain tubercle bacilli.

Tubercle of the testes is most likely to be confounded with syphilis. In the latter the body of the organ is most often affected, there is less pain, and the outlines of the growth are more nodular and irregular. In obscure peritoneal disease the detection of tubercle in the epididymis may lead to a correct diagnosis. The two conditions may be associated. The lesion in the testis or epididymis may heal completely or the disease may become generalized. Death from tuberculous meningitis is more common than in tuberculous lesions elsewhere. General infection has followed operation. Too much stress can not be laid on the importance of a routine examination of the testes and epididymes.

Fallopian Tubes, Ovaries, and Uterus.—The *Fallopian* tubes are a frequent seat of genital tuberculosis. The disease may be primary and produce a characteristic salpingitis, in which the tubes are enlarged, the walls thickened and infiltrated, and the contents cheesy. Adhesion takes place between the fimbriae and the ovaries, or the uterus may be invaded. The condition is usually bilateral and may occur in young children. Although, as a rule, evident to the naked eye, there are specimens resembling ordinary salpingitis, which show on microscopic examination numerous miliary tubercles. Tuberculous salpingitis may cause serious local disease with abscess formation, and be the starting-point of peritonitis. Tuberculosis of the *ovary* is always secondary. There may be an eruption of tubercles over the surface in an extensive involvement of the stroma with abscess formation. Tuberculosis of the *uterus* is very rare. Only four examples have come under our observation, all with pulmonary tuberculosis. It may be primary. The mucosa of the fundus is thickened and caseous, and tubercles may be seen in the muscular tissue. Occasionally the process extends to the vagina. Tuberculosis of the *placenta* is more common than has been supposed. Of 20 placentas from tuberculous women, 9 were affected; 5 of these were from cases of advanced disease of the lung. The lesions are easily overlooked.

TUBERCULOSIS OF THE MAMMARY GLAND

There may be solitary or disseminated nodules, a sclerosing mastitis or caseation with abscess formation. The disease is most common between the fortieth and sixtieth years. The breast is frequently fistulous, unevenly indurated, and the nipple is retracted. The fistulae and ulcers present a characteristic tuberculous aspect. There is also a cold tuberculous abscess of the breast. The axillary glands are affected in about two-thirds of the cases. The disease runs a chronic course of months or years. The diagnosis is made by the general appearance of the fistulae and ulcers, and the finding of tubercle bacilli. The prognosis is favorable if total eradication is possible.

In 1836 Bedor described *hypertrophy* of the breast in the subjects of pulmonary tuberculosis. As a rule, if one gland is involved, the condition is one of chronic interstitial mammitis and is not tuberculous.

TUBERCULOSIS OF THE CIRCULATORY SYSTEM

Myocardium.—Miliary tubercles are sometimes met with in the acute disease. Larger caseous tubercles are excessively rare. There is also a sclerotic tuberculous myocarditis. The infection may pass from a mediastinal gland.

Endocardium.—Endocarditis was present in only 151 among more than 11,000 autopsies on tuberculous cases (G. W. Norris). As a rule, it is a secondary form, the result of a mixed infection, so common in pulmonary tuberculosis. A true tuberculous endocarditis does occur and, as a rule, is a vegetative form. In rare cases caseous tubercles develop.

Arteries.—Primary tuberculosis of the larger blood vessels is very rare and usually the result of invasion from without. The disease may occur in a large artery and not result from external invasion. Adams (1929) found 36 cases of tuberculosis of the aorta, in 20 of which the aorta was involved from without by extension of a tuberculous process. Aneurism may form and rupture. In the lungs and other organs attacked by tuberculosis the *arteries* are involved in an acute infiltration which usually leads to thrombosis, or tubercles may develop in the walls, caseate and soften, frequently with a resulting hemorrhage. By extension into vessels, particularly veins, the bacilli are widely distributed with the production of miliary tuberculosis.

THE PROGNOSIS IN TUBERCULOSIS

The parable of the sower already referred to expresses better than in any other way the question of individual predisposition. There are five groups of cases of tuberculous infection. 1. Those who become infected and recover spontaneously without knowing they have been infected. 2. Mild infections with slight symptoms, recovery following after a few months. Many of the primary forms (childhood) belong here. 3. Those with well-marked signs of lung disease in whom thorough treatment is followed by complete recovery. 4. Those with extensive local disease and cavity formation in whom arrest takes place and the patients live for many years. 5. Those in whom the infection is of such a type that death follows no matter what is done.

The following may be considered favorable circumstances: An early diagnosis, a good family history, previous good health, a strong digestion, a suitable environment, and an insidious onset, without high fever, and without extensive pneumonic consolidation. Cases beginning with pleurisy seem to run a more protracted and more favorable course. Repeated attacks of hemoptysis are unfavorable. When well established the course of tuberculosis is usually marked by intervals in which the fever lessens, the symptoms subside, and there is improvement in the general health.

In pulmonary cases the duration is extremely variable. Much depends on the condition when the diagnosis is made and the possibilities for thorough treatment. The response of the patient to treatment is important. Much depends on whether proper treatment can be carried on for a sufficient time. The psychical reactions of the patient are important as these may favor or hinder recovery.

Tuberculosis and Marriage.—The following brief statements may be made:

(*a*) Subjects with healed lymphatic or bone tuberculosis marry with personal impunity and may beget healthy children.

(*b*) The question of marriage of a person who has arrested or cured lung tuberculosis is more difficult to decide. In a male the personal risk is not so great; and when the health and strength are good, the external environment favorable, and the family history not extremely bad, the experiment—for it is such—is often successful, and many healthy families are begotten under these circumstances. In women the question is complicated with that of childbearing, which increases the risks enormously. As a rule, pregnancy should be avoided. With a localized lesion, absence of hereditary taint, good physique, and favorable environment marriage might be permitted. When tuberculosis has existed in a girl whose family history is bad, and whose physique is below the standard, the physician should, if possible, place his veto upon marriage. If married, then the prevention of pregnancy is indicated.

(*c*) With existing disease, fever, bacilli, etc., marriage should be prohibited. Pregnancy usually hastens the process, though it may be held in abeyance. After parturition the disease may advance rapidly. There is much truth in the remark of Dubois: "If a woman threatened with phthisis marries, she may bear the first accouchement well; a second, with difficulty; a third, never." Conception may occur in an advanced stage of the disease. The decision as to a therapeutic abortion requires careful consideration.

PROPHYLAXIS IN TUBERCULOSIS

General.—Among the more important measures may be mentioned the following: *First,* education of the public. Much has been done by the anti-tuberculosis crusade, which has resulted in the formation of many active societies and has stimulated widespread interest in the disease. *Second,* making tuberculosis a reportable disease. This gives the board of health control of the situation and is a most helpful measure. *Third,* improved conditions of living, particularly as regards food and housing. *Fourth,* direct preventive measures, such as the enactment of laws against spitting in public, the disinfection and cleaning of rooms which have been occupied by tuberculous patients, the inspection of cattle and pasteurization of milk. *Fifth, organization* of sanatoria and hospitals for early curable and late incurable cases, and the establishment of dispensaries with a system of visiting the patients at their homes by specially trained nurses. *Sixth,* the care of the sputum of the tuberculous. The patient should expectorate into a paper sputum cup held close to the mouth and wipe the lips afterwards with a paper napkin which is folded with the soiled surface inside and placed in a paper bag. A paper napkin should be held before the mouth during coughing. The used cups and napkins should be burned. These measures are important for the patient himself and for others. In hospitals it is well to have printed directions as to the care of the sputum, and printed cards for outpatients, giving the important rules. It should be explained to the patient that the only risk, practically, is from this source. *Seventh,* the careful study of all those who have been in contact with patients having tuberculosis.

Individual.—Individual prophylaxis with delicate children is most important. An infant born of tuberculous parents, or of a family in which tuberculosis prevails, should be brought up with great care and guarded against infections of all kinds. There should be no contact with persons who have open tuberculosis. Special attention should be given to the throat and nose, and on the first indication of mouth-breathing, or any obstruction of the nasopharynx, a careful examination should be made for adenoid vegetations. The child should be clad in flannel and live in the open air as much as possible, avoiding close rooms. It is a good practice to sponge the throat and chest night and morning with cold water. Special attention should be paid to the diet. The meals should be at regular hours and the food plain and substantial. From the outset the child should be encouraged to drink freely of milk. As the child grows older, systematically regulated exercise or a course of pulmonary gymnastics may be taken. In the choice of an occupation preference should be given to an out-of-door life. Immunization of infants by the use of *Bacillus Calmette-Guérin* (B-C-G) is under trial and final judgment can not be passed. If efficient, it or some other such method would be indicated in children born of parents with open pulmonary tuberculosis or who are in contact with tuberculous persons.

The examination of children who have been in contact with tuberculous individuals is important. Four groups of suspects come to tuberculosis dispensaries: (1) The underfed, anemic, badly developed child, without local lesions; the question is one of mulnutrition. (2) Cases of thymolymphatism usually having adenoids and enlarged tonsils. These children may not be anemic, but they have stunted, badly formed chests, and the superficial lymph nodes may be enlarged. (3) Children with enlarged lymph nodes, usually cervical; it may not be easy to determine whether the adenopathy is due to throat infection or bad teeth, or whether it is tuberculous. (4) Children with signs in the chest pointing to a definite lesion, the tuberculous nature of which may not at first be easy to determine.

The trifling ailments of children should be carefully watched. In the convalescence from the fevers the greatest caution should be exercised to prevent catching cold. An open air life, a generous diet, especially in fats and vitamins and iron, if there is anemia, are important aids. Care of the throat is important; enlarged tonsils and adenoids should be removed.

To ensure proper disposal of the sputum is one of the most important points in prevention. The dishes used by a patient with bacilli in the sputum should be boiled and those used by others should not be washed in the same water or dried with the same cloth as those used by the patient.

TREATMENT OF TUBERCULOSIS

The Natural or Spontaneous Cure.—The spontaneous healing of local tuberculosis is an every-day affair. A majority of those infected never have the clinical disease, *i.e.*, they recover without symptoms, without the slight lesion having disturbed the health. Many cases of adenitis and disease of the bone or joints terminate favorably. The healing of pulmonary tuberculosis is shown clinically by the recovery of patients in whose sputum elastic tissue and bacilli have been found; anatomically, by the presence of lesions in all stages of repair. In the granulation products and associated pneumonia a scar tissue is formed, while the smaller caseous areas become impregnated with lime salts. To such alone should the term healing be applied. When the fibroid change encapsulates but does not involve the entire tuberculous tissue, the tubercle may be termed quiescent, but is not destroyed. As to *cavities* we have had to alter the older views and recognize that healing is possible in a certain number of cases. The X-ray evidence seems conclusive. What limit there is as to the size of a cavity which may heal it is difficult to state. Cavities may be greatly reduced in size—indeed, an entire series of them may be so contracted by sclerosis of the tissue about them that a lobe may be reduced to a third of its ordinary dimensions.

There is an old German axiom, *Jedermann hat am Ende ein bischen Tuberculose,* a statement partly borne out by the statistics showing the proportion of persons dying of all disease in whom quiescent tuberculous lesions are found. We find at the apices the following conditions, which have been held to signify healed tuberculous processes: (*a*) Thickening of the pleura, usually at the posterior surface, with some subadjacent induration. This has, perhaps, no greater significance than a milky patch on the pericardium. (*b*) Puckered cicatrices at the apex, depressing the pleura, and showing a pigmented, fibrous scar. The bronchioles in the neighborhood may be dilated, but there are neither tubercles nor cheesy masses. This may sometimes, but not always, indicate a healed tuberculous lesion. (*c*) Puckered cicatrices with cheesy or cretaceous nodules, and with scattered tubercles in the vicinity. (*d*) The *cicatrices fistuleuses* of Laënnec, in which fibrosis has reduced the size of cavities which communicate directly with the bronchi.

General Measures.—The question of nutrition is most important; digestion and assimilation play a large part. There are three indications: First, to place the patient in surroundings most favorable for a maximum degree of rest and nutrition; second, to take such measures as, in a local or general way, influence the tuberculous processes; third, to alleviate symptoms.

The psychology of the patient should be carefully studied. The frequency of fear in the psychical processes must always be remembered. The mental side may require careful handling. There is often "deliberate cheerfulness", which may be deceptive. Tuberculosis with its long duration and many possibilities for worry favors emotional stress and strain. The view that the toxin (or toxemia) is responsible is not proved. The problem of readjustment may require time and much help. The diagnosis should be given in the best way for each patient. There is the danger of making too light of the condition and on the other side of being too serious as to the outlook. There should be no concealment as relatives too often request.

Rest.—If in doubt—*more rest.* The patient has to learn to relax both mentally and physically. When activity is allowed this should be begun very gradually and closely supervised. The amount of rest and exercise should be prescribed as carefully as a drug.

Open-air Treatment.—The value of fresh air and out-of-door life is well established. A patient confined to the house—particularly in the close, stuffy dwellings of the poor—has less chance than a patient living in the fresh air or sunshine for the greater part of the day. The open-air treatment may be carried out at home, by change of residence or in a sanatorium.

At Home.—In a majority of cases the patient has to be cared for in his own home, and, if in the city, under disadvantageous circumstances. Much may be done even in cities to promote arrest by insisting upon systematic treatment as is shown by the success of J. H. Pratt's *tuberculosis classes.* As not 5 per cent of the patients can be dealt with in sanatoria, it is gratifying to see how successful the home treatment may be. Even in cities the patients may sleep out of doors, and the results obtained by Pratt, Millett, and others are as good as any that have been published. *While there is fever the patient should be at rest in bed,* and night and day the windows should be open, so that he may be exposed freely to the fresh air. Low temperature is not a contra-indication. If there is a balcony or a suitable yard or garden, on the brighter days the patient may be wrapped up and put in a reclining chair or on a sofa. The important thing to emphasize is the fact that cough, fever, night sweats or hemoptysis do not contra-indicate full exposure to fresh air. In country places this can be carried out much more effectively. In the summer the patient should be out of doors for at least eleven or twelve hours, and in winter six or eight hours. At night the room should be cool and thoroughly well ventilated. With a sleeping porch the patient may spend nearly all the time in the open air. It may require several months of rest treatment in the open air before the temperature falls to normal.

In Sanatoria.—An important advance has been the establishment of institutions in which patients live according to strict rules. To Brehmer, of Göbersdorf, we owe the successful execution of this plan, which has been followed with most gratifying results. In the United States the zeal, energy, and scientific devotion of Edward L. Trudeau demonstrated its feasibility and the Saranac institution is a model of its kind. The results at hundreds of institutions demonstrate the great importance of system and discipline in carrying out successful treatment. Much has been done to promote the sanatorium treatment and the good results have justified the heavy expenditure of money. In many places it has been demonstrated that with an inexpensive plant excellent results may be obtained. The all-important matter is the establishment near the larger cities of public sanatoria for treatment in the early stages. The large general hospitals should have out-patient departments for tuberculous patients, from which suitable cases could be sent to the sanatoria. Much discussion has taken place as to the result of sanatorium treatment but there is no doubt of its benefits in suitable cases.

Climatic Treatment.—This, after all, is only a modification of the open-air method. The first question to be decided is whether the patient is fit to be sent from home. In many instances it is a positive hardship. A patient with active disease is much better at home, and the physician should not be too much influenced by the importunities of the sick man or his friends. The requirements of a suitable climate are a *pure atmosphere,* an *equable temperature* not subject to rapid variations, and a *maximum amount of sunshine.* Given these, it makes little difference *where* a patient goes, so long as he lives *an outdoor life.* The different climates may be grouped into the high altitudes, the dry, warm climates, and the moist, warm climates. Among high altitudes in the United States, the Colorado, Arizona and New Mexico resorts are the most important. The high altitudes may cause dilatation of the air-vesicles and a permanent increase in the size of the chest which is a disadvantage when such persons attempt subsequently to reside at sea-level. In Europe the chief resorts at high altitudes are in Switzerland. Of resorts at a moderate altitude, Asheville and the Adirondacks are the best known in America. One advantage is that after arrest of the disease the patient can return to sea-level without any special risk. The cases most suitable for high altitudes are those in which the disease is limited, without much cavity formation, and without much emaciation. The thin, irritable patients with chronic tuberculosis and a good deal of emphysema are better at sea-level. A cold winter climate seems to be of decided advantage in tuberculosis and the patients are able to lead an out-of-door life throughout the entire winter.

Other considerations which should influence the choice of a locality are good accommodations and good food and, most important of all, a competent physician. Very much is said concerning the choice of locality in the different stages of pulmonary tuberculosis, but when the disease is limited, in a patient of fairly good personal and family history, the chances are that he may fight a winning battle if he lives out of doors in any climate, whether high, dry, and cold, or low, moist, and warm. With bilateral disease and cavity formation the mild or warm climates are preferable.

Heliotherapy.—Both natural and artificial heliotherapy is of value in some forms of tuberculosis, especially of the bones, glands, intestines, and peritoneum. It has to be carefully supervised and may be harmful in pulmonary disease.

Measures which Influence the Tuberculous Process.—Under this heading we may consider the specific, dietetic, and general medicinal treatment.

Specific Treatment.—Introduced by Koch in 1890, the tuberculin treatment soon fell into disfavor, but, in spite of the bad results from its injudicious use, certain men continue to use it. In suitable cases it may have a beneficial influence; the difficulty is to decide which they are. In certain surgical forms of tuberculosis it has some usefulness but in the vast majority of cases of pulmonary tuberculosis it has no place. Tuberculin is a remedy potent for harm if improperly used and it should be given only to carefully selected cases by those experienced in its use. It is contra-indicated in patients with fever, hemoptysis, and pleurisy or acute features. It is not desirable—quite the contrary in fact—to get a general reaction, particularly as this may be associated with marked focal reactions. The aim is to get as high a grade of tuberculin tolerance as possible. It may require many months of the small dose, nonreaction method to accomplish this. Treatment with tuberculin should not be begun unless it can be continued for some months.

Dietetic Treatment.—The outlook in tuberculosis depends much upon the digestion and it is rare to see recovery in a patient in whom there is persistent gastric trouble. Basal metabolism may be normal or slightly above normal. Excessive feeding may increase it and so exaggerate respiration. Probably 2,500 calories a day are enough with 60 grams of protein. The early nausea and loss of appetite in many cases are serious obstacles. Many patients loathe food of all kinds. A change of air may promptly restore the appetite. When this is impossible, and if, as is almost always the case, fever is present, the patient should be at absolute rest, kept in the open air as much as possible, and fed at stated intervals with small quantities of milk, buttermilk, or koumyss, alternating if necessary with meat juice and egg albumen. Raw eggs are suitable for some patients and may be taken between meals. The diet should be as varied as possible and care taken to give sufficient vitamins. Overfeeding should be guarded against, especially in toxic patients. The use of *insulin* (5 unit doses at first and increased if indicated) may be of value, especially in undernourished patients.

In many cases the digestion is not at all disturbed and the patient can take an ordinary diet. It is remarkable how rapidly the appetite and digestion improve with the fresh air treatment, even in a city. Care should be taken that drugs do not disturb the stomach. Not infrequently cough mixtures, cod-liver oil and creosote produce irritation, and do more harm than good. On the other hand, the bitter tonics, with acids, and malt preparations are often satisfactory. A routine administration of alcohol is not advisable, and there is no evidence that its use promotes fibroid processes. In advanced stages, particularly when the temperature is low between eight and ten in the morning, whisky and milk, or whisky, egg, and milk may be given with advantage.

Rest and Exercise.—One month in bed is a minimum period for all patients beginning treatment, whether febrile or afebrile. Fever is an indication for absolute rest. Greater emphasis is being placed on the importance of prolonged rest, meaning rest in bed. The duration of rest must be decided for each patient, and better too long than too short. The febrile patient is regarded as one in whom auto-inoculation is excessive. To overcome this the patient is immobilized in bed as far as possible. The effect of this is often remarkable in reducing the fever. The pulse rate is important in deciding the safe amount of activity.

Immobilizing the Lung.—Years ago Cayley induced *pneumothorax* in a case of hemoptysis. The method did not come into general use; but later was advocated in pulmonary tuberculosis by Forlanini and J. B. Murphy. Air is introduced into the pleural cavity. At first from 200 to 300 cc., later as much as 500 cc. are introduced, so that the lung is completely collapsed, and there is a neutral or slightly positive interpleural pressure. It is used in patients with unilateral or predominately unilateral lesions who do not respond to the usual treatment, in patients with hemorrhage, especially if repeated; and in case of cavities which show no tendency to close. The presence of adhesions limits its usefulness but in some cases these can be divided. Many patients can carry on their usual activity with an induced pneumothorax. Pneumothorax should be done only by those skilled in its use. There are dangers, as serous effusion, pleural shock and empyema. The duration of the treatment has to be prolonged as the collapse should be for long periods and the pleural cavity requires to be refilled every few weeks.

Other methods of immobilizing the lung include postural rest by having the patient lie on the affected side (Webb), controlled and slow diaphragmatic breathing (Knopf) and fixation of the chest wall by strapping or apparatus. *Oleothorax*, using mineral oil to produce collapse, has a limited field. *Phrenic evulsion* or *phrenicotomy* produces paralysis of the diaphragm on the side involved and has a definite place. Crushing the phrenic nerve should be done first. Scaleniotomy, with or without phrenicotomy, does not seem to be of much value. *Thoracoplasty* is useful when pneumothorax has failed or is impossible; marked fibroid change and thickened pleura are favorable conditions for it.

General Medical Treatment.—No drugs have any special or peculiar action upon tuberculous processes. In glandular and bone tuberculosis *cod-liver oil* itself or as a concentrate is undoubtedly beneficial. The concentrates are easier to take than oil. The vitamins are useful in all forms of tuberculosis.

Tonics.—There is no general tonic more satisfactory in tuberculosis than Fowler's solution. It may be given in 5 minim (0.3 cc.) doses three times a day, stopping its use whenever unpleasant symptoms arise, and in any case intermitting it every third or fourth week. Some prefer dilute hydrochloric acid or tincture of nux vomica before meals. Iron should be given freely for anemia.

Sanocrysin.—There is no agreement as to the value of this and opinion in Europe seems more favorable than in North America. It should be used with care and only by those who have had experience in its use.

Treatment of Special Symptoms.—Fever.—The patient should be at absolute rest and, if possible, *in the open air night and day for some weeks.* For continuous pyrexia or the remittent type of the early stages, small doses of mild antipyretic drugs, such as acetylsalicylic acid, may be tried; but they are uncertain and rarely reliable. It is better, when the fever rises above 103° to rely upon sponging. When softening has taken place and the fever assumes the characteristic septic type, the problem becomes still more difficult. The pyrexia, at this stage, lasts only for twelve or fifteen hours and as a rule there are not more than from eight to ten hours in which the fever is high enough to demand antipyretic treatment. Sometimes phenacetine, given in 2-grain (0.13 gm.) doses every hour for three or four hours before the rise in temperature prevents or limits the paroxysm. It answers better in this way than given in single doses. Sponging of the extremities for half an hour during the height of the fever is useful.

Sweating.—Atropine, in doses of gr. 1/120-1/60 (0.0005-0.001 gm.), and aromatic sulphuric acid in large doses are the best remedies. When there are cough and nocturnal restlessness, codein (gr. 1/2, 0.032 gm.) may be given with the atropine. Camphoric acid (gr. x, 0.65 gm.) at bedtime may be tried. The patient should use light flannel garments.

Cough.—The *cough* is a troublesome, though necessary, feature in pulmonary tuberculosis. The patient should endeavor to learn to control the cough as much as possible. The use of a support which compresses the abdomen and elevates the diaphragm may give comfort and lessen cough (Gordon). Unless very worrying and disturbing sleep or so severe as to produce vomiting, it is not well to attempt to restrict it too much. When irritative in character, inhalations are useful, particularly the tincture of benzoin or preparations of menthol or eucalyptus. Some of the most irritable and distressing forms of cough result from laryngeal erosions. The nocturnal cough, which begins just as the patient is preparing to fall asleep, requires, as a rule, preparations of opium. Codein (gr. 1/4-1/2, 0.016-0.03 gm.) may be given. An excellent combination is morphia (gr. 1/8, 0.008 gm.), dilute hydrocyanic acid (♏ iij, 0.2 cc.), and syrup of wild cherry (ʒ j, 4 cc.). The spirit of chloroform, or a mixture of chloroform and sedatives or Hoffman's anodyne, given in whisky before going to sleep, is efficacious. Mild counterirritation or the application of a hot poultice will sometimes lessen the cough. The morning cough is often relieved by taking immediately after waking a glass of hot milk or a cup of hot water, to which 15 grains of sodium bicarbonate are added. In the later stages, when cavities have formed, the accumulated secretion must be expectorated and the paroxysms of coughing are most exhausting. The sedatives should be given cautiously. The aromatic spirit of ammonia may help to allay the paroxysm. When the expectoration is profuse, creosote internally, or inhalations of turpentine and iodine, or oil of eucalyptus, are useful. For the troublesome dysphagia a solution of cocaine (gr. x, 0.6 gm.) with boric acid (gr. v, 0.3 gm.) in glycerine and water (℥ j, 30 cc.) may be used locally.

DIARRHEA.—For this large doses of bismuth with Dover's powder, and small starch enemata, with opium, may be given. The diet should be simple. In some cases, 5 cc. of a 5 per cent solution of calcium chloride injected intravenously is useful.

The treatment of hemoptysis will be considered in the section on hemorrhage from the lungs. Dyspnea is rarely a prominent symptom except in the advanced stages, when it may be very troublesome and distressing. Ammonia and morphia, cautiously administered, may be used.

If the pleuritic pains are severe, the side may be strapped, or painted with tincture of iodine. The dyspeptic symptoms require careful treatment, as the outlook in individual cases depends much upon the condition of the stomach. Small doses of bismuth and soda often allay the distressing nausea.

The treatment of lesions such as of the kidney, epididymis, etc., is surgical if recognized early enough. Disease elsewhere, as in the lungs, is not a necessary contra-indication. The possible harm resulting from ether anesthesia must always be kept in mind. Arsphenamine or its modifications should not be given to tuberculous patients with syphilis. There is doubt as to whether iodide is harmful.

A last word on the subject of tuberculosis to the general practitioner: *The leadership of the battle against this scourge is in your hands. Much has been done, much remains to do. By early diagnosis and prompt, systematic treatment of individual cases, by the prompt recognition of contact cases, by striving in every possible way to improve the social condition of the poor, by joining actively in the work of the local and national antituberculosis societies you can help in the most important and the most hopeful campaign ever undertaken by the profession.*

DISEASES DUE TO RICKETTSIA BODIES

TYPHUS FEVER

Definition.—An acute infectious disease characterized by sudden onset, maculated and hemorrhagic rash, nervous symptoms, and a course terminating by rapid lysis, usually about the end of the second week.

The disease is known by the names of hospital fever, spotted fever, jail fever, camp fever, and ship fever, and in Germany is called *exanthematic* typhus, in contradistinction to *abdominal* typhus (typhoid). The word signifies "smoke" or "mist" in Greek and was used by Hippocrates to describe any condition with a tendency to stupor. In the eighteenth century the name was given by de Sauvages to the common putrid or pestilential fever, and the general use came in through its adoption by Cullen.

Etiology.—Typhus has been one of the great *epidemics* of the world, whose history, as Hirsch remarks, is written in those dark pages which tell of the grievous visitations of mankind by war, famine, and misery. Ireland was terribly scourged by the disease between the years 1817 and 1819, and again in 1846. It prevailed extensively in all the large cities of Great Britain and the Continent. In 1875 in England and Wales there were 1,499 deaths from the disease, but of late years the deaths have been few. It is endemic in many parts of the world.

Sporadic typhus fever offers peculiarities which make its recognition difficult. There may be outbreaks of a few cases, the origin of which may be very difficult to trace. It is not infrequent along the Atlantic coast of the United States. Brill drew attention to this sporadic form in New York. The typhus fever prevailing in Mexico, known as Tabardillo, is more severe, and in its study Ricketts, of Chicago, fell a victim. The European and American forms are similar but not identical. They show certain differences in the results of infection in guinea-pigs. The antigens differ somewhat and cross-immunization occurs. There is a close relationship to Rocky Mountain Spotted Fever, which has probably been regarded as typhus fever at times in the eastern part of the United States. It may be that these sporadic cases occur more frequently than was generally supposed as the diagnosis may be difficult.

The disease is transmitted by the body louse and possibly by the head louse and so is associated with filth and overcrowding. In the Southern United States there were cases in which lice apparently played no part in transmission. The evidence suggests that the rat is the source of infection which is carried by the rat flea (*Xenopsylla cheopis*). It may transmit the disease and the organisms are found in its feces. In epidemics it is one of the most dangerous of all diseases, and those in attendance upon patients are in danger unless special precautions are taken to guard against lice and fleas.

It seems established that *Rickettsia prowazeki* is the causal organism. The Rickettsia have been demonstrated in human and guinea-pig tissues. In the human lesions they have been found in all the tissues in which changes occur. The Rickettsia bodies are bacterium-like, very small, occur in pairs and are difficult to stain. A curious phenomenon is the agglutination of a proteus bacillus (x 19) by the serum of typhus fever patients in high dilutions. This organism is not regarded as a cause of the disease. This reaction appears by the fifth day in almost half the cases.

Pathology.—The gross changes are not characteristic. The hemorrhagic lesions are present in the skin. The viscera show parenchymatous changes but there are no characteristic changes in the bowel. The vessels of the brain may show perivascular hemorrhage. Endothelial proliferation is common in the small arteries and arterioles, often causing thrombosis. The lesions in the skin are marked; in early stages there is swelling of the endothelium in the small vessels. There is a distinctive perivascular infiltration.

Symptoms.—Incubation.—This is placed at about twelve days, but it may be less. There may be ill-defined feelings of discomfort. As a rule, however, the *invasion* is abrupt and marked by chills, followed by fever. The chills may recur during the first few days, and there is headache with pains in the back and legs. There is early prostration, and the patient takes to his bed at once. The temperature is high at first, and may attain its maximum on the second or third day. The pulse is full, rapid, and not so frequently dicrotic as in typhoid. The tongue is furred and white, and there is an early tendency to dryness. The face is flushed and the eyes congested. Vomiting may be distressing. In severe cases mental symptoms are present from the outset, a mild febrile delirium or an excited, almost maniacal condition. Bronchitis is common and the respiration rate is increased.

Stage of Eruption.—From the third to the fifth day the *eruption* appears—first upon the abdomen and upper part of the chest, and then upon the back and extremities; occurring so rapidly that in two or three days it is general. There are two elements in the eruption: a subcuticular mottling, "a fine, irregular, dusky red mottling, as if below the surface of the skin some little distance, and seen through a semi-opaque medium" (Buchanan); and distinct papular rose-spots which change to petechiae. In some instances the petechial rash comes out with the rose-spots. Collie describes the rash as consisting of three parts: rose-colored spots which disappear on pressure, dark-red spots which are modified by pressure, and petechiae upon which pressure produces no effect. In children the rash at first may present a striking resemblance to that of measles and give a curiously mottled appearance. The term mulberry rash is sometimes applied to it. In mild cases the eruption is slight, but even then is largely petechial in character. As the rash is hemorrhagic, it does not disappear after death. Usually the skin is dry, so that sudaminal vesicles are not common. It is stated by some authors that a distinctive odor is present. During the second week the general symptoms are much aggravated. The prostration becomes more marked, the delirium more intense, and the fever rises. The patient lies on his back with a dull, expressionless face, flushed cheeks, injected conjunctivae, and contracted pupils. The pulse increases in frequency and is feebler; the face is dusky, and the condition becomes more serious. Retention of urine is common. Coma-vigil is frequent, a condition in which the patient lies with open eyes, but quite unconscious; with it there may be subsultus tendinum and picking at the bedclothes. The tongue is dry, brown, and cracked, and there are sordes on the teeth. Respiration is accelerated, the heart's action becomes more and more enfeebled, and death takes place from exhaustion. In favorable cases about the end of the second week the temperature falls and reaches normal in two or three days. Although the prostration may be extreme convalescence is rapid and relapse very rare. This fairly rapid termination is in striking contrast to the mode of termination in typhoid fever.

Fever.—The temperature rises steadily during the first four or five days, and the morning remissions are not marked. The maximum is usually attained by the fifth day, when the temperature may be 105° to 107° F. In mild cases it seldom rises above 103° F. After reaching its maximum the fever generally

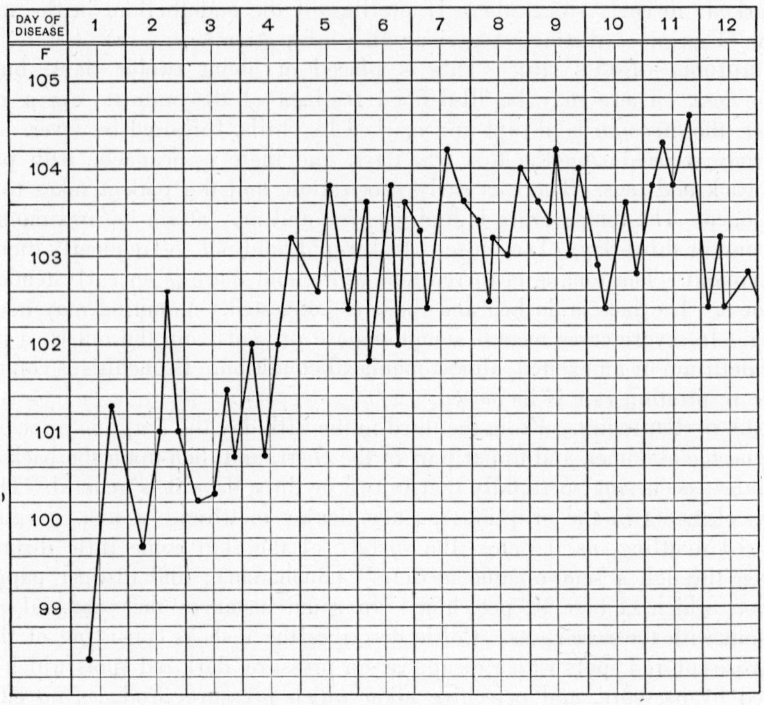

Chart V.—Typhus Fever (Murchison).

continues with slight morning remissions until the twelfth or fourteenth day. Preceding a fatal termination, there is usually a rapid rise in the fever to 108° or 109° F.

The *heart* may show signs of weakness. The first sound becomes feeble and almost inaudible, and a systolic murmur at the apex is not infrequent. Hypostatic congestion of the lungs occurs in severe cases. The brain symptoms are usually pronounced and delirium is frequent. A slight leukocytosis is common and eosinophiles are absent. The frequent arterial thrombosis may involve visceral arteries or cause necrosis and gangrene of the skin.

The urine shows the usual febrile characteristics. Albumin is present in a large proportion of the cases, but nephritis seldom occurs.

Variations in the course of the disease are naturally common. There are malignant cases which rapidly prove fatal within two or three days; the so-called *typhus siderans.* On the other hand, during epidemics, there are extremely mild cases in which the fever is slight, the delirium absent, and convalescence is established by the tenth day.

Sporadic Form.—Beginning with the usual prodromes, the fever increases rapidly and reaches a maximum about the third or fourth day, where it remains fairly constant between 103° and 104°. On the 5th or 6th day an eruption appears, maculopapular in type, dull red in color, rarely hemorrhagic, not appearing in crops, not disappearing on pressure, and neither profuse as in measles nor diffuse as in typical typhus; there may be only a few hundred spots. The rash persists until the crisis and then fades rapidly. The patients are much prostrated, with severe headache, but no abdominal symptoms. Constipation is usually a marked feature. After persisting for 12 to 15 days, the fever declines rapidly, usually with a critical fall, and there is a speedy convalescence. It is rarely fatal and the death rate in these cases is apparently not more than two per cent.

Complications.—Bronchopneumonia is perhaps the most common complication. It may pass on to gangrene. In certain epidemics gangrene of the feet, the hands, or the nose, and in children noma or cancrum oris have occurred. Meningitis is rare. Paralyses, which are probably due to cerebral thrombosis or embolism, are not very uncommon. Septic processes, such as parotitis and abscesses in the subcutaneous tissues and in the joints, are occasionally met with. Hematemesis may occur.

Prognosis.—The mortality ranges in different epidemics from 12 to 50 per cent but is low in the sporadic cases. It is very slight in the young. Children rarely die. After middle age the mortality is high, in some epidemics 50 per cent. Death usually occurs toward the close of the second week and is due to toxemia or pneumonia.

Diagnosis.—During an epidemic there is rarely any doubt, for the disease presents distinctive general characters. Isolated cases and the form described by Brill may be very difficult to distinguish from typhoid fever. While in typical instances the eruption in the two affections is very different, yet taken alone it may be deceptive, since in typhoid fever a roseolous rash may be abundant and there may be occasionally a subcuticular mottling and even petechiae. The difference in the onset, particularly in the temperature, is marked; but cases in which it is important to make an accurate diagnosis are not usually seen until the fourth or fifth day. The suddenness of the onset, the greater frequency of the chill, and the early prostration and toxemia are the distinctive features in typhus. It is easy to put down on paper elaborate differential distinctions, which are practically useless at the bedside. The Widal reaction and blood cultures are important aids. Severe *cerebrospinal fever* may closely simulate typhus at the outset, but the diagnosis is usually clear within a few days. Malignant *variola* also has certain features in common with severe typhus, but the greater extent of the hæmorrhages and the bleeding from the mucous membranes make the diagnosis clear within a short time. The rash at first resembles that of *measles,* but in the latter the eruption is brighter red, often crescentic or irregular in arrangement, and appears first on the face. *Rocky Mountain Spotted Fever* may resemble typhus fever but the onset is more gradual, the rash usually appears first on the ankles and wrists and the course is longer.

Weil-Felix Reaction.—This depends on the agglutinating power of blood serum from typhus fever patients on a strain of *B. proteus* known as x 19, which is found in the urine of patients with the disease. The agglutination occurs in high dilutions and is usually present by the fifth or sixth day. It may be present in Rocky Mountain Spotted Fever.

Prophylaxis.—This involves measures against lice and fleas, and those attending patients should take special precautions to prevent infection by lice and wear louse-proof clothing. The patient's clothing should be sterilized by heat. Removal of the patient to an isolation hospital is important. Convalescent serum has been used.

Treatment.—The general management is like that of typhoid fever. Hydrotherapy should be thoroughly and systematically employed; water should be given freely. Medicinal antipyretics are even less suitable than in typhoid, as the tendency to heart-weakness is often more pronounced. As a rule, the patients require from the outset a supporting treatment. The bowels may be kept open by mild aperients and enemas. The special nervous symptoms and the pulmonary symptoms should be dealt with as in typhoid fever. In epidemics, when the conditions of the climate are suitable, the patients are best treated in tents in the open air.

TRENCH FEVER

This is an acute infection, with a short period of fever, followed by a second rise or by two or three or more paroxysms of one or two days' duration. The causal organism is a form of Rickettsia and is transmitted by the body louse. The disease was first recognized in 1915 during the War.

The disease usually sets in acutely with chilliness, headache, and general pains, the latter sometimes of great severity. The fever is usually not high and of two or three days' duration. After an afebrile period one or more recurrences lasting for one or two days are very characteristic. In some instances the fever lasted for four or five days but there was great variation. The symptoms usually subsided during the afebrile period. The greatest complaint was of *tender shins.* As a rule there was no swelling or redness, and the pain was usually most marked at night. The course of the fever and the tender shins are the two most important aids in diagnosis. Many cases were regarded at first as influenza. There is no specific treatment. Complete rest is important and acetylsalicylic acid usually relieved the pain. A local application of a saturated solution of magnesium sulphate sometimes gave relief.

ROCKY MOUNTAIN SPOTTED FEVER; TICK FEVER

Definition.—An acute disease, occurring in certain of the western states of the United States, and perhaps in the southeastern states, conveyed by ticks, characterized by chills, fever, general pains and a macular rash, becoming hemorrhagic.

Etiology and Pathology.—The disease prevails especially in Montana and Idaho but occurs less frequently in other western and Pacific states. It is most prevalent in the spring and summer and among those who work in the fields and woods. The etiological agent is one of the Rickettsia group which is found in lesions in the patient, in infected animals and in thc tick. It is conveyed by a tick (*Dermacentor andersoni*) which is apparently infected by biting wild animals, squirrels, etc. The "eastern" form may be conveyed by the dog tick. The disease is readily conveyed to monkeys and guinea-pigs. An attack gives immunity which is transmitted to the offspring. The specific microscopic lesions are endothelial proliferation, local necrosis of endothelium and thrombosis. Perivascular accumulation of cells is common.

Symptoms.—After an incubation of three to ten days, the onset is sudden with a chill, fever and severe pains, especially in the arms and legs. The fever is high and with it are the general features of an acute infection. The *rash* appears from the second to the sixth day, is macular, gradually becomes darker and finally hemorrhagic. It often begins on the extremities and then spreads to the body. The skin is often swollen. Hemorrhages from the mucous membranes may occur. There is usually a moderate leukocytosis with an increase in the large mononuclear cells. The course averages about four weeks, the fever falling by lysis. The mortality varies greatly with locality, reaching 70 per cent in Montana but in Idaho being below 5 per cent.

Diagnosis.—Typhus and typhoid fever are the diseases most likely to cause difficulty. The diagnosis from typhus fever may be difficult especially in areas where it occurs, especially as the Weil-Felix reaction may be given by both. The specific findings of typhoid fever are lacking. In some reported cases which suggest this disease, a tick has been found in the auditory canal.

Prophylaxis.—The destruction of ticks and protective measures, by special clothing, against them are important. The use of "tick vaccine" made from infected ticks has proved useful both in humans and animals.

Treatment.—The treatment of the disease is that of typhus fever with special attention to the circulation. Serum from a convalescent would seem worth a trial.

THE MYCOSES

The local and general infections caused by the group of fungoid organisms variously classed as Streptothrix, Actinomyces, Cladothrix and Leptothrix may be grouped under the term Mycoses. Four or five of these diseases are of sufficient importance to be considered in a work of this scope.

ACTINOMYCOSIS

Definition.—A chronic infective disorder produced by the actinomyces or ray-fungus, *Actinomyces bovis*.

Etiology.—The disease is widespread among cattle, and occurs also in the pig. It was first described by Bollinger in the ox, in which it forms the affection known in America as "big-jaw." The first accurate description of the disease in man was given by James Israel, and subsequently Ponfick insisted upon the identity of the disease in man and cattle.

In the United States and England the disease is less common than in Germany. It is nearly three times as common in men as in women.

The *parasite* in both man and cattle can be seen in the pus from the affected region as yellowish or opaque granules from one-half to two millimetres in diameter, which are made up of cocci and radiating threads, presenting bulbous, club-like terminations. The youngest granules are gray in color and semitranslucent; in these the bulbous extremities are wanting. The parasite has been cultivated, and the disease has been inoculated both with the natural and artificially grown organism. A bacillus, *B. actinomycetem comitans,* is frequently associated. It produces no specific effects when inoculated into animals and its significance is not decided.

Mode of Infection.—There is no evidence of direct infection with the flesh or milk of diseased animals. The streptothrix has not been detected outside the body. It seems highly probable that it is taken in with the food. The site of infection in a majority of cases in man and animals is in the mouth or neighboring passages. In cattle, possibly also in man, barley, oats, and rye have been carriers of the germ.

Morbid Anatomy.—As in tubercle, the first effect is the destruction of adjacent cells and the attraction of leukocytes—later the surrounding cells begin to proliferate. After the tumor reaches a certain size there is great proliferation of the surrounding connective tissue, and the growth may, particularly in the jaw, look like, and was long mistaken for, osteosarcoma. Finally suppuration occurs, which in man, according to Israel, may be produced directly by the actinomyces itself.

Clinical Forms.—Digestive Tract.—The fungus has been found in the cavities of carious teeth. The jaw has been affected in a number of cases in man. There is swelling of one side of the face, or a chronic enlargement of the jaw which may simulate sarcoma. The *tongue* may be involved, showing small indolent growths (in which sinuses may form) either primary or following disease of the jaw. The salivary glands have been affected. In the *intestines* the disease may occur as a primary or secondary affection. The most common seat is the region of the cecum and appendix. With involvement of the *appendix* or cecum the process tends to be chronic without marked acute features. There is a mass which increases in size and gradually becomes fixed by spreading induration with marked adhesions. There may be extension to the bones and pelvic organs and metastases to the liver and lungs. Primary actinomycosis of the large intestine with metastases has occurred and Ransom found the actinomyces in the stools. Actinomycotic *peritonitis* due to infection through a gastrostomy wound has been described. Actinomycosis of the *liver* is rare. It forms a most characteristic lesion, an alveolar honey-combed abscess—like a sponge soaked in pus. It is usually secondary to an intestinal lesion, but in a few cases no other focus was found.

Pulmonary.—In 1878 Israel described a mycotic disease of the lungs, which was found to be the affection described the year before by Bollinger in cattle. It is a chronic disorder, characterized by cough, fever, wasting, and a mucopurulent, sometimes fetid, expectoration. The lesions are unilateral in a majority of the cases. Hodenpyl classifies them in three groups: (1) Lesions of chronic bronchitis; the diagnosis has been made by the presence of actinomyces in the sputum. (2) Miliary actinomycosis, closely resembling miliary tubercle, but the nodules are made up of groups of fungi, surrounded by granulation tissue. (3) The cases with more extensive destructive disease of the lungs, bronchopneumonia, interstitial changes, and abscesses, the latter forming cavities large enough to be diagnosed during life. Actinomycotic lesions of other organs are often present; erosion of the vertebrae, necrosis of the ribs and sternum, with node-like formations, subcutaneous abscesses, and occasionally general metastases.

The *fever* is irregular and depends largely on the existence of suppuration. The cough is an important symptom and there may be recurring hemoptysis. Lung involvement is usually basal and there may be marked pleural thickening. Pleurisy with effusion sometimes occurs; the fluid may be purulent. Death results usually with septic symptoms but recovery is possible. Clinically the disease closely resembles pulmonary tuberculosis and fetid bronchitis. The diagnosis is made by finding actinomyces in the sputum. Radiating leptothrix threads from the mouth may present a striking resemblance.

CUTANEOUS.—In about half the recorded cases the disease has involved the skin of the head and neck; the buccal, lingual and pharyngeal structures may be involved also. It is a very chronic affection, which may suggest syphilis or lupus, associated with the growth of tumors which suppurate and leave open sores, which may remain for years. The characteristic yellow granules are found in the pus.

CEREBRAL.—Bollinger reported an instance of primary disease of the brain with the symptoms of tumor. Brain abscesses are usually metastatic. In a case, reported by Keller, there was empyema and actinomyces were found in the pus. Subsequently she had Jacksonian epilepsy, caused by abscesses which contained actinomyces grains. Death occurred after the second operation.

GENITO-URINARY SYSTEM.—Involvement of the kidney is rare and may be primary. The tubes and ovaries may be involved.

Prognosis.—Much depends on early diagnosis and treatment and the situation is of importance as cases with involvement of the face and neck have a relatively favorable outlook. The pulmonary cases are very serious and death usually occurs. Of the cases with abdominal infection about half recover.

Diagnosis.—To remember the possibility of actinomycosis and look for it are essential. The yellow granules are suggestive and microscopic examination gives the diagnosis promptly. Tuberculosis, syphilis and sarcoma have to be kept in mind to be distinguished. The tendency in actinomycosis to chronic suppuration, especially in the pleura and appendix, should excite suspicion. The serum agglutination reaction is of some value. Cultures by special methods may be successful.

Treatment.—This is surgical if suppuration has occurred. Iodine should be applied locally whenever possible and tincture of iodine, 5 drops increased to 20 or 30 drops three times a day, given in milk. This has proved curative in a number of cases. The injection of 1 per cent copper sulphate solution in small amounts into infiltrated areas until softening occurs has been useful. The X-rays and radium have been successful. The use of an autogenous vaccine has proved helpful in chronic cases. With abscess and fistula free drainage and curetting are indicated.

SPOROTRICHOSIS

Definition.—A chronic infection with cutaneous and internal lesions due to various forms of parasitic fungi of the sporotrichosis group.

History.—In November, 1896, a patient presented himself at Finney's out-patient clinic at the Johns Hopkins Hospital with an infection of the right arm, which had lasted for several weeks. There were ulcerations on the hand and indurations on the forearm. The condition was recognized as unusual and Schenck found on culture a branched mycelium with numerous spores or conidia. Its identification was made by Erwin F. Smith, and it was named *Sporotrichum schenckii.* Since then, the disease has been widely recognized, owing chiefly to the studies of Beurmann and Gougerot; it is widely distributed and one of the most clearly defined of the mycoses.

The Parasite.—In the tissues and in the pus the parasite is a large short rod from 3 to 5 μ long and from 2 to 3 μ in breadth. In cultures it grows in filaments of about 2 μ in diameter and forms characteristic ovoid spores. The points of differentiation between the forms are due largely to variation in the modes of sporulation. The parasite is introduced chiefly by accidental inoculation, and possibly through grains and fruit. The spores have been found in the blood. Widal and Abrami determined the agglutinating and fixation properties of the serum and specific reactions occur. There are minor differences between the form described by Schenck and that by Beurmann.

Clinical Forms.—There are several forms: (1) The disseminated *gummatous* form in which in the subcutaneous tissues in various parts of the body there are small, firm, solid nodules, which break down and form small abscesses which may ulcerate. (2) In the *ulcerative* type the lesions are not unlike those of cutaneous tuberculosis, occurring commonly on the hands and arms, though they may appear on the legs or on the body. They may be single or in groups of two or three, and in several cases seen in Paris they resembled very much eroded syphilitic gummata. (3) There is a *localized* lesion, a hard chancroid body, eroded on the surface. Dissemination occurs through the lymphatics, the regional glands become involved and there may be a group of open sores along the arm or on the side of the head. (4) There are certain *extracutaneous forms*—ulcerous lesions of the mucous membranes, gummata of the muscles, glands, lungs and periostitis with osteitis. (5) The disease may generalize in the internal organs and there are acute febrile forms.

The disease is essentially chronic, lasting often for a year or two; sometimes disturbing the health very slightly, and other times leading to anemia.

Diagnosis.—This has to be made from tuberculosis, syphilis, and actinomycosis, which may be done by cultures (as the parasites grow in a very specific way) and by agglutination and the complement fixation reaction.

Treatment.—Iodide or iodine should be given freely and ulcerated lesions painted with tincture of iodine. Closed abscesses may be aspirated and injected with a weak iodide solution. Active surgical interference is not advisable.

NOCARDIOSIS

J. H. Wright of Boston separated this group from the actinomycoses and the streptothrix infections. On the one hand the parasites resemble bacteria, on the other hand the hypomycetes or moulds, in forming branching, thread-like filaments and in the production of fine conidia. They represent a transition between the bacteria and the lower fungi. The majority of reported cases have had the signs and symptoms of pulmonary tuberculosis or of multiple abscesses. In the lungs, nodules, caseous masses and lesions not unlike tubercle have been found. In some cases there was abscess of the brain. The parasite may be recognized by the typically branched filaments and by the growth in cultures.

BLASTOMYCOSIS

Definition.—Under this term various infections due to blastomycetes or yeast-like organisms are included (*Saccharomyces, Oidium, Coccidioides, Monilia* and *Cryptococcus*). The lesions may be local or general.

Pathology.—The essential lesion is a granuloma which may break down with resulting abscess or ulceration. The lungs are involved in some cases; a secondary meningitis has been described and infiltrations have been found in the liver, spleen and lymph nodes.

Forms.—In the skin and mucous membrane infections the early lesions are described as papular or papillomatous in character which gradually enlarge and soften. The skin may be greatly thickened and abscesses are common. Sometimes there are sinuses leading to the deeper structures. The lesions are very chronic and there is always danger of extension to the viscera. In the systemic invasion the special features depend on the organ involved. Fever is common. *Coccidioidal granuloma,* which occurs particularly in California, usually begins in the skin with later involvement of the viscera. In the lungs the picture is like that of tuberculosis. *Histoplasmosis* possibly belongs here. The *prognosis* is serious in all forms. The surface lesions are very chronic and death follows visceral involvement.

Diagnosis.—Syphilis and tuberculosis are suggested and have to be excluded. The finding of the causal organism gives the only certain diagnosis.

Treatment.—Excision, the cautery and the application of tincture of iodine may be tried in local lesions. The use of the X-rays or radium may be effectual, and iodide should always be given in large doses.

TORULOSIS

This is due to infection by *Torula histolytica,* a yeast which multiplies by budding, does not ferment carbohydrates and does not produce a mycelium in tissue or culture. It has the general features of a mild acute or chronic systemic infection in which the local features are usually predominantly *cerebral* or *meningeal.* The clinical features in the nervous system are those of a meningo-encephalitis. Probably a certain number of the cases are regarded as tuberculous meningitis. The torula has been found in the spinal fluid. The symptoms may vary greatly from time to time; the average duration is about four months but has been as long as two years. In the lungs the clinical picture may suggest tuberculosis or tumor. Acute miliary torulosis of the lungs may occur. The *diagnosis* has to be made from blastomycosis, especially oïdiomycosis. There is no special treatment and the prognosis is grave.

MYCETOMA

Vandyke Carter of Bombay, a pioneer in the study of tropical diseases, gave an admirable description of this affection, which prevails largely in certain districts of India, and sporadically in other parts of the world.

The disease, usually involving the foot (hence the term *Madura Foot*), is characterized by great swelling, nodular growths and the formation of multiple abscesses. There are remarkable granules 1 mm. in diameter, usually of a black color, in the discharges; in other cases the granules are yellow or brownish. In the pale variety a streptothrix has been found, which closely resembles actinomyces. It is held by most observers that this streptothrix and actinomyces are distinct species. From the black variety of granules a hypomycete has been grown, closely allied to aspergillus.

The disease begins as a granuloma, with swelling of the foot, generally on the sole. The tumors gradually soften, others form, the foot increases enormously in bulk, becomes much deformed, numerous sinuses pass between the bones, the discharges are mucopurulent and contain the characteristic granules. *Treatment* by the use of the X-rays and the intravenous injection of antimony has been helpful. Sometimes curetting or early excision is useful or, in later stages, amputation of the foot may be necessary.

ASPERGILLOSIS

Bennett in 1842 described the parasite from the lungs, the *Aspergillus fumigatus,* a fungus widely distributed as a harmless parasite, having been found in the auditory canal, nose and throat. In birds, in cattle, more rarely in dogs, the aspergillus may cause lesions of the lungs resembling tuberculosis, and there have been some cases reported in man, particularly in pigeon keepers and hair sorters. The infection is usually secondary to some long-standing affection of the lungs, but it has been met with as a primary disease with lesions resembling bronchopneumonia, which undergo necrosis and softening and the clinical picture is that of ordinary tuberculosis.

The *symptoms* are those of chronic pulmonary disease, cough, fever, and expectoration, in which the aspergillus is found. It is readily recognized by the character of its spores. In the case reported by the senior author, at intervals of two or three months for twelve years the patient coughed up, usually with a good deal of difficulty, a grayish-brown mass the size of a small bean, which was made up entirely of the mycelium and spores of the aspergillus. The interesting point was that the patient had no symptoms, other than the cough, and was in excellent health.

The *diagnosis* depends upon finding the fungus which appears as grayish, downy masses of mycelium frequently the size of a bean. An odorless sputum is always suggestive of mold infection. Tuberculosis must be excluded by the repeated absence of the tubercle bacillus. Roengenograms show an absence of calcified glands with clear apices and dense shadows radiating in coarse lines from the hilum to the periphery of one lobe.

In the majority of cases the outlook is bad, and the treatment is that of chronic tuberculosis.

PROTOZOAN INFECTIONS

PSOROSPERMIASIS

Though widely spread in invertebrates, pathogenic psorosperms are not common in mammals, and in man serious disease is very rarely caused by them. One of the commonest forms is the so-called Rainey's tube, an ovoid body found in the muscle of the pig, filled with small sickle-shaped unicellular organisms, *Sarcocystis miescheri.* In a few instances similar structures have been found in the muscles of man. The only human parasite of this group which has caused serious disease belongs to the *coccidia.* The parasite is *Coccidium oviforme,* which is common in rabbits and mice.

Coccidiosis.—In a majority of the cases of this group the psorosperms have been found in the liver, producing a disease similar to that in rabbits. In Guebler's case there were tumors which could be felt during life, and they were determined by Leuckart to be due to coccidia. A patient of W. B. Haddon's had slight fever and drowsiness, and gradually became unconscious —death occurring on the fourteenth day of observation. Whitish neoplasms were found upon the peritoneum, omentum, and on the layers of the pericardium; and a few were found in the liver, spleen, and kidneys. A case with a very acute course, is reported by Silcott. A woman, aged fifty-three, had a chill six weeks before admission. She showed intermittent fever, slight diarrhea, nausea, tenderness over the liver and spleen, and a dry tongue; death occurred from heart failure. The liver was enlarged, weighed 83 ounces, and in its substance there were caseous foci, around each of which was a ring of congestion. The spleen contained similar bodies. The masses resembled tubercles, but on examination coccidia were found.

The parasites are also found in the kidneys and ureters. In Eve's case the symptoms were hematuria and frequent micturition, and death took place on the seventeenth day. The nodules throughout the pelvis and ureters have been regarded as mucous cysts. There is no special treatment.

AMEBIASIS

(*Amebic Dysentery, Amebic Hepatitis*)

Definition.—Infection by *Endamoeba histolytica* of the intestine which may be without symptoms or cause colitis, acute or chronic, and hepatitis or abscess of the liver.

Distribution.—The disease is wide spread and while most frequent in the tropics it is common in temperate climates. It is estimated that 5 to 10 per cent of the population of the United States is infected. The cases occurring in the tropics tend to be more severe. It is uncommon in Great Britain. There are at least five species of amebae found in man, *Endamoeba histolytica* (pathogenic) and *E. coli, Endolimax nana, Iodamoeba bütschlii* and *Diendamoeba fragilis,* which are nonpathogenic.

Age.—It is not uncommon in children but the greatest number of cases occur between the ages of 20 and 35.

Sex.—Males are much more frequently affected. Of 182 cases at the Johns Hopkins Hospital 171 were males (Futcher).

Race.—The white race is more susceptible, 163 whites to 19 blacks in the Johns Hopkins Hospital series. In the Philippines the whites are more often attacked. In India the disease is common in the native races.

The Ameba.—The *Endamoeba histolytica* was first described by Lambl in 1859 and subsequently by Lösch in 1875. Kartulis in 1886 found them in the stools of the endemic dysentery in Egypt and in the liver abscesses. In 1890 the senior author found them in a case of dysentery with abscess of the liver originating in Panama. Subsequently from his wards a series of cases was described by Councilman and Lafleur. The studies of many workers have put our knowledge of the disease on a firm basis. To find the amebae the flakes of mucus or pus in the stools should be examined or the mucus obtained by passing a soft rubber tube or by the sigmoidoscope.

Endamoeba histolytica is from 15 to 20 μ in diameter, has a clear outer zone (ectosarc) and a granular inner zone (endosarc). The nucleus is seen with difficulty and contains little chromatin. The movements are similar to those of the ordinary pond ameba, consisting of slight protrusions of the protoplasm. They vary a good deal, and usually may be intensified by having the slide heated. Not infrequently the amebae contain red blood corpuscles. In the tissues they are readily recognized by suitable stains. In the pus of a liver abscess they may be very abundant, though in large, long standing abscesses they may not be found until after a few days, when the pus begins to discharge from the wall. In the sputum in the cases of pulmonohepatic abscess they are readily recognized.

The parasite occurs in three forms: (*a*) motile or vegetative (trophozoite) stage, (*b*) precystic stage and (*c*) cystic stage. The recognition of the *vegetative* organism is aided by vital staining with a 1 per cent aqueous solution of neutral red. The vegetative amebae die rapidly after a stool is passed and probably play little part in the transmission of the disease. The *cysts* may be difficult to recognize. Culture methods and sedimentation may aid. Emulsifying the feces in iodine solution or the iodine-eosin method is useful. The cysts are responsible for the spread of the disease and their occurrence in carriers is of great importance. They are rarely present in any number in the stools of patients with acute dysentery. They are resistant and may live for weeks in water or feces. Infection occurs by food or water and flies may convey the infection. Food handlers may be a source of infection. There are numerous *carriers* in temperate climates. They may have loose stools only occasionally but show a variety of symptoms, malaise, anorexia, alternating constipation and diarrhea, abdominal discomfort or pain relieved by a loose stool, abdominal distention, and mucous stools. The *diagnosis* of a carrier is made only by finding amebae or cysts in the stools.

Morbid Anatomy.—Intestines.—The lesions consist of ulceration, produced by preceding infiltration of the submucosa, due to an edematous condition and to multiplication of the fixed cells. In the earliest stage these infiltrations appear as elevations above the level of the mucosa. The mucous membrane over these becomes necrotic and is cast off, exposing the infiltrated submucous tissue as a grayish yellow gelatinous mass, which at first forms the floor of the ulcer, but is subsequently cast off as a slough. The individual ulcers are round, oval or irregular, with infiltrated, undermined edges. The visible aperture is often small compared to the loss of tissue, the ulcers undermining the mucosa, coalescing, and forming sinuous tracts bridged over by apparently normal mucous membrane. The floor of the ulcer may be formed by the submucous, muscular or serous coat of the intestine. The ulceration may affect the whole or some portion only of the large intestine, particularly the cecum, the hepatic and sigmoid flexures and the rectum. In severe cases the whole intestine is thickened and riddled with ulcers, with here and there islands of intact mucous membrane. In 100 autopsies in Manila the appendix was involved in 7; perforation of the colon took place in 19.

The disease advances by progressive infiltration of the connective tissue layers of the intestine, which produces necrosis of the overlying structures. Thus, in severe cases there may be in different parts of the bowel sloughing *en masse* of the mucosa or of the muscularis, and the same process is observed, but not so conspicuously, in the less severe forms. In some cases a secondary diphtheritic inflammation occurs. Healing takes place by the gradual formation of fibrous tissue in the floor and at the edges of the ulcers, which may result in partial and irregular strictures of the bowel.

Microscopic examination shows a notable absence of the products of purulent inflammation. In the infiltrated tissues polymorphonuclear leukocytes are seldom found and never constitute purulent collections. On the other hand, there is proliferation of the fixed connective-tissue cells. Amebae are found more or less abundantly in the tissues at the base of and around the ulcers, in the lymphatic spaces, and occasionally in the blood vessels. The portal capillaries occasionally contain them, and this seems to afford the best explanation for the mode of infection of the liver.

Liver.—The lesions are of two kinds: first, local necroses of the parenchyma, scattered throughout the organ and, secondly, abscesses. These may be single or multiple. There were 37 cases of hepatic abscess among the 182 cases of amebic dysentery in the Hopkins Hospital. Of these, 18 came to autopsy. In 10 the abscess was single and in 8 multiple. When single they are generally in the right lobe, either toward the convex surface near its diaphragmatic attachment or on the concave surface in proximity to the bowel. Multiple abscesses are small and generally superficial. There may be innumerable miliary abscesses containing amebae scattered throughout the organ. Although the hepatic abscess usually occurs within the first two months from the onset of the dysentery, in one case the latter had lasted one and in another six years. In 5 cases the intestinal symptoms had been so slight that no complaint of dysentery had been made. In an early stage the abscesses are grayish yellow, with sharply defined contours, and contain a spongy necrotic material, with more or less fluid in its interstices. The larger abscesses have ragged necrotic walls, and contain a viscid, greenish yellow or reddish yellow purulent material mixed with blood and shreds of liver tissue. The older abscesses have fibrous walls of a dense, almost cartilaginous toughness. There is the same absence of purulent inflammation as in the intestine, except when a secondary infection with pyogenic organisms has taken place.

Lesions in the lungs are seen when an abscess of the liver points toward the diaphragm and extends by continuity through it into the lower lobe of the right lung. This is the commonest situation for rupture to occur. Rupture may occur into the right pleura, causing empyema or a lung abscess may rupture into the pleura, producing a pyopneumothorax. Perforation may occur into *adjacent structures.* In 3 of our cases perforation took place into the inferior vena cava and in another the upper pole of the right kidney was invaded. The abscess may rupture into the pericardium, peritoneum, stomach, intestine, portal and hepatic veins, or externally. The lungs may be involved directly without extension from the liver.

Amebae have been reported as occurring in many parts of the body but many of these are undoubtedly incorrect. Warthin reported a case in which *End. histolytica* was found in the testis and epididymis with tissue lesions.

Symptoms.—Three groups of cases may be recognized:

Mild Form.—The incubation varies and infection may be present for two or three months before the individual is aware of it. There may be vague symptoms—headache, lassitude, weakness, slight abdominal pains and occasional diarrhea. Latency is the feature in a large number of cases. The amebae may be present without exciting symptoms, or there might be slight transient attacks of diarrhea, and yet in these cases hepatic abscess may follow. There is evidence to suggest that infection without symptoms is present in a number (some suggest 10 per cent) of the population.

Acute Amebic Dysentery.—Many cases have an acute onset. There may be general abdominal tenderness or over parts of the colon. Pain and tenesmus are common. The stools are bloody, or mucus and blood occur together. In very severe cases there may be constant tenesmus, with pain of the greatest intensity, and the passage every few minutes of a little blood and mucus. In some cases large sloughs are passed. The temperature as a rule is not high. There may be slight leukocytosis; eosinophilia is rare. The patient may become rapidly emaciated; the heart's action becomes feeble, and death may occur within a week of the onset. *Hemorrhage* from the bowels, and *perforation* of an ulcer with general peritonitis occur in some cases. A majority of the patients recover; in others the disease drags on and becomes chronic, the symptoms often showing a periodicity. In a few cases, after the separation of the sloughs, there is extensive ulceration remaining, with thickening and induration of the colon, and the patient has constant diarrhea, loses weight, and ultimately dies exhausted, usually within three months of the onset. With the exception of cancer of the esophagus and anorexia nervosa, no such extreme emaciation is seen. Extensive ulceration of the cornea may occur.

Chronic Amebic Dysentery.—The disease may be subacute from the onset, and gradually passes into a chronic stage, the special characteristic of which is alternating periods of constipation and of diarrhea. These may occur over a period of from six months to a year or more. Some of our patients were admitted to the hospital five or six times within a period of two years. During the exacerbations there are pain, frequent passages of mucus and blood, and slight fever. Many patients do not feel very ill, and retain their nutrition in a remarkable way; indeed, in the United States it is rare to see the extreme emaciation so common in the chronic cases from the tropics. Alternating periods of improvement with attacks of diarrhea are the rule. The appetite is capricious, the digestion disordered, and slight errors in diet are apt to be followed at once by an increase in the number of stools. The tongue is often red, glazed, and beefy.

Complications and Sequelae.—LIVER ABSCESS.—A presuppurative stage lasting for several weeks or months may occur, characterized by fever of an intermittent type, moderate leukocytosis, and an enlarged and tender liver. Suppuration in the liver is the most serious complication. It may occur in patients who have had no symptoms of dysentery. Abscess of the brain has occurred.

Perforation of the intestine and *peritonitis* occurred in three of our cases. *Intestinal hemorrhage* occurred three times. The infrequency of this complication is probably due to the thrombosis of the vessels about the areas of infiltration. Polypoid colitis may be a late manifestation (Hines). Occasionally an *arthritis,* probably toxic in origin, may occur. Bacillary and amebic dysentery may occur together.

Urinary Amebiasis.—This is very rare. The infection may be of the kidney, bladder, seminal vesicles or urethra. Amebae have been found in the seminal fluid. The process may be a primary infection or secondary to amebic dysentery.

Diagnosis.—The frequency of mild, latent and atypical cases should be kept in mind. From the other forms of dysentery the disease is recognized by the finding of amebae or cysts in the stools. Unless one sees undoubted ameboid movement a suspected body should not be considered an ameba. A nonmotile body containing one or more red cells is probably an ameba, but should lead to further search for motile organisms. Swollen epithelial cells are confusing, but the hyaline periphery is not ameboid. The trichomonads and cercomonads are not likely to give trouble. The *End. histolytica* is distinguished from nonpathogenic forms by its larger size, distinct refractile ectoplasm, faint or invisible nucleus, marked mobility, vacuoles, contained red blood cells, and scanty chromatin in the nucleus. The cysts are small and do not contain more than four nuclei. Various stains are an aid in differentiation. Cultures may be made. Craig devised a complement fixation test. The extent of liver dulness should be watched and any increase should lead to the suspicion of abscess. Hepatic abscess is usually accompanied by fever, sweats, or chills and local pain, but may be entirely latent. A varying leukocytosis occurs in the abscess cases. The highest count in our series was 53,000, the average being 18,350. The average leukocyte count in the uncomplicated dysentery cases was 10,600. Hepatopulmonary abscess is attended by local lung signs and the expectoration of "anchovy sauce" sputum in which amebae are almost invariably found.

Prognosis.—In many cases the disease yields to treatment, especially if begun early, but the tendency to relapse is a striking characteristic. Some patients are very resistant to treatment. Amebic abscess is always serious.

Prevention.—The prevention of contamination of food and drink is the ideal but the individual has small chance in many cases to ensure this, as seen in the Chicago epidemic of 1933. Fortunately it seems that carriers are not often responsible for direct infection.

Treatment.—Rest in bed is very important, even in mild attacks, and materially hastens recovery. The diet should be governed by the severity of the intestinal manifestations. In the very acute cases the patient should be given a liquid diet, consisting of milk, whey, and broths.

The use of emetine is particularly efficacious in the early stages when the infection is acute but it should always be followed by other remedies. Emetine hydrochloride hypodermically is given in doses of ½ grain (0.03 gm.) twice a day for six days or 1 grain (0.06 gm.) daily for twelve days. The patient should be in bed and toxic symptoms watched for. This course should be repeated if necessary. Emetine sometimes causes diarrhea which may be mistaken for the original dysentery. The same treatment should be given to prevent liver abscess when there is a suspicion of hepatitis. Another preparation is emetine bismuth iodide given in keratin capsules in doses of gr. ii-iii (0.12-0.18 gm.) each night for twelve doses. Some patients do well with ipecacuanha given at night in salol coated pills or keratin capsules; the first dose is 60 gr. (4 gm.) reduced by five grains each night until it is down to ten grains (0.6 gm.). Some advise emetine hypodermically and ipecac by mouth at the same time.

To destroy the cysts other remedies may be required, among which are: *Chinofon* (yatren or anayodin) is given orally (gr. iv, 0.25 gm. in keratin coated pills three times a day for eight to ten days) and by enema daily for ten days (200 cc. of a 2 per cent solution in warm water retained for some hours if possible). These may be repeated after an interval of ten days. *Vioform* is given in the same dosage by mouth. *Acetarsone* (stovarsol) is given in doses of gr. iv (0.25 gm.) by mouth three times a day for a week. *Carbasone* is given in doses of gr. iv (0.25 gm.) in capsules twice daily for ten days. These last two are arsenic compounds and should not be given if there is hepatic disease. Symptoms of arsenical overdosage should be watched for. If diarrhea occurs the dose should be reduced to half the amounts. These drugs are the most efficient in the treatment of carriers.

It must be remembered that a quick symptomatic cure may result but the patient may not be free of the disease. He should be followed and an examination for amebae and cysts made every three months for a year and then every six months for another year.

Bismuth probably does more harm than good, as it coats the surface of the ulcers. It is well in the chronic forms to give an occasional dose of saline or castor oil. Injections of silver nitrate solution (1 to 2,000, increased to 1 to 500) are useful in chronic cases. When there is much tenesmus a starch and laudanum enema gives great relief. Hot applications to the abdomen are grateful.

When medical treatment fails, cecostomy may be tried or irrigations given through the appendix.

Hepatic abscess may be drained and the cavity irrigated by quinine solution (1 to 1,000). Emetine should be given as advised for the dysentery. Repeated aspiration of the abscess with the use of emetine has been successful. But care should be taken not to delay operation too long.

MALARIAL FEVER

Definition.—A protozoal disease with: (*a*) paroxysms of intermittent fever of quotidian, tertian, or quartan type; (*b*) a continued fever with marked remissions; (*c*) certain pernicious, rapidly fatal forms; (*d*) a chronic cachexia, with anemia and enlarged spleen.

Sporozoa, genus *Plasmodium*, transmitted to man by the bite of anopheline mosquitoes, are invariably associated with the disease. Malaria occurs as an endemic and epidemic disease, the latter prevailing in the tropics under favoring conditions. No infection except, perhaps, tuberculosis compares with it in the extent of its distribution or its importance as a killing and disabling disease. It has had an important influence on the history of the human race, probably greater than that of any other disease.

Geographical Distribution.—In Europe, southern Russia and parts of Italy and Greece are the chief seats of the disease. It is rare in Germany, France, and England, and is becoming less frequent. In the United States malaria has progressively diminished in extent and severity during the past fifty years. From New England, where it once prevailed extensively, it has disappeared and in New York even the milder forms of the disease are rare. In Philadelphia and along the valleys of the Delaware and Schuylkill Rivers, formerly hot-beds of malaria, the disease has become much restricted. In Baltimore a few cases occur in the autumn, but a majority of the patients are from the outlying districts. Throughout the Southern States there are many regions in which malaria prevails; but here, too, the disease has diminished in prevalence and intensity. In the northwestern states malaria is almost unknown. The St. Lawrence basin remains free from the disease.

In India the disease is very prevalent, particularly in the great river basins. Terrible epidemics occur. In Burma and Assam severe types are met with. In Africa the malarial fevers form the great obstacle to European settlements on the coast and along the river basins. The *black-water* fever is a serious form of malarial hemoglobinuria. The Atlantic coast of Central America is severely infected, and the Isthmus of Panama for centuries was known as the "white man's grave." In the tropics there are minimal and maximal periods, the former corresponding to the summer and winter, the latter to the spring and autumn months.

Etiology: The Parasite.—History.—Parasites of the red blood corpuscles are widespread throughout the animal series. They are met with in the blood of frogs, fish, birds, and among mammals in monkeys, bats, cattle, and man. In birds and in frogs the parasites appear to do no harm except when present in very large numbers.

In 1880 Laveran, a French army surgeon stationed at Algiers, noted in the blood of patients with malarial fever pigmented bodies, which he regarded as parasites, and as the cause of the disease. Richard, another French army surgeon, confirmed these observations. In 1885 Marchiafava and Celli described the parasites with great accuracy, and Golgi made the all-important observation that the paroxysm of fever invariably coincided with the sporulation or segmentation of a group of the parasites. In the following year (1886) Laveran's observations were brought before the profession of the United States by Sternberg. Councilman and Abbott in 1885 described the pigmented bodies in the red blood corpuscles in the blood vessels of the brain in a fatal case, and in 1886 Councilman confirmed the observations of Laveran in clinical cases. Stimulated by his work, the senior author began studying the malarial cases in the Philadelphia Hospital, and soon became convinced of the truth of Laveran's discovery, and confirmed Golgi's statement as to the coincidence of the sporulation with the paroxysm. Among British observers, Vandyke

Carter alone, in India, seems to have appreciated at an early date the profound significance of Laveran's work.

The next important observation was the discovery by Golgi that the parasite of quartan malarial fever differed from the tertian. From this time on the Italian observers took up the work with great energy, and in 1889 Marchiafava and Celli determined that the organism of the severer forms of malarial fever differed from the parasite of the tertian and quartan varieties.

The connection of insects with the disease is an old story suggested in Roman times and revived by John Crawford, of Baltimore (1807), King, of Washington, and settled finally by Ross. The idea that fever was transmitted by the bite of the mosquito prevailed widely in the West Indies and in the Southern States. The important rôle played by insects as an intermediate host had been shown in Texas cattle fever, in which Theobald Smith demonstrated that the hæmatozoa developed in, and the disease was transmitted by, ticks; but it remained for Manson to formulate in a clear and scientific way the theory of infection in malaria by the mosquito. Impressed by this, Ross studied the problem in India, and showed that the parasites developed in the bodies of the mosquitoes, demonstrating conclusively that the infection in birds was transmitted by the mosquito. W. G. MacCallum suggested that the flagella were sexual elements and observed the process of fertilization by them. Studies by Grassi, Bastianelli and Bignami, and many others, confirmed the observations of Ross and demonstrated that the malarial parasites of human beings develop only in mosquitoes of the genus anopheles.

Then came the demonstration by Italian observers, and the interesting experiments on Manson, Jr., of the direct transmission of the disease to man by the bite of infected mosquitoes. And lastly, the antimalarial campaigns so energetically advocated and carried out by Ross showed that by protecting the individual from mosquitoes, by exterminating the insects, or by carefully treating all patients so that no opportunity is offered for the parasite to enter the mosquito, malaria may be eradicated from any locality.

THE PARASITE.—Belonging to the sporozoa, it has received a large number of names. The term *Plasmodium,* inapt though it may be, must, according to the rules of zoological nomenclature, be applied to the human parasite. There are three well-marked varieties which exist in two separate phases or stages: (*a*) The parasite in man, who acts as the intermediate host, and in whom, in the cycle (asexual) of its development, it causes symptoms of malaria; and (*b*) an extracorporeal cycle (sexual), in which it lives and develops in the body of the mosquito, which is its definitive host. The parasites have been grown in artificial media (Bass).

The Parasite in Man.—Tertian Fever (*Plasmodium vivax*).—The earliest form seen in the red blood corpuscles is round or irregular in shape, about 2 μ in diameter and unpigmented. It corresponds very much in appearance with the segments of the rosettes formed during the chill. A few hours later the body has increased in size, is still ring-shaped, and there is pigment in the form of fine grains. It has a relatively large nuclear body, consisting of a well-defined, clear area, in part almost transparent, in part consisting of a milk-white substance, in which there lies a small, deeply-staining chromatin mass. At this period it usually shows active ameboid movements, with tongue-like protrusions. The pigment increases in amount and the corpuscle becomes larger and paler, owing to a progressive diminution of its hemoglobin. There is a gradual growth of the parasite, which, toward the end of forty-eight hours, occupies almost all of the swollen red corpuscle. It is now much pigmented, and is in the stage called the full-grown parasite. Between the fortieth and forty-eighth hours many of the parasites undergo segmentation, in which the pigment becomes collected into a single mass, and the protoplasm divides into fifteen to twenty spores, often showing a radial arrangement. Certain full-grown tertian parasites, however, do not undergo segmentation. These forms, which are larger than the sporulating bodies, and contain very actively dancing pigment granules, represent sexually differentiated forms of the parasite—gametocytes.

Quartan fever (*Plasmodium malariae*).—The earliest form is very like the tertian but as it increases in size the granules are coarser and darker and the movement is not nearly so marked. By the second day the parasite is still larger, rounded in shape, scarcely at all ameboid, and the pigment is more often arranged at the periphery of the parasite. The rim of protoplasm about it is often of a deep yellowish-green color or of a dark brassy tint. On the third day the segmenting bodies become abundant, the pigment flowing in toward the centre of the parasite in radial lines so as to give a star-shaped appearance. The parasites finally break up into from six to twelve segments. Here also, as in the case of the tertian parasite, some full-grown bodies persist without sporulating, representing the gametocytes.

Estivo-Autumnal Fever (*Plasmodium falciparum*).—This parasite is considerably smaller than the other varieties; at full development it is often less than one-half the size of a red blood corpuscle. The pigment is much scantier, often consisting of a few minute granules. At first only the earlier stages of development, small, hyaline bodies, sometimes with one or two pigment granules, are to be found in the peripheral blood; the later stages are ordinarily seen only in the blood of certain internal organs, the spleen and bone marrow particularly. Some workers believe that there are two varieties of this form, tertian and quotidian (*P. falciparum quotidianum*). The corpuscles containing the parasites frequently become shrunken, crenated and brassy-colored. After the infection has existed for about a week, larger, refractive, crescentic, ovoid, and round bodies, with central clumps of coarse pigment granules, begin to appear. These bodies are characteristic of estivo-autumnal fever. The crescentic and ovoid forms are incapable of sporulation; they are analogous to the large, full-grown, nonsporulating bodies of the tertian and quartan parasites and represent sexually differentiated forms—gametocytes. Within the human host they are incapable of further development, but upon the slide, or within the stomach of the mosquito, the male elements (microgametocytes) give rise to a number of long, actively motile flagella (microgametes) which break loose, penetrating and fecundating the female forms—macrogametes (W. G. MacCallum). The fecundated female form enters into the stomach wall of the mosquito, where it undergoes a definite cycle of existence.

A subspecies of *P. vivax* has been described, termed *P. vivax minutum*, and rare forms, *P. tenue*, *P. caucasicum*, and *P. ovale* have been observed.

The Parasite in the Mosquito.—The brilliant researches of Ross, followed by the work of Grassi, Bastianelli, Bignami, Stephens, Christophers, and Daniels, proved that a certain genus of mosquito—anopheles—is the definitive host of the malarial parasite and the usual source of infection. An exception is by *direct inoculation* which may occur in drug addicts by the careless use of needles used for intravenous injections. The more common genera of mosquito in temperate climates are culex and anopheles. The different species of culex form the majority of our ordinary house mosquitoes, and are incapable of acting as hosts of the malarial parasite. All malarial regions which have been investigated contain anopheles but they may be present without the existence of malaria under two circumstances: first, when the climate is too cold for the development of the malarial parasite; and secondly, in a region which has not yet been infected. So far as is known, the parasite exists only in the mosquito and in man.

A large number of species of anopheles have been described in different parts of the world. In North America the varieties most concerned in the spread of the disease are *A. maculipennis* and *quadrimaculatus;* the former is the most important agent in the spread of the disease in Europe. The culex lays its eggs in sinks, tanks, cisterns, and any collection of water about or in houses, while the anopheles lays its eggs in small, shallow puddles or slowly running streams, especially those in which certain forms of algae exist. The culex is essentially a city mosquito, the anopheles a country insect.

Evolution in the Mosquito.—When a mosquito of the genus anopheles bites an individual whose blood contains sex-ripe forms (gametocytes) of the malarial parasite, flagellation and fecundation of the female element occur within the stomach of the insect. The fecundated element (zygote) penetrates the wall of the mosquito's stomach and begins a definite cycle of development in the muscular coat. The zygote becomes motile (oökinete) and penetrates the wall of the stomach forming the oöcyst. The mother oöcyst then bursts, setting free into the body cavity of the mosquito an enormous number of delicate spindle-shaped sporozoites. These make their way to the veneno-salivary glands of the mosquito, and, escaping into the ducts, are inoculated with subsequent bites of the insect. These little spindle-shaped sporozoites develop, after inoculation into the warm-blooded host, into young parasites. The sporozoite which has developed in the oöcyst in the stomach wall of the mosquito is the equivalent of the spore resulting from the asexual segmentation of the full-grown parasite in the circulation. Either one, on entering a red blood corpuscle, may give rise to the asexual or sexual cycle. As a rule the first several generations of parasites in the human body pursue the asexual cycle, the sexual forms developing later. These sexual forms, sterile in the human host, serve as the means of preserving the life of the parasite and spreading infection by the mosquito.

Morbid Anatomy.—The changes result from the disintegration of the red blood corpuscles, accumulation of the pigment set free, and possibly the influence of toxic materials produced by the parasite. Cases of simple malarial infection are rarely fatal, and the morbid antatomy has been studied from pernicious malaria or chronic cachexia. Rupture of the enlarged spleen may occur spontaneously, but more often from trauma. Fatal hemorrhage has followed exploratory puncture of a malarial spleen.

Pernicious Malaria.—The blood is hydremic and the serum may even be tinged with hemoglobin. The red blood corpuscles present the endoglobular forms of the parasite and are in all stages of destruction. The capillaries of the brain may be filled by masses of red cells and parasites, often forming thrombi. The *spleen* is enlarged, often only moderately. In a fresh infection the spleen is usually soft. The *liver* is swollen and turbid. In some acute pernicious cases the capillaries of the gastro-intestinal mucosa may be packed with parasites.

MALARIAL CACHEXIA.—In fatal cases of chronic paludism death occurs usually from anemia or hemorrhage associated with it. The spleen may weigh from five to ten pounds. The liver may be greatly enlarged and of a grayish-brown or slate color, due to the large amount of pigment. In the portal canals and beneath the capsule the connective tissue is impregnated with melanin. The pigment is seen in the Kupffer's cells and the perivascular tissue. The kidneys may be enlarged and present a grayish-red color, or areas of pigmentation may be seen. The peritoneum is usually of a deep slate color. The mucous membrane of the stomach and intestines may have the same hue, due to the pigment in and about the blood-vessels.

ACCIDENTAL AND LATE LESIONS.—*The Liver.*—Malarial hepatitis plays a very important rôle in malaria as described by French writers. Only those cases in which the history is definite, and in which the melanosis of both liver and spleen coexist, should be regarded as of malarial origin.

Pneumonia is believed by some to be common in malaria, and even to depend directly upon the malarial parasite, occurring either in the acute or in the chronic forms of the disease.

Nephritis.—Moderate albuminuria is a frequent occurrence, having occurred in 46.4 per cent of the cases in the Johns Hopkins Hospital. Acute nephritis is relatively frequent in estivo-autumnal infections, having occurred in over 4.5 per cent of our cases. Chronic nephritis occasionally follows long-continued or frequently repeated infections.

Clinical Forms of Malarial Fever.—The relative frequency of the different forms varies in different regions. The tertian is the most common in temperate regions, the estivo-autumnal in the tropics, the quartan generally rare except in certain parts of India.

THE REGULARLY INTERMITTENT FEVERS.—Tertian fever; quartan fever. These forms are characterized by recurring paroxysms, in which, as a rule, chill, fever, and sweat follow in orderly sequence. The *incubation* period in the tertian form is about two weeks and in the quartan form about three weeks. In patients with paresis, inoculated with *P. vivax,* the incubation period varies from 5 to 30 days. The amount of infectious material introduced influences the incubation period. On the other hand, the patient may have a paroxysm months after he has removed from a malarial region but only if he had the disease when living there. The period of latency may be prolonged.

Description of the Paroxysm.—The patient generally knows he is going to have a chill a few hours before its advent by unpleasant feelings and uneasy sensations, sometimes by headache. The paroxysm is divided into three stages —cold, hot, and sweating.

Cold Stage.—The onset is indicated by lassitude and a desire to yawn and stretch, by headache, uneasy sensations in the epigastrium, sometimes by nausea and vomiting. Even before the chill there is a rise in temperature. Gradually the patient begins to shiver, the face looks cold, and in the fully developed rigor the whole body shakes, the teeth chatter, and the movements may be violent enough to shake the bed. Not only does the patient look cold and blue, but a surface thermometer shows a reduction of the skin temperature. The mouth or rectal temperature may, during the chill, be greatly increased, and the fever may rise to 105° or 106°. Of associated symptoms, nausea and vomiting are common. There may be intense headache. The pulse is quick, small, and hard. The urine is increased in quantity. The chill lasts a variable time, ten minutes to an hour, or even longer.

Hot Stage.—The *hot stage* is ushered in by transient flushes of heat; gradually the coldness of the surface disappears and the skin becomes intensely hot. The contrast in the appearance is striking: the face is flushed, the hands congested, the skin reddened, the pulse full and bounding, the heart's action forcible, and the patient may complain of a throbbing headache. There may be active delirium. One patient in this stage jumped through a window and sustained fatal injuries. The rectal temperature may not increase much during this stage; in fact, by the termination of the chill the fever may have reached its maximum. The duration of the hot stage varies from half an hour to three or four hours.

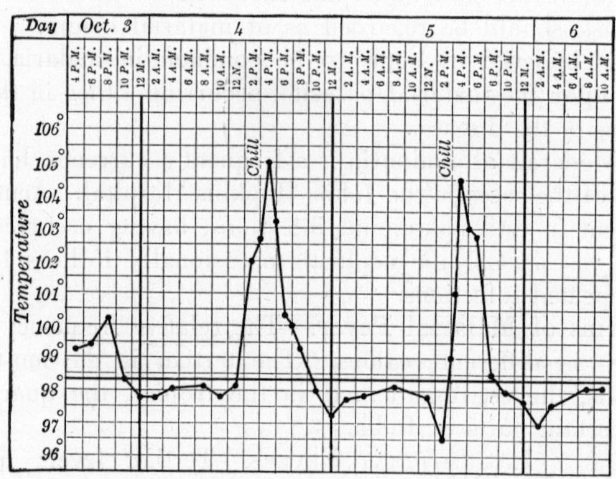

CHART VI.—DOUBLE TERTIAN INFECTION. QUOTIDIAN FEVER.

Sweating Stage.—Beads of perspiration appear upon the face and gradually the entire body is bathed in a copious sweat. The discomfort disappears, the headache is relieved, and within an hour or two the paroxysm is over and the patient usually sinks into a refreshing sleep. The sweating varies much. It may be drenching in character or it may be slight.

The total duration of the paroxysm averages from ten to twelve hours, but may be shorter. Variations are common; the patient may, instead of a chill, experience only a chilly sensation. The most common variation is the occurrence of a hot stage alone or with slight sweating. In the interval or intermission of the paroxysm the patient feels well, and, unless the disease is unusually severe, he is able to be up. Bronchitis is common and herpes, usually labial, is almost as frequent in malaria as in pneumonia.

Tertian Fever.—This type depends upon the presence in the blood of the tertian parasite, an organism usually present in sharply defined groups, whose cycle of development lasts approximately forty-eight hours, segmentation occurring every third day. In infections with one group of tertian parasites the paroxysms occur at remarkably regular intervals of about forty-eight hours, every third day—hence the name *tertian*. Very commonly there are two groups

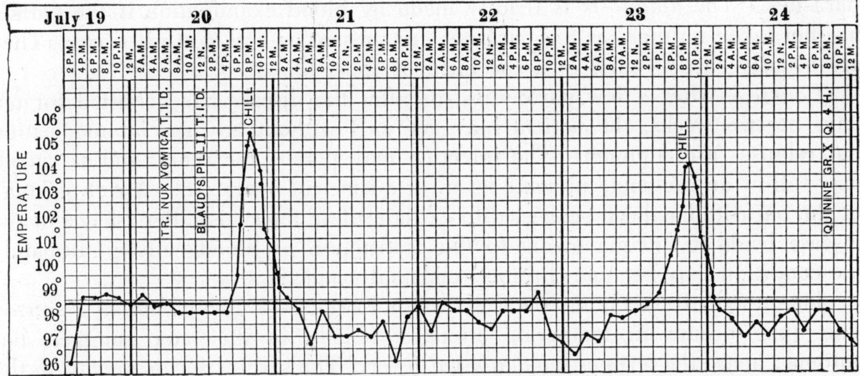

CHART VII.—QUARTAN FEVER.

of parasites which reach maturity on alternate days, resulting in daily (*quotidian*) paroxysms—*double tertian infection.* In young children the fever may be irregular.

Quartan Fever.—The symptoms resemble those of the tertian infection but as a rule are milder. Paroxysms appear on the fourth day and correspond with

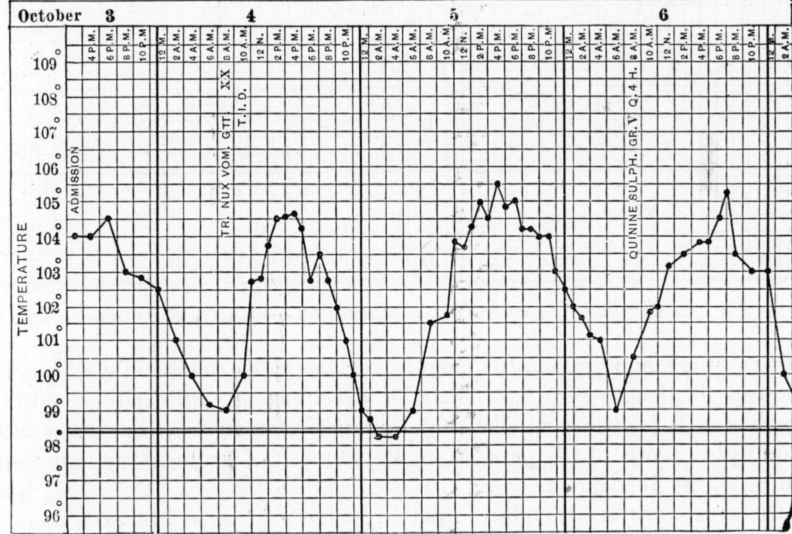

CHART VIII.—ESTIVO-AUTUMNAL FEVER.—QUOTIDIAN PAROXYSMS.

the evolution of a parasitic cycle of seventy-two hours. In recent infections the recurrence of the paroxysm may be almost precisely the same hour every day. The infection may be *double*, in which case there are two paroxysms followed by a day of intermission, or *triple*, in which there is a daily paroxysm. As pointed out by the old Greek physicians, the quartan infection is difficult to cure. Disappearing for a time spontaneously, or yielding to quinine, it has a proneness to relapse, even after energetic treatment.

A daily intermittent fever may be due to infection with tertian or quartan parasites. The *diagnosis* is readily made by blood examination if the patient has not taken quinine, as the parasites are present as a rule at all times. They are usually easily found in a specimen of fresh blood.

Course.—After a few paroxysms, or after the disease has persisted for ten days or two weeks, the patient may get well without any special medication but relapses are common. The infection may persist for years, and an attack may follow an accident, an acute fever, or a surgical operation. A resting stage of the parasite has been suggested to explain these intervals. Persistence of the disease leads to anemia owing to the destruction of blood cells. Ultimately the condition may become chronic—malarial cachexia.

Irregular, Remittent, or Continued Fevers.—*Estivo-autumnal Fever.*—This type occurs in temperate climates, chiefly in the later summer and autumn; hence the term *estivo-autumnal* fever. The severer forms prevail in the

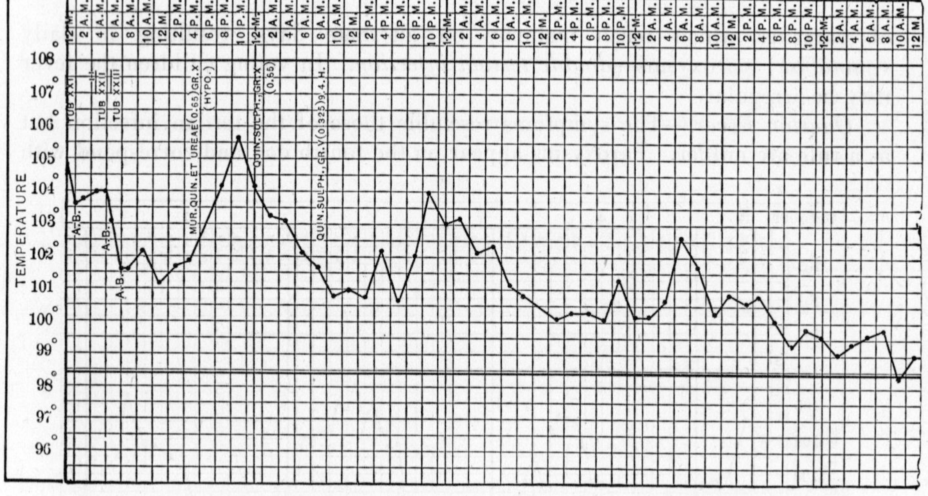

Chart IX.—Estivo-Autumnal Infection.—Remittent Fever.

southern states and in tropical countries. The estivo-autumnal parasite is an organism the length of whose cycle of development, ordinarily about forty-eight hours, is probably subject to considerable variations, while the existence of multiple groups of the parasite, or the absence of arrangement into definite groups, is not infrequent.

The *symptoms* are therefore often irregular. In some instances there may be regular intermittent fever occurring at uncertain intervals of from twenty-four to forty-eight hours, or even more. In the cases with longer remissions the paroxysms are longer. Some of the daily intermittent cases may closely resemble the fever depending upon double tertian or triple quartan infection. Commonly, however, the paroxysms show material differences; their length averages over twenty hours, instead of from ten to twelve; the onset occurs often without chills and even without chilly sensations. The rise in temperature is frequently gradual and slow, instead of sudden, while the fall may occur by lysis instead of by crisis. There may be a marked tendency toward anticipation in the paroxysms, while frequently, from the anticipation of one paroxysm or the retardation of another, more or less continuous fever may result, sometimes without sharp paroxysms. In these cases of continuous and remittent fever the patient has a flushed face and looks ill. The tongue is furred, the pulse is full and bounding but rarely dicrotic. The temperature may range from 102° to 103°, or is in some instances higher. The general appearance is strongly suggestive of typhoid fever—further supported by the splenic enlargement; an initial bronchitis may be present. The course of these cases is variable. The fever may be continuous, with remissions more or less marked; definite paroxysms with or without chills may occur, in which the temperature rises to 105° or 106° F. Intestinal symptoms are usually absent, but a slight jaundice may arise early. Delirium of a mild type may occur. The cases vary greatly in severity; in some instances the condition becomes grave and assumes the pernicious type. It is in this form of malarial fever that so much confusion exists. The similarity to typhoid fever is striking, more particularly the appearance of the facies; the patient *looks* very ill. The cases occur in the autumn when typhoid fever is prevalent. The fever yields, as a rule, to quinine, though cases are met with—rarely indeed in our experience—which are refractory.

The *diagnosis* is definitely made by the examination of the blood. Repeated examinations at short intervals may be required before the parasites are found. The small hyaline forms of the estivo-autumnal parasite are to be found, while, if the course has been over a week, the larger crescentic and ovoid bodies are often seen. The presence of pigmented leukocytes is about as significant as the parasites.

Pernicious Malarial Fever.—This is fortunately rare in temperate climates. Pernicious fever is always associated with the estivo-autumnal parasite. The following are the most important types:

Comatose Form.—In this the patient is struck down with symptoms of intense cerebral disturbance, either acute delirium or, more frequently, a rapidly developing coma. A chill may or may not precede the attack. The fever is usually high, and the skin hot and dry. The unconsciousness may persist for from twelve to twenty-four hours, or the patient may sink and die. After regaining consciousness a second attack may prove fatal. In these instances the special localization of the infection is in the brain, where actual thrombi of parasites with marked secondary changes in the surrounding tissues have been found.

Algid Form.—In this the attack sets in usually with gastric symptoms; there are vomiting, intense prostration, and weakness, out of proportion to the local disturbance. The patient complains of feeling cold, although there may be no actual chill. The temperature may be normal or subnormal; consciousness may be retained. The pulse is feeble and the respirations are increased. There may be severe diarrhea and the urine is often diminished or suppressed. This condition may persist with slight exacerbations of fever for several days and the patient die in profound asthenia. In cases with vomiting and diarrhea the gastro-intestinal mucosa is often the seat of a special invasion by the parasites, thrombosis of the small vessels with superficial ulceration and necrosis occurring.

Hemorrhagic Forms.—Black-water Fever—Hemoglobinuric Fever—Malarial Hemoglobinuria.—There are two types of hemoglobinuria in malaria, the one associated with any severe pernicious attack in which an enormous number of red blood corpuscles are destroyed by parasites, but in the true *black-water fever* there is a solution of red blood corpuscles by an unknown hemolysin, not directly by the malarial parasites themselves. There are many obscure features connected with black-water fever, especially concerning its etiology. Most authorities consider that malaria is concerned, as the majority of patients have had repeated attacks. Various occurrences may precipitate an attack in a predisposed individual. The taking of quinine is apparently one of these, but quinine is not the cause; it may be a *tertium quid* necessary to produce the hemolysin. The *symptoms* may come on rapidly with rigors, restlessness, fever, vomiting and marked prostration. There is the passage of dark urine, often scanty, the fever continues and yellow pigmentation appears. In favorable cases after a few days recovery follows. Ominous features are: severe asthenia with syncope, anuria with uremic manifestations and hyperpyrexia. A rapidly developing severe anemia may occur. If malarial parasites are present in the blood before the attack they usually disappear during it but return later. The prognosis is always serious.

The figures at Panama, based on five years' work at the Ancon Hospital (Deeks and James), show 230 cases in more than 40,000 cases of malaria. Their studies favor the association of black-water fever with malaria, holding that there are three causes superadded to the malarial infection: (i) A renewed malarial attack with production of toxins sufficient to destroy many red blood cells; (ii) a lowering of the bodily resistance; (iii) quinine.

Malarial Cachexia.—The general symptoms are those of secondary anemia —dyspnea on exertion, edema of the ankles, and hemorrhages, particularly into the retina. Occasionally the bleeding is severe, and fatal hematemesis may occur in association with the enlarged spleen. The fever is variable. The temperature may be low for days. In other instances there may be irregular fever, and the temperature rises to 102.5° or 103° F. With careful treatment the outlook is good, and a majority of cases recover. The spleen may reduce in size but may always remain somewhat enlarged.

Latent Malarial Infection.—There may be parasites in the body without any clinical manifestations of the disease. The parasites are present in the spleen in all the stages of the human cycle.

Rarer Complications.—Paraplegia may be due to a peripheral neuritis or to changes in the cord, and hemiplegia may occur in the pernicious comatose form, or occasionally at the very height of a paroxysm. Acute ataxia has been described, and there are remarkable cases with the symptoms of disseminated sclerosis (Spiller). Multiple gangrene may occur. *Orchitis* has been described. Acute pancreatitis has been reported.

Relapse.—It is not easy to explain the relapse. Some think there is a resting stage of the parasite which remains in the spleen or the bone marrow. Schaudinn believed that there is a special parthenogenetic form which may remain latent for an indefinite period. It may be that parasites are present but not in sufficient numbers to cause symptoms. Years may elapse between the primary infection and a relapse occurring under conditions that preclude the possibility of reinfection.

Prognosis.—This is good as regards life except in the cases of pernicious malaria in which much depends on prompt recognition and treatment. As to complete killing of all parasites much depends on perseverance in treatment. Complete cure of the estivo-autumnal forms is often difficult.

Diagnosis.—The endemic index of a country may be determined by the "parasite rate" or by the "spleen rate." It is best sought for in children, in whom the infection may occur without much disturbance of the health. To determine the index by examining the blood for the parasites is a laborious task; the index may be readily gauged by an examination of the spleen. Thus, in Mauritius, of 31,022 children, 34.1 per cent had enlarged spleen. In Bombay, among 50,000 children, the spleen index varied from 5.3 per cent in the Hindoos to 23.2 per cent in the Parsees (Bentley).

The individual forms of malarial infection are readily recognized by examination of the fresh or stained film, but it requires a long and careful training to become an expert in blood examination. Great progress has been made and a diagnosis of malaria is no longer a refuge for our ignorance. One lesson it is hard for the practitioner to learn—namely, that an intermittent fever which resists quinine is not malarial.

The malarial poison is supposed to influence many affections in a remarkable way, giving to them a paroxysmal character. A whole series of minor ailments and some more severe ones, such as neuralgia, are attributed to certain occult effects of malaria. The more closely such cases are investigated the less definite appears the connection with malaria.

Prophylaxis.—In the discovery of Laveran there lay the promise of benefits more potent than any gift science had ever offered to mankind—viz., the possibility of the extermination of malaria. By the persistent efforts of Ross this promise reached the stage of practical fulfilment, and one of the greatest scourges of the race is now under our command. The story of the Canal Zone, Panama, under Gorgas is a triumph of the application of scientific methods. Between 1881 and 1904 among the employees of the French Canal Company, the monthly mortality ranged from 60 to 70, and on seven occasions was above 100, once reaching the enormous figure of 176.97 per 1,000. With the measures given below, the mortality fell below that of temperate regions.

This most successful campaign was carred out on the following lines: (1) The eradication of mosquito progagation areas by drainage, and the filling of places where the larvae exist. This has been done in large districts.

(2) The control of propagation areas that are allowed to exist or that cannot be economically and permanently treated. On small areas the larvae are prevented from arriving at the adult stage by the use of crude oil or kerosene, and in large bodies of water by treating the edges where alone the mosquito larvae exist. A concentrated larvacide is applied to the edges of large pools, ditches, wet areas and streams. A barrel of oil with an automatic drip at the head of a stream has been found to work satisfactorily.

(3) Protection by *screening* of houses. Copper-bronze screens of 18 mesh to the inch are effective. Cotton bar treated with wax is recommended as inexpensive. Screened vestibules decrease the chance of access of mosquitoes. Mosquito nets over the beds are found, as a rule, to be a failure, chiefly because

few persons sleep through a night without an arm or leg coming in contact with the netting on which the anopheles settle.

(4) The *destruction* of adult anopheles. In rooms the mosquitoes are usually in the corners, and very often within a foot of the floor.

Individual.—Every patient with malaria should be regarded as a source of infection (a *carrier*). In the tropics segregation of Europeans may do much to lessen the chances of infection. Every patient should receive thorough and prolonged treatment. There is far too much carelessness on this point in the profession. Malarial infection is difficult to eradicate. Patients should resume treatment in the spring and autumn for several years after the primary infection. In very malarial districts, as many persons harbor the parasites who

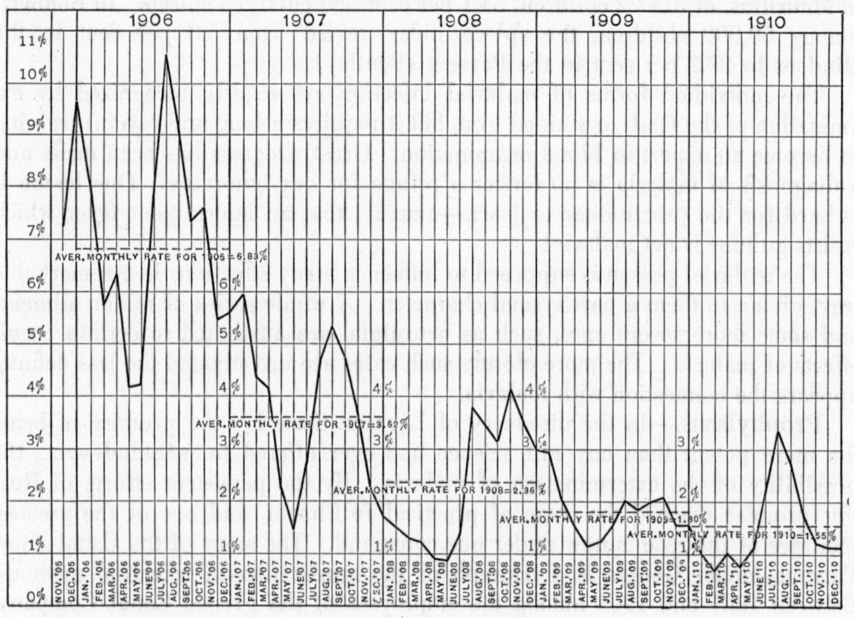

CHART X.—MALARIA CASES AMONG THE EMPLOYEES OF THE ISTHMIAN CANAL COMMISSION, 1906-1910.

do not show any (or at the most very few) signs, a systematic treatment is important, particularly in young children.

Patients with the disease should be protected from mosquitoes as far as possible. As a rule, anopheles are more likely to bite after sundown, so that in regions in which the disease prevails extensively screening should be used. Persons in a malarial region should take 10 to 15 grains (0.6 to 1 gm.) of quinine daily.

Treatment.—The patient should be in bed and given liquid or soft diet. The bowels should be moved freely, for which a calomel and saline purge is best. During the paroxysm the patient should, in the cold stage, be wrapped in blankets and given hot drinks. The reactionary fever is rarely dangerous and sponging gives comfort. In *quinine* we possess a specific remedy and the parasites are most easily destroyed at the stage when they are free in the circulation—that is, during and just after segmentation. While in most instances the parasites of the tertian and quartan forms may be destroyed fairly rapidly, in estivo-autumnal fever this is much more difficult. If the patient comes under observation shortly before an expected paroxysm, the immediate administration of quinine gives a maximum effect upon the group of parasites. The quinine will not prevent the paroxysm, but will destroy the greater part of the group of organisms and prevent its recurrence. In general the best method is to give quinine regularly without special reference to the paroxysms. Small doses may be sufficient to stop the paroxysms but the object is to kill all the parasites. A safe dosage is 30 grains (2 gm.) a day for one to two weeks, 10 grains (0.6 gm.) daily for a month and 5 grains (0.3 gm.) daily for two months. The taking of quinine *every day* is important. In estivo-autumnal fever larger doses may be necessary, though in relatively few instances is it necessary to give more than 30 grains (2 gm.) in the twenty-four hours. It is wise to take a course of quinine (10 grains—0.6 gm.—daily for three weeks) twice a year for three years after an attack.

The quinine should be given in solution or capsules. Pills and compressed tablets may not be dissolved. The use of dilute hydrobromic acid to dissolve the quinine often prevents ringing in the ears. Euquinine or quinidine, in the same dosage, or quinine tannate, double the amount, may be given to patients with whom quinine disagrees. *Plasmochin* (a quinoline derivative) is used, especially to kill the sexual forms, in a daily dosage of gr. 1 (0.06 gm.) for periods of 5 to 7 days. It may be given with quinine. Plasmochin may give toxic symptoms. *Atebrin* (an alkylamino-acridin derivative) is given in doses of gr. 1-1½ (0.06 to 0.1 gm.) three times a day for four or five days. It acts on the sexual forms and may be given with plasmochin. Both have been used for prophylaxis.

In cases of estivo-autumnal fever with *pernicious* symptoms it is necessary to introduce the quinine as rapidly as possible. In these instances the drug should be administered intravenously as the dihydrochloride in 10 grain (0.6 gm.) doses, in a freshly prepared normal saline solution (100 to 150 cc.). Further administration must be decided by the condition. Fifteen grains (1 gm.) of the bimuriate may be given intravenously in 150 cc. of normal saline solution. For extreme restlessness in these cases opium or morphine is indicated, and cardiac stimulants may be necessary. If in the comatose form the temperature is raised, the patient should be sponged or given a tub bath. For malarial anemia iron and arsenic are indicated.

In *hemoglobinuria* if the blood shows parasites quinine may be administered cautiously in small doses. The use of plasmochin has been advised. In the postmalarial forms quinine aggravates the attack. Absolute rest is essential; fluid should be given freely, by bowel or intravenously if necessary. Stimulation may be necessary. In malarial *cachexia* the patient should have a change of climate, be given a liberal diet, and take quinine in small doses with iron and arsenic for some time.

TRYPANOSOMIASIS

Definition.—A chronic disorder characterized by fever, lassitude, weakness, wasting, and often a protracted lethargy—*sleeping sickness. Trypano-*

soma gambiense and *T. rhodesiense* are the active agents in the disease in Africa and *T. cruzi* (*Schizotrypanum cruzi*) in South America. Trypanosomes are flagellate infusoria, parasitic in a great many invertebrates and vertebrates.

History.—In 1843 Gruby found a blood parasite in the frog which he called *Trypanosoma sanguinis.* Subsequently it was found to be a common blood parasite in fishes and birds. In 1878 Lewis found it in the rat—*T. lewisi* —in which it apparently does no harm. The pathological significance was first suggested in 1880 by Griffith Evans, who discovered *trypanosomes—T. evansi—* in the disease of horses and cattle in India known as *surra.* In 1895 Bruce announced that the tsetse fly disease or *nagana* of South Africa, which made whole districts impassable for cattle and horses, was due to a trypanosome—*T. brucei.* Normally present in the blood of the big game animals of the districts, it was conveyed by the tsetze fly to the nonimmune horses and cattle imported into what were called the fly belts. Other trypanosomes are *T. cruzi* (Brazil), the Philippine surra, studied by Musgrave, the *mal de caderas.—T. equinum*—of South America and a harmless infection in cattle in the Transvaal caused by *T. theileri.*

Human Trypanosomiasis.—In 1901 Dutton found a trypanosome in the blood of a West Indian. In 1903 Castellani found trypanosomes in the cerebrospinal fluid and blood of five cases of African sleeping sickness. The Royal Society Commission (Bruce and Nabarro) demonstrated the frequency of the parasites in the cerebrospinal fluid and blood in sleeping sickness, and suggested that it was a human tsetse fly infection.

Distribution.—For many years it had been known that the West African natives were subject to a remarkable malady known as the lethargy or sleeping sickness. The disease prevails in many parts of Africa. The opening up of equatorial Africa has led to intercommunication between districts which were formerly isolated, and the seriousness of the disease may be appreciated from the fact that within three years after its introduction 100,000 negroes died of it in Uganda. In the infected regions a large number of natives, not apparently suffering from the disease, harbor the parasites in the blood and suffer only with occasional attacks of fever, during which the trypanosomes are also found in the cerebrospinal fluid. Persons particularly prone are those who live on the wooded shores of the lakes and rivers, such as fishermen and canoe men.

The *T. gambiense* is introduced by the bite of a fly, the *Glossina palpalis,* and *T. rhodesiense* and *T. brucei* by *Glossina morsitans.* The fly lives on the bushes on the lake shores or river banks, and feeds on the blood of crocodiles, antelopes, etc. The trypanosomes undergo changes in the body of the fly and the infectivity appears in from three to six weeks.

Symptoms.—The *incubation* period is regarded as usually from ten to twenty days. The *acute* stage shows fever which is often irregular and may be absent for weeks, enlargement of the lymph nodes (especially the posterior cervical) and of the spleen, skin rashes, mostly erythematous, and localised areas of edema. After this there may be latent periods of months, rarely years, before symptoms of involvement of the central nervous system appear (sleeping sickness). Before this, tremors, shuffling gait, slurred speech and psychical changes may be present. In the *chronic* stage, headache, extreme weakness, mental dulness, paralyses, contractures, convulsions and coma give the picture of sleeping sickness. The parasites are found in the cerebrospinal fluid, less constantly in the blood. Todd and Dutton recommended puncture of the enlarged lymph nodes for diagnosis. Death is usually caused by some intercurrent infection, as purulent meningitis or suppuration of the lymph nodes. The duration is longer in *T. gambiense* infections; *T. rhodesiense* is much more virulent and kills in a few months. To prevent the spread of the disease will tax the energies of the nations interested in tropical Africa. The hope appears to be in the extermination of the animals upon which the *Glossina palpalis* feeds, just as the killing of the big game in other parts of Africa has saved the cattle from the ravages of the tsetse fly. Though a colossal task, the examination of natives of infected districts should be undertaken, isolation villages established, and the patients kept under observation and treatment.

The South American form (*T. cruzi*) occurs chiefly in Brazil (sometimes termed Chagas' disease). The parasites are found in the peripheral blood for a short time only: in the organs they assume a form like Leishmania. The clinical features are varied; acute forms occur especially in children, in some showing involvement of the nervous system, which is usually fatal, in others the main effect is insufficiency of the endocrine glands, especially the thyroid. The more chronic forms show features due particularly to hypothyroidism, cardiac disease, and varied nervous phenomena—paralyses, idiocy, etc.

Diagnosis.—The trypanosomes may be found in the blood or by puncture of the enlarged glands. In the "sleeping sickness stage" they may be found in the cerebrospinal fluid which shows increase in globulin and lymphocytes. Inoculation of blood or emulsified excised lymph nodes into guinea-pigs is an important aid.

Prognosis.—A few cases in Europeans have been cured, and some of these have been without symptoms for years. The criteria of cure are the absence of symptoms, failure to find the trypanosomes, and negative inoculations into susceptible animals. With early diagnosis and prompt treatment there is a good prospect of recovery. After the nervous system is involved the outlook is always grave.

Treatment.—Every effort should be made to improve the general health. Various drugs have been used. *Tryparsamide*, especially useful if the nervous system is involved, is given intravenously once a week (1 gm. the first week, 2 gm. the second and 3 gm. the third and subsequent weeks) for ten weeks. Some give it weekly for four weeks, discontinue for a month and then resume. Toxic features should be watched for. "Bayer 205" (Germanin) is given intravenously in doses of 1 gram weekly for ten weeks. It may cause nephritis. In the acute stages, atoxyl (in doses of gr. iii, 0.2 gm. intramuscularly twice a week) and potassium or sodium antimony tartrate, intravenously, in doses of gr. ½ (0.03 gm.), increased to gr. iii (0.2 gm.), given two or three times a week, are useful. Combinations of these drugs may be employed.

LEISHMANIASES

Definition.—Under this designation there are two main forms of disease: one is a general infection (Kala-azar and infantile Kala-azar); the other presents cutaneous lesions (tropical or oriental sore in the East and the cutaneous Leishmaniasis of tropical America).

Kala-Azar.—This is characterized by enlargement of the spleen and liver, anemia, irregularly remittent fever and marked emaciation. Leishman, in 1900, discovered the parasite which was subsequently studied by Donovan (*Leishmania donovani*).

Etiology.—The method of transmission is not settled but the sand fly (*Phlebotomus argentipes*) seems to be responsible. Proof of transmission by bed-bugs and fleas is lacking. Dogs and monkeys can be inoculated with the parasite which is an oat-shaped body 2 to 4 μ long by 1 to 2 μ broad, containing two chromatin bodies. It can be cultivated outside the body.

Pathology.—The Leishmania bodies are distributed throughout, especially as intracellular parasites of the endothelial cells. The largest numbers are in the liver, spleen and bone marrow. Ulcers in both the small and large intestine are found. The intestinal villi are enlarged and contain large numbers of the parasites especially in the endothelial cells.

Symptoms.—The onset is with irregular fever and enlargement of the liver and spleen. Anemia is marked with hemorrhages and progressive emaciation. A curious pigmentation appears, from which the name black-fever. Diarrhea and dysentery are not infrequent. The hemoglobin and red cells are reduced to about half the normal figures. Leukopenia is marked; often the white cells number 2,000. Parasites may be found in the leukocytes. The course of the disease without treatment varies from some months to two years and the mortality is about 90 per cent. The *diagnosis* is made by finding the parasite which occurs in the peripheral blood in a large percentage of cases. The blood may be citrated and after centrifugalization the contents of the bottom of the tube examined. Splenic puncture may be done. The formol-gel or aldehyde test of Napier is valuable.

Treatment.—Antimony has almost a specific effect, especially if given early. Potassium or sodium antimony tartrate twice a week intravenously is given in 1 or 2 per cent solution, freshly prepared. The first dose is one-half grain (0.03 gm.) gradually increased to gr. ii or iii (0.13-0.2 gm.), until gr. xxx (2 gm.) have been given. Various pentavalent antimony compounds are also used, such as stibamine and ureastibamine (0.15 gm. a day for 10 doses). The general health should be improved as much as possible and iron given freely.

Infantile Kala-Azar.—This form is the infantile splenic anemia long recognized in the Mediterranean basin formerly thought to be due to *L. infantum* but now regarded as due to *L. donovani.* The clinical features are much like those of the disease in adults. An infection of dogs exists in the endemic areas of infantile kala-azar. The disease may be transmitted by ticks.

Oriental Sore.—(Aleppo Boil, Delhi Boil, Tropical Sore, Bagdad Sore, etc.). Under various names is described a form of Leishmaniasis characterized by a granuloma of the skin which may ulcerate or not and is usually on exposed parts. The parasite (*L. tropica*) was discovered by Homer Wright. This occurs widely distributed in the East; imported cases are occasionally seen in the United States. The first lesion is a papule which extends and may ulcerate. The ulcer somewhat resembles a gumma. The course, if the disease is untreated, is self-limited with a period of six to eighteen months. Marked scars are left. The *diagnosis* is made by finding the parasite, usually in the margin of an ulcer, or in cultures taken from the lesion. The *treatment* is the same as for kala-azar or by the application of a 2 per cent antimony ointment. X-ray and radium treatment has given good results.

The American form (Espundia) occurs in Central and South America and is due to *L. braziliensis.* In its general features it is much like the previous form but often involves the mucous membrane of the nose and mouth. The treatment is the same.

THE RELAPSING FEVERS

Definition.—A group of specific infections caused by spirochetes, characterized by febrile paroxysms which usually last five or six days with remissions of about the same length of time. The paroxysms may be repeated several times, whence the name relapsing, or recurring, fever. European, Indian, American and African forms are described presenting clinically much the same features, but the parasites differ. The organism varies in different countries and insects (lice and ticks) are concerned in its transmission.

Etiology.—The European form, also known as "famine fever" and "seven-day fever," has been known since the early part of the eighteenth century, and at times prevailed extensively especially in Ireland. It is a very rare disease in England. In the United States the disease appeared in 1844, when cases were admitted to the Philadelphia Hospital, described by Meredith Clymer in his work on Fevers. In 1869 it prevailed extensively in New York and Philadelphia; since when it has not reappeared. The European form is due to *Spirochaeta recurrentis* (formerly *Spirillum obermeieri*) the American form is due to *S. novyi;* the Asiatic form to *S. carteri;* and the Persian form to *S. persica.*

The *Central African relapsing fever,* known as *tick fever,* is a widespread affection, the parasite of which is *S. duttoni.* It is transmitted by the tick *Ornithodoros moubata,* but as Leishman has shown, not by direct inoculation with the salivary secretion, but from other secretions voided in the act of gorging. The symptoms are similar to those of European relapsing fever, and from five to seven relapses may take place. The mortality is not high. The North African form is due to *S. berbera* and is transmitted by lice.

The spirochete, described by Obermeier in 1873, was one of the first organisms shown to be definitely associated with a specific fever. It is from 15 to 40 μ in length, spirally arranged like a corkscrew, sometimes curved and twisted. It is actively motile, and it is present in the blood during the febrile paroxysm, disappearing at intervals. Plotz reported the cultivation of the spirochetes directly from the blood. The mode of transmission is by infection through an insect bite or by scratching; the material is rubbed into the wound. Neither age, sex, nor season seems to have any special influence. One attack does not confer immunity, but later infections may be milder and with one febrile period only or with few symptoms.

Morbid Anatomy.—There are no characteristic anatomical appearances in relapsing fever. If death takes place during the paroxysm the spleen is large and soft, and the liver, kidneys and heart show cloudy swelling. There may be infarcts in the kidneys and spleen. The bone-marrow has been found in a condition of hyperplasia. Ecchymoses are not uncommon.

Symptoms.—The *incubation* appears to be short; in some instances the attack occurs within twelve hours after exposure; more frequently, however, from five to seven days elapse.

The *invasion* is abrupt, with chill, fever, and intense pain in the back and limbs. In young persons there may be nausea, vomiting, and convulsions. The temperature rises rapidly and may reach 104° on the evening of the first day. Sweats are common. The pulse is rapid, ranging from 110 to 130. There may be delirium if the fever is high. Swelling of the spleen can be detected early. Jaundice is common in some epidemics. The gastric symptoms may be severe, but intestinal symptoms are rare. Cough may be present. Occasionally herpes is noted, and there may be miliary vesicles and petechiae. During the paroxysm the blood invariably shows the spirochetes and there is usually a

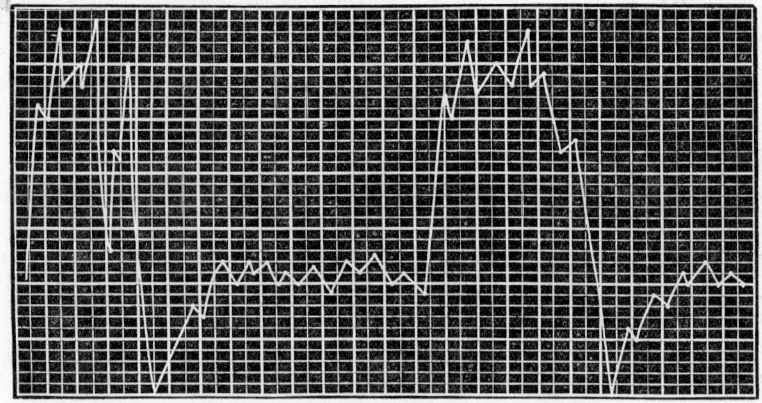

Chart XI.—Relapsing Fever (Murchison).

leukocytosis. After the fever has persisted with severity or even with an increasing intensity for five or six days the crisis occurs. In the course of a few hours, accompanied by profuse sweating, sometimes by diarrhea, the temperature falls to normal or even subnormal. In the African Tick Fever the duration of fever is shorter (three or four days).

The crisis may occur as early as the third day or may be delayed to the tenth; it usually comes, however, about the end of the first week. In delicate and elderly persons there may be collapse. The convalescence is rapid, and in a few days the patient is up and about. Then in a week, usually on the fourteenth day, he again has a rigor, or a series of chills; the fever returns and the attack is repeated. A second crisis occurs from the twentieth to the twenty-third day, and again the patient recovers rapidly. As a rule, the relapse is shorter than the original attack. A second and a third may occur, and even a fourth and a fifth. The number varies in the different forms; there is usually one in the American form. In epidemics some cases terminate by crisis on the seventh or eighth day without the occurrence of relapse. In protracted cases the convalescence is very tedious.

Relapsing fever is not a very fatal disease. The mortality is usually from 2 to 5 per cent, but it has been as high as 30 per cent in India. In the enfeebled and old, death may occur at the height of the first paroxysm.

Complications are not frequent. In some epidemics hematemesis and hematuria have occurred. Pneumonia is not infrequent. The acute enlargement of the spleen may end in rupture. Postfebrile paralyses may occur. Ophthalmia has followed in certain epidemics. In pregnant women abortion usually takes place. Convulsions occasionally follow. Dutton, the well-known worker on tropical diseases, died in *status epilepticus* some weeks after the attack.

Diagnosis.—The onset and general symptoms at first may not be distinctive. At the beginning of an epidemic the cases are usually regarded as anomalous typhoid or influenza; but the typical course makes the diagnosis clear. The blood examination is distinctive during the febrile period.

Prophylaxis.—This is concerned with the avoidance of insects which carry the infection; measures to exterminate them and to prevent them from gaining access to sick and well are in order. In the African form avoidance of infected huts is essential.

Treatment.—The disease should be treated like any other continued fever, by careful nursing, a regular diet, and ordinary hygienic measures. Two doses of neoarsphenamine are usually effective. Pain in the back, limbs and joints may require sedatives. In enfeebled persons the collapse at the crisis may be serious, and ammonia and digitalis should be given freely.

SYPHILIS

HISTORY, ETIOLOGY AND MORBID ANATOMY

Definition.—A specific disease of slow evolution caused by *Treponema pallidum* (Spirochaeta pallida) propagated by inoculation (acquired syphilis) or transmission through the mother (congenital syphilis).

History.—Whether the disease was known in Europe before 1493 is still discussed. One school insists that there is no evidence of pre-Columbian syphilis in the Eastern hemisphere before the return of the Spanish sailors from Hayti from whom it spread among the inhabitants of Barcelona. In 1493 it reached Italy with the army of Charles VIII. His soldiers syphilized Naples; the disease spread throughout Italy, and in a few years Europe was aflame. On the other hand, those who contend for the antiquity of the disease in Asia and Europe rely on certain old Chinese records, on references in the Bible and in old medical writers to diseases resembling syphilis and on suggestive bone lesions in very old skeletons. The balance of evidence seems to be in favor of the American origin. At first it was called the Neapolitan disease, the French pox, or Morbus Gallicus; and in 1530 Fracastorius, in a poem entitled "Syphilis sive Morbus Gallicus," gave it the name by which it is now commonly known. The etymology of the name is uncertain.

At first the disease was thought to be transmitted like any other epidemic, but gradually the venereal nature was recognized, and Fernel, a famous Paris physician of the 16th century, insisted on the necessity of a primary inoculation. Paracelsus observed its congenital character. Throughout the 16th century the symptoms were well described. The disease appears to have been of much greater severity then than at present. Mercury and guaiacum were introduced as the important remedies. In the 18th century Lancisi recognized the relations existing between syphilis and aneurism, and Morgagni described many of the visceral lesions. Hunter, misled by inoculations made on his own person, decided in favor of the unity of gonorrhea, soft chancre and syphilis. Ricord clearly differentiated the soft and hard chancre, and throughout the 19th century the clinical and pathological lesions were so thoroughly studied that scarcely a feature of the disease remained unknown. But all efforts at discovering the cause had failed, until in 1905 Schaudinn demonstrated the presence of a spirochaete in the lesions. Since then his work has been amply verified, and in 1910 Ehrlich announced the discovery of an arsenic compound with special spirochaeticidal power.

Etiology: The Parasite.—The treponema is a spiral, curved organism from 5 to 15 μ in length, showing active movements in fresh specimens. It has been demonstrated in every tissue affected by the disease and has been found in semen. It lives only for a short time under natural conditions outside the body and is killed by weak antiseptics. It may live in the body as long as the host is alive. It is inoculable into monkeys and rabbits can be infected. There is doubt as to whether the parasite has been cultivated. We know little of the life history and nature of the parasite. Has it a complex cycle of which the organism which we know is only one phase? Is the organism filterable in some stage? Has it an intermediate stage in which it is infective? What determines latency or activity of the parasites in those who are treponema carriers?

There are possibly various strains of the treponema and this may explain some of the clinical differences. The spirochaetes from cases of general paresis are said to take 60 to 80 days for propagation and 60 days for lesions to be produced in rabbits, whereas with organisms from early lesions three or four weeks is sufficient. A strain of spirochaetes may result with greater resistance but perhaps less power of reproduction. The infection then does not cause any active symptoms but may persist indefinitely in a latent form to resume activity after a long interval of quiescence. In some cases the tissues, so to speak, become accustomed to the spirochaetes, antibodies are not produced, and in the absence of these the Wassermann reaction is negative. The infection must be active to cause the production of antibodies. In many cases a resistance of the parasite to the usual remedies is apparently established.

A most important result of the discovery of the parasite has been the application of serum diagnosis. The serological tests give a means of determining the presence of antibodies in the blood of a patient suffering from syphilitic infection. A positive result is obtained in from 90 to 95 per cent of cases in the acute stages. It appears from the end of the second to the end of the fourth week, becomes more marked and may continue for an indefinite period. During active treatment it may be absent, to reappear again. Its intensity bears some relation to the activity of the lesions. In visceral and late congenital syphilis it is positive in a smaller percentage.

Modes of Infection.—In a majority of all cases the disease is transmitted by *sexual congress*, but the designation *venereal* disease (*lues venerea*) is not always correct, as there are many other modes of inoculation. In the St. Louis Hospital collection there are illustrations of 26 varieties of extragenital chancres.

Accidental Infection.—In surgical and in midwifery practice physicians are not infrequently inoculated. Infection may occur without a characteristic local sore. Midwifery chancres are usually on the fingers, but may be on the back of the hand. The lip chancre is the most common of these extragenital forms, and may be acquired in many ways apart from direct infection. Mouth and tonsillar sores result as a rule from improper practices. Wet-nurses are sometimes infected on the nipple, and it occasionally happens that relatives of a syphilitic child are accidentally contaminated. Syphilis has been conveyed by blood transfusion.

Congenital Transmission.—The disease is *not inherited* but the fetus is infected through the placenta. It is a question entirely of intra-uterine infection. The mother herself may be, and often is, apparently quite healthy, but the Wassermann reaction is present and it is through her and not directly from the father that the disease is transmitted. We can now understand what is known as Beaumès' or Colles' law, which was thus stated by the distinguished Dublin surgeon: "That a child, born of a mother who is without obvious venereal symptoms, and which, without being exposed to any infection subsequent to its birth, shows this disease when a few weeks old, this child will infect the most healthy nurse, whether she suckle it, or merely handle and dress it; and yet this child is never known to infect its own mother, even though she suckle it while it has venereal ulcers of the lips and tongue."

Morbid Anatomy.—The typical *primary lesion,* or chancre, shows: (*a*) A diffuse infiltration of the connective tissue with small, round cells. (*b*) Larger epithelioid cells. (*c*) Giant cells. (*d*) Changes in the small arteries and veins, chiefly thickening of the intima. The sclerosis is due in part to this acute obliterative endarteritis. The related lymph nodes undergo hyperplasia and become indurated.

The *secondary lesions* of syphilis are too varied for description here. They consist of condylomata, skin eruptions, affections of the eye, etc.

The *tertiary lesions* consist of circumscribed tumors known as gummata, a diffuse infiltration of the tissues, various skin lesions, and a special type of arteritis.

The most characteristic change is in the *blood vessels,* showing marked round cell infiltration in the adventitia and vasa vasorum. The process later involves the other coats of the arteries with fibrous changes in the media and hyaline changes in the intima. The vascular change is the key to the understanding of many of the lesions of syphilis. In the late visceral lesions there are parenchymatous changes and the formation of fibrous tissue.

Gummata.—Syphilomata occur in the bones or periosteum—here they are called nodes—in the muscles, skin, brain, lungs, liver, kidneys, heart, testes, and adrenals. They vary in size from small, almost microscopic bodies to large solid tumors from 3 to 5 cm. in diameter. They are usually firm and hard, but in the skin and on the mucous membranes they tend to break down and ulcerate. On cross-section a medium-sized gumma presents in the centre caseous substance and at the periphery translucent, fibrous tissue.

Pathogenesis.—There are many gaps in our knowledge of what happens in syphilitic infection. The infection is by *inoculation* followed by immediate dissemination of the spirochaetes throughout the body. The spirochaete invades and proliferates in the perivascular lymph spaces. There is a general infection within a few days of inoculation, possibly within twenty-four hours. What is the result? The answer varies and it is tempting to ascribe the variations to possible differences in strains of spirochaetes and to the strength of the individual's resistance. The first evident response to the infection is the appearance of a reaction at the point of inoculation—the chancre—but this does not occur in every case or is not marked in every case. Is this due to the particular spirochaete or to the patient? The local lesion, when typical, represents an exudate of plasma cells and lymphocytes especially around the blood vessels, which show marked changes. It may be said that histologically syphilitic lesions are essentially the same at all stages. The surface of the chancre usually becomes eroded, but not always, with the production of an ulcer, the serum from which contains large numbers of spirochaetes. If untreated, the primary lesion lasts for a month or so and in healing marked induration occurs which may be permanent. Years later, spirochaetes may be found in the scar of the primary lesion.

The *general infection* results in evident changes after an interval of six to eight weeks. These show great variety, from severe general manifestations to signs so slight that they are not noted. The evidence of infection, fever, rash, etc., are much like those in the acute exanthemata but requiring a longer period for development. Hence the designation of syphilis as "a fever diluted by time." Does an active response in this stage of acute general infection represent a stronger resistance? It may, and when we compare the percentage of patients in this stage who show evidence of involvement of the nervous system with the much smaller percentage who show later involvement, there is basis for the suggestion that the body resistance may be able to overcome the spirochaetes to some extent. Can the body overcome the infection entirely by its own resistance? We do not know.

This *acute* or secondary stage lasts for an uncertain time, usually months and rarely a year, and then in the majority of cases the manifestations of infection disappear forever in some patients, for varying periods in others. The surmise is that the spirochaetes and body cells settle down to a relationship which may be amicable or the reverse. There does not seem any doubt that in some individuals the spirochaetes live in certain tissues for the rest of the patient's life without causing any evident disease. The patient has the spirochaetal infection but does not have clinical syphilis. In a smaller number the infection progresses so that there is really no interval between the acute secondary features and the usual late chronic involvement. In fact the two may be present together. In the majority, after the acute stage a period of quiescence results, usually for years, and subsequently more chronic manifestations appear, especially in the viscera. As to what determines their appearance we know very little; trauma may do it. In some cases there may not be any quiescent stage; the process advances very slowly and years are required before the damage is sufficient to be recognized clinically.

ACQUIRED SYPHILIS

Primary Stage.—This extends from the appearance of the initial sore until the onset of the constitutional symptoms, and has a variable duration of six to twelve weeks. The initial sore usually appears in about a month after inoculation, and shows first as a small red papule, which gradually enlarges and breaks in the centre, leaving a small ulcer. The tissue about this becomes indurated so that it ultimately has a gristly, cartilaginous consistence—hence the name, hard or indurated chancre. The size attained is variable, and when small the sore may be overlooked, particularly if it is just within the urethra. The initial lesion has no invariable characteristic and may not be indurated. It must be emphasized that infection may occur without any marked primary lesion which may be only a superficial erosion or ulceration. A negative history as to the occurrence of a chancre is of no value in excluding infection. There are a considerable number of extragenital infections. Syphilitic infection may occur with a chancroid. The glands in the lymph district of the chancre enlarge and become hard. Suppuration both in the initial lesion and in the glands may occur as a secondary change. The general condition of the patient in this stage is good. There may be no fever and no impairment of health. Even at this stage there is a general infection; in 49 of 221 cases with chancre, changes in the spinal fluid were found (Wile and Hasley); in 8.83 per cent of 283 cases (Mills, 1927).

Secondary Stage.—The constitutional symptoms usually appear within three months of the appearance of the primary sore. They rarely occur earlier than the sixth or later than the twelfth week:

Fever, slight or intense, and very variable in character, may occur before the skin rash; more frequently it is the "fever of invasion" with the secondary symptoms, or it may occur at any period. It may be a mild continuous pyrexia or with marked remissions, but the most remarkable form is the intermittent, often mistaken for malaria. The fever may reach 105° and the paroxysms persist for months.

Anemia.—Some patients show a muddy pallor of the skin. A moderate grade of secondary anemia is common and occasionally this becomes severe. The red cells do not show any special alterations. In some patients mercury causes a rapid anemia, the hemoglobin falling more rapidly than the red cells. There may be a moderate leukocytosis with lymphocytosis.

Cutaneous Lesions.—The earliest and most common is a *macular syphilide* or *syphilitic roseola,* which occurs on the trunk and on the front of the arms. The face is often exempt. The spots, which are reddish-brown and symmetrically arranged, persist for a week or two. There may be multiple relapses of roseola, sometimes at long intervals, even eleven years (Fournier). The *papular syphilide,* which forms acne-like indurations about the face and trunk, is often arranged in groups. Other forms are the *pustular rash,* which may closely simulate variola, and a *squamous syphilide* not unlike ordinary psoriasis, except that the scales are less abundant. The rash is more copper-colored and not specially confined to the extensor surfaces. The rash tends to be polymorphous.

In the moist regions of the skin, such as the perineum and groins, and at the angles of the mouth, the so-called *mucous patches* occur, which are flat, warty outgrowths, with well-defined margins and surfaces covered with a grayish secretion. They are among the most distinctive lesions of syphilis.

The hair may fall out (alopecia), either in patches or by a general thinning. Occasionally the nails become affected (syphilitic onychia).

Mucous Lesions.—With the fever and the roseolous rash the throat and mouth become sore. The pharyngeal mucosa is hyperemic, the tonsils are swollen and often present small, kidney-shaped ulcers with grayish-white borders. Mucous patches are seen on the inner surfaces of the cheeks and on the tongue and lips. There may be a smooth glossitis with glistening areas over which the papillae disappear. Hypertrophy of the papillae in various portions of the mucous membranes produces the syphilitic warts or condylomata which are most frequent about the vulva and anus.

Adenitis.—This is often general. The glands are hard, painless and not much enlarged. Involvement of the epitrochlear and posterior cervical glands is specially significant.

Arthritis is not rare and may occur in the acute and like stages, also in the congenital form. It is often symmetrical, likely to be of long duration, if untreated, apt to relapse, may be quite acute but rarely causes serious damage. It may be so acute that rheumatic fever is suspected. *T. pallidum* has been found in the synovial fluid.

The *bones* may be attacked and periostitis occur. Involvement of the spine, especially in the cervical region, may be found. Syphilitic spondylitis is not uncommon.

Nervous System.—Even at the time of the primary lesion changes may be found in the spinal fluid. In the secondary stage the percentage showing meningeal involvement increases; some studies give 80 per cent but probably 30 to 40 per cent is more correct. Of symptoms *headache* is common, often occipital and passing up to the top of the head; it is usually worse at night. There may be frequent acute general pains, possibly due to meningeal irritation.

Other Lesions.—*Iritis* is common, and usually affects one eye before the other. It comes on from three to six months after the chancre. There may be only slight ciliary congestion in mild cases, but in severer forms there is great pain, and the condition is serious. *Choroiditis* and *retinitis* are rare secondary manifestations. Pupillary changes are not uncommon in the early stages. *Ear* affections are not common in this stage, but sudden deafness occurs, which may be due to labyrinthine disease or to the extension of inflammation from the throat to the middle ear. The *spleen* may be enlarged. Orchitis and parotitis are rare. Jaundice may occur, even in the primary stage, the *icterus syphiliticus praecox.* The acute nephritis will be referred to later. Disease of the cardiovascular system is not common.

Tertiary Stage.—No hard and fast line can be drawn between the lesions of the secondary and those of the tertiary period; and, indeed, in exceptional cases, manifestations which usually appear late may appear before the primary sore has properly healed. In all the late lesions the importance of the involvement of the arteries must be remembered. *Fever* is common with tertiary lesions.

The late *syphilides* show a great tendency to ulceration and destruction of the deeper layers of the skin, so that in healing scars are left. They are also more scattered and seldom symmetrical. One of the most characteristic is *rupia,* the dry stratified crusts of which cover an ulcer which involves the deeper layers of the skin and in healing leaves a scar.

Gummata.—These may occur in the skin, tissues of the mouth, subcutaneous tissue, muscles, or internal organs. In the skin they tend to break down and ulcerate, leaving ugly sores which heal with difficulty. In the solid organs they undergo fibroid transformation and produce puckering and deformity. On the mucous membranes these lesions lead to ulceration, in the healing of which cicatrices are formed; thus, in the larynx great narrowing may result, and in the rectum ulceration with fibroid thickening and retraction may lead to stricture. Gummatous ulcers may be infective.

Amyloid Degeneration.—Syphilis plays a most important rôle in the production of this affection. Of 244 instances analyzed by Fagge, 76 had syphilis, and of these 42 had no bone lesions. It follows the acquired form and is common in association with rectal syphilis in women. In congenital lues amyloid degeneration is rare.

Syphilis of the Bones.—This is not uncommon and should be searched for by radiography in doubtful cases. The commonest lesions are periostitis and osteoperiostitis which may exist without any symptoms. Occasionally a gumma is found. *Bursitis* occurs rarely and is usually very chronic and without pain. The bone lesions occur both in the acquired and congenital form. *Pain* is common, often nocturnal and relieved by exercise. It may occur only on pressure over small areas. Involvement of the *spine* is not unusual. There may be periostitis, osteomyelitis with necrosis, and sometimes the formation of exostoses, which may be felt. The cervical region is most often involved and the process is generally limited to a small number of vertebrae. The main features are pain, tenderness, rigidity, and sometimes deformity. In a number of patients neural symptoms are present and root pains may be marked. The degree of deformity varies. There is often marked muscle spasm in the region involved and hypotonicity in other parts of the spine. The *diagnosis* of involvement of the spine may not be easy. Careful search should be made for luetic lesions elsewhere; for example, ulceration of the larynx has been found in some cases of involvement of the cervical region. In the skull, caries may occur in the frontal and temporal bones.

Syphilitic *myositis* affects the calf and sternomastoid muscles especially. There are vascular lesions and interstitial myositis with sclerosis.

Quaternary Stage.—Long years it may be from the primary sore and from any active manifestations, certain forms of syphilis may appear, the chief of which are tabes dorsalis and general paresis.

Latent Syphilis.—In many cases there is a persistence of the spirochaetal infection without evident clinical signs of the disease, proved (postmortem) by the presence of the spirochaetes in certain tissues, especially the aorta and testicles. The essential lesion is a chronic inflammatory process with an accumulation of lymphocytes and plasma cells about the lymphatics and blood vessels leading to fibrosis and atrophy of the parenchyma. Warthin drew especial attention to this and demonstrated the organisms in about one-third of autopsies on adults. Careful examination may show evidence in the form of aortitis or induration of the testicle. The serological reactions and examination of the spinal fluid are useful in the recognition of these cases. They have the spirochetal infection but often no clinical evidence of disease.

CONGENITAL SYPHILIS

With the exception of the primary sore, every feature of the acquired disease may be seen in the congenital form. The intra-uterine conditions leading to the death of the fetus do not here concern us. The child may be born healthy-looking or with well-marked evidences of the disease. In the majority of instances the former is the case and within the first month or two the signs of the disease appear.

At Birth.—When the disease exists at birth the child is feebly developed and wasted, and a skin eruption is usually present, commonly in the form of bullae about the hands and feet (pemphigus neonatorum syphiliticus). The child snuffles, the lips are ulcerated, the angles of the mouth fissured, and there is enlargement of the liver and spleen. The bone changes may be marked, and the epiphyses may be separated. Osteochondritis is common. In such cases the children rarely survive long.

Early Manifestations.—When born healthy the child thrives, is fat and plump, and shows no abnormality; then from the fourth to the eighth week, rarely later, a nasal catarrh occurs, *syphilitic rhinitis,* which impedes respiration, and produces the characteristic *snuffles.* The discharge may be seropurulent or bloody. The child nurses with great difficulty. In severe cases ulceration takes place with necrosis of the bone, leading to a depression at the root of the nose and a characteristic deformity (saddle nose). This coryza may be mistaken for an ordinary catarrh, but the coexistence of other manifestations usually makes the diagnosis clear. The disease may extend into the Eustachian tubes and middle ears and lead to deafness.

The *cutaneous* lesions arise with or shortly after the onset of the snuffles. The skin often has a sallow, earthy hue. The eruption is first noticed about the nates. There may be an erythema or an eczematous condition, but more commonly there are irregular reddish-brown patches with well-defined edges and a papular syphilide is not uncommon. A desquamative dermatitis of the palms of the hands and soles of the feet may occur. Fissures occur about the lips, either at the angles of the mouth or in the median line. These *rhagades* are very characteristic. There may be marked ulceration of the mucocutaneous surfaces. The secretions from these mouth lesions are very virulent, and it is from this source that the wet-nurse is usually infected. Not only the nurse, but members of the family, may be infected; other children have been accidentally inoculated from a syphilitic infant. The hair of the head or of the eyebrows may fall out. The syphilitic *onychia* is not uncommon. Enlargement of the glands is not so frequent in the congenital as in the acquired disease. When the cutaneous lesions are marked the contiguous glands can usually be felt. The *spleen* is enlarged in many cases. Enlargement of the *liver,* though often present, is less significant, since in infants it may be due to various causes. The child may be restless and wakeful, particularly at night. Some writers describe a peculiar hoarse syphilitic cry. Among rare manifestations are hemorrhages—the *syphilis haemorrhagica neonatorum.* The bleeding may be subcutaneous, from the mucous surfaces, or, when early, from the umbilicus. All of such cases, however, are not syphilitic, and the disease must not be confounded with the acute hemoglobinuria of newborn infants. E. Fournier described a remarkable enlargement of the subcutaneous veins. Acute infections may stir up latent congenital syphilis.

Late Manifestations.—Children with congenital syphilis may present a wizened, wasted appearance, and a prematurely aged face. In patients who recover the general nutrition may remain good and the child show no further manifestations; commonly, however, at the second dentition or puberty the disease reappears. Although the child may have recovered from the early lesions, it does not develop normally. Growth is slow, development tardy, both mental and physical, and there are facial and cranial characteristics which often render the disease recognizable at a glance. A young man of nineteen or twenty may neither look older nor be more developed than a boy of ten or twelve—infantilism. The forehead is prominent, the frontal eminences are marked, and the skull may be very asymmetrical. The bridge of the nose is depressed, the tip *retroussé*. The lips are often prominent, and there are striated lines running from the corners of the mouth. The *teeth* are deformed and may present appearances which Jonathan Hutchinson claimed are specific and peculiar. The upper central incisors of the permanent set are peg-shaped, stunted in length and breadth, and narrower at the cutting edge than at the root. On the anterior surface the enamel is well formed, and not eroded or honeycombed. At the cutting edge there is a single notch, usually shallow, sometimes deep, in which the dentine is exposed. The upper first large molar may have a supernumerary cusp on the inner side which forms a protuberance but this is not peculiar to syphilis.

Among late manifestations, apt to appear about puberty, is interstitial *keratitis,* which usually begins as a slight steaminess of the corneae, which present a ground-glass appearance. It affects both eyes, though one is attacked before the other. It may persist for months and leave opacities, which prevent clear vision. *Strabismus* is relatively common. *Iritis* and *choroiditis* may occur. Of *ear affections,* apart from those which follow the pharyngeal disease, a form occurs, about the time of puberty or earlier, in which deafness comes on rapidly and persists in spite of treatment. It is unassociated with obvious lesions, and is probably labyrinthine in character. *Bone lesions* are not rare. Epiphysitis may occur with swelling and occasionally separation follows. It may simulate paralysis. Chronic *periostitis,* affecting especially the tibiae, usually appears after the sixth year and may cause marked deformity with great thickening of the bone (sabre-tibia). Nodes of congenital syphilis may be diffuse and affect the bones of arms and legs. They are generally symmetrical, rarely painful, may occur late, even after the twentieth year, and are often mistaken for rickets. *Dactylitis,* usually in the second or third year, causes fusiform swelling of the fingers, rarely of the toes. *Arthritis* may occur at any age; it is often symmetrical with swelling but comparatively slight disability or pain, and tends to be chronic.

Visceral lesions occur much as in the acquired form except that involvement of the central nervous system may result in lack of mental development. General paresis may result. Symptoms much like those of acute infectious *chorea* appear in some children. Enlargement of the *spleen,* sometimes of the lymph nodes, may be a late manifestation, with or without disease of the liver. Much interest attaches to the influence of congenital syphilis on the *endocrine glands.* They may be disturbed leading to disorders of development and function. It is a good rule to consider congenital syphilis in any obscure abnormality in a child.

Is syphilis transmitted to the third generation? The discovery of the treponema answers this question. The disease can be carried through as many generations as are able to reproduce. This makes a thorough study of the family for several generations an important aid in the diagnosis of congenital syphilis.

VISCERAL SYPHILIS

Cerebrospinal Syphilis

The nervous system is frequently involved in the early stages as shown by changes in the cerebrospinal fluid. In the great majority there are no later manifestations. Mattauschek and Pilcz followed 4,143 cases of syphilis for from 20 to 30 years with special reference to this point: 4.7 per cent developed paresis, 3.2 per cent cerebrospinal syphilis and 2.7 per cent tabes dorsalis. The figures were highest in those who had little or no treatment.

Pathology.—The process may involve the meninges, the arteries and the parenchyma. In the majority of cases the lesions are not limited to one of these structures. Predominant involvement of one alone is probably most common in the arteries—endarteritis. With this the cerebrospinal fluid shows little if any change and the symptoms are due to the vascular disease. It is a mistake to carry any classification too far because vascular and meningeal lesions of some grade occur in practically all cases. In all forms marked perivascular changes are common. The exudate due to these interferes with the lymphatic circulation. This with the endarteritis often results in marked interference with nutrition. In general the lesions may be classified as (1) parenchymatous, which include tabes and paresis, and (2) interstitial, which comprise the forms usually termed cerebrospinal syphilis.

The parenchymatous lesions appear as a rule later than the interstitial, but there is often a history of earlier nervous symptoms which responded quickly to treatment. These are usually due to a basilar meningitis. The interval suggests that there has been a slow process gradually advancing which gives time for degenerative processes to develop. The majority of the cases of the interstitial type appear within five years of infection.

Meninges.—Meningitis is common and occurs particularly at the base, about the chiasm and along the Sylvian fissures. *Gummata* form, attached to the pia mater, sometimes to the dura; they are most common in the cerebrum. They form definite tumors varying in size from a pea to a walnut and are usually multiple. They are rarely found unassociated with the meninges. When small they have a uniform, translucent appearance, but when large the centre undergoes a fibrocaseous change with a firm grayish tissue at the periphery. They may resemble tuberculous tumors and occasionally undergo cystic degeneration. Large growths are not so common in the cord. Intense encephalitis or myelitis may occur in the neighborhood of a gumma. There are cases of acute syphilitic meningitis, some with a negative Wassermann reaction, which are rapidly fatal.

In the brain, gummatous arteritis is a common cause of softening, which may be extensive, as when the middle cerebral artery is involved, or when there is a large patch of meningitis. In such cases the process is really a meningo-encephalitis and the symptoms are due to the secondary changes.

Arteries.—A common lesion is the typical progressive endarteritis. Perivascular changes are common. There may be a marked inflammatory reaction with edema and resulting interference with the lymphatics or small nodular tumors on the vessels which may break down or lead to rupture. Arterial disease is often combined with lesions in the meninges.

Parenchyma.—The changes here are largely degenerative and are due partly to interference with nutrition by the vascular lesions and partly to the direct action of toxins from spirochetes in the tissues (especially in paresis). It is evident that lesions of the meninges and vessels offer much more hope of benefit from treatment than those of the parenchyma.

Cerebrospinal Fluid.—The examination of this is of great value in diagnosis and in estimating the effect of treatment. The special points in cerebrospinal syphilis are:

Cell Content.—A lymphocytosis occurs in 85-90 per cent of cases. The cells are often over 100 and may reach 1,000 per c.mm., the number being some guide to the intensity of the meningitis. With endarteritis alone the cells may be normal.

Globulin.—An increase is present in 90-95 per cent of cases. It probably represents abnormal transudation from damaged vessels and may occur in a great variety of conditions. An increase in globulin may be the only change in the fluid in the early secondary period.

Wassermann Reaction.—This is positive in 85-90 per cent, and indicates some active process in the cerebrospinal tissues. In the early secondary period it may be absent even with increase in cells and globulin.

Colloidal Gold Reaction.—This is present in 75-80 per cent of cases. The type of curve, a mid-zone reaction, is useful in distinguishing paresis from tabes and cerebrospinal syphilis.

Symptoms.—The onset is usually within one to five years after infection but it may be earlier. *Headache,* often worse at night, irritability and mental fatigue may be prodromal symptoms. The clinical features are many, occur in various combinations and naturally vary depending on the relative degree of involvement of meninges and vessels. The multiplicity of signs is often a great aid in diagnosis. Headache is usually marked. *Ocular* features are common and often show remarkable variations from time to time. The pupils may be unequal or irregular and react sluggishly to light. Ptosis, weakness of the eye muscles, diplopia and optic neuritis may be present. As a rule there is involvement of more than one of the cranial nerves.

Psychical Features.—A sudden and violent *delirium* may be the first symptom or prior to the delirium there may have been headache, alteration of character, and loss of memory. The condition may be accompanied by convulsions. There may be no neuritis, no palsy, and no localizing symptoms.

More commonly following headache, giddiness, or an excited state which may amount to delirium, the patient has convulsion or a hemiplegic attack, or there is involvement of the nerves of the base. Some display a prolonged torpor or *coma,* a special feature of brain syphilis to which Buzzard and Huebner referred, which may persist for a month.

In some cases the clinical picture is that of general paresis.

Some cases of cerebral syphilis display features suggestive of brain tumor. They may be due to a gumma. Of these convulsions are most important, and both Fournier and Wood laid great stress on the value of this symptom in persons over thirty. The first symptoms may, however, be those of embolism or thrombosis; thus there may be sudden hemiplegia, with or without loss of consciousness. The hemiplegia usually develops slowly and there may be weakness rather than paralysis.

The symptoms of *spinal syphilis* are extremely varied and may be caused by large gummatous growths attached to the meninges, in which case the features are those of tumor, by gummatous arteritis with secondary softening, by meningitis with secondary cord changes, or by late scleroses. Syphilitic myelitis will be considered under affections of the spinal cord.

Diagnosis.—The history is of the first importance, but it may be extremely difficult to get a trustworthy account. Careful examination should be made for traces of a primary sore, for scars on the skin and for bone lesions. The oculocardiac reflex may be absent. The character of the signs is often of great assistance. They are multiform, variable, and often such as could not be explained by a single lesion; thus there may be anomalous spinal symptoms or involvement of the cranial nerves on both sides. The study of the spinal fluid and the Wassermann reaction in it and in the blood are of the greatest aid. The result of treatment has a bearing as the symptoms may disappear with the use of antisyphilitic remedies.

Prognosis.—This is always uncertain and depends largely on the extent of arterial disease. With marked arteritis and secondary softening the possibilities of restoration are slight. Meningeal disease is much more hopeful. Much depends on early recognition and prompt treatment. The tendency to relapse is marked. In the case of large gummata the problem is practically that of brain tumor.

Syphilis of the Respiratory Organs

Trachea and Bronchi.—L. A. Conner analyzed 128 recorded cases of syphilis of the trachea and bronchi. In 52 per cent of the cases the trachea was alone involved. In only 10 per cent were characteristic lesions of syphilis found in the lungs. Bronchial dilatation below the lesion was found in 15 per cent of the cases. In 10 cases the lesion occurred in congenital syphilis. The *symptoms* are often of obstruction, dyspnea, often paroxysmal, stridor, prolonged inspiration and a hard paroxysmal cough. *Tracheo-esophageal fistula* occurs very rarely; Bucher and Ono (1934) found 12 cases reported.

Lung.—This is a rare disease. In 2,800 postmortems at the Johns Hopkins Hospital there were 12 cases with syphilitic disease in the lungs; in 8 of these the lesions were in congenital syphilis. In 11 cases there were definite gummata. Clinically, syphilis of the lung was suspected in three cases. Fowler, in the museums of the London hospitals and the Royal College of Surgeons, found only 12 specimens of syphilitic lesions of the lungs, two of which are doubtful. It occurs under the following forms:

The "White Pneumonia" of the Fetus.—This may affect large areas or an entire lung, which then is firm, heavy, and airless, even though the child may have been alive. On section it is grayish-white—the so-called white hepatization of Virchow. The chief change is in the alveolar walls, which are greatly thickened and infiltrated, and the section is like one of the pancreas. In the early stages, for example in a seven or eight months' fetus, there may be scattered miliary foci of this induration chiefly about the arteries. The air cells are filled with desquamated and swollen epithelium.

In the form of *gummata*, which vary in size from a pea to an egg. They occur irregularly through the lung, but, as a rule, are more numerous toward the root. They present a grayish-yellow caseous appearance, are dry and usually imbedded in a translucent, more or less firm, connective tissue. In rare instances there are extensive caseous gummata with softening and formation of *bronchiectatic* cavities, and clinically a picture of pulmonary tuberculosis without the presence of tubercle bacilli. Bronchiectasis in children may be due to syphilis.

A Form Suggesting Tuberculosis.—Areas may be involved either at the root, or at the apex or base of the lung. The physical signs are much as in tuberculosis. There may be cough, possibly with a good deal of sputum, sometimes blood-streaked, loss of weight and fever, with signs at one apex or base. The picture may suggest tuberculosis but tubercle bacilli are not found. The condition may persist for a considerable time without very marked change. The *diagnosis* is difficult. C. P. Howard gives the following points as important: (1) Symptoms out of proportion to the physical signs; (2) absence of tubercle bacilli; (3) history; (4) a positive Wassermann reaction; (5) evidence of syphilis elsewhere; and (6) the therapeutic test. The signs may suggest advanced tuberculosis. In one case, a man aged twenty-seven had cough and bloody expectoration for a year and died of severe hemoptysis. There were extensive caseous gummata throughout both lungs, with much fibrous thickening, and in a lower lobe a cavity 3 by 5 cm. in diameter, on the wall of which a branch of the pulmonary artery was eroded.

A majority of authors follow Virchow in recognizing the fibrous interstitial pneumonia at the root of the lung and passing along the bronchi and vessels as probably syphilitic. This much may be said, that in certain cases gummata are associated with these fibroid changes. Again, this condition alone is found in persons with well-marked syphilitic history or with other visceral lesions. It seems in many instances to be a purely sclerotic process, advancing sometimes from the pleura, more commonly from the root of the lung, and invading the interlobular tissue, gradually producing a more or less extensive fibroid change. It rarely involves more than a portion of a lobe or portions of lobes at the root of the lung. The bronchi are often dilated.

Diagnosis.—Physicians and pathologists the world over bear witness to the extreme rarity of lung syphilis. The therapeutic test upon which so much reliance is placed is by no means conclusive. With pulmonary tuberculosis there should be no confusion, owing to the readiness with which tubercle bacilli are found. Bronchiectasis in a lower lobe, dependent upon an interstitial fibrosis of syphilitic origin, could not be distinguished from any other form of the disease. Tuberculosis in a syphilitic subject has no special peculiarities and the lesions of syphilis and tuberculosis can coexist in a lung.

Prognosis.—Evidently this depends on the character of the lesions as fibrosis cannot be greatly influenced. In general the patients can be markedly helped if not made well.

Syphilis of the Liver

Varieties.—*Congenital.*—Gubler in 1852 described the diffuse hepatitis which occurs in a large percentage of all deaths in congenital lues. While there may be little or no macroscopic change, the liver preserves its form and is usually enlarged, hard and resistant, and has a yellowish color, compared by Trousseau to sole-leather. Small grayish nodules may be seen on the section. In other cases there are definite gummata with extensive sclerosis. The spirochaetes are present in extraordinary numbers.

The child may be still-born, die shortly after birth, or may be healthy when born and the liver enlarges within a few weeks. The organ is firm; the edge may be readily felt, usually far below the navel. The spleen is also enlarged. The features are those of cirrhosis, but jaundice and ascites are not common. Hochsinger states that of 45 cases recovery took place in 30.

Delayed Congenital Syphilis.—The condition is by no means rare. Of 132 cases of syphilis hereditaria tarda collected by Forbes, in 34 the liver was involved. The children are nearly always ill-developed, sometimes with marked clubbing of the fingers and showing signs of infantilism. Jaundice is rare. The liver is usually enlarged or it may show nodular masses.

Acquired Syphilis.—In the *secondary* and sometimes in the *primary stage* the liver may be slightly enlarged. Jaundice may occur coincident with the rash and the adenitis. Rolleston thinks it is probably due to a catarrhal condition of the smaller ducts, part of a general syphilitic hepatitis. There are cases in which it has passed on to acute yellow atrophy. The prognosis is generally good.

Tertiary Lesions.—The frequency of syphilis of the liver in adults is variously estimated. J. L. Allen found 37 cases of hepatic gummata among 11,629 autopsies at St. George's Hospital; in 27 cases cicatrices alone were present. Flexner at the Philadelphia Hospital found 88 cases of hepatic syphilis among 5,088 autopsies. Among 2,300 autopsies at the Johns Hopkins Hospital there were 47 cases of syphilis of the liver, gummata in 19, scars in 16, cirrhosis in 21 cases; 6 of the cases were congenital. Some hold that syphilis is an important factor in the etiology of portal cirrhosis.

Anatomically the lesions may be gummata, scars or a syphilitic sclerosis. The gummata range in size from a pea to an orange. When small they are pale and gray; the larger ones present yellowish centres; but later there is a "pale, yellowish, cheese-like nodule of irregular outline, surrounded by a fibrous zone, the outer edge of which loses itself in the lobular tissue, the lobules dwindling gradually in its grasp" (Wilks). They may form enormous tumors, as in the remarkable one figured in Rolleston's work on Diseases of the Liver. They may be felt as large as an orange in the epigastrium and may disappear with the same extraordinary rapidity as the subcutaneous gumma. Macroscopically they may look like a massive cancer. Extensive caseation, softening and calcification may occur. The syphilitic scars are usually linear or star-shaped. They may be numerous and divide the liver into small sections—the so-called botryoid organ, of which a remarkable example is figured in the Lectures on Abdominal Tumors (Osler).

Symptoms.—In the first place, the clinical picture may be that of cirrhosis —slight jaundice, fever, portal obstruction, ascites. The liver is enlarged and may be smooth. There may not be the slightest suspicion of the syphilitic nature of the case. One of our patients had been tapped thirteen times before admission to the hospital. The diagnosis was made by finding gummata on the shins. She recovered promptly.

In a second group the liver is enlarged, sometimes with a marked round prominence. The surface may be smooth throughout or with nodular enlargement in places. In a number of these cases amyloid change may have occurred.

Thirdly, in a very important group the symptoms are those of tumor of the liver, causing pain and distress, and on examination an irregular or nodular mass is discovered. A *friction rub* may be heard over it. Naturally carcinoma is thought of, as there may be nothing to suggest syphilis. Lastly, irregular fever with enlargement and irregularity of the liver may suggest suppuration or gallbladder disease, or the uniform great enlargement of the organ hypertrophic biliary cirrhosis, while in some cases the spleen is so greatly enlarged, the anemia so pronounced and the liver so contracted that the diagnosis of splenic anemia is made.

Diagnosis.—Syphilis of the liver is much commoner clinically than the autopsy figures suggest. It should be considered in every case of hepatic disease in which the diagnosis is obscure and in some in which it seems clear. The liver may show a great variety of changes. Relatively greater enlargement of the *left lobe* is always suggestive of syphilis. The spleen is often enlarged. Signs of syphilis elsewhere are important and the therapeutic test is of value because the response is usually so marked. This applies particularly to the fever which usually disappears within two or three days after iodide is begun. The Wassermann reaction is *negative* in a proportion of the cases and no weight should be given to its absence. It may be given by the ascitic fluid when the blood is negative.

Prognosis.—This is better than in other forms of visceral syphilis if recognized before marked damage is done. The recurrence of symptoms after thorough treatment is rare. Arsenic compounds should not be given on account of the danger of severe damage to the liver cells.

Syphilis of the Digestive Tract

The base of the *tongue* may show obliteration of the usual surface markings with smoothness of the surface and induration of the tissues due to fibroid change. Gummata and diffuse glossitis may occur. The *salivary glands* are rarely involved, the parotid most often. The *esophagus* may show esophagitis in the acute stage. Later a gumma may be present followed by ulceration, infiltration, fibrosis and stenosis. There is pain with difficulty in swallowing and, if there is obstruction, malignant disease may be diagnosed. Examination with the *esophagoscope* and the serological tests are important. The frequency of syphilis of the *stomach* is difficult to estimate. There is no definite clinical picture, the symptoms depending on the site and extent of the lesion. There may be the usual features of dyspepsia or ulcer, or the findings may suggest carcinoma. Hemorrhage is rare. A positive serological test and rapid improvement under specific treatment are suggestive, but gastric disease and ulcer in patients with syphilis are not necessarily due to it. The X-ray study usually shows a circumscribed or diffuse involvement which may lessen peristalsis and cause contraction. The frequency of syphilis of the *pancreas* is uncertain. Warthin regarded interstitial pancreatitis as common in latent syphilis. The *spleen* is often enlarged with or without liver involvement. Syphilis of the intestine is very rare. The jejunum is usually affected; the lesions may be multiple, tend to encircle the bowel and cause stenosis. The diagnosis is difficult as the signs suggest neoplasm.

Syphilis of the *rectum* is most common in women, and results from the growth of gummata in the submucosa above the internal sphincter. The symptoms are usually those of narrowing of the lower bowel. The condition is recognized by rectal examination. The history of gradual oncoming stricture, the state of the patient, and the fact that there is a hard, fibrous narrowing, not an elevated crater-like ulcer, usually render easy the diagnosis from malignant disease. These cases may come under observation for other symptoms, particularly amyloid degeneration; the rectal disease may be overlooked and only discovered postmortem. A rare condition is multiple fissures of the anus.

Circulatory System

Syphilis of the Heart.—A fresh *endocarditis* due to syphilis is not recognized, though occasionally in persons dead of the disease this form is present, as is not uncommon in conditions of debility. The frequent involvement of the aortic valves is due to extension from the aorta.

Involvement of the *myocardium* may occur in the secondary stage or within two or three years of the primary lesion. Epicardial changes, with peri-arteritis, are common. The *symptoms* are those of slight cardiac insufficiency with a varying amount of precordial pain, sometimes vague, sometimes severe and localized. There may be increase in rate and some irregularity with a soft apex systolic murmur, not transmitted, and increased by exercise. Later the signs are those of more marked myocarditis with pain and precordial tenderness; the pain may suggest angina pectoris. The association of pain with signs of myocarditis in a young adult should suggest the possibility of syphilis. The pain differs in position from that of acute aortitis which may be associated with it. Dyspnea is often marked. There may be definite myocardial failure. Treatment often results in rapid improvement. Rupture or sudden death may take place.

The frequency of late syphilitic involvement of the *myocardium* is difficult to state. Warthin held that it was common but the weight of opinion is against this view. How often are fibroid areas due to syphilis? Some regard these as often of syphilitic origin; others consider them as more often the result of coronary artery sclerosis. The coronary arteries are not often the seat of syphilitic disease in their course; syphilis of the aorta often involves them at their origin. The most important effect of syphilis on the heart is secondary to syphilitic aortitis with extension to the aortic valves and the production of aortic insufficiency.

Syphilis of the Arteries.—Syphilis plays an important rôle in aortitis and aneurism. Its connection with these processes will be considered later; here we refer to the syphilitic affection of the pulmonary arteries and smaller vessels, which occurs in two forms:

An *obliterating endarteritis,* characterized by a proliferation of the subendothelial tissue. The basic lesion is a periarteritis to which the endarteritis may be secondary. The new growth lies within the elastic lamina, and may gradually fill the entire lumen; hence the term obliterating. The media and adventitia are also infiltrated with small cells. This form of endarteritis is not characteristic of syphilis, and its presence alone in an artery could not be considered pathognomonic.

Gummatous Periarteritis.—Nodular gummata may develop in the adventitia of the artery, producing globular or ovoid swellings, which may attain considerable size. They are not infrequent in the cerebral arteries, which seem to be specially prone to this affection. This form is distinctive of syphilis. *Treponema pallidum* has been found in the syphilitic aortitis and also in gummatous arteritis of the cerebral vessels.

Pulmonary arteries.—Syphilis of these vessels is apparently rare and is not often recognized. The main clinical features are dyspnea and cyanosis with hemoptysis occurring occasionally. Emphysema and chronic bronchitis are marked. The right heart is enlarged and aortitis is usually present. In the *diagnosis,* absence of previous bronchial, pulmonary or cardiac disease which might cause the symptoms is important. In the later stages there is progressive myocardial failure with a regular pulse. There are so many other causes for a similar picture that a positive diagnosis is not often possible. There is no agreement as to whether Ayerza's disease in all cases represents syphilis of the pulmonary arteries.

Syphilis of the Urinary Tract

Kidney.—Acute nephritis is estimated to occur in the secondary stage in 3 to 4 per cent, and may appear in from three to six months, sometimes later, from the initial lesion. The outlook is good, though often the albuminuria may persist for months; more rarely chronic nephritis follows. In a few instances syphilitic nephritis has proved rapidly fatal in a few weeks. Both in congenital and acquired syphilis there may be a marked localization of the spirochetes in the kidneys with evidence of excretion, chiefly in the convoluted tubules. The spirochaetes have been found in the urine in a few cases. Rich (1932) described minute areas beneath the capsule and in the cortex in the secondary stage and later scars of varying size are found. Dense accumulations of round cells in the interstitial tissue may obliterate adjoining tubules. *Gummata* occasionally are found in the kidneys, particularly in cases with extensive gummatous hepatitis. Clinically the affection is not recognizable.

Bladder.—This is not common, but should be considered with unexplained frequency of painful urination and hematuria. Papilloma may be simulated and a gumma may suggest carcinoma. Involvement of the *prostate* is very rare. Warthin found the spirochaetes in one case in the prostate.

Syphilis of the Reproductive Organs

Testicle and Epididymis.—The testicle is a favorite site for the spirochaetes to settle. Orchitis occurs in congenital syphilis but is specially frequent in the acquired form. It occurs in two forms, interstitial and nodular (gumma), which may exist together. In the *interstitial* form the testicle (usually one only) is painless, enlarged, smooth, not tender, the testicular sensation often being absent, heavy and with a distinct feeling of induration. Atrophy may follow. In the *nodular* form the testicle is irregular and if necrosis occurs the walls of the scrotum are involved with ulceration. The diagnosis has to be made from tuberculosis and neoplasm. The *epididymis* is involved rarely, with or without orchitis. A subacute process of short duration may occur in the secondary stage and later there may be induration or a gumma. Syphilis of the *cord* is very rare.

Syphilis of the *ovary* in the form of a gumma has been reported. Gummata and marked vascular changes occur in the uterus but are rare.

Mammary Gland.—Syphilitic mastitis is found most often in women, is usually unilateral and occurs in acquired and congenital cases. There is a chronic diffuse hard infiltration or local nodules. The skin is rarely involved. The axillary glands may be enlarged. The condition is very like carcinoma; the Wassermann reaction and thereapeutic test are important.

In *pregnancy* the manifestations may be mild and some have found the serological tests variable during pregnancy and after delivery.

DIAGNOSIS, TREATMENT, ETC.

Diagnosis.—GENERAL DIAGNOSIS.—There is seldom any doubt concerning the recognition of syphilitic lesions; but the number of persons, without any evident sign of the disease, in whom a positive serological reaction is found proves that a negative diagnosis cannot be based on the absence of history and clinical manifestations. Syphilis is common in the community, and is no respecter of age, sex, or station in life. The primary sore may have been of trifling extent, or urethral and masked by a gonorrhea, and the patient may not have had severe secondary symptoms, or the infection may occur without any chancre and the secondary lesions may be so slight that they are not noticed. Inquiries should be made into the history to ascertain if the patient has had skin rashes, sore throat, or if the hair has fallen out. Careful inspection should be made of the throat and skin for signs of old lesions. Skin lesions with induration or scarring and a crescentic shape should excite suspicion. The cicatrices on the legs are often copper-colored, though this cannot be regarded as peculiar to syphilis. The bones should be examined for nodes. The scar of the primary sore may be found or there may be atrophy or induration of the testes. In women the occurrence of miscarriages and the bearing of stillborn children are always suggestive. In doubtful cases the study of the spinal fluid is important.

In the congenital disease, the occurrence within the first three months of snuffles and skin rash is conclusive. Later, the characters of the syphilitic facies often give a clew to the nature of some obscure visceral lesion. Other distinctive features are the symmetrical development of nodes on the bones and the interstitial keratitis. With a suspicion of congenital syphilis, a complete study of the family history may give valuable aid.

The *Treponema pallidum* may be found in the fresh lesion. After cleaning carefully, serum is sucked out and the living spirochaetes may be seen in the special "dark field" apparatus.

SERUM DIAGNOSIS.—The complement fixation test in good hands is a most valuable aid. It is obtained in the great majority of cases of syphilis with manifestations. The results in tabes and general paresis are very constant. But too much dependence should not be placed on the serological tests, especially if negative. It is only one piece of evidence even if a valuable one. In congenital syphilis and in visceral disease it may be negative. Great caution should be used in the interpretation of "weakly positive" serological tests.

Much harm has resulted from a conclusion that such mean a positive diagnosis of syphilis.

THERAPEUTIC TEST.—In a doubtful case, as, for example, an obstinate skin rash or an obscure tumor in the abdomen, antisyphilitic treatment may prove successful, but this cannot always be relied upon.

Prognosis.—As regards life, a fatal result is rare in the early stages in the acquired but frequent in the congenital form. When manifestations are present at birth or appear shortly after it the outlook is always serious. As regards the ultimate result in general who can say? We are certain that the more efficient the early treatment, the better is the ultimate outlook. To completely rid the body of the spirochetal infection is probably possible only early in the course of the infection. As regards the later lesions prognosis should always be guarded. To estimate the possible late dangers of a syphilitic infection is impossible.

Prophylaxis.—Irregular intercourse has existed from the beginning of recorded history, and unless man's nature wholly changes—and of this we can have no hope—will continue. Resisting all attempts at solution, the social evil remains a great blot upon our civilization, and inextricably blended with it is the question of the prevention of syphilis.

Personal purity is the prophylaxis which we, as physicians, are especially bound to advocate. Continence may be a hard condition (to some harder than to others), but it can be borne, and it is our duty to urge this lesson upon young and old who seek our advice in matters sexual. Certainly it is better, as St. Paul says, to marry than to burn, but if the former is not feasible there are other altars than those of Venus upon which a young man may light fires. He may practise at least two of the five means by which, as the physician Rondibilis counseled Panurge, carnal concupiscence may be cooled and quelled —hard work of body and hard work of mind. Idleness is the mother of lechery; and a young man will find that absorption in any pursuit will do much to cool passions which, though natural and proper, cannot in the exigencies of our civilization always obtain natural and proper gratification.

To carry out successfully any administrative measures seems hopeless, at any rate in our Anglo-Saxon civilization. The state accepts the responsibility of guarding citizens against smallpox or cholera, but in dealing with syphilis the problem has been too complex and has baffled solution. Inspection, segregation, and regulation are impossible to carry out, and public sentiment is bitterly opposed to this plan. The compulsory registration of every patient with gonorrhea and syphilis, with greatly increased facilities for thorough treatment, offers a more acceptable alternative. Tracing the source of infection and the effort to find possible contacts, as would be done with the other pox, with proper treatment of the infected is important. With this goes the need of "follow-up" measures to ensure that treatment is carried out for a sufficient time. The need of care to prevent accidental infection should be emphasized to nurses and ever present in the minds of physicians. The prevention of congenital syphilis is largely a matter of proper treatment of syphilitic women, especially when pregnant. Children born of parents who have had syphilis should be carefully examined and treated if necessary—sometimes on suspicion only.

The patient should be warned of the various ways in which he may spread the disease and given directions regarding this. Measures for the prevention of infection after exposure in males can be carried out in the military and naval services more efficiently than in civil life. Thorough cleansing followed by the application of calomel ointment after exposure seems to be the most efficient.

Treatment.—That the later stages which come under the charge of the physician are so common results, in great part, from the carelessness of the patient, who, wearied with treatment, cannot understand why he should continue to take treatment after all the symptoms have disappeared; but, in part, the profession also is to blame for not insisting more urgently that acquired syphilis is not cured in a few months, but takes at least three years, during which time the patient should be under careful supervision.

Certain general principles may be stated regarding treatment when the diagnosis is made early. Active treatment should be kept up for eighteen months. Arsenic should be given first and while arsphenamine is more efficient, for the general practitioner the use of neoarsphenamine is to be preferred. A total of 20 to 30 injections of an arsenic preparation should be given. These may be alternated with the use of a heavy metal, bismuth or mercury, and it is well to let whichever one is used overlap the use of the arsenic preparation. The weight of opinion to-day is that arsenic and bismuth are more efficient than arsenic and mercury. Treatment should be on a regular plan and not governed by the serological tests for one year at any rate after the symptoms disappear. The patient should be followed for at least three years with studies of the blood and spinal fluid.

The patient should lead a regular life, avoiding excess of all kinds. If there is fever rest in bed is advisable. The usual diet can be taken and the patient should drink large quantities of water. The use of alcohol and tobacco should be forbidden during active treatment. When mercury is being taken special care must be given to the mouth, a mouth wash and a potassium chlorate tooth paste being used frequently. Treatment to rid the body of spirochetes consists in the use of arsenic, bismuth and mercury preparations; iodide influences certain of the tissue changes resulting from the infection.

Energetic treatment in the early stages should be started as soon as the diagnosis is made.

There is a marked difference between the early and late stages. In the former the object is to kill the spirochaetes and, for this, treatment should be prompt, energetic and thorough. With ordinary care there is slight danger of injuring the patient. In the late stages the problem is very different. There is a chronic spirochaetal infection, which in many cases, perhaps the majority, can not be "cured" but there is also a patient who may be injured by too vigorous treatment. The patient must be considered more than his disease. The Wassermann reaction must be considered as one of several indications and not the only one. A negative reaction is not always an indication to stop treatment. Insufficient treatment, especially with arsenic, may do more harm than good.

Treatment should be continuous and for at least eighteen months. Rest periods favor relapse. The combination of arsenic and bismuth compounds seems the most efficient. They may be given concurrently or in alternate courses. A total of 30 injections each of an arsenic and bismuth compound may be regarded as an average amount. After this bismuth or mercury may be given without arsenic.

Many things influence the dose of *arsphenamine*. In general the weight of the patient is a good guide. For young children doses of 0.1 to 0.15 gm. are used and for infants 0.02 to 0.1 gm. Changes in the eye grounds and severe circulatory and renal lesions always suggest caution and may be contraindications. In such cases doses of 0.2 gm. are the usual maximum. In general the dose of *neoarsphenamine* may be considered as slightly less than double that of arsphenamine. Many modifications of the original preparation have been introduced. Sulpharsphenamine has the advantage of intramuscular injection.

BISMUTH.—There is considerable difference of opinion as to the use of soluble or insoluble preparations. In general, the use of the former seems preferable. All administration should be intramuscular, not intravenous. Present opinion is that bismuth is preferable to mercury in the early stages when arsenic preparations are being given.

MERCURY.—Salivation is to be avoided and mercury should be used very cautiously if there is nephritis. *Inunction* is the most effective means of administration. One-half to a dram (2-4 gm.) of mercurial ointment or oleate of mercury is thoroughly rubbed into the skin, on areas free from hair, daily for six days; on the seventh a warm bath is taken. It is well to apply the ointment to different places on successive days. The sides of the chest and abdomen and the inner surfaces of the arms and thighs are the best positions. Thirty inunctions is an average number for each course. *Intramuscular* injection is also satisfactory, care being taken to avoid infection and to give the injections deeply. Mercury salicylate (gr. i-ii, 0.06-0.12 gm.) in a 10 per cent solution is probably the best, an injection being given every five to seven days. Bichloride of mercury (gr. 1/20-1/10, 0.003-0.006 gm.) in olive oil and biniodide of mercury (gr. 1/6, 0.01 gm.), are also used. A course of twenty to thirty injections should be given. *Intravenous* injections are sometimes given, usually of the bichloride (♏ xv, 1 cc. of a 0.1 to 0.2 per cent solution in sterile salt solution). By *mouth* the gray powder, hydrargyrum cum creta, in one grain (0.065 gm.) doses with a grain of Dover's powder, may be given. The bichloride (gr. 1/16-1/8, 0.004-0.008 gm.), the biniodide (gr. 1/16, 0.004 gm.) and the protoiodide (gr. 1/4, 0.016 gm.) may also be used. It is well for the profession not to forget that mercury is still in existence; some men seem to have forgotten it. It is particularly useful in the late stages.

The Wassermann reaction should be tried every three months for three years and active treatment resumed if it is positive. No one can be regarded as free of the disease from a negative blood test alone; the spinal fluid should be studied also. While the Wassermann reaction is a helpful guide in treatment it is not always possible to secure a negative reaction. In such cases the character and duration of treatment must be decided for each patient. In later stages harm may be done by too energetic treatment. If mercury by mouth or the "mixed" treatment is used, it should be only after a thorough course of arsenic and bismuth. These have their place in the intervals between or after more intensive treatment.

In *congenital syphilis* the treatment of patients born with bullae and other signs of the disease is not satisfactory, and the infants usually die within a short time. The child should be nursed by the mother alone, or, if this is not feasible, should be hand-fed, but under no circumstances should a wet-nurse be employed. Neoarsphenamine is generally used. The child is most rapidly and thoroughly brought under the influence of mercury by inunction. The mercurial ointment may be smeared on the flannel binder. This is not a very cleanly method, and sometimes rouses the suspicion of the mother. The drug may be given by mouth, in the form of gray powder, half a grain (0.03 gm.) three times a day. In the late manifestations associated with bone lesions the combination of mercury and iodide of potassium is suitable and is well given in the form of Gilbert's syrup, which consists of biniodide of mercury (gr. j, 0.065 gm.), potassium iodide (℥ss, 15 gm.), and water (℥ij, 60 cc.). Of this the dose for a child under three is from five to ten drops three times a day, gradually increased. The medication should be continued at intervals for many months, and it is well to watch these patients carefully during the period of second dentition and at puberty, and give them treatment again.

In the treatment of the *visceral lesions*, iodide is of great value. The iodide saturates the unsaturated fatty acid radicals which inhibit autolysis. The ferments then become active, autolysis follows and the necrotic tissue is absorbed. Under its use ulcers rapidly heal and gummatous tumors melt away. It is as a rule well borne in an initial dose of 10 grains (0.6 gm.); given in milk the patient does not notice the taste. It should be gradually increased to 30 or more grains three times a day if necessary. In syphilis of the nervous system it may be used in still larger doses. For neurosyphilis, tryparsamide and fever therapy (as by malaria or typhoid vaccine intravenously) probably give the best results.

In *aortic* syphilis it is wiser not to give arsenic at first. Mercury or bismuth may be given for a time, always with iodide. If neoarsphenamine is given it should be in a very small dose (0.1 gm.) at first. For *hepatic* syphilis the combination of mercury and iodide is most satisfactory; *arsenic should not be given.* If there is ascites, Addison's or Guy's pill (as it is often called) of mercury, digitalis, and squill will be found useful. Occasionally the iodide of sodium is more satisfactory than the potassium salt. It is less depressing and agrees better with the stomach.

Syphilis and Marriage.—Upon this question the family physician is often called to decide. He should insist upon the necessity of at least three years elapsing between the infection and marriage. This is the earliest possible limit, and marriage should be allowed only if the treatment has been thorough, at least two years have passed without any manifestations, and the serological test is negative in the blood and spinal fluid.

Syphilis and Life Insurance.—An individual with syphilis can not be regarded as a first-class risk unless he can furnish evidence of prolonged and thorough treatment and of immunity for two or three years from all manifestations. Even then, when we consider the extraordinary frequency of the cerebral and vascular complications in persons who have undergone thorough treatment, the risk to the company is certainly increased.

Yaws (*Framboesia*).—This is a disease much like syphilis, prevalent in Africa, parts of Asia, the West Indies and tropical America, caused by *Treponema pertenue* (*Spirochaeta pertenuis* or *pallidula*). Its relation to syphilis is in dispute. The disease may have been present and unrecognized in the Southern States. It is particularly a disease of children and is readily communicated from one to another. The primary lesion is a papule which later shows a fungoid appearance; in the secondary stage similar lesions develop generally. The skin lesions consist of raspberry-like growths from which a seropurulent fluid exudes, or they are covered by a yellow crust. The secondary general eruption has the same character and is widespread. The mucous membranes are not involved. There may be fever, headache and general malaise. The course is from a few months to three years. Late lesions, such as gummatous nodules and deep ulceration, may occur. A positive Wassermann reaction is given. The mortality is low. Neoarsphenamine is specific and its use results in a rapid cure, usually after one injection. Bismuth preparatons and sulpharsphenamine are also effectual. Stovarsol (0.25 gm.) is given by mouth.

SPIROCHAETOSIS ICTEROHAEMORRHAGICA

An acute disease, due to a spirochaete and also termed spirochaetal jaundice, characterized by jaundice in the majority of cases and occasionally by hemorrhages or purpura. This infection was first discovered in Japan in 1914 by Inada and Ido. It occurred during the Great War in various areas and was extensively studied. The organism is *Spirochaeta icterohaemorrhagicae*, which is found in rats, the infection possibly occurring by contamination of earth and water by their urine. It appears to be a disease of temperate climates.

Pathology.—Death apparently results from toxemia, and changes sufficient to cause death are not found in the organs, except in a few cases showing acute yellow atrophy of the liver. Marked duodenitis has been found in some cases. Nephritis with hemorrhagic and degenerative changes may be present. This is probably associated with the occurrence of the spirochaetes in the urine.

Symptoms.—The onset is usually acute with chills, headache, general pains, vomiting, diarrhea and marked prostration. Fever follows, reaching 102° or higher. *Jaundice* appears about the fourth day, reaching its maximum about the tenth day, and may be intense. In some cases it does not appear. The stools are usually clay-colored. The liver is enlarged and there is tenderness in the upper abdomen. The spleen is not enlarged. Herpes is common and often becomes hemorrhagic. There may be other hemorrhagic features, bleeding from the mucous membranes or purpura. Acute bronchitis is common; the pulse rate may be slow in proportion to the fever. *Myositis* is common, the muscles being tender and sometimes swollen. *Nephritis* has occurred in some series with marked renal insufficiency. Meningitis may occur. The course varies; the fever persists for about ten days; the jaundice usually lessens as the fever diminishes. The *mortality* is high in Japan, 30 per cent, but in some of the army series only 4 or 5 per cent.

Diagnosis.—The spirochaetes are found in the blood for the first five or seven days. They may be found on examination or the infection may be conveyed to guinea-pigs by the intraperitoneal injection of blood. The guinea-pig is very susceptible; a severe infection results and the spirochaetes are easily demonstrated. Spirochaetes are found in the patient's urine after the tenth day and sometimes for weeks. They are agglutinated by the patient's blood after the second week. From other forms of infectious jaundice the marked features of this form, the presence of spirochaetes and the agglutination test, usually present by the second week, are diagnostic.

Treatment.—Rest, fluid diet, water freely, alkalies and open bowels by salines and enemata comprise the general management. Serum treatment has been used apparently with benefit. The giving of neoarsphenamine has not proved of value.

RAT-BITE FEVER (SODOKU)

An infection, following rat-bite, characterized by febrile paroxysms which may recur at intervals for months.

The disease has been known in China and Japan for several centuries. The features are very unusual. There is a prolonged period of incubation, lasting in some cases for many months. The wound, which has run the ordinary course and perhaps healed, becomes swollen, red, and eroded; an ulcer forms and the regional lymph glands are involved. The *fever* sets in suddenly with a chill and lasts three or four days. With its onset there is a skin rash, either erythema or a blotchy eruption somewhat resembling measles. The patient feels very ill, there may be pains in the muscles and joints and sometimes delirium. After persisting for a few days, usually seven or eight, the temperature falls and the patient feels well. After a varying interval of from a few days to a couple of weeks the attack is repeated, and this may go on for several months or, according to the Japanese reports, for several years. The intervals may be very regular in a given case. The outlook is favorable; the mortality is highest in Japan, 10 per cent.

Various organisms have been described but the weight of evidence is in favor of *Spirillum minus* being the causal agent. Its exact nature is in dispute. Patients recovered after treatment by mercury or arsphenamine. Schotmüller, Blake, and Tileston each found a streptothrix in their cases. In Tileston's case the organisms were found in fresh smears by dark-field illumination. Blake isolated a streptothrix in a case which at autopsy showed endocarditis, in the vegetations of which the same organism was found.

Treatment.—The wound should be cauterized, neoarsphenamine given intravenously, and the febrile paroxysms treated symptomatically.

DISEASES DUE TO PARASITIC INFUSORIA

Flagellate Dysentery.—Several varieties of flagellates may cause disease. The main features are recurrent attacks of colic and diarrhea, the passage of mucus and sometimes blood, tenderness of the bowel, sometimes leukocytosis and eosinophilia, and neurasthenia. Mucus passed from the bowel may contain large numbers of flagellates. Cases of infection with several flagellates are common. In treatment, liquid diet should be given, the bowels moved freely, and a course of thymol given, followed by irrigation of the colon with weak solutions of quinine. Later, bismuth iodide (gr. i, 0.06 gm.) is given once a day and the dose increased to gr. ii, 0.12 gm.

Trichomoniasis.—This infection (*Trichomonas hominis*) is common and flagellates are found in many parts of the body. They occur in the bronchi and are found in bronchitis and bronchiectasis. In the intestinal tract they may cause indigestion and diarrhea. Secondary anemia may result. In one of

Dock's cases the parasites were associated with a hemorrhagic cystitis without bacteria.

Giardiasis.—The parasite, *Giardia lamblia,* may be responsible for intermittent diarrhea or dysentery. The onset is often insidious and the condition tends to become chronic. The general condition of the patient may be markedly affected. It is often found in the duodenum and gallbladder. Flagellates have been found in the sputum in cases of gangrene of the lung and bronchiectasis, and in the exudate of pleurisy. Mercurochrome in enteric coated capsules, gr. 1½-iii (0.1-0.2 gm.), may be given three times daily for two weeks.

Ciliate Dysentery.—*Balantidium coli,* oval, 70 μ to 100 μ long and 50 μ to 70 μ broad, may be pathogenic. The parasites are found in the stools and on the mucous membrane, and also in the mucosa and submucosa. Apparently they do not extend beyond the wall of the bowel. They cause diarrhea and dysentery and anemia may result. In *treatment* good results are reported from oil of chenopodium, 15 cc. in 150 cc. of olive oil, introduced into the bowel with the patient in the knee-chest position, and retained for two hours.

DISEASES DUE TO METAZOAN PARASITES

DISEASES DUE TO FLUKES—DISTOMATOSIS

The Trematoda or flukes have flat or leaf-shaped bodies. The term *Distomatosis* (*Distomiasis*) is based upon Distoma, the term being used to designate the trematodes.

The following are the important clinical forms:

Pulmonary Distomatosis; Parasitic Hemoptysis.—*Paragonimus westermanii,* the Asiatic lung or bronchial fluke, is from 8 to 16 mm. in length by 4 to 8 mm. broad, and of a pinkish or reddish-brown color.

It is found extensively in China and Japan, Formosa, and the Philippines; cases are occasionally imported into Europe and America, and have been met with in the oriental population of the Pacific coast. It has been found in the United States in the cat, dog and hog.

Clinically the disease is characterized by a chronic cough, with rusty-brown sputum, and occasional attacks of hemoptysis, usually trifling, but sometimes very severe. The disease is easily mistaken for tuberculosis, but the diagnosis is readily made by microscopic examination of the sputum. The ova, which are abundant in the sputum, are oval, smooth, and measure from 80 μ to 100 μ in length by 40 μ to 60 μ in breath. The parasites may affect other organs—the liver, the brain, and eyelid.

Hepatic Distomatosis.—Several species of liver flukes occur in man. (1) The common liver fluke—*Fasciola hepatica*—is common in ruminants. It is a rare and accidental parasite in man, but in Syria a disease called *Halzoun* is caused by eating raw goat-liver infected with the parasite. (2) The lancet fluke—*Dicrocoelium lanceatum.* (3) *Opisthorchis felineus,* found in Prussia and Siberia, and by Ward in cats in Nebraska. (4) *Opisthorchis noverca*—the Indian liver fluke described in man by McConnell. (5) *Clonorchis sinensis* and *C. endemicus,* the most important of the liver flukes, occur extensively in Japan, China, and India. The eggs are oval, 27 μ to 30 μ by 15 μ to 17 μ, dark brown, with sharply defined operculum. Imported cases have been found in Canada and the United States. White found 18 cases in San Francisco.

The *symptoms* of hepatic distomiasis are best described in connection with the last form. Young children are the chief sufferers and many members of a family are usually affected. In some villages a large proportion of the inhabitants are attacked. Among important symptoms is an irregular, intermittent diarrhea; at first there may or may not be blood. The liver enlarges and cirrhosis gradually comes on. There may be pain and intermittent jaundice. There is not much fever. After two or three years dropsy comes on, with anasarca and ascites. Even then transient recovery may take place, but as a rule there is a recurrence, and the patient dies after many years of illness. The ova of the parasite are readily found in the stools. In *treatment*, gentian violet is given by mouth (gr. i, 0.065 gm. in enteric coated pills) three times a day for some weeks.

Intestinal Distomatosis.—In India and China the *Fasciolopsis buskii* is found in the small intestines. A progressive anemia, weakness, diarrhea, edema and ascites are the main clinical features. Thymol, beta-naphthol and carbon tetrachloride have been used in treatment.

Hemic Distamotosis; Bilharziasis.—This is an important parasitic disease, caused by the flood fluke, *Schistosoma haematobium* (*Bilharzia haematobia*). Endemic hematuria has been known for many years, particularly in Egypt, where in 1851 Bilharz discovered the parasite of the disease. It prevails in Africa, Arabia, Persia, India, China, Japan, the West Indies and South America. Imported cases are found in Europe and occasionally in the United States. In Egypt, among 11,698 patients admitted to the Cairo Hospital, 1,270 were infected (Madden). Of 500 autopsies at this hospital, in 8 per cent death was due to the effects of Bilharzial disease. The seriousness of the condition in Egypt is illustrated by the fact that in 7.5 per cent of army recruits the ova are found in the urine.

Other forms are *Schistosoma mansoni,* found in the veins, and *S. japonicum* found in the blood vessels and intestine.

The *parasite* has the sexes separate, and the male usually carries the female in a gynecophorous canal. The eggs are characteristic, oval in shape, 0.16 mm. by 0.06 mm., and one end has a terminal spine. The eggs hatch in water, and emerging from the egg the miracidium enters a snail and becomes transformed into sporocysts and daughter sporocysts, in which numbers of cercariae develop. These escape into the water, penetrate the skin of man, travel to the portal veins and liver, where in six to ten weeks they mature to adult trematodes. They travel to various parts of the body, particularly to the veins of the bladder and rectum, mate and produce the terminal spined eggs which escape with the urine. A majority of the parasites remain in the tissues and cause irritation, fibroid changes, and papillomata in the bladder and rectum. Collecting in the bladder as foreign bodies they form the nuclei of calculi.

Symptoms.—They may cause no inconvenience. Irritability of the bladder, dull pain in the perineum and hematuria are the most frequent symptoms. A chronic cystitis follows when the walls of the bladder are much thickened by the irritation caused by the ova. The anemia caused by the hemorrhage is slight in comparison with that of uncinariasis. There is leukocytosis with eosinophilia. When the rectum is involved there are straining and tenesmus, with the passage of mucus and blood; in severe cases large papillomata form and a chronic ulcerative proctitis. There may be a chronic vaginitis. Calculi form in the kidney and bladder and periurethral abscess and perineal fistulae are common in chronic cases.

Few symptoms are caused by the presence of the parasites in the portal veins, but there may be an advanced *cirrhosis* of a Glissonian type due to an enormous thickening of the periportal tissues (Symmers). This author also reported an instance of Bilharzia in the pulmonary blood in a case of Bilharzial colitis, and the worms were found living in the pulmonary circulation. The *diagnosis* is made by finding the characteristic ova in the bloody urine or in the blood and mucus from the rectum.

Schistosoma mansoni involves the rectum especially. After a period of abdominal symptoms with leukocytosis and eosinophilia, dysentery appears with hepatic and pancreatic cirrhosis and splenomegaly. The rectal mucous membrane becomes very vascular with soft growth formation. Prolapse of the rectum is common and septic infection may result. *Fever* may be high and irregular (Pons and Hoffmann). Some time may elapse after infection before ova appear in the stools.

Schistosoma japonicum.—In China, Japan and the Philippines there is a disease characterized by cirrhosis of the liver, splenomegaly, ascites, dysentery, progressive anemia, and sometimes by focalized epilepsy. Dermatitis and angioneurotic edema may occur. It occurs extensively in one district of Japan, and is known as the "Katayama" disease. The so-called urticarial fever, not very uncommon in China and Japan, seems to be associated with the presence of this parasite, and an eosinophilia with fever and urticaria should lead to a careful examination of the stools for its eggs. The parasite lives in the intestinal wall; the ova are smaller than those of *S. haematobium,* and have not the characteristic spine. The parasite develops in a snail and the disease is acquired by working in wet rice fields.

Treatment.—Antimony is the most successful remedy. Potassium or sodium antimony tartrate is given in doses of gr. ½ (0.03 gm.) intravenously, increased to gr. iii (0.2 gm.), every two or three days until a total of 30 grains is given. Emetine has been used as in amebic dysentery.

DISEASES CAUSED BY CESTODES—TENIASIS

Man harbors the adult parasites in the small intestine, the larval forms in the muscles and solid organs.

INTESTINAL CESTODES; TAPEWORMS

Taenia solium (Pork Tapeworm).—This is not a common form in the United States and is more frequent in Europe and Asia. When mature it is about 6 feet in length. The head is small, round, not so large as the head of a pin, and provided with four sucking disks and a double row of hooklets; hence it is called the *armed* tapeworm. To the head succeeds a narrow, thread-like neck, then the segments, or proglottides, which possess both male and female generative organs; at about the four-hundred-and-fiftieth they become mature and contain ripe ova. The worm attains its full growth in about three months, after which time the segments are continuously shed and appear in the stools. The segments are about 1 cm. in length and from 7 to 8 mm. in breadth. Pressed between glass plates the uterus is seen as a median stem with about eight to twelve lateral branches. There are many thousands of ova in each ripe segment, and each ovum consists of a firm shell, inside of which is a little embryo, provided with six hooklets. The segments are continuously passed, and if the ova are to attain further development they must be taken into the stomach of a pig or of man. The shells are digested, the six-hooked embryos become free, and by the vessels reach various parts of the body (the liver, muscles, brain, or eye), where they develop into the larvae or cysticerci. A hog under these circumstances is said to be *measled,* and the cysticerci are spoken of as measles or bladder worms.

Taenia solium received its name because it was thought to exist as a solitary parasite in the bowel, but two or more worms may occur.

Taenia saginata (Unarmed, Fat, or Beef Tapeworm).—This is a longer and larger parasite than *T. solium.* It is the common tapeworm of North America. It may attain a length of 15 or 20 feet, or more. The head is large in comparison with that of *T. solium,* and measures over 2 mm. in breadth. It is square-shaped and provided with four large sucking disks, but there are no hooklets. The ripe segments are from 17 to 18 mm. in length and from 8 to 10 mm. in breadth. The uterus consists of a medium stem with from fifteen to thirty lateral branches, which are given off more dichotomously than in *T. solium.* The ova are somewhat larger and the shell thicker, but the two forms can scarcely be distinguished by their ova. The ripe segments are passed and ingested by cattle, in the flesh or organs of which the eggs develop into cysticerci.

Of other forms of tapeworm may be mentioned:

Dipylidium caninum.—A small parasite common in the dog and occasionally found in man; the larvae develop in the lice and fleas of the dog.

Hymenolepis diminuta.—This small cestode is common in mice and rats. The larvae develop in beetles.

Hymenolepis nana is frequent in Italy and not very uncommon in the United States (Stiles). It occurs in mice and rats.

Diphyllobothrium latum (Broad Tapeworm).—This is widely distributed in fresh-water fish, especially in northern Europe, and has become an established parasite in lakes of the North West in the United States and Canada, especially in pike, pickerel and perch. Dogs are infected frequently from eating fish. The parasite is large and long, measuring from 25 to 30 feet or more. Its head is different from that of the taenia, as it possesses two lateral grooves or pits and has no hooklets. The larvae develop in the peritoneum and muscles of the infected fish, and grow into the adult worm when raw or insufficiently cooked fish is eaten by man. Infection is common in children. This tapeworm is becoming more important as a cause of disease and infestation with it promises to become more frequent and more widely distributed. The transportation of fish for long distances carries it widely. The principal feature is a severe *anemia* of a secondary form, so severe that in some cases Addisonian anemia is suggested. The hemoglobin may be 25 or 30 per cent with 1,500,000 to 2,000,000 red cells. There is usually leukopenia with eosinophilia. Digestive disturbances and edema may occur.

Symptoms.—Tapeworms are found at all ages, are not uncommon in children and are occasionally found in sucklings. The parasites may cause no disturbance and are rarely dangerous. A knowledge of the existence of the worm is generally a source of worry and anxiety; the patient may have considerable distress and complain of abdominal pains, nausea, diarrhea, and sometimes anemia. Occasionally the appetite is ravenous. In nervous patients the constitutional disturbance may be considerable with marked mental depression. Various nervous phenomena, such as convulsions, are believed to be caused by the parasites but such effects are very rare. *T. saginata* has been found in the gallbladder. Eosinophilia may occur.

Diagnosis.—This is never doubtful as the presence of the segments is distinctive and the ova may be recognized in the stools. The patient's diagnosis should be proved; the laity mistake many things for tapeworm segments.

Prophylaxis.—This is most important and attention should be given to three points. First, all tapeworm segments should be burned and never be thrown into a water closet or outside; secondly, careful inspection of meat; and, thirdly, cooking meat and fish sufficiently to kill the parasites.

In the case of the beef infection, the muscles of the jaw are much more frequently affected than other parts. Sometimes the infection is general. Cold storage kills the cysticercus usually within three weeks. There is a danger with *T. solium* of auto-infection, as during vomiting, with the production of cysticercosis. Special care should be taken in handling this worm or its eggs.

In the examination of hogs for cysticerci "particular stress should be laid upon the tongue, the muscles of mastication, and the muscles of the shoulder, neck, and diaphragm" (Stiles). They may be seen very easily on the under surface of the tongue. American hogs are comparatively free. Specimens have been found alive twenty-nine days after slaughtering. In the examination of 1,000 hogs in Montreal, 76 instances of cysticerci were found.

Treatment.—Three days should be given to preparation for whatever drug is employed. For two days the patient should take soft food and the third day liquids only. The bowels should be well moved by a laxative each evening and a saline in the morning if necessary. Unless the bowels have moved freely an enema should be given. There are many drugs, but male fern is usually the most reliable, given in the form of oleoresin or ethereal extract. This is given early in the morning before any food is taken. The usual dose is ʒi (4 cc.), which is repeated in an hour. It may be given in capsules or in glycerine (℥ss, 15 cc.). If there is fear of nausea a cup of coffee may be taken before the drug. The drug may be given by the duodenal tube. After taking the male fern the patient should remain quiet and resist any desire to vomit. One hour after the second dose of male fern a full dose of saline is taken (magnesium or sodium sulphate, or magnesium citrate), and an hour later a second dose if the bowels have not moved. Castor oil should not be given. Great care should be taken during the expulsion of the worm, which should be passed into a chamber containing water at about the body temperature, a practice recommended by Celsus.

Pomegranate root is an efficient remedy, and may be given as an infusion of the bark, 3 ounces of which may be macerated in 10 ounces of water and reduced to one-half by evaporation. This is taken in divided doses. It occasionally produces colic, but is very effective. The active principle, pelletierine, is employed as the tannate, given in doses of 6 to 8 or even 10 grains (0.4 to 0.6 gm.), and followed in an hour by a purge.

Pumpkin seeds are sometimes efficient. Three ounces should be carefully bruised, macerated for twelve or fourteen hours, the entire quantity taken and followed in an hour by a purge. Of other remedies, carbon tetrachloride (2-3 cc.) naphthalein (gr. v, 0.3 gm.), and thymol (gr. v, 0.3 gm. daily for a week) may be mentioned. Sometimes a combination of remedies is effectual when one fails. In children the use of pumpkin seeds or pelletierine is generally best. One cause of failure is the use of drugs which are old and inert.

Unless the head is brought away, the parasite continues to grow, and within about three months the segments appear again. Some cases are extraordinarily obstinate. Doubtless much depends upon the exposure of the worm. The head and neck may be thoroughly protected beneath the valvulae conniventes, in which case the remedies may not act. Owing to its armature *Taenia solium* is more difficult to expel. It is probable that no degree of peristalsis can dislodge the head, and unless the worm is killed it does not let go its firm hold. Owing to the danger of cysticercosis, treatment should not be delayed in case of infection with *Taenia solium.*

SOMATIC TENIASIS

Whereas adult taenia may give rise to little or no disturbance, and rarely prove directly fatal, the affections caused by the larvae or immature forms in the solid organs are serious. There are two chief cestode larvae known to frequent man: the *Cysticercus cellulosae,* the larva of *Taenia solium,* and (*b*) the *Echinococcus,* the larva of *Taenia echinococcus.* Infection with bothriocephalid larvae is infrequent.

Cysticercosis.—When man accidentally takes into his stomach the ripe ova of *T. solium* he is likely to become the intermediate host, a part usually played by the hog. This may occur in an individual the subject of *T. solium,* in which case the mature proglottides enter the stomach or are forced into it by attacks of vomiting. The accidental ingestion of a few ova is possible, and this should be borne in mind in handling the segments of the worm.

The *symptoms* depend entirely upon the number of ova ingested and the localities reached. In the hog the cysticerci produce very little disturbance. The muscles, the connective tissue, and the brain may be swarming with the "measles," as they are called, and yet the animal does not appear to be seriously incommoded. In the invasion period, if large numbers of the parasites are taken, there is, in all probability, constitutional disturbance; certainly this is seen in the calf, when fed with the ripe segments of *T. saginata.* Carelessness in this may have serious consequences.

In man a few cysticerci lodged beneath the skin or in the muscles give no trouble, and in time the larvae die and become calcified. They are occasionally found in dissection subjects or in postmortems as ovoid white bodies in the muscles or subcutaneous tissue. In America they are very rare. We have seen but two instances in postmortem experience. The symptoms may be grouped into *general, cerebrospinal,* and *ocular.* In 155 cases the parasite in 117 was found in the brain, in 32 in the muscles, in 9 in the heart, in 3 in the lungs, subcutaneously in 5, in the liver in 2 (Stiles).

General.—As a rule the invasion of the larvae in man, unless in very large numbers, does not cause very definite symptoms but occasionally a striking picture is produced. A patient was admitted very stiff and helpless, so much so that he had to be assisted into bed. He complained of numbness and tingling in the extremities and general weakness, so that at first he was thought to have a peripheral neuritis. On examination, however, a number of painful subcutaneous nodules were discovered, which proved on excision to be *cysticerci.* Altogether 75 could be felt subcutaneously, and from the soreness and stiffness they probably existed in large numbers in the muscles. There were none in his eyes and he had no brain symptoms.

Cerebrospinal.—Remarkable symptoms may result from the presence of the cysticerci in the brain and cord. In the silent region they may be abundant without producing any symptoms. In the ventricles of the brain the cysticerci may attain a considerable size, owing to the fact that in regions in which they are unrestrained in their growth, as in the peritoneum, the bladder-like body grows freely. When in the fourth ventricle remarkable irritative symptoms may be produced. In 1884 the senior author saw in Berlin a case in which during life there had been diabetes and anomalous nervous symptoms. Postmortem, the cysticercus was found pressing upon the floor of the fourth ventricle. *Epileptiform* seizures, with many nervous and mental symptoms, may occur, usually years after the entrance of the parasites and possibly due to death of the cysticerci, after which they act as irritants.

Ocular.—Since von Graefe demonstrated the presence of the cysticercus in the vitreous humor many cases have been recorded.

Except in the eye, the diagnosis can rarely be made; when the cysticerci are subcutaneous one may be excised. It is possible that when numerous throughout the muscles they may be seen under the tongue.

Echinococcus or Hydatid Disease.—The hydatid worms or echinococci are the larvae of *Taenia echinococcus* of the dog. This is not more than 4 or 5 mm. in length, consisting of only three or four segments, of which the terminal one alone is mature, and has a length of about 2 mm. and a breadth of 0.6 mm. The head is small and provided with four sucking disks and a rostellum with a double row of hooklets. The worms are so small that they are readily overlooked, since they form small, threadlike bodies closely adherent among the villi of the small intestines. The ripe segment contains about 5,000 eggs, which attain their development in the solid organs of various animals, particularly the hog and ox, more rarely the horse and the sheep. Man may be an intermediate host, owing to accidental ingestion of the ova.

Development.—The little six-hooked embryo, freed from the egg-shell by digestion, burrows through the intestinal wall and reaches the lymphatic vessels or the veins; it may enter the portal vessels and be carried to the liver. It may enter the systemic vessels, and, passing the pulmonary capillaries, as it is protoplasmic and elastic, may reach the brain or other parts. It then undergoes the following changes: The hooklets disappear and the little embryo is gradually converted into a small cyst which presents two distinct layers—an external, laminated, cuticular membrane or capsule, and an internal, granular, parenchymatous layer, the endocyst. The cyst contains a clear fluid. There is more or less reaction in the neighboring tissues, and the cyst in time has a fibrous investment. When this *primary* cyst has attained a certain size, buds develop from the parenchymatous layer, which are gradually converted into cysts, presenting a structure identical with that of the original cyst, namely, an elastic chitinous membrane lined with a granular parenchymatous layer. These *secondary* or daughter cysts are at first connected with the lining membrane of the primary cyst, but are soon set free. In this way the parent cyst as it grows may contain a dozen or more daughter cysts. Inside these daughter cysts a similar process may occur, and from buds in the walls granddaughter cysts are developed. From the granular layer of the cysts buds arise which develop into brood capsules. From the lining membrane the little outgrowths arise and gradually develop into scolices, which represent in reality the head of the *T. echinococcus* and present four sucking disks and a circle of hooklets. Each scolex is capable when transferred to the intestines of a dog of developing into an adult tapeworm. The difference between the ovum of *T. solium*, and *T. echinococcus* is in this way very striking. In the former the ovum develops into a single larva whereas the egg of *T. echinococcus* develops into a cyst which is capable of multiplying enormously. Ordinarily in man the development of the echinococcus is as above mentioned and by an *endogenous* form in which the secondary and tertiary cysts are contained within the primary; but in animals the formation may be different, as the buds from the primary cyst penetrate between the layers and develop externally, forming the *exogenous* variety. A third form is the *multilocular* echinococcus, in which form the primary cyst buds are cut off completely and surrounded by thick capsules of a connective tissue, which join together and ultimately form a hard mass represented by strands of connective tissue inclosing alveolar spaces about the size of peas or a little larger.

The fluid is limpid, nonalbuminous; specific gravity 1.005 to 1.009, occasionally higher. It may contain chlorides, sugar and succinic acid, and, after repeated tapping of the cyst, albumin. When not degenerated the hydatid heads or the characteristic hooklets are found in the contents of the cyst.

Changes in the Cyst.—The echinococcus may remain alive, probably many years, possibly as long as twenty years. The most common change is death with gradual inspissation of the contents and conversion of the cyst into a mass containing putty-like granular material which may be partially calcified. Remnants of the chitinous cyst wall or hooklets may be found. These obsolete hydatid cysts are not infrequent in the liver. A more serious termination is rupture, which may take place into a serous sac, or perforation may take place externally when the cysts are discharged, as into the bronchi, alimentary canal or urinary passages. More unfavorable are the instances in which rupture occurs into the bile passages or the inferior cava. Recovery may follow the rupture and discharge of the hydatids externally. Sudden death has followed the rupture. A serious termination is suppuration, which is most frequent in the liver.

Geographical Distribution.—The disease prevails most extensively in those countries in which man is brought into close contact with the dog, particularly when, as in Australia, the dogs are used for herding sheep, the animal in which the larval form of *T. echinococcus* is most often found. In Iceland the cases are numerous. In Europe the disease is not uncommon. In Great Britain it is rare, and a majority of the cases are in foreigners. The disease is not infrequent in the United States and appears to be increasing.

Distribution in the Body.—Of 1,634 cases in the statistics of Davaine, Böcker, Finsen, and Neisser, the parasite existed in the liver in 820; in the lung or pleura in 137; in the abdominal organs, including the kidneys, bladder, and genitalia, in 334; in the nervous system in 122; in the circulatory system in 42; in other organs 179. Of the 241 cases in Lyon's series in America the liver was the seat in 177, and the omentum, peritoneal cavity, and mesentery in 26. In 11 cases cysts were passed per rectum, in 7 cases cysts or hooklets were expectorated, and in 2 cases passed per urethram.

Symptoms.—*Hydatids of the Liver.*—Small cysts may cause no disturbance; large and growing cysts produce signs of tumor of the liver with great increase in the size of the organ. Naturally the physical signs depend much upon the situation of the growth. Near the anterior surface in the epigastric region the tumor may form a distinct prominence and have a tense, firm feeling, sometimes with fluctuation. A not infrequent situation is to the left of the suspensory ligament, the resulting tumor pushing up the heart and causing an extensive area of dulness in the lower sternal and left hypochondriac regions. In the right lobe, if the tumor is on the posterior surface, the enlargement of the organ is chiefly upward and the vertical area of dulness in the posterior axillary line is increased. Superficial cysts may give what is known as the *hydatid fremitus.* If the tumor is palpated lightly with the left hand and percussed by the right, there is felt a vibration or trembling movement. It is not always present, and it is doubtful whether it is peculiar to the hydatid tumors or due to the collision of the daughter cysts. Very large cysts are accompanied by feelings of pressure or dragging in the hepatic region, sometimes actual pain. The general condition of the patient is at first good and the nutrition little, if at all, interfered with.

Historically, one of the most interesting cases is that of the first Lord Shaftesbury (Achitophel), who had a tumor below the costal border for many years. It suppurated and was opened by John Locke, his physician, who describes with great detail the escape of the bladder-like bodies. Among the Shaftesbury papers in the Record Office are other cases collected by Locke; the disease may have been more common in England at that period.

Suppuration of the cyst changes the picture into one of pyemia. There are rigors, sweats, more or less jaundice, and rapid loss of weight. Perforation may occur into the stomach, colon, pleura, bronchi or externally, and in some instances recovery has taken place. Perforation has occurred into the pericardium and inferior vena cava; in the latter case the daughter cysts have been found in the heart, plugging the tricuspid orifice and pulmonary artery. Perforation of the bile passages causes intense jaundice, and may lead to suppurative cholangitis.

An interesting symptom connected with the rupture of hydatid cysts is the occurrence of *urticaria,* which may also follow aspiration of the cysts. Brieger separated a highly toxic material from the fluid, and to it the symptoms of poisoning may be due.

Diagnosis.—Cysts of moderate size may exist without producing symptoms. Large multiple echinococci may cause great enlargement with irregularity of the outline, and such a condition persisting for any time with retention of the health and strength suggests hydatid disease. An irregular, painless enlargement, particularly in the left lobe, or the presence of a large, smooth, fluctuating tumor in the epigastric region is suggestive, and in this situation, when accessible to palpation, it gives a sensation of a smooth elastic growth and possibly also the hydatid tremor. When suppuration occurs the clinical picture is really that of abscess, and only the existence of previous enlargement of the liver with good health would point to the fact that the suppuration was associated with hydatids. *Syphilis* may produce irregular enlargement without much disturbance in the health, sometimes also a very definite tumor in the epigastric region, but this is usually firm and not fluctuating. The clinical features may simulate *cancer* very closely but, as a rule, the course separates it clearly. Dilatation of the gallbladder and hydronephrosis have been mistaken for hydatid disease. In the former the mobility of the tumor and its shape usually suffice for the diagnosis. In some instances of hydronephrosis the X-ray study and ureteral catheterization may be necessary. More frequent is the mistake of confounding a hydatid cyst of the right lobe pushing up the pleura with *pleural effusion* of the right side. The heart may be dislocated, the liver depressed, and dulness, feeble breathing and diminished fremitus are present in both conditions. In echinococcus cyst the upper limit of dulness presents a curved line, the maximum of which is usually in the scapular region. Suppurative pleurisy may be caused by perforation of the cyst. If adhesions result, the perforation takes place into the lung, and fragments of the cysts or small daughter cysts may be coughed up. For diagnosis the exploratory puncture should be used and the fluid is usually characteristic. Hooklets may be found in the clear fluid or in the suppurating cysts. They are sometimes absent, however, as the cyst may be sterile. The complement fixation test is of value and the intradermal test for which sterile hydatid fluid is used.

Respiratory System.—Of 809 cases of single hydatid cysts collected by Thomas in Australia, the lung was affected in 134 cases. Of 241 American cases, in 16 the pleura or lung was affected. The larvae may develop primarily in the pleura and attain a large size. The symptoms are at first those of compression of the lung and dislocation of the heart. The physical signs are those of fluid in the pleura. The line of dulness may be quite irregular. The general condition may be excellent in spite of extensive disease. Pleurisy is rarely excited. The cysts may become inflamed and perforate the chest wall. Death results in a majority of the cases from toxemia following the rupture and absorption of the fluid or from sepsis following suppuration.

Echinococci occur more frequently in the lung than in the pleura. If small, they may exist for some time without causing serious symptoms. In their growth they compress the lung and sooner or later lead to inflammatory processes, often to gangrene, and the formation of cavities which connect with the bronchi. Fragments of membrane or small cysts may be expectorated. Hemorrhage is not infrequent. Perforation into the pleura with empyema is common. A majority of the cases are regarded as tuberculosis or gangrene, and it is only the detection of the characteristic membranes or hooklets which leads to the diagnosis. The X-ray study is of aid. Of a series of 21 cases, 17 recovered; 5 of the cases suppurated (C. H. Fleming, Victoria).

Kidneys.—In the collected statistics the genito-urinary system comes second as the seat of hydatid disease, though here the affection is rare in comparison with that of the liver. Of 241 American cases, there were 17 in which the kidneys or bladder were involved. The kidney may be converted into an enormous cyst resembling a hydronephrosis. The *diagnosis* is only possible by puncture and examination of the fluid. The cyst may perforate into the pelvis of the kidney, and portions of the membrane or cysts may be discharged with the urine, sometimes producing renal colic.

Nervous System.—The common cystic disease of the choroidal plexuses has been mistaken for hydatids. The symptoms, very indefinite, as a rule are those of tumor. Persistent headache, convulsions, either limited or general, and gradually developing blindness have been prominent features in many cases.

Multilocular Echinococcus.—This merits a brief description, as it differs so remarkably from the usual type. It has been met with in Bavaria, Württemberg, the adjacent districts of Switzerland, and in the Tyrol. In the United States a few cases have been described, chiefly in Germans. Delafield and Prudden's patient for a year before his death had been jaundiced. A fluctuating tumor was found in the right flank, apparently connected with the liver. This was opened, and death followed from hemorrhage. In Oertel's case the patient was deeply jaundiced, and had a tumor mass at the right border of the liver, which was enlarged. Bacon resected a cyst from the left lobe of the liver. The primary tumor presents irregularly formed cavities separated from each other by strands of connective tissue, and lined with the echinococcus membrane. The cavities are filled with a gelatinous material, so that the tumor has very much the appearance of an alveolar colloid cancer. It is possible that a special form of *T. echinococcus* represents the adult type of this peculiar parasite. This form is almost exclusively confined to the liver, and the symptoms resemble those of tumor or cirrhosis. The liver is, as a rule, enlarged and smooth. Jaundice is common and the spleen is usually enlarged; there is progressive emaciation and toward the close hemorrhages are common.

Treatment of Echinococcus Disease.—Medicines are of no avail. Postmortem reports show that in a considerable number of cases the parasite dies and the cyst becomes harmless. Operative measures should be resorted to when the cyst is large or troublesome. Aspiration has been successful but incision and evacuation of the cysts are to be preferred. Suppuration has followed puncture. Injections into the sac should not be practised. Surgeons open and evacuate echinococcus cysts with great boldness, and the Australian records show that recovery is the rule in a large proportion of the cases. Suppurative cysts in the liver should be treated as abscess.

Sparganum mansoni is the larval stage of *Diphyllobothrium mansoni* of dogs. It may occur in many parts of the body.

Sparganum proliferum was first found in Japan. One case was reported in Florida. The infection was generalized.

DISEASES CAUSED BY NEMATODES

ASCARIASIS

Ascaris lumbricoides, the most common human parasite, is found chiefly in children. The female is from 7 to 12 inches in length, the male from 4 to 8 inches. In form it is cylindrical, pointed at both ends, with a yellowish-brown, sometimes a slightly reddish color. Four longitudinal bands can be seen, and it is striated transversely. The ova, which are sometimes found in large numbers in the feces, are small, brownish-red in color, elliptical, and have a very thick covering. The life history has been demonstrated to be "direct"—*i.e.,* without intermediate host. The ovum develops into a larva which is retained in the shell and in a month has reached the infective stage. If swallowed, in water or on infected raw vegetables, the larva is set free by the digestive juices, pierces the wall and passes to the liver and lungs. Here the larvae escape from the capillaries, causing hemorrhage, pass from the air sacs to the bronchi, travel up the trachea and are swallowed. In the intestine they grow to the adult form. Heavy infections in mice, and perhaps in pigs, cause pneumonia. In some cases of human infection there are respiratory tract symptoms due to the larvae in the lungs which are 1-2.5 mm. in length. The mature parasite occupies the upper portion of the small intestine. Usually only a few are present, but occasionally they occur in enormous numbers. The migrations are peculiar. They may pass into the stomach, whence they may be vomited or they may crawl up the esophagus and enter the pharynx, from which they may be withdrawn. This is frequent in children with fever. In other instances the worm reaches the larynx, and has produced fatal asphyxia, or, passing into the trachea, caused gangrene of the lung. They may go through the Eustachian tube and appear at the external meatus. The worms have been found in the bile ducts and gallbladder. They have caused abscess of the liver in which they have been found. They have entered the pancreatic duct and caused acute pancreatitis. The bowel may be obstructed by a mass of the worms or in rare instances an ulcer may be perforated. Even the healthy bowel wall may be penetrated. They have passed through the body wall, especially at the umbilicus.

A peculiarly irritating substance, often evident to the sense of smell in handling specimens, is formed by the round worms and it is suggested that the nervous symptoms, sometimes resembling those of meningitis, are due to this. Some associate a condition with fever, intestinal symptoms, foul breath, and intermittent diarrhea with the presence of lumbricoides. There may be eosinophilia to 25 to 30 per cent, and in some cases a marked anemia. The question of the toxins produced by these parasites is an open one. A condition of "Ascaris Sensitization" has been described.

Symptoms.—A few parasites may cause no disturbance. In children many irritative symptoms are attributed to worms, such as restlessness, irritability, picking at the nose, grinding of the teeth, twitchings, or convulsions. The *diagnosis* is made by finding the worms or eggs in the stools. It may be made in a gastro-intestinal X-ray study by the barium entering the worms and giving a string-like shadow.

Treatment.—It is well to give soft diet on the day previous and a dose of castor oil the night before treatment. *Santonin* is usually efficient given in the morning in doses of one grain (0.065 gm.) for a small child, and three to five grains (0.2 to 0.3 gm.) for an adult. One to two grains of calomel should be given with it. Three hours later a good dose of saline should be given. This should be done two mornings in succession and repeated in a week if worms or eggs are again passed. The occasional effects of santonin (yellow vision, vertigo) should be explained beforehand. Oil of chenopodium is useful in doses of 10 to 15 drops in an ounce of castor oil, followed in an hour by a second dose of castor oil. Carbon tetrachloride may be given in the morning (no food being allowed after 4 P. M. of the day before) in doses of 30 to 45 minims (2 to 3 cc.) and followed by a purgative. Crystalline hexylresorcinol is efficient; it is given in hard gelatine capsules (gr. xv, 1 gm. for adults and gr. vii, 0.5 gm. for children) in the early morning with the stomach empty. No food should be taken for six hours afterwards. Magnesium sulphate should be given the next morning.

Oxyuriasis.—The worm, *Enterobius* (formerly *Oxyuris*) *vermicularis*, known as the pinworm or seatworm, lives in the small intestine when young and is often found in the appendix. The fertilized females wander to the colon and outside the anus. In females they may enter the vagina. The male measures about 4 mm. in length, the female about 10 mm. They produce great irritation and itching, particularly at night, symptoms which become intensely aggravated by their nocturnal migration. The worms may traverse the intestinal wall and reach the peritoneal cavity, where they may form verminous tubercles in Douglas' fossa or perirectal abscesses.

The patients become extremely restless and irritable, the sleep is often disturbed, and there may be loss of appetite and anemia. Though most common in children, the parasite occurs at all ages.

The worm may be detected in the feces or the eggs found about the anus. Infection probably takes place through water or possibly through salads.

Treatment.—Every care should be taken to avoid auto-infection or the infection of others, by care in cleansing the anus and perineum, and thorough washing of the hands after defecation. Auto-infection is often responsible for the persistence of the disease. Treatment must be directed to the removal of the worms both from the small intestine and rectum. Santonin and calomel are useful, given as in ascaris infection for several days. Thymol and naphthalein are also used. Crystalline hexylresorcinol may be used as in ascariasis. To remove the worms from the rectum injections are required which should be retained as long as possible; it is well to wash out the bowel before giving them and the injection need not be over six ounces. Cold solutions of salt and water, copper sulphate solution (1-2,500), glycerine, infusion of quassia (one ounce of quassia chips to a pint of water), or lime water may be employed and should be used daily for two weeks. For the itching, carbolated vaseline or menthol (5 per cent) in vaseline may be employed.

TRICHINIASIS

The *Trichinella spiralis* in its adult condition lives in the small intestine. The disease is produced by the embryos, which pass from the intestines and reach the voluntary muscles, where they finally become encapsulated larvae—muscle trichinae. It is in the migration of the embryos (possibly from poisons produced by them) that the symptoms are produced.

The ovoid cysts were described in human muscle by Tiedemann in 1822; the parasite was figured and named by Richard Owen (1835). Leidy in 1845 described it in the pig. For a long time the trichina was looked upon as a pathological curiosity; but in 1860 Zenker discovered both the intestinal and muscle forms, and established their connection with the disease.

Description of the Parasites.—(*a*) Adult or intestinal form. The female measures from 3 to 4 mm.; the male, 1.5 mm., and has two little projections from the hinder end. (*b*) The larva or muscle trichina is from 0.6 to 1 mm. in length and lies coiled in an ovoid capsule, which is at first translucent, but subsequently opaque and infiltrated with lime salts. The worm presents a pointed head and a somewhat rounded tail.

When flesh containing the trichinae is eaten by man or by any animal in which the development can take place, the capsules are digested and the trichinae set free. They pass into the small intestine, and about the third day attain their full growth and become sexually mature. On the sixth or seventh day the embryos are fully developed. The young produced by each female worm have been estimated at several hundred. Leuckart thought that various broods are developed in succession, and that as many as a thousand embryos may be produced by a single worm. The time from the ingestion of the flesh containing the muscle trichinae to the development of the brood of embryos in the intestines is from seven to nine days. The female worm penetrates the intestinal wall and the embryos are probably discharged directly into the lymph spaces, thence into the venous system, and by the blood stream to the muscles, which constitute their seat of election. J. Y. Graham gives strong arguments in favor of the transmission through the blood stream. They have been found in the *blood* early in the infection and since the demonstration of their presence by Herrick and Janeway have been seen by a number of observers. They are found also in the *spinal fluid* in some cases. They have occurred in the fluid of a pleural exudate, in the milk of a nursing woman and in the pus from a furuncle. After a preliminary migration in the intermuscular connective tissue they penetrate the primitive muscle-fibres, and in about two weeks develop into the full-grown muscle form. In this process an interstitial *myositis* is excited and gradually an ovoid capsule develops about the parasite. Two, occasionally three or four, worms may be seen within a single capsule. This process of encapsulation has been estimated to take about six weeks. Within the muscles the parasites do not undergo further change. Gradually the capsule becomes thicker, and ultimately lime salts are deposited within it. This change may take place in man within four or five months. In the hog it may be deferred for many years. The calcification renders the cyst visible, and these small, opaque, oat-shaped bodies are familiar objects to demonstrators of anatomy. The trichinae may live within the muscles for an indefinite period and have been found alive and capable of developing even twenty-five years after their entrance into the system. In many instances the worms are completely calcified. The trichina has been found or "raised" in twenty-six different species of animals (Stiles). Medical literature abounds in references to its presence in fish, earthworms, etc., but these parasites belong to other genera. In fecal examinations for the parasite it is well to remember that the "cell body" of the anterior portion of the intestine is a diagnostic criterion of the *T. spiralis*. Experimentally, guinea-pigs and rabbits are readily infected by feeding them with muscle containing the larval form. Dogs are infected with difficulty; cats more readily. In the hog the trichinae, like the cysticerci, cause few if any symptoms. In the hog the capsule is not readily calcified, so that the parasites are not visible as in human muscles.

The *anatomical* changes are chiefly in the voluntary muscles. The trichinae enter the primitive muscle bundles, which undergo granular degeneration with marked nuclear proliferation. There is a local *myositis,* and gradually about the parasite a cyst wall is formed. Cohnheim described a fatty degeneration of the liver and enlargement of the mesenteric glands. If death occurs, in the fourth week or later, the adult trichinae may be still found in the intestines.

Infection.—Man is infected by eating the flesh of trichinous hogs. In America inspections have been made since 1892 and the percentage of animals found infected has ranged from 1 to 2. In 1883, with A. W. Clement, the senior author examined 1,000 hogs at the Montreal abattoir, and found only 4 infected.

The danger of infection depends entirely upon the mode of preparation of the flesh. Thorough cooking, so that all parts of the meat reach the boiling point, destroys the parasites; but in large joints the central portions are often not raised to this temperature. The frequency of the disease in different countries depends largely upon the habits of the people in the preparation of pork. In North Germany, where raw ham and *Wurst* are freely eaten, the greatest number of instances have occurred. In South Germany, France, and England cases are rare. In the United States H. U. Williams made a thorough study of the muscle from 505 unselected autopsies, and found 27 cases of trichiniasis, 5.3 per cent. The subjects had all died of causes other than trichiniasis. Riley and Schleifley found 20 instances in 117 cadavers (17 per cent). These studies show how widespread is the disease, and that we frequently overlook the sporadic form. Salting and smoking the flesh are not always sufficient, and animals are readily infected when fed with pickled or smoked meat as prepared in America.

The disease occurs in groups in which from a few to several hundred individuals are attacked, and in sporadic cases which are not infrequent. In the epidemics a large number of persons are infected from one source; in the two famous outbreaks of Hedersleben and Emersleben 337 and 250 individuals were attacked. The discovery by T. R. Brown of the eosinophilia has led to the much more frequent detection of the sporadic cases.

Symptoms.—The ingestion of trichinous flesh is not necessarily followed by the disease. When a limited number are eaten only a few embryos pass to the muscles and may cause no symptoms. Well-characterized cases present a gastro-intestinal period and a period of general infection.

In the course of a few days after eating the infected meat there are signs of *gastro-intestinal* disturbance—pain in the abdomen, loss of appetite, vomiting and sometimes diarrhea. The preliminary symptoms, however, are by no means constant, and in some of the large epidemics cases have been observed in which they have been absent. In other instances the gastro-intestinal features have been marked from the outset, and the attack has resembled food poisoning. Pain in different parts of the body, general debility, and weakness have been noted in some epidemics.

The *invasion* symptoms occur between the seventh and the tenth day, sometimes not until the end of the second week. Chills are not common. There is fever, except in very mild cases, rising to 102° or 104° F.; the fever is usually remittent or intermittent. The migration of the parasites into the muscles excites a more or less intense *myositis,* which is characterized by pain on pressure and movement, and by swelling and tension of the muscles, over which the skin may be edematous. The limbs are placed in the positions in which the muscles are in least tension. The involvement of the muscles of mastication and of the larynx may cause difficulty in swallowing and change in the voice. In severe cases the involvement of the diaphragm and intercostal muscles may lead to intense dyspnea. Chemosis of the bulbar conjunctiva, marked edema of the lids, ecchymosis and retinal hemorrhages may occur. *Edema,* a feature of great importance, may be early in the face, particularly about the eyes. Later it occurs in the extremities when the swelling and stiffness of the muscles are at their height. Profuse sweats, tingling and itching of the skin, and in some instances urticaria, have been described. Kernig's sign is usually present and the leg reflexes may be absent. There may be various signs of central nervous system involvement.

A marked *leukocytosis,* which may reach above 30,000, is usually present. A special feature is the extraordinary increase in the eosinophile cells, which may comprise more than 50 per cent of the leukocytes. Eosinophilia may be absent in very severe cases.

The general nutrition is much disturbed and the patient becomes emaciated and often anemic, particularly in protracted cases. The patients are usually conscious, except in cases of great severity in which the toxemia, dry tongue, and tremor suggest typhoid fever. In addition to the dyspnea in the severer cases, there may be bronchitis, and in the fatal cases pneumonia or pleurisy. In some epidemics polyuria has been common. Albuminuria is frequent. Myocarditis may be marked.

The intensity and duration of the symptoms depend entirely upon the grade of infection. In mild cases the duration is from ten to fourteen days. In the severe forms convalescence is not established for six or eight weeks, and it may be months before the patient recovers his strength. Of 72 fatal cases in the Hedersleben epidemic, the greatest mortality occurred in the fourth and fifth and sixth weeks, namely 52 cases. The mortality has ranged in different outbreaks from 1 or 2 to 30 per cent. Among 456 cases reported in the United States there were 122 deaths.

The **prognosis** depends much upon the quantity of infected meat eaten and the number of trichinae which mature in the intestines. In children the outlook is more favorable. Early diarrhea and moderately intense gastrointestinal symptoms are, as a rule, more favorable than constipation.

Diagnosis.—The disease should always be suspected when a large party is followed by cases of apparent typhoid fever. The parasites may be found in the remnants of the ham or sausages used on the occasion. The worms may be found in the stools or in the duodenal contents. The stools should be spread on a glass plate or black background and examined with a low-power lens, when the trichinae are seen as small, glistening, silvery threads. In doubtful cases the diagnosis may be made by the removal of a piece of muscle. The disease may be mistaken for rheumatic fever, particularly as the pains are so severe on movement, but there is no arthritis. The great increase of the *eosinophiles* in the blood is a most suggestive point. The tenderness is in the muscles both on pressure and on movement. The intensity of the gastro-intestinal symptoms has led to the diagnosis of cholera. Many epidemics have been described as typhoid fever, which the severer cases, with prolonged fever, sweats, delirium, dry tongue, and gastro-intestinal symptoms, somewhat resemble. The spleen is enlarged in some cases. The pains in the muscles, with tension and swelling, edema, particularly about the eyes, and shortness of breath, are important diagnostic points. The Bachman intradermal test, in which a 1 per cent solution of dried powder prepared from isolated larvae is used, has not been tried extensively.

Prophylaxis.—Prophylaxis in the human must depend on the proper cooking of pork for which a temperature of 137° F. is sufficient. "In the last analysis the responsibility for trichiniasis lies in the kitchen" (Stiles). This is especially important for the sausages which are cooked before being sold. Meat inspection apparently has little value in prevention.

Treatment.—If it has been discovered within twenty-four or thirty-six hours or even later that persons have eaten infected pork, the indications are to thoroughly evacuate the gastro-intestinal canal. Calomel (gr. ii, 0.13 gm.) should be given at once and four hours later half an ounce of castor oil or magnesium sulphate and repeated if necessary. An enema should be given unless the bowels move freely. Glycerine has been recommended in large doses, in order that it may by its hygroscopic properties destroy the worm. Male fern, santonin, and thymol have been recommended in this stage. Turpentine may be tried in full doses. There is no doubt that diarrhea in the first week or ten days of the infection is distinctly favorable. The indications in the stage of invasion are to relieve the pains, to secure sleep, and to support the patient's strength. There are no medicines which have any influence upon the embryos in their migration through the muscles. The use of arsphenamine has been advised but proof of its value is lacking.

ANCYLOSTOMIASIS

This is one of the most important and widespread of all metazoan infections, also known as hookworm disease, uncinariasis, anemia of miners, bricklayers, tunnel-workers; tropical and Egyptian chlorosis.

History—For three centuries the disease, but not its nature, was recognized under various names. Dubini, in 1838, first described the worms, and gave the name from the curved appearance of the mouth. In 1853 and 1854 Bilharz and Griesinger recognized the relation of the parasites to the anemia and dropsy. In South America in 1866 Wucherer called attention to the frequency of the disease in negro slaves. In the "seventies" and "eighties" of the last century the anemia of brickworkers in Italy and of miners and tunnel diggers was shown to be due to this parasite. Occasional statements were made as to the occurrence of the disease in the United States, but it was not until the extensive investigations of Stiles in 1901, and later, that it was shown that the hookworm was widely prevalent, that it was responsible for an enormous amount of ill health and that it was directly connected with the old and long-ago described practice of dirt-eating. It was gradually realized how widespread the disease was in the southern states. Ashford and King studied the disease in Porto Rico, and carried out one of the most successful of modern sanitary campaigns. In 1898 Looss discovered the cardinal fact of the penetration of the skin by the larvae and of the route by which they reach the intestine.

Distribution.—The parasite exists in many parts of the world, and there is scarcely a tropical country in which it does not prevail. The prevalence varies in different localities and it is very widespread in the tropics. In Europe it is chiefly an affection of miners in Germany, Hungary, France, and Belgium. In England there was a small out-break in Cornwall but the disease has not extended. Stiles showed that more than 12 per cent of cotton-mill employees in the Southern United States were infected, and the examination of recruits, college students, and school children in different parts of the country gave a percentage of infection of from 20 to 70 or even 80. Among 18,390 white troops examined, hookworm was found in 13.7 per cent. In the West Indies the Rockefeller Commission found 97,632 infected among 165,866 examined.

Parasites.—There are two chief forms, *Ancylostoma duodenale,* the old world species, and *Necator americanus,* the new world species. The former is a small cylindrical nematode, the male about 10 mm. and the female from 8 to 18 mm. in length. The mouth has chitinous plates, and is provided with two pairs of sharp, hook-shaped teeth, with which they pierce the mucosa of the bowel. The male has a prominent, umbrella-like caudal expansion. The new world worm has much the same characters, but it is more slender, the mouth globular, and the arrangement of the teeth quite different. The eggs are from 52 μ to 60 μ by about 34 μ in width in the European form, and from 64 μ to 76 μ by about 36 μ in breadth in the American form. They are very characteristic bodies in the feces of infected individuals. When passed they are already in process of segmentation. Complete desiccation and direct sunlight, or much water in the feces kills the eggs; but they are sometimes very resistant, and may survive freezing followed by a gentle thawing. The rapidity of development depends upon favoring conditions and temperature, and the larvae after escaping from the eggs may live for months in the mud or water of mines, and pass through a series of moults before they reach what is called the ripe stage. They then show a remarkable tenacity of life, and may live in water or slime for many months; and in this, which is the infective stage, they have a tendency to wander.

Modes of Infection.—An extraordinary number of eggs are passed with each stool of a badly infected person; it has been estimated as many as four millions. They develop most readily in feces mixed with sand or earth at a temperature of from 70° to 90°. The eggs are not infective; after moulting they develop into filariform larvae which are infective. Infection takes place either by the mouth directly, which is rare, or by the skin. Looss showed experimentally that the larvae entering the skin are carried by the veins to the heart, and thence to the lungs, in which they escape from the pulmonary vessels, pass up the bronchi and trachea, and so to the gullet, stomach and intestines. These observations of Looss have been abundantly confirmed. As C. A. Smith's work has shown, it takes about seven weeks before the ova appear in the stools, and in the process of infection there may be sore throat and fever. The skin is the common channel of entrance, and usually shows signs of irritation—*ground itch.* Ashford and King give a history of ground-itch in more than 90 per cent of their cases. Larvae accidentally swallowed may pass through the stomach and develop in the intestines.

Morbid Anatomy and Pathology.—The worms are chiefly in the jejunum; Sandwith found 1,353 of 1,524 worms in the first six feet of the bowel.

They are also occasionally found in the stomach. A variable number of worms are found attached to the mucosa. Very characteristic lesions are ecchymoses and small erosions of the mucosa, in the centre of which may be a pale area, slightly raised, to which the worm is attached; it may be almost buried in the mucosa. There are usually more bites or holes than worms. Blood cysts occur in the submucosa, in which, occasionally, worms are found (Whipple). The contents of the bowel are often blood-stained. In long-standing cases the mucosa may show many areas of pigmentation. Other lesions are those of chronic anemia with fatty degeneration. The loss of blood is largely direct, but it has been shown by Loeb and A. J. Smith that the head-glands of the worm secrete a substance which retards coagulation, probably a hemolytic poison, the presence of which Whipple demonstrated. Another feature is the liability to infection through the bites; the anemia may in part, at any rate, be due to poisonous products absorbed through the bowel lesions.

Symptoms.—Hookworm disease presents a very variable picture, nor does the severity of the symptoms seem to depend always upon the number of worms. There have been fatal cases in which only ten or twelve worms were found, while recovery has followed after more than 4,000 worms have been expelled (Dock). In infected districts, the hook-worm disease causes a wide-spread degeneration, the children and young adults showing pallor, under-development and failure of nutrition. With the infection, too, are associated apathy and lack of energy, so that the common opinion in the South is that the hookworm is the cause of laziness. There is no question that the infection is responsible for a great deal of ill health and physical incapacity, often without any actual illness. In more severe cases the anemia is pronounced, the hemoglobin being from 40 to 50 per cent; the child is stunted and puberty is long delayed, and the patient may belong to the group of dirt-eaters. The retardation of growth is remarkable, and the individual may continue to grow until he is 25 or 26 years of age. In the severest type of all the anemia is still more pronounced; the hemoglobin below 25 or 20 per cent; edema occurs, the patient is bedridden, and death occurs from exhaustion, diarrhea, or some inter-current affection. The *anemia* is of a secondary type, averaging from 50 to 60 per cent of the corpuscles, with, as a rule, a low color index. Leukocytosis is not often present, and the differential count shows nothing unusual except the great increase in the eosinophiles, ranging from 15 to 26 or even 30 per cent. The eosinophilia bears no relation to the severity of the infection. Myocardial and vasomotor disturbance are common and may be severe. They probably result largely from the anemia.

"Ground-itch," the local lesion through which the parasites enter, is most common on the feet and legs in children, or on the arms and hands in gardeners and miners. The most common region is between and beneath the toes. The eruption is vesicular at first; then pustules form with a sticky exudate, and sometimes with much swelling of the skin. The vesicles and pustules gradually dry, and in eight or ten days heal with exfoliation.

The digestive symptoms are remarkable. In the mild cases there are slight epigastric pain and discomfort; in the severer ones there are anorexia and remarkable perversions of appetie; the patients eat earth, paper, chalk, starch, hair and clay. The dirt-eaters of the southern states are subjects of hookworm disease. With the apathetic, listless expression there is dilatation of the pupils, and Stiles has remarked upon the "dull, blank, almost fish-like or cadaveric stare," which gives a characteristic appearance.

Diagnosis.—In tropical and subtropical regions slight anemia and ill health should lead to the examination of the stools, from which a certain diagnosis may be made by finding the eggs. "The combination of anemia with underdevelopment, weakness, dilated heart, and the history of ground-itch is not likely to be confused with anything else" (Stiles). In badly infected regions a fairly accurate diagnosis may be made on inspection alone, and this may be confirmed by the examination of the feces and by the rapid improvement after treatment. The *eggs* are characteristic structures, usually containing 4 or 8 segments, sometimes the complete embryo nearly ready to burst its shell. Various estimates have been made of the number of worms based on the number of eggs found. It is to be remembered that the eggs vary greatly in number, and the stools may be negative one day and contain many a few days later. Grassi states that 150 eggs per centigram of feces represent about 1,000 worms. The adult worms may be found in the stools after giving an anthelmintic. The eosinophilia is an important diagnostic aid, but is not invariably present. Boycott and Haldane found that 94 per cent of infected persons had over 8 per cent of eosinophiles.

Prophylaxis.—Destruction of the adult worms, removing conditions suitable to the growth of the embryos, and a campaign of sanitary education are the three essentials. The proper disposal of feces and decreasing the chance of infection by wearing shoes and stockings are important points. The work of the Porto Rico commission shows what can be done in the tropics, even in the most unfavorable surroundings. The International Health Board of the Rockefeller Foundation introduced the intensive method, which is an attempt as nearly as possible to relieve and control hookworm disease within a given area by sanitary and therapeutic measures. A census of the population is taken, a microscopic examination made of the stools, all infected persons are treated, and the treatment continued until a cure has resulted. The people are educated both as to the method of cure and dangers of soil pollution.

In mines care should be taken to prevent local conditions favoring the growth of the embryos. Oliver has found that cinder and slag are destructive of the larvae. New workers should be examined and proved not to have the disease before being admitted.

Treatment.—It is not safe to conclude too soon that all the worms have been removed, as a latent period, during which eggs are not produced, may last for some weeks after treatment. The bowels should be opened before treatment and liquid diet given the day before. A dose of saline, such as sodium sulphate, is given the night before. *Thymol* is given twice in the morning, two hours apart, and a dose of saline two hours after the second dose. The dose of thymol is graduated according to the age of the patient, seven grains (0.5 gm.) for children under five, and increasing the dose according to age and strength to sixty grains (4 gm.) for adults. Very few ill effects follow its use, but it sometimes is irritating to the bowels, and occasionally it is toxic. This treatment should be carried out on one day of each week until the patient is cured. No alcohol or oil should be given at the time of administration of thymol. It must be remembered that toxic effects may follow the administration of many of the remedies used for intestinal parasites.

Oil of chenopodium (wormseed oil) is often efficient, given in doses of 15 drops in castor oil every two hours for two or three doses. Two hours later a full dose of castor oil is given. *Carbon tetrachloride* is given in doses of 2 minims (0.13 cc.) per year of age in children and in doses of 45 minims (3 cc.) to adults, followed in two hours by a saline. Alcohol should not be taken for some time before or after. Crystalline *hexylresorcinol* is given in hard gelatine capsules in the early morning with the stomach empty in doses of gr. xv, 1 gm. for adults and less amounts for children. No food should be taken for six hours afterwards. Magnesium sulphate is given the next morning. *Tetrachlorethylene* is given in doses of 3 cc. in the morning after sodium sulphate the night before and again two hours after the drug is given. For young children the dose is 2 minims for each year of age. The anemia should receive the usual treatment.

FILARIASIS

The important species are:

Loa loa.—This is the eye-worm of tropical West Africa which causes "Calabar swellings." It occurs in the peripheral circulation during the day. The adults move about in the subcutaneous tissues.

Filaria bancrofti (*Wuchereria bancrofti*) (Cobbold, 1877).—This is the most important blood filaria. The embryos are found in the peripheral circulation only during sleep or at night. The mosquito is the intermediate host. The embryos measure 200 to 300 μ long by 7 to 10 μ broad; tail pointed. The adult male measures 83 mm. long by 0.407 mm. broad; the tail forms two turns of a spiral. The adult female measures 155 mm. long by 0.715 mm. broad; eggs 38 μ by 14 μ. The adult worms live in lymphatics, lymph spaces and glands. This is the species to which hematochyluria and elephantiasis are attributed. It is common in Central America and parts of South America. There are many cases in the West Indies and it is prevalent in some of the Pacific islands.

The female produces an extraordinary number of embryos, which enter the blood current through the lymphatics. Each embryo is within its sheath, which is scarcely perceptible and in no way impedes the movements. They are about the ninetieth part of an inch in length and the diameter of a red blood corpuscle in thickness, so that they readily pass through the capillaries. They move with the greatest activity, and form very striking objects under the microscope. A remarkable feature is the periodicity in the occurrence of the embryos in the blood. In the daytime they are almost or entirely absent, whereas at night, in typical cases, they are present in large numbers. There is no agreement as to the explanation of this. Lothrop and Pratt calculated the number of embryos per cc. of blood hourly during the night; it rose steadily from four o'clock in the afternoon till midnight, when 2,100 per cc. were present, then fell, none being found at ten o'clock the following morning. The further development of the embryos is associated with the mosquito, which sucks the blood and in this way frees them from the body. They develop in the mosquito and reach the proboscis from which they pass to the human host. The filariae may be present in the body without causing any symptoms. In the blood of animals filariae are very common and rarely cause inconvenience. It is only when the adult worms or the ova block the lymph channels that definite symptoms occur. Manson suggests that it is the ova (prematurely discharged), which are considerably shorter and thicker than the full-grown embryos, which block the lymph channels. Dead calcified filariae may appear in X-ray films of the tissues as small dots.

The effects produced may be described under the following conditions:

HEMATOCHYLURIA.—Without any external manifestations, and in many cases without special disturbance of health, the subject from time to time passes urine of an opaque white, milky appearance, or bloody, or a chylous fluid which on settling shows a slightly reddish clot. The condition indicates dilatation and rupture of dilated lymphatics in some part of the urinary tract and obstruction of the thoracic duct. In a case described by Stephen Mackenzie the renal and peritoneal lymph plexuses were enormously enlarged, extending from the diaphragm to the pelvis. The thoracic duct above the diaphragm was impervious. The urine may be normal in quantity or increased. The condition is usually intermittent, and the patient may pass normal urine for weeks or months at a time. Microscopically, the chylous urine contains minute molecular fat granules, and usually red blood cells in various amounts. The embryos were first discovered by Demarquay, at Paris (1863), and in the urine by Wucherer, at Bahia, in 1866. It is remarkable how long the condition may persist without serious impairment of the health. Chyluria is not always due to filaria; there is a nonparasitic form.

ELEPHANTIASIS is common in countries in which the filariae prevail. The parasites are not always found in the blood. The condition is more common in the legs, one or both, beginning below the knee, but gradually involving the entire limb. Next in frequency is *lymph-scrotum* and other forms involving the genitalia. The *scrotal* tumor may reach an enormous size, and 40 to 50 pounds in weight. The onset may be painless and slow, or sudden with fever, rapid swelling and redness of the part (lymphangitis). There may be a series of such attacks, each one leaving the part more swollen. The so-called "elephantoid fever" may occur in all forms of the infection.

Among other conditions are: *varicose groin glands* which lessen or disappear when the patient lies down and are easily mistaken for hernia; *orchitis* which may appear and subside rapidly; *hydrocele* often follows it; *filarial abscesses* which may be deeply seated and contain dead adult worms.

Sporadic Elephantiasis.—A nonparasitic type may be mentioned here, which is not very uncommon in temperate regions, characterized by a progressive enlargement of a limb or portion of the body, with a hyperplasia of the skin and subcutaneous tissues, due apparently to an obstructive inflammation of the lymph vessels. It may arise spontaneously without any obvious cause, or follow an inflammation of the skin of the part, occasionally removal of the lymph glands. The legs are most frequently involved, beginning usually in one leg, about the foot or ankle, and gradually extending until the whole leg is greatly enlarged. The skin is usually smooth, but it may be hard and indurated or warty and nodular. Most of the cases are in young women, in whom the affection has come on without any obvious cause and progressed slowly until the leg was greatly enlarged. In one case eight years elapsed before the other leg became involved, and in another case more than ten years passed with the disease still confined to one leg. The outlook in these cases is not good unless some cause of obstruction can be found and removed.

Diagnosis.—The filaria larva may be found in the blood, urine or chylous fluid. A negative finding does not exclude filarial infection. Adult worms may be found in lymph glands or in abscesses. Eosinophilia is present.

Treatment.—So far as known, no drug destroys the embryos in the blood with certainty. In infected districts protection of the infected and well from mosquitoes is essential. In cases of chyluria the patients should use a dry diet and avoid excess of fat. The chyle may disappear quite rapidly from the urine under these measures, but it does not necessarily indicate cure. So long as clots and albumin are present the leak in the lymphoid varix is not healed, although the fat, not being supplied to the chyle, may not be present. A single tumblerful of milk will at once give ocular proof of the patency or otherwise of the rupture in the varix (Manson).

Elephantoid fever demands rest, liquid diet, free purgation and sedative applications to painful areas. In *elephantiasis* during periods with acute symptoms the patient should be at rest and the legs firmly bandaged. Good results are reported from the use of fibrolysin. The surgical treatment of some cases is most successful, particularly in the removal of adult filariae from the enlarged lymph glands, especially in the groin. Surgical measures may be advisable in elephantiasis and lymph-scrotum. The treatment has to be decided by the particular problem presented by each patient.

Dracontiasis (Guinea-worm Disease)

Dracunculus medinensis is a widely spread parasite in parts of Africa, India and Brazil. In the United States instances occasionally occur. Chitwood (1933) discusses the reported cases and doubts if any have arisen in the United States. The parasite has been found in the fox, mink and raccoon in the United States and Canada.

The female develops in the subcutaneous and intermuscular connective tissues and produces vesicles and abscesses. In the large majority of the cases the parasite is found in the leg. Of 181 cases, in 124 the worm was found in the feet, 33 times in the leg, and 11 times in the thigh. It is usually solitary, though there are cases on record in which six or more have been present.

In water the embryos develop in a cyclops—a small crustacean—and it seems likely that man is infected by drinking the water containing these developed larvae. It is probable that both male and female are ingested; but the former dies and is discharged, while the latter after impregnation penetrates the intestine and attains its full development in the subcutaneous tissues, where it may remain quiescent for a long time and can be felt beneath the skin like a bundle of string. The worm contains an enormous number of living embryos, and to enable them to escape she travels slowly downward head first, and usually reaches the foot or ankle. The head then penetrates the skin and the epidermis, forms a little vesicle, which ruptures, and a small ulcer is left, at the bottom of which the head often protrudes. The distended uterus ruptures and the embryos are discharged in a whitish fluid.

When the worm first appears it should not be disturbed, as after parturition it may leave spontaneously. When the worm begins to come out a common procedure is to roll it round a portion of smooth wood and in this way prevent retraction, and each day wind a little more until the entire worm is withdrawn.

Special care must be taken to prevent tearing of the worm, as severe inflammation may follow this.

The parasite may be excised entire, or killed by injections of bichloride of mercury (1 to 1,000). Asafetida in full doses is said to kill the worm.

OTHER NEMATODES

Trichocephaliasis.—*Trichuris trichiura* (whipworm) is not infrequently found in the cecum and large intestine of man. It measures from 4 to 5 cm. in length, the male being somewhat shorter than the female. The worm is readily recognized by the remarkable difference between the anterior and posterior portions. The former, which forms at least three-fifths of the body, is extremely thin and hair-like in contrast to the thick hinder portion of the body, which in the female is conical and pointed, and in the male more obtuse and usually rolled like a spring. The eggs are oval, lemon-shaped, 0.05 mm. in length, and provided with a button-like projection.

The number of the worms is variable, as many as a thousand having been counted. It is a widely spread parasite. In parts of Europe it occurs in from 10 to 30 per cent of all bodies, but in the United States it is not so common. The whipworm rarely causes symptoms. French and Boycott found ova in 40 of 500 Guy's Hospital patients. They found no etiological relationship of the parasite to appendicitis. Several cases have been reported in which profound anemia occurred with this parasite, usually with diarrhea. Urticaria and eosinophilia may occur. Enormous numbers may be present without any symptoms. The *diagnosis* is made by the examination of the feces, which contain the characteristic lemon-shaped, hard, dark-brown eggs. In *treatment*, thymol, oil of chenopodium or crystalline hexylresorcinol may be used as in ascariasis.

Dioctophyme renale (*Eustrongylus gigas*).—This enormous nematode, the male of which measures about a foot in length and the female about three feet, occurs in many animals and has occasionally been found in man. It is usually found in the renal region and may entirely destroy the kidney.

Anguillula aceti.—The vinegar eel is sometimes present in urine and has been found in the bladder. It may be mistaken for a filarial parasite.

Strongyloides stercoralis.—This is a common parasite in tropical diarrhea and has a wide distribution in tropical and subtropical countries. It is found in the Southern and occasionally in the Northern United States. The mother worm burrows in the mucous membrane and deposits ova. The parasite is found in the upper parts of the small intestines. With light infections there may be alternating diarrhea and constipation; in heavy infections the diarrhea may be severe. Urticaria and edema sometimes occur, and there may be moderate anemia. The *diagnosis* is made by finding the larvae in the stools. In *treatment*, gentian violet is given in a keratin-coated pill (gr. ii, 0.13 gm.) three times a day for ten days.

PARASITIC ARACHNIDA AND TICKS

Pentastomes.—LINGUATULA RHINARIA (*Pentastoma taenioides*) has a somewhat lancet-shaped body, the female being from 3 to 4 inches in length, the male about an inch in length. The adult worm infects the frontal sinuses and nostrils of the dog, more rarely of the horse. The larval form, known as *Linguatula serrata* (*Pentastomum denticulatum*), is seen in the internal organs, particularly the liver, but has also been found in the kidney. The adult worm has been found in the nostril of man, but is rare and seldom occasions any inconvenience. The larvae are not uncommon, particularly in parts of Germany. The parasite is very rare. Flint refers to a Missouri case in which from 75 to 100 parasites were expectorated. The liver was enlarged and the parasites probably occupied this region.

The ARMILLIFER ARMILLATUS (*Pentastomum constrictum*) has the length of half an inch, with twenty-three rings on the abdomen. It is found in the Congo district and in parts of Asia. The larvae, found in cysts in the lungs and liver, cause disease as they wander. The adult form lives in the nasal cavities and lungs of pythons and other snakes and man is infected probably through the drinking water.

Arachnidism (*Spider poisoning*).—The bite of the black widow spider (*Lactrodectus mactans*) may cause severe symptoms and death in some cases (17 deaths in 380 cases, Bogen, 1933). The bite may be on different parts of the body or extremities and the mark may be very slight. Locally there may be a stinging sensation or severe pain. Later there are anxiety, sweating, dyspnea, nausea, vomiting, retention of urine, and sometimes delirium. Tremors, convulsions and paralysis have followed. A remarkable point is the occurrence of abdominal features suggestive of an acute lesion with extreme rigidity of the abdominal muscles. There may be fever and leukocytosis. Sometimes the lumbar and thigh muscles show marked rigidity. In other cases tetanus has been suggested. The diagnosis may be rendered more difficult if the patient does not know that he has been bitten. Tenderness is often less than the muscular rigidity. The *treatment* will depend on the condition. Stimulation by caffeine and epinephrine is indicated for shock. The intravenous injection of magnesium sulphate (25 per cent solution) has been suggested. Sedatives may be advisable in some cases.

Demodex (Acarus) folliculorum (var. hominis).—A minute parasite from 0.3 mm. to 0.4 mm. in length, which lives in the sebaceous follicles, particularly of the face. It is doubtful whether it produces any symptoms. Possibly when in large numbers they excite inflammation leading to acne.

Sarcoptes (Acarus) scabiei (*Itch Insect*).—This is the most important of the arachnid parasites. The male is 0.23 mm. in length and 0.19 mm. in breadth; the female is 0.45 mm. in length and 0.35 mm. in width. The female can be seen readily with the naked eye and has a pearly-white color. It is not so common in the United States and Canada as in Europe.

The insect lives in a small burrow, about 1 cm. in length, which it makes for itself in the epidermis. At the end of this burrow the female lives. The male is seldom found. The chief seat of the parasite is in the folds where the skin is most delicate, as in the web between the fingers and toes, the backs of the hands, the axilla, and the front of the abdomen. The head and face are rarely involved. The lesions which result from the presence of the itch insect are very numerous and result largely from the irritation of scratching. The commonest is a papular and vesicular rash, or, in children, an ecthymatous eruption. The irritation and pustulation which follow the scratching may completely destroy the burrows, but in typical cases there is rarely doubt as to the diagnosis.

The *treatment* consists of warm baths with a thorough scrubbing and use of a soft soap, after which the skin should be anointed with sulphur ointment, which for children should be diluted. An ointment of naphthol (dram to the ounce) is very efficacious. The clothing should be sterilized.

Leptus autumnalis (*Harvest Bug*).—This reddish-colored parasite, about half a millimenter in size, is often found in large numbers in fields and in gardens. They attach themselves to animals and man with their sharp proboscides, and the hooklets of their legs produce a great deal of irritation. They are most frequently found on the legs. They are readily destroyed by sulphur ointment or corrosive-sublimate lotions.

Ixodiasis (*Tick-fever*).—In certain parts of Africa there is a disease known by this name, believed to be transmitted by a tick—the *Ornithodorus* or *Argas moubata.* The ticks live in old houses, and their habits are very much like those of the common bed-bug. This tick transmits the *Spirochaeta duttoni*, the cause of the African form of relapsing fever.

Dermacentor andersoni is present in the northwestern states from California to Montana. The bites may cause severe lymphangitis. It is a medium of transmission of Rocky Mountain spotted fever.

Otobius megnini (spinose ear tick) is widely spread over the western and southwestern states. The tick enters the ear in the larval stage and buries itself between folds of skin. Animals are frequently infected. The local symptoms are marked. Chloroform vapor followed by syringing or the introduction of oil is effective in removal. Several other varieties of ticks are occasionally found on man—the *Ixodes ricinus* and the *Dermacentor americanus,* which are met with in horses and oxen.

Tick Paralysis.—In connection with the bites of ticks of the genus Ixodes and the genus Dermacentor a flaccid paralysis of the legs has been described, particularly in British Columbia, Wyoming, Montana, and possibly in Australia. Children are usually affected, and, curiously enough, if the tick is found and removed promptly, the child gets well within twenty-four hours, but if not, the paralysis may spread to the arms, stupor may come on, and the child may die of a widespread paralysis. In adults sometimes there are pain, an erythematous rash, and vertigo. It appears to be a toxic effect of the parasite and not an infection.

PARASITIC INSECTS

Pediculi (*Phthiriasis; Pediculosis*).—There are three varieties:

Pediculus capitis (*Head Louse*).—The male is from 1 to 1.5 mm. in length and the female nearly 2 mm. The color varies somewhat with the different races of men. It is light gray with a black margin in the European, and very much darker in the negro and Chinese. They are oviparous, and the female lays about sixty eggs, which mature in a week. The ova are attached to the hairs and are known popularly as nits. The symptoms are irritation and itching of the scalp. When numerous, the insects may excite an eczema or a pustular dermatitis, which causes crusts and scabs, particularly at the back of the head. In extreme cases the hair becomes tangled in these crusts and matted together, forming a firm mass which is known as *plica polonica,* as it was not infrequent among the Jewish inhabitants of Poland.

Pediculus corporis (*vestimentorum*).—This is larger than the head louse. It lives on the clothing, and in sucking the blood causes minute hemorrhagic specks, which are very common about the neck, back, and abdomen. The irritation of the bites may cause urticaria and the scratching is usually in linear lines. In long-standing cases, particularly in old dissipated characters, the skin becomes rough and greatly pigmented, a condition which has been termed the vagabond's disease—*morbus errorum*—which may be mistaken for the bronzing of Addison's disease. The pigmentation may be extreme and extend to the face and buccal mucosa.

Pediculus pubis (*crab louse*) differs somewhat from the other forms, and is found in the parts of the body covered with short hairs, as the pubes; more rarely the axilla and eyebrows.

The *taches bleuâtres, maculae ceruleae,* or peliomata, excited by the irritation of pediculi, are subcuticular bluish or slate-colored spots from 5 to 10 mm. in diameter seen about the abdomen and thighs, particularly in febrile cases. The spots are more marked on white thin skins. They are stains caused by a pigment in the secretion of the salivary glands of the louse.

Treatment.—For the head louse, when the condition is very bad, the hair should be cut short, as it is very difficult to destroy all the nits. Repeated saturations of the hair in coal-oil or in turpentine are usually efficacious, or with lotions of carbolic acid, 1 to 50. The application of a mixture of equal parts of xylene, alcohol and ether is useful. Scrupulous cleanliness and care are sufficient to prevent recurrence. In the case of the body louse, the clothing should be thoroughly disinfected. To allay the itching a warm bath containing 4 or 5 ounces of bicarbonate of soda is useful. For the *Pediculus pubis* white precipitate or ordinary mercurial ointment should be used, and the parts thoroughly washed two or three times a day with soft soap and water. Phenol (2 per cent solution) may be applied.

Cimex lectularius (*Bed-bug*).—The tropical and subtropical variety is *Cimex rotundalius.* It lives in the crevices of the bedstead and in the cracks in the floor and in the walls. It is nocturnal in its habits. The peculiar odor of the insect is caused by the secretion of a special gland. The parasite possesses a long proboscis, with which it sucks the blood. Individuals differ remarkably in the reaction to the bite of this insect; some are not disturbed by them, in others the irritation causes hyperemia and often intense urticaria. Fumigation with sulphur or scouring with corrosive sublimate solution or kerosene destroys them. Iron bedsteads should be used.

Pulex irritans (*Common Flea*).—The male is from 2 to 2.55 mm. in length, the female from 3 to 4 mm. The flea is a transient parasite on man. The bite causes a circular red spot of hyperemia in the centre of which is a little speck where the boring apparatus has entered. The amount of irritation caused by the bite is variable. Many persons suffer intensely and a diffuse erythema or an urticaria develops; others suffer no inconvenience.

The *Tunga penetrans* (*sand-flea, jigger*) is found in tropical countries, particularly in the West Indies and South America. It is much smaller than the common flea, and not only penetrates the skin, but burrows and produces an inflammation with pustular or vesicular swelling. It most frequently attacks the feet. It is readily removed with a needle. Where they exist in large numbers the essential oils are used on the feet as a preventive.

PARASITIC FLIES

The accidental invasion of the body cavities and of the skin by the larvae of the diptera is known as *myiasis* or *myiosis*.

The larvae of the *Compsomyia macellaria,* the so-called screw-worm, have been found in the nose, in wounds, and in the vagina after delivery. They can be removed readily with forceps; if there is any difficulty, thorough cleansing and the application of an antiseptic solution are sufficient to kill them. The ova of the blue-bottle fly may be deposited in the nostrils, ears, or conjunctiva. This rarely takes place unless these regions are the seat of disease. In the nose and in the ear the larvae may cause serious inflammation. Even the urethra has not been spared in these dipterous invasions.

Gastro-intestinal myiasis may result from the swallowing of the larvae of the common house-fly or of other species. There are many cases on record in which the larvae of the *Musca domestica* have been discharged by vomiting. Instances in which dipterous larvae have been passed in the feces are less common. Finlayson, of Glasgow, reported a case in a physician, who, after protracted constipation and pain in the back and sides, passed large numbers of the larvae of the flower-fly—*Anthomyia canicularis.* Among other forms of larvae or gentles, as they are sometimes called, found in the feces are those of the common house-fly, the blue-bottle fly, and the *Techomyza fusca.* The larvae of other insects are rare. It is stated that the caterpillar of the taby moth has been found in the feces. A specimen of *Homalomyia scalaris,* one of the privy flies, was sent by Dr. Hartin, of Kaslo City, B. C., the larvae of which were passed in large numbers in the stools of a native of Louisiana. There are cases in which the larvae have been passed for years. Although no grave results necessarily follow the invasion by these larvae, yet they may be the cause of serious intestinal ulceration manifesting itself by a dysenteric disease with fatal result. In treatment, the bowels should be cleared by castor oil.

Cutaneous Myiasis.—The most common form is that in which an external wound becomes "living," as it is called due to the larvae of the blue-blottle or the common flesh-fly. The skin may also be infected by the larvae of the *Musca vomitoria,* but more commonly by the bot-flies of the ox and sheep which occasionally attack man. This is rare in temperate climates. Matas described a case in which estrus larvae were found in the gluteal region. In parts of Central America the eggs of another bot-fly, the *Dermatobia,* may be deposited in the skin and produce a swelling very like the ordinary boil.

Dermamyiasis linearis migrans estrosa is a remarkable cutaneous condition, observed particularly in Russia and occasionally in other countries, in which the larva of *Gastrophilus,* the horse bot-fly, makes a slightly raised pale red "line" which travels over the body surface sometimes with great rapidity. It has been referred to as Larva migrans and as Creeping Eruption. Corrigan reported cases from Lampman, Sask., Canada, in which he obtained the larva from the skin.

In Africa the larvae of the Cayor fly are not uncommonly found beneath the skin in little boils. In the Congo region Dutton, Todd, and Christy found a troublesome blood-sucking dipterous larva, known as the floor maggot, the fly of which is the *Anchmeromyia luteola.*

Caddis Flies (*Trichoptera*).—These have a wide distribution and their emanations (epithelium and hairs) cause allergic manifestations in susceptible persons. Parlato (1934) found 5 per cent of 850 allergic patients hypersensitive to this fly. An aqueous extract of the whole fly is used for the usual tests. Desensitization can be done by subcutaneous injection beginning with very small doses.

Caterpillar Rash.—In some districts in Europe the hairs of the procession caterpillar, particularly of the species *Cnethocampa,* cause an intense urticaria, the so-called *U. epidemica.* In parts of the United States the caterpillar of the brown-tailed moth has caused much discomfort. The hairs are widely distributed and the barbs readily work into the skin. There may be an intense eruption which has been mistaken for that of smallpox. In England, Thresh called attention to the frequency of these caterpillar rashes due to the yellow-tailed moth, *Porthesia similis.*

Harvest Rash (*Erythema Autumnale*).—In parts of England during the autumn many people are attacked by the harvest bug or harvesters, which may cause an obstinate and distressing malady. Usually attributed to the harvest spider, it is in reality caused by a mite, parasitic upon it, the hexapod larva of the silky trombidian. It is so small as to be scarcely visible and is brick-red in color. They chiefly attack persons with delicate skins, on the ankles and legs, but also attack the arms and neck. The mite attaches itself to the skin by its claws, sucks the blood, and the swollen red abdomen may sometimes be seen as a bright-red dot. A papulovesicular, sometimes a pustular, eruption with an intolerable itching is caused by it. So intense may the eruption be, with perhaps an entire family attacked, that suspicion of poisoning is aroused. The parasite is readily killed by benzine.

INFECTIOUS DISEASES OF DOUBTFUL OR UNKNOWN ETIOLOGY

SMALLPOX (Variola)

Definition.—An acute infectious disease, characterized by a cutaneous eruption which passes through the stages of papule, vesicle, pustule, and crust. A secondary streptococcus infection is an important feature.

History.—The existence of the disease in ancient Egypt is suggested by the eruption on the skin of a mummy of the 20th dynasty—1,200 to 1,100 B. C. (Rüffer and Ferguson). The disease existed in China many centuries before Christ. The *pesta magna* described by Galen (of which Marcus Aurelius died) is believed to have been smallpox. In the sixth century it prevailed, and subsequently, at the time of the Crusades, became widespread. It was brought to America by the Spaniards early in the sixteenth century. The first accurate account was given by Rhazes, an Arabian physician who lived in the ninth century, and whose description is available in Greenhill's translation for the Sydenham Society. In the seventeenth century Sydenham differentiated measles from smallpox. Special events in the history of the disease are the introduction of inoculation into Europe, by Lady Mary Wortley Montagu, in 1718, and the discovery of vaccination by Jenner in 1796.

Etiology.—Smallpox is one of the most virulent of infectious diseases, and persons exposed, if unprotected by vaccination, are almost invariably attacked. Instances of natural immunity are rare. It is said that Diemerbroeck, a celebrated Utrecht professor in the seventeenth century, was not only himself exempt, but likewise many members of his family. An attack may not protect for life. There are undoubted cases of a second, reputed instances, indeed, of a third attack. Louis XV of France died of a second attack of smallpox.

Age.—Smallpox is common at all ages, but is particularly fatal to young children. Of 3,164 deaths in the Montreal epidemic of 1885-'86, 2,717 were of children under ten years of age. The *fetus in utero* may be attacked, but only if the mother is the subject of the disease. The child may be born with the rash out or with the scars. In the case of twins, only one may be attacked; Kaltenbach records an instance of triplets, only two of which were affected (Comby). Children born in a smallpox hospital, if vaccinated immediately, may escape the disease; usually, however, they die early.

Sex.—Males and females are equally affected.

Race.—Among aboriginal races smallpox is terribly fatal. When the disease was first introduced into America the Mexicans died by thousands, and the North American Indians have also been frequently decimated by this plague. It is stated that the negro is especially susceptible, and the mortality is greater—about 42 per cent in the black, against 29 per cent in the white (W. M. Welch).

The disease smoulders here and there and when conditions are favorable becomes epidemic. This was well illustrated by the Montreal outbreak of 1885. For several years there had been no smallpox in the city, and a large unprotected population grew up among the French-Canadians, many of whom were opposed to vaccination. On February 28 a Pullman-car conductor, who had traveled from Chicago, was admitted into the Hôtel-Dieu, the civic smallpox hospital being closed at the time. Isolation was not carried out, and on the 1st of April a servant in the hospital died of smallpox. Following her decease, the authorities of the hospital dismissed all patients presenting no symptoms who could go home. The disease spread like fire in dry grass, and in nine months 3,164 persons died in the city of smallpox.

Variations in Virulence.—Sydenham states that "smallpox also has its peculiar kinds, which take one form during one series of years, and another during another"; and not only does what he called the epidemic constitution vary greatly, but one sometimes sees the most extraordinary variations in the intensity of the disease in members of a family all exposed to the same infection. A striking illustration of this variability has been given in recent epidemics, which have been of so mild a character that in many localities it has been mistaken for chickenpox. Very often a correct diagnosis is not reached until a fatal case has occurred. Even in unvaccinated children the disease has been exceedingly mild. In 1922, in the north of England among 821 cases there were 3 deaths and in London 74 cases with 24 deaths. This is an old story in the history of the disease. John Mason Good, in commenting on this very point, refers to the great variability in the epidemics, and states that he himself as a child of six (1770) passed through smallpox with "scarcely any disturbance and not more than twenty scattered pustules"!

Anomalous Forms.—In Africa, Australia, Brazil and the West Indies, an infection occurs known as alastrim, amaas or varioloid varicella, which is regarded as a mild form of smallpox. It attacks adults especially; the lesions are superficial and may appear in crops; the course is short and the mortality slight.

Recent Prevalence.—In the United States in 1930 there were 165 deaths in the registration area. The mild type of the disease continues, but in places there have been virulent outbreaks. In England and Wales there were 250 deaths in ten years (1922-1931 inclusive). In California in 1916 there were 248 cases; in 1917, 329; in 1918, 1,100; in 1919, 2,053; and in 1920, 4,486 cases. Of 4,226 of the 1920 cases in which a vaccination history was obtained, 1 per cent had been vaccinated in the preceding five years, 7 per cent had been vaccinated over five years before, and 92 per cent had never been vaccinated.

Nature of Infection.—Protozoön-like bodies were described in the skin lesions by Guarnieri—*Cytoryctes variolae.* These may be the same as the "Paschen bodies." Infection occurs probably by the respiratory tract and may be direct or indirect. It has been contracted from the body of one dead from the disease. The dried scales are an important element, and as a dust-like powder are distributed in the room during convalescence, becoming attached to clothing and articles of furniture. The disease is probably infectious from a very early stage, though it has not been determined whether the infection is active before the eruption develops. The agent is of unusual tenacity and clings to infected localities. It is conveyed by persons who have been in contact with the sick and by fomites. During epidemics it is no doubt widely spread in street cars and public conveyances. An unprotected person may contract a very virulent form of the disease from a patient with a mild attack. The virus is filterable; its nature is unknown.

Morbid Anatomy.—The cutaneous lesions are in the deeper epidermal layers. The pustules may be seen on the tongue, the buccal mucosa and the palate; sometimes also in the pharynx. In some cases the lesions are present in the esophagus and even in the stomach. Swelling of the Peyer's follicles is not uncommon; the pustules have been seen in the rectum.

In the larynx the eruption may be associated with a fibrinous exudate and sometimes with edema. Occasionally the inflammation penetrates deeply and involves the cartilages. In the trachea and bronchi there may be ulcerative erosions, but true pocks, such as are seen on the skin do not occur.

The heart may show myocardial changes; endocarditis and pericarditis are uncommon. French writers have described an endarteritis of the coronary vessels. The spleen is markedly enlarged. Apart from the cloudy swelling and areas of coagulation-necrosis, lesions of the kidneys are not common. Nephritis may occur. The reticulo-endothelial system shows marked alterations.

In the *hemorrhagic* form extravasations are found on the serous and mucous surfaces, in the parenchyma of organs, in the connective tissues, about the nerve-sheaths and in the muscles. In one instance the entire retroperitoneal tissue was infiltrated with a large coagulum, and there were also extensive extravasations in the course of the thoracic aorta. Hemorrhages in the bone marrow have been described and it may show marked changes. The spleen is firm and hard in hemorrhagic smallpox.

Symptoms.—Different forms of smallpox are described, but they only represent various degrees of severity.

Ordinary Smallpox or Variola Vera.—The period of *incubation* is from nine to fifteen days, usually twelve. The senior author saw it as early as the eighth day after exposure, and there are authenticated instances in which it was prolonged to twenty days. It is unusual for patients to complain of any symptoms during this period.

Invasion.—In adults a chill and in children a convulsion are common initial symptoms. There may be repeated chills within the first twenty-four

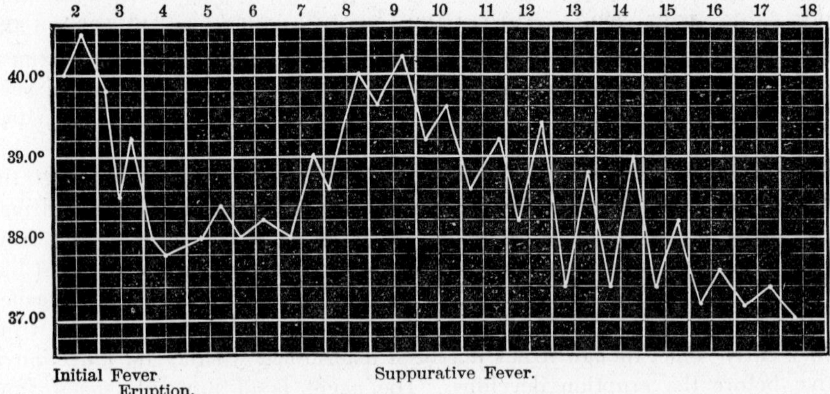

Chart XII.—Smallpox (Strümpell).

hours. Intense frontal headache, severe lumbar pains, and vomiting are very constant features. The pains in the back and in the limbs are more severe in the initial stage of this than of any other eruptive fever, and their combination with headache and vomiting is so suggestive that precautionary measures may often be taken before the eruption appears. The temperature rises quickly, and may on the first day be 103° or 104°. The pulse is rapid and full, not often dicrotic. In severe cases there may be marked delirium, particularly if the fever is high. The patient is restless and distressed, the face flushed, and the eyes bright and clear. The skin is usually dry, though occasionally there are profuse sweats. One cannot judge from the initial symptoms whether a case is likely to be discrete or confluent, as convulsions, severe headache, and high fever may precede a mild attack.

Initial Rashes.—Two forms can be distinguished: the diffuse, *scarlatinal*, and the *macular* or measly form; either of which may be associated with petechiae and occupy a variable extent of surface. In some instances they are general, but as a rule are limited to the lower abdominal areas, to the inner surfaces of the thighs, to the lateral thoracic region or to the axillae. Occasionally they are found over the extensor surfaces, particularly in the neighborhood of the knees and elbows. These rashes, often purpuric, are often associated with an erythematous or erysipelatous blush. The scarlatinal rash may come out as early as the second day, and be as diffuse and vivid as in scarlet fever. The measly rash may also be diffuse and resemble closely that of measles. Urticaria is seen only occasionally. The initial rashes are more abundant in some epidemics and occur in from 10 to 15 per cent of cases.

Eruption.—In the *discrete form,* usually on the third or fourth day, *macules* appear on the forehead, preceded sometimes by an erythematous flush, and on the anterior surfaces of the wrists. Within the first twenty-four hours from their appearance they occur on other parts of the face and on the extremities, and a few are seen on the trunk. The spots are from 2-3 millimetres in diameter, of a bright red color, and disappear completely on pressure. On the second day of the eruption the macular eruption becomes *papular.* As the rash comes out the temperature falls, the general symptoms subside, and the patient feels comfortable. On the third day of the eruption the papules change into *vesicles* with clear summits. Each one is elevated, circular, and presents a little depression or umbilication in the centre. They are divided into compartments and do not collapse if a single opening is made. They are *in the skin* rather than *on the surface.* About the fifth day of the eruption the vesicles change into *pustules,* the umbilication disappears, the flat top assumes a globular form and becomes grayish-yellow in color, owing to the contained pus. There is an areola of injection about the pustules and the skin between them is swollen. This maturation first takes place on the face, and follows the order of the appearance of the eruption. The temperature now rises—*secondary* fever—and the general symptoms return. The swelling about the pustules is attended with a good deal of tension and pain in the face; the eyelids become swollen and closed. In the discrete form the temperature of maturation does not usually remain high for more than twenty-four hours, so that on the tenth or eleventh day of the disease the fever disappears and the stage of convalescence begins. The pustules rapidly dry, first on the face and then on the other parts, and by the fourteenth or fifteenth day desquamation may be far advanced on the face. The distribution of the rash is often most characteristic. The abdomen, groins, axillae and the legs are least affected. The rash is often copious on the upper part of the back, scanty on the lower. Vesicles in the mouth, pharynx, and larynx cause soreness and swelling in these parts, with loss of voice and the formation of shallow ulcers. Whether pitting takes place depends a good deal upon the severity of the disease. In a majority of cases Sydenham's statement holds good, that "it is very rarely the case that the distinct smallpox leaves its mark." The odor of a smallpox patient is very distinctive even in the early stages, and has been a help in the diagnosis of a doubtful case.

The Confluent Form.—With the same initial symptoms, though usually of greater severity, the rash appears on the third or fourth day. The more the eruption shows itself before the fourth day the more sure it is to become confluent (Sydenham). The papules at first may be isolated, and it is only later in the stage of maturation that the eruption is confluent. But in severer cases the skin is swollen and hyperemic and the papules are very close together. On the feet and hands, too, the papules are thickly set; more scattered on the limbs; and quite discrete on the trunk. With the appearance of the eruption the symptoms subside and the fever remits, but not to the same extent as in the discrete form. Occasionally the temperature falls to normal and the patient may be comfortable. Then, usually on the eighth day of the disease, the fever again rises, the vesicles change to pustules, the hyperemia becomes intense, the swelling of the face and hands increases, and by the tenth day the pustules have fully maturated, many have coalesced, and the entire skin of the head and extremities is a superficial abscess. The fever rises to 103° or 105°, the pulse is from 110 to 120, and there is often delirium. Salivation in adults and diarrhea in children are common in this stage. There is usually much thirst. The eruption may be present in the mouth, and usually the pharynx and larynx are involved and the voice is husky. Great swelling of the cervical lymphatic glands occurs. At this stage the patient presents a terrible picture, which fully justifies the horror and fright with which smallpox is associated in the public mind. Even when the rash is confluent on the face, hands, and feet, the pustules remain discrete on the trunk. The danger, as pointed out by Sydenham, is in proportion to the number upon the face. "If upon the face they are as thick as sand, it is no advantage to have them few and far between on the rest of the body." In fatal cases by the tenth or eleventh day the pulse gets feebler and more rapid, the delirium is marked, there is subsultus, sometimes diarrhea, and with these symptoms the patient dies. In other instances between the eighth and eleventh day hemorrhagic features occur. When recovery takes place, the patient enters on the eleventh or twelfth day the period of desiccation.

Desiccation.—The pustules break and the pus exudes or they dry and form crusts. In the third week the desiccation proceeds and in cases of moderate severity the secondary fever subsides; in others it may persist until the fourth week. The crusts in confluent smallpox adhere for a long time and the process of scarring may take three or four weeks. On the face they fall off singly, but the tough epidermis of the hands and feet may be shed entire.

Blood.—There is a marked leukocytosis, 10-15 thousand, about the eighth day, then a slight decline and a rise again about the twelfth or fourteenth day, sometimes to 18,000 or 20,000. There is an increase in the mononuclear elements. The blood platelets are diminished in the early stages in all forms and continue to decrease in the purpuric forms. In ordinary variola they show a rapid increase after the vesicular stage.

HEMORRHAGIC SMALLPOX occurs in two forms. In the *hemorrhagic* or black smallpox the special features appear early and death follows in from two to six days. In the other form the case progresses as one of ordinary variola, and in the vesicular or pustular stage hemorrhages take place into the pocks or from the mucous membranes—*variola hemorrhagica pustulosa.*

Hemorrhagic smallpox is more common in some epidemics than in others. It is less frequent in children than in adults and young and vigorous persons seem more liable to it. Men are more frequently affected than women. The influence of vaccination is shown in the fact that of 27 cases 14 were unvaccinated, while not one of the 13 who had scars had been revaccinated. The illness starts with the usual symptoms, but with more intense constitutional disturbance. On the second or the third day there is a diffuse hyperemic rash, particularly in the groins, with small punctiform hemorrhages. The rash extends, becomes more distinctly hemorrhagic, and the spots increase in size. Ecchymoses appear on the conjunctivae, and as early as the third day there may be hemorrhages from the mucous membranes. Death may take place before the papules appear. In this truly terrible affection the patient may present a frightful appearance. The skin may have a uniformly purplish hue and the unfortunate victim may even look plum-colored. The face is swollen and large conjunctival hemorrhages with the deeply sunken corneae give a ghastly appearance. The mind may remain clear to the end. Death occurs usually from the third to the sixth day. The earliest death was on the third day and there were no traces of papules. Hematuria is perhaps most common, next hematemesis, and melena was noticed in a third of the cases. The pulse is rapid and often hard and small. The respirations are greatly increased in frequency and out of all proportion to the intensity of the fever.

In *variola pustulosa haemorrhagica* the disease progresses as a severe case, and the hemorrhages do not occur until the vesicular or pustular stage. The first indication is hemorrhage into the areolae of the pocks, and later the maturated pustules fill with blood. The earlier the hemorrhage the greater is the danger. Bleeding from the mucous membranes is common and the great majority prove fatal, usually on the seventh, eighth, or ninth day, but a few recover. In patients with the discrete form, if allowed to get up early, hemorrhage may take place into the pocks on the legs.

Varioloid.—This term is applied to the modified form in persons who have been vaccinated. It may set in with abruptness and severity, the temperature reaching 103°. More commonly it is in every respect milder in its initial symptoms, though the headache and backache may be very distressing. The papules appear on the third or fourth day. They are few in number and may be confined to the face and hands. The fever drops at once and the patient feels comfortable. The maturation of the pocks takes place rapidly and there is no secondary fever. There is rarely any scarring. As a rule, when smallpox attacks a person who has been vaccinated within five years the disease is mild, but it may prove severe, even fatal.

Abortive Types.—Recent epidemics have been characterized by the large number of *mild cases.* Even in unvaccinated children only a few pustules may appear and the disease is over in a few days. Even with a thickly set eruption the vesicles, instead of filling, dry and abort, forming the so-called horn-, crystalline-, or wartpox. *Variola sine eruptione* is described. Bancroft observed twelve cases in a Boston outbreak, all among physicians and attendants. The symptoms are headache, pain in the back, fever, and vomiting. The pocks may be very scanty and easily overlooked, even in unvaccinated persons. One of Bancroft's cases was of special interest—a pregnant woman who had slight symptoms after exposure, but no rash. Her child showed a typical eruption when two days old.

There has been much discussion about *variola minor* and whether there may be a disease with features like mild smallpox but which is not the true disease. It seems safer to hold that smallpox, like other acute exanthemata, may occur in a very mild form.

Complications.—Considering the severity of many of the cases and the character of the disease, associated with multiple foci of suppuration, the complications in smallpox are remarkably few.

Laryngitis is serious in three ways: it may produce a fatal edema of the glottis; it is liable to extend and involve the cartilages, producing necrosis; and by diminishing the sensibility of the larynx it may allow irritating particles to reach the lower air passages, where they excite bronchitis or bronchopneumonia. *Bronchopneumonia* is almost invariably present in fatal cases. *Lobar pneumonia* is rare. *Pleurisy* is common in some epidemics.

Cardiac complications are rare. At the height of the fever a systolic murmur at the apex is not uncommon; but endocarditis is rare and pericarditis is uncommon. Myocarditis seems to be more frequent, and may be associated with endarteritis of the coronary vessels.

Of complications in the *digestive* system, parotitis is rare. In severe cases there is extensive pseudodiphtheritic angina. Vomiting, so marked in the early stage, is rarely persistent. Diarrhea is not uncommon, particularly in children. *Albuminuria* is frequent, but true *nephritis* is rare. Inflammation of the testes and ovaries may occur.

Among the serious complications are those pertaining to the *nervous system,* among which *encephalitis* is important. In children convulsions are common. In adults the delirium of the early stage may persist and become violent, and finally subside into a fatal coma. Postfebrile insanity is occasionally met with during convalescence, and very rarely epilepsy. Many of the old writers spoke of paraplegia with the intense backache of the early stage, but it is probably associated with the severe lumbar and crural pains and is not a true paraplegia. It must be distinguished from the form occurring in convalescence, which may be due to peripheral neuritis or diffuse myelitis. The neuritis may involve the pharynx alone or be multiple. Of this nature, in all probability, is the so-called pseudotabes, or *ataxie variolique.* Hemiplegia and aphasia have occurred in a few instances, the result of *encephalitis.*

Among the most constant and troublesome complications are those involving the *skin.* During convalescence boils are very frequent and may be severe. Acne and erythma are also met with. Alopecia may follow. Local gangrene in various parts may occur. A remarkable secondary eruption (recurrent smallpox) occasionally occurs after desquamation.

Arthritis may occur, usually in the period of desquamation, and may pass on to suppuration. Osteomyelitis is sometimes met with in the ordinary form and there is also a nonsuppurative variety which may cause deformity of the long bones. There may be injury to the epiphyses resulting in inequality of growth.

Special Senses.—The eye affections are not now so frequent, owing to the care taken to keep the conjunctivae clean. A catarrhal and purulent conjunctivitis is common in severe cases. Unless great care is taken a diffuse keratitis occurs which may go on to ulceration and perforation. Iritis is not very uncommon. Otitis media may result from an extension of the disease through the Eustachian tubes.

Prognosis.—In unprotected persons smallpox is a very fatal disease, the death rate ranging from 25 to 35 per cent. In the recent mild epidemics the mortality has been very slight, often less than 1 per cent. At the Municipal Hospital, Philadelphia, of 2,831 cases of variola, 1,534—*i.e.*, 54.18 per cent—died, while of 2,169 cases of varioloid only 28—i.e., 1.29 per cent—died (W. M. Welch). Purpura variolosa is invariably fatal, and a majority of those with the severer confluent forms die. The intemperate and debilitated succumb more readily. As Sydenham observed, the danger is directly proportionate to the intensity of the disease on the face and hands. "When the fever increases after the appearance of the pustules, it is a bad sign; but if it is lessened on their appearance, that is a good sign" (Rhazes). Very high fever, delirium and subsultus are signs of ill omen. The disease is particularly fatal in pregnant women and abortion usually takes place but is not inevitable. Severe cases may recover after miscarriage. Very severe pharyngitis, laryngitis and bronchopneumonia are serious complications.

Death results in the early stage from the action of the disease upon the nervous system. In the later stages it usually occurs about the eleventh or twelfth day, at the height of the eruption from the secondary infection.

Diagnosis.—During an epidemic the initial chill, the headache and back ache, and the vomiting at once put the physician on his guard.

Certain general points may be mentioned. The nature of any prevailing epidemic, the possibility of exposure, previous vaccination and an exact history of the onset are important. The patient should be properly stripped and examined in good daylight, with careful inspection of the mouth and pharynx. The student should remember that, in the diagnosis of the acute exanthemata, the very elect have gone astray, that hasty judgment may mean long repentance, that twenty-four hours later the question is often answered and that doubtful cases should be isolated and reported promptly to the health authorities.

The *initial rashes* may lead to error. The scarlatinal rash has rarely the extent and never the persistence of the rash in scarlet fever. The rash of measles has been mistaken for the initial rash of smallpox. The general condition of the patient, the coryza, conjunctivitis and Koplik's sign, may be better guides than the rash itself.

Malignant hemorrhagic smallpox may prove fatal before the characteristic rash appears. Of 27 cases of purpura variolosa, in only one, in which death occurred on the third day, did inspection fail to show the papules. In 3 patients dying on the fourth day the characteristic papular rash was noticed. It may be difficult or impossible to diagnose this form of hemorrhagic smallpox from *hemorrhagic scarlet fever* or *measles*, but in the latter there is rarely so constant involvement of the mucous membranes.

Naturally enough, as they are allied affections, *chickenpox* is the disease which most frequently leads to error. Particularly is this the case in mild epidemics. Any large number of cases of an infectious disease with a pustular eruption occurring in adults is strongly in favor of smallpox. The following points are important. The rash of chickenpox appears usually in the first 24 hours of illness, first on the trunk, is chiefly on the face and body and is rare on the extremities of the arms and legs. In smallpox the eruption first appears, after 3 to 4 days of illness, on the face and wrists and is more profuse on the limbs than on the body (not if there are very few pocks). Many lesions on the palms and soles are in favor of smallpox. In chickenpox the eruption comes out in successive crops for 3 to 5 days and pocks of all stages of development are found on the same area. In smallpox the eruption is in one crop over a given area and the lesions appear steadily for 24 to 48 hours (in a general way from above downwards). The lesion in chickenpox develops rapidly and is mature in 24 hours; several days are required in smallpox. The pock in chickenpox is thin walled, tense, translucent (at the height), easily broken, and the collapsed vesicle is soft, hence many broken down vesicles are significant. The vesicles are unilocular and are emptied by one puncture;

they are more superficial and sometimes look as if they were placed *on* the skin. The areola about them is not so intense or constant. In smallpox the lesion is firm, deep-seated (*in* the skin), not easily ruptured; the vesicle is multilocular and not emptied by one puncture. There is usually a definite areola about it. The shape (chickenpox more oval, smallpox round) is not a safe guide. The chickenpox vesicle is rarely umbilicated, the smallpox vesicle often is but this disappears on pustulation. A rash which has matured in 2 days, or is unchanged for some days is not smallpox.

Successful vaccination within five years is against smallpox. But there are mild epidemics in which the diagnosis is only confirmed by the appearance of a severe case of the confluent or hemorrhagic form.

The disease may be mistaken for *cerebrospinal fever,* in which purpuric features are not uncommon. A four-year-old child was taken suddenly ill with fever, pains in the back and head, and on the second or third day petechiae appeared. There were retraction of the head and marked rigidity of the limbs. The hemorrhages became more abundant; finally hematemesis occurred and the child died on the sixth day. At autopsy there was no meningitis and in the hemorrhagic skin the papules could be readily seen. The postmortem diagnosis was confirmed by the mother taking smallpox and dying of it.

Pustular Syphilides.—A copious pustular rash may resemble variola, particularly if accompanied by fever, but the history and distribution, particularly the polymorphous character, leave no question as to the diagnosis.

Pustular glanders has been mistaken for smallpox. In an instance in Montreal there was a widespread pustular eruption, thought at first to be smallpox, but the course and the fact that there was glanders among the horses in the stable led to the correct diagnosis.

Impetigo contagiosa is stated to have been mistaken for variola.

Specific Test.—Rabbits sensitized to vaccine virus give a marked reaction in 24 to 48 hours after the intradermic injection of smallpox vesicle contents. The result of inoculation of material from the pocks in the cornea of the rabbit is helpful when positive. The virus of smallpox gives a specific complement fixation and flocculation with an antivariola serum. The reaction is done with a suspension of the crusts from a suspected case and a specific flocculating serum from a rabbit.

Prophylaxis.—Thorough vaccination and revaccination are the most important preventive measures. All those exposed to infection should be vaccinated at once, as four days after exposure a successful vaccination may protect from the disease. During epidemics general vaccination of the community should be done and special care taken to recognize mild cases. Those who have been exposed should be isolated for sixteen days. Isolation of those with the disease should be rigid and they should be placed in a special hospital. The attendants should wear gowns and caps; rubber gloves are an advantage. The linen should be placed in phenol solution (2 per cent) and boiled afterwards. Dressings should be burned. The patient should not be discharged until all the crusts are removed; a thorough sponging with phenol solution (2 per cent) is advisable.

Treatment.—General Considerations.—Segregation in special hospitals is imperative. In local outbreaks temporary barracks or tents may be used. We have no specific treatment. There should be abundance of fresh air; the diet should be liquid and large amounts of water and cold drinks given. A calomel and saline purge is advisable at the onset and later the bowels should be kept open by salines. In the early stages two symptoms call for treatment: the pain in the back, which, if not relieved by phenacetine or acetylsalicylic acid (gr. v, 0.3 gm.), requires opium in some form, as advised by Sydenham; and the vomiting, which is very difficult to check. Nothing should be given except a little ice, and it usually stops with the appearance of the eruption.

For the fever, cold sponging or the tub bath may be used; when there is much delirium with high fever the latter or the cold pack is preferable. In some cases, particularly with severe toxemia and marked eruption, the continuous warm bath is advisable.

The treatment of the *eruption* is important. After trying all sorts of remedies, such as puncturing the pustules with nitrate of silver, or treating them with iodine and various ointments, Sydenham's conclusion that in guarding the face against being disfigured "the only effect of oils, liniments, and the like was to make the white scurfs slower in coming off" seems correct. The constant application on the face and hands of lint soaked in solutions, such as phenol (2 per cent), potassium permanganate (1 per cent) or bichloride of mercury (1 to 5,000) is perhaps the most suitable local treatment. Equal parts of tincture of iodine and alcohol may be applied daily. When the crusts begin to form, the chief point is to keep them thoroughly moist with oil or glycerine. This prevents the desiccation and diffusion of the flakes of epidermis. Vaseline is useful and may be freely used upon the face. Phenol (3 to 5 per cent) in oil or vaseline may be used and also relieves the itching. For the odor, the dilute phenol solutions are best. When suppuration is marked the continuous warm bath (95°) is useful. Boric acid, alum or potassium permanganate may be added to the water.

The papules do not maturate so well when protected from the light, and for centuries attempts have been made to modify the course of the pustules by either excluding the light or by changing its character. In the Middle Ages John of Gaddesden recommended wrapping the patient in red flannel, and treated in this way the son of Edward I. It was an old practice of the Egyptians and Arabians to cover the exposed parts of smallpox patients with gold-leaf. The red-light treatment of the disease has been advocated by Finsen, but the statements do not agree as to its value. Exposure to violet rays has been advised.

Complications.—If the diarrhea is severe, paregoric may be given. When the pulse becomes feeble and rapid, stimulants may be freely given. The maniacal delirium may require chloroform or morphia, but for less intense nervous symptoms the bath or cold pack is the best. For the severe hemorrhages of the malignant cases nothing can be done, and it is only cruel to drench the patient with iron, ergot, and other drugs. Symptoms of obstruction in the larynx, usually from edema, may call for tracheotomy. In the late stages, if the patient is debilitated and the subject of abscesses and bed sores, he may be placed on an air bed or treated in the continuous bath.

The care of the *eyes* is most important. The lids should be thoroughly cleansed and the conjunctivae washed with a warm solution of boracic acid. In the confluent cases the eyelids are swollen and glued together, and only constant watchfulness prevents keratitis. The edges of the lids should be smeared with vaseline. The mouth and throat should be kept clean, a potassium permanganate mouth wash and gargle used, and treatment of the nose with glycerine or oil should be begun early, to prevent the formation of crusts. Douching the nose with a warm alkaline solution is helpful.

The treatment in the stage of convalescence is important. Frequent bathing helps to soften the crusts, and the skin may be oiled daily. Convalescence should not be considered established until the skin is perfectly smooth and clean and free from any trace of scabs.

VACCINIA (Cowpox)—VACCINATION

Definition.—An eruptive disease of the cow, the virus of which, inoculated into man (vaccination), produces a local pock with constitutional disturbance, which affords protection, more or less permanent, against smallpox.

History.—For centuries it had been a popular belief among farmer-folk that cowpox protected against smallpox. The notorious Duchess of Cleveland, replying to some joker who suggested that she would lose her occupation if she was disfigured with smallpox, said that she was not afraid of the disease, as she had had a disease that protected her against smallpox. Jesty, a Dorsetshire farmer, had had cowpox, and in 1774 vaccinated successfully his wife and two sons. Plett, in Holstein, in 1791, successfully vaccinated three children. When Jenner was a student at Sodbury, a young girl, who came for advice, when smallpox was mentioned, exclaimed, "I cannot take that disease, for I have had cowpox." Jenner subsequently mentioned the subject to Hunter, who in reply gave the famous advice: "Do not think, but try; be patient, be accurate." As early as 1780 the idea of the protective power of vaccination was firmly impressed on Jenner's mind. The problem was brought to a practical issue when, on May 14, 1796, he took matter from the hand of a dairy-maid, Sarah Nelmes, who had cowpox, and inoculated a boy named James Phipps, aged eight years. On July 1st, matter was taken from a smallpox pustule and inserted into the boy, but no disease followed. In 1798 appeared An Inquiry into the Causes and Effects of the Variola Vaccinae, a Disease Discovered in Some of the Western Counties of England, Particularly Gloucestershire, and Known by the Name of Cowpox (pp. iv, 75, four plates, 4to. London, 1798).

In the United States cowpox was introduced by Benjamin Waterhouse, Professor of Physic at Harvard, who on July 8, 1800, vaccinated seven of his children. In Boston on August 16, 1802, nineteen boys were inoculated with the cowpox. On November 9th twelve of them were inoculated with smallpox; nothing followed. A control experiment was made by inoculating two unvaccinated boys with the same smallpox virus; both took the disease. The nineteen children of August 16th were again unsuccessfully inoculated with fresh virus from these two boys. This is one of the most crucial experiments in the history of vaccination, and fully justified the conclusion of the Board of Health—*cowpox is a complete security against the smallpox.*

Nature of Vaccinia.—Is cowpox a separate independent disease, or is it smallpox modified by passing through the cow? After long controversy it seems established that cowpox and horsepox are variola modified by transmission through the animal. The smallpox virus is altered or attenuated so that its usual course, when inoculated into the human individual, is to produce a local lesion only. It is also altered in that its infective powers are altered and it can be conveyed only by inoculation. The histology of the vaccine lesion is like that of smallpox.

The "Paschen bodies" are found in the lesions of vaccinia and Ledingham has shown that these bodies are agglutinated by the immune sera of rabbits. Some regard these bodies as the virus of the disease. Vaccinia and smallpox may have a common antigen but different antibodies are produced in response to each virus. The vaccine virus has been cultivated on artificial media. This tissue culture lymph is free of contamination by bacteria.

Normal Vaccination.—Period of Incubation.—At first there may be a little irritation at the site of inoculation, which subsides.

Period of Eruption.—On the third day, as a rule, a papule is seen surrounded by a reddish zone. This gradually increases, and on the fifth or sixth day shows a definite vesicle, the margins of which are raised while the centre is depressed. By the eighth day the vesicle has attained its maximum size. It is round and distended with a limpid fluid, the margin hard and prominent, and the umbilication is more distinct. By the tenth day the vesicle is still large and is surrounded by an extensive areola. The contents have now become purulent. The skin is also swollen, indurated, and often painful. On the eleventh or twelfth day the hyperemia diminishes, the lymph becomes more opaque and begins to dry. By the end of the second week the vesicle is converted into a brownish scab, which gradually becomes dry and hard, and in about a week (that is, about the twenty-first or twenty-fifth day from the vaccination) separates and leaves a circular pitted scar. If the points of inoculation have been close together, the vesicles fuse and may form a large combined vesicle. Constitutional symptoms of a more or less marked degree follow the vaccination. Usually on the third or fourth day the temperature rises, and may persist, increasing until the eighth or ninth day. There is a marked leukocytosis. In children it is common to have with the fever restlessness, particularly at night, and irritability; but as a rule these symptoms are trivial. If the inoculation is made on the arm, the axillary glands may become large and sore; if on the leg, the inguinal glands. Immunity is not necessarily complete at once after vaccination; it may take as long as three weeks; on the other hand, a person exposed to smallpox and successfully vaccinated at once may escape entirely, or the two diseases may run concurrently, with the smallpox much modified. The duration of the immunity is extremely variable. In some instances it is permanent, but a majority of persons within ten or twelve years again become susceptible. With the intracutaneous methods of vaccination the period of immunity is shorter.

Revaccination should be performed about the ninth or tenth year, and whenever smallpox is epidemic. The susceptibility to revaccination is very general. In 1891-'92 vaccination pustules developed in 88.7 per cent of the newly enrolled troops of the German army, most of whom had been vaccinated twice in their lives before. The vesicle in revaccination is usually smaller, has less induration and hyperemia, and the resulting scar is less perfect. Particular care should be taken to watch the vesicle of revaccination, as it not infrequently happens that a spurious pock is formed, which reaches its height early and dries to a scab by the eighth or ninth day.

Irregular Vaccination.—Local Variations.—In occasional instances the vesicle develops rapidly with much itching, has not the characteristic flattened appearance, the lymph early becomes opaque, and the crust forms by the seventh or eighth day. The evolution of the pocks may be abnormally slow and in such cases the operation should again be performed. The contents of the vesicles may be watery and bloody. Bruising or irritation of the pocks may lead to ulceration and inflammation. A very rare event is the recurrence of the pock in the same place. Sutton reported four such recurrences within six months.

Accidental Vaccinia.—The virus may be inoculated in other parts by the fingers: the eyelids, face and genitals are the most common sites. Occasionally, by sucking the vaccinated area to prevent "a take," the lips are inoculated.

Generalized Vaccinia.—Vesicles may occur in the vicinity of the primary sore. Less common is a true generalized pustular rash, developing in different parts of the body, often beginning about the wrists and on the back. The secondary pocks may continue to make their appearance for five or six weeks after vaccination. They may be most abundant on the vaccinated limb, and occur usually about the eighth to the tenth day.

Complications.—In unhealthy subjects, or as a result of uncleanliness, or sometimes injury, the vesicles inflame and ulcers result. Sloughing and deep cellulitis may follow. In debilitated children there may be a purpuric rash with this.

(1) During the first three days: Erythema; urticaria; vesicular and bullous eruptions; invaccinated erysipelas.

(2) After the third day and until the pock reaches maturity: Urticaria; lichen urticatus, erythema multiforme; accidental erysipelas.

(3) About the end of the first week: Generalized vaccinia; impetigo; vaccinal ulceration; glandular abscess; septic infections; gangrene.

(4) *Encephalitis.*—Cases of this have been reported in recent years and the cause can not be regarded as proved. The incubation period is ten to twelve days with a sudden onset of symptoms, fever, delirium, strabismus and occasionally paralysis of the limbs. The mortality has been high, over 50 per cent in some series, but complete recovery may occur. The etiology is in doubt; it does not seem to be due to the vaccine virus alone. There is a perivascular infiltration and marginal demyelination in the form of a zone around the veins, along the ventral fissure of the cord and beneath the pia and ependyma. The histological picture is the same as that in encephalitis in other eruptive fevers, such as measles. *Age* plays a part as it usually occurs in those vaccinated for the first time between the ages of 3 and 13 years. In *treatment,* the blood serum from one recently vaccinated has been given intravenously, apparently with benefit.

Transmission of Diseases by Vaccination.—*Syphilis* has very rarely been transmitted by arm to arm vaccination, but a large number of the cases of alleged vaccinosyphilis must be thrown out. The question is now of *no importance* since the general use of animal lymph.

Tuberculosis.—"No undoubted case of invaccinated tubercle was brought before the Royal Commission on Vaccination" (Acland). The risk of transmitting tuberculosis from the calf is so slight that it need not be considered. The transmission of leprosy by vaccination is doubtful. Actinomyces has been found in vaccine virus in the past.

Tetanus.—The occurrence of *tetanus* due to vaccination is most unlikely with the care taken in the preparation of vaccine matter. The vaccination area may be infected subsequently with tetanus organisms as any wound.

Influence of Vaccination upon Other Diseases.—A quiescent malady may be lighted into activity by vaccination. This has happened with congenital syphilis, occasionally with tuberculosis. An old idea was prevalent that vaccination had a beneficial influence upon existing diseases. Thomas Archer, the first medical graduate in the United States, recommended its use in whooping cough, and said that it had cured several cases in his hands.

Technique.—That part of the arm about the insertion of the deltoid or the back and inner side of the upper arm is usually selected. Some mothers prefer to have girl babies vaccinated on the leg. The skin should be thoroughly cleaned, best with acetone on sterile gauze or cotton. If an antiseptic is used, it should be washed off with sterile water. If the incision method is used, only one should be made, if possible without drawing blood in large drops. The virus is applied to the incision and allowed to dry. A simple dry dressing may be applied. Another method is to place the virus on the skin and with the point of a sterile needle passed through the virus, a slight scratch is made or several punctures. With the side of the needle the virus is gently rubbed across the scratch. With the pressure method, the virus is placed on the skin and the needle is held parallel to the surface. The side of the point of the needle is then pressed quickly up and down about 30 times through the virus. By the elasticity of the skin a portion of epidermis is pulled over the point of the needle each time and introduces the virus. The skin is then wiped dry and no dressing should be applied. The vaccination should be observed in 7 and 11 days. In revaccination at the end of 48 hours, the reaction of immunity may appear.

Vaccination is usually performed between the fourth and sixth month. If unsuccessful, it should be repeated from time to time. It should be postponed if the child has any ailment or suffers from syphilis or a skin disease. Revaccination should be done at the age of nine years. A person exposed to smallpox should always be revaccinated. This, if successful, will usually protect; but not always. Multiple insertions—not less than one inch apart—should be done in case of exposure to smallpox, if there has been failure of previous vaccinations and in conditions in which the potency of the virus may be in question. The cases in which smallpox is taken within a few years after vaccination are probably instances of spurious vaccination.

The Value of Vaccination.—Sanitation cannot account for the diminution in smallpox and for the low rate of mortality. Isolation is a useful auxiliary but it is no substitute. Vaccination is not claimed to be an invariable and permanent preventive of smallpox, but in an immense majority of cases successful inoculation renders the person for many years insusceptible. Communities in which vaccination and revaccination are thoroughly and systematically carried out are those in which smallpox has the fewest victims. On the other hand, communities in which vaccination and revaccination are persistently neglected are those in which epidemics are most prevalent.

Although the effects of a single vaccination may wear out, as we say, and the individual again becomes susceptible to smallpox, yet the mortality in such cases is very much lower than in persons who have never been vaccinated.

There is evidence that the greater the number of marks the greater the protection; thus, the English Vaccination Report states that out of 4,754 cases the death rate with one mark was 7.6 per cent; with two marks, 7 per cent; with three marks, 4.2 per cent; with four marks, 2.4 per cent. W. M. Welch's statistics of 5,000 cases on this point give with good cicatrices 8 per cent; with fair cicatrices, 14 per cent; with poor cicatrices, 27 per cent; post-vaccinal cases, 16 per cent; unvaccinated cases, 58 per cent.

VARICELLA (Chickenpox)

Definition.—An acute infectious disease, characterized by an eruption of vesicles on the skin which appear in successive crops.

History.—Ingrassias, a distinguished Neapolitan professor, first recognized the disease as differing from smallpox (1553). Heberden gave it the name chickenpox (1767).

Etiology.—The disease occurs in epidemics, but sporadic cases are also met with. Infection is usually direct but may be by fomites. It is a disease of childhood; a majority of the cases occur between the second and sixth years. Adults who have not had the disease in childhood may be attacked.

Varicella is an affection distinct from variola and without any relation to it. An attack of the one does not confer immunity to the other. The cause of the disease is not determined. There is much to suggest that it is a virus, in which connection there is the curious association with herpes zoster. Certain elementary bodies are described as found in the fluid of the vesicles of varicella. These are agglutinated by the serum of convalescent patients. The results of animal inoculation give results much like those in vaccinia.

Symptoms.—After a period of incubation of ten or fifteen days the child becomes feverish and in some instances has a slight chill. Prodromal rashes may occur, usually erythematous but sometimes like measles. There may be vomiting, and pains in the back and legs. Convulsions are rare. The eruption usually appears within twenty-four hours. It is first seen upon the trunk, either on the back or on the chest. It may begin on the forehead and face. At first in the form of macules, then raised red papules, these are in a few hours transformed into hemispherical vesicles containing a clear or turbid fluid. Many are translucent and seem to be *on* rather than *in* the skin. As a rule there is no umbilication, but in rare instances the pocks are flattened, and a few may even be umbilicated. They are often ovoid in shape and look more superficial than the variolous vesicles. The contents are in one chamber and the pock collapses on puncture. The skin in the neighborhood is not often infiltrated or hyperemic. At the end of thirty-six or forty-eight hours the contents of the vesicles are purulent. They begin to shrivel, and during the third and fourth days are converted into dark brownish crusts, which fall off and as a rule leave no scar. Fresh crops appear during the first two or three days of the illness, so that on the fourth day one can usually see pocks in all stages of development and decay. They are always discrete, and the number may vary from eight or ten to several hundreds. The rash is most profuse on the trunk, particularly on the back. On the arms and legs it is scanty on the distal portions. The eruption may occur on the mucous membrane of the mouth, and occasionally in the larynx. In adults the disease may be severe, the initial fever high, the rash very widespread, and the constitutional symptoms marked, so that the diagnosis of smallpox may be made. The fever in varicella is slight, but it does not as a rule disappear with the appearance of the rash. The blood in early stages may show leukocytosis with a high lymphocytosis (over 80 per cent) suggesting leukemia. The course is favorable in a large majority of the cases and no ill effects follow. The disease may recur in the same individual.

There are occasional modifications of the rash. The vesicles may become very large and develop into *bullae,* looking not unlike ecthyma or pemphigus (varicella bullosa). The irritation of the rash may be excessive, and if the child scratches the pocks ulcerating sores may form, which leave scars on healing. Cicatrices after chickenpox are more common than after varioloid. In delicate children, particularly the tuberculous, *gangrene* (varicella escharotica) may occur about the vesicles, or in other parts, as the scrotum. Cases of *hemorrhagic* varicella have been described with cutaneous ecchymoses and bleeding from the mucous membranes.

Nephritis may occur. Infantile hemiplegia has occurred during an attack and neuroretinitis has been noted. Death has followed from extensive involvement of the skin. Encephalitis and meningitis have been reported.

Diagnosis.—The diagnosis is as a rule easy, particularly if the patient has been seen from the onset. When a patient comes under observation for the first time with the rash well out, there may be considerable difficulty. The abundance of the rash on the trunk in varicella is most important. The pocks in varicella are more superficial, more bleb-like, have not so deeply an infiltrated areola about them, and may usually be seen in all stages of development. They rarely at the outset have the hard, shotty feeling of those of smallpox. The general symptoms, the greater intensity of the onset, the prolonged period of invasion, and the more frequent occurrence of prodromal rashes in smallpox are important points in the diagnosis.

Prognosis.—Death is very rare, and, unless from the complications, raises a suspicion of the correctness of the diagnosis. Thus of the 152 deaths in the United States in 1930 ascribed to chickenpox, it is probable that some were from unrecognized smallpox.

Vaccination from the vesicles seems to have decreased the incidence in those exposed to infection. Convalescent serum (10-15 cc. intramuscularly) obtained within a month of an attack is an efficient preventive.

No special *treatment* is required. The child should be isolated and in bed until the acute features are over. The application of equal parts of tincture of iodine and alcohol to the lesions is useful. Care should be taken to prevent the child from scratching the pustules. A soothing lotion or powder should be applied.

MEASLES (Morbilli)

Definition.—An acute, highly infectious fever with specific localization in the upper air passages and in the skin.

As a cause of death measles ranks high among the fevers of children. In 1915 there were 16,445 deaths from this disease in England and Wales, but only 3,288 deaths in 1931. In the U. S. registration area there were 3,820 deaths in 1930. The death rate is highest in the second year.

History.—Rhazes, an Arabian physician, in the ninth century described the disease with smallpox, of which it was believed to be a mild form until Sydenham separated them in the seventeenth century.

Etiology.—The liability to infection is almost universal in persons unprotected by a previous attack. It is a disease of childhood, but in the widespread epidemics in the Faroe and Fiji Islands, unprotected adults of all ages were attacked. Within the first three months of life there is a relative immunity. Occasionally infants of a month or six weeks take the disease. Intra-uterine cases have been described, and a mother with measles may give birth to a child with the eruption, or the rash may appear in a few days.

The disease is endemic in cities, and becomes epidemic at intervals of a few years, prevailing most extensively in the cooler months, though this is by no means a fixed rule.

The germ of the disease is unknown. J. F. Anderson has shown that the blood of a patient inoculated into the Rhesus monkey produces after eight days a fever of short duration with a well-marked slight exanthem. The agent is present in the blood, the secretions of the mouth and nose, and in the skin. In the eighteenth century Monro and others demonstrated the inoculability of the disease. Direct infection is the most common. The agent is probably not in the expired air, but in the particles of mucus and in the sputum and secretions of the mouth and nose, which, dried, are conveyed with dust. An important point is the infectiousness of the disease in the pre-eruptive stage. A child with catarrhal symptoms only may be at school and a source of active infection. Indirect infection by means of fomites is not very common. The work of Tunnicliff suggests a diplococcus as the causal organism. Others hold that it is a virus.

Recurrence is rare. Many cases of supposed second and third attacks represent mistakes in diagnosis. Relapse is occasionally seen, the symptoms recurring at intervals from ten to forty days.

Morbid Anatomy.—The catarrhal and inflammatory appearances seen postmortem have nothing characteristic. Fatal cases show, as a rule, bronchopneumonia and an intense bronchial catarrh. The lymphatic elements all over the body are swollen, the tonsils, the lymph glands, and the solitary and agminated follicles of the intestines. The spleen is rarely much enlarged. During convalescence latent tuberculous foci may become active. Encephalitis with punctate hemorrhages may occur.

Symptoms.—Incubation.—"From seven to eighteen days; oftenest fourteen." The child shows no special changes, but coryza and swelling of the cervical lymph glands may be present. A polymorphonuclear leukocytosis may be present.

Invasion.—In this period, lasting from three to four days, very rarely five or six, the child presents the symptoms of a feverish cold. The onset may be insidious, or it may start with great abruptness, even with a convulsion. There is not often a definite chill. Headache, nausea, and vomiting may usher in the severe cases. Abdominal symptoms may suggest *appendicitis* and operation has been done. The common catarrhal symptoms are sneezing and running at the nose, redness of the eyes and lids, and cough.

Bronchitis may be marked. The fever is slight at first, but gradually the skin is hot with turgescence of the face. Prodromal rashes occur in a few cases, usually a blotchy erythema or scattered macules. The tongue is furred and the mucous membranes of the mouth and throat are hyperemic, and frequently show a distinct punctiform rash. The fever may rise abruptly; more frequently it takes 24 or 48 hours to reach the fastigium. The pulse-rate increases with the fever (104-105°), and may reach 140 or 160 per minute, gradually falling with defervescence.

Eruption.—The general features become more severe as the time of eruption approaches and especially if the eruption is delayed. The respirations may be rapid and slight cyanosis may be present. The rash appears first on the forehead and behind the ears. It spreads rapidly over the neck, body and extremities and is usually fully developed in two or three days. The first stage is a *macular* eruption which becomes *maculopapular* and the lesions often join to form irregular crescentic areas. The rash has a mottled blotchy character. The face is usually swollen and congested and with the catarrhal features has a characteristic appearance. Photophobia is common at this stage. The rash is often more intense on the face than on the trunk and extremities but it may be confluent over the greater part of the body. The general features do not lessen with the appearance of the rash but persist until the fifth or sixth day; the temperature then falls rapidly. The rash usually persists for two or three days and fades rapidly, but instances of longer duration are not uncommon. It is hyperemic and disappears on pressure, but in the malignant cases it may become of a deep rose, inclining to purple. Among peculiarities of the rash are the occurrence of numerous miliary vesicles and of petechiae, seen occasionally even in cases of moderate severity. Recession of the rash, so much dwelt upon by older writers, is rarely seen. In reality it is the failing circulation which causes the rash to fade.

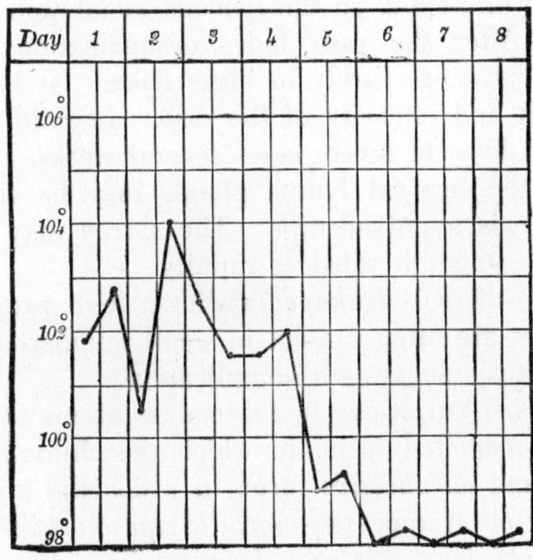

Chart XIII.—Measles.

Measles Line.—About the time of the onset of fever a line of congestion may be found on the lower eyelid about the margin of the cartilage (Stimson,

1928). It should be well marked to be suggestive and it is soon obscured by the general conjunctivitis.

Buccal spots were described by Filatow in 1895, and by Koplik in 1896. They are seen on a level with the bases of the lower milk molars on either side, or at the line of junction of the molars when the jaws are closed. They are white or bluish-white specks, surrounded by red areolae, and are best seen by daylight. Their importance depends upon their early appearance, three days before the skin rash, and remarkable constancy—six-sevenths of all cases. Macules may be seen on the soft palate.

The fauces may be injected, and there is sometimes an eruption of scattered spots over the entire mucous membrane of the mouth. Ringer called attention to opaque white spots on the mucous membrane of the lips.

Desquamation.—After the rash fades desquamation begins, usually in the form of fine scales, more rarely in large flakes. It bears a definite relationship to the extent and intensity of the rash. In mild cases desquamation may take only a few days, in severe cases several weeks.

The tonsils and the cervical lymph glands may be slightly swollen and sore; sometimes there is a polyadenitis. The *spleen* may be enlarged at the height of the eruptive stage; it subsides rapidly.

During the course there is *leukopenia* with a high proportion of mononuclears, and myelocytes are often present in small numbers during the eruption (Tileston). Leukocytosis suggests a complication.

Atypical Measles.—Variations in the course of the disease are not common. There is an *attenuated* form, in which the child may be well by the fourth or fifth day, and an *abortive* form, in which the initial symptoms may be present, but no eruption appears—*morbilli sine morbillis.*

Malignant or *black measles* is most frequent in widespread epidemics, but it is also met with in institutions, and occasionally in general practice. Hemorrhages occur into the skin and from the mucous membranes, there is high fever, and profound toxemia, often with cyanosis, dyspnea, and extreme cardiac weakness. Death may occur from the second to the sixth day.

Complications.—Those of the air passages are the most serious. The *coryza* may become chronic and lead to irritation of the lymphoid tissues of the nasopharynx, causing enlarged tonsils and adenoids. *Epistaxis* is sometimes serious. *Laryngitis* is not uncommon: the voice becomes husky and the cough croupy in character. Edema of the glottis and pseudomembranous inflammation are rare. Ulceration, abscess, and perichondritis may occur.

Bronchitis and Bronchopneumonia.—In every severe case there is the possibility of the bronchitis extending to the small tubes and causing bronchopneumonia. It is more apt to occur at the height of the eruption or as desquamation begins. The high mortality in institutions is due to this complication, which, as Sydenham remarked, kills more than the smallpox. *Lobar pneumonia* is less common. Venous *thrombosis* has occurred.

Severe *stomatitis* may follow the slight catarrhal form. In institutions *cancrum oris* or *gangrenous stomatitis* is a terrible complication. *Parotitis* occasionally occurs. *Enteritis* and *acute colitis* occur in some epidemics.

Nephritis is less rare than is stated and occasionally cases of chronic nephritis date from an attack of measles. Inflammation of the genitals may occur in girls but is usually not severe.

Endocarditis is rare. *Arthritis* may be general and severe, and in one instance ankylosis of the jaw followed an attack of measles in a child of four years. The conjunctivitis may be followed by *keratitis*. Optic neuritis and atrophy may occur. *Otitis media* is not uncommon and may lead to perforation of the drum or mastoid disease. *Hemiplegia* is a serious complication and usually persists. *Encephalitis* may occur early but usually after the rash has disappeared; it has no relation to the severity of the attack. It shows drowsiness or stupor, possibly with convulsions, and signs of meningitis. With special spinal involvement there may be paraplegia with loss of sphincter control. *Polyneuritis* may occur with widespread atrophy. Acute mania, convergent squint, *meningitis, abscess of the brain*, and *multiple sclerosis* are among the rare complications or sequelae. *Scarlet fever* may occur with measles. *Whooping cough* not infrequently follows measles.

Diagnosis.—During the prevalence of an epidemic the disease is easily recognized. At the onset the catarrhal symptoms may be regarded as a simple coryza or if laryngitis is marked, diphtheria may be suspected. In early stages, edema of the palpebral conjunctivae is important. Physicians to isolation hospitals appreciate the difficulties and patients with measles may be sent to the smallpox hospital; it is well to bear in mind that in adults, especially negroes, the beginning of the eruption on the face, its nodular character, and the isolation of the spots may be suggestive of variola. From *scarlet fever* measles is distinguished by the longer initial stage with characteristic symptoms, and the blotchy irregular character of the rash, so unlike the diffuse uniform erythema. In measles the mouth (with the early Koplik sign), in scarlet fever the throat, is chiefly affected. Occasionally in measles, when the throat is very sore and the eruption diffuse, there may at first be difficulty in determining which disease is present, but a short interval makes the diagnosis clear. As a rule there is no leukocytosis. It may be extremely difficult to distinguish from *rubella*. The shorter prodromal stage, the absence of oculonasal catarrh, and the slighter fever in many cases are perhaps the most important features. It is difficult to speak definitely about distinctions in the rash, though perhaps the more uniform distribution and the absence of the crescentic arrangement are more constant in rubella in which adenitis is more marked. The distribution of the rash, the coryza, and the rash in the mouth are important points. Of *drug* eruptions, that due to copaiba is very like measles, but is distinguished by the absence of fever and catarrh. Antipyrin, chloral and quinine rashes rarely cause any difficulty. A serum exanthem may be difficult to distinguish. In adults acute malignant measles may resemble typhus fever, especially when the rash is dusky, but in typhus fever the rash is rarely on the face and always is in measles. Occasionally erythema multiforme simulates measles.

The lesions of Fordyce's disease may be mistaken for Koplik spots. This is a chronic disease of the mucous membrane of the mouth and lips, with white and yellow lesions, pin-point to pin-head in size, on the buccal mucous membrane opposite the line of the teeth back to the last molar.

Prognosis.—The mortality from the disease itself is not high, but the pulmonary complications render it one of the most serious of the diseases of children. In some epidemics, the death rate may be high, not so much from the disease itself as from the bronchopneumonia. Imported in 1875 from

Sydney to the Fiji Islands, 40,000 of 150,000 inhabitants died in four months. Panum, a Danish physician, described the widespread epidemic which decimated the inhabitants of the Faroe Islands in 1846. In private practice the mortality is from 2 to 3 per cent; in hospitals from 6 to 10 per cent. The greatest danger is from bronchopneumonia but epidemics vary in severity.

Prophylaxis.—The difficulty is inherent in the prolonged incubation and the period of invasion, during which the catarrhal symptoms are marked, and the disease is infectious, and one often finds that quarantine has been in vain. From contact with cases in the stage of invasion and mild cases with scarcely any fever the disease is readily disseminated through schools and conveyed to healthy children in the everyday contact with each other. The patient should be carefully quarantined and all possible precautions taken against the spread of the disease in the house. The deliberate exposure of children to infection should be strongly forbidden. The usual quarantine period is for fourteen days after the appearance of the rash, unless there is cough or discharge from the nose or ears. The blood serum of convalescents gives passive immunity and is used in prevention, 5 cc. being given intramuscularly for the first four days after exposure. If given from the sixth to the ninth day after exposure it may modify the attack. Larger doses should be given for children over three years of age.

Treatment.—Confinement to bed in a well-ventilated room, a liquid diet with fruit juices, ice cream and abundance of water and a simple fever mixture are the only measures necessary in ordinary cases. If there is photophobia the light should be cut off and the eyes bathed with boric acid solution. The fever rarely reaches a dangerous height. If it does it may be lowered by sponging or by the tepid bath gradually reduced. If the rash does not come out well, warm drinks and a hot bath will hasten its maturation. The bowels should be freely opened. If the cough is distressing compresses should be applied to the chest and inhalations of the compound tincture of benzoin or small doses of paregoric or codein given. There is no drug with any special influence. The patient should be kept in bed for a few days after the fever subsides. During desquamation the skin should be oiled daily, and warm baths given to facilitate the process. The mouth and nostrils should be carefully cleansed, even in mild cases. The reports of the use of convalescent serum (10-20 cc.) suggest that it has some value. It apparently does not influence the complications. The convalescence is a most important stage and watchfulness and care may prevent serious pulmonary complications. The frequency of the history in simple or tuberculous bronchopneumonia that "the child caught cold after measles," and the contemplation of the mortality should make us extremely careful in our management of this affection.

RUBELLA (German Measles)

Definition.—This is an exanthem with features resembling both scarlet fever and ordinary measles but is a distinct and separate disease.

Etiology.—It is propagated by infection and spreads with great rapidity. It frequently attacks adults, and the occurrence of measles or scarlet fever in childhood is no protection against it. The epidemics of it are often very extensive. The causal organism is not known, but it is probably given off from the respiratory tract and mouth.

Symptoms.—These are usually mild, and it is altogether a less serious affection than measles. Very exceptionally, the symptoms are severe. The stage of incubation is from two to three weeks. There may be a short prodomal stage, not over 24 hours, with slight catarrhal symptoms, perhaps headache and malaise. The rash appears on the first or second day, usually first on the face or neck, spreading rapidly to the trunk and limbs and being general within 24 hours. The eruption consists of round or oval, slightly raised spots, pinkish red in color, sometimes discrete but often confluent. The rash resembles that of measles in its early stages and later may become more like that of scarlet fever. At times it has some resemblance to both diseases. The rash commonly lasts for two or three days, fades gradually, and there is usually a fine desquamation. The throat shows a macular, rose-red eruption, which may involve the soft palate, and the tonsils may be swollen and red. Koplik's spots do not occur. *Adenitis* is a characteristic feature, the occipital and posterior cervical glands being enlarged and tender. Occasionally the axillary and inguinal glands are involved also. The swelling may persist for some time. The *fever* is usually slight and rarely persists for more than two or three days.

There are no special complications but encephalitis and purpura have occurred. The disease usually progresses favorably but in rare instances the symptoms are of greater severity. Albuminuria, arthritis or nephritis may occur. Pneumonia and colitis have been present in some epidemics. Icterus has been seen.

Diagnosis.—The slightness of the prodromal symptoms, the mildness or the absence of the fever, the more diffuse character of the rash, its rose-red color, and the early enlargement of the cervical glands, are the chief points of distinction from measles. From scarlet fever, it is distinguished by the absence of the severe symptoms of onset and specific skin tests, slight fever, absence of a rapid pulse rate, adenitis, and mixed character of the rash.

The treatment is that of a simple febrile affection.

"Fourth Disease."—Clement Dukes described a "fourth disease," in which the body is covered in a few hours with a diffuse exanthem of a bright red color, almost scarlatiniform in appearance. The face may remain quite free. The desquamation is more marked than in rubella. There is doubt as to this being a distinct disease.

Erythema Infectiosum.—This is a feebly infectious disease occurring usually in children but also in adults. The incubation is from seven to fourteen days. The onset is with malaise, headache, and vomiting. The rash is variable and polymorphous. The face may be specially involved but there may be circumoral pallor. There is erythema with swelling of the skin, suggesting urticaria. The distribution over the trunk and limbs is variable. The eruption may disappear and recur. There may be slight bronchitis and conjunctivitis. Fever is usually slight. The spleen may be enlarged. The blood shows a leukopenia with lymphocytosis and sometimes eosinophilia. The treatment is symptomatic.

EPIDEMIC PAROTITIS (Mumps)

Definition.—A specific infectious disease, characterized by swelling of the salivary glands, especially the parotid, and a liability to orchitis in males.

Hippocrates described the disease and its peculiarities—an affection of children and young male adults, the absence of suppuration, and the orchitis.

Etiology.—The nature of the virus is not proved; various organisms have been described. It is endemic in large centres of population, and at certain seasons, particularly spring and autumn, the cases increase rapidly. It is met most frequently in childhood and adolescence. Very young infants and adults are seldom attacked. Males are somewhat more frequently affected than females. In institutions, barracks, and schools the disease has been known to attack over 90 per cent of the residents. It may be curiously localized in a city or district, or even in one part of a school or barrack. Mumps was very prevalent in the U. S. Army during the great war with 231,490 cases. The infection may persist as long as six weeks. It is probably conveyed by droplet infection from the mouth and nose. It may be congenital, and Hale White reported a case in which the mother and her newborn child were attacked at the same time.

A remarkable idiopathic, nonspecific parotitis may follow injury or disease of the abdominal or pelvic organs (see Diseases of the Salivary Glands).

Foci of acute interstitial inflammation have been found postmortem.

Symptoms.—The period of incubation is from two to three weeks, but may be longer and there are rarely any symptoms during this stage. The invasion is marked by *fever*, which is usually slight, rarely rising above 101°, but an exceptionally severe case reaches 103° or 104° F. The child complains of pain just below the ear on one side, most often the left, where a slight swelling is noticed, which increases gradually, and within forty-eight hours there is great enlargement of the neck and side of the cheek. The swelling passes forward in front of the ear, the lobe of which is lifted, and back beneath the sternomastoid muscle. It fills the space between the jaw and the mastoid process. The other side usually becomes affected within a day or two, and the whole neck is surrounded by a collar of doughy infiltration. Only one gland is involved in about one-third of the cases; an interval of four or five days may elapse before the other side is involved. The submaxillary and sublingual glands may become swollen; in a few cases they may be alone attacked. The lachrymal glands may be involved and the tonsils swollen. The greatest inconvenience is experienced in taking food, for the patient is unable to open the mouth, and even speech and deglutition become difficult. There may be an increase in the secretion of the saliva, but the reverse is sometimes the case. The mucous membrane of the mouth and throat may be slightly inflamed. The opening of the parotid duct may be swollen. There is seldom great pain, but an unpleasant feeling of tension and tightness. There may be earache, even otitis media, and slight impairment of hearing. There is usually a slight leukocytosis with relative increase in the lymphocytes, changing to a polymorphonuclear increase with orchitis.

After persisting for from seven to ten days, the swelling gradually subsides and the child rapidly regains his strength. Occasionally the disease is very severe and characterized by high fever, delirium, and great prostration. The patient may even lapse into a typhoid condition.

Relapse is rare, but there may be two or three slight recurrences within a few weeks, in which the cervical glands may enlarge. A second or even a third attack may occur but one attack usually gives immunity.

Orchitis.—Excessively rare before puberty, it occurs usually about the eighth day, and more particularly if the boy is allowed to leave his bed. One or both (5 to 10 per cent) testicles may be involved. The swelling may be great, and occasionally effusion takes place into the tunica vaginalis. The orchitis may occur before the parotitis, or in rare instances may be the only manifestation of the infection (*orchitis parotidea*). The inflammation increases for three or four days, and resolution takes place gradually. There may be acute urethritis with a mucopurulent discharge. In severe cases atrophy may follow, fortunately as a rule only in one organ; occurring in both before puberty, the natural development is usually checked. The atrophy is often slight and may be transient. Even when both testicles are atrophied and small, sexual vigor may be retained. The proportion of cases of orchitis varies in different epidemics from 10 to 20 per cent; 103 cases of atrophy followed 163 instances of orchitis (Comby). No satisfactory explanation of this metastasis has been given. The transference of the virus to the penis with the fingers and its transmissions along the urethra has been suggested. A vulvovaginitis sometimes occurs in girls and the breasts may become enlarged and tender. Mastitis has been seen in boys. Involvement of the ovaries is rare but suppurative ovaritis has occurred. Acute *pancreatitis* occurs rarely and has been found at operations and autopsy. Acute abdominal pain, nausea and vomiting, tenderness and possibly swelling in the epigastrium, with occasionally fatty stools, are the features. Transient glycosuria has followed. Fortunately recovery is the rule.

Complications and Sequelae.—Of these the cerebral affections are perhaps the most serious. There may be delirium with meningo-encephalitic phenomena and changes in the spinal fluid, but actual meningitis is rare. Hemiplegia and aphasia may occur. A majority of the fatal cases are associated with meningeal symptoms which are rare in comparison with the frequency of the disease. Acute mania has occurred, and there are instances on record of insanity following the disease.

Arthritis, albuminuria, nephritis, with uremia and convulsions, jaundice, endocarditis, pleurisy, facial paralysis, and peripheral neuritis are occasional complications. Suppuration of the gland is extremely rare. Gangrene has occasionally occurred. The special senses may be seriously involved. Deafness may occur and be permanent. Affections of the eye are rare, but optic neuritis with atrophy has been described. Thyroiditis may occur.

Chronic hypertrophy of the gland may follow.

Diagnosis.—During an epidemic this is usually easy except in cases in which other salivary glands are involved or orchitis occurs before the parotitis. The nonspecific forms of parotitis rarely cause difficulty. Marked swelling of the cervical glands with cellulitis has been mistaken for mumps but the position of the swelling should prevent error. Inflammation of the parotid in children is rare apart from mumps. In adults in whom the onset is with severe general symptoms, the diagnosis is usually in doubt until the parotitis appears.

Treatment.—It is well to keep the patient in bed for two weeks. This is especially important in males to lessen the chance of orchitis. Isolation for four weeks is advisable. Special care should be given to the mouth by cleaning after feeding and the use of alkaline antiseptic solutions. The bowels should be freely opened, and the patient given a liquid diet. No medicine is required unless the fever is high, in which case acetylsalicylic acid may be given. Cold compresses may be placed on the gland, but children, as a rule, prefer hot applications. Belladonna or ichthyol ointment is sometimes useful. With delirium and head symptoms the ice cap may be applied and sedatives given. For the orchitis, rest, with support and protection of the swollen gland with cotton wool, is usually sufficient. Nonimmune contacts should be isolated for three weeks. Blood serum from convalescents (20 to 40 cc.) has been used as a preventive.

YELLOW FEVER

Definition.—A fever of tropical and subtropical countries, characterized by a toxemia of varying intensity, with jaundice, albuminuria, and a marked tendency to hemorrhage, especially from the stomach, causing the "black vomit." The disease is usually transmitted through the bite of a mosquito, the *Aëdes aegypti* (*Stegomyia fasciaba*) but by other varieties in West Africa. There is one yellow fever; the African and American forms are the same. The disease can be communicated to certain monkeys and to white mice.

Distribution.—Yellow fever is endemic over large areas of West Africa. The northern parts of South America, parts of Central America and the West Indies, and southern parts of North America comprise the areas of recent American prevalence. Formerly it occurred extensively in the United States. In the latter part of the eighteenth century and the beginning of the nineteenth frightful epidemics prevailed in Philadelphia and other northern cities. The epidemic of 1793, in Philadelphia, so graphically described by Matthew Carey, was the most serious that ever visited any city of the middle states. There were 4,041 deaths from August to November, 3,435 being in September and October. The population of the city at the time was only 40,000. Epidemics occurred in the United States in 1797, 1798, 1799, and in 1802, 1803 and 1805; then for many years the outbreaks were slight and localized. In 1853 the disease raged throughout the southern states. There were moderately severe epidemics from 1867 to 1899. In September, 1903, yellow fever became epidemic along the Mexican side of the Rio Grande. It crossed into Texas and prevailed in several border towns. In Laredo there were 1,014 cases with 107 deaths. The efficient work of the public health service is shown by the difference between New Laredo on the Mexican border, just across the river, where 50 per cent of the population contracted the disease, and Laredo, Texas, in which only 10 per cent of a population of 10,000 was attacked. In Europe it has occasionally gained a foothold, but there have been no widespread epidemics. Yellow fever is a disease in which the parasites live a short time in the human host, unlike malaria. The infective period lasts only about four days, so that, unless the stegomyia index is high, the disease has no chance to reach epidemic form. The epidemics in the United States have been in the summer and autumn months, disappearing rapidly with cold weather.

Mode of Transmission.—No belief was more strong among the laity than that the disease is transmitted by infected clothing, and quarantine efforts were chiefly directed to the disinfection of articles shipped from infected ports. The Yellow Fever Commission of the United States Army, consisting of Drs. Walter Reed, Carroll, Lazear, and Agramonte, demonstrated conclusively that the disease can not be conveyed in this way. In their experiments, seven nonimmune subjects during a period of sixty-three days lived in contact with fomites and remained perfectly well. These experiments, conducted in the most rigid scientific manner, completely discredited the belief in the transmission of the disease by fomites.

We must bear testimony to the heroism of the soldiers who voluntarily, without compensation and purely in the interests of humanity, submitted to the experiments, and also to the zeal with which members of our profession, at great personal risk, attempted to solve the riddle of this serious disease. The deaths of Lazear, Myers, Noguchi, Stokes, Young and Lewis from yellow fever added their names to the long roll of the martyrs of science.

The American Commission demonstrated conclusively that yellow fever is transferred by a mosquito, *Aëdes aegypti*, previously fed on the blood of infected persons. The Commission showed that in nonimmunes the disease could be produced by the subcutaneous or the intravenous injection of blood taken from patients suffering with the disease.

An interval of about ten days or more after biting the patient is necessary before the mosquito is capable of transmitting the disease. As Reed pointed out, the mosquito theory fits in with well-recognized facts in connection with epidemics. After the importation of a case into an uninfected region, a definite period elapses, rarely less than two weeks, before a second case occurs. The disease prevails most during the mosquito season and disappears with the appearance of frost. Probably, the disease is kept up by its prevalence in a very mild form among children. In all probability the immunity which is acquired by prolonged residence in a locality in which the disease is endemic is due to the occurrence of very slight attacks. One attack does not always confer immunity.

The cause of yellow fever is probably a filterable virus. The disease can be transmitted to certain *Macacus* monkeys. Convalescent serum protects the monkeys against infection. The virus is present in the blood of a patient with yellow fever on the first four days of the disease and possibly in the incubation period. A mosquito when infected probably remains so for the duration of its life, which may be as long as sixty days. There may be *direct infection* from contact with the blood of man or animals with the disease or from the organs at autopsy. Yellow fever virus can penetrate the unbroken skin. Infection has resulted from the examination of blood from yellow fever patients without adequate protection of the hands. Such cases have occurred in England.

Morbid Anatomy.—The skin is more or less jaundiced, even though the patient did not appear yellow before death. Cutaneous hemorrhages may be present. Degenerative changes in the capillary endothelial cells cause the hemorrhages. The myocardium shows degenerative changes; fatty degeneration is constant and vacuolar and hyaline alterations are common. The sino-auricular node and the bundle of His may be affected. The stomach presents more or less hyperemia of the mucosa with petechiae. There is often general glandular enlargement; the cervical, axillary and mesenteric groups are most involved. The liver is usually of a pale yellow or brownish-yellow color, and the cells are in various stages of necrosis. Inclusion bodies are found in the liver cells. Hemorrhagic and necrotic areas are common. The toxin has a selective toxic effect on the liver cells without any inflammatory process. The kidneys show acute parenchymatous inflammation. The epithelium of the convoluted tubules is swollen and very granular; there may also be necrotic changes. The spleen is not enlarged but there is degeneration of its endothelial cells. The adrenal glands may show fatty degeneration. Hemorrhages may be found in the serous membranes and in the meninges. None of the lesions can be regarded as absolutely specific. The character of the changes suggests the effect of toxins rather than acute inflammatory lesions.

Symptoms.—The incubation is usually three or four days; it was ten days in two cases in London contracted by handling the blood of a patient. The onset is sudden, as a rule, without premonitory symptoms, and in the early hours of the morning. Chilly feelings are common, and are usually associated with headache and very severe pains in the back and limbs. The fever rises rapidly and the skin feels very hot and dry. The tongue is furred, but moist; the throat sore. Nausea and vomiting are not constant, and become more intense on the second or third day. The bowels are usually constipated. There are divergent statements as to the leukocytes; some report leukopenia, others leukocytosis. The following are the more important characteristics:

FACIES.—Even as early as the first morning the patient may present a characteristic facies, one of the three distinguishing features of the disease, which Guitéras describes as follows: The face is flushed, more so than in any other acute infectious disease at such an early period. The eyes are injected, the color is a bright red, and there may be a slight tumefaction of the eyelids and of the lips. Even at this early date there is to be noticed in connection with the injection of the superficial capillaries of the face and conjunctivae a slight icteroid tint, and "the early manifestation of jaundice is undoubtedly the most characteristic feature of the facies of yellow fever."

FEVER.—On the morning of the first day the temperature may range from 100° to 106° F., usually it is between 102° and 103° F. During the evening of the first day and the morning of the second day the temperature keeps about the same. There is a slight diurnal variation on the second and third day. In very mild cases the fever may fall on the evening of the second or on the morning of the third day, or in abortive cases even at the end of twenty-four hours. In cases that are to terminate favorably the defervescence takes place by lysis during a period of two or three days. The remission is succeeded by a febrile reaction or secondary fever, which lasts one to three days, and in favorable cases falls by a short lysis. In fatal cases the temperature is continuous, becomes higher than in the initial fever, and death follows shortly.

PULSE.—On the first day the pulse is rarely more than 100 or 110. On the second or third day, while the fever still keeps up, the pulse begins to fall, as much perhaps as 20 beats, while the temperature has risen 1.5° or 2°. On the evening of the third day there may be a fever between 103° and 104° with a pulse of 70 to 80. This important feature was first described by Faget, of New Orleans. The bradycardia is due to injury of the sino-auricular node and disturbance of conduction. During defervescence the pulse may fall to 50 or even as low as 30; a slow pulse at this period is not the special circulatory feature of the disease, but *the slowing of the pulse with a steady or even rising temperature.*

ALBUMINURIA.—This, the third characteristic feature, occurs as early as the third day. "Even in the mild cases that do not go to bed—cases of 'walking yellow fever'—on the second, third, or fourth day of the disease albuminuria will show itself." It may be quite transient. In the severer cases the amount of albumin is large, and there may be numerous casts and the signs of acute nephritis; or complete suppression may supervene, and death occurs in convulsions or coma within twenty-four or thirty-six hours.

GASTRIC FEATURES.—*"Black Vomit."*—Irritability of the stomach is present from the outset, and the vomitus consists of the contents of the stomach, and subsequently of mucus and a grayish fluid. In the third stage the vomiting becomes more pronounced and in severe cases is characterized by the presence of blood. It may be copious and forcible with pain in the abdomen and along the gullet. There is nothing specific in this "black vomit," which consists of altered blood, and it is not necessarily a fatal symptom, though occurring only in the severer attacks. Other hemorrhagic features may be present—petechiae on the skin and bleeding from the gums or other mucous membranes. The bowels are usually constipated, the stools not clay-colored, except late in the disease; they sometimes contain blood.

MENTAL FEATURES.—In very severe cases the onset may be with active delirium. "As a rule, in a majority of cases, even when there is black vomit, there is a peculiar alertness; the patient watches everything going on about him with a peculiar intensity and liveliness" (Guitéras).

Relapses occasionally occur. Among the varieties it is important to recognize the mild cases, characterized by slight fever, continuing for one or two days, and succeeded by a rapid convalescence. In the absence of an epidemic they would scarcely be recognized as yellow fever. Cases of greater severity have high fever and the features of the disease are well marked. And, lastly, in the malignant form the patient is overwhelmed by the intensity of the disease and death takes place in two or three days.

In severe cases convalescence may be complicated by parotitis, abscesses in various parts of the body, and diarrhea.

Diagnosis.—FROM DENGUE.—The difficulty in the differential diagnosis of these two diseases may lie in their coexistence. In a majority of cases the three diagnostic points—the facies, the albuminuria, and the slowing of the pulse with maintenance or elevation of the fever—are sufficient. Jaundice, which sometimes occurs in dengue, rarely appears as early as the second or third day, and on this much stress should be laid. Hemorrhages are much less common in dengue but do occur. There is a marked leukopenia in dengue.

FROM MALARIAL FEVER.—In the early stages of an epidemic cases may be mistaken for malarial fever. In the southern states the outbreaks have usually been in the late summer months, when estivo-autumnal fever prevails. Among the points to be specially noted is the absence of early jaundice. Even in the most intense types of malarial infection the color of the skin is rarely changed within four or five days. Albumin is rarely present in the urine so early in a malarial infection. The spleen in yellow fever is not much enlarged. Hemorrhages, particularly the black vomit, epistaxis, and bleeding gums are very rare in malaria. In the so-called hemorrhagic malarial fever the patient has usually had previous attacks of malaria. Hematuria is a prominent feature, while in yellow fever it is not frequent. The point of greatest importance is the finding of malarial parasites.

Spirochetal jaundice may cause difficulty. The finding of spirochetes in the blood or urine, or the injection of the patient's blood intraperitoneally into a guinea-pig causes a marked infection; nothing results in yellow fever.

The "protection test" is done by injecting monkeys or mice with serum from a recovered patient, or from the individual being tested, and then with a lethal dose of yellow fever virus. By this method mild cases can be recognized.

Prognosis.—The mortality has ranged from 10 to 85 per cent. In heavy drinkers and those exposed to hardships the death-rate is much higher than among the better classes. In the epidemic of 1878, in New Orleans, while the mortality in hospitals was over 50 per cent of the white and 21 per cent of the colored patients, in private practice it was not more than 10 per cent among the white patients.

Prophylaxis.—The objects are: (1) To prevent the breeding of stegomyia mosquitoes. (2) To destroy those that have become infected. (3) To prevent mosquitoes becoming infected by protecting the sick so that they can not be bitten by mosquitoes. If the patient is protected from mosquitoes for the first four days of the attack infection is prevented.

The greatest care should be taken in any blood work done with patients or infected animals and in autopsy work (there is very little danger if death occurred on the fifth day or later) to prevent any chance of skin infection. The use of convalescent serum gives temporary immunity. "Vaccination" with the virus fixed for mice combined with immune serum apparently gives immunity.

Treatment.—The patient should be at rest in bed and for the first few days the diet should consist of very simple fluids. Elimination is an important part of treatment. Water should be given as freely as possible, best in the form of cold carbonated alkaline water. The bowels should be opened by a calomel and saline purge and enemata used if necessary. If there is vomiting, fluid should be given by the bowel or subcutaneously. Ice in small quantities or cocaine (gr. 1/4, 0.016 gm.) may be tried. The fever should be treated by hydrotherapy, sponges, packs or baths being used. The alkaline treatment is favorably regarded, sodium bicarbonate in full doses being given at short intervals and as much alkaline water as possible. Glucose solution should be given freely, intravenously, in severe cases. Uremic symptoms are best treated by hot baths or packs, the free administration of fluid and hot bowel irrigations. Stimulants, especially strychnine, caffeine and epinephrine, should be used when the heart becomes feeble and rapid.

DENGUE

Definition.—An acute disease of tropical and subtropical regions, characterized by febrile paroxysms, pains in the joints and muscles, an initial erythematous and a terminal polymorphous eruption. It is known as *breakbone* fever from the atrocious character of the pain, and *dandy fever* from the stiff, dandified gait. The word dengue is supposed to be derived from a Spanish, or possibly Hindostanee, equivalent of the word dandy.

History and Geographical Distribution.—The disease was first recognized in 1779 in Cairo and in Java, where Bylon described the outbreak in Batavia. There have been widespread epidemics in India and China. The description by Benjamin Rush of the epidemic in Philadelphia in 1780 is one of the first and best accounts of the disease. Between 1824 and 1828 it was prevalent at intervals in India and in the southern states. S. H. Dickson gives a graphic description of the disease as it appeared in Charleston in 1828. Since that date there have been widespread epidemics in tropical countries and in North America along the Gulf States. There were 30,000 cases in Galveston in 1922. None of the recent epidemics extended into the northern states, but in 1888 it prevailed as far north as Virginia.

Etiology.—The rapidity of diffusion and the pandemic character are two important features of dengue. There is no disease, not even influenza, which attacks so large a proportion of the population. The specific cause is a filterable virus present in the blood for at least the first three days of the attack. The disease is transmitted by a mosquito, *Aëdes aegypti.* Biting experiments are successful (after eleven days from infection of the mosquito) and it is transmitted by injecting the blood subcutaneously. The virus is present in the whole blood, the serum and the fluid part of citrated blood.

Pathology.—The changes are not striking. Cloudy swelling in various organs with petechial hemorrhages are found. The liver cells may show considerable cloudy swelling and fatty change.

Symptoms.—The period of incubation is from three to seven days, during which the patient feels well. The attack sets in suddenly with headache, chilly feelings, and intense aching pains in the joints and muscles. The temperature rises gradually, and may reach 106° or 107°. The pulse is rapid, and there are the other phenomena associated with acute fever—loss of appetite, coated tongue, slight nocturnal delirium, and concentrated urine. The face has a suffused, bloated appearance, the eyes are injected and painful, and the mucous membranes are flushed. There is a congested erythematous state of the skin. Rush's description of the pains is worth quoting, as in it the epithet break-bone occurs in the literature for the first time. "The pains which accompanied this fever were exquisitely severe in the head, back, and limbs, the pains in the head were sometimes in the back parts of it, and at other times they occupied only the eyeballs. In some people the pains were so acute in their backs and hips that they could not lie in bed. In others the pains affected the neck and arms, so as to produce in one instance a difficulty of moving the fingers of the right hand. They all complained more or less of a soreness in the seats of these pains, particularly when they occupied the head and eyeballs. A few complained of their flesh being sore to the touch in every part of the body. From these circumstances the disease was sometimes believed to be a rheumatism, but its more general name among all classes of people was the break-bone fever." The large and small joints are affected, sometimes in succession, and become swollen, red, and painful. In some cases cutaneous hyperesthesia has been noted. Hemorrhage from the mucous membranes was noted by Rush, and black vomit has been described.

The fever gradually reaches its maximum by the third or fourth day; the patient then enters upon the apyretic period, which may last from two to four days, and in which he feels prostrated and stiff. A second paroxysm of fever then occurs, and the pains return. In a large number of cases an *eruption* is common, which, judging from the descriptions, has nothing distinctive, being sometimes macular, like that of measles, sometimes diffuse and scarlatiniform, or papular, or lichen-like. In other instances the rash has been described as urticarial, or even vesicular. The rash may persist for a month after the symptoms have disappeared. Certain writers describe inflammation and hyperemia of the mucous membrane of the nose, mouth and pharynx. Enlargement of the lymph nodes is not uncommon, and may persist for weeks after the attack. The *leukocytes* diminish early and may fall to 2000 by the fifth or sixth day. There is a relative lymphocytosis. Convalescence is often protracted, and there is marked mental and physical prostration. The pains in the joints or muscles, sometimes very local, may persist for weeks. The average duration of a moderate attack is from seven to eight days. Dengue is seldom fatal but in 1928 there were 20 deaths reported in the United States.

Complications are rare. Insomnia and occasionally delirium have been observed, and convulsions in children. Atrophy of the muscles may occur after the attack. A relapse may occur even as late as two weeks.

Diagnosis.—The diagnosis of the disease, prevailing as it does in epidemic form and attacking all classes indiscriminately, rarely offers any special difficulty. Isolated cases might be mistaken at first for rheumatic fever. The seven-day fever of East Indian ports is believed to be dengue. It is a sporadic fever of the hot weather, attacking a large proportion of Europeans within the first year or two of their arrival. It is characterized by early and severe pains in the back and limbs, and a fever of six to seven days' duration. Care may be required to distinguish dengue from yellow fever and influenza.

Treatment.—The patients should be protected from mosquitoes during the febrile period. The treatment is entirely symptomatic. Hydrotherapy may be employed to reduce the fever. The salicylates or antipyrin may be tried for the pains, which usually, however, require opium or morphine. During convalescence iodide of potassium is recommended for the arthritic pains, and tonics are indicated.

RABIES (Lyssa; Hydrophobia)

Definition.—An acute disease of warm-blooded animals, dependent upon a filterable virus which is communicated by inoculation to man.

Distribution.—Rabies is very variously distributed. In Russia it is common. In England the muzzling order has been followed by a complete disappearance of the disease and there were no deaths from 1912-1931. In the decennium ending with 1890 the deaths averaged 29 annually (Tatham). In the United States there has been a yearly average of 64 deaths in the registration area from 1911-1920 and 107 deaths in 1928.

Etiology.—Dogs are especially liable to the disease. It also occurs in the wolf, fox, skunk, cat, horse and cow. Most animals are susceptible; and it is communicable by inoculation to the rabbit and pig. The disease is propagated chiefly by the dog. The virus is filterable. It is contained chiefly in the nervous system and in some of the secretions, particularly in the saliva. Bartarelli has shown that the virus reaches the dog's salivary glands by way of the nerves and not through the blood vessels.

A variable time elapses between the introduction of the virus and the appearance of the symptoms. Horsley stated that this depends upon the following factors: "(*a*) Age. The incubation is shorter in children than in adults. For obvious reasons the former are more frequently attacked. (*b*) Part infected. The rapidity of onset of the symptoms is greatly determined by the part of the body which has been bitten. Wounds about the face and head are especially dangerous; next in order come bites on the hands, then on the other parts of the body. This relative order is, no doubt, greatly dependent upon the fact that the face, head, and hands are usually naked, while the other parts are clothed; it also appears to depend somewhat upon the richness in nerves of the part. (*c*) The extent and severity of the wound. Puncture wounds are the most dangerous; the lacerations are fatal in proportion to the extent of the surface afforded for absorption of the virus. (*d*) The animal conveying the infection. In order of decreasing severity come: the wolf; the cat; the dog; and other animals." Only a limited number of those bitten by rabid dogs become affected by the disease; according to Horsley, not more than 15 per cent. The death rate of those persons bitten by wolves is higher, not less than 40 per cent. Babes gives the mortality as from 60 to 80 per cent.

The *incubation* period in man is extremely variable. The average is from six weeks to two months. In a few cases it has been under two weeks. It may be prolonged to three months. It is stated that the incubation may be prolonged for a year but this has not been definitely settled.

Morbid Anatomy.—The important lesions consist in the accumulation of leukocytes around the blood vessels and the nerve cells, particularly the motor ganglion cells, of the central nervous system (rabic tubercles of Babes). Especial importance in the rapid diagnosis of rabies is attached to the accumulation of lymphoid and endothelioid cells around nerve cells of the sympathetic and cerebrospinal ganglia. Negri described in the central nervous system irregular bodies varying from 4 to 10 microns in size, widespread, frequently in the cells of the cerebellum, cerebral cortex and pons, and in the spinal cord. They furnish a rapid and trustworthy means of diagnosis. The virus is not present in the liver, spleen, or kidneys, but is abundant in the spinal cord, brain, and peripheral nerves. In the spinal fluid the globulin is increased and often the cells, polymorphonuclear or mononuclear.

Symptoms.—Three stages of the disease are recognized:

PREMONITORY STAGE, in which there may be irritation about the bite, pain, or numbness. The patient is depressed and melanchoy; and complains of headache and loss of appetite. He is irritable and sleepless, and has a sense of impending danger. There is often greatly increased sensibility. A bright light or a loud voice is distressing. The larynx may be injected, the voice becoming husky, and the first symptoms of difficulty in swallowing are experienced. There is a slight rise in the temperature and pulse.

STAGE OF EXCITEMENT.—This is characterized by great excitability and restlessness, and an extreme degree of hyperesthesia. "Any afferent stimulant—*i.e.*, a sound or a draught of air, or the mere association of a verbal suggestion—will cause a violent reflex spasm. In man this symptom constitutes the most distressing feature of the malady. The spasms, which affect particularly the muscles of the larynx and mouth, are exceedingly painful and are accompanied by an intense sense of dyspnea, even when the glottis is widely opened or tracheotomy has been performed" (Horsley). Any attempt to swallow is followed by an intensely painful spasm of the muscles of deglutition and respiration. These spasmodic attacks may be associated with maniacal symptoms. In the intervals the patient is quiet and the mind unclouded. The temperature in this stage is usually elevated and may reach from 100° to 103°. In some instances the disease is afebrile. The patient rarely attempts to injure his attendants, and in the intense spasms may be particularly anxious to avoid hurting any one. There are, however, occasional fits of furious mania, and the patient may, in the contractions of the muscles of the larynx and pharynx, give utterance to odd sounds. This stage lasts from a day and a half to three days and gradually passes into the—

Paralytic Stage.—In herbivora and rodents the preliminary and furious stages are absent, as a rule, and the paralytic stage may be marked from the outset—the so-called dumb rabies. This stage rarely lasts longer than from six to eighteen hours. The patient then becomes quiet; the spasms no longer occur; unconsciousness gradually supervenes; the heart's action becomes more and more enfeebled, and death follows. Some cases, which may occur in epidemics, have marked paralytic features suggestive of poliomyelitis or Landry's paralysis.

Diagnosis.—In man this offers no special difficulties. *Tetanus* is distinguished by trismus, the presence of persistent and not intermittent muscle spasm and the absence of special involvement of the muscles of deglutition and respiration. Lyssophobia should not cause difficulty if a careful examination is made. Whenever possible the animal should be secured and kept; if it has rabies death will soon follow and the diagnosis can be established beyond doubt. The recognition of the Negri bodies in smears of brain substance enables the diagnosis to be made promptly.

Prophylaxis.—By a systematic muzzling of dogs the disease can be practically eradicated. In case of a bite from a suspicious animal, bleeding should be encouraged, the wound freely opened and washed with bichloride of mercury solution (1 to 1,000). Thorough cauterization should be done as soon as possible, for which pure phenol or nitric acid should be used, being applied to every part of the wound. The wound is washed with a saturated solution of bicarbonate of soda and then with alcohol.

Preventive Inoculation.—Pasteur found that the virus, when propagated through a series of rabbits, increases in its virulence; so that whereas subdural inoculation of the brain of a mad dog takes from fifteen to twenty days to produce the disease, in successive inoculation in a series of rabbits the incubation period is gradually reduced to seven days (*virus fixé*). The spinal cords of these rabbits contain the virus in great intensity, but when preserved in dry air this gradually diminishes. If dogs are inoculated from cords preserved for from twelve to fifteen days, and then from cords preserved for a shorter period, *i. e.*, with a progressively stronger virus, they gradually acquire immunity against the disease. Relying upon these experiments, Pasteur began inoculations in the human subject, using, on successive days, material from cords in which the virus was of varying degrees of intensity. Myelitis with paralysis has occurred with the treatment and has been fatal, but the risk of this is small. Polyneuritis has also followed.

Treatment.—When once established the disease is hopelessly incurable. No measures have been found of the slightest avail, consequently the treatment must be palliative. The patient should be kept as quiet as possible in a darkened room. To allay the spasm, chloroform may be administered and morphia given hypodermically. It is best to use these remedies from the outset, and not temporize with less potent drugs. By the local application of cocaine, the sensitiveness of the throat may be diminished sufficiently to enable the patient to take liquid nourishment. Sometimes he can swallow readily. Fluid can be given by the bowel.

Pseudohydrophobia.—(*Lyssophobia*).—This may closely resemble hydrophobia, but is nothing more than a neurotic or hysterical manifestation. A nervous person bitten by a dog, either rabid or supposed to be rabid, has within a few months, or even later, symptoms somewhat resembling the true disease. He is irritable and depressed, and constantly declares his condition to be serious and that he will inevitably become mad. He may have paroxysms in which he says he is unable to drink, grasps at his throat, and becomes emotional. The temperature is not elevated and the disease does not progress. It lasts much longer than the true rabies, and is amenable to treatment. Probably a majority of the cases of alleged recovery in rabies have been of this hysterical form. Certain cases of acute bulbar paralysis may resemble hydrophobia, and there is a form of tetanus with hydrophobic symptoms.

RHEUMATIC FEVER

Definition.—An acute infection with an unknown etiology, characterized by arthritis, myocarditis, and a marked tendency to inflammation of the endocardium of the valves of the heart.

Etiology.—Distribution and Prevalence.—It prevails in temperate and humid climates, and is apparently rare in the tropics. In England and Wales in 1931 there were 1,260 deaths from the disease and 2,920 deaths in the U. S. registration area for 1930. The disease prevails more in the northern latitudes. In the Montreal General Hospital there were, for the twelve years ending 1903, 2 deaths in 482 cases among 12,044 admissions; at the Royal Victoria Hospital, Montreal, for ten years ending 1903, 3 deaths in 285 cases among 9,286 admissions (John McCrae). At the Johns Hopkins Hospital for the fifteen years ending 1904 there were 360 admissions (330 patients) and 9 deaths. The general impression is that the disease prevails more in the British Isles than elsewhere; but the returns are imperfect (this holds good everywhere).

Season.—In London the cases reach the maximum in the months of September and October. In Montreal the largest number was admitted in February, March, and April. The same is true in Baltimore; 55 per cent of the cases were admitted in the first four months of the year. The disease prevails most in dry years or a succession of such, and is specially prevalent when the subsoil water is abnormally low and the temperature of the earth high (Newsholme).

Age.—The disease occurs most often in childhood and a first attack rarely occurs after the age of 25 years. The cardiac involvement is the most striking feature in children in whom severe arthritis is less common than in adults. The disease is rare in children below the age of 3 years; it has occurred in the fetus.

SEX.—If all ages are taken, males are affected oftener than females. Of our series of 330 patients, 239 were males, 91 females. In the Collective Investigation Report there were 375 males and 279 females. Up to the age of twenty, however, females predominate. Between the ages of ten and fifteen girls are more prone to the disease.

HEREDITY.—It is a deeply grounded belief that this is a family disease. The occurrence in several members of one family is used by those who believe in the infectious origin as an argument in favor of its being a house disease.

CHILL.—Exposure to cold, a wetting, and a sudden change of temperature are among the factors in determining the onset of an attack, but they were present in only 12 per cent of our cases.

Not only does an attack not confer *immunity*, but, as in pneumonia, predisposes the subject to further manifestations of the disease. One view is that a condition of allergy is established. In general it may be said that subsequent attacks cause more cardiac damage than the initial one.

The Nature of Rheumatic Fever.—The view is gaining ground that the manifestations of the disease represent a condition of hypersensitiveness to various forms of streptococci. With this conception there are points of resemblance to tuberculosis and syphilis in the allergic response and in the fact that the lesion is a granuloma. There is an initial lesion with more serious manifestations occurring elsewhere in the body. The initial lesion may be in the tonsils with resulting sensitization and subsequent attacks may be due to fresh infection or to areas of chronic infection (tonsils, sinuses). Organisms are recovered from patients with the disease only in a small proportion of cases. The organisms found are usually nonhemolytic streptococci with no immunological relationship. This suggests that rheumatic fever may represent a response to a number of organisms and not be caused by a specific organism. The work of Swift is suggestive of this. Patients once infected may react to filtrates of many types of streptococci. This hypersensitiveness may be due to two products, (1) a neutralizable toxin and (2) some nonneutralizable substance. The disease can not be reproduced in animals but inoculations in rabbits with the organisms obtained show various allergic reactions. In the human infection, the lesions are exudative at first and later proliferative. A hypersensitive state once established, a chronic infection or repeated slight infections may serve to prolong it and an acute infection may precipitate another attack. Long after an acute attack there may be active lesions in the body.

The tonsils are culture centres for many organisms, particularly of the streptococcus type. The association of rheumatic fever and arthritic affections generally with infected tonsils is an old story insisted on by Lasague and other French writers years ago. Some cases of rheumatic fever begin with tonsillitis. There is considerable evidence against the view that it is simply a pyogenic infection. Salicylates have no effect on the ordinary streptococcus infections, and the clinical course in the streptococcus arthritis is very different; rheumatic joints never suppurate. The endocarditis caused by a pyogenic streptococcus is of a very different character from that of rheumatic fever.

Morbid Anatomy.—The affected joints show hyperemia and swelling of the synovial membranes and of the ligamentous tissues. The fluid in the joint is turbid, albuminous, and contains leukocytes and a few fibrin flakes. Rheumatic fever rarely proves fatal, except with complications, such as pericarditis, endocarditis, myocarditis, pleurisy, or pneumonia. The changes in the myocardium are regarded as characteristic by many workers. The *submiliary nodules,* described by Aschoff, are most often in the wall of the left ventricle, but may be in the auricle, aorta and elsewhere. The lesions in the aorta may occur in all the coats and the Aschoff bodies have been found in the adventitia. Fibrosis and calcification may occur. There are fan-shaped collections of giant cells, perivascular fibrous nodules, and infiltration of small cells into the surrounding tissue. Klotz has drawn attention to the frequency of arterial lesions, especially in the aorta. Changes in the coronary arteries, an inflammatory fibrosis, are common.

Symptoms.—As a rule, the disease sets in abruptly, but it may be preceded by irregular pains in the joints, slight *malaise,* sore throat, and particularly by tonsillitis. A definite rigor is uncommon; more often there is slight chilliness. The fever rises quickly, and one or more of the joints may become painful. Within twenty-four hours from the onset the disease is fully manifest. The temperature range is from 102° to 104°. The pulse is frequent, soft, and usually above 100. The tongue is moist and covered with a white fur. There are the ordinary symptoms associated with an acute fever, such as loss of appetite, thirst, constipation, and scanty, highly acid urine. In a majority of the cases there are profuse, acid sweats, of a peculiar sour odor. Sudaminal and miliary vesicles are abundant, the latter usually surrounded by a minute ring of hyperemia. The mind is clear, except with hyperpyrexia. The affected joints are painful to move, soon become swollen and hot, and present a reddish flush. The order of frequency of involvement of the joints in our series was knee, ankle, shoulder, wrist, elbow, hip, hand, foot. The joints are not attacked together, but successively. For example, if the knee is first affected, the redness may disappear from it as the wrists become involved. The disease is seldom limited to a single joint. The amount of swelling is variable. Extensive effusion into a joint is rare, and much of the enlargement is due to the infiltration of the periarticular tissues with serum. Corresponding joints are often affected. In attacks of great severity every one of the larger joints may be involved. Perhaps no disease is more painful; the inability to change the posture without agonizing pain, the drenching sweats, the prostration and helplessness, combine to make it a most distressing affection. A special feature is the tendency of the inflammation to subside in one joint while increasing in another. In children there may be no arthritis whatever or if present only in a mild form.

The temperature range in an ordinary attack is between 102° and 104° F. In only 18 of our cases did the temperature rise above 104° F. In 100 it reached 103° F. or over. It is peculiarly irregular, with marked remissions and exacerbations, and defervescence is usually gradual. The profuse sweats materially influence the temperature curve.

The *blood* is profoundly altered and there is no acute febrile disease in which an anemia occurs with greater rapidity. The average leukocyte count in our cases was about 12,000 per c. mm. Epistaxis is not uncommon.

With the high fever a murmur may often be heard at the apex region.

Endocarditis is also a common cause of an apex *bruit.* The heart should be carefully examined at the first visit and subsequently each day.

The urine is, as a rule, reduced in amount, of high density and high color. It is very acid, and, on cooling, deposits urates. The chlorides may be greatly diminished or even absent. Formic acid is present (Walker). Febrile albuminuria is not uncommon. Hematuria occurs occasionally.

Subacute rheumatic fever represents a milder form of the disease, in which all the symptoms are less pronounced. The fever rarely rises above 101° F.; fewer joints are involved; and the arthritis is less intense. The cases may drag on for weeks or months. It should not be forgotten that mild or subacute forms may be associated with endocarditis or pericarditis.

The influence of *age* on the manifestations is marked. While the usual description applies to the disease as seen in adults, in young children there may not be any pronounced arthritis or any arthritis at all, and the discovery of endocarditis often suggests the diagnosis. Endocarditis and myocarditis are the prominent features in children in whom the picture may be very variable. The onset may be so insidious that it can hardly be termed even subacute. Ill health without any evident cause, loss of weight, anorexia, fatigue, complaint of slight pains and fever with no apparent cause should suggest the possibility. Acute arthritis is the exception in the child; cardiac involvement of some kind is the rule. Arthritis in a young child is probably not due to rheumatic fever. Recognition of this fact would save some serious errors.

Cardiac Affections.—*Endocarditis* occurs in a considerable percentage of all cases. A child may come under observation with a well-marked endocarditis. Of 889 cases, 494 had signs of old or recent endocarditis (Church). The liability to endocarditis diminishes as age advances and increases directly with the number of attacks. Of 116 cases, in the first attack 58.1 per cent had endocarditis, 63 per cent in the second attack, and 71 per cent in the third attack (Stephen Mackenzie). Thirty-five per cent of our cases showed organic valve lesions; in 96 per cent the mitral was involved, in 27 per cent the aortic, and in 23 per cent the lesions were combined. The mitral segments are most frequently involved and the affection is usually of the simple, verrucose variety. Ulcerative endocarditis is very rare. The valvulitis in itself is rarely dangerous, producing few symptoms, and often overlooked. Unhappily, though the valve at the time may not be seriously damaged, the inflammation starts changes which lead to sclerosis of the segments, and so to chronic valvular disease. Venous thrombosis is an occasional complication.

Pericarditis may occur independently of or with endocarditis. It may be simple fibrinous, serofibrinous, or purulent. It was present in 20 cases of our series—6 per cent—in only four of which did effusion occur. The physical signs are very characteristic. The condition is described under Pericarditis. A peculiar form of delirium may accompany rheumatic pericarditis.

Myocarditis is probably always present in some degree and is especially marked with endopericardial changes. As Sturges insisted, the term *carditis* is applicable to many cases. The anatomical condition is a degeneration of the heart muscle, which leads to weakening of the walls and dilatation. There is dilatation of the heart in the majority of cases during the acute period and practically always in children. The rate is increased, there is often a diffuse impulse, the dulness is increased, especially to the right, the first sound may be soft and murmurish or completely replaced by a murmur. It may be difficult for some weeks to make the diagnosis from endocarditis.

Many *electrocardiographic* changes are found (in over 90 per cent of cases) such as extra systoles, various degrees of auriculoventricular block, auricular paroxysmal tachycardia and changes in various waves. These are often transient. Delayed auriculoventricular conduction is frequent and is an important diagnostic point of rheumatic fever in the absence of any other cause for it.

AORTITIS.—This is especially common in children and particularly with aortic endocarditis. The enlargement of the aorta may be marked. In some cases the acute condition results in permanent dilatation. *Arteritis* should be carefully looked for; there may be marked tenderness on pressure over the artery.

Complications.—These are important and serious.

HYPERPYREXIA.—The temperature may rise rapidly a few days after the onset, and be associated with delirium. It is most apt to occur during the second week. Delirium may precede or follow its onset. In our series there was no instance of hyperpyrexia; it seems rare in the United States.

PULMONARY AFFECTIONS.—Pneumonia and pleurisy occurred in 9.94 per cent of 3,433 cases (Stephen Mackenzie). They frequently accompany the cases of endopericarditis. According to Howard's analysis of a large number of cases, there were pulmonary complications in only 10.5 per cent of cases of rheumatic endocarditis; in 58 per cent of cases of pericarditis; and in 71 per cent of the cases of endopericarditis.

NERVOUS COMPLICATIONS.—They may be grouped as follows: (*i*) *Cerebral,* characterized by (*a*) *delirium,* associated with hyperpyrexia or toxemia. It may be excited by sodium salicylate. It was present in only 5 of our cases, and in 4 of these we thought the salicylate at fault. A peculiar delirium occurs with rheumatic pericarditis. (*b*) *Coma* may occur without preliminary delirium or convulsions and prove rapidly fatal. Certain cases occur with hyperpyrexia but others are evidently uremic. (*c*) *Convulsions* are less common, though they may precede the coma. (*ii*) *Chorea.* The relations of this disease and rheumatic fever will be subsequently discussed. In only 88 of 554 cases from the Infirmary for Diseases of the Nervous System, Philadelphia, were chorea and rheumatism associated. It is most apt to develop in the slighter attacks in childhood. (*iii*) *Meningitis* is extremely rare, though undoubtedly it does occur. (*iv*) *Polyneuritis* has been described and may follow hyperpyrexia. In one case free venesection saved the patient's life. After many months the patient recovered, but with ataxia.

CUTANEOUS AFFECTIONS.—Sweat vesicles are extremely common and a red miliary rash may also develop. Scarlatiniform eruptions are occasionally seen. Depressions on the nails may follow rheumatic fever or chorea. Purpura, with or without urticaria, and various forms of erythema may occur. It is doubtful whether the cases of extensive purpura with urticaria and arthritis—peliosis rheumatica—belong to rheumatic fever.

RHEUMATIC NODULES.—These structures, described originally by Meynet, occur in the form of small subcutaneous nodules. They vary in size from a small shot to a large pea, and are most numerous on the fingers, hands, and wrists. They also occur about the elbows, knees, the spines of the vertebrae, and the scapulæ. They are not often tender. They are more common after the decline of the fever and in children with endocarditis. In only 5 of our patients were they noted during the acute attack. The nodules may grow with great rapidity and usually last for weeks or months. They are more common in children than in adults, and in the former their presence may be regarded as an indication of rheumatic fever. Subcutaneous nodules occur also in migraine, gout, and arthritis deformans. Histologically they are made up of round and spindle-shaped cells and may contain Aschoff bodies. They suggest a proliferative response to the infection.

Swelling or tenderness of the *thyroid* gland may be present.

Course.—This is extremely variable. Rheumatic fever is, as Austin Flint first showed, self-limited, but this does not mean that it follows a regular course. A usual average of symptoms in uncomplicated cases is from two to three weeks, but with endocarditis the illness may last for months. Relapse and recrudescence are common and the period of rest should be prolonged. The frequency of myocarditis is an additional reason for caution. In patients with previous endocarditis the course is usually protracted.

Prognosis.—Rheumatic fever is the most serious of all diseases with a low death-rate. The mortality is rarely above 2 or 3 per cent. Only 9 of our 330 patients died, 2.7 per cent, all with endocarditis and 6 with pericarditis. The ultimate prognosis depends largely on the injury to the heart.

Sudden death in rheumatic fever is due most frequently to myocarditis. Herringham has reported a case in which on the fourteenth day there was fatty degeneration and acute inflammation of the myocardium. In a few rare cases it results from embolism. Symptoms of depression sometimes follow excessive doses of sodium salicylate.

Diagnosis.—Practically, the recognition of rheumatic fever is usually easy; but there are several affections which closely resemble it.

(*a*) Multiple Secondary Arthritis.—Under this term may be embraced the forms of arthritis which occur with or follow tonsillitis, scarlet fever, dysentery, cerebrospinal meningitis, etc. The associated features usually make the diagnosis clear.

(*b*) Septic arthritis, which occurs in the course of septicopyemia from any cause, and particularly in puerperal fever. No hard and fast line can be drawn between these and the cases in the first group: but the inflammation often passes on to suppuration and there is more or less destruction of the joints. The conditions under which the arthritis occurs give a clue to the nature of the case. Under this section may be mentioned:

(1) *Acute necrosis or acute osteomyelitis* may be mistaken for rheumatic fever. Sometimes it is multiple. The greater intensity of the local symptoms, the involvement of the epiphyses rather than the joints, and the more serious constitutional disturbances are points to be considered. The condition is unfortunately often mistaken for acute arthritis, and, as the treatment is essentially surgical, the error may cost the life of the patient. Rheumatic fever is extremely rare in very young children.

(2) *The acute arthritis of infants* is usually confined to one joint (the hip or knee), the effusion in which rapidly becomes purulent. The affection is most common in sucklings and undoubtedly pyemic in character. It may also occur with the gonorrheal ophthalmia or vaginitis of the newborn.

(*c*) Gonococcus Arthritis.—This may give difficulty at the onset, but there is not the rapid shifting from joint to joint and there is usually some thickening about the most affected joints in a short time. A careful search for gonococci is important and the complement fixation test may aid.

(*d*) Gout.—While the usual localization in a single joint, the age, the history, and the mode of onset enable us to recognize acute gout, there are everywhere cases of acute arthritis, called rheumatic fever, which are in reality gout. The involvement of several of the larger joints is not infrequent in gout, and unless tophi are present or bursitis occurs, the diagnosis may be difficult. The dusky red color of the skin over the affected joints, severe pain when the joint is at rest, less fever relatively than the intensity of the arthritis and increased uric acid in the blood are helpful points in gout.

(*e*) Acute Arthritis deformans.—This may easily be mistaken for rheumatic fever. It may come on with fever and multiple arthritis, and for weeks there may be no suspicion of the true nature of the disease. Gradually the fever subsides, but the periarticular thickening persists. As a rule, in the acute febrile cases the involvement of the smaller joints, the persistence and the changes in the articulations suggest arthritis deformans.

In *children* the diagnosis of rheumatic fever may be very difficult, as arthritis may be slight or entirely absent. The possibility of rheumatic fever should be considered in all febrile attacks in children for which no definite cause can be found. Special care should be given to the examination of the heart and aorta, particularly for any signs of dilatation or endocarditis.

Prognosis.—The immediate outlook is usually good; death comes usually from extensive cardiac disease. In the acute attack the mortality is about 3 per cent. For the majority the danger lies in the future and is increased by every subsequent attack. Recurrence is the important factor. The great majority of those with marked cardiac damage ultimately die from it.

Treatment.—The main object should be to bring the patient through the attack with an undamaged heart or with as little injury as possible. The first essential is complete rest, which should be begun at once and insisted upon for as long as is necessary. This is especially important for children. The duration of rest has to be decided for each patient. Special thought should be given to the myocardium. Until it is restored to the best possible condition rest is indicated, frequently for months. Convalescence should never be hurried and the safe rule is to increase exertion very slowly—if in doubt, delay. The bed should have a smooth, soft, yet elastic, mattress. The patient should wear a flannel nightgown, which may be opened all the way down the front and slit along the outer margin of the sleeves. Three or four of these should be made, so as to facilitate the frequent changes required after the sweats. He may wear also a light flannel cape about the shoulders. He should sleep in blankets, not in sheets, so as to reduce the chance of being chilled.

Milk is the most suitable diet and may be diluted with alkaline mineral waters. Fruit juices, lemonade and oatmeal or barley water should be freely given. The thirst should be fully satisfied. As convalescence is established a fuller diet may be allowed, but meat should be used sparingly.

Local treatment is usually necessary. It often suffices to wrap the affected joints in cotton. If the pain is severe, hot cloths may be applied, saturated with Fuller's lotion (carbonate of soda, 6 drams, 24 gm.; laudanum, 1 oz., 30 cc.; glycerine, 2 oz., 60 cc.; and water, 9 oz., 270 cc.) or the lead and opium lotion. Oil of wintergreen is useful, the joint being gently rubbed with it or small amounts sprinkled over flannel, which is then applied. Chloroform liniment is also a good application. Fixation of the joints is of great service in allaying the pain. Splints, padded and bandaged with moderate firmness, will often give comfort. Cold compresses are sometimes useful. The application of blisters above and below the joint often relieves the pain but this is not to be compared with the light application of the cautery. If there is much effusion, aspiration of the joint is useful.

Salicylates.—Introduced by Maclagan in 1876 in the form of salicin, the salicylates in some cases may be regarded as having an action which is almost specific. They relieve pain, often seem to shorten the course, and lessen the chances of relapse. Certainly the occurrence of hyperpyrexia and pericarditis seems to have greatly decreased since their use. There is no proof that they influence endocarditis unless by shortening the febrile period its chance of development is lessened. The best preparation is sodium salicylate, usually given with sodium bicarbonate. The drug should be given in amounts of 120 grains (8 gm.) in the twenty-four hours as an average. An excellent plan is to give a large dose (60 to 90 grains, 4 to 6 gm.) by rectum once a day, reducing the dose by mouth if this is done. If administration by mouth causes gastric disturbance, the drug can be given by rectum. In severe cases it is well to give 90 gr. (6 gm.) by rectum at once and an equal amount by mouth in the first twenty-four hours. Children as a rule stand the drug well and depressing effects are rarely seen. The natural has no advantage over the synthetic product. Of other salicylate preparations acetylsalicylic acid may be given, but none is equal to the sodium salt. After the fever has lessened and the pain decreased the dose can be gradually reduced. It is wise not to discontinue the drug until the danger of relapse is over. Small doses may be given for a long period. The giving of salicylate intravenously is not advised. The occasional occurrence of delirium due to salicylate should be remembered.

Alkaline Treatment.—The urine should be rendered alkaline as soon as possible. Potassium acetate and citrate in doses of 15 grains (1 gm.) each are given every three hours until the urine is alkaline and then enough to keep it so. Potassium or sodium bicarbonate may be given with the salicylate.

To allay the *pain* opium may be given in the form of Dover's powder, or morphia hypodermically. The coal tar products are sometimes useful for the purpose. During convalescence iron is indicated in full doses. Of the complications, hyperpyrexia should be treated by the bath or the cold pack. The treatment of endocarditis and pericarditis and the pulmonary complications will be considered under their respective sections. In all the cardiac complications the importance of prolonged rest must be remembered. The value of streptococcus vaccine given intravenously to lessen the chance of further attacks, perhaps by desensitization, is not decided.

Tonsils.—With disease of these and the possibility that they are the portals of entry for the infective agent, the question arises as to their removal. In patients with diseased tonsils in whom rheumatic fever has occurred removal is advisable and should be complete. In patients with endocarditis and fever this can be done without risk in many cases. Sodium salicylate should be given for some days before the operation and afterwards.

ERYTHEMA NODOSUM

This can not be regarded as a specific disease and its exact position in any classification is not settled. There are various views as to its nature: (1) that it is an acute specific fever ("nodal fever") which may occur in epidemics; (2) that it is a manifestation of rheumatic fever; (3) that it is a manifestation of tuberculosis; and (4) that it represents an allergic manifestation which may result from various bacterial allergens, those of the tubercle bacillus and streptococci being the most frequent. There is no doubt that many of the patients develop frank tuberculosis later. It occurs usually below the age of twenty years and much more often in females than in males.

Clinical Features.—The onset may be with malaise, sore throat, more or less general pains and slight fever. The last is rarely high but may persist for some time. The local lesions consist of round or oval areas, slightly raised, dusky red in color, tender and rarely more than two inches in diameter. There may be some edema of the surrounding tissue. They are usually bilateral and occur most often on the legs, especially over the tibia, but may be on the arms or over the scapula. They may come out in crops and the total number is variable. Suppuration may be suspected but does not occur. The duration of each node is about ten days and discoloration is left behind. The attack may last for two or three weeks. The *diagnosis* is not difficult but they have been mistaken for syphilitic nodes. By the laity they may be mistaken for bruises and unjust charges of cruelty have resulted.

Treatment.—The patient should be in bed until the nodes have disappeared. The salicylates sometimes relieve the pain and should be tried. Local sedative applications to the lesions are useful. Careful search should be made for any focus of infection and, in view of the possibility of tuberculosis, for any sign of that disease.

ACUTE TONSILLITIS

Definition.—An acute infection, sporadic or epidemic, involving the structures of the tonsillar ring, usually due to organisms of the streptococcus class.

Etiology.—Acute tonsillitis occurs in sporadic and epidemic forms. The *sporadic* variety occurs in young persons particularly. Infants are rarely attacked. Chronic enlargement of the lymphatic structures of the throat is a predisposing cause. Exposure to cold and wet may predispose to an attack. It is directly communicated from one to another. It may be followed by endocarditis, erythema nodosum, chorea, and acute nephritis. Felty and Hodges, from an extensive study, regard the causal organism as the *Streptococcus haemolyticus* of the beta type. While not absolutely identical in all cases the organisms are intimately related forms of beta-hemolytic streptococci. With this view the disease is regarded as a specific disease rather than as an infection which may be caused by various organisms. In some cases the predominating organism seems to be the pneumococcus. The source of infection is usually a *carrier* of the organism and the conditions of indoor life in cold seasons naturally favor infection.

Epidemic tonsillitis is not infrequent, the cases increasing in the community to epidemic proportions. As a rule it is impossible to trace it to any special cause. There are remarkable localized outbreaks, sometimes in institutions, which have been traced to milk infection. The one in Boston in 1911 was exceptionally severe, involving more than 1,000 persons, and the connection with the milk from one dairy seems to have been proved.

Morbid Anatomy.—The lacunae of the tonsils become filled with exudation products, which form cheesy-looking masses, projecting from the orifices of the crypts. Not infrequently the exudations from contiguous lacunae coalesce. The intervening mucosa is usually swollen, deep red in color, and may present herpetic vesicles, or, in some instances, even membranous exudation, in which case it may be difficult to distinguish from diphtheria. The contents of the crypt are made up of organisms and epithelial débris.

Symptoms.—Chilly feelings, or even a definite chill, and aching pains in the back and limbs may precede the onset. The fever rises rapidly and in a young child may reach 105° F. on the evening of the first day. The patient complains of soreness of the throat and difficulty in swallowing. The appearance is that of acute illness. On examination the tonsils are seen to be swollen and the crypts present the characteristic exudate. The pharynx is usually inflamed and the uvula may be edematous. The tongue is furred, the breath is heavy and foul, and the urine is highly colored and loaded with urates. In children the respirations are usually rapid and the pulse increased in rapidity. Swallowing is painful and the voice often becomes nasal. Slight swelling of the cervical glands is present. There is usually a moderate leukocytosis. About the third to fifth day the temperature falls, often by crisis, and the symptoms lessen rapidly.

In epidemic cases the fever may be very high, the adenitis considerable, and even the deeper tissues may be involved. The complications are very serious: endocarditis, pericarditis, pneumococcic peritonitis, and pneumonia. A peritonsillar abscess may follow or there may be septicemia. In the Boston epidemic the clinical sequence was not unlike that in rheumatic fever—sore throat, adenitis, multiple arthritis, endocarditis, and pneumonia. Febrile albuminuria is common and acute nephritis may follow. A diffuse erythema may simulate scarlet fever. Acute otitis media is a frequent complication in children. Sinus infection may occur. Phlebitis is an occasional complication. Relapses are not uncommon and the tonsils may remain enlarged. Occasionally paralyses follow the streptococcus tonsillitis which are identical with those of diphtheria. In some years *acute pleurisy* is a common complication; it may be fibrinous or serofibrinous. As a rule, its duration is not prolonged and little or no thickening of the pleura results.

In the sporadic and mild epidemic form it is rare to see a fatal case, but in severe outbreaks the mortality from complications may be three or four per cent. There were about 50 deaths in the Boston epidemic.

A *necrotic* form is described, usually in young adults, with fever for some weeks; adenitis and enlargement of the liver and spleen are found. There may be a marked increase in the mononuclear cells. In the tropics a form of acute tonsillitis due to *mycotic* infection is described; monilia, saccharomyces, oïdium, etc., may be responsible. There are creamy white patches on the tonsils which may extend to the soft palate, pharynx and larynx.

Diagnosis.—It may be difficult to distinguish tonsillitis from diphtheria. In the follicular form, the individual yellowish-gray masses, separated by the reddish tonsillar tissue, are very characteristic; whereas in diphtheria the membrane is ashy-gray and uniform, not patchy. A point of the greatest importance in diphtheria is that the membrane is not limited to the tonsils, but creeps up the pillars of the fauces and appears on the uvula. The diphtheritic membrane, when removed, leaves a bleeding, eroded surface; whereas the exudation of lacunar tonsillitis is easily separated, and usually there is no erosion beneath it. In all doubtful cases cultures should be made. The distinction from Vincent's angina rarely gives difficulty; smears should be examined and a culture made.

Treatment.—The patient should be in bed and stay there until the attack is over. The diet should be liquid with soft foods added if desired. Water should be taken in large amounts. The bowels should be moved freely by a calomel and saline purge and kept open by daily doses of saline, if required. Aconite in full doses often acts beneficially in children. The combination of salol and phenacetine (of each, gr. iii-v, 0.2-0.3 gm.) can be given every three hours. Acetylsalicylic acid (gr. v, 0.3 gm.) is often useful in relieving symptoms. Ten grains (0.6 gm.) of Dover's powder or codein (gr. ½, 0.03 gm.) may be given at night. One of the best applications to the throat is a 10 per cent solution of silver nitrate. Gargles should only be used if they do not cause pain. Solutions of iodine, acetylsalicylic acid, phenol (1 per cent), hydrogen peroxide (25 per cent) or an alkaline antiseptic mixture may be employed. The application of sodium bicarbonate directly to the tonsils sometimes gives relief. An ice bag to the neck is usually an advantage. In convalescence abundant nourishment and a tonic, such as the tincture of nux vomica (♏ xv, 1 cc.), are useful. As a rule it is wise to have the tonsils removed after the attack is over; recurrence is probable. With repeated attacks removal is advisable.

ACUTE CATARRHAL FEVER

(*Acute Coryza*)

Definition.—An acute infection of the mucous membrane of the upper air passages associated with the presence of various organisms.

Etiology.—The cause is probably a filterable virus with which other organisms are associated especially streptococci, staphylococci and pneumococci. *Micrococcus catarrhalis* and the influenza bacillus are found in cultures but they may be secondary invaders. In some cases there seems to be a definite susceptibility which in certain cases is associated with chronic sinus infection or chronic tonsillar or nasal infection. A sensitive mucous membrane may be a factor.

Prevailing most extensively in the changeable weather of the spring and early winter, coryza may occur in epidemic form, many cases arising in a community within a few weeks, outbreaks which are very like though less intense than the epidemic influenza. It is often a local outbreak in a house or school. The infection is spread by coughing, sneezing, etc.

Symptoms.—The patient feels indisposed, perhaps chilly, has slight headache, and sneezes frequently. In severe cases there are pains in the back and limbs. There is usually slight fever, the temperature rising to 101° F. The pulse is quick, the skin is dry, and there are all the features of a feverish attack. At first the mucous membrane of the nose is swollen, "stuffed up," and the patient has to breathe through the mouth. A thin, clear, irrigating secretion flows, and makes the edges of the nostrils sore. The mucous membrane of the tear-ducts is swollen, so that the eyes weep and the conjunctivae are injected. The sense of smell and, in part, the sense of taste are lost. With the nasal catarrh there is slight soreness of the throat and stiffness of the neck; the pharynx looks red and swollen, and sometimes the act of swallowing is painful. The larynx also may be involved and the voice becomes husky or is even lost. If the inflammation extends to the Eustachian tubes the hearing may be impaired. In more severe cases the infection extends to the bronchi. Occasionally there is labial or nasal herpes. Usually within thirty-six hours the nasal secretion becomes turbid and more profuse, the swelling of the mucosa subsides, the patient gradually becomes able to breathe through the nostrils, and within four or five days the symptoms disappear, with the exception of the increased discharge from the nose and upper pharynx. There may be infection of the ears or sinuses. When the attacks are frequently repeated the disease may become chronic.

Diagnosis.—This is usually easy, but caution must be exercised lest the initial catarrh of measles or influenza be mistaken for a simple coryza.

Prophylaxis.—Avoidance of contact with infected persons and of places where people are crowded together should be of value. The use of sprays and gargles is not often effectual. Vaccine therapy is of value in some cases, but often fails, especially when stock vaccines are used; autogenous vaccines in patients with repeated attacks are more successful. The removal of foci of infection is important, especially in the tonsils and sinuses.

Treatment.—Many attacks are so mild that the patients are able to be about and attend to their work. If there are fever and constitutional disturbance, the patient should be kept in bed and take a simple fever mixture, and at night a drink of hot lemonade and a full dose of Dover's powder. For the local discomfort ephedrine solution (3 per cent) is useful and sometimes gives immediate relief. Methenamine in full doses or active alkaline treatment by giving sodium bicarbonate may be useful. Ointments containing menthol and camphor may be applied locally. When the secretion is profuse atropine can be given in doses sufficient to lessen this. Acetylsalicylic acid or phenacetine (gr. v, 0.3 gm.) with codein (gr. ¼, 0.015 gm.) is often useful. A combination of codeine and papaverine (of each gr. ¼, 0.015 gm.) every 2 or 3 hours may be helpful. Simple saline or oily sprays if employed should be used very gently.

FEBRICULA—EPHEMERAL FEVER

Definition.—Fever of slight duration, probably depending upon a variety of causes, some autogenous, others extrinsic and bacterial.

A febrile paroxysm lasting for twenty-four hours and disappearing completely is spoken of as ephemeral fever. If it persists for three, four, or more days without local affection it is designated febricula.

The cases may be divided into several groups:

(*a*) Those which represent mild or abortive types of the infectious diseases. It is not very unusual, during an epidemic of typhoid, scarlet fever, or measles, to see patients with some of the prodromal symptoms and slight fever, which persist for two or three days without any distinctive features. Possibly some of the cases are due to mild streptococcus infections.

(*b*) In a larger group of cases the symptoms develop with dyspepsia. In children indigestion and gastro-intestinal catarrh are often accompanied by fever. There may be headache, malaise, fever, vomiting and diarrhea or constipation. Slight fever has been known to follow the eating of decomposing substances; but the gastric juice has remarkable antiseptic properties, and the frequency with which persons take articles which are "high" shows that poisoning is unlikely unless there is existing gastro-intestinal disturbance.

(*c*) Cases which follow exposure to foul odors. The cases described are of two kinds: an acute, severe form with nausea, vomiting, colic, and fever; secondly, a form of low fever with or without chills.

(*d*) Many cases doubtless depend upon slight unrecognized lesions, such as tonsillitis or occasionally an abortive or larval pneumonia. Children are much more frequently affected than adults. The possibility of pyelitis should be kept in mind; in children there may be few urinary symptoms.

The *symptoms* set in, as a rule, abruptly, though in some instances there may have been preliminary *malaise* and indisposition. Headache, loss of appetite, and furred tongue are present. The urine is scanty and high-colored, the fever ranges from 101° to 103°; sometimes in children it rises higher. The cheeks may be flushed and the patient has the outward manifestations of fever. In children there may be bronchial catarrh with slight cough. Herpes on the lips is common. Occasionally in children the cerebral symptoms are marked and there may be irritation, restlessness and nocturnal delirium. The fever terminates abruptly by crisis from the second to the fourth day; in some instances it may continue for a week.

The *diagnosis* generally rests upon the absence of local manifestations, particularly the skin rashes of the eruptive fevers, and the rapid disappearance of the pyrexia. The cases most readily recognized are those with acute gastro-intestinal disturbance. *Pyelitis* should always be kept in mind and its occurrence excluded. Careful search should be made for tonsillitis or sinusitis. Some of the cases may be due to mild attacks of *food poisoning*, in which thorough cultural studies of the stools are important. Mild attacks of *colon bacillus* infection have been suggested in some cases.

The *treatment* is that of mild pyrexia—rest in bed, a laxative, and a fever mixture containing nitrate of potassium and sweet spirit of nitre.

INFECTIOUS JAUNDICE

There are several forms of infectious jaundice which may occur in epidemic form. Outbreaks have occurred in many parts of the world and it was common in the great war. Certain forms may be separated.

(1) *Epidemic Catarrhal Jaundice.*—This seems to be a definite entity, the cause of which is obscure but due to a common source rather than to infection from one to another. There have been many localized epidemics in the United States which have been studied by Blumer. No proved etiological organism has been found. The early features are abdominal discomfort, gastric symptoms, diarrhea, or constipation, fever for two to four days, and malaise. Jaundice appears about the fourth day with pale stools and bile in the urine. The jaundice reaches a maximum in about ten days. There is enlargement of the liver and spleen, with tenderness of the former. Dilatation of the right heart is not uncommon but usually is present for a few days only. The mortality in a large series in soldiers was only 0.4 per cent. In some cases severe toxemia or icterus gravis occurred.

(2) *Spirochaetosis icterohaemorrhagica.*—(See page 275).

(3) *Weil's Disease.*—It is difficult to know where to classify the disease described by Weil in 1886. It is usually regarded as synonymous with spirochetal jaundice. It would be an advantage if the designation "Weil's Disease" was dropped.

(4) A form of *hemorrhagic jaundice* with severe features has been described in some districts on the Mediterranean. The etiology is unknown. There is acute fever with jaundice appearing about the fourth day. The liver is enlarged and hemorrhagic features are marked. The mortality is high, death usually occurring in the second week.

In *treatment,* rest is important with milk diet and large amounts of water, which should be given by bowel or by duodenal tube if there is vomiting. Alkalis should be given freely as potassium citrate and sodium bicarbonate. The bowels should be kept open by salines and enemata. Judging from the excellent results in ordinary catarrhal jaundice Lyon's method of bile duct drainage should be most useful. The duodenum should be irrigated with mild antiseptic solutions.

MILK-SICKNESS

This disease prevails in certain districts of the United States, mostly west of the Alleghany Mountains, and is connected with the affection in cattle known as the *trembles.* It prevailed extensively in the early settlements in certain of the western states and proved very fatal. The general opinion is that it is communicated to man only by eating the flesh or drinking the milk of diseased animals. The butter and cheese are also poisonous. In animals, cattle and young horses and sheep are most susceptible. It is stated that cows giving milk do not themselves show marked symptoms unless driven rapidly, and, according to Graff, the secretion may be infective when the disease is latent. When a cow is very ill, food is refused, the eyes are injected, the animal staggers, the entire muscular system trembles, and death occurs in convulsions, sometimes with great suddenness. Fortunately, the disease has become rare. No definite pathological lesions are known. Jordan and Harris studied a New Mexico epidemic (1908) and found a bacillus (*B. lactimorbi*) with cultures of which the disease may be reproduced in other animals. Another view is that animals fed on white snake-root or the ragless goldenrod may develop "trembles" and that the disease can be contracted by drinking the milk from affected cows. Bulger *et al.* state that experimental animals show ketosis, lipemia and a tendency to hypoglycemia.

In man the *symptoms* are those of a more or less acute intoxication. After a few days of uneasiness and distress the patient is seized with pains in the stomach, nausea and vomiting, fever and intense thirst. There is usually obstinate constipation. The tongue is swollen and tremulous, the breath is extremely foul, and, according to Graff, is as characteristic of the disease as is the odor in smallpox. Cerebral symptoms—restlessness, irritability, coma, and convulsions—are sometimes marked, and a typhoid state may gradually be produced in which the patient dies.

The duration is variable. In the most acute form death occurs within two or three days. It may last for ten days, or even for three or four weeks. Graff states that insanity occurred in one case. The *treatment* is symptomatic, rest, liquid diet, abundance of fluid and carbohydrates, and free elimination.

GLANDULAR FEVER: INFECTIOUS MONONUCLEOSIS

Definition.—An infectious disease, usually in children, characterized by slight redness of the throat, high fever, swelling and tenderness of the lymph nodes of the neck, particularly those behind the sternocleidomastoid muscles. The fever is of short duration but the enlargement of the glands persists for ten days to three weeks. In children acute adenitis of the cervical and other glands with fever had been noted by many observers, but Pfeiffer in 1889 called special attention to it under the name of *Druesenfieber*.

Etiology.—The disease usually occurs sporadically but may be in epidemics. Most commonly in children, adults may be affected. The causative organism is not known. Infection is probably by the respiratory tract and by contact although conveyance from a healthy carrier has occurred. In schools a large proportion of those exposed may be infected. The incubation period is usually about 7 days but may vary from 5 to 12 days.

Symptoms.—The onset is sudden and the first complaint is of pain on moving the head and neck. There may be nausea and vomiting and abdominal pain. The temperature ranges from 101° to 103° F. The tonsils may be a little red and the lymphatic tissues swollen, but the throat symptoms are transient and unimportant. On the second or third day the enlarged glands appear, and during the course they vary greatly in size. They are painful to the touch, but there is rarely any redness or swelling of the skin, though at times there is some puffiness of the subcutaneous tissues of the neck, and there may be difficulty in swallowing. A rash, variable in character, may occur. The liver and spleen are enlarged and tender in many cases. The leukocytes are increased, 15,000 to 20,000, due to an increase (75 to 90 per cent) in mononuclear cells of a lymphoblastic type. The return to normal may take weeks. The enlarged mesenteric glands may be felt. In some instances there has been discomfort in the chest and a paroxysmal cough, indicating involvement of the mediastinal glands. The swelling of the glands persists from two to three weeks. Among the serious features are the termination of the adenitis in suppuration, which seems rare (though Neumann met with it in 13 cases), septicemia and hemorrhagic nephritis. Acute otitis media and retropharyngeal abscess have been reported. There may be an aseptic meningitis with increase of globulin and lymphocytes in the spinal fluid. The outlook is generally favorable.

The disease in *adults* may show different features from those in children as pointed out by Tidy (1931). Three stages are described: invasion, eruption; and glandular enlargement. The onset is acute with headache, malaise, fever (102° to 103°) and occasionally chills. There may be symptoms suggestive of meningitis. In a few days a *rash* appears, a pinkish-brown maculopapular eruption, usually scanty, which fades in a few days. The character of the rash is variable; it has been mistaken for that of measles and typhus fever, and in some cases is like urticaria. Later there is glandular enlargement which may not appear until the third week and is usually less marked than in children. The spleen may be enlarged. The blood may show varying changes and for a time may not show any increase in the mononuclears. The fever gradually lessens. The duration may be several weeks.

Diagnosis.—The situation of the swelling excludes mumps. The similarity to leukemia may require time to make a diagnosis but the severe features of leukemia are lacking. Adenitis secondary to local infection can be excluded by the absence of a local focus and the differential count. The blood findings exclude Hodgkin's disease and are also against acute tuberculous adenitis. Time may be required in addition. The *treatment* is symptomatic.

MILIARY FEVER—SWEATING SICKNESS

The disease is characterized by fever, profuse sweats, and an eruption of miliary vesicles. It prevailed and was very fatal in England in the fifteenth and sixteenth centuries, and was made the subject of an important memoir by Johannes Caius, 1552. Hirsch gives a chronological account of 194 epidemics between 1718 and 1879, many of which were limited to a single village or to a few localities. Occasionally the disease has become widely spread. The most recent epidemics have been in France. They are usually of short duration, lasting only for three or four weeks—sometimes not more than seven or eight days. A large number of persons are attacked in rapid succession. In the mild cases there is only slight fever, with loss of appetite, and erythematous eruption, profuse perspiration, and an outbreak of miliary vesicles. The severe cases present the symptoms of intense infection—delirium, high fever, profound prostration, and hemorrhage. The death rate at the outset of the epidemic is usually high, and, as is so graphically described in the account of some epidemics of the Middle Ages, death may occur in a few hours. The treatment is symptomatic.

FOOT-AND-MOUTH DISEASE—EPIDEMIC STOMATITIS—APHTHOUS FEVER

Foot-and-mouth disease is an acute infectious disorder met with chiefly in cattle, sheep, and pigs, but attacking other domestic animals. It is of extraordinary activity, and spreads rapidly. The nature of the ultramicroscopic virus has not been determined. In cattle, after a period of incubation of three or five days, the animal becomes feverish, the mucous membrane of the mouth swells, and little grayish vesicles develop on the tongue, on the gums, and on the mucous membrane of the lips. They contain at first a clear fluid, which becomes turbid, then they enlarge and become converted into superficial ulcers. There is ptyalism and the animals lose flesh rapidly. In the cow the disease is also seen about the udder, and the milk becomes yellowish-white in color and of a mucoid consistency.

The transmission to man is by no means uncommon by drinking the milk, eating milk products or by contact. The onset is with chilly sensations, general malaise, fever, and discomfort in the mouth. Vesicles appear in the mouth and pharynx, on the lips and occasionally on other parts—such as the fingers and toes. The vesicles rupture and shallow ulcers result which gradually heal. There is considerable discomfort from the mouth condition and sometimes salivation. In some epidemics there has been a hemorrhagic tendency. Severe toxemia is unusual. The ordinary course is from ten days to three weeks. Recovery is the rule but a mortality of 8 per cent occurred in one epidemic. When the disease is prevalent in cattle, all milk should be boiled. Patients should be isolated and the secretions from the mouth destroyed. The *treatment* is symptomatic for the general condition, with potassium permanganate solution as a mouth wash and the application of silver nitrate to the ulcers.

PSITTACOSIS

Definition.—A disease in birds, characterized by loss of appetite, weakness, diarrhea, convulsions, and death; in man characterized by an atypical pneumonia, great weakness and depression, and a profound infection.

Etiology.—The disease occurs especially in parrots and parrakeets. Originating in the tropics, it has been widely distributed and seems to be endemic among birds in some parts of the United States. It is conveyed to humans from infected birds and is highly infectious. A number of laboratory workers have contracted the disease. The causal agent is a filterable virus.

Pathology.—There is a pneumonitis which is primarily focal or lobular but not closely related to the bronchioles. There is a remarkable swelling of the alveolar epithelium with proliferation. There is an extensive exudate which may obstruct the bronchioles and result in collapse. There may be also a bronchopneumonia from secondary infection. The spleen may be enlarged.

Clinical Features.—The onset is sudden after an incubation period of about 10 days. Malaise, headache, perhaps a chill, fever (up to 102° or 103°), dullness and the picture of a general infection are present. The cough varies in severity and sputum is scanty. The lung signs are variable and change from day to day. They vary from those of diffuse bronchitis to consolidation with collapse, the last probably often causing variation. The pulse rate remains relatively low. There is no change in the blood. In fatal cases the signs of toxemia increase. The attack may be over in 2 weeks or prolonged for 3 or 4 weeks. The mortality has varied; sometimes it is 25 to 30 per cent.

Diagnosis.—This is difficult if no suspicion is aroused by an epidemic or by association with sick birds. *Influenza* may cause difficulty. *Typhoid fever* may be suggested and in some cases a positive agglutination test is said to have been given in psittacosis. Negative blood and stool cultures should be helpful.

Prophylaxis.—Careful quarantine of imported birds is essential. The destruction of all parrots might be an advantage for more reasons than because they may have psittacosis. Sick birds should be promptly killed and burned.

Treatment.—This should be symptomatic and as for a general infection. The use of convalescent serum is of doubtful value but, if available, should be tried.

SWINE FEVER

A few cases have been described from accidental inoculation in the preparation of cultures and in making postmortems upon pigs. In the course of from twelve hours to three days there is swelling of the fingers of the affected hand, which have a blue-red color, and small nodules form. In some of the instances the course has been like that of a painful erythema migrans, with swelling of the lymph-glands. A specific serum has been used with success.

EPIDEMIC DIAPHRAGMATIC PLEURODYNIA

Finsen observed in 1856 and 1863 an epidemic disease in Iceland which he reported in 1874 as pleurodynia or muscular rheumatism of the chest. Daae and Homann described cases in Norway. It was termed the "Bamle disease" from the locality of the first cases. Dabney described an outbreak in Virginia in 1888, calling it "devil's grip." Later it was termed *epidemic diaphragmatic spasm.* Epidemics have been described in many countries. Recently the disease has been specially studied in the Danish island of Bornholm and the designation "Bornholm disease" has been applied.

The disease occurs as a rule in epidemic form, usually in the summer and autumn. All ages are attacked but children from 5 to 15 years seem most susceptible. The cause is not known; transmission seems to be by contact. The *onset* is sudden, sometimes with a chill, and there is usually fever. The main symptom is pain in the upper abdominal muscles, sometimes also in the thorax and back. There may be pain on inspiration even with shallow breathing. The painful muscles are tender on pressure and this may persist after the pain has gone. Hiccough may occur. The blood may show leukocytosis with increase in the eosinophiles in convalescence. Headache, sweating and rapid heart action may occur. There are no signs of lung or pleural involvement. The duration of severe pain is usually short, one or two days. Relapses are common and an attack does not give immunity. As *complications,* otitis media, pneumonia and pleurisy, and orchitis have been reported.

The *diagnosis* of acute thoracic or upper abdominal conditions may be suggested but careful study should exclude these. The *prognosis* is good and the *treatment* is symptomatic.

SIX (SEVEN) DAY FEVER

This is a fever like dengue of about a week's duration, probably caused by a spirochete, *Leptospira hebdomadis.* It occurs chiefly in India and Japan. The spirochete is found in the blood from the second to the fourth day and also in the urine, where it may be found for some weeks after the fever has gone. The disease begins suddenly, the temperature shows marked remissions, skin rashes are common, usually a blotchy erythema, sometimes with petechiae. It terminates on the sixth or seventh day by crisis, and when the date of onset is known the defervescence may be predicted within a few hours. The treatment is symptomatic.

LYMPHOGRANULOMA INGUINALE

(*Climatic or Tropical Bubo*)

This is a specific venereal disease with involvement of the inguinal lymph nodes usually followed by suppuration and fistulae. (It is to be distinguished from *granuloma inguinale* which is a disease of the skin and subcutaneous tissues, usually about the genitals). It occurs mostly in Africa and Asia but is extending its occurrence to Europe and North America. It probably is unrecognized not infrequently. The cause is unknown but a virus is suggested. It usually results from intercourse with a colored woman.

Clinical Features.—The incubation period is from 10 to 30 days. The primary lesion, which is usually transitory and easily overlooked, takes various forms: (1) papular; (2) ulcerative (sometimes herpetic); (3) nodular; and (4) urethral with urethritis. The adenitis appears in from 10 days to 6 weeks, usually in about 3 weeks. There is swelling with brawny infiltration, in the majority of cases unilateral. Pain may be absent or severe. The skin over the area becomes dark red; if suppuration occurs without incision, fistulae form with a thin fluid discharge. In women there may be fistulae about the anus with a purulent rectal discharge. The general features include fever, weakness and loss of weight, anemia, and a moderate leukocytosis with an increase in the mononuclear cells. The *course* is from weeks to months; the rectal cases are more prolonged.

Diagnosis.—The various causes for inguinal bubo have to be considered, chancroidal bubo especially. The Frei test uses an emulsion of a suppurating gland or the pus, heated to 60° C. on two days, diluted 1 to 10 with saline solution; 0.1 cc. of this is used for an intradermal test, which if positive shows a papule in 24 hours. (An autogenous vaccine is of no value.) This test may be positive for years.

Treatment.—The patient should be at rest. Antimony and potassium tartrate may be given in doses of 5 to 10 cc. of a 1 per cent solution, intravenously twice a week for 10 to 15 doses. Protein therapy (typhoid vaccine, intravenously every 3 to 5 days, beginning with 50 million bacilli and increasing the dose to 250 million) has been useful especially in chronic cases. X-ray therapy has been employed. The local treatment depends on conditions. Applications may be made to relieve pain. With signs of suppuration, drainage should be done. Some practise excision of the affected nodes and when possible this would seem to be indicated. Iron should be given for anemia.

MISCELLANEOUS INFECTIONS

Phlebotomus Fever.—(*Sandfly Fever; Three-day Fever*). This is due to a filtrable virus conveyed by the sandfly, *Phlebotomus papatassii.* The disease occurs in India, Persia, Mesopotamia, Egypt and southeastern Europe. The onset is sudden and the features are those of an acute febrile illness with fever for two to three days. There is a leukopenia. Bradycardia is common in convalescence. Death is very rare. Influenza and malaria are the diseases most likely to cause difficulty in diagnosis. The treatment is symptomatic.

Verruga peruviana.—This is a febrile disease occurring in parts of the Andes in Peru characterized by tubercles of the skin much like yaws. This is regarded by some as the eruptive stage of oroya fever in those with a strong resistance; others hold that they are distinct diseases. The attacks begin with malaise, fever, marked pains in the joints and muscles, followed by a severe anemia. There is difference of opinion as to the occurrence of rod-shaped bodies (Barton's bodies) in the red cells. The eruption appears as papules or tubercles varying in size from that of a pea to a chestnut. They gradually assume a warty form. The face, neck, and extremities are the common sites but the eruption may be general. The mucous membranes may be involved. Successive crops appear for a time. Ulceration is common; healing occurs gradually leaving a scar. The duration is 2 or 3 months to a year. Death occurs in from 10 to 25 per cent. In the prevention avoidance of infected areas is important. Local treatment is indicated for the lesions.

Oroya Fever.—This occurs in Peru, is possibly transmitted by an insect, and presents fever, marked anemia and adenitis with a high mortality. The causal organism is *Bartonella bacilliformis.* The disease shows irregular fever, severe pains and adenitis. There is extreme anemia of the pernicious type with the red cells reduced to a million and a considerable leukocytosis. The mortality is 25 to 40 per cent. There is no specific treatment.

Tsutsugamushi Fever (Japanese River Fever).—This is an acute disease occurring in Japan transmitted by the bite of a trombidium (mite). The organism is one of the Rickettsia group. At the site of the bite a small area of necrosis results. The regional lymph nodes enlarge, fever follows with the general symptoms of an acute infection. About a week after the onset a rash appears on the face and spreads to the trunk and limbs. It is macular and papular, becoming hemorrhagic. The fever lasts two to three weeks. The mortality is given as 20 to 50 per cent. Treatment is symptomatic.

Gangosa.—This is characterized by an ulcerative process which involves the pharynx, larynx, mouth and nose. It occurs in the West Indies and some of the Pacific islands. There is doubt as to the nature of the disease; some regard it as akin to yaws, others to dermal Leishmaniasis. The process begins usually in the palate and gradually spreads with ulceration until the mouth, nose, palate and sometimes the larynx and eyes are destroyed. Leprosy, syphilis, yaws and Leishmaniasis have to be considered. The process may stop or go on until death from sepsis and exhaustion. Arsphenamine and antimony should be used, with local treatment of the ulceration.

Exanthema Subitum.—This has an acute onset. There is high fever for three to five days. As the temperature falls a morbilliform rash appears mostly on the trunk and little on the mucous membranes. It lasts about four days. There is leukopenia with 80-85 per cent of lymphocytes. The course is mild with no complications or sequels described.

SECTION II

DISEASES DUE TO PHYSICAL AGENTS

SUNSTROKE; HEAT EXHAUSTION

(Insolation, Thermic Fever, Siriasis)

Definition.—Under these terms are comprised certain manifestations following exposure to excessive heat, of which thermic fever or sunstroke, heat exhaustion, and heat cramps are the common forms.

History.—It is one of the oldest of recognized diseases. The case of the son of the Shunammite woman (2 Kings, IV) is perhaps the oldest on record. The Arabians called the symptoms due to excessive heat "Siriasis," after Sirius, the Dog Star. Cardan recognized it in the sixteenth century and thought it was apoplexy due to heat—morbus attonitus. In the eighteenth century Boerhaave regarded it as phrenitis. It was not until the nineteenth century that the Anglo-Indian surgeons and the physicians of the United States gave us a full knowledge of the different affections due to excessive heat. Various classifications have been suggested, but two chief forms are everywhere recognized—heat exhaustion and thermic fever or sunstroke—to which Edsall added the remarkable heat cramps which occur in persons working under very high external temperatures.

Distribution.—Sunstroke occurs in the tropics and in temperate regions during protracted heat waves. High humidity and exertion are predisposing causes. Heat exhaustion is frequently met with in conditions similar to those in which sunstroke takes place, and it is not infrequent in the engine rooms of steamships, less often in foundries. In the U. S. Navy in 35 years (to 1913) there were 20 deaths and 33 invalided on account of heat prostration (Fiske).

Heat Exhaustion.—In the tropics and in temperate regions during protracted heat waves many persons become depressed physically and are unable to work or take nourishment. In children the condition is very often associated with gastro-intestinal disturbances and fever. The true heat syncope is specially seen in persons who have not been in good health or who are intemperate. The heat may be that of the sun or artificial heat. The symptoms begin with giddiness, nausea, an uncertain, staggering gait; there is pallor, the pulse is small, the heart's action weak, the respirations rapid, and the patient may quickly become unconscious. Muscular spasms, often painful, are common. Externally the body may be clammy, with sweat, but as a rule the rectal temperature is decreased. In the axilla it may be as low as 95° or 96° F. From slight attacks, the patients recover rapidly when brought into a cooler atmosphere; in other cases the unconsciousness may end in deep coma and death.

Sunstroke.—This is more common in men than in women and children, and is principally seen in persons exposed to the sun, who are too heavily clad, or who are addicted to alcohol. High humidity favors its occurrence. It is more common in Europeans than in the dark races, but in the United States negroes are often attacked. Some regard a decrease in the alkaline reserve with high lactic acid content of the blood and acidosis as important.

MORBID ANATOMY.—Rigor mortis occurs early and putrefactive changes may come on rapidly. The venous engorgement is extreme, particularly in the cerebrum. The left ventricle is contracted and the right chamber dilated. The blood is usually fluid; the lungs are intensely congested. Parenchymatous changes occur in the liver and kidneys. There may be punctate hemorrhages in the nervous system and changes in the nerve cells.

SYMPTOMS.—The patient may be struck down and die within an hour, with symptoms of circulatory failure, dyspnea, and coma. This form, sometimes known as the asphyxial, occurs chiefly in soldiers. Death may be almost instantaneous, the victims falling as if struck upon the head. The more usual form comes on during exposure, with pain in the head, dizziness, a feeling of oppression, absence of sweating, and sometimes nausea and vomiting. Visual disturbances are common and a patient may have colored vision. Diarrhea or frequent micturition may supervene. Insensibility follows, which may be transient or deepen into profound coma. The patients are usually admitted to hospital in an unconscious state, with the face flushed, the skin hot, the pulse rapid and full, and the temperature from 107° to 110° F., or even higher. The breathing is labored and deep, sometimes stertorous. Usually there is complete relaxation of the muscles, but twitchings, jactitation, or very rarely convulsions may occur. The pupils may at first be dilated, but by the time the patients are admitted to hospital they are (in a majority) contracted. Petechiae may be present upon the skin. In the fatal cases the coma deepens, the pulse becomes more rapid and feeble, the breathing hurried and shallow and of the Cheyne-Stokes type. The fatal termination may occur within twenty-four or thirty-six hours. Favorable indications are the return of consciousness and a fall in the fever. The recovery in these cases may be complete. In other instances there are remarkable after-effects, the most constant of which is a permanent inability to bear high temperatures. Such patients become very uneasy when the thermometer reaches 80° F. in the shade. Loss of the power of mental concentration and failure of memory are troublesome sequelae. Such patients are always worse in the hot weather. Occasionally there are convulsions, followed by marked mental disturbance. Dercum described peripheral neuritis as a sequence.

Many observers have called attention to a fever in the tropics which lasts for a few days, with no special symptoms other than those of pyrexia and weakness and which may be heat exhaustion.

DIAGNOSIS.—It is rarely difficult to distinguish thermic fever from the malignant types of malaria and other forms of coma. The diagnosis of heat exhaustion from sunstroke is readily made. In the one the skin is moist, pale and cool, the pulse small and soft, and consciousness may remain till near the end; in the other there is high fever with early unconsciousness.

PROGNOSIS.—In the old, the infirm, and alcoholic subjects the mortality from sunstroke during a hot wave may be as high as 30 or 40 per cent.

TREATMENT.—In heat exhaustion stimulants (ammonia, epinephrine and caffeine) should be given freely, and if the temperature is below normal the hot bath should be used. In *sunstroke* the indications are to reduce the temperature as rapidly as possible. Rubbing the body with ice is an excellent procedure to lower the temperature rapidly. The wet pack with an electric fan blowing on the patient or the bath may be used until the rectal temperature falls to 103°. Iced-water enemata may also be employed. Alkaline solutions should be given by bowel or intravenously. In the cases with intense asphyxia, and in which death may take place in a few minutes, free bleeding should be practised, a procedure which saved Weir Mitchell when a young man. For

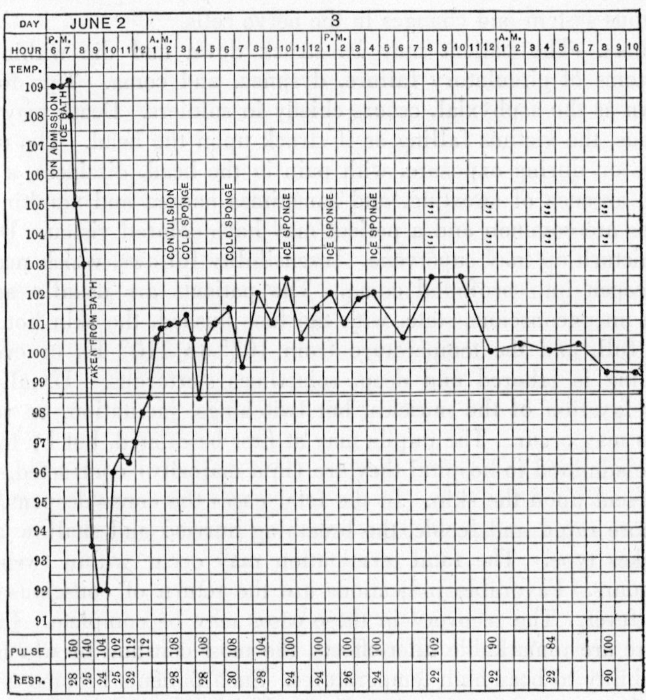

CHART XIV.—CASE OF SUNSTROKE TREATED BY THE ICE-BATH; RECOVERY.

the convulsions, chloroform should be given at once. Antipyretics should not be employed. Lumbar puncture is useful.

Heat Cramps.—Persons doing heavy muscular work while exposed to a very high temperature are liable to attacks of severe cramp. The condition, which was described by Edsall, occurs principally in stokers in the furnace rooms of steamships and in workers in iron foundries. The spasms occur chiefly in the muscles of the calves, the arms, and sometimes in the abdomen; they are often of great intensity and very painful. A movement, pressure, or any stimulus, as electricity, may send the muscle into spasm at once. In addition to ordinary cramps there are sometimes fibrillary contractions. The attacks may last for from 12 to 34 hours and are followed by muscular soreness and sometimes by great weakness. Warm baths with massage and morphia hypodermically give relief. Dehydration and loss of sodium chloride are important factors so that physiological salt solution should be given intravenously and subcutaneously. Milk should be given freely. In prevention the taking of sodium chloride and water freely should be helpful.

CAISSON DISEASE

(Compressed Air Disease; Diver's Paralysis)

Definition.—A disease of caisson workers and divers, due to a saturation of the tissues with nitrogen under the increased pressure. If decompression takes place quickly, a too-rapid escape of bubbles of nitrogen occurs into the tissues and into the blood causing air embolism.

Etiology.—The cases are met with chiefly in workers in caissons and tunnels and in divers. Fat subjects are specially susceptible. "The higher the pressure and the shorter the period of decompression the greater is the risk" (Hill). In caissons the pressure is rarely 30 to 35 pounds, but in the St. Louis bridge the pressure reached as high as 45 to 50 pounds. Divers go down to 20 fathoms with a pressure of 53 pounds; U. S. Navy divers did useful work at 275 feet (Honolulu). The disease may occur in very deep mines. In building the St. Louis bridge across the Mississippi, among 352 workers there were 50 cases of paralysis and 14 deaths. In constructing the East River tunnels in New York, among 10,000 men employed there were 3,692 cases and 20 deaths resulted.

Pathology.—To Hoppe-Seyler, Bucquoy, and Paul Bert we owe a rational explanation of the disease. During compression the blood passing through the lungs becomes saturated with nitrogen, which is carried to the tissues until the whole body is saturated. "The mass of blood is about 5 per cent of the body, and the capacity of the tissues to dissolve N is estimated by Boycott as 35 times that of the blood—in a fat man considerably more" (Hill). With active work it does not take long to effect complete saturation. During decompression the process is just the reverse. "The blood gives up N to the alveolar air and returns to the tissues for more. Those organs in which the circulation is rapid will yield up their N quickly, and those with a sluggish circulation slowly . . . and at the end of decompression a condition may be set up in which the slow tissues still hold, say 3 per cent of N, while the blood can dissolve only 1 per cent. Herein we have a danger of bubbles forming" (Hill). The nitrogen in the body fluids begins to dissolve out as soon as the pressure is lowered. This is only harmful if the nitrogen separates in the form of bubbles. These form first in the venous blood and fatty tissues, in the synovial fluid of the joints and in the nervous system. As a rule a rapid reduction in pressure must occur before bubbles form. The spinal cord may contain many air emboli, usually more numerous in the white matter. This was the lesion determined by Leyden, who found fissuring and laceration of the cord, which explains the paraplegia. Pulmonary air embolism also occurs. In an analysis of gas from the right heart, Erdman found 80 per cent of N and 20 per cent of CO_2.

Symptoms.—In slight cases within from half an hour to two hours after leaving the caisson, the patient has headache, giddiness and feels faint, symptoms which may pass off and leave no further trouble. In other instances the patients have severe pains in the extremities, usually the legs and the abdomen, sometimes associated with nausea and vomiting—attacks which the workmen usually speak of as "the bends." The pains may be of the greatest intensity and associated with giddiness and vomiting. Paralysis, usually of the legs, comes on rapidly, and varies in degree from weakness to complete loss both of motion and sensation. This occurred in 15 per cent of A. H. Smith's cases and in 61 per cent of the St. Louis cases. Monoplegia and hemiplegia are rare. In extreme instances the attacks resemble apoplexy; the patient rapidly becomes comatose and death occurs in a few hours. The paraplegia may be permanent, but in slight cases it gradually disappears and recovery may be complete. Late resulting features are spinal cord changes, chronic arthritis and deafness.

Prophylaxis.—The only safeguard is properly conducted decompression, which obviates the risk of rapidly setting free the nitrogen from the tissues. Haldane and his colleagues introduced the "Stage Method," which is now widely adopted with the most beneficial results. For work in very high pressures the shifts should be short, not more than two hours.

Treatment.—The caisson workers found very early that the best remedy was immediate recompression, and A. H. Smith of New York introduced a medical air-lock for the Brooklyn bridge workers. The workers should live and sleep not far from the works, where such an air-lock is available for immediate treatment. Patients with severe symptoms may be saved by recompression. Hot fomentations, massage and hypodermics of morphia may be necessary for the extreme pains.

MOUNTAIN OR ALTITUDE SICKNESS: ANOXEMIA

Definition.—An illness associated with exposure to low atmospheric pressures and due to lack of oxygen, characterized by cyanosis, nausea, headache, intestinal disturbances, hyperpnea and sometimes syncope.

Etiology.—The symptoms are due to want of oxygen produced by the diminished pressure of the atmosphere. Haldane, Douglas and Henderson made an exhaustive study of the process of accommodation in a five weeks' residence at the top of Pike's Peak. After acclimatization the symptoms disappeared, but dyspnea, blueness and periodic breathing are apt to follow exertion. The alveolar carbon dioxide pressure was reduced from about 40 mm. to about 27 mm. during rest, which corresponded to an increase of about 50 per cent in the ventilation of the lung alveoli. This process of accommodation is associated with a marked increase in the red blood cells and hemoglobin to 120 to 150 per cent. These authors conclude that acclimatization is largely due to increased secretory activity of the alveolar epithelium, to greater lung ventilation and to increased hemoglobin.

The disturbance known as "Aviators' Sickness" also involves the problem of a low barometric pressure. The pressure of the oxygen in the arterial blood in high altitudes may be higher than in the alveolar air. Active secretion of oxygen occurs in the lungs; that is, the passage of oxygen is accelerated and this apparently has a selective action. There is a tendency to bradycardia in aviators after a sudden descent, probably part of a vagobulbar syndrome.

Symptoms.—These usually begin at altitudes of 12,000-15,000 feet. Dyspnea is usually the first symptom, made markedly worse by exertion and accompanied by cyanosis. Headache, nausea, vomiting, hyperpnea, epistaxis and frequent micturition follow with marked muscular weakness, so that even slight exertion is difficult. The muscular weakness has been particularly marked in mountain climbing at high altitudes. Of special interest are the *mental changes,* which are common in aviation, especially when a high altitude is reached quickly. There is mental inaccuracy with lethargy and disturbance of the psychical functions, especially judgment and memory. Syncope may result. Ringing in the ears followed by deafness is common. Death has occurred in balloon ascents.

Treatment.—The condition may be prevented by the use of apparatus to supply a proper amount of oxygen. If symptoms have appeared the patient should be kept as quiet as possible, given oxygen if available, and brought down to a lower altitude.

GAS POISONING

Carbon Monoxide.—*Acute* poisoning is comparatively frequent and due especially to illuminating gas, with many cases caused by the exhaust from motor cars in closed or poorly ventilated places. It is a common method of suicide. The so-called "water gas" contains much more carbon monoxide than that manufactured by dry distillation. There is difference of opinion as to whether the only effect of carbon monoxide is through its combination with hemoglobin and the resulting lack of oxygen or whether in addition it has a toxic effect apart from anoxemia. Damage to the brain cells results fairly quickly—within a few hours—and hence continued coma is probably due to edema of the brain and degenerative processes rather than to lack of oxygen, as the greater part of the carbon monoxide is given off in four or five hours. The frequency of *chronic* poisoning is difficult to state. In occupations about furnaces in many trades, in mining (carbon monoxide is derived from the explosive) and in garages there are possibilities of poisoning.

The main *symptoms* are a general feeling of illness, headache, vertigo, nausea and vomiting, and marked muscular weakness. If the dose is large the subject becomes drowsy and then unconscious. Muscular twitchings and convulsions often occur. At this stage the respiration is usually rapid; the pulse is rapid and usually weak. Cyanosis is marked, accompanied by a peculiar redness of the skin. The blood has a bright red color. Pulmonary complications are important, particularly pneumonia (less frequent if the carbon dioxide-oxygen treatment is used) and they may appear some time after the poisoning. Recovery may result after coma has lasted for many hours but its duration for twenty-four hours is usually fatal. A great variety of nervous sequels have resulted, neuritis, tremor, paralyses, psychoses, visual disturbances, etc. In *chronic* poisoning, headache, vertigo, nausea, weakness and sometimes mental disturbance are common.

The *diagnosis* is rarely in doubt in the acute cases. The odor of the breath may be characteristic and the spectroscopic test is positive. In chronic cases the estimation of the amount of carbon monoxide in the blood may be necessary.

Treatment.—The patient should be removed from the poisoned air at once and then the essential need is vigorous breathing "to draw oxygen in and wash the carbon monoxide out." Oxygen inhalation is required. Venesection and transfusion are not helpful and may be harmful. Artificial respiration is useful in starting breathing if this has stopped. Henderson and Haggard showed that the best stimulus for deep breathing is to supply enough carbon dioxide (5 per cent) with oxygen for this purpose. The special apparatus should be kept ready for use by the emergency crews of gas companies and in large hospitals. The mask may be held over the face while artificial respiration is carried on if the breathing is feeble. The results have been very satisfactory. If the apparatus is not available, the best method is to introduce oxygen into the pharynx by a small tube passed through the mouth or nose, using artificial respiration if the breathing is feeble. The less one does in addition the better. The use of apparatus to aid respiration is advised against. If coma continues, lumbar puncture is useful.

Carbon Bisulphide.—This is used to treat rubber and poisoning may occur. Headache, vertigo, insomnia and depression are common. Subsequently areas of anesthesia and paresthesias of various kinds may be found. Vision and taste may both show changes. A great variety of symptoms from disturbance of the nervous system results and organic nervous diseases may be closely simulated. The diagnosis may be made on a history of exposure, peripheral neuritis, hysterical and psychic symptoms. Poisoning by various ingredients in rubber solvent solutions may make the picture extremely complex. Prophylactic measures are usually successful and the treatment is symptomatic.

Benzene (Benzol) Poisoning.—Benzene is used extensively in trades for its solvent qualities, especially in rubber manufacture, in dry cleaning and in quick drying paints. (*Benzine* is a petroleum distillate and much less toxic than benzene.) A commonly used material called "solvent naphtha" is a combination of crude benzene, toluene and xylene. *Acute* poisoning from benzene usually occurs in the refining works, death resulting rapidly. *Chronic* poisoning results from continued exposure with absorption by the skin or respiratory tract. The symptoms are headache, general malaise, nausea, vomiting, and abdominal pain. Hemorrhages may occur from the nose, mouth, stomach and uterus. Extreme *anemia* develops in which the red cells may fall to a million or less with marked leukopenia. The platelets are greatly reduced. Aplastic anemia may follow. The outlook in the severe cases is grave. *Prophylaxis* consists in preventing the possibility of absorbing the material but this is difficult and small amounts may cause poisoning. Those exposed to benzene should have periodical blood examinations so that anemia or leukopenia may give warning of danger. In the chronic cases with anemia the usual treatment and blood transfusion are indicated.

Gas-poisoning in War.—Our interest is now concerned with the after-effects in those who were gassed. Several possibilities exist. (1) The psychical result is a factor in some cases. (2) Actual damage to the respiratory tract. Some show this but the exact effects are sometimes difficult to estimate; chronic bronchitis, emphysema and fibroid changes are the most important. (3) Changes in the respiratory exchange which may be permanent. (4) There is no evidence of any increased liability to tuberculosis.

CAR SICKNESS AND SEASICKNESS

These are not diseases but combinations of symptoms which have much in common. The causes are various and in different individuals the factors are not necessarily the same. The disturbance due to the movements and the difficulty of adjustment to them are important factors, in which the eyes, the labyrinths and the general sensorium are concerned. The disturbance of orientation is important, but other factors, such as unpleasant odors or poor ventilation, play a part. A psychical factor operates in some patients, as when seasickness occurs before the vessel has sailed or from the sight or hearing of others who are ill. Some persons suffer when riding in a closed motor car for more than a short time but not in an open car. In many cases the absence of fresh air is certainly a factor. The necessity of exertion has sometimes a marked effect in prevention. Constipation is apparently a factor in many people. The subjects of migraine are prone to all these forms of disturbance. The individual reaction varies greatly; some are never ill on a large steamer but suffer in a sail boat or launch if there is much motion, and *vice versa*. Many succumb on a voyage only if rough weather comes on early in the trip; after a couple of days with ordinary weather they have their "sea legs" and are immune.

Symptoms.—These are divided into those affecting particularly the nervous system and the digestive tract. One or other may predominate but both usually occur. There is generally some disturbance of the nervous system. In train and motor car sickness there are usually distress, headache, nausea and often vomiting. In some persons the passing of a long train of cars on another track is apt to cause symptoms, pointing to ocular disturbance as responsible. In train sickness there may be persistent retching and vomiting, sometimes followed by marked prostration. In seasickness there is general discomfort, perhaps with headache, salivation and nausea, soon followed by retching and vomiting. Usually there is constipation but occasionally there may be frequent stools, at first fecal and later composed largely of mucus. The vomiting may be continuous and, as the contents of the stomach are soon disposed of, the vomitus consists of mucus, bile and watery fluid. Anorexia is common and there is marked pallor. Headache, vertigo and marked depression may occur. In extreme cases, as in rough Channel crossing, there may be severe collapse. After some days the loss of fluids is marked; there is obstinate constipation and scanty urine, and acidosis may result. The exhaustion and prostration may be marked. The duration is rarely more than a few days, unless rough weather continues, and recovery is rapid. Some suffer for the whole voyage but death probably never results.

Prevention.—For those who are subject to train sickness the diet should be very simple for a day before the journey and the bowels should be freely opened. The use of bromide (gr. xv. 1 gm.) three times a day for two days before the journey is often effectual. If the journey is a long one the bromide should be taken during it. The securing of good ventilation is important. To lessen the chance of seasickness, the diet should be very simple for several days before sailing and the bowels freely opened. As constipation is common it is well to take laxatives and drink freely of water. Many drugs are employed. Of these the bromides are useful, taken for two or three days before and during the first half of the voyage. Chloretone (gr. v to x, 0.3 to 0.6 gm.) is useful, taken in the same way. On the ship some are better to stay in the berth if the weather is rough; others do better on deck. There is no rule. A hot drink before getting up in the morning is useful.

Treatment.—With sea sickness the patient is better in bed and kept warm. Bromide or chloretone may be taken if vomiting does not prevent. Atropine in full dosage is sometimes useful. The bowels should be kept open if possible, for which salines are usually best. Care should be taken to give very simple food after the vomiting ceases but sometimes most unusual food is desired. The taking of alkaline fluid freely is important. In very severe cases the giving of morphine and atropine hypodermically is useful. Alcohol is regarded by many as helpful but for the majority it is not of value. Recovery is usually aided by the patient being on deck after the acute features are over. In severe cases with acidosis, the administration of fluids and dextrose solution (intravenously or by bowel) is useful.

POISONING FROM RADIOACTIVE SUBSTANCES

There is great danger in handling radioactive substances (mesothorium and radium) and in those exposed to the rays from these substances, there are deposits of radioactive substances in the bones which are fixed and give off emanations, 95 per cent of which are alpha rays. These injure the adjoining bone marrow with the production of a severe anemia and occasionally leukemia. The anemia is often clinically of the aplastic form but may be more like ordinary pernicious anemia. There is a marked leukopenia. Necrosis of bones often results, especially in the jaw, and is probably a radiation osteitis with secondary infection. Osteosarcoma occurs in some cases. The *diagnosis* is made by finding emanations in the expired air or from the body by means of the gamma electroscope. After death the diagnosis is made by special photographic methods from the bones or the bone ash. In the organs the radioactivity can be demonstrated by the alpha electroscope. The *prognosis* is very grave but better in the mesothorium than in the radium cases. The *treatment* is symptomatic, every care being taken to keep the mouth clean and prevent sepsis. The usual treatment for anemia is given. The prevention depends on the kind of exposure. In industrial poisoning the habit of moistening a brush, used in painting luminous dials, in the mouth has been responsible for a number of cases.

SECTION III

THE INTOXICATIONS

ALCOHOLISM

Acute Alcoholism.—When a large quantity of alcohol is taken, the influence is chiefly on the nervous system, and is manifested in muscular incoordination, mental disturbance, and, finally, narcosis. The individual presents a flushed, sometimes slightly cyanosed face, the pulse is full, respirations deep but rarely stertorous. The pupils are dilated. The temperature is frequently subnormal, particularly if the patient has been exposed to cold. Perhaps the lowest reported temperatures have been in cases of this sort. In one instance the patient on admission to hospital had a temperature of 24° C. (ca. 75° F.), and ten hours later the temperature had not risen to 91° F. The unconsciousness is rarely so deep that the patient can not be roused to some extent and in reply to questions he mutters incoherently. Muscular twitchings may occur, but rarely convulsions. The breath has a heavy alcoholic odor. The respirations may be slow, as low as six in the minute.

The *diagnosis* is not difficult, yet mistakes are frequently made. Persons are brought to a hospital by the police supposed to be drunk when in reality they are dying from apoplexy or uremia. Too great care can not be exercised, and the patient should receive the benefit of the doubt. In some instances the mistake arises from the fact that a person who has been drinking has been stricken with apoplexy or fractured the skull. In apoplexy the coma is usually deeper, stertor is present, and there may be evidence of hemiplegia in the greater flaccidity of the limbs on one side. The diagnosis is considered in the section on uremia. The amount of alcohol in the blood may be estimated.

Dipsomania is a form of acute alcoholism seen in persons with a strong hereditary tendency to drink. Periodically the victims go "on a spree," but in the intervals they are entirely free from any craving for alcohol.

Chronic Alcoholism.—The harmful effects of alcohol are manifested (1) as a functional poison, as in acute narcosis; (2) as a tissue poison, in which its effects are seen on the parenchymatous elements, producing a slow degeneration; (3) in the formation of a habit with disastrous results on the moral character; and (4) as a checker of tissue oxidation. This leads to fatty changes and sometimes to a condition of general steatosis. Acidosis may occur. The chief effects may be thus summarized:

Nervous System.—Functional disturbance is common. Unsteadiness of the muscles in performing any action is a constant feature. The tremor is best seen in the hands and in the tongue. The mental processes may be dull, particularly in the early morning and the patient is unable to transact any business until he has had his accustomed drink. Irritability of temper, forgetfulness and a change in the moral character gradually come on. The judgment is seriously impaired, the will enfeebled, and in the final stages dementia may supervene. An interesting combination of symptoms in chronic alcoholics is characterized by peripheral neuritis, loss of memory, and pseudoreminiscences—that is, false notions as to the patient's position in time and space, and fabulous explanations of real occurrences. The peripheral neuritis is not always present; there may be only tremor and jactitation of the lips, and thickness of the speech, with visual hallucinations. Korsakoff designated it as a *psychosis polyneuritica*, and the symptom complex is sometimes called by his name. The relation of chronic alcoholism to insanity has been much discussed. It is one of the important elements in the strain which leads to mental breakdown. Epileptiform attacks may result directly from chronic drinking. It is a hopeful form, and may disappear entirely with a return to habits of temperance.

There is a remarkable condition in chronic alcoholism termed "*wet brain*," in which a heavy drinker, who may perhaps have had attacks of delirium tremens, is drowsy or a little more befuddled than usual; gradually the stupor deepens until he becomes comatose, in which state he may remain for weeks. There may be slight fever, but there are no signs of paralysis and no optic neuritis. The urine may be normal. The lumbar puncture yields a clear fluid but under high pressure. In one patient who died at the end of six weeks, there were the anatomical features of a serous meningitis.

No characteristic changes are found in the nervous system. Hemorrhagic pachymeningitis is not very uncommon. There are opacity and thickening of the pia-arachnoid membranes, with more or less wasting of the convolutions. These are in no way peculiar to chronic alcoholism, but are found in old persons and in chronic wasting diseases. In the very protracted cases there may be chronic encephalomeningitis with adhesions of the membranes. Finer changes in the nerve cells, their processes, and the neuroglia have been described. The alcoholic neuritis will be considered later.

Digestive System.—Catarrh of the stomach is common. The toper has a furred tongue, heavy breath, and in the morning a sensation of sinking until he has had his dram. The appetite is usually impaired and the bowels constipated. In beer-drinkers dilatation of the stomach is common.

Alcohol produces changes in the liver, favoring the production of cirrhosis. The effect is a primary degenerative change in the liver cells. A special vulnerability of the liver cells may be necessary in the etiology of alcoholic cirrhosis. There are cases in which comparatively moderate drinking for a few years has been followed by cirrhosis; on the other hand, the livers of persons who have been steady drinkers for thirty or forty years may show only a moderate grade of sclerosis. For years, heavy drinkers may have an enlarged and tender liver, with at times swelling of the spleen. With the gastric and hepatic disorders the facies often becomes very characteristic. The venules of the cheeks and nose are dilated; the latter becomes enlarged, red, and may present the condition known as *acne rosacea*. The eyes are watery, and conjunctivae hyperemic and sometimes bile-tinged.

The *heart* and *arteries* in chronic topers show degenerative changes, and alcoholism is a factor in causing myocardial degeneration. Steel pointed out the frequency of cardiac dilatation in these cases.

Kidneys.—The influence of chronic alcoholism upon these organs is by no means so marked. The occurrence of renal disease does not seem to be greater in the drinking class. Formad pointed out that in a large proportion of chronic alcoholics the kidneys are increased in size. The Guy's Hospital statistics support this, and Pitt noted that in 43 per cent of the bodies of hard drinkers the kidneys were hypertrophied without showing morbid change. A granular kidney may result through vascular changes.

It was formerly thought that alcohol was in some way antagonistic to tuberculous disease, but the reverse is the case and chronic drinkers are more liable to both acute and pulmonary tuberculosis. It is probably a question of altered tissue-soil, the alcohol lowering the vitality and enabling the bacilli to develop and grow more readily.

Delirium tremens, an incident in chronic alcoholism, results from the long-continued action of the poison. The condition was first accurately described early in the 19th century by Sutton, of Greenwich, who had numerous opportunities for studying it among sailors. A spree in a temperate person, no matter how prolonged, is rarely if ever followed by delirium tremens; but in a habitual drinker a temporary excess may bring on an attack or it follows the sudden withdrawal of alcohol. An accident, a sudden shock or an acute inflammation, particularly pneumonia, may determine the onset. It is especially apt to occur in drinkers admitted to hospitals for injuries, especially fractures, and, as this seems most likely to occur when alcohol is withdrawn, it is well to give such patients a moderate amount. At the outset of the attack the patient is restless and depressed and sleeps badly; after a day or two the characteristic *delirium* sets in. The patient talks constantly and incoherently; he is incessantly in motion, and desires to go out and attend to some imaginary business. Hallucinations of sight and hearing develop. He sees objects in the room, such as rats or mice, and fancies that they are crawling over him. The terror inspired by these imaginary objects is great and the patients need to be watched constantly, for in their delusions they may jump out of the window or escape. Auditory hallucinations are not so common, but the patient may complain of hearing animals or the threats of imaginary enemies. There is much muscular tremor; the tongue is covered with a thick white fur and is tremulous. The pulse is soft, rapid and readily compressed. There is usually fever but the temperature rarely registers above 102° or 103°. In fatal cases it may be higher. *Insomnia* is a constant feature. On the third or fourth day in favorable cases the restlessness abates, the patient sleeps, and improvement gradually sets in. The tremor persists for some days, the hallucinations gradually disappear and the appetite returns. In more serious cases the insomnia persists, the delirium is incessant, the pulse becomes more frequent and feeble, the tongue dry, the prostration extreme, and death results.

Some regard *mania à potu* as a distinct form in which the onset is sudden and the patients are very violent, but hallucinations and terror are rare.

There is a condition termed *acute hallucinosis,* in which auditory hallucinations are marked, orientation is retained, and the mental disturbances are fixed. Ideas of persecution are common. There are intermediate forms between this and the ordinary delirium tremens.

Diagnosis.—The clinical picture can scarcely be confounded with any other. Cases with fever may be mistaken for meningitis. The most common error is to overlook some local disease, such as pneumonia, or an injury, as a fractured rib, which in a chronic drinker may precipitate an attack of delirium tremens. In every instance a careful examination should be made, particularly of the lungs. It is to be remembered that in the severer forms, particularly the febrile cases, congestion of the bases of the lungs is by no means uncommon. Another point is that pneumonia of the apex may be accompanied by similar delirium.

Prognosis.—Recovery takes place in a large proportion of the cases in private practice. In hospital practice, particularly in large city hospitals to which debilitated patients are taken, the death-rate is higher. Recurrence is frequent, indeed, the rule, if the drinking is kept up.

Treatment.—*Acute* alcoholism rarely requires any special measures, as the patient sleeps off the effects of the debauch. In the case of profound alcoholic coma it is advisable to wash out the stomach, and if collapse symptoms occur the limbs should be rubbed, hot applications made to the body and stimulation given by ammonia and epinephrine. Should convulsions supervene, chloroform may be carefully administered. In the acute, violent alcoholic mania the hypodermic injection of apomorphia, one-eighth of a grain (0.008 gm.), is usually very effectual, causing nausea and vomiting, and rapid disappearance of the maniacal symptoms.

Chronic alcoholism is very difficult to treat, and once fully established the habit is rarely abandoned. The most obstinate cases are those with marked hereditary tendency. Withdrawal of the alcohol is the first essential. This is most effectually accomplished by placing the patient in an institution, in which he can be carefully watched. The absence of temptation in institution life is of special advantage. For the sleeplessness the bromides or hyoscine may be employed. Strychnine in tonic doses may be given. Prolonged seclusion in a suitable institution is in reality the only effectual means of cure. When a hereditary tendency exists a lapse into the drinking habit is almost inevitable.

In *delirium tremens* the patient should be confined to bed and carefully watched night and day. The danger of escape is very great, as the patient imagines himself pursued by enemies or demons. Flint mentions the case of a man who escaped in his nightclothes and ran barefooted for fifteen miles on frozen ground before he was overtaken. If possible the patient should not be strapped in bed, as this aggravates the delirium; sometimes some form of restraint is advisable which should be as simple as possible; a sheet tied across the bed may be sufficient or a jacket may be required. This is better than violent restraint by attendants. The giving or withdrawal of alcohol has to be decided for each patient; small amounts may be helpful for a few days.

Delirium tremens is a disease which, in a large majority of cases, runs a course very slightly influenced by medicine. The indications for treatment are to procure sleep and to support the strength. In mild cases half a dram (2 gm.) of bromide of potassium with tincture of capsicum may be given every three hours. Chloral is often of service (15 grains, 1 gm.) and may be given without hesitation. Good results sometimes follow the hypodermic use of hyoscine (gr. 1/100, 0.00065 gm.). Opium must be used cautiously. A special merit of Ware's work was the demonstration that with expectant treatment the percentage of recoveries was greater than with the indiscriminate use of sedatives, which had been in vogue for many years. When opium is indicated it should be given as morphia, hypodermically. The effect should be carefully watched, and, if after three or four quarter-grain doses have been given the patient is still restless and excited, it is best not to push it farther. Repeated doses of barbital (gr. x, 0.6 gm.) or phenobarbital (gr. i, 0.065 gm.) may be tried. Lambert advises ergotin hypodermically in both acute and chronic alcoholism. With acidosis alkalies and water should be given freely. When fever is present the effects of a bath or wet packs may be tried. The large doses of digitalis formerly employed are not advisable. Lumbar puncture is often useful.

Careful feeding is a most important element in the treatment. Milk and concentrated food should be given at stated intervals. If the pulse becomes rapid and weak, alcohol may be given with aromatic spirit of ammonia.

Methyl (Wood) Alcohol Poisoning.—Methyl alcohol is used extensively in trade but its importance as a toxic agent is due to its use as an adulterant in spirits for internal use and applications for external use, such as bay-rum, etc. It is not oxidized or excreted as rapidly as ethyl alcohol and is much more toxic. Poisoning usually results from drinking methyl alcohol but may result from external application or from inhalation. It has a selective toxic effect on the optic nerve and retina, resulting in a partial or complete blindness.

Symptoms.—These are much like those of ethyl alcohol with the addition of the injury to the optic nerve or retina. The coma due to wood alcohol is often deeper and of longer duration and delirium, nausea, vomiting and collapse are usually more marked. There may be marked dyspnea and respiratory failure. Acidosis may be present, due partly to the production of formic acid. The outlook is serious if the coma is marked. In *treatment* the stomach should be washed and an ounce of Epsom salts given by the tube, the colon washed out and stimulation used as indicated. Gastric lavage should be repeated for some days. Alkaline treatment is advisable by mouth and rectum, and intravenous injection of saline solution. Lumbar puncture should be done daily for 4 or 5 days.

Ginger or Jake Paralysis.—Outbreaks of peripheral neuritis have occurred in the United States due to drinking a fluid extract of Jamaica ginger which contained an adulterant, a phenol ester. The symptoms were those of peripheral neuritis.

OPIUM (MORPHIA, HEROIN) HABIT

Taken at first for various reasons, a craving for the drug is gradually engendered, and the habit acquired. The effects of the constant use of opium vary very much. In the East, where opium-smoking is quite common, the ill effects are, according to good observers, not very striking. Taken as morphia and hypodermically, as is the rule, it is very injurious but a moderate amount may be taken for years without serious damage. The habit is particularly prevalent among women and physicians who use the hypodermic syringe for the alleviation of pain, as in neuralgia or sciatica. The acquisition of the habit as a pure luxury is rare.

In the United States the use of *heroin* has been important. In many cases the habit begins in youths below the age of twenty. The "neurotic" seems especially prone to acquire the habit. The alcoholic as a rule does not take to these drugs. There is no evidence of the use of codein leading to a habit.

Symptoms.—The symptoms at first are slight and for months there may be no disturbance of health. There are exceptional cases in which for years excessive amounts have been taken without deterioration of mind or body. As a rule, the necessary dose has gradually to be increased. As the effects wear off the victim experiences lassitude and mental depression, accompanied often with slight nausea and epigastric distress, or recurring colic, which may be mistaken for appendicitis. The confirmed opium-eater usually has a sallow, pasty complexion, is emaciated, and becomes prematurely gray. He is restless, irritable, and unable to remain quiet for any time. Itching is a common symptom. The sleep is disturbed, the appetite and digestion are deranged, and except when directly under the influence of the drug the mental condition is one of depression. Occasionally there are profuse sweats, which may be preceded by chills. The pupils, except when under the direct influence of the drug, are dilated, sometimes unequal. In one case there was a persistent edema of the legs without renal changes or anemia to account for it. Persons addicted to morphia or heroin are inveterate liars, and no reliance whatever can be placed upon their statements. In many instances this is not confined to matters relating to the vice. In women the symptoms may be associated with those of pronounced hysteria or neurasthenia. The practice may be continued for an indefinite time, usually requiring increase in the dose until ultimately enormous quantities may be needed to obtain the desired effect. Finally a condition of asthenia is induced, in which the victim takes little or no food and dies from bodily debility. An increase in the dose is not always necessary, and there are *habitués* who are satisfied with a daily amount of 2 or 3 grains of morphia, and who are able to carry on successfully for many years the ordinary business of life. They may remain in good physical condition, and indeed often look ruddy. The general effects of heroin addiction are less marked than those of morphinism.

Treatment.—This is extremely difficult, and can rarely be successfully carried out by the general practitioner. Isolation, systematic feeding, and gradual withdrawal of the drug are the essential elements. As a rule, the patients must be under control in an institution and should be in bed for the first ten days. It is best in a majority of cases to reduce the morphia gradually and replace it by codein for a time. The sufferings of the patients are usually very great, more particularly the abdominal pains, sometimes nausea and vomiting, and the distressing restlessness. Insulin is useful in some cases, beginning with 5 or 10 units three times a day and watching carefully for hypoglycemia. A high carbohydrate diet should be given. Usually within a week or ten days the drug may be entirely withdrawn. In all cases the pulse should be carefully watched and, if feeble, aromatic spirit of ammonia and digitalis should be given. For the restlessness a hot bath is serviceable. Insomnia is a distressing symptom, and various drugs may have to be used, particularly hyoscine and one of the barbiturates, and sometimes, if the insommia persists, morphia itself.

It is essential to be certain that the patient has no means of obtaining morphia. Even under the favorable circumstances of seclusion in an institution and constant watching, patients may practise deception. After an apparent cure the patients are only too apt to relapse.

Physicians should exercise the utmost caution in prescribing morphia, particularly to female patients and to those with chronic diseases. Under no circumstances should a patient be allowed to use the hypodermic syringe.

COCAINISM

The addiction may be acquired through curiosity or by the use of cocaine to relieve fatigue. Habitués seem to take pleasure in teaching the habit to others. The use of cocaine solutions in sprays may be responsible. The subjects are often of the "neurotic" class and the habit is frequently acquired by minors. The drug is usually taken by snuffing, sometimes hypodermically. As a rule the dose is increased rapidly.

Symptoms.—These are much like those of morphinism but the effects of the drug are of shorter duration and are followed by marked depression and weakness. Sometimes there are temporary periods of marked exhilaration. Later the general health suffers: weakness, digestive disturbances, tremor, disturbances of sensation and mental features appear. If present, hallucinations are often associated with the skin and the patient imagines that insects cover him or are in the skin. The delusions are often of persecution and may lead to criminal acts. The moral degradation is often greater than from morphinism and the chance of ending the habit is less. The *treatment* is along the same general lines as in morphinism.

LEAD POISONING

(*Plumbism, Saturnism*)

Etiology.—The disease is widespread, particularly in the lead industries and among plumbers, painters and storage battery workers. In the United States it is not easy to get accurate statistics. In the registration area there were 101 deaths in 1930. The metal is introduced into the system in many forms. Miners usually escape, but those engaged in the smelting of lead ores are often attacked. Animals in the neighborhood of smelting furnaces have suffered with the disease, and even the birds that feed on the berries in the neighborhood may be affected. Men engaged in the white-lead factories are particularly prone to plumbism. Dusty lead trades are especially dangerous. Accidental poisoning may come in many ways; most commonly by drinking water which has passed through lead pipes or been stored in lead-lined cisterns. Wines and cider which contain acids quickly become contaminated in contact with lead. It was the frequency of colic in certain of the cider districts of Devonshire which gave the name of Devonshire colic, as the frequency of it in Poitou gave the name *colica Pictonum.* Among the innumerable sources of accidental poisoning may be mentioned milk, various sorts of beverages, cosmetics containing lead, hair dyes, false teeth, and thread. A few cases have followed the retention of lead bullets in gun-shot wounds. Given medicinally, lead may cause poisoning. It has followed the use of Emplastrum Diachylon to produce abortion, and there is a case reported in an infant from the application of lead-water on the mother's nipples. One grain every three hours for three days, and two grains every three hours for one day, have caused signs of poisoning. A serious outbreak of lead-poisoning occurred in Philadelphia, owing to adulteration of a baking powder with chromate of lead, used to give a yellow tint to cakes. Poisoning has followed the use of snuff to which chromate of lead has been added. Children may be poisoned by swallowing paint from toys, etc.

All ages are attacked; the largest number of cases occur between thirty and forty. According to Oliver, females are more susceptible than males. They are much more quickly brought under its influence, and in an epidemic in which 1,000 cases were involved the proportion of females to males was four to one. Miscarriage is common and it is rare for a woman working in lead to carry a child to term. It also destroys the reproductive power in man.

The lead gains *entrance* through the lungs, the digestive organs or the skin. Through the lungs it is freely absorbed. The chief channel, according to Oliver, is the digestive system. It is carried in the body as a phosphate and stored in the calcareous parts of the bones. An excess of calcium favors harmless storage in the body and a deficiency favors excretion. It is rapidly eliminated by the gastro-intestinal tract and kidneys. The susceptibility is remarkably varied. The symptoms may be manifest within a month of exposure. On the other hand, Tanquerel (des Planches) saw a case in a man who had been a lead-worker for fifty-two years. E. R. Hayhurst examined 100 painters, not one of whom had symptoms of acute plumbism, but 70 showed in varying degrees symptoms, signs or after-effects of chronic plumbism; a lead-line on the gums was present in 19 cases. *Tetra-ethyl lead,* used in motor fuel, causes severe poisoning, affecting the nervous system particularly. It is rapidly absorbed through the skin.

Morbid Anatomy.—Small quantities of lead occur in the body in health. Of 287 deaths in subjects of plumbism 32 were due to an encephalopathy, 43 to nephritis, 47 to cerebral hemorrhage, 43 to paralysis, 44 to lead poisoning, 38 to tuberculosis, and 40 to various maladies, pneumonia, heart disease, aneurism, etc. (Legge). In chronic poisoning lead is found in the various organs. The affected muscles are yellow, fatty and fibroid. The nerves present the features of a peripheral degenerative neuritis. In the primary atrophic form the ganglion cells of the anterior horns are implicated. In acute fatal cases there may be intense enterocolitis.

Symptoms.—ACUTE FORM.—We do not refer here to the accidental or suicidal cases, which present vomiting, pain in the abdomen, and collapse symptoms. There are manifestations which follow a short time after exposure and set in acutely. There may be severe *colic* with constipation or diarrhea with enteritis and a rapidly developing anemia. Acute neuritis has been described, and convulsions, epilepsy, and a delirium, not unlike that produced by alcohol. There are cases in which the gastro-intestinal symptoms are intense and rapidly prove fatal. These acute forms occur more often in persons recently exposed, and more often in winter than in summer. Da Costa reported the onset of hemiplegia after three days' exposure to lead.

CHRONIC POISONING.—*Blood Changes.*—A moderate grade of *anemia* is usually present. There is marked pallor perhaps due to vasoconstriction. The corpuscles do not often fall below 50 per cent. Many of the red cells show a remarkable stippling when stained with Wright's stain or polychrome methylene blue. Pepper (tertius) and White showed that they were constantly present in lead poisoning. Such granulations are found in the blood in a variety of conditions, even in normal blood, but they are most numerous in lead poisoning, in which their occurrence in large numbers is of value in diagnosis. Cadwalader showed the constant presence of *nucleated red blood corpuscles* even when the anemia is slight.

The blue line on the gums is a valuable indication but is not invariably present. Two lines must be distinguished: one, at the margin between the gums and teeth, is *on*, not *in* the gums, and is removed by cleansing the teeth. The other is the characteristic blue-black line at the margin of the gum. The color is not uniform, but being in the papillae of the gums the line is, as seen with a magnifying glass, interrupted. The lead is converted in the tissues into a black sulphide by the action of sulphuretted hydrogen from the tartar of the teeth. The line may form in a few days after exposure (Oliver) and disappear within a few weeks, or persist for months. A black line may occur in miners, due to the deposition of carbon, and bismuth may give a line much like lead.

The most important symptoms of chronic poisoning are *colic*, *palsy*, and *encephalopathy*. Of these, the colic is the most frequent. Of Tanquerel's cases, there were 1,217 of colic, 101 of paralysis, and 72 of encephalopathy.

Colic is the most common symptom of chronic lead poisoning. It is often preceded by gastric or intestinal symptoms, particularly constipation. The pain is over the whole abdomen. The colic is usually paroxysmal and relieved by pressure. There is often a dull, heavy pain between the paroxysms. There may be vomiting. During the attack, as Riegel noted, the pulse is increased in tension and the heart's action is retarded. Attacks of pain with acute diarrhea may recur for weeks or even for three or four years.

Certain of the cases with colic may present the features of an acute intra-abdominal inflammatory condition. A patient may be admitted with a diagnosis of appendicitis or intestinal obstruction. Localized pain, slight fever, and moderate leukocytosis may be present. The history, the blue line on the gums and the blood changes are of importance in diagnosis.

Lead palsy.—This is rarely a primary manifestation. Among 54 cases of lead poisoning in the J. H. H. there were 30 cases of lead paralysis (H. M. Thomas). The upper limbs are most frequently affected. In 26 cases the arms alone were affected, and 18 of these showed the typical double wrist-drop. In 7 the right arm alone was involved, and in one the left. In 4 cases both arms and legs were attacked. The onset may be acute, subacute, or chronic. It usually occurs without fever. In its distribution it may be partial, limited to a muscle or to certain muscle groups, or generalized, involving in a short time the muscles of the extremities and the trunk. The muscles most used are often attacked. Dejerine-Klumpke described the following *localized forms:* (1) *Antebrachial* type, paralysis of the extensors of the fingers and of the wrist. In this the musculospiral nerve is involved, causing the characteristic wrist-drop. The supinator longus usually escapes. In the long-continued flexion of the carpus there may be slight displacement backward of the bones, with distention of the synovial sheaths, so that there is a prominent swelling over the wrist known as Gruebler's tumor. (2) *Brachial* type, which involves the deltoid, the biceps, the brachialis anticus, and the supinator longus, rarely the pectorals. The atrophy is of the scapulohumeral form. It is bilateral, and sometimes follows the first form but may be primary. (3) The Aran-Duchenne type, in which the small muscles of the hand and of the thenar and hypothenar eminences are involved. The atrophy is marked, and may be the first manifestation. Möbius has shown that this form is particularly marked in tailors. (4) The *peroneal* type. According to Tanquerel, the legs are involved in the proportion of 13 to 100 of the arms. The lateral peroneal muscles, the extensor communis of the toes, and the extensor proprius of the big toe are involved, producing the *steppage* gait. (5) *Laryngeal* form; adductor paralysis may occur in lead-palsy.

Generalized Palsies.—There may be a slow, chronic paralysis, gradually involving the extremities, beginning with the classical picture of wrist drop. More frequently there is a rapid generalization, producing complete paralysis in all the muscles of the parts in a few days. It may pursue a course like an ascending paralysis, associated with rapid wasting of all four limbs but such cases are rare. Death has occurred by involvement of the diaphragm. In one patient with generalized paralysis this began in the legs after but two weeks' work as an enameler. It spread rapidly, so that in a little over a week he was bedridden, and on admission to the hospital nearly every muscle below the neck was involved. The diaphragm was completely paralyzed. He was walking when he left the hospital, though there was still some weakness. Dejerine-Klumpke also recognized a febrile form of general paralysis which may closely resemble the subacute spinal paralysis of Duchenne.

There is also a primary saturnine muscular atrophy in which the weakness and wasting come on together. It is this form, according to Gowers, which most frequently assumes the Aran-Duchenne type.

The electrical reactions are those of lesions of the lower motor segment. The reaction of degeneration in its different grades may be present, depending upon the severity. Usually with the onset of the paralysis there are pains in the legs and joints. Sensation may, however, be unaffected.

Cerebral Symptoms.—*Headache* is common and there may be marked depression; delusions and maniacal excitement may follow. In other cases transient delirium, attacks of unconsciousness and convulsions result. Optic neuritis or neuroretinitis may occur. Hysterical symptoms occasionally occur in girls. *Convulsions* are not uncommon and in an adult the possibility of lead-poisoning should always be considered. True epilepsy may follow the convulsions. An acute delirium may occur with hallucinations. The patients may have trance-like attacks, which follow or alternate with convulsions. There may be marked edema of the brain. A few cases of lead encephalopathy finally drift into asylums. Tremor, especially of the lips, eyelids, tongue and fingers, is a common manifestation.

Arteriosclerosis.—Lead-workers are notoriously subject to arteriosclerosis with contracted kidneys and hypertrophy of the heart. Some show gouty deposits but in the United States acute gout in lead-workers is rare.

Diagnosis.—In marked cases this offers no difficulty. The occupation is of aid if it is one in which lead is handled. It is in the cases of "accidental" poisoning that difficulty arises. In women the use of certain face powders and applications is not an uncommon cause and should be kept in mind. The amount of lead in the skin may be determined by removal of a portion of skin and the estimation made by special methods. A careful study of the blood and a search for lead in the urine are important; excretion may continue long after ingestion has ceased. In children the diagnosis may be aided by an X-ray study, showing areas of increased density in the growing ends of the long bones.

Prognosis.—In the minor manifestations this is good. According to Gowers, the outlook is bad in the primary atrophic form of paralysis. Convulsions are, as a rule, serious, and the mental symptoms which succeed may be permanent. Occasionally the wrist drop persists. Encephalopathy always has a grave prognosis. With vascular or renal disease, the prognosis depends largely on the degree of damage in these systems.

Treatment.—Prophylactic measures should be taken at all lead works, but, unless employees are careful, poisoning is apt to occur even under favorable conditions. Cleanliness of the hands and of the finger nails, frequent bathing, and the use of respirators when necessary should be insisted upon. The patient should be in bed on liquid and soft diet; water should be taken freely and the bowels kept open. This last is difficult to accomplish; mineral oil in full doses and sodium or magnesium sulphate (one ounce once or twice a day) should be given. Smaller doses of the salines (ʒi-ii, 4-8 gm.) several times a day may be more effectual. Belladonna or atropine in full doses often seems to be of advantage. In *acute* cases it is well to try and hold the lead in the bones and for this calcium should be given freely as calcium lactate 60 grains (4 gm.) daily. Two quarts of milk a day should be taken. After the acute features are over a diet low in calcium should be given (meat, potatoes, rice, macaroni, milk-free bread, sugar, apples, bananas; avoiding milk, eggs and green vegetables). Ammonium chloride ʒii-iii (8-12 gm.) a day, sodium bicarbonate gr. 30-60 (2-4 gm.) a day or dilute phosphoric acid in doses of ʒ v (20 cc.) may be given to aid the excretion. Iodide can be given in from 5 to 10-grain (0.3-0.6 gm.) doses three times a day unless the poisoning is severe. For the colic hot applications, amyl nitrite, atropine and, if severe, morphia may be used. For the anemia iron should be used. In acute cases it is well not to give iodide, as the liberation of the lead deposited in the tissues may increase the severity of the symptoms. For the local palsies massage and the constant current should be used. With encephalopathy lumbar puncture should be done and repeated as indicated. After recovery the need of change in occupation should be considered.

The intravenous administration of sodium thiosulphate (0.5 gm. being the average dose) daily for four days and afterwards every other day for as long as necessary is advised and seems useful in some cases.

BRASS AND ZINC POISONING

Brass, a compound of copper and zinc, is not harmful itself; poisoning is due to the inhalation of zinc oxide fumes. The cause is not clear; an anaphylactic reaction due to destruction of protein in the respiratory tract is suggested. Brass polishers and those exposed to the dust have the hair stained somewhat green and there is often a slight greenish deposit in the teeth and gums. It is said that there may be a green tint to the perspiration, even after a thorough bath.

The dust may cause an itching of the skin, the so-called "brass itch." The fumes from molten brass cause peculiar symptoms, the so-called "brass-workers' ague," "metal fume fever," "smelters' shakes" and "zinc chills." The *symptoms* are an acute chill, which comes on some hours after exposure to the molten metal, sweating and a feeling of nausea; there may be vomiting, great thirst, a rapid, feeble pulse, fever, leukocytosis, and in a couple of hours very profuse sweating. The entire attack may last for six or eight hours, or the patient may be ill for a day. Many of our patients used to say that they were more liable to it on Monday, after Sunday's rest. A large percentage of the workers are susceptible. It does not seem to impair the health very much. A decrease in vital capacity has been found. The malady is widespread among the workers in zinc in the United States.

In *treatment* an emetic and a brisk purge may give relief. The drinking of milk and taking of sodium bicarbonate are advised.

ARSENICAL POISONING

Acute poisoning by arsenic is common, particularly by Paris green and such mixtures as "Rough on Rats," which are used to destroy vermin and insects. The chief symptoms are intense pain in the stomach, vomiting, and, later, colic, with diarrhea and tenesmus; occasionally the symptoms are those of collapse. If recovery takes place, paralysis may follow. The *treatment* is similar to that of other irritant poisons—rapid removal with the stomach tube, the promotion of vomiting and the use of milk and eggs. Moist ferric hydroxide (half an ounce of Tct. ferri chloridi in a glass of water and add magnesia to excess) should be given freely. Morphia should be given for pain and stimulation used for collapse.

Toxic effects from the *arsenobenzol* compounds are not infrequent. Among them are: (1) Dermatoses of various kinds. Erythema is not uncommon and its appearance is a signal to stop the therapy. Purpura and ecchymoses occur. (2) Encephalitis hemorrhagica with which purpura may be associated. (3) Injury to the liver cells of varying grade, with jaundice, toxemia and possibly rapid atrophy. (4) A severe anemia with the features of aplastic anemia. The coagulation time of the blood may be prolonged. (5) Attacks of marked vasomotor disturbance with low blood pressure. (6) Symptoms described as "anaphylactoid" or "nitritoid crisis" in which there are sudden dyspnea, cyanosis, dilatation of the pupils, local edema and erythematous or urticarial eruptions. The blood pressure may be low. The injection of epinephrine is indicated (15 min., 1 cc. of a 1-1000 solution).

Arseniuretted hydrogen poisoning has occurred in submarines and from the gas given off from "ferro-silicon." There is a special toxic action on the liver and kidneys. Symptoms appear in a few hours, nausea, vomiting, and headache; jaundice, hematuria and anemia follow. The anemia may be severe. Delirium followed by coma may result in death.

Chronic Arsenical Poisoning.—Arsenic is used extensively in the arts, particularly in the manufacture of colored papers, artificial flowers and in many fabrics. The glazed green and red papers used in kindergartens also contain arsenic. It is present in many wall-papers and carpets. The arsenic compounds may be in the form of solid particles detached from the paper or as gaseous volatile bodies formed from arsenical organic matter by the action of several moulds. In moisture, and at a temperature of from 60° to 95° F., a volatile compound is set free, probably "an organic derivative of arsenic pentoxide" (Sanger). The chronic poisoning from fabrics and wall-papers may be due to the ingestion of minute continued doses of this derivative. Contaminated glucose, used in manufacturing beer, caused a widespread epidemic of poisoning at Manchester. The associated presence of selenium compounds may have played a part in the production of the poisoning (Tunnicliffe and Rosenheim). Arsenic is eliminated in all the secretions and has been found in the milk. J. J. Putnam showed that it is not uncommon to find traces of arsenic in the urine of many persons in apparent health. The effects of moderate quantities of arsenic are not infrequently seen in medical practice. Flushing and hyperemia of the skin, puffiness of the eyelids or above the eyebrows, nausea, vomiting, and diarrhea are the most common symptoms. Redness and sometimes bleeding of the gums and salivation occur. In the protracted administration of arsenic patients may complain of numbness and tingling in the fingers. Cutaneous *pigmentation* and keratosis are very characteristic, and, as a late rare sequence of the latter, epithelioma. Perforation of the nasal septum may occur. Care should be exercised to avoid the therapeutic overdosage of arsenic, especially in chorea. It is advisable to reduce the dose occasionally for a few days when arsenic is given for long periods.

In the Manchester epidemic nearly all cases presented signs of neuritis and lesions of the skin. In some the sensory disturbances predominated, in others the motor, the individuals being unable to walk or to use their hands. In a certain number there was muscular incoördination, resembling that of tabes dorsalis. Rapid muscular atrophy characterized some cases. In not a few a condition of erythromelalgia was present. Occasionally a catarrh of the respiratory and alimentary tracts was the chief feature. Pigmentation, keratosis and herpes were the most characteristic cutaneous manifestations.

Arsenical paralysis has the same characteristics as lead palsy, but the legs are more affected than the arms, particularly the extensors and peroneal group, so that the patient has the characteristic *steppage* gait of peripheral neuritis. The electrical reaction in the muscles may be disturbed before there is any loss of power, and when the patient is asked to extend the wrist fully and to spread the fingers slight weakness may be detected early.

Treatment.—Active elimination by the bowels and kidneys is advisable and the treatment of special conditions as indicated. The use of sodium thiosulphate (0.5 gm.) intravenously is advised as in lead poisoning.

MERCURIAL POISONING

Acute Poisoning.—This is comparatively common in mild forms from the use of mercury compounds in therapy, especially calomel by mouth and ointment by inunctions. The commonest results are salivation and stomatitis. There is usually a curious foul metallic odor to the breath for some days before stomatitis appears. This should be watched for as prompt treatment may prevent later manifestations. The patient may complain of a metallic taste, tenderness on chewing or bringing the teeth forcibly together, or of tenderness of the gums. The secretion of saliva increases, the gums swell, ulceration may follow, the teeth may be loosened and fall out, and in severe cases extensive necrosis may result which may involve the carotid artery.

The most acute form results from the taking of *bichloride of mercury*, sometimes accidentally, often for suicide. The symptoms usually appear in a short time. Corrosive effects on the mouth or throat may give pain. Vomiting with abdominal pain, frequent bowel movements often containing blood, and sometimes collapse follow promptly. Severe stomatitis usually appears in a short time and the signs of colitis usually increase. The movements are bloody and may contain shreds of necrotic tissue. *Nephritis*, usually of a severe form, results also, the urine being very scanty or complete suppression resulting. In some cases the signs of colitis may be delayed for some days. There is much difference in the severity of the symptoms, largely due to the amount absorbed. If vomiting occurred promptly or lavage can be done soon after the ingestion of the poison, the symptoms may be mild and the outlook is more favorable. The prognosis depends largely on the extent of renal damage. There may be almost complete suppression for several days followed by recovery. Edema is not common but there is marked retention of the nitrogenous substances in the blood, which is an important aid in prognosis. Patients may do well for some days and then renal insufficiency becomes more marked. If there is any doubt as to the diagnosis confirmation may be obtained by the demonstration of mercury in the saliva, excreta, urine and vomitus. This demonstration is not easy and should be carried out by a trained chemist. It should be remembered that mercury appears periodically in the urine.

Treatment.—Care should be taken in the administration of mercury to recognize the earliest signs of salivation and stop the drug. Patients should be told which signs to watch for and instructed to report. Any form of mercury used for purgation should be followed by a saline. For *stomatitis* the diet may have to be liquid, water should be given freely and the bowels kept open by salines and enemata. Mouth washes should be used freely and often, such as potassium chlorate solution, hydrogen peroxide solution (1 to 4) or potassium permanganate (2 per cent). The gums should be painted daily with silver nitrate solution (5 per cent). Atropine in sufficient dosage usually controls the salivation. In patients taking mercury for syphilis particular care should be given to the state of the gums and teeth.

In *bichloride* poisoning, the whites of several eggs and a pint of milk should be given at once and the stomach emptied by the tube, after which one ounce of Epsom salts is given through the tube. An enema should then be given and the colon emptied. Saline solution (1,000 cc.) should be given intravenously. The stomach should be washed and the colon irrigated twice a day, using sodium bicarbonate solution (5 per cent), as mercury is excreted by the gastric and intestinal mucous membrane. A hot pack should be given twice a day. It is important to give fluid freely. Milk or orange juice is given every two hours (8 ounces) and alternately every two hours 8 ounces of the following (Lambert and Patterson): Potassium bitartrate and cane sugar, each ʒ ii (8 gm.), lactose ℥ i (30 gm.), lemon juice ℥ ii (60 cc.) and water to one quart (1,000 cc.). As much alkaline solution as possible is given by the bowel; potassium citrate gr. xv, 1 gm. to the pint (500 cc.) either by the drop method or 250 cc. every two hours. Saline solution should be given subcutaneously or intravenously as long as there is vomiting. The administration of fluid should be kept up through the twenty-four hours, the patient being waked if necessary.

Good results are reported from the intravenous administration of sodium thiosulphate (0.5 gm.) as in lead poisoning. In case of poisoning by absorption from the vagina, douches of 5 per cent sodium thiosulphate solution should be used. The use of sodium formaldehyde sulphoxylate has been advocated (Rosenthal). Gastric lavage is done, using a 5 per cent solution of the sulphoxylate and 200 cc. are left in the stomach. Then 10 grams in 200 cc. of distilled water are given intravenously, 20-30 minutes being taken for this. In a severe case this may be repeated in 4 to 6 hours, 5 to 10 gm. being given. For the colitis, colon irrigations (1-1000 solution) are given once or twice daily. Immediate cecostomy, if the condition permits, with constant lavage of the colon has been done, apparently with advantage.

Chronic Poisoning.—This occurs chiefly among workers with the metal (in making instruments, electric bulbs, and mirrors), workers in furs and makers of hats in which nitrate of mercury is used. There have been cases due to the vapor and also from long continued medicinal use, as bichloride vaginal douches. It is occasionally a sequel of acute poisoning. The *local* features include stomatitis and salivation, marked fetor of the breath, an extreme condition of mouth infection, sometimes a blue line on the gums, dyspepsia, colitis, which may be ulcerative, and nephritis. The *nervous system* manifestations are important; tremors are common, usually fine and involving the tongue, face, arms and hands, and even the trunk and legs. Psychical changes may occur and general weakness, loss of weight and anemia. If there is any doubt of the diagnosis, mercury should be searched for in the stools. In *treatment*, the patient should be removed from exposure to mercury; elimination aided by giving water freely and keeping the bowels open by salines and enemata; and necessary symptomatic measures used.

MANGANESE POISONING

Manganese does not seem to be highly poisonous and does not accumulate in the body. The cause is the inhalation of dust or fumes. The clinical picture seems to depend on lesions in the basal ganglion, which are much like those in Parkinson's disease. As a rule a history of working in manganese dust for at least three months is the rule. The first complaints are of weakness and drowsiness. The patients develop a masklike facies with disturbance of speech, the voice being monotonous. Later there is muscular twitching which varies from a fine tremor of the hands to gross movements of the arms, legs, head and trunk. There may be cramp-like pains in the calves of the legs with stiffness in the muscles of the legs. The cramps usually come on at night and are worse after exertion. The deep reflexes are increased and ankle and patellar clonus appear. There is no definite incoordination. Later there may be emotional disturbance. The process apparently involves some part of the neuromuscular system.

METHYL CHLORIDE POISONING

Methyl chloride is used in refrigeration and poisoning occurs from leaking pipes. The main symptoms are headache, vertigo, drowsiness, mental confusion, convulsions, coma, stupor, weakness, cyanosis, nausea, vomiting and abdominal pain. Fever occurs about 36 hours after the poisoning with rapid pulse and respiration, and low blood pressure. The pupils are dilated and occasionally strabismus, ptosis and nystagmus are found. The blood shows anemia with leukocytosis. There is an acetone odor to the breath and acetone is found in the urine, unless there is anuria, which is common. The coma may persist for two to three days. Death is due to respiratory paralysis and may be preceded by convulsions. Sequelae may be in the form of mental changes or ataxia. The diagnosis has to be made from food poisoning, methyl alcohol and carbon monoxide poisoning, mercury and strychnia poisoning, encephalitis and meningitis. In *treatment* the acidosis should be met by sodium bicarbonate freely by mouth or bowel with dextrose, alkaline solution intravenously and oxygen. Caffeine and digitalis may be needed for the circulation.

FOOD POISONING

There may be "death in the pot" from many causes. Food poisons may be *endogenous* or *exogenous.* Those articles in which the poison is of endogenous origin can scarcely be designated as foods. The poisonous mushroom, for example, is often mistaken for the edible form. The former is injurious because it normally contains a highly poisonous alkaloid, muscarine. Certain fish also produce normal physiological but toxic products. When eaten by mistake, as occurs in the West Indies and Japan, these fish may cause illness. The *exogenous* origin of food poisons is by far the commonest. Under this head come those foods which are rendered poisonous by accidental contamination from outside sources. This may be from metal containers or the food may contain specific organisms, especially the Salmonella group; milk and other foods may become infected with typhoid bacilli, streptococci, etc., and so convey disease.

Animals (or insects, as bees) may feed on substances which cause their flesh or products to be poisonous to man. The grains used as food may be infected with fungi and cause epidemics of ergotism, etc. Foods of all sorts may become contaminated with the bacteria of putrefaction, the products of which may be highly poisonous.

The term "ptomaine poisoning" has been popularized to such an extent that it is used synonymously with food poisoning but true ptomaine poisoning is very rare and the use of the term should be stopped. The term *ptomaine* was introduced by the Italian chemist, Selmi, to designate basic alkaloidal products formed in putrefaction. Mytilotoxin, found in poisonous mussels, is of this class, and is by far the most poisonous of the known ptomaines.

Among the more common forms are the following:

Poisoning from Fungi.—Poisonous fungi are eaten in error for edible mushrooms. The most poisonous varieties are the *Amanita muscaria* and *phal-*

loides. The former contains muscarine, and the symptoms usually appear within an hour after ingestion. They are largely gastro-intestinal, salivation, vomiting, pain and diarrhea with collapse, sweating and delirium. The *treatment* consists in promoting free vomiting or washing out the stomach, washing out the colon, giving atropine freely and general stimulation. The *A. phalloides* contains a toxin which produces degeneration in the liver and kidney especially. The symptoms do not appear for some days. There are vomiting, diarrhea, marked prostration, jaundice and suppression of urine. Death usually occurs in a few days. The *treatment* consists in free elimination and symptomatic measures.

Food Poisoning Due to Infection.—Outbreaks of disease of bacterial origin are not uncommon.

Acute Epidemic Food Poisoning.—The organisms causing this belong to the "Salmonella" group and those most often responsible are *B. aertrycke, B. enteritidis* and *B. suipestifer.* The identification of these organisms depends on their sugar reactions and on specific serum reactions. The infection is usually carried by meat, especially pork. The incubation period varies from a few hours to 3 or 4 days. The onset may be with a chill followed by fever or the temperature may be subnormal. Vomiting, abdominal pain and frequent offensive stools, sometimes bloody, follow, frequently with severe muscular pains and marked collapse. Skin rashes, erythema, urticaria and even purpura, are not uncommon. Individuals react very differently; some have slight symptoms while in others death may result in twenty-four hours. Some cases of paratyphoid fever B have a close resemblance to this group and there may be a double infection. Food poisoning due to *Staphylococcus aureus* occurs, with the onset in 2 to 4 hours. There is severe vomiting and diarrhea with great prostration but apparently little mortality. The *diagnosis* is usually clear from the clinical picture but metallic poisoning and acute dysentery may have similar features. The organism may be isolated from the stools, rarely from the blood and the serum reactions may be diagnostic. The possibility of *carriers* must be kept in mind. In *treatment,* if seen early, gastric lavage should be done or vomiting produced or encouraged if it has already occurred. Absolute rest, little food by mouth for a day (albumen water only), aerated water, hot applications to the abdomen and colon irrigations are important. Morphia hypodermically (gr. 1/4, 0.016 gm.) is often useful. Bismuth and soda may be given by mouth in full dosage (gr. xxx, 2 gm. of bismuth). In case of collapse, heat, saline injections and stimulation should be used.

The question of *chronic* bacterial food poisoning is an obscure one. In case of persistent infection by a carrier such a condition may occur. The symptoms are those of chronic gastro-intestinal disturbance, perhaps colitis. Stool cultures and serum tests are essential for diagnosis.

Meat poisoning associated with putrefaction.—Here alterations of appearance, of smell and taste are usually present. The products are those of protein hydrolysis, various aromatic compounds, but particularly putrescine, cadaverine and sepsin. How far these bodies are responsible for the symptoms, how far they are due to infection with associated organisms, particularly colon bacilli, has not been definitely settled. Cases of food poisoning have been due to the proteus bacillus. This organism was the cause of a severe outbreak due to eating potato salad.

Botulism (Allantiasis).—Poisoning due to the toxins of the *Bacillus botulinus.* Kuner, the Swabian physician and poet, described "sausage poisoning" in 1817. The organism was found by Van Ermengen in a ham, the eating of which caused 50 cases of botulism. There are various strains, and the organism is widely distributed in the soil. Formerly regarded as exclusively a form of meat poisoning, Dickson and his associates showed that the toxin may be formed in vegetable products, especially when "home-canned." Botulism is a true *intoxication,* the toxin being formed in the food and absorbed in the gastro-intestinal tract. It is destroyed by heating to the boiling point. Instances of poisoning seem to be increasing in the United States, the majority caused by canned vegetables. The presence of bubbles of gas, a rancid odor and a softened appearance of the solid parts are suggestive of *B. botulinus* in canned materials. Uncooked or freshly cooked vegetables or fruits do not contain the toxin. The *pathological* lesions show marked thrombus formation in the arteries and veins with hyperemia and hemorrhages in the meninges and central nervous system. There is an absence of inflammatory reaction. Edmunds holds that the peripheral changes are important, that it is a "curare-like" reaction, not necessarily complete, a paralysis of the motor nerve endings. He states that the nuclei most affected do not give the most marked clinical findings. The results are motor, not sensory.

Symptoms.—The onset is from 4 to 48 hours (usually 12 to 24) after ingestion of the toxin. There are weakness, dizziness, disturbance in vision, diplopia, ptosis, paralyses of the eye muscles, and difficulty in swallowing and respiration. Vertigo and incoördination are common. Cranial nerve paralyses are always present; all the cranial nerves except the first and second have been involved. Dryness of the mouth and throat and constriction of the throat with difficulty in speaking and swallowing follow. There is no headache or sensory disturbance. There may be retention of urine and occasional paralyses of the arms and legs. The deep reflexes are not altered. There are retention of food in the stomach and obstinate constipation. In the later stages *bulbar* symptoms are common, rapid respiration with dyspnea and a slow pulse. There is no fever. Death occurs in from 1 to 8 days from cardiac or respiratory failure. There are grades of severity—mild or abortive cases may be recognized only by the association with more severe forms. The mortality in the United States has been about 66 per cent but lower in Europe. In *diagnosis* the evidence of food poisoning from a common source is important but the onset of symptoms varies and the victims may be widely scattered before symptoms appear. The cranial nerve paralyses seem to be a constant feature. Epidemic encephalitis may give difficulty, in which the history is perhaps the greatest aid. There are special methods of diagnosis by feeding suspected food material to chickens, susceptible to the A strain, but not to B, and its intraperitoneal injection into mice. Individual *prophylaxis* lies in the avoidance of suspicious canned material and the various forms of potted meat preparations. In *treatment* the stomach should be promptly washed out, a purgative given and the colon irrigated; water should be given freely. Artificial respiration should be kept up as long as possible. The use of the antitoxin depends on early diagnosis; it may be useful up to 24 hours after ingestion and should be used when it is available.

Certain game birds, particularly the grouse, are poisonous in special districts and at certain seasons. It is interesting to note that mutton and lamb have thus far not been implicated as a cause of food poisoning.

Poisoning by Milk Products.—(*a*) The poisonous effects which follow the drinking of milk infected with saprophytic bacteria are considered in the section on the diarrhea of infants.

(*b*) Various milk products, ice cream, custard and cheese, may prove highly poisonous. In one epidemic Vaughan and Novy isolated from cheese a substance belonging to the poisonous albumins. The symptoms are those of acute gastro-intestinal irritation.

Poisoning by Shell-fish and Fish.—*Mussel Poisoning.*—Brieger separated a ptomaine—mytilotoxin—which exists chiefly in the liver of the mussel. Schmidtmann and Cameron showed that the mussel from the open sea only becomes poisonous when placed in filthy waters.

Dangerous, even fatal, effects may follow the eating of either raw or cooked mussels. The symptoms are those of an acute poisoning with profound action on the nervous system, and without gastro-intestinal manifestations. There are numbness and coldness, no fever, dilated pupils, and rapid pulse; death occurs sometimes within two hours with collapse symptoms. In an epidemic at Wilhelmshafen, Germany, in 1885, nineteen persons were attacked, four of whom died. Salkowski and Brieger isolated the *mytilotoxin* from the mussels. Poisoning occasionally follows the eating of oysters which are stale or decomposed. The symptoms are usually gastro-intestinal.

Fish Poisoning.—There are two distinct varieties: in one the poison is a physiological product of certain glands of the fish, in the other it is a product of bacterial growth. The salted sturgeon used in parts of Russia has proved fatal to large numbers of persons. In China and Japan various species of the *tetrodon* are toxic, sometimes causing death within an hour, with symptoms of intense disturbance of the nervous system. Canned fish may cause poisoning by infection before the canning; after the cans are opened, canned fish is very liable to bacterial infection.

Grain and Vegetable Food Poisoning.—*Ergotism.*—The prolonged use of meal made from grain contaminated by the ergot fungus (*Claviceps purpurea*) causes a series of symptoms known as ergotism, epidemics of which have prevailed in parts of Europe. In acute ergotism there is acute enteritis with nervous system manifestations. Two forms of chronic ergotism are described—the one, *gangrenous,* is believed to be due to sphacelinic acid, the other, *convulsive* or spasmodic, is due to cornutin. In the former gangrene affects the extremities—usually the toes and fingers, less commonly the ears and nose. Preceding the gangrene there are usually anesthesia, tingling, pains, spasmodic movements and blood stasis in certain territories.

The *nervous* manifestations are very remarkable. After a prodromal stage of ten to fourteen days, in which the patient complains of weakness, headache, and tingling sensations in different parts of the body, perhaps accompanied with slight fever, symptoms of spasm develop, producing cramps in the muscles and contractures. The arms are flexed and the legs and toes extended. These spasms may last from a few hours to many days and relapses are frequent. In severer cases convulsive seizures develop and the patient may die in them. Mental symptoms are common, manifested sometimes in a preliminary delirium, but more commonly as melancholia or dementia. *Posterior spinal sclerosis* occurs in some cases. In a group of 29 cases (Tuczek and Siemens) 9 died at various periods after the infection, and four showed degeneration of the posterior columns. A condition similar to tabes dorsalis is gradually produced by this slow degeneration in the spinal cord.

Lathyrism (*Lupinosis*).—An affection produced by the use of meal from certain vetches, chiefly *Lathyrus sativus* and *L. cicera*, popularly known as the chick-pea. The grains are usually powdered and mixed with the meal from other cereals in the preparation of bread. As early as the seventeenth century it was noticed that the use of flour with which the seeds of the *Lathyrus* were mixed caused stiffness of the legs. The subject did not attract much attention until the studies of James Irving, in India, who, between 1859 and 1868, described a form of spastic paraplegia due to the use of meal made from the *Lathyrus* seeds. It also produces a spastic paraplegia in animals. The Italian observers describe a similar paraplegia, and it has been observed in Algiers. The condition is a spastic paralysis, involving chiefly the legs, which may proceed to complete paraplegia. The arms are rarely, if ever, affected. It is evidently a slow lateral sclerosis.

Potato poisoning.—Potatoes contain normally a very small amount (about 0.06 per cent) of the poisonous principle solanin, and, under certain circumstances, it may be in amounts sufficient to cause grave disturbance. The increase is due to the action of at least two species of bacteria, *B. solaniferum non-colorabile* and *B. solaniferum colorabile*, and occurs in tubers which, during growth, have lain partially exposed above ground, and in those which, during storage, have become well sprouted. In one outbreak fifty-six persons, after eating sprouted potatoes, had chills, fever, headache, vomiting, diarrhea, colic and great prostration. Many were jaundiced and several collapsed, but all recovered. The remaining potatoes yielded 0.38 per cent of solanin, indicating that a full portion contained about 5 grains.

The "Vomiting Sickness" of Jamaica is due to poisoning by immature or spoiled ackees—the fruit of *Blighia sapida*. Children are especially susceptible; the main features are vomiting, convulsions and coma; the average duration is twelve hours; the death rate is 85 per cent (Scott). In *treatment* alcohol has reduced the mortality greatly. It precipitates the poison.

Favism.—This is a syndrome caused by inhalation from the bean plant (*Vicia fava*) when in blossom or by ingestion of the beans. It is characterized by an acute febrile anemia with jaundice, hematuria and hemoglobinuria. It occurs most frequently in Sicily and southern Italy. It is apparently due to an idiosyncrasy to the pollen of the plant or to the ingested bean. Heredity, apparently, plays a part in some cases. Of the reported cases, about 40 per cent are due to inhalation from the blossom and 60 per cent to ingestion of the beans. The incubation period is from 2 to 6 hours when due to inhalation and usually 1 to 2 days following ingestion of the beans.

The *clinical features* are fever, sometimes with chills, vomiting, marked weakness with vertigo and unconsciousness in many cases. The fever varies greatly, is usually irregular and rarely above 103°. There is jaundice which comes on quickly and increases for about three days. Usually within an hour after the onset large quantities of bile are found in the urine. There may be nausea, vomiting and diarrhea. Hematuria occurs promptly and large amounts of blood and hemoglobin are passed in the urine. The anemia is acute; the red cells may fall rapidly to below 2,000,000. The blood platelets are considerably reduced. The blood serum of the patient has no hemolytic action on the patient's blood or on that of normal individuals. The *diagnosis* has to be made from other causes for hemoglobinuria. The history is important.

In *treatment* in the early stages with marked shock, epinephrine is indicated. In very severe anemia blood transfusion should be done. Large doses of iron are indicated in convalescence.

Anaphylaxis.—Some individuals have a hypersusceptibility to certain proteins and this may result in very diverse phenomena. The sensitization may be natural or acquired and may be due to absorption from the digestive tract. The features are very variable; in an infant susceptible to cow's milk there may be vomiting, diarrhea, urticaria, or erythema, dyspnea and prostration with a weak and rapid pulse. Angioneurotic edema results in some individuals. Some chronic skin affections, such as eczema, perhaps psoriasis, certain forms of erythema and urticaria, and some cases of asthma are due to this cause. Milk, eggs, meat, shell fish, strawberries, etc., are among the foods concerned. Duke has drawn attention to the importance of recognizing that severe *abdominal pain* may be due to food allergy. The use of skin tests made with the isolated protein is an important diagnostic measure.

In the *treatment* it may be possible to avoid the particular food to which the patient is sensitized. Otherwise an immunity may be obtained by giving very minute doses of the protein concerned, insufficient to produce a reaction, and gradually increasing the amount. Children often lose the hypersusceptibility as they grow older.

SECTION IV

DEFICIENCY DISEASES

PELLAGRA

Definition.—A deficiency disease, with periodical manifestations characterized by gastro-intestinal disturbances, skin lesions, and a tendency to changes in the nervous system.

Historical.—The disease appears to have been endemic in Spain by 1735 and the first description is by Cazal, who named it *mal de la rosa.* It existed in Italy in 1750 and was described in 1771 by Frapolli, who named it pellagra (rough skin). By the eighteenth century it had spread over northern Italy and appeared in France and Roumania. It is probable that there have been sporadic cases in the United States for the last hundred years.

Distribution.—The disease is prevalent in parts of southern Europe, particularly in Italy and Roumania. It exists in Spain, Portugal, France, Egypt and the United States, in the southern part of which country it spread with extraordinary rapidity some years ago. In 1930 there were 6,333 deaths in the U. S. registration area. The disease is sometimes one of particular localities, as beri-beri; it is a disease of the country more than of the cities in Europe, but in the United States many towns and villages show a number of cases. As regards the influence of place, the number of cases in asylums is significant. A few cases have occurred in England.

Etiology.—This has been the subject of much controversy and finality has not been reached. Diet plays a most important rôle in the causation, perhaps partly in the food balance and also in the lack of a pellagra preventive (P. P.) factor, vitamin G (B_2), but this is not proved to be a specific substance capable of curing pellagra. As regards the protein supply, "the dominating rôle of diet in the development of the disease would seem referable to a specific quality of the amino-acid makeup of the protein supply (Goldberger)." It may be that the deficiency is multiple and variable rather than single and constant. There may be interference with absorption both of proteins and vitamins from the intestinal tract. "Secondary pellagra" has appeared in patients who have taken a limited diet for some time on account of gastro-intestinal disease. The serum albumin in the blood is low, probably due to poor absorption of proteins. Yeast contains the largest amount of the preventive factor so far as known at present. It is possibly present in foods which contain the antineuritic vitamin. The view that an infection may have some influence can not be altogether discarded. Sensitization to light may play a part.

Age.—The disease occurs at any age, but the majority of cases are between twenty and forty years. As regards races, the negro is more susceptible than the white, and women are, as a rule, slightly more susceptible than men.

Occupation.—In Europe the disease is almost confined to laborers of the poorer classes, but this is not true of the United States.

Season.—The disease occurs particularly in the spring and sometimes in the autumn, both in its onset and recurrences.

Pathology.—There is nothing characteristic in the morbid anatomy. In the acute cases there may be atrophy of the walls of the intestines, fatty degeneration of the internal organs and changes in the nervous system. The alterations in the cord are fairly constant. There is degeneration of the lateral columns in the dorsal region and of the posterior columns in the cervical and dorsal regions. In the brains of patients with mental deterioration atrophy of the cerebrum is found. Osteoporosis may be present.

Symptoms.—These vary markedly in severity, usually appearing in the spring and sometimes in the autumn. There is always a tendency to recurrence, and with each succeeeding attack more damage is done, particularly to the nervous system. The onset is usually in the spring with indefinite symptoms, such as weakness, headache, and depression.

Digestive Tract.—Disturbance of the alimentary tract is usually an early symptom. In the mouth there may be sensations of heat, with loss of taste. Stomatitis and salivation are common, the mucous membrane is very red, ulcers may appear and the epithelium is stripped off, leaving a raw surface so that chewing is painful. Anorexia, nausea and vomiting are frequent; there is also diarrhea, sometimes dysentery, often severe and accompanied by pain, the stools being serous or bloody. It may alternate with constipation. Hydrochloric acid in the stomach is often absent or greatly reduced.

Skin.—The *erythema* usually begins on the backs of the hands and at first resembles an ordinary sunburn. There may be puffy swelling. The affected areas are symmetrical and sharply defined as a rule, extending above the wrist and down to the last finger joint. The face, neck and feet may be affected in the same way. The process may not advance any further, the skin becomes darker and desquamates, some pigmentation remaining. In other cases vesicles and bullae form, containing serum or pus. These dry gradually, with the production of fissures. After drying and desquamation the skin may have a dry appearance and a deep red color. With repeated attacks the skin may become indurated, thickened and dark; later atrophy and thinning follow. Exposure to the sun may have an influence on the eruption but is not the sole cause. The erythema occurs sometimes on protected parts. The pigmentation is supposed to be due to some substance of the phenyl group.

Nervous System.—Headache and vertigo are common. *Mental* features are often marked, among which are confusion, dullness, lassitude, irritability, feelings of anxiety and depression, change in the disposition, and hallucinations of sight and hearing. These may progress to profound depression and ultimately to dementia. Mania occurs sometimes and suicidal tendencies are not uncommon. The symptoms due to changes in the *cord* vary with the lesion. A spastic condition, disturbances of sensation, paralysis of the sphincters, or loss of the reflexes of the legs may be found.

The blood shows no special features beyond those of a secondary anemia. The temperature is usually normal except in some of the acute cases.

Clinical Forms.—The disease occurs in two main forms, an acute and a chronic recurrent form. In the *acute* form there are fever, marked prostration, severe diarrhea, delirium or stupor and a rapid downward course. Death may occur in a few weeks from the onset. These cases seem to be more frequent in the United States than in Europe. In the *chronic* form the manifestations are not severe, but tend to recur each year, and each attack leaves the patient in a worse condition. There is always the tendency to mental deterioration which occurs in fully 10 per cent of the cases. Death occurs from exhaustion and cachexia, or some intercurrent disease. Fortunately, succeeding attacks are not necessarily more severe than the preceding ones. There are instances of this form persisting for twenty-five years.

Cases without the skin lesions—pellagra sine pellagra—have been described.

Diagnosis.—A typical case offers no difficulties, but in the absence of the skin lesions considerable difficulty may be experienced. Scurvy might give difficulty, but the absence of the other features of pellagra should be conclusive. Skin lesions of the nature of erythema might cause confusion, but the absence of the general features removes doubt. The study of the stools differentiates it from sprue. The psychical features might suggest general paresis, but the skin lesions and digestive disturbance should make the diagnosis clear. The acute cases might be mistaken for various infections, but the erythema and gastrointestinal features should prevent this.

Prognosis.—In the United States the outlook is regarded as serious, if not as regards death, certainly as regards ultimate recovery. In Europe, the prognosis is more favorable, and in Italy in some years the mortality is only 4 per cent. In cases with acute features or fever the prognosis is grave and signs of severe toxemia or of mental involvement are ominous. Erythema of a moist character is regarded as a grave sign. Any complications should be regarded seriously. The prognosis is best in the chronic cases without mental features. The outlook is serious in asylum cases.

Prophylaxis.—Improvement in the living conditions and good sanitation are important. Too much corn or maize should not be used, particularly in institutions. A diet rich in animal protein food is the essential with a sufficient amount of milk, eggs, meat and vegetables, especially beans.

Treatment.—The patient should be placed in the best general conditions and a change of diet and climate is advisable. Rest in bed is necessary while the symptoms are acute. The diet should be as nutritious as possible and the diarrhea need not interfere with sufficient nourishment. Fresh milk, buttermilk, eggs, fresh meat, fresh or dried vegetables and tomato juice should be taken in full amounts. Yeast in some form should be given freely (℥½-1, 15-30 gm. of dried brewer's yeast) and also salt. Dilute hydrochloric acid (ʒ i, 4 cc. twice after each meal) should be taken. Arsenic by mouth, as Fowler's solution, is useful. Large doses of liver extract intramuscularly have given good results. It is specially indicated if there is difficulty in giving sufficient food by mouth. The use of autoclaved yeast and desiccated hog stomach has a marked effect on the mouth lesions. Sodium thiosulphate (0.5 gm.) may be given intravenously daily for at least 20 injections with liver extract intramuscularly. Transfusion of blood, both from healthy individuals and those who have recovered from the disease, has apparently given good results. Symptomatic treatment and a proper diet seem to have been as successful as any special measure.

Any other disease, such as hookworm infection, should receive treatment.

BERI-BERI

(*Kakke, Endemic Multiple Neuritis*)

Definition.—A disease due to deficiency of the antineuritic vitamin, and characterized by multiple neuritis, anasarca, and muscular atrophy.

It seems probable that several forms of multiple neuritis have been described under the term beri-beri. The form which is particularly common in China and Japan is due to a diet deficient in the antineuritic vitamin (water soluble B) which occurs in the outer layer of rice.

History.—The disease is believed to be of great antiquity in China and is possibly mentioned in the oldest known medical treatise. In the early years of the nineteenth century it attracted much attention among the Anglo-Indian surgeons, and we may date the modern scientific study of the disease from Malcolmson's monograph, published at Madras in 1835. The work of many investigators established the etiology.

Distribution.—It is specially prevalent among the Malays, Chinese and Japanese. It prevails in the Philippines. In India it is less common. Localized outbreaks have occurred in Australia. It prevails in parts of South America, and in the West Indies. It is met with among the fishermen of Norway and of the Newfoundland Banks. It occurs also in asylums, in which there have been severe outbreaks in the United States.

Etiology.—The deficiency is in the lack of the antineuritic vitamin which is present in the germ and pericarp of cereals, in peas, beans, carrots and potatoes, in milk, eggs, certain meats and in yeast. There is no special association with rice; in the areas where the disease is most prevalent, a large source of the vitamin is from rice in which it is situated in the pericarp. The occurrence of the disease on ships, in institutions and elsewhere is due to the same deficiency in the diet. Crowding, poor hygienic conditions and hot moist seasons seem to favor the occurrence of the disease. Some believe that infection is necessary in addition to the vitamin deficiency. Deficiency of protein may be a factor in the edema.

Morbid Anatomy.—The most constant and striking features are changes in the peripheral nerves and degenerative inflammation involving the axis cylinder and medullary sheaths. In acute cases this is found not only in the peripheral nerves, but also in the vagus and phrenic. The fibres of the voluntary muscles, as well as of the myocardium, are much degenerated. Myocardial degeneration is usually marked. The changes are regarded as due largely to water retention and swelling, especially in the nerves and striated muscles.

Symptoms.—The disease occurs in various forms:

The INCOMPLETE OR RUDIMENTARY FORM sets in with catarrhal symptoms, followed by pains and weakness in the limbs and a lowering of the sensibility in the legs, with the occurrence of paresthesia. Slight edema sometimes appears. After a time paresthesia is felt in other parts of the body, and the patient may complain of palpitation of the heart, uneasy sensations in the abdomen, and sometimes shortness of breath. There may be weakness and tenderness of the muscles. After a few days to months, these symptoms disappear, but there may be a recurrence.

The ATROPHIC FORM sets in with much the same symptoms, but the loss of power in the limbs progresses more rapidly, and soon the patient is no longer able to walk or to move the arms. The atrophy, which is associated with a good deal of pain, may extend to the muscles of the face. The edematous symptoms and heart disturbance play a minor rôle in this form, which is known as the dry or paralytic variety.

WET OR DROPSICAL FORM.—Setting in as in the rudimentary variety, *edema* becomes the most marked feature, extending over the whole subcutaneous tissue, and with effusions into the serous sacs. The edema may be due largely to low plasma protein with added myocardial weakness. The electrocardiographic findings suggest myocardial change. The atrophy of the muscles and disturbance of sensation are not so prominent but palpitation and rapid action of the heart and dyspnea are common. The wasting may not be apparent until the dropsy disappears.

The ACUTE, PERNICIOUS, OR CARDIAC FORM is characterized by acute cardiac failure, especially of the right heart, coming on rapidly after the existence of slight symptoms. Degeneration of the vagi may be responsible. Death may follow within twenty-four hours; more commonly the symptoms extend over several weeks. Widespread paralysis with anesthesia may be present.

The mortality varies greatly, from 2 or 3 per cent to 40 or 50 per cent among the coolies in certain settlements of the Malay Archipelago.

Diagnosis.—In tropical countries there is rarely any difficulty. In cases of peripheral neuritis, associated with edema, coming from tropical ports, the possibility of this disease should be remembered. The peculiar epidemic dropsy of Calcutta and Bengal is probably beri-beri. Greig has shown it to be a nutritional disorder associated with the use of polished rice.

Prophylaxis.—Much has been done to prevent the disease by diets containing sufficient amounts of vitamins such as beans, peas, barley, potatoes, eggs and fresh meat. Polished rice should not be used for food.

Treatment.—It is a very chronic and obstinate malady. A nutritious diet rich in the lacking vitamin, rest in bed, purgation for the dropsy, cardiac stimulants, and the usual measures for the neuritis are the important factors. Dry powdered yeast (one ounce a day) or the concentrated form and malt extract are especially useful. Salicylates and saline laxatives are used in Japan. If the cardiac features are marked the usual treatment with active stimulation should be employed. Prolonged rest is important if myocardial changes are present. When the edema has subsided massage, passive movements, and electricity may be used for the atrophic muscles.

SCURVY

Definition.—A disorder of metabolism due to deficiency of antiscorbutic vitamin C, characterized by great debility, with anemia, a spongy condition of the gums, and a tendency to hemorrhages.

Etiology.—The disease has been known from the earliest times, and has prevailed particularly in armies in the field and among sailors on long voyages. It has been well called "the calamity of sailors." Owing largely to the efforts of Lind and to a knowledge of the etiological conditions, scurvy has disappeared from the naval service. In the mercantile marine cases still occasionally occur, owing to the lack of proper food.

In parts of Russia scurvy is endemic. In the United States scurvy is not a very rare disease. To the hospitals in the seaport towns sailors are now and then admitted with it. In large almshouses outbreaks occasionally occur. A great increase of foreign population of a low grade has made the disease not uncommon in certain districts. In the mining districts of Pennsylvania the Hungarian, Bohemian and Italian settlers are sometimes attacked. Their diet may be composed largely of bread, coffee and meat. Occasionally one meets with scurvy among quite well-to-do people. In Great Britain and Ireland it has become rare. It is not uncommon in the South African natives.

The essential cause is a lack of the antiscorbutic vitamin C. This is present in green vegetables, fresh fruit juices, especially of oranges and lemons, in roots and tubers, in tomatoes and in small amounts in milk. It is very sensitive to oxidation, heat and drying and is destroyed by alkalies (hence the effect of sodium bicarbonate when used in cooking vegetables).

Other factors may play a slight part, particularly bad hygienic conditions —overcrowding, cold, damp quarters, and prolonged fatigue under depressing influences. Exposure to scorbutic conditions for four to six months is usually necessary. The disease attacks all ages. Sex has no influence, but during the siege of Paris the males attacked were greatly in excess of the females.

Morbid Anatomy.—The anatomical changes are marked but not specific, and are chiefly those associated with hemorrhage. The skin shows the ecchymoses evident during life. There are hemorrhages into the muscles, under the periosteum, and occasionally about or even into the joints. Hemorrhages occur particularly on the serous membranes and in the kidneys and bladder. The gums are swollen and sometimes ulcerated. Ulcers are occasionally met with in the ileum and colon. Hemorrhages into the mucous membranes are extremely common. The spleen is enlarged and soft. Parenchymatous changes are constant in the liver, kidneys, and heart. Fragility of the bones may be found and changes in the bone marrow.

Symptoms.—The disease is insidious in its onset. Early symptoms are loss in weight, progressive weakness, pains in the legs and pallor. Swelling of the pinna of the ear, which may extend to the scalp, has been noted early. Very soon the gums become swollen and spongy, bleed easily, and in extreme cases present a fungous appearance. These changes, regarded as characteristic, are sometimes absent. The teeth may become loose and even fall out. Actual necrosis of the jaw is not common. The breath is excessively foul. The tongue is swollen, but may be red and not much furred. The salivary glands are occasionally enlarged. *Hemorrhages* beneath the mucous membranes of the mouth, especially on the hard palate, are common. The skin becomes dry and rough, and ecchymoses soon appear, first on the legs and then on the arms and trunk, and particularly into and about the hair-follicles. They are petechial, but may become larger, and when subcutaneous may cause distinct swellings. In severe cases, particularly in the legs, there may be effusion between the periosteum and the bone, forming irregular nodes, which may break down and form foul-looking sores. The slightest bruise or injury causes hemorrhages into the injured part. Edema about the ankles is common. The "*scurvy sclerosis*," seen oftenest in the legs, is a remarkable infiltration of the subcutaneous tissues and muscles, forming a brawny induration, the skin over which may be blood-stained. Hemorrhages from the mucous membranes are less constant; epistaxis is, however, frequent. Conjunctival hemorrhage is not uncommon and retinal hemorrhage may occur. Hemoptysis and hematemesis are uncommon. Hematuria, often microscopic, is common and bleeding from the bowels may occur in severe cases.

Palpitation of the heart with a feeble and irregular impulse is common. The heart may be enlarged, especially the right ventricle, and the rate increased. A murmur can usually be heard at the base. Lowered capillary resistance is sometimes found. Secondary anemia is usual; the leukocytes vary and there may be a leukopenia or an increase with lymphocytosis. Hemorrhagic infarction of the lungs and spleen has been described. Respiratory symptoms are not common. The appetite is impaired, and owing to the soreness of the gums the patient is unable to chew. Constipation is more frequent than diarrhea. The urine is often albuminous, the amount usually reduced and the specific gravity high.

There are mental depression, indifference, in some cases headache, and in the later stages delirium. Cases of convulsions, or hemiplegia, and of meningeal hemorrhage have been described. Remarkable ocular symptoms are occasionally met with, such as night-blindness or day-blindness, associated with anemia of the retina. Changes in the optic disk have been found.

In advanced cases necrosis of the bones may occur, and in young persons even separation of the epiphyses. There are instances in which the cartilages have separated from the sternum. The callus of a recent fracture may undergo destruction. Fever is not present, except in the later stages, or when secondary inflammations in the internal organs appear. The temperature may be below normal. Acute arthritis is an occasional complication.

Diagnosis.—No difficulty is met in the recognition of scurvy when a number of persons are affected together. In isolated cases the disease is distinguished with difficulty from certain forms of purpura. Mercurial stomatitis does not show the other features of scurvy and acute leukemia is recognized by the blood picture. The association with manifest insufficiency in diet and the rapid amelioration with suitable food are helpful points.

Prognosis.—The outlook is good, unless the disease is far advanced and the conditions persist which led to its occurrence. Death results from heart-failure, occasionally with sudden syncope. Meningeal hemorrhage, gangrene of the lung, extravasation into the serous cavities, enterocolitis, and intercurrent affections may prove fatal.

Prophylaxis.—This depends on a proper supply of antiscorbutic vitamin. The fresh juice of oranges and lemons, fresh uncooked vegetables, tomatoes (fresh or canned), cabbage, potatoes, meat and milk are the most useful.

Treatment.—The juice of two or three lemons or oranges daily and a full diet of meat and fresh vegetables suffice to cure all cases unless far advanced. When the stomach is much disordered, small quantities of scraped meat and milk should be given at short intervals, and orange juice in increasing quantities. Mashed potato, mixed with milk, is useful. As the patient gains in strength the diet may be more liberal, and he may eat freely of potatoes, cabbage, water-cress and lettuce. For the stomatitis a permanganate of potash (1-2 per cent) or dilute phenol (0.5 per cent) solution forms a good mouth-wash. A solution of nitrate of silver applied to the gums is useful. Ascorbic acid (cevitamic acid) acts as vitamin C and is given intravenously in doses of 40 mg. in 3 cc. of normal saline solution daily. The constipation is best treated by enemata. For conditions such as hemorrhage and ulceration suitable measures must be employed.

INFANTILE SCURVY (*Barlow's Disease*)

A special form of scurvy occurs in children which differs from the adult form only in the changes occuring in structures which are different in early life. W. B. Cheadle and Gee, in London, described in very young children a cachexia associated with hemorrhage. Cheadle regarded the cases as scurvy ingrafted on a rickety stock. Gee called his cases periosteal cachexia. The condition had previously been regarded as acute rickets. Barlow made an exhaustive study of the affection with careful anatomical observations and it is now recognized as infantile scurvy and called Barlow's disease.

Etiology.—The disease usually appears between the sixth and twelfth month and is rare after the second year. The essential cause is the absence of the antiscorbutic vitamin. A diet of condensed or malted milk seems to be most often responsible, sometimes sterilized or boiled milk, pasteurized milk rarely. In the rare cases in which the child has been breast fed, the mother's diet was insufficient in the antiscorbutic vitamin.

Symptoms.—The following summary is taken from Barlow:

"So long as it is left alone the child is tolerably quiet; the lower limbs are kept drawn up and still; but when placed in its bath or otherwise moved there is continuous crying, and it soon becomes clear that the pain is connected with the lower limbs. At this period the upper limbs may be touched with impunity, but any attempt to move the legs or thighs gives rise to screams. Next, some obscure swelling may be detected, first on one lower limb, then on the other, though it is not absolutely symmetrical. . . . The swelling is ill-defined, but is suggestive of thickening round the shafts of the bones, beginning above the epiphyseal junctions. Gradually the bulk of the limbs affected becomes visibly increased. . . . The position of the limbs becomes somewhat different from what it was at the outset. Instead of being flexed they lie everted and immobile, in a state of pseudoparalysis. . . . About this time, if not before, great weakness of the back becomes manifest. A little swelling of one or both scapulae may appear, and the upper limbs may show changes. These are rarely so considerable as the alterations in the lower limbs. There may be swelling above the wrists, extending for a short distance up the forearm, and some swelling in the neighborhood of the epiphyses of the humerus. There is symmetry of lesions, but it is not absolute; and the limb affection is generally consecutive, though the involvement of one limb follows very close upon another. The joints are free. In severe cases crepitus in the regions adjacent to the junctions of the shafts with epiphyses may be found. The upper and lower extremities of the femur, and the upper extremity of the tibia, are the common sites of such fractures; but the upper end of the humerus may also be so affected. . . . A very startling appearance may be observed at this period in the front of the chest. The sternum, with the adjacent costal cartilages and a small portion of the contiguous ribs, seems to have sunk bodily back, *en bloc*, as though it had been subjected to some violence which had fractured several ribs in the front and driven them back. Occasionally thickenings of varying extent may be found on the exterior of the vault of the skull, or even on some of the bones of the face. . . . There develops a rather sudden proptosis of one eyeball, with puffiness and very slight staining of the upper lid. Within a day or two the other eye presents similar appearances, though they may be of less severity. The ocular conjunctiva may show a little ecchymosis, or may be quite free. With respect to the constitutional symptoms the most important feature is the profound anemia. . . . The anemia is proportional to the amount of limb involvement. As the case proceeds there is a certain earthy-colored or sallow tint, which is noteworthy in severe cases, and when once this is established bruise-like ecchymoses may appear, and more rarely small purpura. Emaciation is not a marked feature, but asthenia is extreme and suggestive of muscular failure. The temperature is very erratic; it is often raised for a day or two, when successive limbs are involved, especially during the tense stage, but is rarely above 101° or 102° F. At other times it may be normal or subnormal."

If the teeth have appeared the gums may be spongy.

The essential lesion is a subperiosteal blood extravasation, which causes the thickening and tenderness in the shafts of the bones. In some instances there is hemorrhage in the intramuscular tissue. There may be intracranial hemorrhage. Petechiae and subcutaneous hemorrhages are rare; *hematuria* is the only common hemorrhage.

Diagnosis.—In young children with difficulty in moving the legs, or in whom paralysis is suspected, the condition should always be looked for. What is known sometimes as Parrot's disease, or syphilitic pseudoparalysis, may be confounded with it. In it the loss of motion is more or less sudden in the arms or legs or in both, due to a solution of continuity and separation of the cartilage at the end of the diaphysis. There are usually crepitation and much pain on movement. The diagnosis from osteomyelitis or epiphysitis may be difficult but high fever is against scurvy and the X-ray study is of aid. Rheumatic fever is rare below the age of two years. In mild forms of scurvy the tenderness on handling or a puzzling hematuria may be the most marked features.

A study of the diet and the results of treatment are important aids.

The *prophylaxis* is most important. The proprietary forms of condensed milk and preserved foods for infants should not be used. The fresh or pasteurized cow's milk should be given and a teaspoonful of meat-juice or gravy may be added with a little mashed potato. After the first month every infant on artificial feeding should be given one teaspoonful of orange juice (with a little sugar if sour), increased to half an ounce at three months of age.

Treatment.—The child should be handled carefully, carried on a pillow and the affected part supported by light splints or wrapped in cotton wool with a light bandage. Orange juice or lemon juice should be given freely and foods containing the antiscorbutic vitamin. Ascorbic acid may be given by mouth in doses of 20-40 mg. daily. Recovery is usually prompt and satisfactory.

RICKETS (RACHITIS)

Definition.—A disease of infants and young children, characterized by impaired general nutrition and alterations in the growing bones.

Glisson accurately described the disease in 1650. The name is derived from the old English word *wrickken*, to twist. Glisson suggested to change the name to rachitis, from the Greek ϱ ἄ χ ι ς , the spine, as it was one of the first parts affected, and also from the similarity in the sound to rickets.

Etiology.—Rickets exists in all parts of the world, but particularly among the poor of the larger cities, who are badly housed and ill fed. In the cities of the United States it is prevalent, particularly among the children of the negro and Italian races. There is a seasonal incidence associated with the amount of sunlight; rickets increases in the autumn and through the winter reaching its maximum in March. Rickets affects male and female children equally. It is particularly a disease of the first and second years of life. Jenner described a late rickets, in which the disease may not appear until the ninth or even the twelfth year, or later (the osteomalacia of puberty). There is no evidence that the disease is hereditary or due to syphilis. Poor hygienic conditions, apart from lack of sunlight, probably play a part. The disease is often seen in children in whose diet there is a large amount of carbohydrate but little animal fat. The essential factor is lack of vitamin D. There may be interference with absorption of the vitamin from the intestinal tract.

There is a failure of calcification of the bones associated with a change in the proportions of calcium and phosphorus in the blood. Normally there is 10 mg. of calcium in 100 cc. of blood and the calcium content is normal in rickets but the phosphorus content of 5 mg. usually falls below 3 mg. per 100 cc. of blood. The diminished phosphorus content is associated with a decrease of vitamin D in the diet or insufficient formation of this vitamin in the body. This vitamin is present in animal fats in various amounts and in human milk; cod-liver oil is an abundant source. It is also formed in the skin by the influence of ultra-violet radiations, from sunlight or from artificial ultraviolet rays, on cholesterol in the skin. Ergosterol, after treatment with ultraviolet rays (viosterol), is powerfully antirachitic.

Morbid Anatomy.—Glisson's original description of the external appearances of a rickety child is remarkably complete; indeed, his monograph is an enduring monument to the skill and powers of observation of this great physician. "(1) An irregular or unusual proportion of its parts. The head is evidently larger than normal, and the face fatter in respect to the other parts. . . . (2) The external members and muscles of the whole body are seen to be delicate and emaciated, as though consumed by atrophy or tabes, and this (so far as we know) is always observed in those dead of this affection. (3) The whole skin, both the true and the fleshy and fatty layers, is flaccid and rather pendulous, like a loose glove, so that you think it could hold much more flesh. (4) About the joints, especially in the wrists and ankles, there are certain protuberances which, if opened, are seen to arise, not in the fleshy or membranous parts, but in the ends of the bones themselves, especially in their epiphyses. (5) The joints, limbs, and habitus of all these external parts are less firm and rigid, less inflexible than in other dead bodies, and the neck scarcely becomes rigid, *a frigore*, postmortem, or to a less extent than in other cadavers. (6) The chest externally is thin and much narrowed, especially beneath the scapulae, as though compressed from the sides, and the sternum acuminated like the keel of a ship or the breast of a fowl. (7) The ends of the ribs which join with the cartilages of the sternum are nodular, like the ends of the wrists and ankles." He also described the prominent abdomen, the enlarged liver, and the changes in the mesenteric glands.

The *bones* show the most important changes, particularly the ends of the long bones and the ribs. Between the shaft and epiphyses a slight bulging is apparent, and, on section the zone of proliferation, which normally is represented by two narrow bands, is greatly thickened, bluish in color, more irregular in outline, and very much softer. The width of this cushion of cartilage varies from 5 to 15 mm. The line of ossification is irregular and more spongy and vascular than normal. The periosteum strips off readily from the shaft, and beneath it there may be a spongy tissue not unlike decalcified bone. The outcome is imperfect ossification, so that the bone has neither the natural rate of growth nor the normal firmness. In the cranium there may be areas, particularly in the parieto-occipital region, in which ossification is delayed, so that the bone yields readily to pressure. There are localized depressed spots of atrophy, which give the so-called "parchment crackling." Flat hyperostoses arise on the outer table, particularly on the frontal and parietal bones, producing the characteristic broad forehead with prominent frontal eminences, sometimes mistaken for hydrocephalus. The analysis of rickety bones shows a marked diminution in calcium, which may be as low as 25 or 35 per cent instead of the normal 60 per cent.

The liver and spleen are usually enlarged, and sometimes the mesenteric glands. As Gee suggested, these conditions probably result from the general state of the health associated with rickets. Beneke has described a relative increase in the size of the arteries in rickets.

Symptoms.—The disease comes on insidiously about the period of dentition, before the child begins to walk. Mild grades of it are often overlooked. In many cases digestive disturbances precede the appearance of the characteristic lesions, and the nutrition is impaired. There is usually slight fever, the child is irritable and restless, and sleeps badly. If he has already walked, he now shows a marked disinclination to do so, and seems feeble and unsteady in his gait. Sir William Jenner called attention to three features of importance: First, a diffuse *soreness* of the body, so that the child cries when an attempt is made to move him and prefers to keep perfectly still. Secondly, *slight fever* (100° to 101.5° F.), with nocturnal restlessness and a tendency to throw off the bedclothes. This may be due to the fact that the general sensitiveness is such that their weight is distressing. Thirdly, profuse *sweating*, particularly about the head and neck, so that the pillow is soaked with perspiration.

The tissues become soft and flabby; the skin is pale; and from a healthy, plump condition the child becomes puny and feeble. The muscular weakness may be marked, particularly in the legs, and paralysis may be suspected. This so-called pseudoparesis of rickets results in part from the flabby, weak condition of the legs and in part from the pain associated with the movements. Coincident with, or following closely upon, the general symptoms the characteristic *skeletal lesions* are observed. Among the first are the changes in the ribs, at the junction of the bone with the cartilage, forming the so-called *rickety rosary*. When the child is thin these nodules may be distinctly seen, and in any case can be easily felt. They rarely appear before the third month. They may increase in size up to the second year, and are rarely seen after the fifth year. The thorax undergoes important changes. Just outside the junction of the cartilages with the ribs there is an oblique, shallow depression extending downward and outward. A transverse curve, called Harrison's groove, passes outward from the level of the ensiform cartilage toward the axilla, and may be deepened at each inspiration. It is rendered more prominent by the eversion and prominence of the costal border. The sternum may project, particularly in its lower half, forming the pigeon or chicken breast. These changes in the thorax are not peculiar to rickets, and may be associated with hypertrophy of the tonsils, or anything which interferes with the free entrance of air into the lungs. The spine is often curved posteriorly, the processes are prominent; lateral curvature is not so common.

The *head* of a rickety child usually looks large in proportion to the body and the face, and the fontanelles remain open for a long time. There are areas, particularly in the parieto-occipital regions, in which ossification is imperfect; and the bone may yield to the pressure of the finger, to which the term *craniotabes* has been given. Coincidentally with this, hyperplasia proceeds in the frontal and parietal eminences, so that these increase in thickness, and may form irregular bosses. In one type the skull may be large and elongated, with the top considerably flattened. In another, and perhaps more common, case the shape of the skull, when seen from above, is rectangular—the *caput quadratum.* The forehead is broad and square, and the frontal eminences marked. The anterior fontanelle is late in closing, and may remain open until the third or fourth year. The skin is thin, the veins are full and prominent, and the hair is often rubbed from the back of the skull.

A systolic murmur may frequently be heard over the anterior fontanelle or in the temporal region. This, first described by John D. Fisher, of Boston, in 1883, is heard with the greatest frequency in rickets, but its presence in healthy infants has been amply demonstrated. The murmur is rarely present after the fifth year. A knowledge of the existence of this murmur may prevent errors. A case was reported as an instance of tumor of the brain.

Changes occur in the bones of the face, chiefly in the maxillae, which are reduced in size. The normal process of dentition is much disturbed and late teething is a marked feature. The teeth may be small and badly formed.

Changes in the scapulae are not common. The clavicle may be thickened at the sternal end and near the attachment of the sternocleidomastoid muscle. The most noticeable changes are at the lower ends of the radius and ulna. The enlargement is at the junction-area of the shaft and epiphysis. Less evident enlargements may occur at the lower end of the humerus. In severe cases the natural shape of the bones of the arm may be much altered, since they have had to support the weight of the child in crawling on the floor. The changes in the pelvis are of special importance, particularly in female children, as in extreme cases they lead to great deformity. In the legs, the lower end of the tibia first becomes enlarged; and in slight cases it may alone be affected. In the severe forms the upper end of the bone, the corresponding parts of the fibula, and the lower end of the femur become greatly thickened. If the child walks, slight bowing of the tibiae inevitably results. In more advanced cases the tibiae, and even the femora, may be arched forward. In other instances knock-knee occurs. Unquestionably the chief cause of these deformities is the weight of the body, but muscular action takes part in it. The green-stick fracture is not uncommon in the soft bones of rickets.

These changes in the skeleton proceed slowly, and the general symptoms vary a good deal with their progress. The child may become emaciated, though "fat rickets" is by no means uncommon, and a child may be well nourished but "pasty" and flabby. Fever is not constant, but in actively progressing changes in the bone there is usually a slight pyrexia. The abdomen is large, "pot-bellied," due partly to flatulent distention, partly to enlargement of the liver, and in severe cases to diminution of the volume of the thorax. The spleen is often enlarged and readily palpable. The urine is stated to contain an excess of lime salts. There is usually some secondary anemia; a leukocytosis may or may not be present; it is more common with enlargement of the spleen (Morse). Many rickety children show marked nervous symptoms; irritability and sleeplessness are present. Jenner called attention to the close relationship between rickets and infantile convulsions, particularly to the fits which occur after the sixth month. Tetany is by no means uncommon. Laryngismus stridulus is a common complication and more frequent in rickety children. Rachitic children are very susceptible to respiratory-tract infections. Severe rickets interferes seriously with the growth of a child. Extreme examples of rickety dwarfs are not uncommon.

Late Rickets.—The disease may set in from the tenth to the fourteenth year, either for the first time or in a child rickety in infancy. The long bones are involved, with enlargement of the epiphyses and a marked tendency to deformity.

Diagnosis.—The condition exists before we can diagnose it clinically. In ordinary cases, the open fontanelle, delayed dentition and the changes in the bones are characteristic, but it is often overlooked because not looked for. The radiographic picture is characteristic, especially of the lower ends of the radius, ulna and femur. The bones show a diminished shadow due to imperfect ossification. The ends of the bones are broadened, the surface irregular with a shadowy fringe, and concave and irregular. Development of the carpal bones may be delayed.

Prognosis.—The disease is rarely in itself fatal, but the condition of the child is such that it is readily carried off by intercurrent affections, particularly those of the respiratory organs. The loss of rigidity in the thorax results in a reduction in its size and loss of the power of expansion. Spasm of the larynx and convulsions occasionally cause death. In females the deformity of the pelvis is serious, as it may lead to difficulties in parturition.

Prevention.—The better the condition of the mother during pregnancy the less likelihood there is of rickets in the child. Of the general treatment, attention to the feeding of the child is important. If the mother is unhealthy, or can not nurse the child, a suitable wet-nurse should be provided, or the child must be artificially fed, in which case cow's milk, diluted according to the age of the child, should constitute the chief food. Later sufficient fat should be given and too much starchy food avoided. Cereals should not be given until the child is nine months of age and small amounts only for the first two years. Egg yolk is useful; half the yolk of a raw egg can be given to infants of one or two months and the whole yolk after this age. Small amounts of cod-liver oil (10 drops three times a day) and exposure to sunlight for two hours a day are preventive. Viosterol may be given in doses of 10 drops a day. Some advise this during the winter months, others at all times until the child is taking a mixed diet. *Ultraviolet radiation* given for 15 minutes a month prevents rickets in infants up to eight months of age. The intervals between exposures should not be over two weeks. At first exposures of one minute anteriorly and posteriorly may be given and increased by one minute each exposure up to five minutes front and back with a total of ten minutes per week.

Treatment.—The child should be warmly clad and in the open air and sunshine as much as possible. The child should be bathed daily in warm water. Careful friction with sweet oil is advantageous, and, if properly performed, allays rather than aggravates the sensitiveness. Special care should be taken to prevent deformity. The child should not be allowed to walk, and for this purpose splints applied so as to extend beyond the feet are very effective. There are three specifics—cod-liver oil, sunlight or ultraviolet light rays and irradiated ergosterol (viosterol). The cod-liver oil does not require to be given in large doses—10 drops three times a day is enough. The exposure to sunlight for two hours a day is sufficient. The ultraviolet rays should be given for gradually increasing periods (one to twenty minutes). Care should be taken not to blister the skin. The dose of viosterol is 10 drops per day. There seems to be a possibility of harm from overdosage in young children. The syrup of the iodide of iron may be given if there is anemia. The digestive disturbances, together with the complications, should receive appropriate treatment. Orthopedic treatment may be required for the deformities.

SECTION V

DISEASES OF METABOLISM

GOUT (PODAGRA)

Definition.—A disorder of metabolism associated with retention of uric acid and of other purin bodies in the body, characterized clinically by attacks of acute arthritis, the deposition of sodium urate in and about the joints, and by the occurrence of irregular constitutional symptoms.

Etiology.—The purin bodies, adenin, guanin, hypoxanthin, xanthin, and uric acid, result from the transformation of the nucleoproteins of the food and of the tissues by ferments or enzymes, each one of which has its own specific action. Among the proteolytic enzymes nuclease has a universal distribution, and, no matter what the source of the nucleoprotein, it sets free adenin and guanin. Specific enzymes also liberate uric acid from the nucleoproteins of the tissues and from the purins of the food. Once formed, the difficulty is to get rid of uric acid, and this appears to be one essential factor in the etiology of gout. Birds and serpents, unable to oxidize it, excrete large quantities. "All mammals, with the important exception of man, are able to destroy uric acid rapidly and in considerable quantities. This destruction is an oxidation accomplished by a specific enzyme called uricase, and the reaction seems to consist of the removal of one of the carbon atoms from the uric acid, thus converting it into the more readily soluble allantoin" (Wells). These transforming enzymes are variously distributed in the body; nuclease is present in all cells, adenase and the xanthin enzyme are not so widely distributed. Uricase, on which the uricolytic power of the different tissues depends, is present chiefly in the liver and kidneys of mammals, and to a less degree in the muscles. Man alone seems to have a difficulty in oxidizing uric acid. Even on a purin-free diet he excretes daily a certain amount, and purin-rich food is followed by a rise. In other mammals it is oxidized into allantoin, of which human urine never contains more than a trace.

Gout, then, can not be regarded as loss of the power of a given individual to destroy uric acid, since this does not appear to be an active function in the human body. Loss of power to *eliminate* favors the deposition of uric acid, and individuals who can not get rid easily of their purins, endogenous or exogenous, may be said to be gouty.

There is a form of gout in swine, characterized by a deposit of guanin in the muscles—the chalky flakes so often seen in Virginia and Westphalian hams—and the pig's liver is deficient in the enzyme guanase, which in other animals oxidizes this purin body. We can not say how great is the part played by uric acid in human gout and how much by the other purin bodies, but the tendency is to regard *imperfect elimination* rather than imperfect oxidation of the purin bodies as the chief factor.

The normal daily output of uric acid is from 0.4 to 1.5 gm., and it is greater by day than by night. The amount from the intake of the exogenous oxypurins varies from 40 to 60 per cent of the total purin content. The more active the functions of the body the greater the discharge. Severe exertion, fever and exposure to cold increase the output. The amount is greatly influenced by food, particularly when rich in purin bases; after a meal containing sweetbread the amount may be doubled. In gouty persons the output is low, and there are cases of gout in which, in the intervals between attacks, the excretion was nil (Futcher). With an attack the output rises, and the phosphoric acid is greatly increased (Chart XV).

Predisposing Factors.—*Heredity* is important. In from 50 per cent to 75 per cent of all cases the disease existed in the ancestors, and the transmission is more marked on the male side. Males are more subject than females. It is rarely seen before the thirtieth year, though cases have occurred before puberty, and even in infants at the breast.

Alcohol is an important factor in the etiology. Fermented liquors are more apt to cause it than distilled spirits, and the disease is more common in England and Germany, the countries which consume the largest amount of beer *per capita.* The disease is not uncommon in the United States and, as Futcher pointed out, gout is only one-third less frequent at the Johns Hopkins Hospital than at St. Bartholomew's Hospital, London. Among 18,000 patients (J. H. H.) there were 59 cases of gout; all but three in whites, and all in males but two (Futcher).

Food plays a rôle of importance and overeating without exercise is a predisposing cause. But the disease is by no means confined to the well-to-do. A combination of poor food, defective hygiene and the excessive consumption of malt liquors makes "poor man's gout" not infrequent.

Occupation is of great importance, and the disease is much more common in workers in breweries, and in persons who deal in any way with alcohol.

It is not uncommon in persons of great mental and bodily vigor. Among distinguished members of our profession who have been terrible sufferers were the elder Scaliger, Jerome Cardan and Sydenham. The statement of the last, that "more wise men than fools are victims" does not hold good to-day. The celebrated Pirckheimer wrote a famous "Apology for Gout" (1521), and there is much truth in what Podagra says: "For I take no pleasure in those hard, rough, rusticke, agresticke kind of people, who never are at rest, but always exercise their bodies with hard labors, are ever moyling and toyling, do seldom or never give themselves to pleasure, do endure hunger, which are content with a slender diet." (English Edition, 1617.)

Among the direct *exciting causes* of an attack is a meal with large quantities of rich food and alcohol; worry, or a mental shock, and in sensitive persons a slight injury or accident may be followed by an acute attack.

Pathology.—The *blood* contains an excess of uric acid. The normal figures are 2 to 4 mg. per 100 cc. of blood by the new method of Folin and Benedict. Figures above 5 mg. per 100 cc. are definitely abnormal. The high uric acid content is generally constant and the amount is apparently greater during an attack than in the intervals. This excess is not peculiar to gout, but occurs in leukemia, lead poisoning and severe nephritis. The red cells in the "lead-gout" cases may show basophilic granular staining.

The important changes are in the articular tissues. The first joint of the great toe is frequently involved but not always; then the ankles, knees, and the small joints of the hands and wrists. The deposits may be in all the joints of the legs and absent from those of the arms (Moore). If death takes place during an acute paroxysm, there are signs of inflammation, hyperemia, swelling of the ligamentous tissues, and effusion into the joint. The primary change, according to Ebstein, is a local necrosis, due to the presence of an excess of urates in the blood. This is seen in the cartilage and other articular tissues in which the nutritional currents are slow. The excess of uric acid in the serum may act as a potential exciting cause capable of determining a local reaction, with urate deposit, when some provocative agent is associated. The articular cartilages are first involved with the gouty deposit uniform or in small areas. Though it looks superficial, the deposit is invariably interstitial and covered by a thin lamina of cartilage. The deposit is thickest at the part most distant from the circulation. The ligaments and fibrocartilage ultimately become involved and are infiltrated with urate deposits, the so-called chalk-stones or tophi. These are usually covered by skin; but in some cases, particularly in the metacarpophalangeal articulations, this ulcerates and the chalk-stones appear externally. The synovial fluid may also contain crystals. In long-standing cases, owing to an excessive deposit, the joint becomes immobile. The marginal outgrowths in gouty arthritis are true exostoses (Wynne). The cartilage of the ear may contain tophi, which are seen as whitish nodules at the margin of the helix. The cartilages of the nose, eyelids, and larynx are less frequently affected.

The changes in the *renal* and *vascular* systems are important. The kidney changes are: (*a*) A deposit of urates chiefly in the region of the papillae but this is less common than usually supposed; Moore found it in only 12 of 80 cases. The apices of the pyramids show lines of whitish deposit. Ebstein described areas of necrosis in both cortex and medulla, in which were crystalline deposits of sodium urate. (*b*) An interstitial nephritis, either the ordinary "contracted kidney" or the arteriosclerotic form, neither of which is in any way distinctive. (*c*) Arteriosclerosis and cardiac hypertrophy are frequent. Concretions of sodium urate may occur on the valves. Myocarditis is common.

Changes in the respiratory system are rare. Deposits have been found in the vocal cords, and uric-acid crystals have been found in the sputum of a gouty patient (J. W. Moore).

Symptoms.—Gout is divided into acute, chronic, and irregular forms.

Acute Gout.—Premonitory symptoms are common—twinges of pain in the small joints of the hands or feet, nocturnal restlessness, irritability of temper and dyspepsia. The urine is acid, scanty and high-colored and there may be transient albuminuria. There may be traces of sugar (gouty glycosuria). Before an attack the output of uric acid is low and is also diminished in the early part of the paroxysm. The relation of uric and phosphoric acids to the acute attacks is represented in Chart XV, prepared by Futcher. Both may be extremely low in the intervals, but reach normal limits shortly after the onset of the acute symptoms. The phosphoric acid and uric acid show almost parallel curves. The patient was on a very light fixed diet at the time the determinations were made. In some instances the throat is sore, and there may be dyspnea. The *attack* sets in usually in the early morning hours. The patient is aroused by a severe pain in the affected joint or joints. The tarsus is often involved, sometimes alone. The pain is agonizing, and, as Sydenham says, "insinuates itself with the most exquisite cruelty among the numerous

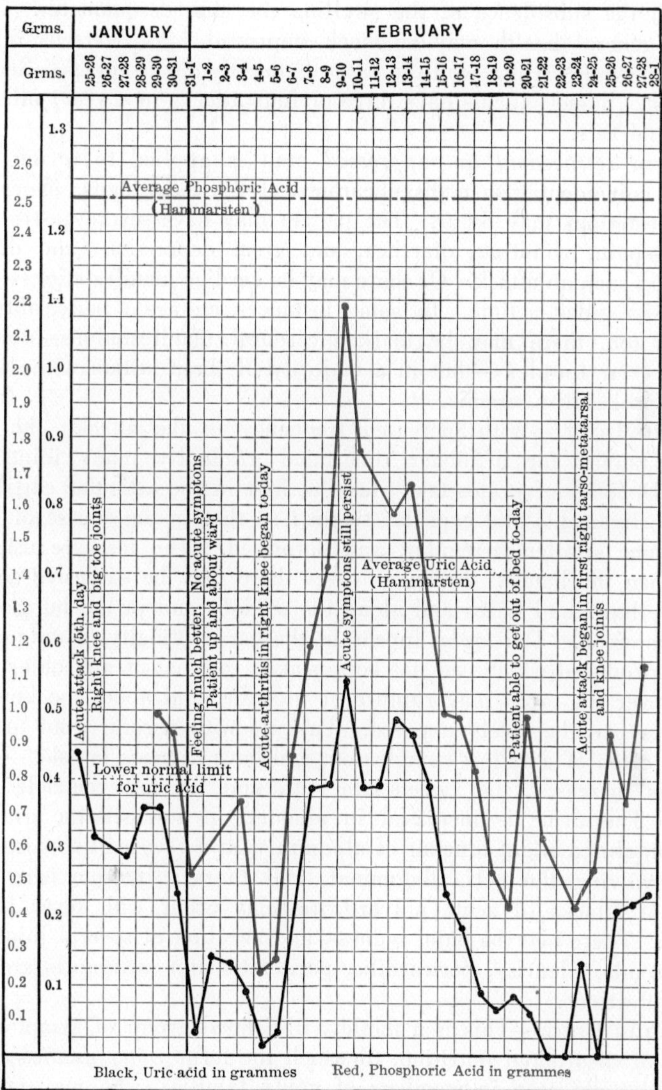

Chart XV.—Uric Acid and Phosphoric Acid Output in Case of Acute Gout.

small bones of the tarsus and metatarsus, in the ligaments of which it is lurking." The joint swells rapidly, and becomes hot, tense and shiny. The sensitiveness is extreme, and the pain makes the patient feel as if the joint were being pressed in a vice. There is fever and the temperature may rise to 102° to 103° F. Toward morning the severity of the symptoms subsides, and, although the joint remains swollen, the day may be passed in comparative comfort. The symptoms recur the next night, and the "fit," as it is called, usually lasts for from five to eight days, the severity of the symptoms gradually abating. There is usually a polymorphonuclear leukocytosis during the acute manifestations. The inflammation, however intense, never goes on to suppuration. With the subsidence of the swelling the skin desquamates. After the attack the general health may be much improved. As Aretaeus remarks, a person in the interval has won the race at the Olympian games. Recurrences are frequent. Some patients have three or four attacks in a year; others suffer at longer intervals.

The term *retrocedent* or *suppressed* gout is applied to serious internal symptoms, coincident with a disappearance of the local signs. Very remarkable manifestations may occur. The patient may have severe gastro-intestinal symptoms—pain, vomiting, diarrhea, and great depression—and death may occur during such an attack. Or there may be cardiac manifestations—dyspnea, pain, and irregular action. In some instances an acute pericarditis proves fatal. So, too, there may be marked cerebral manifestations—delirium or coma, and even apoplexy—but in a majority of these instances the symptoms are, in all probability, uremic.

Chronic Gout.—With increased frequency in the attacks, the articular symptoms persist for a longer time, and gradually many joints become affected. Deposits of urates take place, at first in the articular cartilages and then in the ligaments and capsular tissues; so that in the course of years the joints become swollen, irregular, and deformed. The feet are usually first affected, then the hands. In severe cases there may be extensive concretions about the elbows and knees and along the tendons and in the bursae. *Bursitis* is fairly common. The *tophi* appear in the ears. Finally, a unique clinical picture is produced which can not be mistaken for that of any other affection. The skin over the tophi may rupture or ulcerate, and about the knuckles the chalk-stones may be freely exposed. Patients with chronic gout are usually dyspeptic, often of a sallow complexion, and have arteriosclerosis. The blood pressure is increased, the vessels are stiff, and the left ventricle is hypertrophied. The urine is increased in amount, of low specific gravity, and usually contains a slight amount of albumin with a few hyaline casts. Severe cramps involving the calf, abdominal, and thoracic muscles are common. Intercurrent attacks of acute polyarthritis may occur with fever from 101° to 103° F. There may be pain, redness, and swelling of several joints without fever. Uremia, pleurisy, pericarditis, peritonitis and meningitis are common terminal affections.

Irregular Gout.—This is a motley, ill-defined group of symptoms, manifestations of disordered nutrition, to which the term *gouty diathesis* has been given. Cases are seen in members of gouty families, who may never themselves have suffered from the acute disease, and in persons who have lived not wisely but too well, who have eaten and drunk largely, lived sedentary lives, and yet have been fortunate enough to escape an acute attack. It is interesting to note the various manifestations in a family with marked hereditary disposition. The daughters often escape, while one son may have gouty attacks of great severity, even though he lives a temperate life and tries in every way to avoid the conditions favoring the disorder. Another son has, perhaps, only the irregular manifestations and never acute arthritis. While the irregular features are perhaps more common in the hereditary form, they occur in persons who appear to have acquired the disease. The tendency in some families is to call every affection gouty. Even infantile complaints, such as eczema, nasopharyngeal vegetations, and enuresis, are often regarded, without sufficient grounds, as evidences of the family ailment. Among the manifestations of irregular gout are the following:

Cutaneous Eruptions.—Garrod and others called special attention to the frequent association of eczema with the gouty habit. This may be shown particularly by the children in gouty families.

Gastro-intestinal Disorders.—Attacks of what is termed "biliousness," in which the tongue is furred, the breath foul, and the bowels constipated, are not uncommon in gouty persons. A gouty parotitis is described.

Cardiovascular Symptoms.—With gout arteriosclerosis is frequently associated. The blood pressure is high, the vessel walls become stiff, and cardiac and renal changes gradually occur so that the symptoms may be renal and dropsical features supervene. The manifestations may be cardiac, when the left ventricle fails, or they may be vascular and thrombosis of the coronary arteries may cause sudden death, or, more frequently, cerebral hemorrhage occurs. It makes little difference whether we regard this condition as primarily arteriosclerosis or nephritis; the point is that the disorder with which an excess of uric acid is associated induces in time increased tension, arteriosclerosis, chronic nephritis and changes in the myocardium. Pericarditis is not an infrequent terminal complication. Phlebitis is not very uncommon and may arise in connection with varicose veins or occur in many venous districts in succession or simultaneously.

Nervous Manifestations.—Headache, migraine attacks, neuralgias, sciatica and paresthesias are not uncommon. A common gouty manifestation, upon which Duckworth laid stress, is the occurrence of hot or itching feet at night. Plutarch mentions that Strabo called this "the lisping of the gout." Cramps in the legs may be very troublesome. Hutchinson called attention to hot and itching eyeballs. Associated or alternating with this symptom there may be attacks of episcleral congestion. Apoplexy is a common termination and meningitis may occur, usually basilar.

Urinary Disorders.—The urine is acid and high colored, and may deposit crystals of uric acid on standing. In many cases of chronic gout the amount of uric acid is diminished, and increased only at certain periods, forming the so-called uric acid showers. A sediment of uric acid in a urine does not necessarily mean an excess. It is often dependent on the inability of the urine to hold it in solution. Sugar is found occasionally in the urine of gouty persons—gouty glycosuria. It may pass into true diabetes, but is usually very amenable to treatment. Oxaluria may also be present. Gouty persons are specially prone to calculi, Jerome Cardan to the contrary, who reckoned freedom from stone among the chief of the *dona podagrae.* Small quantities of albumin and casts are common. Urethritis, with a purulent discharge, may arise, so it is stated, usually at the end of an attack. It may occur spontaneously or follow a pure connection.

Pulmonary Disorders.—There are no characteristic changes, but chronic bronchitis occurs with great frequency in persons of a gouty habit.

Of eye affections, iritis, glaucoma, hemorrhagic retinitis, and suppurative panophthalmitis have been described.

X-rays.—The changes in the bones, which are not typical but suggestive, consist of small dark areas on the plates, circular in outline, with clear, sharp borders. They are usually found in the epiphysis of the affected joints, especially of the fingers, and are due to the absorption of calcium in areas in which sodium urate has been deposited.

Diagnosis.—Recurring attacks of arthritis, limited to the big toe or to the tarsus, occurring in a member of a gouty family, or in a man who has lived too well, leave no question as to the nature of the trouble. There are many cases of gout, however, in which the feet do not suffer most severely. After an attack or two in one toe, other joints may be affected, and it is just in such cases of polyarthritis that the difficulty in diagnosis is apt to arise. The presence of tophi may settle the nature of an arthritis which in the previous attacks has been regarded as rheumatic. The following are suggestive points: (1) The patient's habits and occupation. Workers in breweries and barkeepers are often affected. (2) The presence of *tophi.* The ears should always be inspected in a case of polyarthritis. The diagnosis may rest with a small tophus. The student should learn to recognize, on the ear margin, Woolner's tip, fibroid nodules and small sebaceous tumors. The last are easily recognized microscopically. The needle shaped sodium urate crystals are distinctive of the tophi. (3) The urine. The uric acid output is usually very low during the intervals and at the height of the attack the elimination, as a rule, is greatly increased. (4) The amount of uric acid in the blood. If this is increased above normal limits constantly, leukemia and nephritis being excluded, it is important evidence. The gouty polyarthritis may be afebrile. A patient with several red, swollen and painful joints in rheumatic fever has pyrexia, and, while it may be present and often is in gout, its absence is a valuable sign. Many cases go a-begging for a diagnosis. A careful study of the patient's habits, of the location of the initial arthritic attacks, and the examination for tophi and bursitis will prevent cases being mistaken for rheumatic fever or arthritis deformans.

Prognosis.—"Once gouty, always gouty" is usually true, but by care the frequency and intensity of attacks can be reduced. As regards the duration of life, the circulation and kidneys are the important factors.

Treatment.—Hygienic.—Individuals with gout should live temperately, abstain from alcohol and eat moderately. The bowels should be kept open. An open-air life, with plenty of exercise and regular hours, does much to counteract an inborn tendency to the disease. The skin should be kept active and an occasional Turkish bath is advantageous. The patient should dress warmly, avoid rapid alterations in temperature, and be careful to avoid sudden chilling. Overweight should be avoided.

Dietetic.—With few exceptions, persons over forty eat too much, and the first injunction to a gouty person is to keep his appetite within reasonable bounds, to eat at stated hours, and to take plenty of time at his meals. In the matter of food, quantity is a factor of more importance than quality with many gouty persons. As Sir William Roberts well said, "Nowhere perhaps is it more necessary than in gout to consider the man as well as the ailment, and very often more the man than the ailment."

The weight of opinion leans to a modified nitrogenous diet, without excess in starchy and saccharine foods. In some patients restriction of carbohydrates is important. Foods rich in purins, such as bouillon, beef extracts, sweetbreads, liver, kidneys, and brain, should be avoided. Milk and eggs are particularly useful, owing to their being purin free. Fresh vegetables and fruits may be used freely but strawberries and bananas should be avoided.

Ebstein urged strongly the use of fat in the form of fresh butter, from 2½ to 3½ ounces in the day. He held that stout gouty subjects not only do not increase in weight with plenty of fat in the food, but that they lose weight and the general condition improves. Hot bread of all sorts and the articles of food prepared from Indian corn should, as a rule, be avoided. Roberts advised gouty patients to restrict the use of common salt, since the sodium urate readily crystallizes out in tissues with a high percentage of sodium salts. In diet each individual must receive separate consideration.

Alcohol in any form is harmful; if some must be taken whisky is the least injurious. Some forms are especially harmful, particularly malted liquors, champagne, port, and a large proportion of all the light wines.

Mineral Waters.—All forms may be said to be beneficial in gout, as the main element is the water, and the ingredients are usually indifferent. Much humbuggery still lingers about mineral waters. The question of the utility of *alkalies* in the treatment of gout is closely connected with this subject of mineral waters. This deep-rooted belief was shaken by Sir William Roberts, who claimed that alkalescence as such has no influence whatever on the sodium urate and that the sodium salts are particularly harmful. In spite of the theoretical denunciation of the use of sodium salts, the gouty from all parts of the world flock to those very Continental springs in which these salts are most predominant. Of the mineral springs best suited for the gouty may be mentioned, in the United States, those of Saratoga, Bedford, and White Sulphur; Buxton and Bath, in England; in France, Aix-les-Bains and Contrexeville. Excellent results are claimed for mineral waters with special radioactive properties. The efficacy in reality is in the water, in the way it is taken, on an empty stomach, and in large quantities; and the important accessories in the modified diet, proper hours, regular exercises, with baths, douches, etc., play an important rôle.

Medical Treatment.—In an acute attack the patient should be at rest, on a milk diet, and take water freely. The limb should be elevated and the affected joint wrapped in cotton-wool. Warm fomentations or Fuller's lotion may be used. A brisk mercurial purge is advantageous at the outset. The wine of colchicum, in doses of 20 to 30 minims (1.2 to 2 cc.) may be given every four hours with citrate of potassium. The action of the colchicum should be carefully watched; its effect is most marked when free purgation follows. It has in a majority of the cases a powerful influence over the symptoms—relieving the pain, and reducing, sometimes with great rapidity, the swelling and redness. It should be stopped as soon as the pain is relieved. Cinchophen (atophan) is more useful in subacute attacks and chronic conditions than in acute attacks. The dosage is 5 to 10 grains (0.3-0.6 gm.) three or four times a day. It is sometimes useful in smaller doses given on two days each week as a preventive. It increases the excretion of uric acid. In view of the danger to the liver, one hesitates to give this drug without careful consideration. If used it should not be given for more than two days in succession. Neocinchophen is apparently safer; it is given in the same dosage. In cases in which the pain and sleeplessness are distressing and do not yield to treatment, morphia is necessary. During convalescence the diet should be increased slowly and the taking of large amounts of water should be continued.

In some acute and subacute attacks sodium salicylate or acetylsalicylic acid may be useful. The chronic and irregular forms are best treated by dietetic and hygienic measures. Potassium iodide is sometimes useful. Albu speaks favorably of lemon-juice as a remedy. The vegetable acids are converted in the system into alkaline carbonates, enabling the blood to keep the uric acid compounds in solution and facilitating their elimination.

Where the arthritic attacks are confined to the great toe joint, surgical interference may be considered. The entire joint capsule of the big-toe joint has been removed with permanent relief.

Calcium Gout.—This is very rare and occurs principally in young women. It is suggested that there is disturbance of calcium metabolism due to altered function of the parathyroid glands. The deposits occur in the peri-articular tissues of the joints of the fingers and toes and are described as tophi. These contain a chalklike substance which contains a large amount of calcium salts with traces of uric acid salts and phosphates. The *diagnosis* may be made by analysis of the contents of a tophus and by X-ray study which shows the circular shadows in the periarticular structures and not in the bones. In *treatment* the intake of calcium should be reduced as far as possible. The tophi may be removed if indicated.

DIABETES MELLITUS

Definition.—A disease of metabolism, especially of the carbohydrates, in which the normal utilization of carbohydrate is impaired with an increase in the sugar content of the blood and glycosuria. There is a tendency to subsequent disturbance of the fat metabolism with resulting ketosis.

History.—The disease was known to Celsus. Aretaeus first used the term diabetes, calling it a wonderful affection "melting down the flesh and limbs into urine." He suggested that the disease got its name from the Greek word signifying a syphon. Willis in the seventeenth century gave a good description and recognized the sweetness of the urine "as if there has been sugar and honey in it." Dobson in 1776 demonstrated the presence of sugar, and Rollo in 1797 wrote an admirable account and recommended a meat diet. The modern study dates from Claude Bernard's demonstration of the glycogenic function of the liver in 1857. The studies of von Mehring and Munkowski in 1889 on the results of the removal of the pancreas were followed by advances in the general knowledge of metabolism by many workers. In 1922 came the discovery of insulin by Banting and his coworkers.

Etiology.—The digestive enzymes convert the starches and sugars of the food into monosaccharides which pass into the portal circulation, but the major portion remains in the liver, where it is converted into glycogen. The percentage of sugar in the systemic blood remains constant—0.08 to 0.12 per cent. The figures depend on the method used. These are for the Folin-Wu method. With the Benedict method the values are 0.06 to 0.1 or 0.11 per cent. Part of the sugar passes to the muscles, where it is stored as glycogen. The total storage capacity of the liver is estimated at about one-tenth of its weight, *i.e.*, about 150 gms. for an organ weighing 1,500 gms.

Glucose is also derived from protein, of which 58 per cent is converted into glucose, and from fat, of which 10 per cent is converted into glucose. This applies both to exogenous and endogenous protein and fat.

The following conditions influence the appearance of sugar in the urine:

Carbohydrate Intake.—Normally the blood sugar is from 0.08 to 0.12 per cent. An intake of 100 grams of dextrose causes a rise to about 0.18 per cent. This reaches its maximum ordinarily in about 40-60 minutes after ingestion and then in about two hours falls to the normal figure. The percentage and times vary in different individuals. In normal individuals this does not result in the appearance of sugar in the urine but we find great variation depending on the renal threshold for sugar ("the leak point"). The kidney cells excrete sugar at different concentrations in the blood, in one at 0.15 per cent and in another at 0.2 per cent. In diabetes the percentage is usually from 0.18 to 0.25. Like the balance at the mint, which is sensitive to the correct weight of the gold coins passing over it, the renal cells only react at a certain point of saturation. There is no constant relation between the amount of sugar in the blood and that in the urine, although the figures are often comparative. There may be a high blood sugar and a small amount in the urine. The renal threshold for sugar seems to rise with the duration of diabetes and as age increases, so in old persons it is specially important to know the amount of blood sugar. It rises also in nephritis.

Nervous System.—Bernard showed that there was an area in the medulla puncture of which is followed by hyperglycemia due to an increased outflow of sugar from the liver. He demonstrated that the efferent path of this influence was through the splanchnic nerves and the afferent through the vagi. Many lesions of the nervous system cause glycosuria—tumors, particularly in the neighborhood of the medulla, injuries to the brain and to the upper part of the spinal cord, meningitis and hemorrhage. These probably disturb the internal secretion of the pituitary gland.

The influence of *functional nervous disturbance* is difficult to estimate. There does not seem proof that this may be the sole primary factor but there is no doubt that, once established, diabetes mellitus is influenced by the general state of the nervous system. Worry, mental strain, anxiety, etc., may have a marked influence. Severe nervous strain may cause temporary glycosuria possibly through increased action of the adrenal glands.

Internal Secretions.—Four of the glands of internal secretion influence the amount of sugar in the blood. Of these the pancreas (islands of Langerhans) is the most important and is alone in its action, being opposed by the suprarenal, thyroid and pituitary (posterior lobe) glands. Overactivity of these three glands tends to cause glycosuria; underactivity increased sugar tolerance. Underactivity of the pancreas (internal secretion) results in hyperglycemia and glycosuria. There may be a condition of hypoglycemia due to overproduction of insulin.

Pancreas.—Diabetes mellitus can be produced experimentally by removal of the pancreas. This results from lack of the internal secretion, derived from the islands of Langerhans, which is necessary for carbohydrate metabolism. The essential factor in diabetes mellitus is a disturbance of this function of the pancreas. The cells of the islands of Langerhans contain specific granules in the beta cells (Bensley) which disappear if overworked by excessive carbohydrate or total food intake. The granules may disappear and the cells show hydropic degeneration. Many diseases of the pancreas are associated with glycosuria, some with permanent diabetes. Hemorrhagic pancreatitis, cancer, calculus and chronic interstitial pancreatitis may be associated with disurbance in the carbohydrate metabolism. The islands of Langerhans have the ability to produce increased amounts of insulin when this is required. But it is not clear how insulin acts. One view is that it aids the oxidation of glucose but there is no evidence that there is interference with the oxidation of glucose in the muscles in diabetes. The increase in metabolism in diabetes by insulin may be due to its action on the glucose in the blood enabling it to be used or to be converted to glycogen.

Pituitary Gland.—It was long known that glycosuria occurred in tumors of the region of the pituitary, particularly in acromegaly, and it follows fractures of the base of the skull. Experimentally, Cushing and his students have shown that the pituitary gland has an important influence in carbohydrate metabolism. Any operative disturbance of it, or of the infundibulum, is followed by glycosuria, and by a lowering of the carbohydrate tolerance. On the other hand, a deficiency of this secretion is followed by an increased tolerance for carbohydrates. Houssay has demonstrated a diabetogenic factor in the anterior lobe.

A tumor which at first irritates the gland, as in the early stages of acromegaly, may cause glycosuria, but later there is an extraordinarily high carbohydrate tolerance, and associated with it a great increase in the deposition of fat in the body.

Adrenals and Thyroid.—Glycosuria does not necessarily follow lesions of the *adrenals,* but epinephrine has a powerful influence on the carbohydrate metabolism, and glycosuria may be readily produced in animals by subcutaneous injection and by the local application of epinephrine to the pancreas. Clinically, we know practically nothing of an adrenal glycosuria. It has occasionally been noticed in the prolonged use of epinephrine. Puncture of the floor of the fourth ventricle does not cause glycosuria after removal of the adrenal glands. The influence of the adrenal secretion is antagonistic to that of the pancreas. In disturbances of the *thyroid* gland glycosuria is not uncommon. The use of thyroid extract is occasionally followed by glycosuria. Hyperthyroidism and glycosuria are often associated, and the hyperthyroid patient is more prone to diabetes for the rest of life. In myxedema the carbohydrate tolerance may be increased and the blood sugar is usually low. This results also after complete thyroidectomy.

The glycosuria with pregnancy may be due to disturbance of the pituitary gland or to a lower renal threshold for sugar. It is transient, usually disappearing with parturition, and rarely leads to diabetes. It may recur in successive pregnancies.

Liver Function.—A remarkable feature is that the great warehouse of the sugars may be damaged to any degree without causing hyperglycemia or glycosuria. Whether there is a form of disease to which the name "liver diabetes" may be given is doubtful. There are cases of cirrhosis of the liver and of gall stones—particularly those with enlargement of the organ—in which glycosuria is present, but they are probably all associated with coincident affections of the pancreas. In hemochromatosis, which is accompanied by great enlargement of the liver, the glycosuria is probably pancreatic.

Renal Function.—Disease of the kidneys is rarely associated with glycosuria. Occasionally one finds it and increased blood sugar in chronic nephritis. There is a remarkable experimental glycosuria of great interest. If phloridzin, a glucoside from the bark of the apple tree, is given by mouth or subcutaneously to man or animals glycosuria results, and even continues on a nitrogenous diet, and in man when fasting. The glycosuria may be marked, yet there is no hyperglycemia. In the condition termed "renal glycosuria," in which the blood sugar is normal but the kidney threshold for sugar is low, there may be glycosuria but this is not diabetes mellitus.

Obesity.—Joslin has specially emphasized the importance of overweight in the etiology, especially in adult and mature life.

Miscellaneous Disturbances.—The carbohydrate metabolism may be upset in acute fevers with a transient glycosuria. In septic conditions, sometimes with carbuncle, glycosuria may occur as a *secondary* phenomenon and disappear after recovery. It is not uncommon after the administration of ether, less so after chloroform. Metabolic disturbances in gout may show glycosuria, and cachexias and profound anemias have a transient glycosuria. There are patients, usually with marked arteriosclerosis, in whom there is apparently no lack of insulin and little or no response to its administration. The difficulty seems to be in the utilization of sugar in some way apart from lack of insulin. Patients suffocated by smoke or poisoned by coal gas may have glycosuria. Syphilis does not play a marked rôle.

Incidence.—The disease is on the increase in all civilized countries, due partly to overnutrition and less exercise, in which the motor car plays a part. In England and Wales the deaths increased from 8.6 per 100,000 population in 1900 to 15.3 in 1932. In the United States the statistics for 1870 gave 2.1; for 1890, 3.8; for 1900, 9.3; and for 1915, 17.5 deaths to 100,000 population. The rate for 1932 is 22.

Hereditary influences play an important rôle and the disease may occur in many members of the same family. Morton, who calls the disease *hydrops ad matulam* (Phthisiologia, 1689), records a family in which four children were affected, one of whom recovered on a milk diet and diascordium. The family dietary and obesity are factors in this. There are instances of the coexistence of the disease in man and wife. Similarity in habits of diet probably accounts for this.

Sex and Age.—There has been an increase in the number of cases in women over 45 years of age. In Joslin's series, of 2,440 cases from 1898 to 1922, 45 per cent were females, but of 2,646 cases from 1922 to 1927, 55 per cent were females. It is a disease of adult life; a majority of the cases occur from the third to the sixth decade. Over half of the cases occur between the ages of 40 and 60. The death rate in women exceeds that of men by 76 per cent. In childhood and early adult life there is little difference in the incidence or death rate in the sexes. There has been a decline in the deaths in the young of both sexes and in males of middle life.

Diabetes in Children.—This usually occurs among the better classes. Hereditary influences are marked. While the disease is usually severe there are not infrequent cases of a mild type. One case is mentioned of a child apparently born with glycosuria, who recovered in eight months.

RACE.—Hebrews seem especially prone to it; one-fourth of Frerichs' patients were of the Semitic race. Diabetes is not as rare in the colored race as was formerly supposed. Of 329 patients at the Pennsylvania Hospital, 80 were negroes.

Metabolism in Diabetes.—Glycosuria may be a simple overflow of sugar over the renal threshold, but the essence of true diabetes is a waste of the carbohydrates, which hurry through the body, in great part never warehoused as glycogen. It is suggested that there is a difference in the form of glucose in the normal person and in the diabetic. The result is a failure of the normal oxidation of the carbohydrates. The polyuria is a result of the diuretic action of the sugar which requires considerable water to carry it off. The thirst is a result of the polyuria. There is a very considerable daily loss of energy in warming the liquids taken to the temperature of the body, according to Benedict and Joslin nearly 6 per cent of the total heat of the day. The excess of sugar renders the body a favorable culture medium for pus organisms. There is loss of energy with the waste of sugar; every gram of sugar excreted in the urine means a loss of 4.1 calories, so that a diabetic patient excreting 100 grams of sugar and 20 grams of β-oxybutyric acid loses 500 calories in this way, so that the patients are underfed, unless this loss is made up by other food (Benedict and Joslin). The respiratory quotient in diabetics shows a decrease from normal owing to impairment in the utilization of carbohydrate. A respiratory quotient above 0.74 indicates a fairly liberal supply of glycogen stored in the body; while a respiratory quotient of 0.70, or below, indicates that the patient has no available carbohydrates and has lost in a measure the power of storing them. Here is a special danger; as the carbohydrates pass through the body unburned, the energy must be provided from protein and fat. The metabolism of the former does not appear to be seriously disturbed, and the carbohydrate portion of the protein molecule in part supplies the lost sugars. The danger is in the metabolism of the fats. The carbohydrates are not used as fuel; the proteins are easily utilized, but apparently it takes so much draught to burn them that not enough is left to consume the fats completely; and the products of incomplete combustion accumulate and suffocate the patient as effectually as does the CO of a charcoal stove. The chief products of this incomplete combustion of the fats are β-oxybutyric acid, diacetic acid and acetone, and one danger in the disease is the production of ketosis.

The CO_2 combining power of the blood is reduced. In slight acidosis it is between 40 and 50, in moderate acidosis between 25 and 40 and in severe acidosis below 25 volumes per cent (normal 55 to 75 volumes per cent).

Lipemia.—The blood contains an excess of fat in severe cases; fat, lecithin and cholesterol may all be increased. Some emphasize the importance of the amount of blood cholesterol as an indication of the condition of the patient. In *lipemia retinalis* the vessels are white against a pink background. This may be due to a film of fatty lymph in the perivascular spaces or to fat deposits in the adventitia.

Renal Glycosuria.—This is a better term than "renal diabetes" to designate a condition in which there is glycosuria without increase of the blood sugar. In it the glycosuria is independent of the carbohydrate intake and the blood sugar is normal or decreased in amount. The blood sugar tolerance curve is normal. The kidney threshold for sugar is low. As a rule it is discovered accidentally as there are rarely any symptoms. In some cases exercise immediately after meals prevents the glycosuria and removal of infected tonsils has influenced it (Schneiderman). It may be associated with an absolute decrease in the proportion of calcium in the blood plasma.

Morbid Anatomy.—The *nervous system* shows no constant lesions. In a few instances there have been tumors or sclerosis in the medulla, or a cysticercus has pressed on the floor. A secondary multiple neuritis is not rare and changes occur in the posterior columns of the cord similar to those in pernicious anemia. In the sympathetic system the ganglia have been enlarged and in some instances sclerosed. *Arteriosclerosis* is usually marked in the older patients and coronary artery sclerosis is common, with relatively frequent coronary artery occlusion. The *myocardium* often shows degeneration. Endocarditis is very rare. The *lungs* show important changes. Bronchopneumonia or lobar pneumonia (either of which may terminate in gangrene) and tuberculosis are common. In rare cases there is a chronic fibroid pneumonia. Fat embolism of the pulmonary vessels may occur with diabetic coma.

The *liver* is usually enlarged; fatty degeneration is common. In the so-called diabetic cirrhosis—the *cirrhosis pigmentaire*—the liver is enlarged and sclerotic, and cachexia develops with melanoderma. Dilatation of the stomach with enlargement of the duodenum and colonic stasis are common.

Pancreas.—There may be no macroscopic changes but the gland is often small. Histologically there may be chronic interstitial fibrosis, hyalinization, a decreased number of the islands of Langerhans and hydropic degeneration. In the islands of Langerhans the specific granules may be absent and the cells show changes.

The *kidneys* may show a diffuse nephritis with fatty degeneration. Glycogen may be found in the renal tubules.

Symptoms.—*Acute* and *chronic* forms are recognized, but there is no essential difference between them, except that in the former the patients are, as a rule, younger, the disease is more severe and emaciation is usually more marked. The *onset* is usually gradual, and either frequent micturition or inordinate thirst first attracts attention. The glycosuria is often discovered in an insurance or routine examination. Very rarely it sets in rapidly, after sudden emotion, an injury or a severe chill. When fully established the disease is characterized by great thirst, the passage of large quantities of saccharine urine, a voracious appetite, and, as a rule, emaciation.

Among the GENERAL SYMPTOMS *thirst* is one of the most distressing. Large quantities of water are required to keep the sugar in solution and for its excretion in the urine. The amount of fluid intake bears a definite ratio to the quantity excreted. Instances, however, are not uncommon in which the thirst is not excessive; but in such cases the amount of urine is never large. The thirst is most intense an hour or two after meals. As a rule, the digestion is good and the appetite may be inordinate. Lumbar pain is common.

The tongue is usually dry, red, and glazed, and the saliva scanty. The gums may become swollen, and in the later stages aphthous stomatitis is common. Constipation is the rule.

In spite of a large intake of food a patient may become rapidly emaciated.

This loss of flesh bears some ratio to the polyuria, and when the sugar is reduced, the patient may gain in flesh. The skin is dry and harsh, and sweating is rare, except when tuberculosis coexists. Drenching sweats have alternated with excessive polyuria. General *pruritus* or pruritus pudendi may be very distressing, and occasionally is one of the earliest symptoms. The temperature is often subnormal; the pulse is usually frequent, and the tension may be increased. Many diabetics do not show marked emaciation. Patients past the middle period of life may have the disease for years without much disturbance of the health, and may remain well nourished.

URINE.—The amount varies from 3 to 5 litres in mild cases to 10 litres in severe cases. In rare instances the quantity is not much increased. Under treatment the amount is much lessened, and in intercurrent febrile affections it may be reduced to normal. The specific gravity is high, ranging from 1.025 to 1.045; but in exceptional cases it may be low, 1.010 to 1.020. The highest specific gravity recorded is by Trousseau—1.074. Very high specific gravities—over 1.070—suggest fraud. The urine is pale in color almost like water, and has a sweetish odor and taste. Sugar is present in varying amounts. In mild cases it does not exceed 1 or 2 per cent, but it may reach from 5 to 10 per cent. The total amount excreted in twenty-four hours may be 10 to 20 ounces (320 to 640 grams).

Ketonuria.—The ketone bodies, acetone, diacetic acid and β-oxybutyric acid are present, sometimes in small amounts in mild cases but increasing with the severity of the disease; they are indications of ketosis. In coma the excretion of β-oxybutyric acid may be as much as 100 gm. or more a day. Functional renal insufficiency may develop with ketosis.

Glycogen has been found in the urine, and in rare instances sugars other than glucose occur, lactose, levulose, and pentose, and to these conditions the term *melituria* is sometimes applied. *Albumin* is not infrequent.

Pneumaturia, gas in the urine, due to fermentation in the bladder, is occasionally met with. Fat may be passed in the urine in the form of a fine emulsion (lipuria).

BLOOD.—Polycythemia may be present and towards the end with complications (especially coma) there may be a leukocytosis and the leukocytes may contain glycogen. The blood sugar is rarely above 0.4 per cent. An increase in the blood sugar may persist after glycosuria has disappeared.

The alkalinity is lessened and the specific gravity reduced. *Lipemia* is present in many cases. The blood lipoids are increased from the normal figure of about 0.6 per cent to 0.8 per cent in mild cases, to 0.9 in moderately severe and even 2 per cent in severe cases. Lipemia may be present without ketosis.

Complications.—COMA (*Ketosis*).—In the typical dyspneic coma, the air-hunger of Kussmaul, there are loud and deep in- and expirations and the breath very often has the fruity odor of acetone. It may come on without any premonition and the patient may waken out of sleep in dyspnea. An acyanotic dyspnea is one of the best indications of ketosis. Dyspepsia, constipation, abdominal pain, marked irritability and restlessness may precede the onset of coma and should suggest its possibility. Other features are marked signs of *dehydration*, a soft eyeball, probably due to lowered intraocular tension, low blood pressure, a marked reduction in the carbon dioxide combining power of the blood and rarely convulsions. There may be a marked leukocytosis (with a normal differential count) which may suggest an acute inflammatory abdominal condition, especially if the abdominal pain is severe and the existence of the diabetes is not known.

Difficulty may arise in the diagnosis of coma from insulin reaction (hypoglycemia) especially without a clear history. The blood sugar estimation is important, but takes time and may not be possible. The dry skin and soft eyeball in coma and a low temperature, usually below 97° F., in insulin hypoglycemia are important. An extensor plantar response has been obtained in hypoglycemic coma. Some patients present a form of coma which is not typical diabetic coma; the blood sugar may be normal or nearly so without ketonuria or glycosuria, yet coma persists. There may be features suggestive of uremia but there is no marked nitrogen retention. Death usually follows.

Cutaneous.—Boils and carbuncles are common and painful onychia may occur. Eczema is also met with, and at times an intolerable itching. In women there may be the most intense pruritus pudendi, and in men a balanitis. Rarer affections are xanthoma and purpura. *Gangrene* is common, associated usually with arteriosclerosis. In the prevention of gangrene it is important to watch for early changes in the legs. Kramer has emphasized the occurrence of small red areas, which may feel nodular and leave a brown pigmented area or a small depression. There may be blebs which appear suddenly and may show bluish or black discoloration with scar formation. Small painless areas of gangrene may appear or there may be deep seated cellulitis or osteomyelitis. Perforating ulcer of the foot may occur. Bronzing of the skin (*diabète bronzé*) occurs in *hemochromatosis*.

Necrobiosis Lipoidica Diabeticorum or *Dermatitis Atrophicans Lipoides Diabetica*.—In this the early lesions are usually papules and the later ones plaques. The papules are sharply marked, elevated and 1 to 3 cm. in diameter. Later there are irregular plaques with well defined borders which may have a glazed appearance. The cause is regarded by some as a fatty degeneration and by others as a necrobiosis of the connective tissues. There are quite marked lipoid deposits. This does not seem to be a typical form of xanthoma. Trauma may play a part. In some cases the process advances to gangrene.

Pulmonary.—*Acute pneumonia,* lobar or lobular, may cause death. *Gangrene* is apt to supervene but the breath does not necessarily have the foul odor of ordinary gangrene. Abscess may follow lobar pneumonia. *Tuberculosis bronchopneumonia* may occur and run a rapid course.

Renal.—*Albuminuria* is tolerably frequent. The amount varies greatly, and, when slight, is not of much moment. Edema of the feet and ankles is not infrequent but general anasarca is rare. It occasionally precedes diabetic coma. Marked edema may occur apart from renal disease; sometimes it is due to large doses of sodium bicarbonate. Occasionally cystitis is troublesome.

Nervous System.—*Peripheral Neuritis.*—Neuralgia, numbness and tingling, uncommon in diabetes, are probably minor neuritic manifestations. The involvement may be general of the arms and legs. Sometimes it is unilateral, or the neuritis may be in a single nerve—the sciatic or the third nerve. Herpes zoster may occur. The so-called "*diabetic tabes*" is a peripheral neuritis, characterized by pains in the legs, loss of knee jerk—which may occur without the other symptoms—and a loss of power in the extensors of the feet. Changes in the posterior columns of the cord have been found. *Diabetic paraplegia* is probably due to neuritis. There are cases with loss of power in both arms and legs.

Mental Symptoms.—The patients are often morose, and there is a strong tendency to become hypochondriacal. Some patients display an extraordinary degree of irritability, restlessness and anxiety.

SPECIAL SENSES.—Cataract is likely to occur, and rapidly in young persons. Diabetic retinitis closely resembles the albuminuric form and is probably due to vascular changes. Hemorrhages are common. Sudden amaurosis, similar to that in uremia, may occur or temporary visual disturbances, possibly due to osmotic changes in the lens. They disappear with proper treatment. Paralysis of the muscles of accommodation and atrophy of the optic nerves may be present. *Lipemia retinalis* may occur; the retinal vessels are white against a pink background. Aural symptoms may come on with great rapidity, an otitis media or inflammation of the mastoid cells. Ocular tension may be lowered in coma.

REPRODUCTIVE FUNCTIONS.—Impotence is common and may be an early symptom. Conception is rare; if it occurs, abortion is apt to follow. A diabetic mother may bear a healthy child; there is no instance of a diabetic mother bearing a diabetic child. If there is not strict control of the diabetes during pregnancy the disease is usually aggravated after delivery.

CIRCULATION.—The *myocardial* condition is important and tracings may show changes. Attacks of *precordial pain* are fairly common. Hypoglycemia is a danger if there is coronary artery disease and the frequency of *coronary artery occlusion* is important. Overdosage of insulin may result in precordial pain. *Arteriosclerosis* is common in elderly diabetics and in the arteries of the legs increases the danger of gangrene of the feet. Hypertension is relatively common; Kramer found it in nearly 40 per cent of his series. The association of obesity probably plays a part. There may be a possible causal influence in arteriosclerosis of the pancreatic vessels.

Diabetes mellitus may occur with Addisonian anemia. Achlorhydria is common in diabetes.

Diagnosis.—There is no difficulty in determining the presence of sugar in the urine if proper tests are applied. Alcapton may prove deceptive, and in one reported case of ochronosis (Osler) a diagnosis of diabetes was made by five leading physicians in Europe, one of whom was an authority on diabetes. Deception may be practised. Levulose, lactose and pentose should be kept in mind as possible causes of error. Certain drugs, especially salicylates, yield reducing substances in the urine.

To determine whether the case is one of simple alimentary glycosuria or diabetes is not always easy, as the one readily merges into the other. It is well to test the assimilation limit; 100 grams of glucose given to a fasting patient should not give glycosuria. The determination of the blood sugar is an important aid; a blood sugar above 0.12 per cent, taken when fasting, usually means diabetes. To preserve blood for this test add one drop of 40 per cent formaldehyde solution to each 5 cc. The specimen can be used within 3 days. A thorough test of the sugar tolerance is of great value in a doubtful case. The diagnosis of *renal glycosuria* depends on a persistent glycosuria independent of the amount of carbohydrate intake, a low or normal amount of sugar in the blood, a normal glucose tolerance test and the absence of the usual features of diabetes. *Hemochromatosis* should not cause difficulty. The detection of a little sugar in the urine may have the great advantage of frightening the patient into a more rational mode of life. The forms following anesthesia, accidents, business worries, fright and that which occurs in pregnancy are, as a rule, readily controlled.

Prognosis.—This has been materially improved by the discovery of insulin, but the same general rules still apply and there is the same need of intelligent care. The social condition, the intelligence of the patient and his or her capacity to obey orders, the ability to obtain a proper diet and, above all, the physician himself are important factors. The patient who will not do as he is told has a heavy handicap. The occurrence of complications and infections influences the outlook materially. Complete restoration of normal carbohydrate tolerance is very rare and usually occurs only in mild cases. The results of treatment and the carbohydrate tolerance which the patient acquires are important factors.

Treatment.—In families with a predisposition to the disease the use of starchy foods and particularly sugar should be restricted. It is important to reduce overweight especially in those over forty years of age. The personal hygiene is of the first importance. Sources of worry should be avoided, and he should lead an even, quiet life, if possible in an equable climate. The heat waste should be prevented by wearing warm clothes and avoiding cold. A warm, or, if robust, a cold, bath should be taken every day. An occasional Turkish bath is useful. Systematic, moderate exercise should be taken. When this is not feasible, massage should be given. Special attention should be given to the care of the feet to reduce the danger of gangrene. The patient should be told to report any skin lesion at once.

Each patient presents an individual problem and should be studied as such. Exact records should be kept of the food intake and of the urine examinations. It is an advantage, certainly early in treatment, to examine single specimens. The endeavor is to keep the urine sugar free, the blood sugar as near normal as possible, and the patient in the best general condition. Physicians and students are often puzzled by the various methods employed, which seem to differ so markedly. It is not possible here to do more than indicate the general principles. There is abundant literature which can be consulted; Joslin's book is excellent. The majority of patients do well on any proper treatment *carefully supervised.* In the more difficult cases the physician may have to try different methods to find the one best adapted to that patient. Education of the patient is essential; he should know the nature of his disease and its dangers, and must learn food values as thoroughly as he knows the value of coins. He should learn to weigh his food and test his urine.

DIET.—There are several methods and, in general, the one employed should be as simple as possible. Sudden changes in diet should not be made without careful consideration and if in doubt it is safer to have a patient on too low than too high a diet. Effort should be made to avoid monotony and there are many changes which can be made by careful study of food tables. The intelligence of the patient should be studied and we should be sure that he understands the instructions. If possible the patient should be in a hospital for study and instruction for a sufficient period. The severity of the disease influences the treatment. Mild cases do with simple dietary restrictions.

Moderately severe and severe cases require more rigid treatment. The ratio of the ketone forming elements to the antiketone forming elements should be such that acidosis will not result. In this 1 gram of carbohydrate represents 1 gram of glucose, 1 gram of protein 0.58 gram of glucose, and 1 gram of fat 0.1 gram of glucose. Difficulty should be rare, especially with the use of more carbohydrate in the diet than formerly. One gram of glucose used in the body results in the utilization of 1.5 to 2.5 grams of fatty acid. Nitrogen balance should be maintained, for which 0.66 gram of protein per kilogram of weight is a minimum if there are sufficient total calories, but the protein should not exceed 1 gram per kilogram of weight. Larger amounts of protein are required for children. A total of 25-30 calories per kilogram of weight is sufficient at rest.

There is now less tendency to restrict the total intake. Formerly, special emphasis was placed on undernutrition, so that the patient was at a lower level of weight and metabolism than his normal. This spares the metabolic functions. With undernutrition and loss of weight, the tolerance is increased. The studies of Allen proved the value of this method. To-day there is sometimes a tendency to go too far the other way. Any system should not be followed too rigidly and modifications should be made as the study of the patient indicates. In general it may be said that a conservative course is usually the best. As a rule it is well to keep the patient a little below his normal weight. How far his nutrition should be below the normal is a problem in each patient. When a patient comes under treatment, unless the condition is severe or there is some complication, a moderate diet may be given, such as 80 to 100 grams of carbohydrate, 60 grams of protein and enough fat to make up the total calories. The result in a few days gives a guide as to the severity. It may be possible to control the disease by diet alone. Whether we should endeavor to return to a diet with practically normal proportions of foods is a subject on which there is difference of opinion. It seems wiser to keep up a decreased amount of carbohydrate. The use of insulin permits much greater flexibility in the diet.

The treatment by *high fat diet* was introduced by Newburgh and Marsh. In this there is a large proportion of fat and a small proportion of protein and carbohydrate. An adult patient may begin with 15 to 20 grams of protein, 85 to 95 grams of fat and 10 to 12 grams of carbohydrate. After sugar disappears from the urine the diet is gradually increased until ⅔ of a gram of protein and 30 to 40 calories per kilogram of weight are given, with not more than 35 grams of carbohydrate. If the urine is sugar free, it is safe to give fat in three times the amount of carbohydrate if the protein is not more than 1 gram per kilogram of weight.

The following course may be followed in cases other than severe forms. The patient is given a maintenance diet calculated for his weight and age. This can be calculated from the proper weight for the height and sex, on a basis of 25 to 30 calories per kilogram, or the standards of DuBois or Dreyer may be used. The amount of protein should be 0.7 to 1 gram per kilogram of weight in an adult and more in a child.

The present tendency is to give larger amounts of carbohydrate. In patients not requiring insulin 70 to 100 grams of carbohydrate may be given, while those needing insulin from the outset are given 100 to 120 grams of carbohydrate. Sufficient fat is given to supply the calories required in addition to those supplied by carbohydrate and protein. High carbohydrate diets (over 200 grams) are given by some; others give high carbohydrate with a minimum of fat and restricted total calories; others use a diet between the extremes. The carbohydrate and fat should be given in proportions to prevent ketosis. The ratio of 3 grams of fat to 1 gram of carbohydrate is safe but with higher carbohydrate diets the ratio is usually less than this. If the patient becomes sugar free on this diet, the tolerance is studied and the best diet found. The fatty acid content = 0.46 protein + 0.9 fat. The glucose content = carbohydrate + 0.58 protein + 0.1 fat. If the patient is not sugar free in six or seven days insulin should be given. We must remember that all the food eaten is not necessarily absorbed.

Saccharine may be used for sugar. It is an advantage in using vegetables which are boiled in cooking, to do the boiling in three different waters, all the water being removed after each boiling. This reduces the amount of carbohydrate, an advantage for patients who demand bulk in diet. There should be sufficient vitamins and salts, especially calcium.

Insulin.—The discovery of insulin by F. G. Banting, working with C. H. Best and J. B. Collip, in association with J. J. R. MacLeod, revolutionized the treatment of diabetes. It is an aqueous solution of the active principle of the islands of Langerhans. One unit causes an average utilization of 1 to 5 grams of glucose. The glucose-insulin ratio increases with increasing amounts of carbohydrate in the diet, that is, the more carbohydrate taken the less insulin is required for each gram. There are certain precautions to be taken in its use. The first is to be sure that the patient has diabetes mellitus; "renal glycosuria" should be excluded. Blood sugar estimations are of great importance in controlling its administration and should be obtained if possible. The regulation of diet should be even more careful when insulin is being given, which should be administered hypodermically and in most cases half an hour before meals. Modifications may be needed; some do best with one dose before breakfast, one before the evening meal and a small dose on going to bed; some are best with the insulin an hour before breakfast, half an hour before lunch and one or two hours after supper; and others may do best with four doses. Two doses a day are usually best before breakfast and supper; at lunch little carbohydrate should be taken.

Dosage.—In ordinary cases it is best to begin with one to five units, two or three times a day before meals, gradually increasing by one unit, either with each successive dose or one unit a day, until the required dosage is found. The daily amount required in many patients runs between 10 and 20 units a day. The best adjustment between the amount of carbohydrate and insulin requires good judgment. The danger of *hypoglycemia* is important. Every patient should be given careful instruction as to its symptoms and treatment. The minor symptoms are restlessness and nervousness, sudden weakness, perhaps with a feeling of hunger, headache, vasomotor disturbance shown by flushing or pallor, and vertigo. The more severe features are sweating, tremor, anxiety or excitement, psychical disturbance, diplopia, aphasia, transient hemiplegia, convulsions and collapse. Insulin shock may cause severe precordial pain. For the minor features the patient should take a lump of sugar, some candy, the juice of an orange or three ounces of milk. In more severe cases

20 grams of glucose or corn syrup can be given by mouth or by stomach tube, or by rectum if the patient can not swallow. In a very severe case 10 to 20 cc. of a 50 per cent solution of dextrose should be given intravenously. Epinephrine (♏ 5-15 of the 1-1000 solution) should be given hypodermically. Unusual exercise, digestive disturbance, a meal delayed or omitted, or increase in carbohydrate tolerance may be responsible, as well as too large a dose of insulin. Depending on the cause of the hypoglycemia, the insulin should be reduced or the carbohydrate increased to prevent a recurrence.

Some patients are *resistant* to insulin so that enormous doses have little or no effect. This may be due to progressive destruction of the pancreas, hepatic disease (especially cirrhosis), or very severe infection and toxemia. It is seen with infectious disease, ketosis, increased metabolism, sometimes in pregnancy, with certain skin disturbances such as sunburn and reaction to X-ray therapy, and with certain endocrine disturbances. Some elderly patients with marked arteriosclerosis show very little effect from insulin. *Allergic reactions* from insulin occur rarely in a general form, more often locally. A change in the particular preparation used is advisable. Local edema and sometimes atrophy of the subcutaneous fat may occur at the site of injection.

Coma.—It is well to warn the patient to regard any unusual symptom, especially fever or loss of appetite, as a possible warning of coma. He should go to bed at once and notify the physician. Fluid should be taken as freely as possible and it is well to take the juice of one orange. Treatment should be carried out energetically: (1) *Rest* should be absolute and the patient should be kept warm. (2) *Fluid* should be given as freely as possible by the mouth, by the bowel or subcutaneously. Care should be taken not to cause vomiting by too large amounts by mouth. The fluid by bowel can be given by the drop method or by injecting 300 to 500 cc. of salt solution. It is well to give salt solution subcutaneously (750 to 1000 cc.) at once. (3) An *enema* should be given as soon as possible so that fluid can be given by the bowel if necessary. (4) *Food.* The only form necessary is carbohydrate and not more than 150 grams in the 24 hours is required. This can be given as orange juice, gruel, ginger ale and glucose. If there is constant vomiting, 25 grams of glucose can be given by rectum or, if this is not possible, intravenously. (5) *Insulin.* Before this is given there should be certainty that the condition is diabetic coma. The dose of insulin should be carefully considered and no set rules can be given. The danger of over-dosage should always be kept in mind. It is usually safe to give 50 units (20 intravenously and 30 subcutaneously) for the first dose. Then 10 to 20 units are given subcutaneously each half hour or hour until the patient becomes conscious or the glycosuria and blood sugar are greatly reduced. After this the repetition and dosage must depend on the results. Small frequent doses are more effective than large doses at longer intervals. The urine should be examined frequently and the blood sugar estimated if possible. Carbohydrate should be given in amounts of half to one gram for each unit of insulin. Insulin should be given in doses above 50 units for some days. The dosage is to be governed by urine analysis and blood sugar determinations. The diet should be relatively high in carbohydrate and given in five or six meals with insulin before each of them. This should be done for some days and then a gradual return made to the usual rules.

(6) *Alkalies.* There is much difference of opinion as to their value. The

COMPOSITION OF FOOD SUITABLE FOR DIABETICS

Food	*Wt. Gms.*	*Approx. Meas.*	*P.*	*F.*	C.	Cal.
Cereal						
Cooked	120	½ c.	3	—	16	76
Dry	20	½ c.	3	—	16	76
Shredd. Wheat	28	1 biscuit	3	—	21	96
Bread	30	1 slice	3	—	16	76
Bread	15	½ slice	1.5	—	8	38
Crackers, soda	6	2 biscuits (2″x2″)	1	1	4	29
Milk, whole	240	1 c.	7	10	12	166
Milk, skimmed	240	1 c.	7	—	12	76
20% Cream	120	½ c.	4	24	4	248
40% "	120	½ c.	2	48	2	448
3% Vegetable	100	½ c. 1 serving	2	—	3	20
6% "	100	½ c. "	2	—	6	32
9% "	100	½ c. "	3	—	9	48
12% "	100	½ c. "	4	—	12	64
15% "	100	½ c. "	4	—	15	76
18% "	100	½ c. "	5	1	18	101
3% Fruit	100	½ c. "	—	—	3	12
6% "	100	½ c. "	—	—	6	24
9% "	100	½ c. "	—	—	9	36
12% "	100	½ c. "	—	—	12	48
15% "	100	½ c. "	—	—	15	60
18% "	100	½ c. "	—	—	18	72
Egg	50	1	7	5	—	73
Meat and Chicken	30	1 oz.	7	5	—	73
Fish, fresh	30	1 oz.	6	2	—	42
Cheese, Am.	30	1 oz.	9	11	—	135
" Cream	30	1 oz.	8	10	1	126
" Cottage	30	1 oz.	6	—	1	28
Gelatin	3	1 tsp.	3	—	—	12
Bacon, lean	15	3 thin strips, crisp	3	8	—	84
Butter	10	2 tsp.	—	8.5	—	77
Oil	10	2 tsp.	—	10	—	90
Mayonnaise	14	1 tbsp.	—	12	—	108
Cocoa	5	2 tsp.	1	1	2	21

c: cup tsp: teaspoon tbsp: tablespoon

1 gram protein contains 4 calories
1 " carbohyrate contains 4 calories
1 " fat contains 9 calories
1 " alcohol contains 7 calories

1 kilogram—2.2 pounds
6.25 grams protein contain 1 gram nitrogen.
A patient "at rest" requires 25 to 30 calories per kilogram of body weight.

DIABETIC FOOD TABLE, INCLUDING THE COMPARATIVE WEIGHTS AND MEASURES OF AVERAGE SERVINGS WITH THE FOOD VALUES

30 grams = 1 oz. } 2 Tablespoonfuls

THE CARBOHYDRATE PERCENTAGE OF FRUITS AND VEGETABLES

	3 per cent	6 per cent	9 per cent	12 per cent	15 per cent	18 per cent
VEGETABLES	Asparagus, fresh or canned Beans, green, wax, fresh or canned Beet greens Broccoli Cabbage Cauliflower Celery Chard Cucumbers Dock Endive Fennel Lettuce Mung bean sprouts Mustard greens Okra, canned Radishes Romaine Sauerkraut, fresh or canned Sorrel Spinach Squash, summer Tomatoes, fresh or canned Tomato juice, fresh or canned Turnip tops Watercress	Beans, scarlet runner " snap Beets, canned Chives Collards Dandelion greens Egg plant Kohlrabi Lambsquarters Leeks Okra Peppers, green or red Pumpkin Squash, winter Tomato pureed, canned Turnips	Artichokes, Globe or French Beets Brussels Sprouts Carrots Onions Peas, very young " canned Rutabagas	Beans, lima, canned	Corn, green, very young Parsnips Peas, medium Salsify	Beans, baked " red kidney, cooked Corn, canned Potatoes Succotash, canned
FRUITS	Blackberry juice Muskmelon, including cantaloupe and honeydew Rhubarb Strawberries Strawberry juice Watermelon		Blackberries Cranberries Currants Currant juice Gooseberries Grapefruit Grapefruit juice Lemons Lemon juice Limes Lime juice Loganberry juice Raspberry juice Tangerines	Apple juice Apricots Cherries, sour Oranges Orange juice Peaches Peach juice Pineapple Pineapple juice, fresh Plums (excluding prunes), Raspberries	Apples Blueberries Blueberry juice Grapes Loganberries Nectarines Pears	Cherries, sweet Crabapples Figs Grape juice, unsweetened

From the Bulletin of the United States Department of Agriculture opinion of Joslin, who does not use them, must carry great weight. If employed the dosage should not be over 10 grams a dav of sodium bicarbonate. (7) *Circulation.* This should be supported by digitalis and caffeine if necessary. (8) *Gastric lavage.* This should be done if there is abdominal pain or vomiting. Normal saline solution can be used.

Complications.—The use of insulin is of great aid. In acute infections the danger of acidosis should be remembered. In conditions requiring surgery the patient should be carefully treated until he is in the best possible condition. Fluids should be given freely. If an emergency operation has to be done carbohydrate can be given as orange juice, gruel and ginger ale. With infection it is not wise to adopt too rigid a diet. As to the anesthetic, nitrous oxide with oxygen, spinal anesthesia or a local anesthetic is best. Carbuncles should be operated on early. The patient with *gangrene* should be given insulin and a surgical opinion secured at once. In general, early operation is wise. With coexisting pulmonary tuberculosis the usual diabetic treatment can be employed.

MEDICAL TREATMENT.—Phenobarbital or bromide is sometimes useful for irritable patients. The bowels should be kept open and for this mineral oil, cascara, senna and phenolphthalein are most useful. Purging should be avoided. *Pruritus* is best treated by controlling the diabetes and by lotions of boric acid or hyposulphite of soda, or sedative ointments.

Synthalin.—Certain guanidine derivatives (synthalin and neosynthalin) though contra-indicated in the presence of hepatic and renal disease, and severe ketosis, are effective in reducing glycosuria and blood sugar. Though most useful in mild diabetes (given orally in doses of 10 mg. three times daily, before meals, omitting every third day, owing to the cumulative effect) the tendency to morning hyperglycemia and the necessity of a fourth daily dose of insulin in severe diabetics are frequently avoided by giving 10 mg. before the evening meal. Loss of weight, anorexia, nausea, diarrhea and distaste for fat are indications for discontinuance or reduction of the dosage.

CHRONIC HYPERINSULINISM—HYPOGLYCEMIA

Definition.—A syndrome in which there is excessive secretion of insulin resulting in hypoglycemia.

Etiology.—This is varied and there are probably many causes. Functional overactivity of the islands of Langerhans may be responsible. Adenoma and carcinoma of the islands have been found in some cases. *Pancreatitis* is suggested as a cause. This may be due to a general infectious disease, to focal infection or to some area of infection in the abdomen. A diet deficient in vitamins (especially A and B) may play a part. Other suggested factors are: hepatic disease with deficient glycogenesis; disturbance due to adrenal insufficiency; and disturbed function of the thyroid or pituitary gland. Heredity, trauma and functional disturbance of the nervous system are also suggested causes.

Pathology.—The pancreas may be normal. Hyperplasia of the islands of Langerhans has been found. Adenoma and carcinoma are rare findings.

Clinical Features.—In *mild* forms, weakness, anxiety or irritability, and hunger occur particularly before meals. Fatigue, tremor, sweating and vertigo may be common. In more severe forms the symptoms are marked, especially fatigue, and there may be attacks suggesting *petit mal.* In *severe* cases there may be convulsions, delirium and loss of consciousness, or the picture may suggest alcoholic intoxication. Abdominal pain may occur during the attacks and suggest an acute emergency. There may be tenderness over the pancreas. In the mild cases the fasting blood sugar is from 0.060 to 0.075, in moderate cases from 0.050 to 0.060 and in severe cases below 0.050 per cent. The glucose tolerance test gives a low curve which may not go above 0.110 per cent and falls rapidly.

Diagnosis.—Careful and repeated blood sugar studies should be made. A persistent low blood sugar is suggestive. The symptoms are increased by fasting or exercise. The condition has been mistaken for alcoholic intoxication, epilepsy, psychosis, aphasia and intracranial vascular lesions. The result of giving sugar may be an aid.

Prognosis.—This depends on the cause. There is a tendency to obesity which is unfavorable.

Treatment.—If there is an adenoma of the pancreas, the attempt to remove it is indicated. Part of a normal pancreas has been removed. Otherwise the treatment is largely by diet with frequent feedings of slowly absorbable food. The amount should depend somewhat on the weight. Vitamins should be given freely. It is well to have these patients carry dextrose tablets or lump sugar with them so that they can be taken at once on the appearance of symptoms. Internal secretion therapy may be useful.

Von Gierke's disease is due to a congenital disturbance of glycogen metabolism. There is inability to mobilize glycogen and slight response to the injection of epinephrine. The glycogen content of the blood is high and it is split with difficulty. The persistence of a fetal type of glycogen metabolism has been suggested. Changes in the adrenal glands have been found and some patients show hirsutism and pigmentation. The *clinical* features are (1) infantilism, (2) a large smooth liver (without splenomegaly), (3) adiposity and (4) a low blood sugar and ketosis when fasting. The blood cholesterol is increased. Other organs than the liver may show increased glycogen content which is given as the cause for hypertrophy of the heart and pylorus. The infantilism may result from the low blood sugar.

DIABETES INSIPIDUS

Definition.—A chronic affection characterized by the passage of large quantities of urine of low specific gravity. It is to be distinguished from polyuria, which is frequent in hysteria and some forms of nephritis. There may be polyuria with abdominal tumors and aneurism, tuberculous peritonitis and carcinoma. Willis in 1674 first recognized the distinction between a saccharine and nonsaccharine form of diabetes.

Etiology.—The disease is most common in young persons and may begin at about two years of age. Males are more frequently attacked than females. The affection may be congenital. A hereditary tendency has been noted in many instances. Weil found among 91 members in four generations that 23 had persistent polyuria without any deterioration in health.

There are two main views as to the cause. In one it is regarded as a disturbance of the hypothalamus with failure to regulate the output of water and chloride by the kidney. The other view stresses disturbance of the function of the pituitary gland probably due to inhibition or arrest of secretion of an antidiuretic principle. A number of conditions seem to stand in an etiological relationship—injury to the base of the skull, tumors, lesions of the pituitary gland and medulla, and syphilis (basal and meningitic, a gumma in the fourth ventricle, endarteritis with changes). Hemianopsia is found in a number of the cases. In general, irritation or injury in the region of the fourth ventricle, of the tuber cinerium or hypothalamus (possibly from pressure on the pituitary gland), and of the region bounded in front by the optic chiasm and posteriorly by the peduncle prominence may be responsible. It is possible that the mechanism is not always the same. In some cases the capacity of the kidney to eliminate salt and urine is diminished. Cushing suggested that disturbance of the pituitary function through its autonomic nervous connections may explain the polyuria in functional nervous disturbance.

Morbid Anatomy.—There are no constant anatomical lesions. The *kidneys* have been found enlarged and congested. The *bladder* has been found hypertrophied. Dilatation of the ureters and of the pelves of the kidneys has been present. Death has not infrequently resulted from chronic pulmonary disease. Very varied lesions have been met with in the nervous system.

Symptoms.—The disease may come on rapidly, as after a fright or an injury; more commonly it is gradual. A copious secretion of urine, with increased thirst, is the prominent feature. The amount of urine in the twenty-four hours may be 15 litres or even more. Trousseau speaks of a patient who consumed 50 pints of fluid and passed about 56 pints of urine in the twenty-four hours. In some cases the amount passed is greater than that ingested in liquids and solids. The specific gravity is low, 1.001 to 1.005; the color is extremely pale and watery. The total solid constituents may not be reduced. The amount of urea has sometimes been found in excess. Abnormal ingredients are rare. Muscle-sugar, inosite, has been found. Albumin is rare. Traces of sugar have been met with.

Naturally, with the passage of such enormous quantities of urine, there is a proportionate thirst, and a great inconvenience is the necessity for frequent micturition and frequent drinking. Water intoxication may be responsible for convulsive seizures. This may result if the patient has not been allowed fluid for some hours. The appetite is usually good, rarely excessive as in diabetes mellitus; but Trousseau tells of the terror inspired by one of his patients in the keepers of eating-houses where bread was allowed without extra charge to the extent of each customer's wishes, and says that the man was paid to stay away. The patients may be well nourished and healthy looking and the disease in many instances does not interfere with the general health. The amount of saliva is small and the mouth usually dry. The tolerance for alcohol is remarkable.

Course.—This depends largely upon the nature of the primary trouble. Sometimes, with organic disease, the general health is much impaired; the patient becomes thin, and rapidly loses strength. The affection has persisted for fifty years. Spontaneous cure may take place.

Diagnosis.—A low specific gravity and the absence of sugar in the urine distinguish the disease from diabetes mellitus. Hysterical polyuria may simulate it; the amount of urine may be enormous, and only the development of other hysterical manifestations may enable the diagnosis to be made. This condition is, however, always transitory. In certain cases of chronic nephritis a very large amount of urine of low specific gravity may be passed, but the presence of albumin and casts, high blood pressure, stiff vessels, and hypertrophied left ventricle make the diagnosis easy. Careful search should be made for syphilis and an X-ray study done of the sella turcica.

Treatment.—No attempt should be made to reduce the amount of liquid. In some cases gradual reduction of the protein and salt intake is useful. This should be done gradually. Administration of pituitrin or pitressin subcutaneously usually has a prompt effect which lasts for some hours. In some cases the application to the nasal mucous membrane has been successful. Some patients improve under large doses of thyroid extract. Lumbar puncture has been followed by marked improvement and should be tried. Theocin is sometimes useful in doses of 5 grains (0.3 gm.) three times a day. Antisyphilitic treatment should be given in patients with a suspicious history or a positive Wassermann reaction.

OBESITY

Definition.—A disorder of metabolism characterized by excessive deposit of fat in the body.

Etiology.—Corpulence, an overgrowth of the bodily fat, an "oil dropsy," as Byron termed it, is a common condition which may be a source of great bodily and mental distress. There are a number of factors to consider:

Heredity.—This figures in a considerable number of cases but there is no proof that we inherit a habit of metabolism. The basal metabolism may be normal. The specific dynamic action of protein may be less marked than normal. Sometimes the eating habits of the family may be responsible rather than any factor of heredity.

Simple obesity is due to disproportion between the food intake and the bodily activity. In these cases the basal metabolism is normal. The increased weight, especially if there is anemia, renders exercise difficult and a vicious circle is established. Too much food and too little exercise are the causes in this group. Alcohol may play an important part, especially the malt liquors, both in the extra intake and perhaps through interference with metabolism. The lack of exercise results in less oxygen supply and decreased oxidation.

Metabolism.—Some patients show a *marked retention of water.* This may be responsible for a gain in weight when tissue is being consumed. Decreased oxidation results from lack of exercise and anemia. The latter may be important as the oxygen-carrying capacity is reduced.

Internal Secretions.—The influence of the *gonads* is seen in the increased fat in eunuchs, castrated animals, in some women after the menopause and during pregnancy, and in girls at puberty. The influence of the *thyroid* gland is seen in hypothyroidism. A low basal metabolism seems to be due to hypothyroidism and evidence is lacking that it is a feature of obesity alone. In the obesity of hypothyroidism the patients have a round fat face ("moon face") and a fat neck. The *pituitary gland* apparently has less influence than we formerly thought. In cases attributed to it the face and neck are not fat, the deposit of fat being particularly about the lower part of the trunk, around the pelvis and on the upper parts of the thighs. Tumors of the gland or in its neighborhood may be associated with adiposity and sexual infantilism (Fröhlich's syndrome). *Juvenile obesity* may be due in a large proportion of cases to endocrine disturbance.

Diencephalon.—What part disturbance of nervous centres in this region, which may regulate weight, plays in obesity is difficult to state with certainty. Lesions of various kinds which may not involve the pituitary gland may be responsible.

We must acknowledge that in some cases of obesity the cause is obscure. To say that there is one essential cause—overeating—does not explain all cases, granting that many patients have erroneous ideas of the amount of food they take. In many cases an accurate estimate of the intake of food can be obtained only with the patient in a hospital.

Pathology.—The fat is deposited in the subcutaneous tissues, mesentery, omentum and about the organs, especially the heart and kidneys. The pericardial fat may be greatly increased and penetrate between the muscle fibres. The liver may contain large amounts of fat.

Symptoms.—Inconvenience caused by the bulk, and loss of good looks in women, are the features for which we are usually consulted. While fat is no sign of health, the great bulk may be consistent with remarkable vigor and activity. Shortness of breath, embarrassed cardiac action and difficulty in walking are common complaints. In children obesity is often associated with careless habits in eating and lack of proper control on the part of parents. The condition is increasing, particularly in the United States, where one sees an extraordinary number of very stout children. A remarkable phenomenon associated with excessive fat is an uncontrollable tendency to sleep—like the fat boy in Pickwick. It is probable that this narcolepsy is a manifestation of disturbed pituitary function.

Prognosis.—This depends on the recognition of the cause and the possibility of influencing it. Naturally the character of the patient counts for much as cooperation is essential. In hereditary cases the outlook is always doubtful. Obesity is always a danger, especially if the subject has an acute infectious disease, such as pneumonia. It plays an important part in the etiology of diabetes mellitus and vascular diseases, especially hypertension.

Treatment.—The famous George Cheyne, a man of enormous bulk, reduced himself by dieting from 448 pounds to proper dimensions. One of his aphorisms says: "Every wise man after Fifty ought to begin and lessen at least the quantity of his Aliment, and if he would continue free from great and dangerous Distempers and preserve his Senses and Faculties clear to the last, he ought every seven years to go on abating gradually and sensibly, and at last descend out of life as he ascended into it, even into a Child's Diet." Put in other words, it reads—We eat too much after fifty years of age.

A study of the basal metabolism should be made if possible. Careful records should be kept of the food and liquid intake, amount of urine and the weight. It is best to have the patient at rest in a hospital for a time at the onset of treatment in severe cases. No attempt should be made at rapid reduction; it should not be more than two pounds a week.

Diet.—In mild cases restriction of the carbohydrates and fats may be enough. In severe cases it is well to reduce the calories fairly rapidly. In any case a daily intake of about 1500 calories is usually satisfactory. The reduction should be largely in the carbohydrates and fats; the amount of protein should be kept about 90 grams per day. Sugar and candy should be forbidden; saccharine may be used. The noncarbohydrate flours used in diabetes may be useful. In some patients the total calories may be reduced to 1200; in others larger amounts than 1500 may be required. There should be abundant vitamins; the salt intake should be low. It is well to restrict the fluid intake to about 1200 cc. per day. In children proportionate amounts should be given. Some patients do well on two meals a day; others are better with four small meals. (a) *Fast days.* One day a week when only tea or coffee and a little bouillon are taken is an advantage. At first the patient should stay in bed for this and later he may be about. (b) *Milk days* on which only milk is taken, up to a quart. Skimmed milk is useful. (c) *Green vegetable days* on which small amounts of these are taken, perhaps with some bouillon. In the method used by B. L. Gordon, the usual intake of starch is reduced one-third and one dextrose lozenge (2 gm.) is taken every half hour from 9–11.30 A. M., 2.30–5 and 8–9.30 P. M. No change is made in the intake of fat or protein.

Harrop (1934) suggests a diet with milk and bananas as the basis. The strict diet consists of six bananas and a litre of skimmed milk, taken in three meals, with a small amount of vegetable salad at one meal. Tea and coffee may be taken without sugar or cream; 1500 cc. of water should be taken. This is followed for 10 to 14 days. Another method is to take one or two bananas with 250 cc. of milk for two meals and a third meal of soup, lean meat, 5 per cent vegetables and fruit.

Exercise.—This must be used with judgment. In severe cases at first it should be by massage or by one of the methods for "local exercise" by special apparatus. Exercises carried on with the patient lying are useful. The amount of walking can be gradually increased; if up grade this should be taken into account. Gymnasium work should be carefully controlled. It is well to examine the patient occasionally after exercise to study the result.

Bathing.—Cold baths with vigorous rubbing or exercises afterwards are an advantage. Very hot baths or Turkish baths may be dangerous.

Drugs.—Thyroid extract should be used only in patients with a low basal metabolism and it should not be given routinely. It is wise to begin with one grain (Thyroideum siccum) daily and gradually increase until the best dosage for the patient is found. It is well to omit it for a few days occasionally and it should be stopped at once if any signs of disturbance appear. In some cases the addition of a small amount of pituitary gland extract seems helpful. In fat children in whom hypopituitarism seems present, a combination of pituitary and thyroid may be tried, or either alone. The best dosage or combination has to be found for each patient. Thyroid gland administration is useful in some cases of obesity about the menopause. *Dinitrophenol* has come into use but there is danger of poisoning which should be clearly understood by patient and physician. If given, the patient should be under close observation. The usual dose is 3 to 5 mg. per kilogram of weight with an average dose of 5 grains (0.3 gm.). It causes a great increase in metabolism (but is of no value in myxedema). The related substance dinitrocresol has been used and may be less dangerous. *Cathartics* are given as required, salines usually being best. Drastic purgation is not wise. *Anemia* should be treated by iron and arsenic.

THE LIPOMATOSES

Various forms of localized deposits of fat may be considered here, and we follow the division in Lyon's thorough study of these conditions.

Adiposis Dolorosa (*Dercum's Disease*).—This is characterized by irregular symmetrical deposits of fat in various portions of the body, preceded or attended by pain, and associated sometimes with asthenia and psychical changes.

The lipomatous masses are diffuse and symmetrical, involving the abdomen, chest, arms or legs; or localized on the limbs or trunk. The hands, face and feet are usually spared. The pain is sometimes spontaneous and is easily excited by pressure. Asthenia, not always present, may be a marked feature. The patients are often irritable and there are cases with mental changes. Sometimes the skin over the areas of infiltration is markedly hyperesthetic. The affection is more common in females. Autopsies have not thrown clear light on the pathology. Quite probably it is disturbance of the pituitary gland and the structures lying over it.

Nodular Circumscribed Lipomatosis.—The cases are common. The lipomata are distributed in various localities and vary in size from small encapsulated nodules to large circumscribed tumors, solitary or multiple, sometimes symmetrically placed. They may be painful, and Lyon notes that the accessory features of asthenia and psychical changes may be present.

Diffuse Symmetrical Lipomatosis of the Neck.—This remarkable affection, also called *adenolipomatosis,* is characterized by symmetrical fatty infiltrations, either simple or lobulated, of the subcutaneous tissues, forming a huge collar about the neck. It may occur in this part alone or other limited lipomata are found elsewhere. Males have it more frequently than females. The tumors interfere little with health, but may be very disfiguring. There are sometimes constitutional symptoms. The name "*adenolipomatosis*" has been given because scattered throughout the fatty masses are small firm nodules of lymphatic tissue—sometimes hemolymph glands.

Cerebral Adiposity (*Dystrophia Adiposogenitalis, Fröhlich*).—A condition of obesity may occur with disturbance of the hypophysis, or adjacent parts, associated with a hypoplasia of the genital organs and infantilism. The condition is discussed in the section on internal secretions.

Pseudolipoma.—Sydenham made the keen observation that in hysterical patients there were sometimes swellings, which neither yielded to the impress of the finger nor left a mark. Charcot described the condition as "hysterical edema," of which there is both a blue and a white variety.

Many of these subcutaneous infiltrations, just as in the soft, supraclavicular pad, so common in stout women, are due to fat, and French writers describe all grades of transition from a pseudo-edema to a true lipoma.

Treatment.—This is not satisfactory. A trial of thyroid extract in small doses is advisable, but it is well to suspend its use for a week in every month. Extracts of other glands may also be tried. In patients with signs of tumor of the hypophysis surgical measures should be considered. In adiposis dolorosa large doses of thyroid gland may be advisable and pituitary extract may be tried. Sedatives are generally advisable.

HEMOCHROMATOSIS

Definition.—A disorder of metabolism characterized by a deposition of an iron-containing pigment in the glandular organs, and by an increase in the normal pigmentation with which is associated a progressive sclerosis of various organs, and, in a large proportion of the cases, diabetes. The disease was first described by von Recklinghausen.

Etiology.—Of the cases on record the great majority had diabetes. It very rarely occurs in females. In the majority of the patients, middle-aged men, there seemed to be no marked predisposing causes, though Blumer maintains that alcohol plays an important part. The ingestion of copper has been suggested and large amounts may be found in the liver (140 mg. per kilogram in one of our cases), but this is probably due to deficient excretion and the influence is not proved. Primary carcinoma of the liver may occur with it (in 12 of 128 cases reported in 1927). There is no evidence of excessive hemolysis; it may be a disturbance in iron metabolism. There may be an inborn error of metabolism not evident until middle life. There is a familial incidence in some cases.

Pathology.—On autopsy the ochre or bronze color of the organs is the striking feature. The liver is large and sclerotic; the spleen also enlarged and the pancreas either small and atrophic or fatty and fibroid. The lymph nodes are also pigmented. The pigment is *hemosiderin* or iron-reacting. It is chiefly in the cells of the glands, in the muscle cells of the heart, and in the lymph nodes. The amount in the various organs is enormous, a hundred times the normal in the liver, for example. The *hemofuscin,* the noniron-reacting pigment, has a yellow tint, and is found chiefly in the connective tissue cells. The blood shows no special changes.

Rous and Oliver produced an identical condition in rabbits by repeated transfusions of blood, so that large amounts were being constantly destroyed.

Clinical Features.—There are two groups of cases, the larger one in which diabetes is present, and the smaller in which there is no sugar in the urine. The former group is spoken of by the French as *diabète bronzé,* which has the features of a severe diabetes with weakness, progressive pigmentation of the skin, and an enlarged liver. The pigmentation of the skin varies in color from a dark brown to a leaden or bluish black. Dr. Maude Abbott's case was known as *Blue Mary.* Purpura occurs in some cases. The liver shows cirrhosis with a smooth and uniform enlargement. The spleen may be enlarged secondarily. It was very large in two of our cases. The diabetes is usually severe, and runs a rapid course.

The ultimate *prognosis* is hopelessly bad, most patients dying in the course of months after the establishment of the diagnosis.

There is no special *treatment* beyond measures for the general health; in the patient with diabetes the usual treatment should be carried out, but insulin therapy may cause severe reactions with rapid changes in the blood sugar. There may be resistance to insulin. There is a strong tendency to acidosis.

OCHRONOSIS

Definition.—A rare disorder of metabolism associated with blackening of the cartilages and fibrous tissues and pigmentation of the skin, and the presence of dark urine due to alcapton or to derivatives of carbolic acid.

Etiology.—There are two groups of cases: (*a*) There is a congenital lifelong chemical anomaly in which there is a failure to burn homogentisic acid (alcapton body) formed from tyrosine and phenylalanine with the result that some is excreted in the urine (alcaptonuria) and some stored in the tissues. It may be present in three generations.

(*b*) In the other group the dark urine and the blackening of the tissues are due to the prolonged use of phenol, usually the application of strong solutions externally. There may be a third group with melanuria. In 1929, Goldberg found 51 cases, of which 12 were carbolochronosis.

Symptoms.—When well developed, ochronosis presents a striking picture. The discoloration of the fibrous tissues is best seen about the knuckles, and in thin persons the tendons of the hands and feet show a bluish-gray appearance. The cartilage of the ear has a bluish tint, and there may be symmetrical black patches on the sclerotics. Widespread pigmentation of the skin has been observed. In one patient there was a coal-black discoloration of the skin over the nose and cheeks, and the same was beginning in the hands. This may occur also in the carboluria group. Several of the reported cases had arthritis, and two brothers in the Maryland family had a curious anterior inclination of the trunk with a peculiar waddling gait. There are few symptoms directly due to the chemical malformation. There is usually marked arteriosclerosis. Postmortem, the cartilages, ligaments and fibrous structures are everywhere of a brown-black color.

Treatment.—For the congenital form the intake of protein should be kept to low amounts (0.5 gram per kilogram of body weight). The use of phenol applications should be avoided for any prolonged period.

ACIDOSIS

Definition.—Acidosis is the condition in which acids are absorbed or formed in excess of their elimination or neutralization, or in which there is an excessive loss of bases from the body. This involves a decrease in the alkali reserve of the body and hence a disturbance of the acid-base equilibrium. This alters the pH, the bicarbonate content or the carbon dioxide tension. The free carbon dioxide in the body converts the bases not bound by other acids to bicarbonate and hence the bicarbonate represents the excess of base remaining after non-volatile acids have been neutralized. Hence acidosis involves a depletion of the bicarbonate in the blood which has been termed the "first line of defence" against acidosis. A definite acid-base equilibrium is essential to life and any marked departure from it results in difficulty. This equilibrium is kept at a very constant level and any increase of acid or alkali is automatically guarded against. Under ordinary conditions of diet there is production of acid radicals. These are disposed of by oxidation, elimination, excretion and neutralization.

The means by which the normal ratio is maintained are as follows: (1) Elimination of carbon dioxide by the lungs, in which sodium bicarbonate plays a large part as a carrier; (2) elimination of acid by the kidneys; (3) neutralization of acid by ammonia, and (4) intake of fixed bases with the food. It is evident that oxidation plays a large part in the process. In disturbance of the usual acid-base relations the body endeavors to protect itself by an increase in the normal processes. One important means is increased neutralization of acid by ammonia. The ratio of this to the total N of the urine, which normally is 2 to 5 per cent, may rise to 25 or even 40 per cent. By an increased respiration rate the effort is made to excrete more carbon dioxide by the lungs. The kidneys may excrete more acid than in normal conditions. The reserve of alkali is used so far as it is available. These means may not be sufficient and a decrease in the amount of sodium bicarbonate will result in less CO_2 being carried from the tissues and hence an accumulation of it there. From this dyspnea and air hunger result. So long as the reduction in the alkali reserve is not marked the condition is not serious, but if this does result many changes follow, disturbance in oxidation, disturbed renal function, altered N metabolism, dyspnea, etc.

The mechanism of this decreased alkaline reserve is various. In diabetes mellitus there is excessive formation of ketone bodies. In certain diarrheal diseases it may be that alkali is excreted by the bowel; this probably occurs in cholera. In conditions with loss of fluids there may not be sufficient fluid available. The kidneys may not excrete the normal amount of acid phosphates or may be unable to increase the excretion to meet an emergency. Dehydration is an important element in many cases.

Occurrence.—Acidosis may occur in many diseases, in some of which it is of slight significance only, in others of extreme gravity. The more important are as follows:

STARVATION.—This applies particularly to the absence of carbohydrates from the diet. It is probably a factor in the production of acidosis in acute infections in which there is difficulty in giving sufficient food, and may contribute to the acidosis after anesthesia, especially in cases in which little or no food has been taken for some time beforehand.

ANESTHESIA.—Slight grades of acidosis are common and in the majority unimportant, but in a critical case the incidence of acidosis may be enough to determine a fatal outcome. Hence the wisdom of taking measures to prevent it so far as possible.

PREGNANCY.—Here the acidosis is rarely of serious moment.

IN CHILDREN.—In certain of the diarrheal diseases of children, acidosis may be marked and be sufficient to determine a fatal result. The cyclic vomiting of children is often associated with acidosis. An acid intoxication may be due to a disturbance in the metabolism of the fats and proteins. The condition may come on in a perfectly healthy child, with gastro-intestinal symptoms, vomiting, diarrhea and slight fever. On the second or third day dyspnea appears with abdominal distention, the child becomes drowsy, and may go into coma. The urine usually contains acetone and diacetic acid.

INFECTIOUS DISEASES.—Rheumatic fever, pneumonia, Asiatic cholera and typhoid fever are examples.

DIABETES MELLITUS.—In this ketosis is a serious factor.

Renal and Cardiorenal Disease.—In this group the decrease in the ability of the kidney to excrete acids is an important factor.

Diagnosis.—Increase in the Respiration Rate.—In all cases of hyperpnea for which no other cause is found, the possibility of acidosis should be considered. If the ketone bodies are responsible there is usually a fruity odor to the breath.

The CO_2 combining power of the plasma (method of Van Slyke). The normal is usually 55 to 70 volumes per cent. Figures between 40 and 55 indicate mild acidosis. Symptoms, such as headache, malaise and hyperpnea, usually appear when below 40, and drowsiness appears below 30 with coma at about 20.

Blood.—(*a*) Lowering of the CO_2 content. (*b*) The H-ion concentration. (*c*) Determination of the oxygen-containing power of the hemoglobin.

Urine.—(*a*) Increase in the ammonia. (*b*) Excess of acid or the presence of abnormal acids. (*c*) Change in the fixed bases.

Tolerance.—Tolerance to alkalies, especially bicarbonate, measured by the amount of sodium bicarbonate required to render the urine alkaline.

Prognosis.—As acidosis is not a disease in itself, it is difficult to speak of prognosis, but the outcome of the disease which it complicates may depend on the acidosis, as for example in the diarrheal diseases of children.

Treatment.—Prevention should be used whenever possible. In diabetes mellitus this is essential and should always be considered in the treatment. In general the useful measures in acidosis are: (1) The giving of water freely. (2) The administration of carbohydrate. This may be by mouth, by bowel as by the use of a 2 to 5 per cent solution of glucose or intravenously. (3) The giving of moderate amounts of sodium bicarbonate by mouth, bowel or intravenously until the urine is alkaline. This is important in the early stages, as for instance in children. In some cases the giving of sodium, calcium, potassium and magnesium salts may be of advantage. With established acidosis the treatment must depend on the underlying condition. In general the giving of sodium bicarbonate intravenously (2-5 per cent solution which should not be boiled) even up to 50 grams is advisable in severe cases. In milder ones the administration may be by mouth or by rectum. Large amounts of water should be given.

ALKALOSIS

In *alkalosis* there is the loss of large amounts of acid without a comparable loss of alkali or base, or alkali is supplied to or formed in the body in amount greater than its excretion or neutralization. The condition is often one of compensated alkalosis which may go on to uncompensated alkalosis in which the pH is above 7.5. The means by which the acid-base relation is kept constant have been given under acidosis. The blood is a complex fluid in which the salts, with protein and hemoglobin, act as "buffers" and keep the reaction constant. In this regulation the sodium bicarbonate, carbon dioxide and the respiratory centre are important. Alkalosis may arise from various causes. Increased respiration, which may be voluntary, with increased respiration rate, or due to high altitudes, results in greater excretion of carbon dioxide and the alkali reserve increases. Clinical alkalosis is either alkali excess or carbon dioxide deficit. In either case the results are much the same; the urine becomes alkaline. The alveolar carbon dioxide is increased in alkali excess, decreased in carbon dioxide deficit. Ketosis of a mild degree may occur with alkalosis.

A frequent cause of alkalosis is the excessive administration of alkali, usually sodium bicarbonate, as in the treatment of peptic ulcer, acetate or citrate. It may result from loss of hydrochloric acid by vomiting. The removal of the parathyroid glands produces it. The *symptoms* are headache, restlessness, numbness and tingling, tremor of the eyelids, anorexia, nausea, vomiting and excessive dryness of the mouth. Tetany and convulsions may follow. The facial muscles may be tense and show tremor; Chvostek's sign may be present. General edema may be a striking feature. Ammonia and chloride are greatly reduced in the urine. The blood urea may be greatly increased. There is danger if there is renal insufficiency. Death has resulted. In *treatment*, the cause should be considered. If due to excessive giving of alkalies these should be stopped and dilute hydrochloric acid given by mouth; also if there has been marked hydrochloric acid loss. Physiological salt solution can be given intravenously (750-1000 cc.). Acid sodium phosphate gr. xv (1 gm.) every 3 hours is useful. Glucose may be given freely. If due to excessive breathing, efforts should be made to reduce this by breathing through a tube, rebreathing into a gas bag or by giving an oxygen-carbon dioxide mixture.

SECTION VI

DISEASES OF THE DIGESTIVE SYSTEM

DISEASES OF THE MOUTH

Acute Stomatitis.—Simple or erythematous stomatitis, the commonest form, results from the action of irritants of various sorts. Frequent at all ages, in children it is usually associated with dentition and with gastro-intestinal disturbance, particularly in ill-nourished, unhealthy subjects; in adults it may follow the abuse of tobacco, or the use of too hot or too highly seasoned food; it is a concomitant of indigestion and of the specific fevers.

The affection may be limited to the gums and lips or may extend over the whole surface of the mouth and include the tongue. There are at first superficial redness and dryness of the membrane, followed by increased secretion and swelling of the tongue, which is furred and indented by the teeth. There is rarely any constitutional disturbance, but in children there may be slight fever. The condition causes discomfort, sometimes actual distress and pain, particularly in mastication.

In infants the mouth should be carefully sponged after each feeding. A mouth-wash of glycerin and borax may be used, and in severe cases a one per cent solution of nitrate of silver may be applied.

Aphthous Stomatitis.—This form, also known as *follicular* or *vesicular* stomatitis, is characterized by the presence of small, slightly raised spots, from 2 to 4 mm. in diameter, surrounded by reddened areolae. The spots appear first as vesicles, which rupture, leaving small ulcers with grayish bases and bright-red margins. They are seen most frequently on the inner surfaces of the lips, the edges of the tongue, and the cheeks. They are seldom present on the mucous membrane of the pharynx. This form is met with most often in children under three years, either as an independent affection or in association with a febrile disease or an attack of indigestion. The vesicles come out with great rapidity and the ulcers may be fully formed within twenty-four hours. The child complains of soreness of the mouth and takes food with reluctance. The buccal secretions are increased and the breath is heavy, but not foul. The constitutional symptoms are usually those of the disease with which the aphthae are associated. The disease must not be confounded with thrush. No special parasite has been found in connection with it. It is not serious and heals rapidly with the improvement of the constitutional state. In severe cases it may extend to the pillars of the fauces and to the pharynx, and produce irritating ulcers which are difficult to heal.

Each ulcer should be touched with nitrate of silver and the mouth should be thoroughly cleansed after taking food. A wash of chlorate of potassium, or of borax and glycerin, may be used. The constitutional symptoms should receive careful attention.

A curious affection occurs in southern Italy sometimes in epidemic form, characterized by a pearly-colored membrane with induration, immediately beneath the tongue on the fraenum (Riga's disease). There may be much induration and ultimately ulceration. It occurs in both healthy and cachectic children, usually about the time of the eruption of the first teeth.

Ulcerative Stomatitis.—This form, also known as *fetid stomatitis* or *putrid sore mouth,* occurs particularly in children after the first dentition. It may prevail as a widespread epidemic in institutions. Insufficient and unwholesome food, lack of cleanliness of the mouth, the presence of carious teeth, and the collection of tartar favor the occurrence of the disease. The affection spreads like a specific disease and in some cases the same organisms as in Vincent's angina have been found.

The process begins at the margin of the gums, which become swollen and red and bleed readily. Ulcers form, the bases of which are covered with a grayish-white, firmly adherent membrane. In severe cases the teeth may be loosened and necrosis of the alveolar process occur. The ulcers extend along the gum-line of the upper and lower jaws; the tongue, lips and mucosa of the cheeks are usually swollen, but rarely ulcerated. There is salivation, the breath is foul and mastication is painful. The submaxillary lymph nodes are enlarged. An exanthem may appear and be mistaken for measles. The constitutional symptoms are often severe, and in debilitated children death sometimes occurs.

In the *treatment* chlorate of potassium has been found to be almost specific. It should be given in doses of 3 grains (0.2 gm.), three times a day, to a child, and to an adult double that amount. Locally it may be used as a mouth-wash, or the powdered salt may be applied to the ulcerated surfaces. When there is much fetor, a solution of potassium permanganate may be used as a wash, and silver nitrate applied to the ulcers. Neoarsphenamine intravenously has proved useful in some cases.

A *variety* of ulcerative sore mouth, which differs entirely from this form, is common in nursing women, and is usually seen on the mucous membrane of the lips and cheeks. The ulcers arise from the mucous follicles, and are from 3 to 5 mm. in diameter. They may cause little or no inconvenience; but in some instances they are very painful and interfere seriously with the taking of food and its mastication. As a rule they heal readily after the application of nitrate of silver, and the condition is an indication for tonics, fresh air and a better diet.

Recurring outbreaks of an *herpetic,* even *pemphigoid,* stomatitis are seen in neurotic individuals (*stomatitis neurotica chronica,* Jacobi). It may precede or accompany the fatal form of *phemphigus vegetans.* Parrot describes the occasional appearance in newborn, debilitated children of small ulcers symmetrically placed on the hard palate on either side of the middle line. They rarely heal, but tend to increase in size and may involve the bone. Bednar's aphthæ consist of small patches and ulcers on the hard palate, caused as a rule in young infants by the artificial nipple or the nurse's finger.

Parasitic Stomatitis (*Thrush; Soor; Muguet*).—This affection, most common in children, is dependent upon a fungus, *Oïdium albicans.* It belongs to the order of yeast fungi and consists of branching filaments, from the ends of which ovoid torula cells develop. The parasite grows in the upper layers of the mucosa, and the filaments form a dense felt-work among the epithelial cells. The disease apparently does not arise in a normal mucosa. Improper diet, uncleanliness of the mouth, fermentation of remnants of food, and the occurrence of catarrhal stomatitis predispose to the growth. In institutions it may be transmitted by dirty feeding-bottles, spoons, etc. Robust, well-nourished children are sometimes affected, but it usually occurs in feeble, emaciated infants with digestive trouble, in whom the disease may persist for months. It is not confined to children, but is met with in adults in the final stages of fever, in chronic tuberculosis, diabetes and in cachectic states. The disease begins on the tongue in the form of slightly raised, pearly-white spots, which increase in size and gradually coalesce. The membrane can be scraped off, leaving an intact mucosa, or, if the process extends deeply, a bleeding, slightly ulcerated surface. The process spreads to the cheeks, lips and hard palate, and may involve the tonsils and pharynx. In very severe cases the entire buccal mucosa is covered by the grayish-white membrane. It may extend into the esophagus and to the stomach and cecum. It is ocasionally found on the vocal cords.

The affection is readily recognized, and must not be confounded with aphthous stomatitis, in which the ulcers, preceded by the formation of vesicles, are distinctive. In thrush the microscopic examination shows the presence of the characteristic fungus in the membrane. In this condition the mouth is usually dry, in striking contrast to the salivation with aphthae.

Treatment.—Thrush is more readily prevented than removed. The child's mouth should be kept scrupulously clean, and, if artificially fed, the bottles should be thoroughly sterilized. Lime-water or a 2 per cent solution of sodium bicarbonate may be employed. When the patches are present the alkaline mouth-washes may be continued after each feeding. A spray of borax or of sulphite of soda (a dram to the ounce) or black wash with glycerine may be employed. Permanganate of potassium solution is also useful. The constitutional treatment is of equal importance, and it will often be found that the thrush persists, in spite of all local measures, until the general health of the infant is improved by change of air, the relief of diarrhea, or, in obstinate cases, the substitution of a natural for artificial diet.

Gangrenous Stomatitis (*Cancrum Oris; Noma*).—An affection characterized by a rapidly progressing gangrene, starting on the gums or cheeks, and leading to extensive sloughing and destruction. No specific organism has been found. This terrible, but fortunately rare, disease is seen only in children under very insanitary conditions or during convalescence from the acute fevers, especially measles, more rarely scarlet and typhoid fever. It is more common in girls than in boys. It is met with between the ages of two and five years. The mucous membrane is first affected, usually of the gums or of one cheek. The process begins insidiously, and when first seen there is a sloughing ulcer of the mucous membrane, which spreads rapidly and leads to brawny induration of the skin and adjacent parts. The sloughing extends and in severe cases the cheek is perforated. The disease may spread to the tongue and chin or invade the bones of the jaws and even the eyelids and ears. In mild cases an ulcer forms on the inner surface of the cheek, which heals or may perforate and leave a fistulous opening. The constitutional disturbance is great, the pulse rapid, the prostration extreme, and death usually takes place within a week or ten days. The temperature may reach 103° or 104° F. Diarrhea is usually present, and aspiration pneumonia is a common complication. Destruction of the sore by the cautery is the most effectual treatment. Antiseptic applications should be used to lessen the fetor. The child should be carefully nourished and stimulation used freely.

Mercurial Stomatitis (*Ptyalism*).—It occurs in persons with a special susceptibility, as a result of the excessive use of the drug, and in those whose occupation necessitates the handling of mercury. It may follow the administration of repeated small doses of calomel or gray powder. The patient complains first of a metallic taste in the mouth, the gums become swollen, red, and sore, mastication is difficult, the salivary glands become enlarged and painful, and there is a great increase in their secretion. The tongue is swollen, the breath is foul, and there may be ulceration of the mucosa, and, in rare instances, necrosis of the jaw. The condition is rarely serious, and recovery usually takes place in a couple of weeks. Instances in which the teeth become loosened or in which the inflammation extends to the pharynx and Eustachian tubes are rare.

The administration of mercury should be suspended so soon as the gums are "touched." Mild cases subside within a few days and require only a simple mouth-wash. In severe cases chlorate of potassium may be given internally in doses of gr. v-x (0.3-0.6 gm.) and used to rinse the mouth. The bowels should be freely opened; the patient should take a hot bath every evening and drink plentifully of alkaline mineral waters. Atropine is serviceable, and may be given in doses of $\frac{1}{100}$ of a grain (0.00065 gm.). When the salivation is severe and protracted the patient becomes much debilitated and anemic, so that a supporting treatment is indicated. The diet is necessarily liquid, for the patient finds great difficulty in taking food. If the pain is severe sedatives may be given at night.

Here may be mentioned the influence of stomatitis, particularly the mercurial form, upon the developing teeth of children. The condition known as *erosion*, in which the teeth are honeycombed or pitted owing to defective formation of enamel, is indicative, as a rule, of infantile stomatitis or of severe illness before the second dentition. Such teeth must be distinguished from those of congenital syphilis, which may coexist, but the two conditions are distinct. The honeycombing is frequent on the incisors; but, according to Jonathan Hutchinson, the test teeth of infantile stomatitis are the first permanent molars, then the incisors, "which are almost constantly pitted, eroded, and of bad color, often showing the transverse furrow which crosses all the teeth at the same level."

Geographical Tongue (*Eczema of the Tongue*).—A remarkable desquamation of the superficial epithelium of the tongue in circinate patches, which spread while the central portions heal. Fusion of patches leads to areas with sinuous outlines. When extensive the tongue may be covered with these areas, like a geographical map. The affection causes a good deal of itching and heat, and it may be a source of much mental worry to the patients, who often dread that it may be a commencing cancer.

The *etiology* is unknown. It occurs in infants and children, and is not infrequent in adults. Transient attacks may accompany indigestion. It is liable to relapse and in adults may prove very obstinate. The application of solutions of nitrate of silver give the most satisfactory results.

There is a superficial *glossitis,* limited usually to the border and point of the tongue, which presents irregular reddish spots, as if the epithelium was removed; the papillae are reddened and swollen. It is sometimes known as Möller's glossitis. Local treatment with nitrate of silver gives relief.

Leukoplakia buccalis.—Samuel Plumbe described the condition as *ichthyosis lingualis.* It has also been called *buccal psoriasis* and *leukokeratosis mucosae oris.* The following forms occur; (*a*) Small white spots upon the tongue, slightly raised, even papillomatous—lingual corns. (*b*) Diffuse thickening of the epithelial coating of the tongue, either a thin, bluish-white color or opaque white, depending upon the thickness. It is patchy and more often upon the dorsum and sides. (*c*) Diffuse oral leukoplakia, a condition in which the roof of the mouth, the gums, lips, and cheeks are covered with an opaque white, sometimes smooth, sometimes fissured, rugose layer. In this form the tongue may be spared. The visible mucosa of the lips, occasionally the genital mucosa and the pelves of the kidneys may be involved.

While appearing spontaneously, the condition is most common in heavy smokers, and has been called smoker's tongue. Epithelioma occasionally starts from the localized patches. Many of the patients have had syphilis, but the condition does not yield, as a rule, to specific treatment.

Leukoplakia is a very obstinate affection. Irritants, such as tobacco and very hot food, should be avoided. Local treatment with corrosive sublimate solution (1-200) or chromic acid solution (1 per cent) has been recommended. The propriety of active local treatment is doubtful. Papillomatous outgrowths should be cut off or cauterized. The X-rays may be tried. The most extensive form may disappear spontaneously.

The *glossy flat atrophy* of the posterior part of the tongue, described by Virchow, is in a majority of instances of syphilitic origin. Scars may give an irregular appearance to the surface. Symmers found this smooth atrophy in 55 of 75 postmortems in syphilitic subjects.

Black Hairy Tongue.—This is due to a yeast (*Cryptococcus linguae pilosae*) and an acid reaction of the mouth seems necessary. The nature of the pigment is doubtful; it may be a product of the fungus.

Hyperesthesia of the Tongue.—A very distressing affection, seen chiefly in women at or beyond the menopause, occurs as a sensation of burning felt at the top over the dorsum, along the edges or sometimes over the entire organ. On examination nothing is to be seen; there is no swelling, and there may be no irritation about the teeth. It is a very obstinate affection. Some cases are due to *chronic streptococcal glossitis* with the organisms in the subepithelial layer and difficult to reach. Painting with iodine or in some cases X-ray therapy may give relief.

Fetor oris.—The practitioner is frequently consulted for foul breath and is daily made aware of its prevalence. All unconscious, he is himself often a subject of the condition, to the disgust of his patients. The following are a few of the more important causes: (*a*) With indigestion and associated catarrhal disturbances in the mouth, pharynx, and stomach. The breath is "heavy." A simple mouth-wash and a mercurial purge suffice to remove it. In more serious disease of the stomach the breath may be foul, and occasionally, in sloughing cancer, horribly offensive. (*b*) Local conditions in the mouth: (1) All forms of *stomatitis*. Smokers should remember that, apart from the smell of tobacco, their breath in the morning is usually, to say the least, "heavy." (2) *Pyorrhea alveolaris*. This is the most common cause of foul breath in adults, and is often present after middle life, causing a distinctive odor. To test for its presence draw a bit of stout thread or the edge of a sheet of paper high up between the teeth and the gums and then smell it. Proper mouth hygiene and treatment by a dentist are needed. (*c*) Tonsillar diseases. In the crypts of the tonsils the epithelial débris accumulates, and, invaded by organisms, forms little round or triangular bodies, which can be squeezed out of the lacunae, and when pressed smell like Limburger cheese. The fetor from this cause is quite distinctive. To test the presence in child or adult, smell the finger after it has been rubbed firmly upon the tonsil. Local treatment is needed. (*d*) *Decayed teeth*, the foul odor of which is quite distinct from that of pyorrhea or chronic tonsillitis. (*e*) *Respiratory*. Many diseases of the nose, larynx, bronchi, and lungs are associated with foul breath. (*f*) Hemic. The halitus—the expired air from the lung—may be impregnated with odors from the blood. Of this there are many instances. Pyorrhea alveolaris and chronic lacunar tonsillitis are the most common causes of foul breath.

Oral Sepsis.—To William Hunter is due the credit of insisting upon the importance of the mouth as the chief channel of entrance of pyogenic organisms, and as itself the seat of septic processes. Necrosed teeth, pyorrhea alveolaris, alveolar or apical abscess, etc., are present in many people. A systemic infection may follow or the general health may be lowered by the continuous production of pus. In extensive pyorrhea alveolaris the daily amount of pus is considerable, and there can be no question that it influences the general health and is sometimes associated with a moderate anemia and a pasty complexion. Hunter describes septic gastritis and septic enteritis as sequences; indeed, he regards appendicular, pleuritic, gallbladder and pyelitic inflammations as forms of "medical sepsis" due largely to infection from the mouth. Severe anemia, myocarditis, endocarditis, nephritis and forms of arthritis may be due to oral or dental infection. Possibly the main result of pyorrhea is to cause infection of the digestive tract, which may be followed by disturbance elsewhere.

There is no question of the importance of the subject, and we should insist upon scrupulous cleanliness of the mouth and teeth. Dental floss should be used as well as the toothbrush. We should have less delicacy in telling our friends in whom the odor of the breath reveals the presence of pyorrhea. It is difficult to cure but much may be done to keep it under control. The patient should be referred to a dentist who is especially competent to deal with it. The tartar should be removed and antiseptic mouth-washes used frequently. Hydrogen peroxide (1 to 4) or equal parts of tincture of iodine and alcohol may be applied locally. A saturated solution of thymol is an effective mouthwash. The toothbrush and dental floss should be used at least twice daily.

Affections of the mucous glands are not very common. In catarrhal troubles in children and in measles they may be swollen. They are enlarged and very prominent in Mikulicz's disease, with chronic symmetrical enlargement of the salivary and lachrymal glands. There is a singular affection of the mucous glands of the lips, chiefly of the lower, with much swelling and infiltration known as *macrochilia.* It was described by Volkmann, and has been called Bälz's disease. The mucous glands are enlarged, the ducts much dilated, and on pressure a mucoid or mucopurulent secretion may exude. The skin over the lips may be reddened and swollen. There may be adenoma of the mucous glands. Some cases of "double lip" are due to syphilis.

Torus palatinus.—This is a protrusion in the midline of the hard palate which probably develops *in utero* or shortly after birth, and is found in females more often than in males, does not cause any symptoms and those having it are unaware of the fact unless they are told. It is easily recognized by inspection. It has been regarded as a sign of tuberculosis, of syphilis, of pulmonary osteo-arthropathy and of degeneracy, without any evidence. It is a congenital anomaly without any particular significance.

DISEASES OF THE SALIVARY GLANDS

Supersecretion (*Ptyalism*).—The normal amount of saliva varies from 2 to 3 pints in the twenty-four hours. The secretion is increased during the taking of food and in the physiological processes of dentition. A great increase (*ptyalism*) occurs (1) occasionally in mental and nervous affections, especially Parkinsonism, and in rabies; (2) occasionally in the acute fevers, particularly smallpox; (3) in stomatitis, mouth infection and painful conditions of the mouth; (4) with irritation of the esophagus, gastric hyperacidity, occasionally with ulcer and disease of the pancreas; (5) during gestation, usually early, though it may persist through the entire course; (6) occasionally at each menstrual period; and (7) it is a common effect of certain drugs, mercury, iodine compounds and jaborandi, also muscarine and tobacco. Salivation may be present without any inflammation of the mouth. In some patients there may be constant spitting or swallowing which becomes a habit. The constant secretion is annoying and if it is swallowed digestive disturbance may follow. In some patients, especially in the neurotic type, there may be complaint of a foul taste to the saliva, apart from that due to drugs.

In *treatment,* correction of the cause is important. Belladonna or atropine controls the secretion; the effective dose has to be found for each patient. Bromides may be helpful. The use of milk of magnesia both internally and as a mouth wash is often useful. Sometimes a bitter solution, such as quinine, as a mouth wash is useful if there is an unpleasant taste. The submaxillary glands have been removed to give relief.

Xerostomia (*Deficient Salivary Secretion; Dry Mouth*).—In this condition, first described by Jonathan Hutchinson, the secretions of the mouth and salivary glands are suppressed. The tongue is red, sometimes cracked, and quite dry; the mucous membrane of the cheeks and of the palate is smooth, shining, and dry; and mastication, deglutition, and articulation are very difficult. There is often an unpleasant taste. A majority of the cases are in women, and in several instances have been associated with nervous phenomena. The general health, as a rule, is unimpaired. In *treatment* the diet should be that which tends to stimulate the flow of saliva. Acids and a bitter tonic before meals are useful. Care should be taken to keep the mouth thoroughly clean. The free use of glycerin or vaseline locally is sometimes of value and jaborandi or pilocarpine can be given cautiously.

Inflammation of the Salivary Glands.—(*a*) *Specific Parotitis.* (See Mumps.) (*b*) *Symptomatic parotitis* occurs:

(1) In the infectious fevers—typhus, typhoid, pneumonia, pyemia, etc. In ordinary practice it occurs oftenest in typhoid fever. It is the result of infection by the blood or the salivary duct. The process is usually severe and may progress to suppuration. It is, as a rule, an unfavorable indication in the course of a fever. Care in keeping the mouth clean is important in prevention. Parotitis may occur in secondary syphilis.

(2) In connection with injury or disease of the abdomen or pelvis. Of 101 cases, "10 followed injury or disease of the urinary tract, 18 were due to injury or disease of the alimentary canal, and 23 were due to injury or disease of the abdominal wall, the peritoneum, or the pelvic cellular tissue. The remaining 50 were due to injury, disease, or temporary derangement of the genital organs." By temporary derangement is meant slight injuries or natural processes—a slight blow on the testis, the introduction of a pessary, menstruation. The infection probably takes place through the duct.

(3) In association with facial paralysis, as in a case of fatal peripheral neuritis described by Gowers; in diabetes and chronic metallic poisoning.

(4) It may occur with a calculus.

Treatment of the gland by radium or X-rays is useful.

Uveoparotitis.—In this there is parotitis with uveitis and iridocyclitis. The cause is in dispute; some regard it as tuberculous. The parotitis is usually bilateral, firm and painless; it may last for days or months. Facial palsy may occur. Some cases have fever (*uveoparotid fever*) and erythema; a severe polyneuritis has occurred in some cases. The course is chronic and recovery is usual.

Treatment.—In the infectious diseases rigid cleanliness of the mouth is an important preventive measure. The use of chewing gum may be helpful. For the parotitis an ice bag often aids or hot fomentations may be applied. A free incision should be made *early* if there are signs of suppuration.

(*c*) *Chronic parotitis,* in which the glands are enlarged, rarely painful, may follow inflammation of the throat or mumps. Salivation may be present. It may be due to lead, mercury or iodide. It occurs also in chronic nephritis and syphilis. The cases at the Johns Hopkins clinic were reported by C. P. Howard (Internat. Clinics, xix, 1). It may be associated with xerostomia. The parotid and submaxillary glands are affected with equal frequency. In one case the swelling recurred over a period of 20 years (Grieg).

Sialolithiasis.—Salivary calculi are not rare and occur most often in the submaxillary gland or ducts (75 per cent), next in the parotid (20 per cent) and rarely in the sublingual gland or ducts (Greeley, 1934). They are composed of calcium, oxalate, globulin and mucin. The *symptoms* are variable; there may be pain usually due to obstruction, which is often temporary or there may be a painful swelling. Infection may occur and pus be found coming from the duct. On palpation the stone may be felt if in the duct. The *diagnosis* may be made by palpation or by X-ray study in the proper plane. The passage of a probe is rarely necessary and may cause damage. If the stone is in a salivary gland the diagnosis is more difficult and the X-ray study is important. In *treatment* the salivary secretion should be increased. Sometimes a stone can be gently moved along the duct to the opening. Otherwise surgical removal is advisable. Removal of the submaxillary or sublingual gland may be advisable, rarely the parotid gland.

Tumors.—*Mikulicz's Disease.*—In this remarkable affection, described in 1888, there is a chronic, indolent, painless, symmetrical enlargement of the *salivary* and *lachrymal* glands which may last for several years. In some cases the process is tuberculous or luetic. The gland substance itself may not be disturbed, but there is a great infiltration of the interstitial connective tissue. In one case the lachrymal glands were replaced by fibrous tissue. In some cases the blood presents the picture of leukemia. In America the disease has been seen chiefly in negroes. The enlargement may subside after an acute fever. Good results have followed the use of arsenic, iodide and the X-rays. There is no tendency to recurrence after removal.

Gaseous Tumors of Steno's Duct and of the Parotid Gland.—In glass-blowers and musicians who play wind instruments Steno's duct may become inflated with air and form a tumor the size of a nut or of an egg. Some have contained a mixture of air, saliva and pus. In rare cases there are gaseous tumors of the glands, which give a sensation of crepitation on palpation.

Mixed Tumor of the Parotid Gland.—A variety of tumors are described, the majority being benign. The parotid is enlarged, firm, painless and enlarges slowly. Occasionally the growth becomes malignant.

DISEASES OF THE PHARYNX

Circulatory Disturbances.—*Hyperemia* is common in acute and chronic affections of the throat, and is frequently seen as a result of the irritation of tobacco smoke, and from the constant use of the voice. Venous stasis is seen in valvular disease of the heart, and in mechanical obstruction of the superior vena cava by tumor or aneurism. In aortic insufficiency the capillary pulse may sometimes be seen, and the intense throbbing of the internal carotid may be mistaken for aneurism.

Hemorrhage is found in association with bleeding from other mucous surfaces, or is due to local causes—granulations or varicosities. It may be mistaken for hemorrhage from the lungs or stomach. Sometimes the patient finds the pillow stained in the morning with bloody secretion. The condition is rarely serious and requires only suitable local treatment. Occasionally hemorrhage takes place into the mucosa, producing a pharyngeal hematoma. A condition of the uvula resembling hemorrhagic infarction may occur.

Edema.—An infiltrated edematous condition of the uvula and adjacent parts is not very uncommon in conditions of debility, in profound anemia, and in nephritis. The uvula is sometimes enormously enlarged from this cause whence may arise difficulty in swallowing or in breathing.

Acute Pharyngitis (*Sore Throat; Angina Simplex*).—The entire pharyngeal structures, often with the tonsils, are involved. The condition may follow cold or exposure. In other instances it is associated with constitutional states, such as gout or digestive disorders. The patient complains of uneasiness and soreness in swallowing, of tickling and dryness in the throat, with a constant desire to hawk and cough. Frequently the inflammation extends into the larynx and produces hoarseness. Not uncommonly it is only part of a general nasopharyngeal catarrh. The process may pass into the Eustachian tubes and cause slight deafness. There may be stiffness of the neck with enlarged and painful lymph nodes. The constitutional symptoms are rarely severe. The disease sets in with a chilly feeling and slight fever; the pulse is increased in frequency. Occasionally the febrile symptoms are more severe, particularly if the tonsils are specially involved. The throat shows general congestion of the mucous membrane, which is dry and glistening, and in places covered with sticky secretion. The uvula may be much swollen.

Acute pharyngitis lasts only a few days and requires mild measures. A calomel and saline purge is useful. The nose and throat may be sprayed with a simple saline solution. Cold compresses or an ice bag may be applied to the neck. If the tonsils are involved and the fever is high, acetylsalicylic acid or sodium salicylate may be given.

There is a form due to the *pneumococcus* which is acute with fever and toxemia. There is severe pain with difficulty in swallowing. There are redness and edema, and often membrane which may be extensive. Necrosis may follow or edema of the larynx. Pneumococcus septicemia is common and the mortality is high. In *treatment,* serum should be used if Type I or II is present. The use of optochin locally (1-2 per cent aqueous solution) has been disappointing.

Vincent's Angina.—Probably the primary seat of infection is about the gums. In some cases the tonsils are most involved; in others it is a diffuse process with marked lesions of the gums. It is associated with the fusiform bacillus and spirillum of Vincent occurring together. The onset is usually gradual with general malaise and fever, and sometimes pain in swallowing. There is usually only slight pain but sometimes this is severe. The breath is offensive and usually one tonsil shows a patch of membrane which can be readily detached, leaving an ulcer. The soft palate or pillars of the fauces may be involved. The glands on the affected side are swollen and tender. It may involve the gums causing an ulcerated stomatitis perhaps with membrane ("trench mouth") with severe discomfort, especially on chewing, and fetor of the breath. The *constitutional* symptoms vary and are sometimes marked with high fever and prostration. There is usually a leukocytosis. The duration is variable; some cases are very obstinate. The infection may spread to the lungs and has been mistaken for tuberculosis. The *diagnosis* is aided by the finding of spirilla and the fusiform bacilli in smears, sometimes the latter in cultures. The absence of the diphtheria bacillus is important in excluding diphtheria. Leukemia and agranulocytic angina are excluded by the blood examination. Syphilis may give difficulty but the more acute features and the course are of assistance, as well as the Wassermann reaction. In *treatment* arsphenamine solution (1-10), silver salts or hydrogen peroxide may be applied locally. A mouth wash of sodium perborate (1-50 solution) or potassium permanganate (1-2500) may be used. Fowler's solution may be applied by a cotton swab and a saline mouth wash used afterwards. Neoarsphenamine intravenously usually has a marked effect but is only necessary in severe cases. Infected teeth and tonsils should be removed after the acute features are over.

Chronic Pharyngitis.—This may follow repeated acute attacks. It is very common in persons who smoke or drink to excess, and in those who use the voice very much, such as clergymen, hucksters, and others. It is frequently associated with chronic nasal catarrh. The nasopharynx and the posterior wall are the parts most frequently affected. The mucous membrane is relaxed, the venules are dilated, and roundish bodies, from 2 to 4 mm. in diameter, reddish in color, project to a variable distance beyond the mucous membrane and represent proliferation of lymph tissue about the mucous glands. The pharyngeal mucosa may be dry and glistening, *pharyngitis sicca.* The pillars of the fauces and the uvula are often much relaxed. Secretion forms on the pharynx and is removed only by repeated hawking. There is usually irritation or discomfort felt in the throat.

In the *treatment* special attention must be paid to the general health. If possible, the cause should be ascertained. The condition is frequent in smokers, and can not be cured without stopping the use of tobacco. The use of food either too hot or too much spiced should be forbidden. When it depends upon excessive exercise of the voice, rest should be enjoined. In many of these cases change of air and tonics help very much. In the local treatment, gargles, sprays and pastilles of various sorts give temporary relief, but when the hypertrophic condition is marked the spots should be destroyed by the galvanocautery. Infected tonsils should be removed, sinus infection treated if present, and any diseased condition of the nose remedied if possible.

Ulceration of the Pharynx.—*Follicular.*—The ulcers are usually small, superficial, and generally associated with chronic catarrh.

Syphilitic.—Most frequently painless and situated on the posterior wall of the pharynx, they occur in the secondary stage as small, shallow excavations with the mucous patches. In the tertiary stage they are due to erosion of gummata, and in healing they leave whitish cicatrices.

Tuberculous.—Not very uncommon in advanced cases of pulmonary tuberculosis, if extensive, they form one of the most distressing features of the disease. The ulcers are irregular, with ill-defined edges and grayish-yellow bases. The posterior wall of the pharynx may have an eroded, worm-eaten appearance. These ulcers are, as a rule, intensely painful. Occasionally the primary disease is about the tonsils and the pillars of the fauces.

Ulcers occur in connection with pseudomembranous inflammation, particularly the diphtheritic. In cancer and lupus ulcers are also present.

Ulcers are met with in certain fevers, particularly typhoid.

In many instances the *diagnosis* of the nature of pharyngeal ulcers is very difficult. The tuberculous and cancerous varieties are readily recognized, but doubt frequently arises as to a syphilitic ulcer. In many instances the local conditions may be uncertain. Other evidences of syphilis should be sought for, and the patient placed on bismuth or mercury and iodide of potassium, under which specific ulcers usually heal with great rapidity. The examination of a portion of tissue may be necessary to make the diagnosis.

Acute Infectious Phlegmon of the Pharynx.—This is a severe infection, usually due to streptococci. There are difficulty in swallowing, soreness of the throat, and sometimes hoarseness; the neck enlarges, the pharyngeal mucosa becomes swollen and injected, the fever is high with severe toxemia and the inflammation passes on rapidly to suppuration. The symptoms are very intense. The swelling of the pharyngeal tissues may early reach such a grade as to impede respiration. Similar symptoms may be produced by foreign bodies in the pharynx. The patient should be at rest and given as much nourishment and water as possible. Hot or cold applications should be made to the neck. Antistreptococcic serum may be given. Tracheotomy may be necessary and incisions should be made if there is pus formation.

Retropharyngeal Abscess.—The *acute* form occurs: (*a*) In children between six months and two years of age. The child becomes restless, the voice changes; it becomes nasal or metallic in tone, and there are pain and difficulty in swallowing. Inspection of the pharynx reveals a projecting tumor in the middle line, or, if not visible, it is felt, on palpation, projecting from the posterior wall. (*b*) As a not infrequent sequel of the fevers, particularly scarlet fever and diphtheria. The *treatment* consists in free incision, avoiding the chance of inspiration of the pus. The *chronic* form occurs with caries of the bodies of the cervical vertebrae. The diagnosis is readily made, as the projecting tumor can be seen or felt with the finger on the posterior wall of the pharynx. This should be opened through the neck.

Angina Ludovici (*Ludwig's Angina; Cellulitis of the Neck*).—This occurs as a secondary inflammation in the specific fevers, particularly diphtheria and scarlet fever; it may occur idiopathically or result from trauma. It is probably always a streptococcus infection which spreads rapidly. The swelling at first is most marked in the submaxillary region of one side. The symptoms are, as a rule, intense, and, unless early and thorough surgical measures are employed, there is great risk of systemic infection. The various acute septic inflammations of the throat—acute edema of the larynx, phlegmon of the pharynx and larynx, and angina Ludovici—"represent degrees varying in virulence of one and the same process" (Semon). The treatment is surgical and free incisions should be made.

DISEASES OF THE TONSILS

SUPPURATIVE TONSILLITIS (QUINSY)

Etiology.—Acute suppuration of the peritonsillar tissues is met with most frequently in young persons with chronic tonsillitis, sometimes as a sequence of the acute form, sometimes as a result of exposure.

Symptoms.—The constitutional disturbance is very great. The temperature rises to 104° or 105° F., and the pulse ranges from 110 to 130. Nocturnal delirium is not uncommon. The prostration may be extreme. There is no local disease of similar extent which so rapidly exhausts the strength of a patient. Soreness and dryness of the throat, with pain on swallowing, are the first symptoms. One or both tonsils may be involved. They are enlarged, firm to the touch, dusky red and edematous, and the contiguous parts are also much swollen. The swelling of the glands may be so great that they meet in the middle line, or one tonsil may even push the uvula aside and almost touch the other gland. The salivary and buccal secretions are increased. The glands of the neck enlarge, the lower jaw is fixed and the patient is unable to open his mouth. In from two to four days the area becomes softer, and fluctuation can be felt by placing one finger on the tonsil and the other at the angle of the jaw. The abscess may burst spontaneously, affording instant relief. Suffocation has followed the rupture of a large abscess and the entrance of pus into the larynx. When the suppuration is extensive, the internal carotid artery may be opened; but this is very rare. The *diagnosis* is usually easy, but a gumma or new growth may be regarded as quinsy.

Occasionally a small focus of deep-seated suppuration causes fever lasting for weeks or months.

Treatment.—Hot applications in the form of poultices and fomentations may be more comfortable than the ice bag. Codein or morphia may be required for pain. Irrigation of the throat with a hot alkaline solution usually gives some relief. The area should be opened when fluctuation is distinct. The progress may be shortened and the patient spared several days of suffering if an incision is made early. A curved bistoury, guarded nearly to the point with plaster or cotton, is the most satisfactory instrument. There are cases in which, before suppuration takes place, the swelling is so great that the patient is threatened with suffocation. In such instances the tonsil must be excised or tracheotomy performed. Patients with this affection require a nourishing liquid diet, and during convalescence iron in full doses.

Early removal of the tonsils should be done after the attack is over and thorough local treatment should be given to the nasopharynx.

CHRONIC TONSILLITIS AND ADENOIDS

(*Chronic Nasopharyngeal Obstruction; Mouth-breathing; Aprosexia*)

Under this heading will be considered also hypertrophy of the adenoid tissue in the vault of the pharynx as the affection usually involves both the tonsils proper and this tissue in children. Chronic disease of these tissues is an affection of great importance and may influence in an extraordinary way the mental and bodily development of children.

The lacunae are really culture tubes in which an extraordinary number of organisms grow, the dominant ones being streptococci. Other organisms are the staphylococcus, pneumococcus, and *Micrococcus catarrhalis.* Normally these organisms are kept at bay by the epithelium and by the leukocytes which constantly stream out from the lymphoid tissues. But in catarrhal conditions or by abrasion, the organisms may spread into the substance of the tonsil or pass the capsule and cause a general infection. Chronic tonsillar infection is a frequent source of metastatic infection.

Etiology.—"Adenoids" have become recognized as a most common affection of childhood, occurring most frequently between the fifth and tenth years. The systematic inspection of school children has more than anything else forced upon the profession and the public the importance of tonsillar infection and adenoids as influencing seriously bodily and mental growth, disturbing hearing and furnishing a focus for the development of pathogenic organisms. Few children escape altogether. In many it is a trifling affair, easily remedied; in others it is a serious and obstinate trouble, taxing the skill and judgment of the specialist. It is not easy to say why the conditions have become so prevalent. In the United States it is attributed to the dry, hot air of the houses, in England to the cold damp climate. In winter nearly all the school children in England have the "snuffles," and a considerable proportion of them adenoids.

American children may be especially prone, but the disease is very prevalent in England.

Adenoids may be associated with slight enlargement of the lymph glands, thymus and spleen in the condition of lymphatism.

Morbid Anatomy.—The tonsils are enlarged, due to multiplication of all the constituents of the glands. The lymphoid elements may be chiefly involved without much development of the stroma. In other instances the fibrous matrix is increased, and the organ is then harder, smaller, firmer, and is cut with much greater difficulty.

The *adenoids,* which spring from the vault of the pharynx, form masses varying in size from a small pea to an almond. They may be sessile, with broad bases, or pedunculated. They are reddish in color, of moderate firmness, and contain numerous blood vessels. "Abundant, as a rule, over the vault, on a line with the fossa of the Eustachian tube, the growths may lie posterior to the fossa—namely, in the depression known as the fossa of Rosenmüller, or upon the parts which are parallel to the posterior wall of the pharynx. The growths appear to spring in the main from the mucous membrane covering the localities where the connective tissue fills in the inequalities of the base of the skull" (Harrison Allen). The growths are most frequently papillomatous with a lymphoid parenchyma. Hypertrophy of the pharyngeal adenoid tissue may be present without great enlargement of the tonsils proper. Chronic catarrh of the nose usually coexists.

Symptoms.—The direct effect of adenoids is the establishment of *mouth-breathing.* The indirect effects are deformation of the thorax, changes in the facial expression, sometimes marked mental alteration, in certain cases stunting of the growth, and deafness in a great many subjects. Woods Hutchinson suggested that the embryological relation of these structures and the pituitary body may account for the interference with development. The establishment of *mouth-breathing* is the symptom which first attracts attention. It is not so noticeable by day, although the child may present the characteristic vacant expression. At night the child's sleep is greatly disturbed; the respirations are loud and snorting, and there are sometimes prolonged pauses, followed by deep, noisy inspirations. The pulse may vary strangely during these attacks, and in the prolonged intervals may be slow, to increase greatly with the forced inspirations. The alae naisi should be observed during sleep, as they are sometimes much retracted during inspiration, due to a laxity of the walls, a condition readily remedied by the use of a soft wire dilator. Night terrors are common. The child may wake up in a paroxysm of shortness of breath. Sometimes these attacks are of great severity and the dyspnea may suggest pressure of enlarged mediastinal glands. Sometimes there is a troublesome nocturnal paroxysmal cough usually excited by lying down. Children with adenoids are specially liable to bronchitis. The thin, ill-nourished mouth-breathing child with deformed chest, cough and scattered bronchial râles is a familiar figure in tuberculosis dispensaries.

When the mouth-breathing has persisted for a long time definite changes result in the face, mouth, and chest. The facies is so peculiar and distinctive that the condition may be evident at a glance. The expression is dull, heavy, and apathetic, due in part to the fact that the mouth is habitually open. In long-standing cases the child is stupid looking, responds slowly to questions, and may be sullen and cross. The lips are thick, the nasal orifices small and pinched-in, the superior dental arch narrowed and the roof of the mouth considerably raised. Carious teeth are common.

The remarkable alterations in the *shape* of the *chest* in connection with enlarged tonsils were first carefully studied by Dupuytren (1828), who fully appreciated the great importance of the condition. He noted "a lateral depression of the parietes of the chest consisting of a depression, more or less great, of the ribs on each side, and a proportionate protrusion of the sternum in front." J. Mason Warren (Medical Examiner, 1839) gave an admirable description of the constitutional symptoms and the thoracic deformities induced by enlarged tonsils. These, with the memoir of Lambron (1861), constitute most important contributions to our knowledge on the subject. Three types of deformity may be recognized:

THE PIGEON OR CHICKEN BREAST is the most common form, in which the sternum is prominent and there is a circular depression in the lateral zone (Harrison's groove), corresponding to the attachment of the diaphragm. The ribs are prominent anteriorly and the sternum is angulated forward at the manubriogladiolar junction. As a mouth-breather is watched during sleep one can see the lower and lateral thoracic regions retracted during inspiration by the action of the diaphragm.

BARREL CHEST.—Some children, the subject of chronic nasopharyngeal obstruction, have recurring attacks of asthma, and the chest may be gradually deformed, becoming rounded and barrel-shaped, the neck short, and the shoulders and back bowed. A child of ten or eleven may have the thoracic conformation of an old man with emphysema.

THE FUNNEL BREAST (*Trichterbrust*).—This remarkable deformity, in which there is a deep depression at the lower sternum, has excited much controversy as to its mode of origin. In some instances, at least, it is due to obstructed breathing due to enlarged tonsils or adenoid vegetations. In two children, seen while the condition was in process of formation, during inspiration the lower sternum was forcibly retracted, so much so that at the height the depression corresponded to that of a well-marked "*Trichterbrust*." In repose, the lower sternal region was distinctly excavated.

The voice is altered and acquires a nasal quality. The pronunciation of certain letters is changed, and there is inability to pronounce the nasal consonants *n* and *m*. Some lay stress upon the association of mouth-breathing with stuttering.

The *hearing* may be impaired, usually from extension of inflammation along the Eustachian tubes and the obstruction of their orifices. In some instances it may be due to retraction of the drums, as the upper pharynx is insufficiently supplied with air. Naturally the senses of taste and smell are impaired. There may be little or no nasal catarrh or discharge, but the pharyngeal secretion of mucus is increased. Children do not notice this, as the mucus is usually swallowed, but older persons expectorate it with difficulty.

Among other symptoms are headache, by no means uncommon, general listlessness, and an indisposition for physical or mental exertion. Habit-spasm of the face has been described in connection with it and permanent relief has been afforded by the removal of the adenoid vegetations. Enuresis is occasionally an associated symptom. The influence upon the mental development is striking. Mouth-breathers are usually dull, stupid and backward. It is impossible for them to fix the attention for long at a time, and to this impairment of the mental function Guye, of Amsterdam, gave the name *aprosexia.* Headaches, forgetfulness, inability to study without discomfort are frequent symptoms of this condition in students. There is more than a grain of truth in the aphorism *shut your mouth and save your life,* which is found on the title-page of Captain Catlin's celebrated pamphlet on mouth-breathing (1861), to which he attributed all the ills of civilization.

A symptom sometimes associated with infected tonsils is fetor of the breath. The inspissated secretion undergoes decomposition and the little cheesy masses may sometimes be squeezed from the crypts of the tonsils. In some cases of chronic enlargement the cheesy masses may be deep in the tonsillar crypts; and if they remain for a prolonged period lime salts are deposited and a tonsillar calculus is produced. The *lingual tonsil* may be a source of infection, excite cough, or cause sensations referred to the nose or larynx. It is often overlooked in a routine examination.

Children with chronic tonsillitis and adenoids are especially prone to take cold and to recurring attacks of acute tonsillitis. They may be more liable to diphtheria, and in them the anginal features in scarlet fever are always more serious. The ultimate results of untreated adenoid hypertrophy are important. In some cases the vegetations disappear, leaving an atrophic condition of the vault of the pharynx. Neglect may lead to the so-called Thornwaldt's disease, in which there is a cystic condition of the pharyngeal tonsil and constant secretion of mucopus.

Other conditions which may result from chronic throat and nose infection, including sinusitis, especially in children, are bronchial asthma, bronchitis and bronchiectasis. In patients over 50 years of age chronic tonsillar infection is often associated with apical infection of teeth.

Diagnosis.—Enlarged tonsils are readily seen on inspection of the pharynx. Infected tonsils may be small; careful local examination should be made. There may be no great enlargement of the tonsils and nothing apparent at the back of the throat even when the nasopharynx is completely blocked with adenoid vegetations.

Treatment.—The decision as to the removal of *tonsils* is sometimes a difficult one. There has been much discussion of the subject and a great deal of nonsense talked. A focus of infection in a tonsil should be regarded exactly as a focus elsewhere. It is a good rule to get rid of any focus of infection if there are no contra-indications. If there is chronic tonsillar infection with local symptoms, recurring acute attacks, injury to the ears or general infection (rheumatic fever, endocarditis, arthritis, nephritis, etc.) it is wise to advise removal. The surface condition is no guide as to the absence of infection in the deeper parts. Age should not be regarded in the decision as to removal if there is infection. Treatment by radium or X-rays cannot be regarded as an equal substitute in the majority of cases. Important complications may follow the removal—hemorrhage, hyperpyrexia, infarction and abscess of the lungs, general sepsis, cerebrothrombosinusitis, subcutaneous emphysema, or death from status lymphaticus. Applications of iodine and solutions of silver salts are of service in the milder grades, but it is a waste of time to apply them to chronically infected glands. The galvanocautery is of service in cases of enlarged tonsils when there is objection to removal, but should not be regarded as an effective substitute inasmuch as the method does not result in a complete extirpation.

The treatment of *adenoid growths* should be thorough. Parents should be told frankly that the affection is serious, one which impairs the mental not less than the bodily development of the child. In spite of the thorough ventilation of this subject, some practitioners do not appear to have grasped the full importance of this disease and are far too apt to temporize and unnecessarily postpone radical measures. Special examination should be made of the thymus gland, as if it is enlarged the operation should be postponed. In the state of lymphatism death during anesthesia has occurred. After removal usually the child soon breathes through the nose but sometimes the habit of mouth-breathing persists. In these cases a chin strap can be readily adjusted, which the child wears at night. In severe cases it may take months of careful training before the child can speak properly. An all-important point in the treatment of lesions of the nasopharynx (and, indeed, in the prevention of this unfortunate condition) is to increase the breathing capacity of the chest by systematic exercises.

Throughout the entire treatment attention should be paid to hygiene and diet, and cod-liver oil and iodide of iron may be administered with benefit.

DISEASES OF THE ESOPHAGUS

CONGENITAL SHORT ESOPHAGUS: THORACIC STOMACH

In this the esophagus is congenitally short and does not reach to the diaphragm, so that there is a projection of the stomach above the diaphragm. In children the main features are dysphagia, regurgitation of food and interference with growth and nutrition. Regurgitation may date from birth. In older patients some indiscretion in diet may begin the symptoms. There may be distress or severe pain, usually after meals, but in some patients only in lying down soon after eating. The pain is referred to the lower part of the sternum and may go to the back. Alkalies usually give prompt relief. Some patients sleep in a half sitting position. Difficulty in swallowing and lodgment of food are fairly common. Ulceration may occur in the thoracic portion of the stomach or at the junction of the esophagus and stomach. *Diagnosis.* The symptoms may excite suspicion but the X-ray study is the most important. The right oblique prone position is usually required. There is often some narrowing at the junction of the esophagus and stomach. The stomach above the diaphragm is larger than the esophagus and rugae can be seen in it. With the esophagoscope some inflammation of the esophagus may be found and ulceration in some cases. In *treatment,* simple food and thorough chewing are important. Alkalies and bismuth often give relief to discomfort. A light meal in the evening is helpful for some patients and nothing should be eaten within four hours of going to bed. A stenosis should be dilated and ulceration receive the usual treatment.

ACUTE ESOPHAGITIS

Etiology.—Acute inflammation occurs: (*a*) In some of the specific fevers; more rarely as an extension from infection of the pharynx. (*b*) As a result of intense mechanical or chemical irritation, produced by foreign bodies, very hot liquids, or strong corrosives. The swallowing of *household lye* is a common cause in young children. (*c*) As a pustular inflammation in smallpox. (*d*) In connection with local disease, particularly cancer of the tube itself or extension to it from without. And lastly acute esophagitis, occasionally with ulceration, may occur spontaneously in sucklings.

Morbid Anatomy.—It is extremely rare to see redness of the mucosa, except when chemical irritants have been swallowed. More commonly the epithelium is thickened and has desquamated, so that the surface is covered with a fine granular substance. The mucous follicles are swollen and occasionally there are small erosions. In the pseudomembranous inflammation there is a grayish exudate, usually limited in extent, at the upper portion. In phlegmonous inflammation the mucous membrane is greatly swollen with purulent infiltration of the submucosa. Gangrene occasionally supervenes. There is a remarkable fibrinous or membranous esophagitis, most frequent in the fevers, in which casts of the tube may be vomited.

Symptoms.—In the milder forms of catarrhal inflammation there are usually no symptoms. Pain in deglutition is always present in severe inflammation. A dull pain beneath the sternum is also common. The presence of a foreign body is indicated by dysphagia and spasm with the regurgitation of portions of food. Later, blood and pus may be ejected. It is surprising how extensive disease in the esophagus may be without producing much pain or great discomfort, except in swallowing. The intense inflammation which follows the swallowing of corrosives, when not fatal, gradually subsides, and often leads to cicatricial contraction and stricture. Severe grades of inflammation with ulceration are followed by cicatricial stenosis. In the cases in which there is danger of contraction preventive treatment should be carried out to lessen the chance of severe stenosis. The possibility of a foreign body should be remembered. An X-ray study and esophagoscopy are important.

Treatment.—This is unsatisfactory, particularly in the severer forms. The slight catarrhal cases should be given fluid diet and bismuth in water. Vaseline may be placed frequently on the back of the tongue and olive oil given in half ounce doses. When the dysphagia is intense it is best not to give food by the mouth, but to give glucose solution (5 per cent) and water by the bowel. Fragments of ice may be given, and later, demulcent drinks. External applications of cold often give relief. With severe injury to the esophagus, gastrostomy should be done at once.

Chronic esophagitis occurs when there is retention of food in the esophagus, and may be associated with chronic pharyngitis or gastritis; ulceration may result. Discomfort or pain is felt, occasionally going through to the back. In *treatment*, irritant substances should be avoided and dry bismuth subnitrate placed on the tongue. Local treatment, especially the use of silver salts, should be applied through the esophagoscope. Mouth infection should be treated.

Ulceration.—This occurs with acute esophagitis. Syphilis, tuberculosis, neoplasm, severe infections and aneurism may be responsible. The majority of cases in adults are due to neoplasm. Sometimes with persistent vomiting, fissure-like lesions are found in the lower esophagus and cardiac orifice. These may lead to ulceration. Rupture into the mediastinum may occur with severe vomiting. *Peptic ulcer* occurs at the lower end of the esophagus. The usual complaints are of substernal pain and difficulty in swallowing; hemorrhage and perforation may occur. The diagnosis is made by the history, general features and direct inspection by the esophagoscope. *Treatment* must depend on the cause to some extent. Rest of the esophagus, bland diet, bismuth on the tongue and local endoscopic treatment are important. Gastrostomy may be necessary.

Esophageal Varices.—Associated with chronic heart disease and more frequently with a cirrhotic liver, the esophageal veins may become distended and varicose. Rupture of these varices is one of the commonest causes of hematemesis in cirrhosis of the liver and in enlarged spleen. The blood may pass *per rectum* alone.

SPASM OF THE ESOPHAGUS

This is met with in nervous patients and hypochondriacs, also in chorea, epilepsy, and especially hydrophobia. It is sometimes associated also with the lodgment of foreign bodies, or with cases in which a patient has swallowed a foreign body and thinks it has stuck. For weeks there may be spasm, due perhaps to autosuggestion, though the bougie passes freely. The idiopathic form is found in females of a marked neurotic habit, but may also occur in elderly men. It may be present only during pregnancy. The patient complains of inability to swallow solid food, and in extreme instances even liquids are rejected. The attack may come on abruptly, and be associated with emotional disturbances and with substernal pain. The condition is rarely serious, though it may persist for years. Spasm of the cricopharyngeus is often the cause of *globus hystericus.* In this spasmodic stenosis there is difficulty in starting the swallowing of the bolus of food. Esophagitis, ulcer and malignant disease are causes of spasm.

The *diagnosis* is not difficult, particularly in young persons with marked nervous manifestations. The X-ray study is important. Great care must be taken to exclude cancer and stenosis.

In patients in whom there is no organic disease a cure may be effected by the passage of the esophagoscope. The general neurotic condition requires special attention. Atropine in full doses is sometimes helpful.

Paralysis of the esophagus is a very rare condition, due most often to central disease, particularly bulbar paralysis. It may occur in myasthenia gravis. It may be peripheral in origin, as in diphtheritic paralysis. Occasionally it occurs in hysteria. The essential symptom is dysphagia.

STENOSIS OF THE ESOPHAGUS

This results from: (*a*) Congenital stenosis of the esophagus. There are several forms of complete stricture; in one there is complete occlusion with the two parts connected by a fibrous cord or with no connection at all. In another the upper portion ends in a pouch and the lower portion opens into the trachea or a bronchus, forming a fistula; in another there may be the upper part only or the esophagus may be closed by a membrane. Vinson (1923) found 146 reported cases and added one. Partial congenital stricture also occurs, often remedied by gradual dilatation. (*b*) The cicatricial contraction of healed ulcers, usually due to corrosive poisons, occasionally to syphilis, and in rare instances after the fevers. Of particular importance is the frequency of stenosis in young children from swallowing lye. (*c*) Tumors in the wall. (*d*) External pressure by aneurism, enlarged lymph glands, enlarged thyroid, other tumors, and sometimes by pericardial effusion. The majority of cases of stenosis of the esophagus in adult and later life are due to carcinoma, usually of the squamous cell form. Adenocarcinoma occurs in the lower esophagus or extends from the stomach.

The *cicatricial stricture* may occur anywhere in the gullet, and the narrowing may be extreme, so that only small quantities of fluid can trickle through, or the obstruction may be quite slight. When the stricture is low down the esophagus is dilated and the walls are usually much hypertrophied. When the obstruction is high in the gullet, the food is usually rejected at once, whereas, if it is low, it may be retained and a considerable quantity collects before it is regurgitated. Any doubt as to its having reached the stomach is removed by the alkalinity of the material ejected and the absence of the characteristic gastric odor. Auscultation of the esophagus is sometimes of service. The patient takes a mouthful of water and the auscultator listens along the left of the spine opposite the seventh dorsal spine. The normal esophageal *bruit* may be heard later than seven seconds, the normal time, or there may be a loud splashing, gurgling sound. The secondary murmur, heard as the fluid enters the stomach, may be absent. The bismuth meal and the fluoroscope make the diagnosis easy. In pressure stenosis, careful clinical and X-ray study usually makes the diagnosis. The esophagoscope determines the locality. A bougie should not be used owing to the danger of perforation. It is well always to examine carefully for aneurism, which may produce the symptoms of organic stricture. When the narrowing is extreme there are always emaciation and marked dehydration. In *treatment* it is important to give sufficient food and water. If the obstruction is marked, gastrostomy should be done. Various methods of dilatation are employed. In pressure stenosis the causal condition should be treated if possible. Gastrostomy should not be delayed too long as is often the case.

CANCER OF THE ESOPHAGUS

This is more frequent in middle life and in males. At first confined to the mucous membrane, the cancer gradually increases and soon ulcerates. The lumen of the tube is narrowed, but when ulceration is extensive in the later stages the stricture may be less marked. Dilatation of the tube and hypertrophy of the walls usually take place above the cancer. There may be marked spasm. The ulcer may perforate the trachea or a bronchus, the lung, the pleura, the mediastinum, the aorta or one of its larger branches, the pericardium, or erode the vertebrae. The recurrent laryngeal nerves may be implicated. Perforation of the lung produces, as a rule, local gangrene.

Clinical Features.—The early symptoms may be indefinite, such as curious "nervous" sensations, a feeling of uncertainty in swallowing, a feeling of a lump in the throat and difficulty if eating rapidly. Such symptoms may come and go as may difficulty in swallowing. *Dysphagia* is usually an early symptom but may be absent until late. If present it is usually progressive and becomes extreme, so that the patient emaciates rapidly. Regurgitation may take place at once after swallowing; or, if the cancer is situated near the stomach, it may be deferred for ten or fifteen minutes, or even longer if the tube is much dilated. The rejected materials may be mixed with blood and may contain cancerous fragments. Feelings of discomfort on swallowing, often regarded as neurotic, increased secretion or cough (sometimes due to the overflow of secretion) may be early symptoms. In persons over fifty years of age persistent difficulty in swallowing accompanied by rapid emaciation usually indicates esophageal cancer. Sudden transient attacks of difficulty in swallowing may occur or there may be no symptoms until there is sudden stenosis with an advanced growth. The cervical lymph nodes may be enlarged and give early indications of the nature of the trouble. Pain may be persistent or present only when food is taken. It may be deep-seated or referred to the back. In certain instances the pain is very great. The latent cases are very rare. Bronchitis and bronchopneumonia are common terminal events. Death usually occurs within 3 to 9 months after the onset of definite symptoms.

Diagnosis.—It is important to exclude pressure from without, as by aneurism or tumor. The history enables us to exclude cicatricial stricture and foreign bodies. In every patient over 40 years of age, esophageal symptoms demand the consideration of neoplasm. The esophagoscope is of great aid and tissue may be removed through the tube for examination. The X-ray study is of service both in showing the presence of a growth and its position. In some cases the symptoms from metastases may be more prominent than those from the primary growth.

Treatment.—In most cases milk and liquids can be swallowed, but supplementary fluid should be given by the rectum. Intubation of the esophagus may be useful for a time. As spasm may play a part, atropine is often useful by causing relaxation. The use of radium and X-rays may prolong life and reduce discomfort but sometimes makes the condition worse. When there is difficulty in feeding the patient gastrostomy should be performed at once, as it gives comfort and prolongs the patient's life. With improved surgical technic and early diagnosis we may hope that cure may be possible in some cases; otherwise the outlook is hopeless.

RUPTURE OF THE ESOPHAGUS

In 1933, Gott found that about 40 cases of spontaneous rupture had been reported. The common cause is increased pressure due to vomiting. Syphilis may play a part especially in patients with general paresis. Any obstruction as from stenosis or a foreign body favors rupture. There are severe pain in the lower thorax, subcutaneous emphysema of the thorax, dyspnea and marked prostration usually followed by sudden death. Boerhaave described the first case in Baron Wassenaer, who "broke asunder the tube of the esophagus near the diaphragm, so that, after the most excruciating pain, the elements which he swallowed passed, together with the air, into the cavity of the thorax, and he expired in twenty-four hours." In a few cases rupture has occurred in a diseased and weakened tube, near the scar of an ulcer, for example. Post-mortem softening must not be mistaken for it. In spontaneous rupture the rent is clean-cut; in malacia it is rounded and the margins are softened. The contents of the stomach may be in the pleura. *Treatment* offers little. Nothing should be swallowed. If rupture has occurred into the pleura, drainage may be done.

DILATATIONS AND DIVERTICULA

Stenosis of the gullet is followed by secondary dilatation of the tube above the constriction and great hypertrophy of the walls. Idiopathic dilatation, so called, is due to phrenospasm (cardiospasm) or associated with contraction of the stomach as in scirrhous cancer. The tube may attain extraordinary dimensions, as in the specimen shown in 1904 to the Association of American Physicians by Kinnicut. Difficulty in swallowing, usually most marked with solids, and regurgitation of food are the most common symptoms. Pain occurs in some patients. There may also be difficulty in breathing from pressure. The *diagnosis* has to be made from cancer, in which the X-ray study and the examination by the esophagoscope are important. It is important to begin *treatment* as early as possible. Certain foods may have a special influence and should be avoided. Atropine, in proper dosage for the patient, may be useful. Special treatment for the causal condition should be given. Gastrostomy should be done before the general nutrition suffers.

Diverticula are of two forms: (*a*) *Pressure* diverticula, which are most common at the junction of the pharynx and gullet, on the posterior wall. Owing to weakness of the muscles at this spot, local bulging occurs, which is gradually increased by the pressure of food, and finally forms a saccular pouch. (*b*) The *traction* diverticula on the anterior wall near the bifurcation of the trachea result, as a rule, from the extension of inflammation from lymph nodes with adhesion and subsequent cicatricial contraction, by which the wall of the gullet is drawn out. The diagnosis of these forms is readily made by the X-rays. They can be successfully extirpated.

A rare condition is the esophago-pleuro-cutaneous fistula. In one patient fluids were discharged at intervals through a fistula in the right infraclavicular region, which communicated with a cavity in the upper part of the pleura or lung. The condition had persisted for over twenty-five years.

DISEASES OF THE STOMACH

ACUTE GASTRITIS

Etiology.—Acute gastritis occurs at all ages, and is usually traceable to errors in diet. It may follow the ingestion of too much food or from taking unsuitable articles, which either themselves irritate the mucosa or decompose, and so excite an acute process. A frequent cause is the taking of food which has begun to decompose, particularly in hot weather. In children these fermentative processes are very apt to excite enteritis as well. Another common cause is the abuse of alcohol, and the acute gastritis which follows a drinking-bout is one of the most typical forms. The tendency to gastric disturbance varies much in individuals, and, indeed, in families.

Morbid Anatomy.—Beaumont's study of St. Martin's stomach showed that in acute catarrh the mucous membrane is reddened and swollen, less gastric juice is secreted, and mucus covers the surface. Slight hemorrhages or even small erosions may occur. The submucosa may be somewhat edematous. Microscopically the changes are chiefly noticeable in the mucous and peptic cells, which are swollen and more granular, and there is an infiltration of the intertubular tissues with leukocytes.

Symptoms.—In mild cases the symptoms are those of slight indigestion—an uncomfortable feeling in the abdomen, headache, depression, nausea, eructations, and vomiting, which usually gives relief. The tongue is heavily coated and the saliva is increased. In children there are intestinal symptoms—diarrhea and colicky pains and often fever. The duration is rarely more than twenty-four hours. In the severer forms the attack may set in with a chill and febrile reaction, in which the temperature rises to 102° or 103° F. The tongue is furred, the breath heavy, and vomiting is frequent. The ejected substances, at first mixed with food, subsequently contain much mucus and bile-stained fluids. There may be constipation, but very often there is diarrhea. The urine presents the usual febrile characteristics and there is a heavy deposit of urates. The abdomen may be somewhat distended and tender in the epigastric region. Herpes may appear on the lips. The attack may last from one to three days, and occasionally longer. The examination of the vomitus shows, as a rule, absence of hydrochloric acid, the presence of lactic and fatty acids, and marked increase of mucus. In some cases large amounts of bile are found in the vomitus or in the fluid obtained by lavage.

Diagnosis.—The ordinary afebrile gastritis is readily recognized. The acute febrile form is so similar to the initial symptoms of some infectious diseases that it is impossible for a day or two to make a diagnosis, particularly in the cases which have come on spontaneously and independently of an error in diet. Some of these resemble closely an acute infection; the symptoms may be intense, and if the attack sets in with severe headache and delirium, the case may be mistaken for meningitis. When the abdominal pains are intense the attack may be confounded with gallstone colic or rupture of an ulcer. Gastric crises in tabes have been mistaken for acute gastritis.

Treatment.—Mild cases recover spontaneously in twenty-four hours, and require no treatment other than a dose of castor oil in children or of blue mass in adults. In severer forms, if there is much gastric distress, vomiting should be promoted by warm water or the stomach tube may be employed. A dose of calomel, 2 to 3 grains (0.13 to 0.2 gm.), should be given, and followed, after some hours, by a saline cathartic. If there is eructation of acid fluid, bicarbonate of soda and bismuth may be given. The stomach should have absolute rest, and it is a good plan to cut off all food for a day or two. The patient may be allowed soda water and ice freely. It is well not to attempt to check the vomiting unless it is excessive and protracted. Recovery is usually complete, though repeated attacks may lead to chronic gastritis.

Acute Suppurative Gastritis.—This is a rare disease due to infection of the submucosa, probably through a minute abrasion. Males are more frequently affected than females, and most of the cases are in comparatively young people. In a majority of the instances in which the examination has been made streptococci have been present, but the pneumococcus has been found in a few cases. There is a widespread suppurative infiltration of the submucosa, with great thickening of the walls. Sometimes there is a localized abscess, with tumor, which may burst into the stomach or into the peritoneum.

The important *symptoms* are pain, high fever, vomiting, dry tongue, all the features of a severe infection, and sometimes jaundice. The vomitus may contain pus. A diagnosis is rarely made; occasionally there is a tumor mass to be felt. The outlook is very serious, as peritonitis usually follows. In *treatment,* little can be done unless a localized abscess can be drained.

Toxic Gastritis.—This intense form is excited by swallowing concentrated mineral acids or strong alkalies, or by such poisons as phosphorus, corrosive sublimate, ammonia, arsenic, etc. In the noncorrosive poisons, the process consists of an acute degeneration of the glandular elements and hemorrhage. With powerful poisons the mucous membrane is extensively destroyed, and may be converted into a brownish-black eschar. In less severe grades there may be areas of necrosis surrounded by inflammatory reaction, while the submucosa is hemorrhagic and infiltrated.

SYMPTOMS.—These are intense pain in the mouth, throat and stomach, salivation, great difficulty in swallowing, and constant vomiting, the vomitus being bloody and sometimes containing portions of the mucous membrane. The abdomen is tender, distended and painful on pressure. In the most acute cases symptoms of collapse supervene; there is restlessness, and sometimes convulsions. There may be albumin or blood in the urine, and petechiae may occur on the skin. When the poison is less intense, the sloughs may separate, leaving ulcers, which too often lead, in the esophagus to stricture, in the stomach to chronic atrophy, and finally to death from exhaustion.

DIAGNOSIS.—The diagnosis of toxic gastritis is usually easy, as inspection of the mouth and pharynx shows, in many instances, corrosive effects, while the examination of the vomit may indicate the nature of the poison.

TREATMENT.—In poisoning by acids, magnesia should be administered in milk or with egg albumen. When strong alkalies have been taken, dilute acids should be administered. If the patient is seen early, lavage should be used. For the severe inflammation which follows the stronger poisons palliative treatment is alone available, and morphia should be given freely.

Diphtheritic or Membranous Gastritis.—This is met with occasionally in diphtheria, but more commonly as a secondary process in typhus or typhoid fever, pneumonia, pyemia, smallpox, and occasionally in debilitated children. The exudation may be extensive and uniform or in patches. The condition is not recognizable during life, unless the membranes are vomited.

Mycotic and Parasitic Gastritis.—Fungi occasionally grow in the stomach and excite inflammation. A remarkable case was reported by Kundrat, in which the favus fungus occurred in the stomach and intestine. In cancer and dilatation of the stomach the sarcinae and yeast fungi probably aid in maintaining the chronic gastritis. As a rule, the gastric juice is capable of killing the ordinary bacteria. Anthrax bacilli may produce swelling of the mucosa and ulceration. Acute emphysematous gastritis may be of mycotic origin. The larvae of certain insects may excite gastritis.

CHRONIC GASTRITIS

Definition.—A condition of disturbed digestion associated with increased mucus formation, qualitative or quantitative changes in the gastric juice, and with alterations in the mucosa. The term "chronic gastritis" has been used loosely to designate a variety of gastric disorders, in some of which there are no actual changes in the mucous membrane.

Etiology.—The causes may be classified as follows: (*a*) *Dietetic.* Unsuitable or improperly prepared food, and the persistent use of irritating articles of diet. The use in excessive quantity of hot bread, hot cakes, and pie is a fruitful cause, particularly in the United States, and also the use in excess of tea or coffee, and, above all, of alcohol. Under this heading come habits of eating at irregular hours or too rapidly, and imperfectly chewing the food. "The platter kills more than the sword." Another cause is the abuse of tobacco, particularly chewing. (*b*) *Constitutional Causes.* Anemia, chronic tuberculosis, gout, diabetes and nephritis are often associated with chronic gastritis. (*c*) *Local Conditions:* (1) of the stomach, as in cancer, ulcer, and dilatation; (2) conditions of the portal circulation, causing chronic engorgement of the mucous membrane, as in cirrhosis, chronic heart disease, and certain chronic lung affections. (*d*) *Oral sepsis,* particularly pyorrhea, is regarded as a common cause, the evidence for which is chiefly of the *propter hoc* kind—the improvement in digestion after attention to the mouth. (*e*) The association of *gastritis* with disease elsewhere, as appendicitis or cholecystitis, may be due to a common source of infection. (*f*) The chronic form may follow acute gastritis. (*g*) How important hematogenous infection may be is difficult to state. In some cases gastritis apparently follows an acute infectious disease. In some cases the etiology may be quite obscure.

Morbid Anatomy.—In simple chronic gastritis the organ is usually enlarged, the mucous membrane pale gray in color, and covered with closely adherent, tenacious mucus. The veins are large, patches of ecchymosis are not infrequently seen, and in the chronic catarrh of portal obstruction and of chronic heart disease small hemorrhagic erosions. Toward the pylorus the mucosa may be irregularly pigmented, and present a rough, wrinkled, mammillated surface, which may be so prominent that writers have described it as *gastritis polyposa.* The membrane may be thinner than normal and much firmer. The minute anatomy shows the picture of a parenchymatous and an interstitial inflammation. The mucous membrane may undergo complete atrophy and be represented by a smooth cuticular membrane.

Symptoms.—The affection persists for an indefinite period, and, as is the case with most chronic diseases, changes from time to time. Many of the symptoms are due to functional disturbance. The disease itself probably does not cause many symptoms. The appetite is variable, sometimes greatly impaired, at others very good. Among early symptoms are feelings of distress or oppression after eating, which may become aggravated and amount to actual pain. When the stomach is empty there may also be a painful feeling. The *pain* differs in different cases, and may be trifling or of extreme severity. When localized and felt beneath the sternum or in the precordial region it is known as heartburn. There may be pain on pressure over the stomach, usually diffuse and not severe. The tongue is coated, and the patient complains of a bad taste in the mouth. The tip and margin of the tongue are very often red and with this there may be an increase in the salivary and pharyngeal secretions. *Nausea* is an early symptom, and is particularly apt to occur in the morning hours. It is not nearly so constant as in cancer of the stomach, and may not occur at all. Eructation of gas, which may continue for some hours after taking food, is a prominent feature in cases of so-called flatulent dyspepsia, and there may be marked distention of the intestines. With the gas, bitter fluids may be brought up. *Vomiting*, which is not very frequent, occurs either immediately after eating or an hour or two later. In the chronic catarrh of old topers a bout of morning vomiting is common, in which a slimy mucus is brought up. The vomitus consists of food in various stages of digestion and mucus; examination shows abnormal acids, such as butyric, or even acetic, in addition to lactic acid, while hydrochloric acid, if present, is much reduced in quantity. In the so-called "acid gastritis" there may be increased hydrochloric acid. The digestion may be delayed, but usually there is not much disturbance of motility.

Constipation is usually present, but in some instances there is diarrhea, and undigested food passes rapidly through the bowels. The urine is often scanty, high-colored, and deposits a heavy sediment of urates. Of other symptoms headache is common, and the patient feels out of sorts, indisposed for exertion, and low-spirited. Trousseau called attention to the occurrence of vertigo, a marked feature in certain cases. The pulse is small, sometimes slow, and there may be palpitation of the heart. Fever does not occur. Cough is sometimes present, but the so-called stomach cough of chronic dyspeptics is probably dependent upon pharyngeal irritation.

Gastric Contents.—The fasting stomach usually contains much mucus. Pathogenic organisms are almost constantly found, of which streptococci are the most important. The hydrochloric acid is usually greatly diminished or absent. It may be found after stimulation by histamine. In advanced cases with atrophy of the mucous membrane, mucus is absent and there may be neither acids nor ferments.

The symptoms of *atrophy* of the mucous membrane of the stomach, without contraction of the organ, are very complex, and do not present a uniform picture. The majority of cases present the symptoms of an aggravated chronic dyspepsia, often of such severity that cancer is suspected. The persistent distress after eating, vomiting, and gradual loss of flesh and strength may lead to the diagnosis of cancer. The clinical picture may be that of a severe anemia which is usually hypochromic in character.

Diagnosis.—It is well in any patient complaining of gastric symptoms to decide first whether there is primary organic disease of the stomach or whether the condition is secondary to disease elsewhere. This involves a general study which should always be made thoroughly. It is easy to fix one's attention on the area of symptoms and fail to recognize the site of the cause. The organic causes of chronic gastric disturbance are usually readily recognized. Carcinoma may give the greatest difficulty, but repeated careful studies of the gastric contents and the X-ray findings usually remove any doubt. With this excluded the problem is to decide whether there is any other organic change in the stomach, such as ulcer or dilatation, or whether the symptoms are purely functional. If evidence of gastritis is found the next problem is whether the condition is primary or secondary. In this the history and the general study of the patient are important.

The study of the gastric contents is usually of great aid. The presence of mucus is evidence for gastritis. The symptoms in functional gastric disturbances are usually more irregular. Careful search should be made for disease elsewhere, either general or local. The relation of symptoms to food is usually marked in gastritis.

Chronic duodenitis is usually secondary to gastritis so that the symptoms are not clearly localized. There is discomfort felt to the right of the midline with nausea. The symptoms are usually some hours after meals. There may be vomiting of mucoid material. There may be signs of pancreatic insufficiency. The study of the duodenal contents is important in diagnosis.

Treatment.—Much of what is said here applies to the group of "dyspepsias" whether due to actual gastritis or not. The discovery and proper treatment of the cause is often the essential point. In many cases the symptoms are secondary to disease elsewhere and in them the treatment is largely of the primary condition. Usually there is no difficulty in differentiating the ordinary catarrhal and the nervous varieties. Two important questions should be asked of every dyspeptic—first, as to the time taken at his meals; and, second, as to the quantity he eats. A number of all cases of disturbed digestion comes from hasty and imperfect mastication and from overeating. Especial stress should be laid upon the former point. In some instances it will alone suffice to cure dyspepsia if the patient will eat slowly. The second point is of even greater importance. People habitually eat too much, and it is probably true that a greater number of maladies arise from excess in eating than from excess in drinking. Chittenden's researches have shown that we require much less nitrogenous food to maintain health.

General and Dietetic.—A careful and systematically arranged dietary is important. It is impossible to lay down rules applicable to all cases but in general the diet should be low in protein and largely carbohydrate. Individuals differ extraordinarily in their capability of digesting different articles of food, and there is much truth in the old adage, "One man's food is another man's poison." The individual preferences for different articles of food should be permitted in the milder forms. Physicians have probably been too arbitrary and have not yielded sufficiently to the intimations given by the appetite and desires of the patient. The amount of fluid depends on the condition of the stomach as regards motility. If there is delay in emptying the amount should not exceed 1500 cc. daily. Usually a glass of hot water before meals, especially breakfast, is advisable.

A rigid milk diet may be tried. "Milk and sweet sound Blood differ in nothing but in Color: *Milk* is *Blood*" (George Cheyne). In the forms associated with nephritis and chronic portal congestion, as well as in many instances in which there is general nervous disturbance this plan in conjunction with rest is most efficacious. If milk is not digested well it may be diluted one-third with soda water or Vichy, or 5 to 10 grains of carbonate of soda, or a pinch of salt may be added to each tumblerful. In many cases milk from which the cream has been taken is better borne. Buttermilk is particularly suitable, but can rarely be taken for so long a time alone, as patients tire of it more quickly than they do of ordinary milk. Not only can the general nutrition be maintained on this diet, but patients sometimes increase in weight, and the gastric symptoms disappear. It should be given at fixed hours and in definite quantities gradually increased. The amount varies, but at least 3 to 5 pints should be given in the twenty-four hours. This diet is not, as a rule, well borne when there is a tendency to dilatation of the stomach. The stools should be carefully watched, and if more milk is taken than can be digested it is well to supplement the diet with eggs and dry toast or biscuits.

In many cases it is not necessary to annoy the patient with strict dietaries. It may be sufficient to cut off certain articles of food. Thus, if there are acid eructations or flatulency the farinaceous foods should be restricted, particularly potatoes and the coarser vegetables. A fruitful source of indigestion is hot bread and this as well as pancakes, pies and tarts, with heavy pastry, and fried articles of all sorts, should be forbidden. As a rule, white bread, toasted, is more readily digested than bread made from the whole meal. Sugar and sweet articles of food should be taken in great moderation or avoided altogether. One of the most powerful enemies of the American stomach is the soda-water fountain, with its many "messes," which has usurped so important a place in the apothecary shop.

Fats, with the exception of a moderate amount of good butter, very fat meats, and thick, greasy soups should be avoided. Ripe fruit in moderation is often advantageous, particularly when cooked. Bananas are not, as a rule, well borne. Alcohol and condiments should be prohibited for a time; it is better if they are given up entirely.

In the matter of special articles of food it is impossible to lay down rigid rules, and it is the common experience that one patient will take with impunity the articles which cause distress to another.

Another detail of importance is the general hygienic management. These patients are often introspective, dwelling in a morbid manner on their symptoms, and much inclined to take a despondent view of their condition. Very little progress can be made unless the physician gains their confidence from the outset. Their fears and whims should not be made too light of or ridiculed. Systematic *exercise*, carefully regulated, particularly when, as at watering places, it is combined with a restricted diet, is of special service. Rest after meals is often useful. Change of air and occupation, a prolonged sea voyage, or a summer in the mountains are sometimes helpful.

TEETH.—These should be put in good condition and mouth infection receive attention. The patient should be taught proper dental hygiene, especially the use of dental floss.

MEDICINAL.—The special measures may be divided into those which attempt to replace elements which are lacking in the digestive juices and those which stimulate the organ. In the first group come the hydrochloric acid and ferments, which are so freely employed. The former is the most important.

It is the ingredient in the gastric juice most commonly deficient. It is best given as the dilute acid taken in somewhat larger quantities than are usually advised. Doses of one-half to one dram (2-4 cc.), in 4 ounces of water may be taken wth meals or immediately after them. Sometimes smaller doses seem as effectual or larger doses may prove more useful. The prolonged use of it does not appear to be hurtful.

The digestive ferments are extensively employed. The use of pepsin may be limited to the cases of advanced mucous catarrh and atrophy of the stomach, in which it should be given, in doses from 10 to 15 grains, with dilute hydrochloric acid after meals. Pancreatin may be given in doses from 15 to 20 grains, with sodium bicarbonate. It is conveniently administered in tablets, each of which contains 5 grains of pancreatin and soda, and of these two or three may be taken fifteen or twenty minutes after each meal.

Of measures which stimulate the glandular activity *lavage* is the most important, particularly in the forms with the secretion of a large quantity of mucus. Lukewarm water should be used, or, if there is much mucus, a 1 per cent salt solution, or a 3 to 5 per cent solution of bicarbonate of soda. The use of a 1 or 2 per cent solution of hydrogen peroxide is often useful. Lavage is best in the morning on an empty stomach or in the evening some hours after the last meal, when there is much nocturnal distress and flatulency. Once a day is, as a rule, sufficient, or, in delicate persons, every second day. The irrigation may be continued until the water comes away quite clear. It is not necessary to remove all the fluid after the irrigation. While in some hands this measure has been carried to extremes, it is of value in certain cases. A substitute may be used in the form of alkaline drinks, taken slowly in the early morning or the last thing at night in case the patient has serious objections to lavage.

Of medicines to stimulate the gastric secretion the bitter tonics are employed but their ability to do this seems doubtful. Of these nux vomica is often employed in doses of ♏ xv (1 cc.) before meals. Histamine hydrochloride (0.25 mg. subcutaneously) is a strong stimulant of gastric secretion.

Treatment of Special Conditions.—*Flatulency.*—For this careful dieting may suffice, particularly forbidding such articles as tea, pastry, and the coarser vegetables. Thorough chewing is also important. If there is much *pain*, spirit of chloroform in 20-minim doses or a teaspoonful of Hoffman's anodyne may be used. In obstinate cases lavage is indicated and is sometimes striking in its effects. Very often flatulency is due to the swallowing of air, a habit which the patient can overcome.

Constipation is a frequent and troublesome feature and every effort should be made to remedy it without the use of purgatives. Regularity in going to stool, the taking of sufficient water especially before meals, proper exercise, and the use of agar-agar or mineral oil may be enough. If drugs are needed the simpler laxatives should be used, such as senna, cascara and phenolpthalein. In the cases secondary to other diseases, such as renal or cardiac, the use of salines is indicated. Glycerin suppositories or the injection of a small amount of glycerin may be efficacious.

Many patients are benefited by the use of mineral waters, particularly a residence at the springs with a careful diet and systematic exercise.

CIRRHOSIS VENTRICULI: LINITIS PLASTICA

Brinton described under the term *linitis plastica* a diffuse sclerosis of the stomach with thickening of the walls and reduction of the lumen. It may be localized, but more commonly involves the whole organ, and a similar condition has been found in the colon, small bowel and rectum. There is enormous hypertrophy of the submucosa, with atrophy of the gland elements and hypertrophy of the muscular layers, so that the wall is six to eight times the normal thickness; but, as Brinton remarks, the layers remain distinct. There are two forms, *benign* and *malignant,* which are not easy to separate without the most careful microscopic examination. There has been much difference of opinion as to the nature of the process; a fibrosing malignant neoplasm, fibromatosis and syphilis are suggested. C. P. Howard (1933) in a careful study concludes that an atypical fibrosing carcinoma is the most frequent cause but the malignant cells may be difficult to find.

The *symptoms* are at first indefinite, anorexia, discomfort and tenderness, but when well established vomiting becomes marked and there is inability to retain even small amounts of food. The presence of a sausage-shaped tumor in the epigastrium is important. Hemorrhage may occur. The X-ray picture is of great help. The protracted history (up to 20 years), the restriction in capacity of the stomach and the tumor give a characteristic picture. In *treatment* food should be taken in the most concentrated form, in small amounts and frequently. Gastric lavage may be useful. Sedatives are necessary. Gastro-enterostomy is helpful if it can be done but in the majority it is impossible; total gastrectomy has been performed.

DILATATION OF THE STOMACH

Acute dilatation is a very serious condition, described by Hilton Fagge, characterized by sudden onset, vomiting of enormous quantities of fluid, and symptoms of collapse. Of 102 cases collected by L. A. Conner 42 followed operation with general anesthesia. The next largest group occurs in the course of severe diseases, especially pneumonia, or during convalescence. Cases have followed injuries, particularly of the head and spine. In 9 cases the symptoms came on after a single large meal; 6 cases were associated with spinal disease, in 3 while the patients were in plaster of Paris jacket, and in a few cases it has come on in persons in good health. There were 74 deaths. In 69 autopsies the duodenum was found dilated in 38 cases. In a majority of cases it is due to a constriction of the lower end of the duodenum by traction on the mesenteric root, which is particularly apt to occur when there is a long mesentery and when the coil of small bowel is empty and falls into the true pelvis. It may be due to complete loss of tone of the stomach. The *diagnosis* is usually easy—repeated vomiting of large quantities of bilious nonfecal fluid, with subnormal temperature, pain, collapse symptoms, and distended abdomen are the common features. In *treatment,* nothing should be taken by mouth and glucose (5 per cent) and sodium bicarbonate (1 per cent) solution given by the bowel. The stomach should be emptied repeatedly by the tube; the small tube may be left in position. Pituitrin hypodermically is worth a trial. If possible the patient should lie on the face or assume the knee-chest position. Operation has not proved very satisfactory.

CHRONIC DILATATION results from: (*a*) *Pyloric obstruction* due to narrowing of the orifice or of the duodenum by the cicatrization of an ulcer, malignant disease, hypertrophic stenosis of the pylorus, congenital stricture, or occasionally by pressure from without of a tumor or of a floating kidney. The pylorus may be tilted up by adhesions to the liver or gallbladder, or the stomach may be so dilated that the pylorus is dragged down and kinked. Adhesions about the gallbladder may extend along the adjacent parts of the stomach and hitch up the pylorus into the hilus of the liver, forming a very acute kink. In some cases there is an *intermittent* retention lasting for some hours, often due to pyloric spasm. In such cases there are usually hyperacidity and the signs of vagotonia. It may be associated with disease of the duodenum, gallbladder or appendix. In some cases it seems as if pyloric spasm may lead to definite dilatation. Syphilis and pedunculated benign tumors at the pylorus are rare causes. Edema, perhaps about an ulcer, with pylorospasm may be responsible. (*b*) *Relative or absolute insufficiency of the muscular power* of the stomach, due to repeated overfilling of the organ or to atony of the coats due to chronic inflammation or the degeneration of impaired nutrition, the result of constitutional affections.

The most extreme forms are met with as a sequence of the cicatricial contraction of an ulcer. There may be considerable stenosis without much dilatation, the obstruction being compensated by hypertrophy of the muscular coats. In the group due to atony of the muscular coats, we must distinguish between instances in which the stomach is simply enlarged and those with actual dilatation. The size of the stomach varies greatly and the maximum capacity of a normal organ is about 1,600 cc. Measurements above this point indicate absolute dilatation.

Atonic dilatation may result from weakness of the coats, due to repeated overdistention, to chronic catarrh of the mucous membrane, or to the general muscular debility associated with chronic wasting disorders. The combination of chronic gastric catarrh with overfeeding and excessive drinking is a common cause of atonic dilatation as is seen in diabetics, the insane, and beer drinkers. In Germany this form is common in men employed in breweries. Possibly muscular weakness of the coats may result from disturbed innervation. It is common in cases of general neurosis, especially with visceroptosis. Dilatation of the stomach is most frequent in middle-aged or elderly persons, but is not uncommon in children, especially with rickets.

Symptoms.—In *atonic dilatation* there may be no symptoms whatever, even with a greatly enlarged organ; more frequently there are the associated features of neurasthenia, enteroptosis and nervous dyspepsia; while in a third group there may be all the symptoms of pyloric obstruction—vomiting of enormous quantities, etc.

The features of *pyloric obstruction,* from whatever cause, are usually very evident. Dyspepsia is present in nearly all cases, and there are feelings of distress and uneasiness in the stomach. The patient may complain much of hunger and thirst and eat and drink freely. The most characteristic sign is the vomiting at intervals of enormous quantities of liquid and of food, amounting sometimes to four or more litres. The material is often of a dark-grayish color, with a characteristic sour odor due to organic acids and contains mucus and remnants of food. On standing it separates into three layers, the lowest consisting of food, the middle of a turbid, dark-gray fluid, and the uppermost of a brownish froth. The microscopic examination shows a large variety of bacteria, yeast fungi, and sarcinae. There may also be fruit stones and seeds. The hydrochloric acid may be absent, diminished, normal or in excess, depending upon the cause of the dilatation. The fermentation produces lactic, butyric, and, possibly, acetic acid and various gases. In the *intermittent* forms with pyloric spasm there is retention often for four to eight hours usually with hyperacidity. Vagotonia is often present and disease of the gallbladder, duodenum or appendix should be considered.

In consequence of the small amount of fluid which passes from the stomach there are constipation, scanty urine and extreme dryness of the skin. The general nutrition suffers greatly; there is loss of flesh and strength, and in some cases most extreme emaciation. The color may be retained and if there is much vomiting, there may be polycythemia. Tetany may occur and in some cases in a severe form.

Physical Signs.—*Inspection.*—The abdomen may be large and prominent, the greatest projection occurring below the navel in the standing posture. In some instances the outline of the distended stomach can be plainly seen, the small curvature a couple of inches below the ensiform cartilage, and the greater curvature passing obliquely from the tip of the tenth rib on the left side, toward the pubes, and then curving upward to the right costal margin. Too much stress can not be laid on the importance of inspection. Very often the diagnosis may be made *de visu. Active peristalsis* may be seen in the dilated organ, the waves passing from left to right. Occasionally antiperistalsis may be seen. In cases of stricture, particularly of hypertrophic stenosis, as the peristaltic wave reaches the pylorus, the tumor-like thickening can sometimes be distinctly seen through the abdominal wall. To stimulate peristalsis the abdomen may be flipped with a wet towel. In many cases the outline of the dilated stomach stands out with great distinctness after inflation and waves of peristalsis are very evident.

Palpation.—The peristalsis may be felt, and usually in stenosis a tumor is evident at the pylorus. The resistance of a dilated stomach is peculiar, and has been aptly compared to that of an air cushion. A splashing sound—*clapotage*—may be obtained which is not distinctive, as it can be obtained whenever there are much liquid and air in the organ. The splashing may be very loud, and the patient may produce it himself by suddenly depressing the diaphragm, or it may be produced by shaking him. The gurgling of gas through the pylorus may be felt.

Percussion.—The note is tympanitic over the greater portion of a dilated stomach; in the dependent part the note is flat. The fluid may be withdrawn from the stomach with a tube, and the dulness so made to disappear, or it may be increased by pouring in more fluid. In cases of doubt the organ should be inflated.

Auscultation.—The *clapotage* can be obtained readily. Frequently a curious sizzling sound is present, not unlike that heard over a soda-water bottle when first opened. It can be heard naturally, and is usually evident when the artificial gas is being generated. The heart sounds may sometimes be transmitted with great clearness and with a metallic quality.

Diagnosis.—This can usually be made without much difficulty. Emphasis should be placed on the value of inspection, particularly in combination with inflation of the stomach. Curious errors are on record, one of the most remarkable of which was the confounding of dilated stomach with an ovarian cyst; even after tapping and the removal of portions of food and fruit seeds, abdominal section was performed and the dilated stomach opened. The diagnosis of ascites has been made and the abdomen opened. The X-ray findings are distinctive. The *prognosis* depends upon the cause; it is good in simple atony, bad in cancerous stricture, fairly good in simple stricture. Surgery usually gives excellent results.

Treatment.—In the cases due to atony careful regulation of the diet and proper treatment of the associated general condition will suffice to effect a cure. Lavage is of great service, though we do not see such striking and immediate results in this form. In cases of mechanical obstruction the stomach should be emptied and thoroughly washed, either with warm water or with an antiseptic solution. Three important things are accomplished: The weight which distends the organ is removed; the fermenting materials are washed out; and we cleanse the mucous membrane. The patient can usually be taught to wash out his own stomach, and in dilatation from simple stricture the practice may be followed with great benefit. The rapid reduction in the size of the stomach is often remarkable, the vomiting ceases, food is taken readily, and in many cases the general nutrition improves rapidly. As a rule, once a day is sufficient, and it may be practised either the first thing in the morning or before going to bed. As soon as the fermentatve processes have been checked lukewarm water alone should be used. Care should be taken in giving alkalies to patients with dilatation of the stomach owing to the danger of alkalosis. In the *intermittent* form the use of atropine with small doses of bromide is often useful. Any lesion elsewhere in the abdomen should be properly treated.

The food should be taken in small quantities at frequent intervals, and as concentrated as possible. Fatty and starchy articles of diet are to be avoided. Liquids should be taken sparingly. In *atonic* cases postural treatment is often helpful and the use of an abdominal support may give great relief. The patient should sleep with the foot of the bed elevated and lie on the right side as much as possible.

Surgery should be resorted to early in cases of organic stricture; in atonic dilatation it is not advisable as the cause usually is not in the stomach.

THE PEPTIC ULCER, GASTRIC AND DUODENAL

The round, perforating, simple or peptic ulcer is usually single, and occurs in the stomach and in the duodenum as far as the papilla. Both postmortem statistics and clinical experience show more duodenal than gastric ulcers but the preponderance is greater clinically, about four to one. Probably more gastric ulcers are unrecognized.

Erosions.—Small abrasions of the mucosa—2 to 4 mm.—usually multiple, are common, extending half way or quite through the layer. They are often called hemorrhagic erosions from their blood-stained appearance. They are met with in the newborn, in cachectic states in children, in chronic heart and arterial disease, in cirrhosis of the liver, etc. Of no clinical importance, as a rule, occasionally an acute hemorrhagic erosion of small size opens an artery with resulting hematemesis. There is no difference between this condition and the acute form of gastric ulcer.

In certain acute infections with the pneumococcus (Dieulafoy) and septic organisms there may be hemorrhagic erosions, which occasionally prove fatal by hematemesis. The postoperative hematemesis, slight or grave, may be due to these erosions. The French have described them as if peculiar to operations for appendicitis but cases occur after all sorts of abdominal operations. It is probable that the gastric hemorrhages which occur in connection with the throbbing aorta in neurotic women are due to these erosions.

Etiology of Peptic Ulcer.—Incidence.—This appears to vary in different localities, and postmortem figures from the United States and Canada show a much lower percentage of cases (1.32) than on the Continent of Europe (5 per cent), and in London (4.2 per cent) (C. P. Howard).

Sex.—Acute simple gastric ulcer occurs in young women more often than in males, but chronic ulcer is much more common in males. The acute forms of gastric ulcer in females seem to have greatly decreased in frequency in the United States. Duodenal ulcer is much more common in males.

Age.—In females the largest number of cases occurred between fifteen and twenty-five; in males between thirty and fifty. It may occur in old people. E. G. Cutler studied a series of 29 cases in children. In 6 the symptoms came on immediately after birth. There were 8 cases under seven years of age, and 9 between eight and thirteen.

Occupation.—Among women, anemic dyspeptic servant girls seem very prone. Shoemakers are thought to be specially likely. The medical profession seems especially prone, especially surgeons, a surprising number of whom have, or think they have, an ulcer.

Trauma.—Ulcers have followed injury and the association seems to be more than coincidence.

Associated Diseases.—Anemia predisposes to ulcer, particularly in women. It has been found in connection with disease of the heart, arteriosclerosis and disease of the liver. The tuberculous and syphilitic ulcers of the stomach have been considered. Many cases are associated with disease of the appendix and gallbladder. *Nervous System.* The influence of severe nervous strain and tension is difficult to estimate but increasing importance is being given to it. The suggestion by Cushing of a "centre" which may play a part is important. The midbrain may play a part.

Burns.—A duodenal ulcer may follow large superficial burns. Perry and Shaw found it in 5 of 149 autopsies in cases of burns of the skin.

Infection.—Any focal infection may be responsible, especially in the teeth or tonsils. The importance of this is difficult to estimate but it seems to play a part in some cases. In cases of associated abdominal infections, as in the gallbladder, both may have come from a common source, or the ulcer may be secondary to the other.

Heredity.—There may be an "ulcer constitution" or diathesis. Some families seem to be particularly susceptible. A hypertonic stomach which empties rapidly, plus hyperchlorhydria, so that the duodenal bulb is kept filled with acid fluid, favors the development of a duodenal ulcer.

There are many suggested factors; disturbances of the *circulation* (embolism, thrombosis or spasm of the artery), *neurogenic* influences acting through the sympathetic system (influence of a centre?), the action of acid, inflammation and the effect of general nervous strain and exhaustion. Several of these may be in combination. We have to recognize that our knowledge of the etiology is by no means definite. Probably various causes operate in different patients. Tobacco and alcohol do not cause ulcer; tobacco apparently aggravates it when present.

Morbid Anatomy and Pathology.—The great majority of gastric ulcers are at the pyloric end; nearly all duodenal ulcers are in the first portion, and more than one-half extend up to or within three-fourths of an inch of the pylorus, while 20 per cent involve the margin of the pyloric ring (Mayo). In explanation of the frequency of ulcer just outside the pyloric sphincter it is stated that this part of the duodenum is deficient in blood supply in comparison with the other. Multiple ulcers may occur. In the stomach, postmortem statistics (Welch) give, in 793 cases, 288 on the lesser curvature, 235 on the posterior wall, 69 on the anterior wall, 95 at the pylorus, 50 at the cardia, 29 at the fundus, and 27 on the greater curvature.

The *acute* ulcer is usually small, punched out, the edges clean-cut, the floor smooth, and the peritoneal surface not thickened. The *chronic* ulcer is of larger size, the margins are no longer sharp, the edges are indurated, and the border is sinuous. It may reach an enormous size, as in one reported by Peabody, which measured 19 by 10 cm., involved all of the lesser curvature and spread over a large part of the anterior and posterior walls. The sides are often terraced. The floor is formed either by the submucosa, by the muscular layers, or sometimes by neighboring organs, to which the stomach has become attached. In healing, if the mucosa is alone involved, the granulation tissue grows from the edges and the floor and the newly formed tissue gradually contracts and unites the margins, leaving a smooth scar. In larger ulcers which have involved the muscular coat the cicatricial contraction may cause serious changes, the most important of which is pyloric narrowing and consequent dilatation of the stomach. From a girdle ulcer hour-glass contraction of the stomach may result. Large ulcers may persist for years without any attempt at healing. Among the changes which may result are the following:

Perforation.—In the anterior wall of the stomach this usually excites an acute peritonitis. On the posterior wall the ulcer penetrates into the lesser peritoneal cavity, in which case it may produce an air-containing abscess with the symptoms of subphrenic pyopneumothorax. In rare instances adhesions and a gastrocutaneous fistula form, usually in the umbilical region. Fistulous communication with the colon or a gastroduodenal fistula may occur. The pericardium may be perforated and even the left ventricle. Perforation into the pleura may also occur. General emphysema of the subcutaneous tissues occasionally follows perforation of a gastric ulcer.

Erosion of Blood-Vessels.—In both forms of ulcer hemorrhage occurs. It is more common in the chronic form. Ulcers on the posterior wall may erode the splenic artery, but perhaps more frequently the bleeding proceeds from the artery of the lesser curvature. In duodenal ulcer the pancreaticoduodenal artery may be eroded, or fatal hemorrhage may result from the opening of the hepatic artery, or more rarely the portal vein. Embolism of the artery supplying the ulcerated region has been met with; in others diffuse endarteritis. Small aneurisms have been found in the floor of the ulcers. A rare event is emphysema of the subperitoneal tissue, which may be extensive and even pass on to the posterior mediastinum. Jurgensen ascribes it to entrance of air into the veins, but Welch thought it represents an invasion with the gas bacillus.

CICATRIZATION.—Superficial ulcers often heal without leaving any serious damage. Stenosis of the pyloric orifice not infrequently follows the healing of an ulcer in its neighborhood. In other instances the large annular ulcer may cause in its cicatrization an hour-glass contraction of the stomach. The adhesion of the ulcer to neighboring parts may cause much pain. The mucosa in the neighborhood of the ulcer frequently shows chronic gastritis.

PERIGASTRIC AND DUODENAL ADHESIONS.—The condition is common, as high as 5 per cent of postmortem records. It follows ulcer, lesions of the gallbladder, pancreatic disease, syphilitic disease of the liver and chronic tuberculosis. In some instances the lesions are quite extensive, and the condition has been called *plastic perigastritis*. It may be associated with hypertrophic thickening of the coats of the stomach and with chronic plastic peritonitis. In some instances the pylorus or duodenum may be narrowed as a result of the adhesions, or a sort of hour-glass stomach may be produced, or the motility of the organ is interfered with. *Pain* is the most constant feature, and may simulate that of gastric ulcer or hyperacidity, and may be present constantly or at intervals. It is much influenced by posture and usually relieved by pressure. Local tenderness is present in a majority of instances. The cases are chronic, the general health is but slightly affected, and there are not, as a rule, signs of gastric dilatation. A definite tumor may be present about the region of the pylorus. Chronic appendicitis and lesions of the gallbladder are found in many cases.

JEJUNAL ULCER.—This may occur after gastrojejunostomy, but in many cases the ulcer involves both stomach and jejunum. The frequency is difficult to state; there is considerable difference of opinion as to how frequently it occurs. Certain statistics give a low incidence.

CARCINOMA AND ULCER.—There has been much difference of opinion as to the number of cases in which carcinoma develops in an ulcer. There is no doubt of its occurrence and the figure is probably between 5 and 10 per cent.

Symptoms.—The condition may be latent and only found postmortem. The first symptoms may be those of perforation. In the *acute* gastric ulcer there is pain which usually comes on very soon after meals, associated with epigastric tenderness. Hematemesis, of some grade, is comparatively common and often gives the diagnosis. In some cases the patient has had gastric disturbance for years and the ulcer may not be suspected until a sudden hemorrhage. The usual *history* is of an illness of long duration, generally of some years, in which there have been remissions often with complete relief from symptoms. The periodicity may be marked; the symptoms are rarely continuous. Many of the symptoms are due to associated conditions of which vagotonia is important. The ulcer alone may give few symptoms in some cases.

Digestive disturbance may be slight and trifling or of a most aggravated character. *Vomiting* occurs in about two-thirds of the cases, often not for two or more hours after eating. It is probably most common when the ulcer is near the pylorus.

Hemorrhage is present in at least one-third of all cases. A patient may feel faint and turn pale and sweat; the next day the stools may be tarry from the blood that has passed into the small bowel. The bleeding may be latent (occult). These concealed hemorrhages are often small, and the blood is not readily seen in the vomitus or stools. Such latent hemorrhages may cause a slowly progressive anemia. The bleeding may be profuse, and the blood in such quantities and brought up so quickly that it is fluid, bright red in color and quite unaltered. When it remains for some time in the stomach and is mixed with food it may be greatly changed, but the vomiting of a large quantity of unaltered blood is suggestive of ulcer. As a rule, there are only one or two attacks but profuse bleeding may occur at intervals for many years. Death may follow directly.

The immediate effect of a severe hemorrhage is anemia, from which it may take months to rally; slight fever is common. Rare and untoward effects are convulsions, sometimes only the usual convulsions of extreme cerebral anemia from which recovery takes place, or they may precede a hemiplegia, due probably to thrombosis. Amaurosis may follow the hemorrhage and unfortunately may be permanent, due to degeneration of the retinal ganglion cells or to a thrombosis of the cerebral arteries or veins.

Pain is perhaps the most constant and distinctive feature. It varies greatly in character: it may be only a gnawing or burning sensation, but the more characteristic form comes on in paroxysms, in which the pain is not only felt in the epigastrium, but radiates to the back and to the sides. In many cases the two points of epigastric pain and dorsal pain, about the level of the tenth dorsal vertebra, are very well marked. The association with the taking of food and the regular recurrence are important points. In some cases the pain has no relation to food. Except in severe attacks the pain does not usually last more than an hour and disappears before the next meal. In many cases it appears with greatest regularity as regards time after the same kind of meal. It occurs during the digestive process and usually disappears when the stomach is empty. It is stated that when the ulcer is near the cardia the pain is apt to set in earlier, but there is no certainty on this point. Vomiting and the taking of alkali usually relieve the pain. The attacks may occur at intervals for weeks or months and then disappear entirely for a prolonged period. The mechanism of the pain is not clear. Probably the tissues involved have increased irritability to stimuli which may be chemical from acid or mechanical from pylorospasm, gastric motility or intragastric pressure.

Tenderness on pressure with rigidity is common and patients wear the waist-band very low. The tender area is often constant in its situation in the same patient. Pressure should be made with great care, as rupture of an ulcer is said to have been induced by careless manipulation.

In old ulcers with thickened bases an indurated mass may be felt in the neighborhood of the pylorus.

Gastric Contents.—There may be evidence of some retention. The findings as to acidity vary and too much importance should not be placed on them. With marked retention there may be high acidity figures. If neoplasm has developed in an ulcer the HCl is reduced but there may be achlorhydria with ulcer alone. Careful search should always be made for blood, either fresh or occult, both in the stomach contents and stools. Certain points relating to the test meal may be noted. Gastric analysis gives information of the motor and secretory functions (which may be altered by organic or functional disease) and of pathological elements, mucus, pus, blood, bacteria and cancer tissue. There is no fixed normal for motility or secretion. We show our personality in gastric function as in other ways. As regards secretion our ideas as to hyperacidity have had to be revised; in general high acid figures are of less importance than low figures. There is no pathognomonic curve in any gastric condition; there are general averages. Great importance should be given to pathological products in the fasting stomach and after the test meal. This is too often overlooked in a routine study.

Loss of weight results from the prolonged dyspepsia, but it rarely, except in association with cicatricial stenosis of the pylorus, reaches the high grade met with in cancer. The *anemia* may be marked, and of 44 cases in the Hopkins Hospital the lowest was 1,902,000 per c.mm. There are instances in which the anemia can not be explained by the occurrence of hemorrhage. In a few instances polycythemia is present, even after a hemorrhage, due to concentration of the blood in association with dilatation of the stomach. *Parotitis* may occur, with perforation sometimes or after a hemorrhage.

Perforation.—The acute, perforating form is much more common in women than in men. The symptoms are those of perforative peritonitis. Particular attention must be given to the prompt recognition of this accident, as early operation is so successful. Perforation may take place into the lesser peritoneum or the general peritoneal cavity, in both of which cases operation is indicated; in rare instances the ulcer may perforate the pericardium as in 10 of 28 cases in which the diaphragm was perforated (Pick). Localized, more frequently subphrenic, abscess may follow perforation.

Urine.—Albumin is occasionally present. Acetone and diacetic acid (with syncopal attacks) were described by Dreschfeld. Phosphaturia is often found.

Hour-glass stomach most frequently results from the cicatrization of an ulcer. It may follow perforation of an ulcer into the liver or pancreas. In a few cases it is congenital. The features, fairly characteristic, are thus given by Moynihan: (*a*) In washing out the stomach part of the fluid is lost. (*b*) If the stomach is washed clean, a sudden reappearance of stomach contents may take place. (*c*) "Paradoxical dilatation"; when the stomach has apparently been emptied, a splashing sound may be elicited by palpation of the pyloric segment. (*d*) After distending the stomach, a change in the position of the distention tumor may be seen in some cases. (*e*) Gushing, bubbling, or sizzling sounds are heard on dilatation with carbon dioxide at a point distinct from the pylorus. (*f*) In some cases, when both parts are dilated, two tumors with a notch or sulcus between are apparent to sight or touch. (*g*) A most characteristic X-ray picture. The occurrence of hour-glass stomach due to *spasm* must be remembered. From a hasty X-ray study it might be mistaken for the organic variety.

Duodenal Ulcer.—There is often a long interval between the onset of symptoms and the diagnosis probably due to the tendency to remission of symptoms and the response to simple treatment. The early symptoms may last for short periods of two to four weeks, followed by months of comfort. A profuse hemorrhage or perforation may be the first indication. Emphasis should be placed on the importance of the history in duodenal ulcer. The occurrence of discomfort or pain before meals with relief on taking food is important. A sudden flow of watery saliva occurs not infrequently with the pain. There is great variation in the severity of the pain which tends to become more severe as the ulcer becomes more chronic. The long periods of freedom from symptoms are often remarkable. The first symptom may be discomfort about three hours after a meal. Later there is *pain* which usually appears two to three hours after meals and tends to persist until the next meal or until food or alkali is taken. It frequently wakens the patient at night. It may be associated with a feeling of hunger. The situation is generally a little above the navel, in the midline or a little to the right, rarely to the left. Vomiting is not common but there may be regurgitation of acid fluid. As a rule occult blood is found in the stools. The appetite is usually good and the general condition does not show much change. The test meal may give evidence of hypermotility, which is common. The acidity of the fasting stomach is often high and after an initial fall there is a rapid rise to high figures which remain. Blood may be found in small amounts. The X-ray study usually shows hypermotility and irregularity in the duodenal cap is significant. The stomach may be the short, high type.

Gross *hemorrhage* occurs in about 25 per cent of the cases. The danger from it increases with the age of the patient and the duration of the ulcer. The resulting anemia may be severe. Fever may occur possibly with retention of blood in the bowel. The frequency of perforation is difficult to state. The picture is that of an acute abdominal accident and the diagnosis is usually made without great difficulty. In some cases there is involvement of the *pancreas* to which the duodenum may be adherent. If the process extends to the pancreas there will be severe pain not relieved by food or alkalies. It may suggest biliary or hepatic colic. *Pyloric stenosis* may result.

Prognosis.—In many statistics the acute and chronic ulcer have been considered together. The former is more amenable to medical treatment, but grave complications may occur even before the symptoms are pronounced. The chronic ulcer may last for years—ten or even twenty—with intervals of good health. Controversy as to the relative results of medical and surgical treatment is futile. Medical treatment is indicated in different conditions than surgical. In the early stages medical treatment is advisable and should have a thorough trial. With a chronic ulcer it may be a waste of time to attempt it. Many patients do well with medical treatment; others are helped but do not become well. The possibility of the development of carcinoma in gastric ulcer, while not marked, should be remembered. Surgery is not always successful, for gastro-enterostomy can not be regarded as a physiological operation. The mortality of the chronic ulcer in the hands of good surgeons is very low.

Diagnosis.—The acute non-indurated gastric ulcer may cause very few symptoms—nothing beyond gastric discomfort with pain. This group of cases is seen chiefly in young girls, and appears to be more common in England than in the United States. Hematemesis may be the first symptom of moment. Its occurrence or the persistent presence of blood in the gastric contents is important, cancer being excluded. A condition which may cause difficulty is *gastrostaxis* described by Hale-White. The stomach symptoms are marked, the bleeding may be profuse, but postmortem or at operation no ulcer is found. Careful inspection must be made, as fatal bleeding may come from a very small erosion.

In chronic gastric ulcer the nutrition at first may remain good, and the patient looks well. The whole complaint is of the stomach, of pain and distress, with belching and nausea or vomiting from two to four hours after meals. The special features of the recurrence of the pain after taking food, its extraordinary *regularity*, and the tenderness and rigidity are significant. In the early stages there is usually no alteration in secretion or motility, but sooner or later both are altered. The rhythm of gastric function is disturbed. With disturbance in motility, usually delay, the secretion is altered. The secretory findings depend partly on the extent and chronicity of the ulcer, the presence of gastritis and the impairment of motility. The postdigestion secretion increases. The X-ray examination is of the greatest aid. In general the diagnosis of gastric is more difficult than of duodenal ulcer.

The presence of *adhesions* between the gallbladder or liver and stomach or duodenum may cause difficulty. The symptoms are long continued, present a great variety and may suggest ulcer but in their irregularity are more like those of gallstones. The taking of food may give relief which suggests duodenal or gastric ulcer close to the pylorus. Blood is not found in the gastric contents or stools. The X-ray study may suggest ulcer.

Gastric Ulcer.—The relief of pain by alkalies is common in ulcer. In *nervous* disturbances the discomfort is apt to be irregular in occurrence and the tenderness less localized. There is absence of blood and the X-ray findings are negative. Much the same points apply to *chronic gastritis* in which pain and tenderness are usually less marked. The symptoms associated with appendicitis and gallbladder disease may cause difficulty, especially as either may occur with ulcer, but a thorough study and especially the test meals and X-ray examination should aid.

Duodenal Ulcer.—The features are usually suggestive and as a rule the diagnosis is not difficult. The later onset of pain, its association with an empty stomach, the relief on taking food or alkali, the situation of tenderness, the test meal, findings of high acidity, and the X-ray study are important, in the diagnosis from gastric ulcer. The diagnosis from gallbladder disease may be difficult at first, but a period of study showing the absence of the usual features of ulcer should clear the difficulty. The occurrence of occult blood in the stools is important evidence of ulcer. The result of treatment may be an aid as the response is usually prompt in ulcer.

Perforation of an ulcer usually gives marked signs suggestive of an acute severe abdominal condition. The occurrence of sharp pain in the region of one or both shoulders is important. It probably results from irritation of the diaphragm. If there is a history suggestive of ulcer the diagnosis is easier but, in any case, time should not be wasted in matters of diagnosis except to recognize that something has happened which demands immediate operation. The onset of diabetic coma with abdominal pain and collapse has been mistaken for perforation of a gastric ulcer, which in tabes dorsalis, on the contrary, has been missed on account of the lack of pain.

There is a condition termed "gastric uremia," probably due to alkalosis, in which the patient shows drowsiness or stupor, sometimes irritability, with an increase in the blood urea and vomiting. It is more likely to occur if pyloric stenosis is present. It is a serious condition for which gastro-enterostomy is indicated if it can be done.

Treatment.—Unless there are definite indications for operation, it seems wise to try the effect of medical treatment, but this should be carried out systematically. The patient should be studied and the problem not regarded as merely that of a local lesion. General nervous strain, anxiety states, focal infection and overuse of tobacco have to be considered. Disturbing factors should be eliminated as far as possible. Mouth infection should be treated, gastric rest should be obtained as far as possible and acidity should be neutralized.

The patient should be at rest in bed and kept there for several weeks if the symptoms are severe. In the method advised by Sippy, food is given every hour from 7 A. M. to 7 P. M. during the day. At first three ounces of a mixture of equal parts of milk and cream are given. After a few days soft eggs and cooked cereals are gradually added. These may be given alternately with and in addition to the milk and cream. The total bulk at one feeding should not exceed six ounces. Later, cream soups, bread and butter, and soft foods may be added.

To control the *acidity*, alkali is given between each feeding. This is done by giving a powder of gr. x (0.6 gm.) each of heavy calcined magnesia and sodium bicarbonate alternating with a powder of gr. x (0.6 gm.) of bismuth carbonate and gr. xxx (2 gm.) of sodium bicarbonate. In addition, after the last feeding of the day, the powders should be given every half hour for four doses or until the stomach is empty. The powders are administered in about two ounces of water. It is well to aspirate the stomach about two hours after the last feeding to be sure that it is empty. If this amount of alkali is not sufficient, more sodium bicarbonate may be given. By examining the stomach contents occasionally it can be determined whether or not the free acidity is being controlled. After some weeks the patient may be given light meals, but the taking of equal parts of milk and cream each hour should be kept up. When the hourly feedings between meals are stopped, the alkaline powder should be taken every hour for three doses after each meal. It is usually well to continue this treatment longer than may seem necessary. Neutral antacids (phosphates of calcium and magnesium—neutral and not acid phosphates) are useful. The calcium salt is slightly constipating and the magnesium salt laxative. The dose is one-half to two teaspoonfuls (Kantor).

If the ulcer has caused pyloric obstruction, as a rule a larger amount of alkali is required and it is well to empty the stomach each night about half an hour after the last powder is taken. The important thing is to give sufficient alkali to control the acidity. A careful watch over the progress should be kept and the amount of retained material noted. The emptying of the stomach the last thing at night lessens the tendency to night secretion. Regular examinations of the stools for occult blood are an important guide as to the value of the treatment. In all cases it is important to obtain the co-operation of the patient so that after he passes from immediate observation he will be careful to follow instructions.

In the method advised by Coleman, the patients are kept in bed and for three to five days no food is given by mouth (if necessary 1-3 ounces of water may be given when required). Glucose is given by the bowel (300 cc. of a 10 per cent solution in physiological salt solution) three or four times a day. An enema is given each morning to empty the bowel. On the fourth to sixth day, the whites of three or four eggs are given alternating with olive oil (45-75 cc. given cold on the first day). The oil is increased to 150 cc. a day and the eggs to six or eight. Unsalted butter may be substituted for the olive oil or cream (690 cc. equals 150 cc. of olive oil) may have to be given. This diet should be given for three or four weeks and food increased very carefully afterward.

Atropine or belladonna is often useful in dosage suitable for each patient and if there is a marked nervous element bromide or phenobarbital (gr. ½, 0.032 gm.) three times a day, should be given. Good results may follow the use of histidine (5 cc. of a 4 per cent solution), given intramuscularly, one dose daily for a period of three weeks. Mucin is useful in some cases. For the bowels salines in the morning or enemata may be used. Mineral oil is often effectual. The artificial Carlsbad salts (sulphate of sodium, 50 parts; bicarbonate of sodium, 6; chloride of sodium, 3) may be given.

The *pain* is usually relieved by rest, proper diet, bismuth and alkalies, and atropine. If not relieved, codein (gr. ¼-½, 0.015-0.03 gm.) may be given. For very severe attacks morphia may be required, best hypodermically (gr. ¼, 0.015 gm.). In the milder attacks Hoffman's anodyne, 20 or 30 drops of spirit of chloroform, or the spirit of camphor, will give relief. Counterirritation over the epigastrium with mustard is often useful.

It is important to stop the use of tobacco and alcohol.

When the stomach is irritable, the patient should be fed *per rectum.* He will sometimes retain food which is passed into the duodenum through a tube. Cracked ice, olive oil, oxalate of cerium, and bismuth may be tried. When *hemorrhage* occurs the patient should be put under the influence of morphine as rapidly as possible. No attempt should be made to check the hemorrhage by giving drugs by mouth; the essential point is to give rest, which is best obtained by opium or morphine. Nothing should be given by the mouth for 48 hours except small quantities of ice. Not infrequently the loss of blood is so great that the patient faints but a fatal result is not very common. Blood serum (15-30 cc.) may be injected intramuscularly. Transfusion is advisable in severe conditions. The patients usually recover rapidly from the hemorrhage and require iron in full doses.

Surgical interference is indicated (1) For perforation; (2) in the chronic indurated ulcer. Experience has shown that after gastro-enterostomy the ulcer may heal rapidly; (3) in all cases when the ulcer has caused persistent, mechanical interference by pyloric obstruction or hour-glass stomach; (4) in cases with recurring hemorrhages. In young girls a single attack of hematemesis may be due to gastrostaxis or from a simple ulcer that heals readily, but in men severe hematemesis is almost always from a chronic ulcer; (5) in the perigastric adhesions after chronic ulcer operation is sometimes helpful; (6) in chronic cases in which medical treatment fails to give relief; (7) when there is evidence of pancreatic involvement; (8) with duodenal ileus; and (9) when there is reason to suspect the development of carcinoma.

The simple nonindurated ulcer is, in the majority of cases, a medical disease. A chronic indurated form is best treated surgically. In general the surgical treatment of gastric ulcer is less satisfactory than that of duodenal ulcer. The occurrence of gastrojejunal ulcer after gastro-enterostomy has to be kept in mind.

Duodenal Ulcer.—The treatment of this is much like that of gastric ulcer but surgery may be advised with much more chance of success. In certain cases, especially if recognized early, ambulant treatment may be successful. There should be as much rest as possible and no violent exercise. The patient takes three meals a day, avoiding irritating food, and takes food between meals (such as milk alone or with an egg or cracker). A glass of milk should be kept by the bedside. If pain occurs food or an alkali should be taken.

The *after care* is important for at least two years both after medical treatment and after operation. A careful watch should be kept over the condition of the mouth. The patient should be kept to a simple diet and always eat slowly. Olive oil may be taken before meals. Patients should keep up the taking of alkali for some months and always carry some with them to take at the first sign of any discomfort. The bowels should be kept regular. It is well for the patient with duodenal ulcer to take a glass of milk in the middle of the forenoon and afternoon, and at bedtime; and also to have food or alkali by the bedside to take in the night if necessary.

CANCER OF THE STOMACH

Etiology.—INCIDENCE.—In an analysis of 30,000 cases of cancer, W. H. Welch found the stomach involved in 21.4 per cent, this organ standing next to the uterus in order of frequency. Among 8,464 medical cases admitted to the Johns Hopkins Hospital, there were 150 cases of cancer of the stomach.

SEX.—The disease is more common in males but there is considerable variation in the ratio in different series.

AGE.—Of 7,000 cases (Martin) the ages were: 10-20 years, 0.08 per cent; 20-30 years, 1.5 per cent; 30-40 years, 8.4 per cent; 40-45 years, 18 per cent; 50-60 years, 28 per cent; 60-70 years, 28 per cent, and over 70 years, 16 per cent. Of the 6 cases occurring under the thirtieth year in our series of 150 cases, the youngest was twenty-two. Congenital cancer of the stomach has been described and cases occur in children.

RACE.—Among our 150 cases, 131 were white, 19 were negroes.

PREVIOUS DISEASES, HABITS, ETC.—A history of dyspepsia was present in only 33 cases; of these, 17 had had attacks at intervals, 11 had had chronic stomach trouble, and 5 had had dyspepsia for one or two years before the symptoms of cancer developed. Napoleon, discussing this point with his physician Antommarchi, said that he had always had a stomach of iron and felt no inconvenience until the onset of what proved to be his fatal illness.

GASTRIC ULCER.—In a small proportion, probably about 5 per cent, carcinoma develops in a previous ulcer. In only 4 cases in our series was there a history pointing to ulcer.

Morbid Anatomy.—The most common varieties of gastric cancer are the cylindrical-celled adenocarcinoma and the encephaloid or medullary carcinoma; next in frequency is scirrhous, and then colloid cancers. With reference to the situation, Welch analyzed 1,300 cases, in which the distribution was as follows: Pyloric region, 791; lesser curvature, 148; cardia, 104; posterior wall, 68; the whole or greater part of the stomach, 61; multiple tumors, 45; greater curvature, 34; anterior wall, 30; fundus, 19.

The medullary cancer occurs in soft masses, which involve all the coats of the stomach and usually ulcerate early. The tumor may form villous projections or cauliflower-like outgrowths. It is soft, grayish-white in color, and contains much blood. The cylindrical-celled epithelioma may also form large irregular masses, but the consistence is usually firmer, particularly at the edges of the cancerous ulcers. Cysts are not uncommon in this form. The scirrhous variety is characterized by great hardness and is most frequent at the pylorus, where it is a common cause of stenosis. It may be combined with the medullary form. It may be diffuse and leading to a condition which can not be recognized macrosopically from cirrhosis. This form has also been seen in the stomach secondary to cancer of the ovaries. With diffuse carcinomatosis there may be involvement of the small and large intestines. The colloid cancer is peculiar in its widespread invasion of all the coats and it spreads with greater frequency to neighboring parts and occasionally causes extensive secondary growths. The appearance is distinctive, and with the naked eye large alveoli can be seen filled with the translucent colloid material. Ulceration is not constant and there are instances in which, with extensive disease, digestion has been but slightly disturbed.

Secondary Cancer of the Stomach.—Of 37 cases collected by Welch, 17 were secondary to cancer of the breast. Among the first 1,000 autopsies at the Johns Hopkins Hospital there were 3 cases of secondary cancer.

Changes in the Stomach.—Cancer at the cardia is usually associated with wasting of the organ and reduction in its size. The esophagus may be greatly dilated. On the other hand, annular cancer at the pylorus causes stenosis with great dilatation but in rare instances the pylorus has been extremely narrowed without any increase in the size of the stomach. In diffuse scirrhous cancer the stomach may be greatly thickened and contracted. It may be displaced or altered in shape by the weight of the tumor, particularly in cancer of the pylorus; in such cases it has been found in every region of the abdomen, and even in the true pelvis. The mobility of the tumors is at times extraordinary and deceptive as they may be pushed into the right hypochondrium or splenic region, beneath the ribs. Adhesions frequently occur, particularly to the colon, liver and anterior abdominal wall.

Secondary growths in other organs are frequent, as shown by the analysis by Welch of 1,574 cases: in the lymphatic glands in 551; in the liver in 475; in the peritoneum, omentum and intestine in 357; in the pancreas in 122; in the pleura and lung in 98; in the spleen in 26; in the brain and meninges in 9; in other parts in 92. The lymph nodes affected are usually those of the abdomen, but the cervical and inguinal glands may be attacked, and give an important clue in diagnosis. Subcutaneous metastatic growths at the navel or beneath the skin in the vicinity are of value in diagnosis.

Perforation.—This occurred into the peritoneum in 17 of 507 cases of cancer of the stomach (Brinton). In our series perforation occurred in 4 cases. When adhesions form, the most extensive destruction of the walls may take place without perforation into the peritoneal cavity. In one instance a large portion of the left lobe of the liver lay within the stomach. Occasionally a gastrocutaneous fistula is established. Perforation may occur into the colon, the small bowel, the pleura, the lung or the pericardium.

Symptoms.—LATENT CARCINOMA.—There may be no symptoms pointing to the stomach, and the tumor may be discovered after death. In a second group the symptoms of carcinoma are present, not of the stomach, but of the liver or some other organ, or there are subcutaneous nodules, or, as in one of our cases, secondary masses on the ribs and vertebrae. In a third group, seen particularly in elderly persons, there is gradual asthenia, sometimes anasarca, without nausea, vomiting or other local symptoms.

ONSET.—As a rule this is gradual with indefinite symptoms. If there has been previous gastric disease the symptoms may be little changed or somewhat increased. If the digestion previously was normal the symptoms usually are not characteristic; anorexia, discomfort after meals and vomiting, perhaps with some general disturbance, such as loss of weight or anemia. In some cases the growth progresses for some time without causing any noticeable symptoms so that when these appear in marked form, an acute onset is suggested. In some patients the onset is suggestive of pernicious anemia. *It is a good rule to suspect cancer in every patient over forty in whom gastric disturbance begins without evident cause.*

GENERAL FEATURES.—*Loss of Weight.*—Progressive emaciation is one of the most constant features. In 79 of our cases in which exact figures were taken: To 30 pounds, 32 cases; 30 to 50 pounds, 36 cases; 50 to 60 pounds, 5 cases; 60 to 70 pounds, 4; over 70 pounds, 1; 100 pounds, a case of cancer at the cardiac end with obstruction to swallowing. The loss in weight is not always progressive and increase occurs under three conditions: (*a*) Proper dieting, with treatment of the associated gastritis; (*b*) in cancer of the pylorus after relief of the dilatation by lavage, operation, etc.; (*c*) after a profound mental impression. The visit of an optimistic consultant may be followed by a gain in weight. In Keen and D. D. Stewart's case there was a gain of seventy pounds after an exploratory operation!

Loss in strength is usually proportionate to the loss in weight. One sees sometimes remarkable vigor almost to the close, but this is exceptional.

Anemia is present in a large proportion and with the emaciation gives the picture of cachexia. There is often a yellow or lemon tint of the skin. The average count in 59 cases was 3,712,186 per c.mm. In only 8 cases was the count below 2,000,000, and in none below 1,000,000; in 3 the red corpuscles were above 6,000,000 per c.mm. This occurs in the concentrated condition of the blood in certain cases of cancer of the pylorus with dilatation of the stomach. The average of the hemoglobin was 45 per cent. In only 9 was it below 30 per cent. In 62 cases there were 18 in which the leukocytes were above 12,000; in only 3 cases were they above 20,000.

Among other general symptoms may be mentioned *fever*, which was present at some time in 74 of our 150 cases. In only 13 of these did the temperature rise above 101°; in 2 it was above 103°. Fifteen presented fairly constant elevation of temperature and 8 had sudden rises. Two patients had *chills*, with elevation to 103° and 104°. Chills may be associated with suppuration at the base of the cancer.

Urine.—Albumin and casts may be found. Glycosuria, peptonuria, and acetonuria have been described. Indican is common.

Edema.—Swelling of the ankles is frequent toward the close. With early anasarca and extreme anemia, the cancer is usually overlooked.

The *bowels* are often constipated but occasionally diarrhea is troublesome. There are no special *cardiac symptoms;* the pulse becomes progressively weaker. Thrombosis of one femoral vein may occur or widespread thrombosis in the superficial veins of the body. Symptoms from the nervous system are rare: *coma* may occur, sometimes due to acidosis.

DIGESTIVE DISTURBANCES.—Anorexia is a frequent and valuable symptom, more constant perhaps than any other. *Nausea* is a striking feature in many cases; there is often a sudden repulsion at the sight of food. In exceptional cases the appetite is retained throughout.

Vomiting may come on early or only after the symptoms have persisted for some time. It occurred in 128 cases in our series. At first it is at long intervals but subsequently it is more frequent and may recur several times in the day. There are cases in which it comes on in paroxysms and then subsides; in other cases it sets in early, persists with great violence, and a fatal termination may follow within a few weeks. Vomiting is more frequent when the cancer involves the orifices, particularly the pylorus, in which case it is usually delayed for an hour or more after taking food. When the cardiac orifice is involved it may follow at a shorter interval. Extensive disease of the fundus or of the walls may be present without vomiting. The food is sometimes very little changed, even after it has remained in the stomach for twenty-four hours.

Hemorrhage occurred in 36 of our 150 cases; in 32 the blood was dark and altered, in 3 it was bright red. In 2 cases vomiting of blood was the first symptom. The bleeding is rarely profuse; more commonly there is a slight oozing, and the blood is mixed with, or altered by, the secretions, and, when vomited, the material is dark, the "coffee-ground" vomit. Occult blood is almost constantly present in carcinoma; in ulcer it may be intermittent. This should be searched for carefully in doubtful cases.

Pain, an early and important symptom, was present in 130 of our cases. It is very variable in situation and, while most common in the epigastrium, it may be referred to the shoulders, the back or the loins. The pain is dragging, burning, or gnawing in character, and rarely occurs in severe paroxysms, as in ulcer. As a rule, it is aggravated by taking food. There is usually marked tenderness on pressure in the epigastric region. The areas of skin tenderness are between the nipple and the umbilicus in front and behind from the fifth to the twelfth thoracic spine.

STOMACH CONTENTS.—The finding of pus and blood in the fasting stomach and pus, blood and mucus two hours after the test meal is suggestive. Diminished motility may be an early finding in pyloric cancer. There is a tendency to a downward trend of gastric secretion, the opposite of the findings in gastric ulcer. The results of secondary infection and gastritis are added to the picture. The protein curve often shows a marked divergence from the acid curve which increases as digestion goes on and is most marked in cases of subacidity or achylia. Bacteria in large numbers occur, one, the Oppler-Boas bacillus—an unusually long nonmotile form—is of diagnostic value. Blood is a most important finding; the persistent presence microscopically of red corpuscles in the early morning washings is always very suspicious. Later, when coffee-ground vomiting takes place, the macroscopic evidence is sufficient. Fragments of the new growth may be vomited or appear in the washings.

Free HCl is decreased or absent in a large proportion of all cases of cancer of the stomach. There are other conditions in which free HCl is absent, such as achylia and gastritis. Repeated studies should be made before drawing conclusions. If there has been a previous ulcer the figures may be high. The presence of lactic acid is of some value.

Examination.—*Inspection.*—An all-important matter is to have the patient in a good light. Fullness in the epigastric region, inequality in the infracostal grooves, the existence of peristalsis, a wide area of aortic pulsation, the presence of subcutaneous nodules or small masses about the navel, and, lastly, a well-defined tumor mass—these, together or singly, may be seen on careful inspection. In 62 of the 150 cases a tumor could be seen and in 52 it descended with inspiration; in 36 peristalsis was visible; in 3 cases movements were visible in the tumor itself. In 10 cases with visible peristalsis no tumor was seen, but could be felt on palpation. The presence of subcutaneous and umbilical nodules may help. They were found in 5 of our series.

Palpation.—In 115 cases a tumor could be felt; in 48 in the epigastric region, in 25 in the umbilical, in 18 in the left hypochondriac, in 17 in the right hypochondriac region, while in 7 cases a mass descended on deep inspiration from beneath the left costal margin. These figures illustrate in how large a proportion of the cases the *tumor* is in evidence when the patient comes under observation. In rare cases examination in the knee-elbow position is of value. *Mobility* of a gastric tumor is of much importance. First, the change with respiration, a mass may descend 3 or 4 inches in deep inspiration; secondly, the communicated pulsation from the aorta, which is often suggestive in its extent; thirdly, the intrinsic movements in the hypertrophied muscularis; and fourthly, mechanical movements, with inflation or change of posture, or communicated by the hand. Tumors of the pylorus are the most movable, and in extreme cases can be displaced to either hypochondrium or pushed far down below the navel (see illustrative cases in Osler's Lectures on the Diagnosis of Abdominal Tumors). Pain on palpation is common; the mass is usually hard, sometimes nodular. Gas can at times be felt gurgling through a tumor at the pyloric region.

Percussion gives less important indications—the note over a tumor is rarely flat, more often a flat tympany. *Auscultation* may reveal the gurgling through the pylorus; sometimes a systolic bruit is transmitted from the aorta, and when local peritonitis exists a friction may be heard.

Complications.—*Secondary growths* are common especially in the lymph nodes, liver and other adjacent organs.

Perforation may lead to peritonitis, but in 3 of our 4 cases there was no general involvement. Cancerous ascites is not uncommon. Dock called attention to the value of the examination of the fluid in such cases. The cells show mitoses and are very characteristic. Chylous ascites may occur. Secondary cancer of the *liver* is very common; the enlargement may be great, and such cases may be mistaken for primary cancer of the organ. Involvement of the *lymph nodes* may give valuable indications. There may be early enlargement of a gland above the inner end of the left clavicle; later adjacent glands may become affected. This occurs also in uterine cancer.

A remarkable picture is presented when the cancer *sloughs* or becomes gangrenous; the vomitus has a foul odor, often of a penetrating nature. In cases in which the ulcer perforates the colon the vomiting may be fecal.

Course.—While usually *chronic* and lasting from a year to eighteen months, an *acute* course is by no means infrequent. Of 69 cases in which we could determine accurately the duration of symptoms, 15 were under three months, 16 from three to six months, 14 from six to twelve months—a total of 45 under one year. Four cases lasted for two years or over. One patient lived for at least two years and a half.

Diagnosis.—Every effort should be made to recognize carcinoma before a tumor is present. Persistent gastric symptoms in an individual over forty require that malignant disease be excluded. Repeated studies of the gastric contents with comparison of the findings and the X-ray examination are the greatest aids. The X-ray picture is modified, the peristaltic waves are interfered with; antiperistalsis and shadows varying in intensity with the degree of induration of the carcinoma may be seen. The constant presence of occult blood in the stools is important. In a doubtful case exploration should be advised without much delay if the findings are suspicious. There are cases in which a positive diagnosis can be reached in no other way.

In 115 of our 150 cases a tumor existed, and with this the recognition is rarely in doubt, but it is usually too late for removal. The chief difficulty is in cases with gastric symptoms or anemia, or both, without the presence of tumor. In the one a chronic gastritis is suspected; in the other a severe anemia. In *chronic gastritis* the long history, the absence of cachexia, the absence of lactic acid in the test meal, and the less striking blood changes are important points. The cases with grave *anemia* may give difficulty but the blood-count is rarely so low as in pernicious anemia. The lower color index, the absence of megaloblasts, and a leukocytosis speak for cancer. With metastases in the bone marrow the blood picture may be that of pernicious anemia (Harrington and Teacher).

From *ulcer of the stomach* malignant disease is, as a rule, readily recognized. The *ulcus carcinomatosum* usually presents a well-marked history of ulcer for years. The greatest difficulty is offered when there is ulcer with tumor due to cicatricial contraction about the pylorus. In 3 such cases we mistook the mass for cancer, and even at operation it may (as in one of them) be impossible to say whether a neoplasm is present.

Treatment.—In early surgical treatment lies the only hope. Operated upon early, complete removal is sometimes possible. In a majority of cases the operation is only palliative. In suitable cases early exploration should be advised; the operation *per se* is sometimes beneficial and the patient is rarely the worse for it. The increasingly favorable results from early operation emphasize the importance of early diagnosis.

The diet should consist of readily digested substances of all sorts. Many patients do best on milk alone. Washing out the stomach, which may be done with a soft tube without any risk, is particularly advantageous when there is obstruction at the pylorus, and is the most satisfactory means of combating vomiting and excessive fermentation. When the pain becomes severe, particularly if it disturbs the rest at night, morphia must be given. One-eighth of a grain (0.008 gm.), combined with bicarbonate of soda (gr. v, 0.3 gm.), bismuth (gr. v-x, 0.3-0.6 gm.), usually gives prompt relief, and the dose does not always require to be increased. Creosote (♏ j-ij, 0.06-0.12 cc.) and one or two drops of phenol in glycerine are useful. The bleeding is rarely amenable to treatment. In cases which are inoperable the use of radium or deep X-ray therapy is worthy of trial.

Other Forms of Tumor.—*Noncancerous tumors* of the stomach rarely cause inconvenience. *Adenoma* occurs in several forms: *polypoid adenomata* are common and are often numerous, one to two hundred; the adenoma may form an area raised above the level of the mucosa; or there may be a rare form of Brunner's glands. Adenoma usually occurs in patients over 50 and gives features suggestive of chronic gastritis which are not distinctive. With *polyposis,* nausea and hemorrhage are common. The X-ray picture is characteristic, showing a mottled area with barium trickling round the masses. There may be carcinomatous degeneration of polyps with features suggestive of malignant disease; there may be intermittent pyloric obstruction and hemorrhage. The X-ray study may suggest the diagnosis. H. B. Anderson described a case of multiple *cysts* in the walls of the stomach and small intestine. *Sarcomata* are rare. There are no definite clinical features different from carcinoma except the occurrence in younger patients. *Fibromata* and *lipomata* have been described. External polypoid tumors, myo- or fibrosarcomata may grow from the peritoneal surface, usually the posterior, of which Sherran collected 18 cases.

Foreign bodies occasionally produce remarkable tumors of the stomach. The most extraordinary is the *hair tumor* which occurs in hysterical women who have been in the habit of eating their own hair. A specimen in the medical museum of McGill University is in two sections, which form an exact mold of the stomach. The tumors are large, very puzzling, and are usually mistaken for cancer. Of 7 cases operated upon, 6 recovered; in 9 cases the condition was found postmortem (Schulten).

HYPERTROPHIC STENOSIS OF THE PYLORUS

In Adults.—Microscopically, the condition is found to be very largely hypertrophy of the muscularis and submucosa of the pylorus. The symptoms are those of dilatation of the stomach. Some of these cases may be congenital, as there have been instances reported in older children and adults. In some cases it may be due to marked pylorospasm.

Congenital.—This remarkable affection was first recognized by Beardsley of Connecticut. There is marked thickening of the pylorus with resulting obstruction and dilatation of the stomach.

Etiology.—There are two possibilities, one that the cause is a congenital hypertrophy of the pylorus and the other that spasm is responsible. The latter is probably the cause in the majority of cases and is due to disturbance in the sympathetic system causing a lack of coordination between the pyloric sphincter and the musculature of the pyloric half of the stomach. There is constant activity of the pyloric sphincter with resulting hypertrophy. The importance of spasm is suggested by the fact that the tumor may persist after the symptoms have disappeared. A large proportion of the cases occurs in first born children and about 80 per cent in boys. The majority of the children are breast fed.

SYMPTOMS.—These are rare in the first week of life and usually appear from the second to the fourth week. Vomiting of food and wasting are constantly present; the former begins, as a rule, during the second or third week, and in a few instances at birth; it occurs usually soon after nursing. It is often of the projectile type; the vomitus often contains mucus, rarely blood. The wasting may be marked, there are marked constipation, great weakness, sometimes severe diarrhea, or a sudden fatal syncope. Probably either acidosis or alkalosis may develop. The latter is more likely.

PHYSICAL SIGNS.—These are distinctive—*visible peristalsis* and *palpable tumor.* The peristalsis is best seen after feeding, when the waves pass at intervals, in characteristic form, from left to right above the navel; two or three waves may be seen at once. The pyloric tumor may be felt as a firm, hard, freely movable body, to the right of the navel and a little above it, which varies in size and consistency, and through which gas may sometimes be felt to gurgle. The X-ray examination adds little. There are no sequels; if the child recovers the hypertrophy of the pylorus disappears.

DIAGNOSIS.—This offers little difficulty if peristalsis is observed. Ordinary vomiting has not a projectile character and mild grades of pyloric spasm do not cause peristalsis or the general features. In congenital stricture of the duodenum the symptoms date from birth and there is bile in the vomitus.

TREATMENT.—Medical treatment consists in feeding with breast or modified milk, 1-2 ounces every 2 or 3 hours. Dextrose solution (200 cc., 4 per cent) can be given by the bowel. Lavage of the stomach should be done twice a day. Atropine is useful in some cases, by its effect on spasm, in dosage carefully studied for each patient. Some suggest giving it hypodermically until the vomiting is controlled and then by mouth. The initial dose may be one drop of a 1-1000 solution, freshly prepared (Haas). There should not be delay in resorting to surgical measures if improvement does not occur. The division of the circular muscular layer (Rammstedt's operation) is a successful procedure. Before operation care should be taken to correct dehydration and acidosis or alkalosis. The after care is important. The child should be kept warm, given fluid by bowel and subcutaneously, and fed carefully with a gradual increase in the amount. Blood transfusion is useful in severe cases.

HEMORRHAGE FROM THE STOMACH

(*Hematemesis*)

Etiology.—Hematemesis may result from many conditions, local or general. In *local disease:* (1) cancer; (2) ulcer; (3) disease of the blood vessels, such as miliary aneurisms, occasionally varicose veins and from telangiectases; (4) acute congestion, as in gastritis, and possibly in vicarious hemorrhage; (5) from esophageal varices; (6) syphilis, and (7) following operations in the abdomen, particularly when the omentum is wounded, erosions of the gastric mucosa may occur, from which hemorrhage takes place.

It is a very fatal complication after appendicitis and is usually associated with peritonitis.

Passive congestion due to obstruction in the portal system. This may be (1) *hepatic,* as in cirrhosis of the liver, thrombosis of the portal vein, or pressure upon the portal vein by tumor, and secondly in chronic disease of the heart and lungs. (2) *Splenic.* Gastric hemorrhage is by no means uncommon with splenomegaly, and is explained by the intimate relations between the vasa brevia and the splenic circulation.

Toxic: (1) In some fevers, as smallpox and yellow fever; (2) unknown poisons, as in acute yellow atrophy; (3) phosphorus.

Trauma: (1) Mechanical injuries, as blows and wounds, and occasionally by the stomach tube; (2) the result of severe corrosive poisons.

Certain constitutional diseases: (1) Hemophilia; (2) profound anemias; (3) purpura, and (4) cholemia.

In certain *nervous affections,* particularly hysteria, and occasionally in general paresis and epilepsy.

The blood may not come primarily from the stomach but from the nose or pharynx. In hemoptysis some blood may pass into the stomach. In bleeding from the esophagus blood may trickle into the stomach, from which it is ejected. This occurs with rupture of an aneurism. A child may draw blood with the milk from the mother's breast and vomit it.

Gastrostaxis: Under this name Hale-White described cases of hemorrhage from the stomach in young girls without any evident lesion of the mucosa. They are often mistaken for ulcer. At operation the blood has been seen oozing from points in the mucosa. There may be no pain or any of the ordinary features of ulcer.

Miscellaneous causes: Aneurism of the aorta or of its branches may rupture into the stomach. There are instances in which a patient has vomited blood once without any recurrence or without developing symptoms pointing to disease of the stomach. In newborn infants hematemesis may occur alone or in connection with bleeding from other mucous membranes.

In medical practice, hemorrhage from the stomach occurs most frequently with ulcer of the stomach or duodenum and from esophageal varices.

Morbid Anatomy.—When death has occurred from the hematemesis there are signs of intense anemia. The lesion is evident in cancer and in ulcer. Fatal hemorrhage may come from a small miliary aneurism communicating with the surface by a pinhole perforation, or the bleeding may be due to the rupture of a submucous vein and the erosion in the mucosa may be small and readily overlooked. It may require a prolonged search to find such lesions. In the group associated with portal obstruction, the mucosa is usually pale, smooth, and shows no trace of any lesion. In cirrhosis, fatal by hemorrhage, one may search in vain for any local lesion and we must conclude that it is possible for profuse bleeding to occur by diapedesis. The stomach may be full of blood and yet the source of the hemorrhage be not apparent. In such cases the esophagus should be examined carefully. In toxic cases there are invariably hemorrhages in the mucous membrane.

Symptoms.—In rare instances fatal syncope may occur without any vomiting. In a case of the kind, in which the woman fell over and died in a few minutes, the stomach contained between three and four pounds of blood.

The sudden profuse bleedings rapidly lead to profound anemia. When due to ulcer or cirrhosis the bleeding may recur for several days. Fatal hemorrhage from the stomach is met with in ulcer, cirrhosis, enlargement of the spleen, and in instances in which an aneurism ruptures into the stomach or esophagus. Gastric hemorrhage may occur in splenic anemia or leukemia before the condition has aroused attention.

The vomited blood may be fluid or clotted; it is usually dark in color, but in the basin the outer part becomes red from the action of the air. The longer blood remains in the stomach the more altered it is when ejected.

The amount of blood lost is very variable, and in a day the patient may bring up three or four pounds, or even more. In a case under the care of George Ross, in Montreal, the patient during seven days lost ten pounds, by weight, of blood. The usual symptoms of anemia develop rapidly, and there may be slight fever and subsequently edema. Syncope, convulsions, and occasionally hemiplegia occur after very profuse hemorrhage. Blindness may follow, the result of thrombosis of the retinal arteries or veins, or an acute degeneration of the ganglion cells of the retina.

Diagnosis.—In a majority of instances there is no question as to the origin of the blood. Occasionally it is difficult, particularly if the patient is not seen during the attack. Examination of the vomitus readily determines whether blood is present or not. The material vomited may be stained by wine, the juice of strawberries, raspberries, or cranberries, which give a color resembling that of fresh blood, while iron, bismuth and bile may produce the blackish color of altered blood. The microscope shows the shadowy outlines of red blood cells, and spectroscopic and chemical tests may be applied.

Deception is sometimes practised by hysterical patients, who swallow and then vomit blood or colored liquids. With a little care such cases can usually be detected. The cases must be excluded in which the blood comes from the nose or pharynx, or in which infants swallow it with the milk.

There is not often difficulty in distinguishing between hemoptysis and hematemesis, though coughing and vomiting are not infrequently combined, by a careful history and thorough study.

Prognosis.—Except in the case of rupture of an aneurism or of large veins, the impression is that hematemesis rarely proves fatal, but among 649 cases of severe hematemesis death followed in 94, 14.5 per cent (Bulmer, 1932). There are great differences in the mortality figures from various hospitals. In our experience death follows relatively more frequently in hepatic cirrhosis than in ulcer or cancer. In the chronic ulcer the bleeding may recur for years. The treatment of hematemesis is considered under gastric ulcer.

NEUROSES OF THE STOMACH

(*Nervous Dyspepsia*)

Serious functional disturbances of the stomach may occur without any discoverable anatomical basis. The cases are most frequent in those who have either inherited a nervous constitution or who have gradually, through indiscretions, brought about a condition of nervous weakness. Not infrequently, the gastric symptoms stand so far in the foreground that the general neuropathic character of the patient quite escapes notice. The variable reaction of individuals to "digestive discomfort" has to be kept in mind; there are varying thresholds for pain and discomfort. Anticipation of trouble seems often to favor its occurrence and the influence of worry, nervous strain and fatigue is often shown. Sometimes the gastric manifestations have a reflex origin depending on organic disturbances in other parts, such as the gallbladder, appendix or colon.

In all disturbances of the digestive tract, attention must be given to the whole and not to one part only. The digestive tube is a complicated mechanism which requires perfect coordination for proper function. Disease of one part may disturb the working elsewhere as, for example, disease of the appendix may cause gastric symptoms. Great importance attaches to proper motor function and many disturbances are due to this being disturbed. Motility may be increased, slowed, reversed or stopped, and any of these may result in symptoms. Contraction of a segment causes inhibition of the segment distal to it and this is particularly important in special zones, *e.g.*, the pylorus and duodenum. Irregularities and blocks may occur as in the heart, especially where one zone passes into another, *e.g.*, at the pylorus and ileocecal valve. The nervous control plays a large part and the importance of disturbance of the sympathetic system must always be kept in mind. Keith divides the digestive tract into neuromuscular sections, each separated from the adjoining one by a sphincter which blocks the passage of waves of contraction. He compares these to the blocks on a railroad, in which if one is blocked, the others are also.

As this group of stomach disorders does not represent a disease or even a symptom-complex there is the greatest variety in the clinical picture, not only in the comparison of one patient with another but in the same patient from time to time. It may require careful study to estimate the various causal factors and the possibility of organic disease manifesting itself as functional gastric disturbance must not be forgotten.

Alvarez has drawn attention to the part played by *reversed peristalsis* in causing symptoms. For example, regurgitation may be due to a distended and overactive colon or irritation from a diseased appendix. Vomiting may be due to increased tone and activity in the jejunum for which an irritable colon may be responsible. Belching of gas may represent reversed peristalsis set up by some organic lesion. Nausea is due more often to intestinal lesions, *e.g.*, in the colon with reversed peristalsis, than to disease of the esophagus and stomach. As to the cause of a coated tongue there is no proof that it is always due to gastric disease. It may be due to regurgitation, as particles of material from the colon may easily reach the tongue. The condition termed "biliousness" is often a result of reversed intestinal activity originating in the colon and when this is emptied relief is obtained.

Clinical Features.—These are so varied that it is difficult to know how best to describe them. The combinations are many and the symptoms change from time to time. It seems best to describe the various disturbances in detail.

Motor Disturbances.—HYPERMOTILITY.—Common with duodenal ulcer, this is usually a secondary disturbance, but sometimes is primary so far as any other condition can be found. There are no characteristic symptoms but some patients are satisfied with small amounts of food and suffer from hunger and discomfort two or three hours later, relieved at once by taking food or liquid. If pyloric spasm is associated with hypermotility there may be attacks of considerable distress with acid regurgitation or vomiting. The *diagnosis* is made by the test meal or by the X-ray study.

PERISTALTIC UNREST.—This is a common and distressing symptom. Shortly after eating, the peristaltic movements of the stomach are increased, and borborygmi and gurgling may be heard, even at a distance. The subjective sensations are most annoying, and it appears as if in the hyperesthetic condition the patient felt normal peristalsis, just as the usual beating of the heart may be perceptible to him. A further analogy is afforded by the fact that emotion increases this peristalsis. It may extend to the intestines, and on palpation the gurgling is marked. The cause is usually reversed peristalsis due sometimes to disease elsewhere, as in the colon.

ERUCTATIONS.—*Aerophagia.*—In this condition noisy eructations, often following one another in rapid succession, occur. When violent they last for hours or days. At other times they occur in paroxysms, depending often upon mental excitement. They are most common in neurotic individuals. The expelled air has usually been swallowed. Contrary to the common belief it does not come from fermentation except when there is pyloric obstruction. Aerophagia is common in general nervous disturbance but also occurs with organic conditions, such as gallbladder disease. The patient feels some gastric discomfort which he regards as due to distention with gas and makes an effort to bring it up. In doing this he swallows air and after a time succeeds in eructing this. The common symptom is a feeling of fullness; if there is actual distention this may press on the diaphragm and cause palpitation and thoracic discomfort. In neurotic patients spasm of the diaphragm may cause pseudodistention with fullness of the abdomen and great distress. This may disappear as rapidly as it came, without belching. Nervous patients often insist that the stomach is distended with gas when there is no evidence of it. If there is any doubt after the physical examination the use of the stomach tube or X-ray will settle the question.

NERVOUS VOMITING.—This may be due to influences acting directly or indirectly upon the vomiting centres. The patients are, as a rule, women and the subject of more or less marked nervous manifestations. A special feature is the absence of preliminary nausea and of the usual straining efforts in vomiting. It is rather a regurgitation, and without visible effort or gagging the mouth is filled with the contents of the stomach, which are then spat out. It comes on, as a rule, after eating, but may occur at irregular intervals. In some cases the nutrition is not impaired, a feature which may give a clue to the true nature of the disease, as there may be no other marked nervous manifestation. It may occur in children, but in many cases this recurring vomiting is associated with acidosis. Nervous vomiting may be a serious condition; we have had at least two fatal cases. In some instances, after persisting for weeks or months at home, the patient gets well in a few days in hospital. In other instances the course is protracted, and the cases are among the most trying we are called upon to treat. The general state of the nervous system should always be carefully investigated.

One type of vomiting is associated with certain diseases of the nervous system—particularly tabes—forming part of the gastric crises. There are cases of primary periodic vomiting usually regarded as a neurosis.

Rumination; Merycismus.—In this remarkable condition the patients regurgitate and chew the cud like ruminants. It occurs in neurasthenic or hysterical persons, epileptics, and idiots. In some patients it is hereditary. In one instance a governess taught it to two children. The habit may persist for years, and does not necessarily impair the health.

Cardiospasm.—Termed also phrenospasm, achalasia of the cardia, preventriculosis and idiopathic dilatation of the esophagus. This is a condition in which, without any obstruction which can be demonstrated, food does not pass from the esophagus to the stomach but remains in the esophagus which usually becomes dilated.

Etiology.—There is no agreement as to the essential lesion. Spasm of the cardia has not been demonstrated. Chevalier Jackson states that the obstruction is where the esophagus passes through the diaphragm (*phrenospasm*). Hurst holds that it is due to lack of the normal relaxation of the sphincter—achalasia (absence of relaxation)—a view supported by the finding of changes in Auerbach's plexus at the lower end of the esophagus. The cardiac sphincter has not been found hypertrophied at operation or autopsy. Essentially there is interference with the mechanism of swallowing. Dilatation of the esophagus, of variable degree, results with hypertrophy of the walls. A closed cardiac sphincter can support a column of water 8 inches high so that with this condition the esophagus contains a column of this height. If more is added the cardia opens and some of the contents enters the stomach. Various causes may operate. A neurosis, neuritis, reflex action from disease above or below the diaphragm and irritation of the esophagus have been suggested. Vagotonia is marked in some patients. In many cases no definite cause can be found. *Sex* apparently has no influence. It may occur at any age but is rare in childhood.

Pathology.—There is large dilatation of the esophagus, spindle-shaped or widest at its lowest part. The walls are grayish-white and wrinkled. There may be erosions. The hiatus-csophagcus is not stenotic.

Clinical Features.—The *onset* is usually gradual but may be sudden. Early there is intermittent resistance to the passage of food but it can be forced through. There is discomfort and possibly pain. Gradually the difficulty increases with more obstruction. Food accumulates and regurgitation occurs with or soon after eating. Later there is regurgitation at irregular intervals. There may be a sensation of weight in the thorax. The patient is unable to belch or vomit, and what is described as vomiting is usually regurgitation. With the collection of gas in the stomach, there may be great distress and anginal attacks. There may be complaint of precordial pain. Dulness to the right of the sternum has been described. The deglutition murmur is not heard. There is usually loss of weight but the general condition may be surprisingly good.

Diagnosis.—This is made by the X-ray study and the passage of the esophagoscope. The X-ray study shows a blunt obstruction about the cardia with dilatation of the esophagus above. The diagnosis has to be made from benign stricture and malignant disease.

Treatment.—Drugs are of no value. Some patients have been cured by the passage of a stomach tube or esophagoscope, but the use of a wide tube containing mercury seems to be most successful. If this is not possible the sphincter can be stretched from below by the finger introduced through the stomach. The results from these methods of treatment have been excellent.

PYLOROSPASM.—This may be due to some irritative lesion of the stomach (ulcer) or elsewhere (gallbladder or appendix), or occurs as part of a neurosis. There may be hypersecretion and hypermotility with it, in which case there may be severe attacks of discomfort and pain. Usually there is pain of the "hunger type," coming on 2 or 3 hours after meals, relieved by emptying the stomach or giving food. The pain is often referred to the region of the pylorus which can sometimes be felt as a hard mass which relaxes at intervals. Sometimes atony with dilatation results. Intermittent stagnation and hyperacidity may occur. It may not be easy to distinguish organic stricture from spasm but the duodenal tube usually passes the latter. The effect of atropine in relaxing spasm may be of aid. The X-ray study is of great assistance, done before and after belladonna or atropine has been given freely.

ATONY.—This occurs in general diseases which cause disturbance of nutrition, in anemia, sometimes following pyloric obstruction, occasionally after an acute infection, but most often when the general nervous system is disturbed, especially if there is visceroptosis. The main symptom is gastric discomfort with a feeling of fullness during and after meals, or it may be continuous. In consequence the amount of food taken is reduced. There may be feelings of weight and pressure, eructations, etc. Pain is not present and vomiting is rare. The test meal shows delay in emptying and variable acidity findings, often low. The X-ray study removes any doubt.

INSUFFICIENCY OR INCONTINENCE OF THE PYLORUS.—This condition may be recognized by the rapid passing of gas from the stomach into the bowel on attempts at inflation of the former, as well as by the presence of intestinal contents in the stomach. There are no distinctive clinical symptoms.

INSUFFICIENCY OF THE CARDIA.—This condition is only recognized by the occurrence of eructations or rumination.

Secretory Neuroses.—HYPERACIDITY; HYPERCHLORHYDRIA.—The studies of Hawk and Rehfuss and their coworkers altered materially our views as to hyperacidity. They have shown that grades of acidity which we thought abnormal are normal in certain healthy individuals. Each has his own figure of gastric acidity and no general standard can be given. It is a question what symptoms are due to hyperacidity. Other disturbances, as in the motor function and pylorospasm, have to be taken into account. Organic disease, especially ulcer and causes lower in the digestive tract, should always be considered. Yet there are some symptoms apparently associated with hyperacidity especially in nervous individuals. They do not, as a rule, immediately follow the ingestion of food, but occur one to three hours later, at the height of digestion. There is a sense of weight and pressure, with burning in the epigastrium, often with acid eructations. If vomiting occurs, the pain is relieved. The patient is usually relatively well nourished, and the appetite is good, though he may be afraid to eat on account of anticipated pain. Constipation is common. Hyperacidity as a rule means hypersecretion.

HYPERSECRETION.—This occurs in two forms, (*a*) continuous and (*b*) paroxysmal or intermittent; the former is the more common. The common causes are ulcer, gastric or duodenal, reflex influences from other abdominal diseases, as in the gallbladder or appendix, and general nervous disturbance. The symptoms are much like those of hyperacidity. In the *continuous* form gastric distress, burning sensations and acid eructations are common. As the secretion continues when the stomach is empty the symptoms may occur during the night. Examination of the fasting stomach shows the presence of varying amounts of highly acid fluid with a high percentage of HCl. If pylorospasm exists there may be more or less gastric dilatation. In the *paroxysmal* form the excessive secretion may continue for hours or days. It occurs especially with tabes, hysteria and migraine. The attack begins with disturbed sensations in the stomach, often headache, and later vomiting of the very acid fluid.

HYPOSECRETION.—It may be difficult to distinguish between hyposecretion and hypo-acidity and the two are probably combined as a rule. Lack of or decreased secretion occurs in many diseases; gastritis, acute and chronic, cancer and atony of the stomach, some cases of gallbladder disease and appendicitis, pernicious anemia and in functional nervous disorders. The influence of emotion, excitement and fear is familiar as a temporary phenomenon; if the condition is permanent the effect on gastric secretion is the same. There are no characteristic symptoms and the patient may have many complaints, mostly of sensory disturbance. If the motility is good there may be no symptoms. The diagnosis depends largely on the study of the stomach contents; repeated tests should be done and the effect of histamine should be determined. The effort should then be made to decide if the conditions are secondary and if so what primary condition is responsible.

ACHYLIA GASTRICA.—This term was given by Einhorn to the condition in which there is a complete absence of gastric secretion. This may occur with atrophy of the gastric mucosa but is sometimes an inborn error of secretion and may be familial. The clinical features are variable and some patients are free from symptoms. There may be loss of appetite, nausea, and discomfort for some time after meals. Vomiting is rare. Diarrhea, which may be chronic, occurs not infrequently. The physical examination shows nothing distinctive and the diagnosis depends on the study of the stomach contents. If atony occurs the symptoms are aggravated. The lack of response to histamine hydrochloride (0.25 mg. subcutaneously) distinguishes true achylia.

Sensory Neuroses.—HYPERESTHESIA.—In this the patients complain of fullness, pressure, weight, burning, and so forth, during digestion, just such symptoms as accompany a variety of organic diseases of the stomach, and yet in other respects the gastric functions appear normal. Sometimes these distressing sensations are present when the stomach is empty. These symptoms are usually associated with hysteria or neurasthenia. The pain often follows particular articles of food. A hysterical patient may apparently suffer severe pain after taking the smallest amount of food of any sort, while anything prescribed as a medicine may be well borne. In severe cases the patient may be reduced to an extreme degree by starvation.

GASTRIC PAIN.—Severe pains in the epigastrium, paroxysmal in character, occur (1) as a manifestation of a functional neurosis, independent of organic disease, and usually associated with other nervous symptoms (it is this form which is here described); (2) in chronic disease of the nervous system, the so-called gastric crises; and (3) in organic disease of the stomach, such as ulcer or cancer, and with disease of the appendix and gallbladder.

This functional neurosis occurs chiefly in women, very commonly with disturbed menstrual function or pronounced nervous symptoms. The affection may set in as early as puberty, but it is more common at the menopause. Anemic, constipated women who have worries and anxieties are most prone to the affection but attacks sometimes occur in robust men. More often it is only one feature in general neurasthenia or a manifestation of that form of nervous dyspepsia in which there is hypersecretion.

The *symptoms* are very characteristic; the patient is suddenly seized with severe pains in the epigastrium, which pass to the back and around the lower ribs. The attack is usually independent of the taking of food and may recur at definite intervals. Vomiting is rare; more commonly the taking of food relieves the pain but to this there are striking exceptions. Pressure upon the epigastrium commonly gives relief but deep pressure may be painful. Stress has been laid upon the occurrence of painful points, but they are so common in nervous states that little importance can be given to them.

The *diagnosis* offers many difficulties. Organic disease of the stomach or of the nervous system, particularly the gastric crises of tabes, must be excluded. Disease elsewhere, such as in the gallbladder or appendix, may be the etiological factor and search should be made for such lesions. The prolonged intervals between the attacks and their independence of diet are important features; but in many instances it is less the local than the general symptoms which enable us to make the diagnosis. In gall stone colic jaundice may be absent, and in any long-standing case of gastralgia the question of cholelithiasis should be considered. Such a case may be treated for months as nervous dyspepsia until a more severe attack is followed by jaundice.

Anomalies of Gastric Sensation; Bulimia.—Abnormally excessive hunger may come in paroxysmal attacks; which cause the patient to commit extraordinary excesses in eating. This may occur in diabetes mellitus and sometimes in gastric disorders, particularly those associated with hypersecretion. It is more commonly seen in hysteria and the psychoses. It may occur in cerebral tumors, in Graves' disease and in epilepsy.

The attacks often begin suddenly at night, the patient waking with a feeling of faintness and pain, and an uncontrollable desire for food. Sometimes such attacks occur immediately after a large meal. The attack may be relieved by a small amount of food, while at other times enormous quantities may be taken. In obstinate cases gastritis, atony, and dilatation frequently result from overfilling the stomach.

Hunger.—There may be a variety of disturbing sensations connected with hunger, especially in nervous patients. The possibility of *hypoglycemia* being responsible should be considered. Some have a sudden sensation of extreme weakness with anxiety and sometimes dizziness and sweating; syncope may follow. This may be part of a neurosis but ulcer should always be excluded. In another form the patient may be very hungry when beginning a meal but after taking a small amount of food there is a feeling of satiety and no more is taken. This is practically always in nervous patients.

Akoria.—An absence of the sense of satiety. This is commonly associated with bulimia and polyphagia, but not invariably. The patient always feels "empty." There are usually other well-marked manifestations of hysteria or neurasthenia.

Parorexia.—This term is applied to the condition in which the patient has a craving for very acid foods, and in hookworm infection for a wide variety of substances, such as earth, string, cloth, etc.

Anorexia nervosa.—This condition, which is a manifestation of a neurotic temperament, is discussed under Hysteria.

Nervous Dyspepsia.—This is not a satisfactory term, but it is difficult to find a better one to designate the condition in a large group of patients who complain of gastric disturbance, without any organic disease of the stomach or elsewhere in the abdomen, apparently secondary to neurasthenia and allied states. There is general fatigue, psychical, emotional and physical. The digestive symptoms are characteristic only in their irregularity and uncertainty. Discomfort is a common complaint, usually worse after meals, but varying in occurrence and severity. It has no special relation to any particular food unless the patient gets the notion that some particular food is responsible and expects trouble. Then it usually comes. In consequence one article of food after another is given up and the nutrition may suffer. Distention and flatulency are common, often associated with air swallowing. Constipation is usual and mucous colitis common. Loss of weight may result from insufficient food. There are no special physical findings in the abdomen except general tenderness and often a spastic colon. There may be atony of the stomach. The stomach contents may be normal but usually show some change, perhaps most often hyposecretion. The *diagnosis* should only be made after organic disease is excluded. The possibility of disease of the gallbladder or appendix should be particularly considered. Evidences of the general condition are usually marked. The gastric symptoms reflect the general state; with worry or depression they are worse while with some new interest for a time they are less or disappear temporarily.

Visceroptosis.—The part played by this may be difficult to determine but in the majority of cases it is probably small. Too often a patient is told that she has a "dropped stomach" with resulting additional worry. In many of these patients the position of the stomach is the same before and after the occurrence of symptoms. Of course gastroptosis may lessen the efficiency of the stomach but that it does so often to any marked degree seems doubtful. This does not mean that an abdominal support is not often of great aid.

Treatment of Neuroses of the Stomach.—The most important part is often that directed toward the improvement of the general physical and mental condition of the patient. The possibility that the symptoms may be of reflex origin should be borne in mind; eye-strain, cholelithiasis, or chronic appendicitis should be considered. Tuberculosis should always be excluded. A large proportion of cases of nervous dyspepsia are dependent upon mental and physical exhaustion or worry, and a vacation or a change of scene will often accomplish what treatment at home has failed to do. The manner of life should be investigated and a proper amount of exercise in the open air and systematic hydrotherapy insisted upon. This in some cases is sufficient to cause the symptoms to disappear. Many patients with marked neurasthenic or hysterical symptoms do well with a period of complete rest.

In "*cardiospasm*" the earlier that treatment is begun the better the outlook. The diet should be simple and atropine may be given. Sometimes the passage of the esophagoscope is sufficient, but usually the use of Plummer's water bag or a mercury tube is necessary. This may only require to be used once or in more obstinate cases more frequently. In cases with esophagitis, the patient should try to empty the esophagus soon after every meal.

Diet.—This should depend in the majority of patients on the individual rather than on the symptoms. Many patients demand a diet and to be put on rigid rules is an advantage, usually through the psychical effect. But as a rule patients do better without many restrictions. The psychology of the patient should be carefully studied. How the patient eats is usually more important than what he eats. Thorough mastication, the taking of liquids slowly and avoiding the taking of food when upset nervously or fatigued are important. In these days of dietary fads it is difficult to persuade many patients that simple measures may be sufficient.

The treatment in *atony* should be similar to that in moderate dilatation—the administration of small quantities of food at frequent intervals; the limitation of fluids, which should be taken in small amounts at a time; lavage. Strychnine in full doses may be of value. A proper abdominal support and sleeping with the foot of the bed elevated are useful aids.

In *hyperacidity*, in addition to the treatment of the general condition, alkalies must be employed, as magnesia, calcium carbonate or bicarbonate of soda. These should be given in large doses and at the *height of digestion.* In hyperacidity and hypersecretion the use of atropine frequently gives relief. It should be given before food and in small doses at first, beginning with $\frac{1}{150}$ grain (0.0004 gm.) and gradually increasing. The combination of bromide and belladonna is sometimes useful. The diet should be mainly of proteins and fats with carbohydrate in small amounts. Meat, chicken, fish, eggs, cheese, milk and cream, and butter form the bulk of the diet. Bread is allowed in small amounts, stale or as toast. Condiments and alcohol should be avoided. Special emphasis should be placed on the need of thorough mastication. Half an ounce of olive oil is useful before meals. The bowels should be kept freely open, for which mineral oil is useful. The diet should be gradually increased with sparing addition of starches. The patient should carry alkali with him to take at the first sign of discomfort.

In *supersecretion* the use of the stomach tube is of the greatest value. In the periodical form it should be used as soon as the attack begins. The stomach may be washed with alkaline solutions. Where this is impracticable the taking of albuminous food may give relief. Alkalies in large doses are indicated. In *continued supersecretion* there are usually atony and dilatation. The diet here should be much as in superacidity, but in smaller quantities at frequent intervals. Lavage with alkaline solutions is of great value. To relieve pain alkalies should be given freely at the height of digestion. Atropine is usually of value.

In *subacidity* a carefully regulated, easily digestible mixed diet, not too rich in protein, is advisable. Prolonged mastication is important. Bitter tonics before meals are sometimes of value. Dilute hydrochloric acid should be given freely and the dosage and best method of administration determined for each patient. Thirty to 60 drops may be taken in a glass of water during the latter part of the meal or doses of 30 drops taken 15 and 30 minutes after meals. In *achylia gastrica* the use of predigested foods and hydrochloric acid in full doses may be of assistance.

In marked *hyperesthesia,* the treatment of the general condition is especially important. Abdominal compresses are useful.

For *pain* alkalies should be given, of which the light magnesia and bicarbonate of soda are the best. A teaspoonful of either or of a mixture of equal parts may be given after food and when required. A combination of potassium bromide (gr. xv, 1 gm.) with codeine (gr. ⅓, 0.02 gm.) or atropine (gr. 1/100, 0.00065 gm.) is sometimes useful. Chloroform in small doses or Hoffman's anodyne will sometimes allay the severe pains. The general condition should receive careful attention, and in many cases the attacks recur until the nervous condition is improved. If there is anemia iron may be given freely.

There are forms of nervous dyspepsia occurring in women who are often well nourished and with a good color, yet who suffer—particularly at night—with flatulency and abdominal distress. The sleep may be quiet for two or three hours, after which they are aroused with painful sensations in the abdomen and eructations. The appetite and digestion may appear to be normal but constipation is usually present. In many of those patients the condition seems rather intestinal and the distress is due to the accumulation of gas and reversed peristalsis. The fats, starches, and sugars should be restricted. Some obtain relief from irrigation of the colon at bedtime. Bromide and small doses of phenobarbital are of value. The state of the nervous system should be carefully studied.

In all forms of gastric neurosis special care should be taken to prevent constipation. As this is often with a spastic colon, purgatives should be avoided. Regularity, the taking of water freely and the use of mineral oil or combinations of it with agar, and an occasional enema are helpful.

DISEASES OF THE INTESTINES

DISEASES OF THE DUODENUM

Congenital obstruction of the duodenum is rare. There is vomiting of fluid containing bile. The X-ray study shows the obstruction. A small catheter may be passed into the stomach which is washed until the fluid comes away clear. If the tube can be passed through the pylorus, bile stained fluid is obtained. If the child's condition permits, a gastro-enterostomy should be done. In *duodenum inversum* the duodenum surrounds the head of the pancreas and its mesentery shows defective attachment. There may be no symptoms or there may be obstruction both of the bowel and of the biliary and pancreatic ducts. The symptoms usually suggest duodenal ulcer and the diagnosis can be made only by X-ray study. *Diverticula* in the true sense are congenital and usually on the mesenteric aspect of the duodenum. The acquired form usually occurs about a healed ulcer or results from the traction of adhesions. The *symptoms* usually suggest duodenal ulcer or gallbladder disease. Duodenal ileus is usually present. There may be a history of "bilious attacks" in childhood. There is usually pain after meals, sometimes with a feeling of distention. The pain is usually relieved by vomiting, less by belching or alkalies.

There is usually a history of long duration without quiescent periods. Ulceration with hemorrhage or perforation may occur. The *diagnosis* depends largely on a careful X-ray study, often better under the fluoroscope than from plates. A period of treatment, much as for duodenal ulcer, should be tried to decide whether a diverticulum is responsible for the symptoms or is only an anatomical anomaly. In *treatment,* medical measures should be tried first. Surgery may be necessary, excision or inversion being done.

Duodenitis.—The *simple* or *catarrhal* form is often associated with acute gastritis. There is colicky pain usually two or three hours after meals, felt to the right of the midline, with frequent nausea but rarely vomiting. By the duodenal tube shreds or streaks of mucus may be obtained which are not mixed with the duodenal contents. The process may be part of a general enteritis. *Suppurative* duodenitis is rare and has followed trauma. A local peritonitis may follow and the signs are those of an acute inflammatory condition. *Ulcerative* duodenitis may follow a burn or occur with infectious diseases.

Dilatation or chronic duodenal ileus is often associated with visceroptosis and compression of the terminal portion of the duodenum by the root of the mesentery. Adhesions, spinal deformity and a movable kidney are responsible in some cases. The history may be of attacks in childhood, with freedom from the age of 12 or 15 years and recurrence in adult life. The symptoms are (1) *pain* in the upper abdomen, sometimes described as a pulling or dragging sensation, sometimes more severe, and suggesting ulcer or gallbladder disease; (2) *vomiting* which is frequent and sometimes persistent; it may occur at long intervals and be regarded as due to a "bilious attack"; (3) constipation; and (4) marked vagotonic features. In some cases the condition is intermittent and "biliousness" or migraine is diagnosed. The X-ray study is an important aid in the diagnosis. In *treatment,* position may be useful, the patient lying on the face with the feet elevated, or on the left side, or taking the knee-chest position. Gastric and duodenal lavage is useful. Correction of the visceroptosis may give relief. Constipation should be corrected. In severe cases surgical intervention is advisable.

Duodenal *adhesions* may simulate ulcer very closely and in the X-ray study it may not be possible to distinguish them. The symptoms are not distinctive and suggest ulcer or gallbladder disease. They often occur intermittently, which suggests that another factor is present. *Treatment* is difficult; symptomatic medical treatment should be given; surgery is not always successful.

Carcinoma of the duodenum is rare. There is usually pain, varying in severity, worse after food and relieved by vomiting. Nausea and vomiting are common and pylorospasm is often present. Jaundice is present in the majority of cases, depending on the situation of the tumor. It may be intermittent. A mass may be felt. Occult blood is often present in the stools. In *diagnosis,* the X-ray study is important. The *treatment* is surgical and can be successful only if an early diagnosis has been made.

Fixation.—There may be bands passing from the gallbladder to the colon which surround the duodenum or are in front of it. By these the duodenum is held high. The onset of symptoms is usually between sixteen and twenty years of age but may be in childhood. There is often pain, which may occur in attacks, with distress and distention from one-half to an hour after meals.

The attacks of pain may simulate cholecystitis. The stomach may be dilated and its contents usually show a high acidity. As the patient grows older, headache and weakness with vasomotor and nervous symptoms become prominent. Constipation is common. The *diagnosis* is made by the X-ray study and usually better by fluoroscopy than by plates. The apex of the duodenum is sharp and held up to the right, looking as if suspended on a hook and making a sharp turn. The duodenum beyond the fixed point may be against the liver and flat. The *treatment* is surgical.

LOCAL ILEITIS

This is a condition of subacute chronic inflammation of the terminal ileum which may cause stenosis. The process is most marked at the ileocecal valve and extends upwards for 8 to 12 inches. Exudation and hyperplasia result in thickening of the wall with narrowing and sometimes perforation which occurs slowly so that an abscess may form and sometimes fistulae. There may be diarrhea with blood and mucus in the stools. Pain is common and a tumor may be felt after some time. Fever is variable and may alternate with afebrile periods. If an abscess forms it may discharge into the sigmoid, cecum or ascending colon, or externally. If operation is done the lower ileum is found thickened with edema and there may be an abscess. In the X-ray study there is delay in the terminal ileum. The *diagnosis* may be difficult—appendicitis, perhaps with abscess, actinomycosis, tuberculosis, neoplasm and ulcerative colitis have to be considered. In *treatment*, complete removal is necessary. If an abscess is drained, there will probably be a persistent fistula.

DISEASES OF THE INTESTINES ASSOCIATED WITH DIARRHEA

ENTERITIS; DIARRHEA

Diarrhea results from too rapid passage of the contents through the intestine, resulting in fluid stools. The term should not be used for the passage of frequent solid stools, which may be due to constipation, or, if the word is used in a restricted sense, for the frequent stools of dysentery.

In the classification of acute enteritis the anatomical divisions of the bowel have been too closely followed, and a duodenitis, jejunitis, ileitis, typhlitis, colitis, and proctitis have been recognized; whereas in a majority of cases the entire intestinal tract, to a greater or lesser extent, is involved, sometimes the small most intensely, sometimes the large bowel; but during life it may be quite impossible to say which portion is specially affected.

Etiology.—The causes may be either *primary* or *secondary*. Among the causes of *primary* enteritis are: (*a*) *Improper food*, one of the most frequent, especially in children, in whom it follows overeating or the ingestion of unripe fruit. In some individuals special articles of diet produce a slight diarrhea, which may not be due to a catarrh of the mucosa, but to increased peristalsis induced by the offending material. (*b*) *Infection.* The cases of food poisoning are fairly common in mild forms; possibly some are instances of colon bacillus infection. Infection from the mouth may be responsible in some cases. There may be chronic or intermittent diarrhea due to fermentative or putrefactive conditions in the bowel. (*c*) Various *toxic* substances. Many toxins, such as those produced in the decomposition of milk and articles of food, excite the most intense enteritis. Certain inorganic substances, as arsenic and mercury, act in the same way. (*d*) *Gastrogenous diarrhea.* This is secondary to the absence of free hydrochloric acid in the stomach. There are three to six stools a day, usually without pain. The stools are loose and unformed, paler than normal and contain no mucus or blood. (*e*) *Changes in the weather.* A fall in the temperature of from twenty to thirty degrees, particularly in the spring or autumn, may induce—how, it is difficult to say—an acute diarrhea. On the other hand, the diarrheal diseases of children are associated with the excessive heat of the summer months. (*f*) *Changes in the intestinal secretions.* We know too little about the *succus entericus* to be able to speak of influences induced by change in its quantity or quality. It has been held that an increase in the amount of bile poured into the bowel might excite a diarrhea. Possibly there are conditions in which an excessive amount of bile is poured into the intestine, increasing peristalsis, and hurrying on the contents; but a scanty secretion, by favoring fermentative processes, more commonly causes an intestinal catarrh. Absence of the pancreatic secretion from the intestine is associated in certain cases with a fatty diarrhea. (*g*) *Nervous influences.* Mental states may profoundly affect the intestinal canal. These probably act through the autonomic system with a result of stimulation of peristalsis. These influences should not properly be considered under catarrhal processes, as they result from disturbed peristalsis and are usually described as *nervous diarrhea.* In children it frequently follows fright. It is common in adults as a result of emotional disturbances. In nervous women it is an occasional occurrence, due to excitement, or a chronic protracted diarrhea, which may last for months or years. It is by no means uncommon under stress in any type of individual.

Among the *secondary* causes may be mentioned: (*a*) *Infectious diseases.* Cholera, typhoid fever, pyemia, septicemia, and tuberculosis may have an associated enteritis. In typhoid fever the ulceration is in part responsible but in cholera it is probably a direct influence of the bacilli or their toxins. (*b*) The extension of *inflammatory* processes from adjacent parts. Thus, in peritonitis, catarrhal swelling and increased secretion are always present in the mucosa. In cases of invagination, hernia, tuberculosis, or cancerous ulceration catarrhal processes are common. (*c*) *Circulatory* disturbances cause a catarrhal enteritis, usually very chronic. This is common in diseases of the liver, such as cirrhosis, and in chronic affections of the heart and lungs—all conditions, in fact, which produce engorgement of the portal vessels. (*d*) In *cachectic* conditions in cancer, profound anemia, Addison's diseases, and nephritis, enteritis may occur as a terminal event.

Morbid Anatomy.—It is rare to see the mucous membrane injected; more commonly it is pale and covered with mucus. In the upper part of the small intestine the tips of the valvulae conniventes may be deeply injected. The entire mucosa may be softened and infiltrated, the lining epithelium swollen, or even shed, and appearing as large flakes among the intestinal contents. This is, no doubt, a postmortem change. The lymph follicles are usually swollen, particularly in children. The Peyer's patches may be prominent and the solitary follicles stand out and present erosions, the so-called follicular ulcers. This may be a striking feature in all forms of catarrhal enteritis in children, irrespective of the intensity of the diarrhea. When the process is more chronic the mucosa is firmer, in some instances thickened, in others thinned, and the villi and follicles present a slaty pigmentation.

Symptoms.—Acute and chronic forms may be recognized. The important symptom of both is *diarrhea,* which, in the majority of instances, is the main indication. Diarrhea is not invariably caused by, or associated with, enteritis, as it may be produced by nervous and other influences. It is probable that catarrh of the jejunum may exist without any diarrhea; indeed, it is common to find postmortem a catarrhal state of the small bowel in persons who have not had diarrhea during life. The *stools* vary extremely in character. The color depends upon the amount of bile which they contain, and they may be of a dark or blackish brown, or of a light yellow, or even of a grayish-white tint. The consistence is usually thin and watery, but in some instances the stools are pultaceous like thin gruel. Undigested food can often be seen (lienteric diarrhea), and flakes of yellowish-brown mucus. Microscopically there are innumerable organisms, epithelium and mucous cells, crystals of phosphate of lime, oxalate of lime, and occasionally cholesterin and Charcot's crystals. In *enteritis* there is unchanged bile, the stools may be green, cellulose is not digested and mucus is intimately mixed with the stool. In *colitis* the stool is usually browner, cellulose is largely digested and the mucus is on the outside of the feces and may be in large masses.

Pain in the abdomen is usually present in *acute* enteritis, particularly when due to food. It is of a colicky character, and when the colon is involved there may be tenesmus. More or less tympanites exists, and there are gurgling noises due to the rapid passage of fluid and gas from one part to another. In very acute attacks there may be vomiting usually due to an associated gastritis. Fever is not, as a rule, present, but there may be a slight elevation. The appetite is lost, there is intense thirst, and the tongue is dry and coated. In very acute cases, when the quantity of fluid lost is great and the pain excessive, there may be collapse symptoms. The number of stools varies from four or five to twenty or more in the day. The attack lasts for two or three days, or may be prolonged for a week or ten days.

Chronic diarrhea may follow the acute form, or come on gradually as an independent affection or as a sequence of obstruction in the portal circulation. It may be with or without colic. The dejections vary; when the small bowel is chiefly involved the diarrhea is of a lienteric character, and when the colon is affected the stools are thin and mixed with much mucus. The most common causes are (1) gastrogenous, (2) tuberculous enteritis, (3) pancreatic disease, (4) fatty or chylous diarrhea with disease of the absorption system, and (5) emotional. A special form of mucous diarrhea will be subsequently described. The general nutrition in these chronic cases is greatly disturbed; there may be much loss of flesh and great pallor. The patients are inclined to suffer from depression or hypochondriasis.

In some individuals there is the passage of a loose stool after meals, probably due to an active *gastrocolic reflex.* This may occur only after breakfast or after every meal. Some of the patients in addition pass a loose stool at once on rising in the morning. There is rarely any abdominal discomfort but there may be a feeling of weakness, slight or marked, after each movement. Disturbance in the sympathetic system is usually responsible. This condition may become a permanent habit.

Carbohydrate Indigestion.—This may involve both the stomach and bowels. The main symptom is distention from gas. The stools are acid and contain much undigested starch. If there is much fermentation the stools in addition are mushy and contain bubbles of gas. The result of a protein-fat diet is an important point in the diagnosis.

Diagnosis.—In acute cases there is rarely much doubt, but dysentery may be confused. The distinction is sometimes difficult but tenesmus with blood and mucus in the stools is fairly characteristic of dysentery. In acute cases cultures from the bowel or stools are important. In subacute or chronic attacks care should be taken to be sure that the contents pass rapidly through the intestine by giving charcoal or some coloring matter. If this appears in a stool within 12 hours or less, there is diarrhea. An X-ray study answers the question very readily. There may be frequent watery stools due to the presence of scybala in the colon. When the large intestine is at fault there may be no pain, as in the cases associated with tuberculosis and nephritis. When present, the pains are intense, and, if the lower portion of the bowel is involved, there may be tenesmus. With the sigmoidoscope the changes in the mucous membrane may be seen. In older patients a persistent or recurring diarrhea should suggest the need of excluding malignant disease in which the seigmoidoscope and X-ray study are important.

Duodenitis is usually associated with acute gastritis and, if the process extends into the bile duct, with jaundice. The study of the duodenal contents aids in the diagnosis.

Celiac Disease.—As the "coeliac affection" Gee described an intestinal disorder, most common in children between the ages of one and five, characterized by the occurrence of pale, loose stools (steatorrhea). They are bulky, not watery, yeasty, frothy, and extremely offensive. There is disturbance in the absorption of fats and carbohydrates. There is no evidence of defective fat-splitting, of pancreatic disease or of enteritis. Lack of vitamins is probably a factor. The affection has received various names, such as *diarrhea alba* or *diarrhea chylosa.* It is not associated with tuberculosis. It begins insidiously and there are progressive wasting, weakness, and pallor. Anemia may be marked, hypo- or hyperchromic, with many nucleated red cells. There is a large loss of calcium in the stools. Tetany may occur, sometimes in a severe form. The belly becomes doughy and inelastic with marked distention. There is often flatulency. Fever is usually absent. The child is irritable and there may be marked weakness. Growth is retarded (infantilism). The *diagnosis* from tuberculous peritonitis may be difficult; the character of the stools is important. The duration is usually prolonged but recovery generally results. In *treatment,* the diet should contain a minimum of fat and carbohydrate. At first buttermilk and orange juice may be given with a gradual addition of protein foods, such as junket, gelatine and white of egg. Carbohydrate is added very carefully. An effort to give vitamins as freely as possible should be made. The giving of bile salts (gr. ii-iv, 0.12-0.24 gm.) is helpful in some cases. Anemia should receive proper treatment. Ultraviolet radiation is useful and may prevent rickets. Calcium should be given freely.

Sprue or Psilosis.—It is difficult to decide where this disease should be placed. It occurs especially in the tropics, but is not infrequent in the United States, a point which Wood emphasized. Ashford regards it as due to the combination of several factors causing glandular insufficiency to which are added infection with *Monilia psilosis.* Lack of amino-acids and vitamins A and B, parathyroid gland disturbance and interference with calcium metabolism are suggested as factors. The anemia is usually megalocytic with a high color index. Disturbance of absorption of fats, glucose and calcium in the bowel with diminished production of HCl and the bone marrow stimulating factor are present but the essential etiological factor is unknown. The *pathology* shows absence of fat, atrophy of the gastro-intestinal mucosa and megaloblastic hyperplasia of the bone marrow.

The preliminary *symptoms* are asthenia, dyspepsia, anorexia, constipation sometimes alternating with diarrhea, reduction in the size of the liver, nervousness and depression, pallor and pigmentation of the skin. Later the more marked features are added: (1) *Diarrhea.* The stools are very large, acid, light in color and contain a large amount of fat. It is a fatty diarrhea, without pain or tenesmus, and the stools are like those of pancreatic insufficiency. The stools are usually passed between midnight and 10 A. M. The loss of fat varies from 30 to 50 per cent. There is marked nitrogen loss in the stools. (2) *Tongue.* This may be inflamed and show eroded patches or superficial cracks. (3) *Anemia.* The color index may be high and the picture resemble that of pernicious anemia. The blood calcium is reduced. (4) The disease is chronic and remissions are common. There may be marked emaciation. There is often reduction or absence of free hydrochloric acid in the stomach contents. The diagnosis from pellagra has given difficulty but a study of the stools should prevent this.

Treatment.—The patient should be in bed. As regards *diet,* a remarkable variety of diets has been advised; a high protein, low fat and low carbohydrate diet is indicated. Skimmed milk may be given every 2 hours with an amount of 2 quarts a day, increased to 3 quarts. In the meat diet amounts of 1 to 2 pounds of lean meat are given daily in feedings every 2 to 3 hours. Two quarts of hot water are given. Certain fruit diets are used which may be given with skimmed milk; strawberries, bananas and peaches are especially useful. With achlorhydria hydrochloric acid should be given freely. Good results are reported from a combination of calcium lactate gr. x-xv (0.6-1 gm.) and parathyroid hormone. The giving of pancreatic ferments and the use of autogenous streptococcus vaccine may be tried. Liver extract should be given as in pernicious anemia and full doses of iron are sometimes useful.

Hill Diarrhea.—This occurs at high elevations, particularly in India, and comes on soon after arrival. The cause is obscure. Loose pale stools are passed in the morning. There is much flatulency. A high protein, low fat and low carbohydrate diet may be helpful, with hydrochloric acid, but treatment is usually not satisfactory and removal to a lower altitude may be necessary.

DIPHTHEROID OR CROUPOUS ENTERITIS

This occurs (*a*) most frequently as a secondary process in the infectious diseases—pneumonia, septicopyemia and typhoid fever; (*b*) as a terminal process in many chronic affections, such as nephritis or cancer; and (*c*) as an effect of certain poisons—mercury, lead, and arsenic.

There are three anatomical pictures. (1) The mucosa presents on the top of the folds a thin grayish-yellow diphtheroid exudate situated upon a deeply congested base. In some cases all grades may be seen between the thinnest film of superficial necrosis and involvement of the entire thickness of the mucosa. In the colon similar transversely arranged areas of necrosis are seen situated upon hyperemic patches. There may be extensive inflammation without involvement of the solitary follicles. (2) The membrane is grayish-white in color, more flake-like and extensive, limited, perhaps, to the cecum or to a portion of the colon; thus, in pneumonia this flaky adherent false membrane may form patches 1 to 2 cm. in diameter, not unlike rupia crusts. (3) The affection is really a follicular enteritis, involving the solitary glands, which are swollen and capped with an area of diphtheroid necrosis or in a state of suppuration. Follicular ulcers are common in this form.

The disease may run its course without any symptoms, and the condition is unexpectedly met with in postmortem. In other instances there are diarrhea and pain, but not often tenesmus or the passage of blood-stained mucus. In the toxic cases the intestinal symptoms may be marked, but in the terminal colitis of fevers and chronic affections the symptoms are often trifling.

PHLEGMONOUS ENTERITIS

As an independent affection this is excessively rare, even less frequent than its counterpart in the stomach. It is seen occasionally in connection with intussusception, strangulated hernia and chronic obstruction. Apart from these conditions it occurs most frequently in the duodenum, and leads to suppuration in the submucosa and abscess formation. Except when associated with hernia or intussusception the affection can not be diagnosed. The symptoms usually resemble those of peritonitis.

ULCERATIVE ENTERITIS

In addition to the specific ulcers of tuberculosis, syphilis, and typhoid fever, the following forms of ulceration occur in the bowels:

Follicular Ulceration.—This is common in the diarrheal diseases of children, and in the secondary or terminal inflammations in many fevers and constitutional disorders. The ulcers are small, punched out, with sharply cut edges, and are usually limited to the follicles.

Stercoral ulcers occur in long-standing cases of constipation. In some cases the sacculi of the colon become filled with rounded small scybala, some of which produce distinct ulcers in the mucous membrane. The fecal masses many have lime salts deposited in them and thus form enteroliths.

Ulcerative Colitis.—Apart from dysentery (bacillary, amebic or terminal) there is a variety of ulcerative colitis, sometimes of great severity, not uncommon in England and the United States. It is a disease of adults and the sexes are equally affected. Some patients have had previous bowel trouble; sometimes there have been intermittent attacks of diarrhea and constipation. Postmortem, the colon is dilated, often without hypertrophied walls; the ulceration, as a rule, limited to it and very extensive, the ulcers ranging in size from a pin's head to large areas, with infiltrated, rarely undermined, edges. The work of Bargen suggests a streptococcus as the specific cause but his conclusions are not generally accepted. The *onset* may be acute but is usually gradual. When established, the main features are: (*a*) *Diarrhea:* The motions are very frequent in the day, up to 20 or 30, usually small, bile-stained, with mucus, pus, and blood, sometimes mixed with the motion or separate. There may be clotted lumps of blood, or the blood is uniformly mixed, and the motions look like anchovy sauce. The pain, while severe, is usually diffuse, abdominal, and colicky, and not frequently in the rectum. Many of the motions pass without pain. (*b*) *Fever* occurs in the majority of cases, though severe forms may be free throughout. (*c*) Wasting, debility, and progressive anemia which may be extreme. (*d*) With the sigmoidoscope the mucous membrane is seen to be red and edematous. Later the edema subsides and ulceration appears.

In *diagnosis* it is important to exclude dysentery and malignant disease. The X-ray study usually shows the extent of the lesions.

The disease may run a very acute course, but most frequently it is chronic, lasting from a few weeks to months. Transient improvement may follow, and a relapse. Death results usually from exhaustion, occasionally from hemorrhage, and in a few instances from perforation.

Treatment.—The patient should be in bed and given as nourishing a diet as possible, with a minimum of anything which might irritate the colon, and abundance of vitamins. The use of irrigations should be decided for each patient. An irrigation with salt solution may give comfort. It is doubtful if antiseptic solutions do much good. Tannic acid solution (1 per cent) may be useful. An autogenous vaccine made from cultures taken from the ulcers may be tried, or a vaccine of Bargen's organism. The question of surgery (ileostomy or appendicostomy) may be considered but is not without risk. Blood transfusion should be done when the patient is seriously ill, especially with marked anemia. Drugs are of little value: charcoal or kaolin may lessen discomfort.

Ulceration from External Perforation.—This may result from the erosion of new growths or, more commonly, from localized peritonitis with abscess formation and perforation of the bowel. This is met with most frequently in tuberculous peritonitis, but it may occur in the abscess which follows perforation of the appendix or suppurative or gangrenous pancreatitis. Fatal hemorrhage may result from the perforation.

Cancerous Ulcers.—In very rare instances of multiple cancer or sarcoma the submucous nodules break down and ulcerate.

Solitary Ulcer.—Occasionally a solitary ulcer in the small bowel, cecum or colon may lead to perforation. The cause is usually obscure; possibly thrombosis may be responsible. With obstruction in the lower colon causing stasis, there may be ulceration in the cecum or ascending colon.

Diagnosis of Intestinal Ulcers.—As a rule, diarrhea is present in all cases, but exceptionally there may be extensive ulceration, particularly in the small bowel, without diarrhea. Very limited ulceration in the colon may be associated with frequent stools. The character of the stools is of importance. Pus, shreds of tissue and blood are most valuable indications. *Pus* occurs most frequently with ulcers in the colon, but when the bowel alone is involved the amount is rarely great, and the passage of any quantity of pure pus is an indication that it has come from without, most commonly from the rupture of an abscess. Pus may be present in cancer of the bowel or due to local disease in the rectum. A purulent mucus may be present in the stools in cases of ulcer, but it has not the same diagnostic value. The swollen, sago-like masses of mucus believed by some to indicate follicular ulceration are found also in mucous colitis. *Hemorrhage* is an important sign of ulcer in the bowels, particularly if profuse. It occurs under so many conditions that alone it may not be specially significant, but with other coexisting circumstances it may be the most important indication of all.

Fragments of *tissue* may be found in the stools in ulcer, particularly in the extensive and rapid sloughing in dysenteric processes. *Pain* occurs in many cases, either of a diffuse, colicky character, or sometimes, in an ulcer of the colon, very limited and well defined. Examination by tubes should always be done, as by them ulcers in the lower bowel may be viewed directly.

Perforation is liable to happen when the ulcer extends deeply. In the small bowel it leads to localized or general peritonitis. In the large intestine, fatal peritonitis may result, or, if in the posterior wall of the ascending or descending colon, a large abscess cavity in the retroperitoneum.

Treatment of the Previous Conditions

Acute Diarrhea.—The patient should be in bed and in acute cases no food should be allowed for twenty-four hours. If there is vomiting the stomach should be washed with an alkaline solution. If the attack has followed the eating of infected or indigestible food, castor oil or calomel is advisable, but is not necessary if the patient has been freely purged. If the pain is severe, 20 drops (1.3 cc.) of laudanum and ʒj (4 cc.) of spirit of chloroform may be given, or, if the colic is very intense, a hypodermic of a quarter of a grain (0.016 gm.) of morphia. It is not well to check the diarrhea unless it is profuse, as it usually stops spontaneously within forty-eight hours. If persistent, the aromatic chalk powder or large doses of bismuth (30 to 40 grains, 2 gm.) may be given. A small enema of starch (2 ounces, 60 c. c.), with 20 drops (1.3 cc.) of laudanum, every six hours, is a valuable remedy. The diet should be increased very gradually during convalescence.

In the intense forms of choleraic diarrhea in adults associated with constant vomiting and frequent stools the patient should be given a hypodermic of a quarter of a grain (0.016 gm.) of morphia, which should be repeated in an hour if the pains return or the purging persists. This gives prompt relief, and is often the only medicine needed. The patient should be stimulated, and, when the vomiting is allayed, given small quantities of milk and lime water.

Chronic diarrhea, including chronic catarrh and ulcerative enteritis. An etiological diagnosis is usually essential for proper treatment. So much in treatment depends upon the careful examination of the stools—as to the amount of mucus, the presence of pus, the occurrence of parasites, and, above, all, the state of digestion of the food—that the practitioner should pay special attention to them. Many patients simply require rest in bed and a restricted diet. Chronic diarrhea of many months' or even of several years' duration may be sometimes cured by strict confinement to bed and a diet of boiled milk and albumen water. The patient should wear a warm abdominal binder and avoid chilling. A very simple diet should be taken. The use of finely powdered charcoal or kaolin in full doses is often helpful.

The *gastrogenous diarrhea* may be promptly relieved by giving dilute hydrochloric acid in full doses. Calcium lactate (gr. xv, 1 gm.) and pancreatin are also useful.

In that form in which immediately after eating there is a tendency to loose evacuations it may be that some one article of diet is at fault. The patient should rest for an hour or more after meals. Sometimes this alone is sufficient to prevent the diarrhea. Arsenic in moderate doses taken at the end of the meal is sometimes helpful. In cases in which this form is due to nervous disturbances attention should be given to their correction. The combination of bromide and belladonna is often helpful. In those forms which depend upon abnormal conditions in the small intestine, bismuth is indicated. It must be given in large doses—from half a dram to a dram (2 to 4 gm.). Salol and the salicylate of bismuth may be tried.

In the form due to *carbohydrate indigestion,* the sugars and free starch, as in flour, may be given but not vegetables and fruit. The usual amounts of protein and fat may be allowed. If the diarrhea lessens, vegetables with a low carbohydrate content should be added gradually. Pancreatic extract is often useful. In diarrhea with putrefaction a diet of milk and its products with vegetables should be given. Meat and eggs should not be eaten. Acidophilus bacilli may be given alone or in specially prepared milk.

An extremely obstinate and intractable form is the diarrhea of hysterical and nervous women. A systematic rest cure will be found most advantageous with milk only for a time. The condition seems to be associated in some cases with increased peristalsis, and in such the bromides may do good, or preparations of opium may be necessary. There are instances which prove most obstinate and resist all treatment, and the patient may be greatly reduced. A change of air and surroundings may do more than drugs.

In a large group the mischief is seated in the *colon* and medicines by the mouth are of little value but tincture of iodine, 10 to 20 drops, is sometimes of value and belladonna may be given if there is spasm. The stools should be carefully watched and a diet arranged which shall leave the smallest possible residue. Boiled or peptonized milk may be given. The starch and laudanum enema may be used for severe pain, but when ulceration is present it is better to use astringent injections. From 1 to 2 pints of nitrate of silver solution (1-5000) may be used. Neutral acriflavin (1-4000) in aqueous or saline solution (500-1000 cc.) may be used twice a day and retained for fifteen minutes. The strength or frequency may be reduced if much mucus appears in the stools. In giving large injections the patient should be in the dorsal position, with the hips elevated, and it is best to allow the injection to flow in gradually from a siphon bag. In this way the entire colon can be irrigated and the patient can retain the injection for some time. The silver injections may be painful, but they are invaluable in some forms of ulcerative colitis. Boracic acid, sulphate of copper, sulphate of zinc, and salicylic acid may be used in 1 per cent solutions. Any ulcers which can be reached should be treated by local applications, of which the silver salts are particularly useful. In obstinate cases appendicostomy or cecostomy should be done and the bowel irrigated through the opening, or an artificial anus made to give rest to the colon.

DIARRHEAL DISEASES IN CHILDREN

Children are particularly susceptible to disorders of the alimentary tract. Although several forms are recognized, they so often merge the one into the other that a sharp differentiation is impossible. Those infections should not be regarded as intestinal only for in many cases the general features are of equal or more importance.

General Etiology.—Certain factors predispose to diarrhea. AGE.—The largest number of cases occur just after the nursing period; the highest mortality is in the second half of the first year, when this period falls in the hot weather; hence the dread of the "second summer."

DIET.—Diarrhea is most frequent in artificially fed babies. Of 1,943 fatal cases collected by Holt, only 3 per cent were breast-fed. The agitation for pure milk has decreased materially the number of diarrhea cases among bottle-fed infants. Among the poor, artificial feeding plays a large part due either to milk ill-suited in quantity or poor in quality, or to indigestible articles of diet. Many of the fatal cases have been fed upon condensed milk.

TEMPERATURE.—The relation of the atmospheric temperature to the prevalence of the disease in children has long been recognized. The mortality curve begins to rise in May, increases in June, reaching the maximum in July, and gradually sinks through August and September. The maximum corresponds closely with the highest temperature, yet we can not regard the heat itself as the direct agent, but only as one factor. Neither barometric pressure nor humidity appears to have any influence.

BACTERIOLOGY.—The discovery by Duvall and Bassett of the dysentery bacillus in the dejecta of children suffering from summer diarrhea awakened renewed interest and the Rockefeller Institute research showed that this organism was present in a large number of cases of so-called "summer diarrhea." The causal connection of this group of bacteria with all the diarrhea diseases of children has not been proved. By some workers they have been found in the feces of a large proportion of all cases examined, and less frequently in sporadic diarrhea throughout the year. These organisms occur in the acute primary intestinal infection in children, in subacute infection without previous symptoms coincident with or following acute diseases such as measles, and in the terminal intestinal infection with malnutrition or marasmus. They have been found in breast-fed infants as well as bottle-babies.

The mode of entrance of the organism can not always be determined. Simultaneous cases in remote parts of a community where there is no common milk supply, and occurrence of the disease in breast- and condensed-milk-fed babies, indicate that cow's milk is not the only conveyor of the infection, and point to other causes, possibly water, as a means of infection.

The importance of other organisms must not be overlooked. There is a remarkable simplicity of bacterial flora in the intestines of healthy milk-fed children, *B. aërogenes* being present in the upper portion of the bowel and *B. coli* in the lower bowel, each almost in pure culture. When diarrhea is set up the number and varieties of bacteria are greatly increased, although no forms bear a constant or specific relationship to the diarrhea. Some diarrheas in children are apparently induced by the lactic acid organisms in milk, others by *colon* or *proteus bacilli,* and others by the *pyogenic cocci* and other forms; all these bacteria may be associated with the dysentery bacilli. Possibly destructive lesions of the intestines may be produced by streptococci after an initial infection with a member of the dysentery group.

Morbid Anatomy.—In mild cases there may be only a slight catarrhal swelling of the mucosa of both small and large bowel, with enlargement of the lymph follicles. The mucous membrane may be irregularly congested; often this is most marked at the summit of the folds. The submucosa is usually infiltrated with serum and small round cells. In more severe cases ulceration may take place. The loss of substance begins, usually, in the mucosa, over swollen lymph follicles. About the ulcer there is a more or less distinctly marked inflammatory zone. The destruction of the tissue is limited to the region of the follicles and becomes progressive by the union of adjoining ulcers. This process is usually confined to the lower bowel, and may be so extensive as to leave only ribbons of intact mucosa. The ulcers never perforate. Rarely there is a general pseudomembranous enteritis. The mesenteric glands are enlarged.

The changes in the other organs are neither numerous nor characteristic. Bronchopneumonia occurs in many cases. The liver is often fatty, the spleen may be swollen. Brain lesions are rare; the membranes and substance are often anemic, but meningitis or thrombosis is very uncommon.

Clinical Forms.—Acute Enteritis.—This form occurs in children of all ages, and is associated with infection or improper food. The symptoms often begin abruptly with nausea and vomiting, or, especially in stronger children, several hours or a day or two after the disturbing diet. The local symptoms are colicky pains, moderate tympanites, and diarrhea. The stools are four to ten in twenty-four hours; at first fecal, then fluid, with more or less mucus and particles from undigested material. There is no blood. The usual intestinal bacteria are found and occasionally dysentery bacilli are present. There is always fever; it is rarely very high, and never continues. The pulse may be rapid and the prostration marked in very young or weak children. These symptoms usually subside shortly after the emptying of the bowel. In weakened infants, when treatment has been delayed or the diet remains unchanged, this disturbance may lead to more serious conditions. The attacks tend to recur.

Fermentative Diarrhea.—This form is characterized by more severe constitutional symptoms. It may begin after an intestinal indigestion of several days in which the stools are fluid and offensive, and contain undigested food and curds. In other cases the disease sets in abruptly with vomiting, griping pains, and fever, which may rapidly reach 104°—105° F.

Nervous symptoms are usually prominent. The child is irritable and sleeps poorly. Convulsions may usher in the acute symptoms or occur later. An increasing drowsiness, ending in coma, has been noted in many cases. The stools, which vary from four to twenty in twenty-four hours, soon lose their fecal character and become fluid. Later they consist largely of green or translucent mucus. An occasional fleck of blood is noticed in the mucus, but this is never present in large amounts. Microscopically, besides the food residue and mucous strands are a moderate number of leukocytes and red blood corpuscles. Epithelial cells are found with numerous bacteria.

The acute symptoms generally pass away in a few days with judicious treatment. Relapses are frequent, following any indiscretion. The attack may be the beginning of severe ileocolitis. These gastro-intestinal intoxications are largely confined to the summer months and form an important group of the summer diarrhea of children.

Cholera Infantum.—This term should be reserved for the fulminating form of the disease. The typical cases are rare and form only a small proportion of the diarrhea diseases of infants. The attack sets in with vomiting, which is incessant and is excited by an attempt to take food or drink. The stools are profuse and frequent; at first fecal in character, brown or yellow in color, and finally thin, serous, and watery. The stools first passed are very offensive; subsequently they are odorless. The thin, serous stools are alkaline. There is fever and from the outset marked prostration; the eyes are sunken, the features pinched, the fontanelles depressed, and the skin has a peculiar ashy pallor. At first restless and excited, the child subsequently becomes heavy, dull, and listless. The tongue is coated at the onset, but subsequently becomes red and dry. As in all choleraic conditions, the thirst is insatiable; the pulse is rapid and feeble, and toward the end becomes irregular and imperceptible. Death may occur within twenty-four hours, with collapse and high fever. Before the end the diarrhea and vomiting may cease. In other instances the intense symptoms subside, but the child remains torpid and semicomatose, with fingers clutched, and there may be convulsions. The head may be retracted and the respirations interrupted, irregular, and of the Cheyne-Stokes type. The child may remain in this condition for some days without any signs of improvement. It was to this group of symptoms in infantile diarrhea that Marshall Hall gave the term "hydrencephaloid," or spurious hydrocephalus. As a rule, no changes in the brain or other organs are found. The condition of *sclerema* is described as a sequel of cholera infantum in which the skin and subcutaneous tissue become hard and firm.

Diagnosis.—The diagnosis is readily made. There is no other intestinal affection in children for which it can be mistaken. The constant vomiting, the frequent watery discharges, the collapse symptoms, and the elevated temperature make an unmistakable clinical picture.

Prognosis.—The outlook in the majority of patients below the age of 2 years is bad, particularly in children artificially fed. Hyperpyrexia, extreme collapse, and incessant vomiting are the most serious features.

Enterocolitis.—In this form there is evidence of an inflammatory alteration of the intestinal wall, usually of the lower ileum and large intestine. Several sub-varieties are recognized according to the nature and site of the lesions. Many of the cases are grafted on the forms above described. The mucous discharges continue, mingled with food residue, often streaked with blood and containing pus cells. The temperature remains elevated or may be remittent. After two or three weeks the symptoms gradually subside, the stools become fewer in number, and the fecal character returns.

In other instances severe involvement seems evident within a few hours of the onset, with abdominal pain, vomiting, and fever. Blood and pus may be present in nearly every stool. Tenesmus is frequent and prolapsus ani is not uncommon. In severe attacks the prostration is marked, the tongue is dry, the mouth covered with sordes, and death may ensue in a few days from profound toxemia, or the patient may continue desperately ill for weeks and gradually recover or die from asthenia.

Hemorrhage of large amount is extremely rare. The appearance of bright red stains on the napkin indicates, usually, ulceration of the lower bowel or rectum. When the blood is dark brown the lesion is in the ileum or near the valve. The extent of the ulceration can not be accurately determined by the quantity of the blood passed.

Membranous colitis is usually only to be distinguished by the discovery of the membrane in the rectum through a speculum or in prolapsus, or by the passage of membrane in the stools. Colitis often occurs in marantic infants. It may consist of a catarrhal or follicular inflammation of the lower bowel without destructive lesion, and is frequently a terminal infection.

Enterocolitis may become chronic and persist for months. The signs of active inflammation subside; there is little pain or fever, but more or less mucus remains in the stools. The general condition suffers. There is a continuous loss in weight; the skin is dry and hangs in folds; nervous symptoms are always present. There may be stiffness and contraction of the extremities, with opisthotonos. The progress is irregular, marked by short periods of improvement. Death is often due to a relapse, asthenia or bronchopneumonia. In many of these cases, both acute and chronic, dysentery bacilli have been found with other organisms. In all these forms *acidosis* may occur and should always be kept in mind. Increase in the respiration rate, for which no other explanation is found, should excite suspicion of this.

Prevention.—Unquestionably, many intestinal disorders of children can be prevented. In many cities the mortality from the summer diarrheas has been greatly reduced by prophylactic measures. The infant should have abundance of air-space with plenty of sunlight and fresh air. In hot weather it may be well for him to sleep out of doors, day and night. The clothing must not be too heavy in midsummer; often only a binder and thin dress. The greatest cleanliness should be demanded in the care and preparation of food, and of the feeding utensils and nurse's hands. Breast-feeding is continued whenever possible.

With bottle-babies, in warm weather, the diet should be reduced in strength —*i. e.*, weaker milk mixtures used and more water given. Whenever possible the milk should be pasteurized and all the water given the baby should be boiled. It is better that a child should be in the country during hot weather, but when this is impossible the parks in the large cities afford much relief.

Treatment.—Even after the illness has begun, much can be done by hygienic measures to diminish the severity. Change of air to seashore or mountain is often followed by marked improvement. The patient must not be too warmly clad. The fever may be lowered and nervous symptoms allayed by hydrotherapy. Baths and packs, warm and cool, are helpful. Colon irrigations are of great value and should be given cool when there is much fever.

Diet.—The dietetic management is of the utmost importance. In acute cases all food must be stopped at once. It is best to give the infant nothing but water for several hours, it may be for two or three days, or until the acute symptoms subside; a cereal water may then be substituted, to which may be added egg albumen, broth, glucose or beef juice. The time at which it is safe to return to a milk diet varies with each patient, and no definite rules can be laid down. It is usually better to defer milk until the temperature is normal. *Dehydration* should be prevented; if sufficient fluid can not be given by mouth, salt solution should be given subcutaneously (15 cc. per pound weight in small children).

If the stools are alkaline, a diet consisting largely of carbohydrates—e. g., barley water—is indicated; whereas protein diet, such as beef juice and egg albumen, is more helpful when the stools are strongly acid.

The ingredient in the milk that is not well borne is the fat; hence skimmed milk, diluted or partially digested, can often be safely given before diluted whole milk. Whey is often helpful. Buttermilk may be used in convalescence from intestinal disturbances. The various proprietary foods, or condensed milk mixed with water, although not to be given over long periods, may be found serviceable in the gradual return to a normal diet.

In children from three to seven years of age these acute derangements are rarely serious, and usually respond promptly after purgation and restricted diet, consisting largely of boiled milk.

It must be borne in mind that injudicious treatment, either in diet or medication, may interrupt what otherwise would be a prompt recovery and bring on the most serious intestinal lesions. The chronic cases, both in infants and older children, especially those with ileocolitis and ulceration, present unusual difficulties. Each case must be studied by itself. Food which is digested in the upper portion of the intestinal tract is preferable. Milk, properly modified with cereal water or predigested, if intelligently prescribed, offers the best chance of success.

Care must be taken not to overfeed, although occasionally, when there is persistent anorexia, gavage may be necessary. This is best accomplished through a nasal tube. Some infants will retain food given through a catheter when they will vomit the same mixture taken from a bottle. Beef juice is frequently useful. It should always be given with considerable fluid.

MEDICINAL.—In all cases of diarrhea there are more or less congestion of the mucosa, hypersecretion of mucus and increased peristalsis. In certain forms toxic symptoms are noticed early. In other instances inflammatory lesions in the bowel are present. The keynote of the treatment is promptness. Nature's effort to remove the cause should be assisted, not checked.

Castor oil and calomel are to be preferred as purgatives, especially for infants. A dram (4 cc.) of the former, repeated, if necessary, will usually sweep the intestinal tract and relieve the irritation. Where there is much nausea or intestinal fermentation, calomel is indicated. It may be given in divided doses at short intervals until one grain (0.065 gm.) has been taken, or until green stools appear. Very early in the attack, if nausea is marked, nothing relieves so quickly as gastric lavage with warm water or a weak soda solution. In older children a large draught of boiled water may be substituted. In many cases irrigation of the lower bowel with salt solution removes the irritating material. It also reduces the fever and allays nervous symptoms. The irrigating fluid should be cool when there is much fever. The infant is placed in the dorsal position or turned a little to the left, with hips elevated, and the fluid from a fountain syringe, about two feet above the patient, is allowed to flow into the rectum through a soft rubber catheter. Usually about a pint can be retained before expulsion. Two or three quarts should be used at one irrigation, which may be repeated several times in twenty-four hours if it is beneficial.

Where there is ulceration of the lower bowel various astringents, as alum, witch hazel (one or two teaspoonfuls to one quart), or a weak solution of potassium permanganate may be used as the irrigating fluid. In great local irritation and tenesmus, enemata (2 ounces, 60 cc.) of flaxseed or starch, with 2 to 5 drops (0.12 to 0.3 cc.) of laudanum, are soothing.

Water should be given freely by whichever method is indicated. With *acidosis,* as much water as possible should be given and sodium bicarbonate in doses of gr. xv-xxx (1-2 gm.) by mouth or by the bowel every two hours, until the urine is alkaline. With much loss of fluid or when toxemia is marked normal salt solution should be given subcutaneously (200-300 cc.).

Of the many drugs vaunted as intestinal astringents and antiseptics, bismuth, either as subgallate or subnitrate, has proved most serviceable. It should not be given until the disturbing material has been removed and the temperature is falling; then it should be administered in doses of 5 to 10 grains (0.3 to 0.6 gm.) every hour, until there is discoloration of the stools. Opium should be very sparingly used, and then only for a specific purpose, to check excessive peristalsis, violent colic or very numerous passages. It may be given to an infant as Dover's powder, ¼-1 grain (0.016 to 0.065 gm.); or paregoric, 5-10 minims (0.3 to 0.6 cc.) every four hours; or morphia, hypodermically, 1/200-1/50 grain (0.0003 to 0.0013 gm.), when prompt action is desired. Occasionally it is well to combine it with atropine, 1/1,000-1/250 grain (0.000065-0.00026 gm.). The bowels should not be locked when the stools are foul or the temperature is high. When there is prostration stimulating treatment is indicated.

Serum Therapy.—The results of serum therapy in infections with dysentery bacilli have been disappointing. The results in adult dysentery should encourage further trial.

Treatment of Cholera Infantum.—In this, serious symptoms may occur with great rapidity, and the incessant vomiting and frequent purging render the administration of remedies extremely difficult. Irrigation of the stomach and large bowel is of great service, and when the fever is high ice-water injections may be used, or a graduated bath. Morphia hypodermically gives the greatest relief, and with extreme vomiting and purging, with restlessness and collapse symptoms, this drug alone commands the situation. A child of one year may be given from 1/100 to 1/80 of a grain (0.00065 to 0.0008 gm.) to be repeated in an hour, and again if necessary.

In all cases of diarrhea convalescence requires careful management. An infant who has had a severe attack should be especially watched throughout the hot weather. During this time it is rarely safe to return to a full diet.

APPENDICITIS

Inflammation of the vermiform appendix is the most important of acute intestinal disorders. Formerly the "iliac phlegmon" was thought to be due to disease of the cecum—typhlitis—or of the peritoneum covering it—perityphlitis; but we now know that with rare exceptions the cecum itself is not affected. The contribution of Fitz in 1886 served to put the whole question on a rational basis. For historical and special details the reader is referred to the monograph of Kelly and Hurdon.

Etiology.—The exciting causes are not always evident. An infection is the essential factor. The lumen of the appendix forms a sort of test tube, in which feces lodge and are discharged with difficulty so that the mucosa is liable to injury from inspissated feces or occasionally foreign bodies. The anatomical features of the appendix render it liable to ulceration, strangulation and perforation. In some instances the appendicitis is a local expression of a general infection. The infection is often hematogenous and has its source in the mouth or throat. The causes of the increase of the disease are not known; one explanation is a lack of cellulose in the diet. Direct injury, as in straining and heavy lifting may be a rare exciting cause. Other conditions, tuberculosis and actinomycosis, may present the features of acute appendicitis. Cancer was found in 22 of 5,000 appendices removed at the Mayo Clinic and in 67 of 45,000 cases (Norment, 1932).

The BACTERIOLOGY is most varied. The *B. coli* is present in a large number of cases, and pyogenic organisms, particularly streptococci. The dominant parasite in appendicitis is the colon bacillus, either alone or with streptococci and staphylococci; the former chiefly in the lumen, the latter in the walls of the tube. Rosenow claims that in most cases appendicitis is a blood infection secondary to a distant focus such as the tonsil: and it is suggested that certain streptococci have an elective affinity for the appendix.

AGE.—Appendicitis is a disease of youth, 50 per cent of the cases occurring before the twentieth year. It has occurred as early as the seventh week, but is rare prior to the fifth year. Of 1,223 cases at the Johns Hopkins Hospital only 9 cases were under 5 years, 59 in children under 10, 140 between 11 and 15, 199 between 16 and 20, and 255 between 21 and 25 (Churchman).

SEX.—It is about equally common in males and in females.

In England since 1901 the mortality has increased from 38 per million to 71 in 1929. The increased frequency does not seem to be a result of changes in diet. There were 18,100 deaths in the registration area of the United States in 1930, a rate of 153 per million and in 30 cities (population 28 million) the death rate was 161.5 per million in 1933. Why does the United States have the highest death rate in the world?

Indiscretions in diet are very prone to bring on an attack, particularly in the recurring form of the disease, in which pain in the appendix region not infrequently follows the eating of indigestible articles of food.

Varieties.—McCarty makes the following classification:

(*a*) APPENDICITIS CATARRHALIS ACUTA, a condition in which the mucosa is infiltrated with leukocytes and congested with inflammatory reaction in the lymph follicles and lymphatic tissues of the submucosa.

(*b*) APPENDICITIS CATARRHALIS CHRONICA, following repeated mild or severe acute catarrh, marked by increase of scar tissue, and distortion of the normal regularity of the structure. Blood pigment is often present.

(*c*) APPENDICITIS PURULENTA NECROTICA, an advanced stage of the acute catarrhal condition, plus intramural abscesses, necrosis, and perforation.

(*d*) PERI-APPENDICITIS ACUTA, an extension to the peritoneum of the conditions just described.

(*e*) Obliteration, a condition of the lumen, the result of destruction of the mucosa and the formation of scar tissue, occurring in about 24 per cent of all cases, and an inflammatory, not an involuntary, process.

There are cases, too, in which the appendix becomes sphacelated *en masse*, and may slough off.

Fecal Concretions.—The lumen of the appendix may contain a mould of feces, which can readily be squeezed out. Even while soft the contents of the tube may be moulded in two or three sections with rounded ends. Concretions are also common. Of 700 cases of foreign bodies there were 45 per cent of fecal concretions (J. F. Mitchell). The enteroliths often resemble date stones in shape. The importance of these concretions is shown by the great frequency with which they are found in acute cases.

Foreign Bodies.—In 1,400 cases of appendicitis (J. F. Mitchell) these were present in 7 per cent; in 28 cases pins were found. Some of the concretions bear a striking resemblance to cherry and date stones.

Clinical Features.—In a large proportion of all cases of acute appendicitis the following features are present: (*a*) Sudden pain in the abdomen, usually referred to the right iliac fossa; (*b*) fever, often of moderate grade; (*c*) gastro-intestinal disturbance—nausea, vomiting, and frequently constipation; (*d*) tenderness or pain on pressure in the appendix region.

Pain.—A sudden, violent pain in the abdomen is the most constant, first, decided symptom of inflammation of the appendix. At the onset the pain may be referred to the epigastrium or about the umbilicus but after a short time is usually felt in the right iliac fossa where it may be from the onset. It may extend toward the perineum or testicle. It is sometimes very sharp and colic-like, and cases have been mistaken for nephritic or biliary colic. Some patients speak of it as a sharp, intense pain—serous-membrane pain; others as a dull ache—connective-tissue pain. In very severe cases, especially in children and with gangrene, there may be very little pain after the onset. While a very valuable symptom, pain is at the same time one of the most misleading. The appendicular colic is believed to be due sometimes to partial occlusion of the lumen, leading to violent and irregular peristaltic action.

Fever.—Fever is usually present in the early stage and is a most important feature. An initial chill is very rare. The fever may be moderate, from 100° to 102°; sometimes in children at the very outset it may be above 103.5°. The thermometer is generally a trustworthy guide in the diagnosis of acute appendicitis but in severe attacks with gangrene, especially in children, there may be no fever at any time. When a localized abscess has formed, and in some virulent cases of general peritonitis, the temperature may be normal, but at this stage there are other symptoms which indicate the gravity of the situation. The pulse is quickened and tends to increase as the condition progresses.

Gastro-intestinal Disturbance.—The tongue is usually furred and moist, seldom dry in early stages. Nausea and vomiting are commonly present in acute cases. The vomiting rarely persists beyond the second day in favorable cases. Constipation is the rule, but the attack may set in with diarrhea, particularly in children. Diarrhea is common if the appendix is in the pelvis.

Lymphoid Hyperplasia.—This occurs in children or young adults, subjects of status lymphaticus, and is marked by repeated attacks of colic without any marked change in temperature or pulse rate, or leukocytosis (Symmers).

Local Signs.—Inspection may show decreased movement of the lower right abdomen; early there is no distention, and the iliac fossae look alike. On palpation there is usually from the outset *rigidity* or *muscle spasm* of the right rectus muscle, with tenderness or pain on deep pressure. There may be hyperesthesia of the skin. The muscular rigidity may be so great that a satisfactory examination can not be made without an anesthetic. McBurney called attention to a localized point of tenderness on deep pressure, situated at the intersection of a line drawn from the navel to the anterior-superior spine of the ileum, with a second, vertically placed, corresponding to the outer edge of the right rectus muscle. Firm, deep, continuous pressure with one finger at this spot causes pain, often very severe. In addition to the tenderness, rigidity, and actual pain on deep pressure, there is to be felt, in some cases, an induration or swelling. This may be a boggy, ill-defined mass in the situation of the cecum; more commonly the swelling is circumscribed and definite, situated in the iliac fossa, two or three fingers' breadth above Poupart's ligament. Some claim to have felt the thickened appendix. The later the case comes under observation the greater the probability of the existence of a well-marked tumor mass. In children the symptoms are often very acute with severe pain, vomiting and high fever. The pain is often increased on urination, defecation or when the child is placed in a sitting position. The pain is more often on the left side than in adults, and urinary symptoms are common, as the appendix is frequently close to the bladder. Rectal examination may be of great aid in diagnosis. In patients in whom the appendix is situated behind the colon the symptoms may be referred to the upper right abdomen and simulate gallbladder disease. There may be marked rigidity in the flank. An appendix pointing towards the midline may give symptoms on the left side.

The attitude is often suggestive; the decubitus is dorsal with the right leg semiflexed. Sometimes in males on palpation of the abdomen the right testicle is drawn to the upper part of the scrotum and returns to its previous position when the pressure is removed (Brittain). Pulling on the right spermatic cord may cause pain. There may be tenderness of skin areas elicited by pinching or traction. The symptoms may be entirely pelvic when the appendix dips over the brim. Rectal or vaginal examination may give important information. There may be marked frequency of micturition, especially in children, which may be an early symptom. The urine is scanty and albuminuria is common. Sometimes there is an acute nephritis.

Leukocytosis.—As a rule, in acute attacks there is a leukocytosis of 12,000 to 15,000, chiefly of the polynuclears. There is an increase in the percentage of young polymorphonuclear cells. In mild catarrhal cases there may be no increase. Usually the degree is an expression of the peritoneal irritation. A low leukocytosis or leukopenia indicates a virulent infection.

Two forms may be distinguished as emphasized by Wilkie. (1) Acute inflammation of the wall. (2) Acute obstructive form, which is really intestinal obstruction of the "closed loop" variety and in which gangrene is likely to occur early. There is severe pain, often colicky, and frequent vomiting, little or no fever, a pulse rate little altered at first, and little or no muscular rigidity early.

There are four possibilities in any case: (1) Gradual recovery, (2) the formation of an abscess, (3) local peritonitis and (4) general peritonitis.

Recovery is the rule in the mild catarrhal cases. The pain lessens at the end of the second or third day, the temperature falls, the tongue becomes cleaner, the vomiting ceases, the local tenderness is less marked, and the bowels are moved. By the end of a week the acute symptoms have subsided.

Abscess Formation.—As a result of ulceration and perforation, sometimes following necrosis, by the fourth or fifth day there is an area of induration in the right iliac fossa, with great tenderness, and operations have shown that at this early date an abscess may have formed. Though as a rule the fever becomes aggravated with the onset of suppuration, this is not always the case. The two most important elements in the diagnosis of abscess formation are a gradual increase of the local tumor and aggravation of the general symptoms. Quite early the pus may lie between the cecum and coils of the ileum, with the general peritoneum shut off by fibrin, or there is a serofibrinous exudate with a slight amount of pus between the lower coils of the ileum. The abscess may be small and lie on the psoas muscle, or at the edge of the promontory of the sacrum, and never reach a palpable size. The sac, when larger, may be roofed in by the small bowel and present irregular processes and pockets leading in different directions. In larger collections the roof is generally formed by the abdominal wall. Some of the localized abscesses are situated entirely within the pelvis. The various directions and positions into which the abscess may pass or perforate are many and left alone, it may discharge externally, burrow in various directions, or empty through the rectum, vagina or bladder. Death may be caused by septicemia, perforation into an artery or vein, or pylephlebitis.

General Peritonitis.—This may be caused by direct perforation or gangrene of the appendix before any delimiting inflammation is excited. In a second group of cases there has been an attempt at localizing the infective process, but it fails, and the general peritoneum becomes involved. In a third group of cases a localized focus of suppuration exists about an inflamed appendix, and from this perforation takes place.

Death in appendicitis is due usually to general peritonitis.

The gravity of appendix disease lies in the fact that from the very onset the peritoneum may be infected; the initial symptoms of pain, with nausea and vomiting, fever, and local tenderness may indicate a widespread infection of this membrane. The onset is usually sudden, the pain diffuse, not always localized in the right iliac fossa, but it is not so much the character as the greater intensity of the symptoms from the outset that makes one suspicious of a general peritonitis. Abdominal distention, diffuse tenderness, and absence of abdominal movements are the most trustworthy local signs, but they are not really so trustworthy as the general symptoms. The initial nausea and vomiting persist, the pulse becomes more rapid, the tongue is dry, the urine scanty. In very acute cases, by the end of twenty-four hours the abdomen may be distended. By the third and fourth days the classical picture of a general peritonitis is well established—a distended and motionless abdomen, a rapid pulse, a dry tongue, dorsal decubitus with the knees drawn up, and an anxious, pinched, Hippocratic facies. The picture may be that of septicopyemia; high fever, chills, sweats, without local signs. These are generally acute, gangrenous cases perhaps with an anomalous position of the appendix, behind the colon or deep in the pelvis. Sometimes there have been gastro-intestinal symptoms before, to which no attention has been paid. In one case, seen by the family physician at 2 p. m. for the first time, by the senior author at 4.30 p. m., at 7 p. m. by a surgeon who refused to operate, death occurred within 12 hours after the physician was first called.

Remote Effects.—The remote effects of perforative appendicitis are interesting. Hemorrhage may occur. In one of our cases the appendix was adherent to the promontory of the sacrum, and the abscess cavity had perforated in two places into the ileum. Death resulted from profuse hemorrhage. The internal iliac artery or the deep circumflex iliac artery may be opened. Suppurative pylephlebitis may result from inflammation of the mesenteric veins. Secondary liver abscess may occur. The appendix may perforate in a hernial sac. Distant disorders attributed to chronic disease of the appendix are various types of gastric dyspepsia, ulcer, spasm of the pylorus, pancreatitis, bile tract infection and cirrhosis of the liver.

After operation, thrombosis of the iliac or femoral veins may occur and death from pulmonary embolism has followed. The leg may be permanently enlarged. Hernia may occur in the wound. Strangulation of the bowel is an occasional sequence and adhesions about the cecum may give trouble.

Chronic Appendicitis.—There may be recurring attacks, acute or subacute, to which this term may be applied, but in addition there is a group of cases in which the symptoms do not suggest disease of the appendix as they appear elsewhere. In such cases there may be a history of an acute attack of appendicitis many years before. The clinical picture may be variable but *gastric* symptoms are usually prominent. These are usually irregular but epigastric discomfort or pain is common after meals. Nausea and flatulence are frequent but vomiting is not common and if it does occur rarely gives relief. The pain is epigastric or general more often than referred to the right iliac fossa. It varies from time to time but the patient is not long free from some discomfort. The *signs* are indefinite; there may be tenderness in the right iliac fossa or on pressure there discomfort is most marked in the epigastrium. Sometimes there is very localized tenderness on deep pressure over a small area. If the appendix is behind the colon the pain from pressure may be felt in the upper right quadrant of the abdomen. The results of test meals are variable, normal, hyper- or hyposecretion. There is usually marked constipation. If the appendix is in the pelvis there may be bladder irritability. The results of the X-ray study are important. When the appendix or its probable position is identified under the fluoroscope, palpation shows that this is the point of greatest tenderness and if the organ can be moved the site of tenderness moves also. Adhesions about the cecum suggest chronic appendicitis. By inflation of the colon with air, tenderness over the appendix appears or is increased (Bastedo). It may be difficult, in fact impossible, to distinguish tenderness of the cecum from that due to disease of the appendix.

Diagnosis.—Appendicitis is by far the most common inflammatory condition in the abdomen in persons under thirty. The surgeons have taught us that, with few exceptions, sudden pain in the right iliac fossa, with fever and localized tenderness, means appendix disease. Pneumonia and pleurisy should always be excluded. There are certain diseases of the abdominal organs characterized by pain which may be confounded with appendicitis. Biliary colic, kidney colic, pyelitis, stricture of the right ureter and colicky pains at the menstrual period in women have to be carefully considered. The Dietl's crises in floating kidney have been mistaken for appendicitis.

Diseases of the tubes, rupture of an extra-uterine pregnancy, hemorrhage into a Graafian follicle, an ovarian cyst with a twisted pedicle and pelvic peritonitis may simulate appendicitis very closely, but the history and the examination under ether in most cases should prevent error. Some cases supposed to be recurring appendicitis prove to be tubo-ovarian disease.

Acute hemorrhagic *pancreatitis* may produce symptoms very like those of appendicitis with general peritonitis. The relation of typhoid fever and appendicitis is interesting. The gastro-intestinal symptoms, particularly the pain and fever, may at the onset suggest appendicitis. Operations have been comparatively frequent. Later in the course of typhoid fever perforation of the appendix may occur, and occasionally in convalescence perforation of an unhealed ulcer of the appendix. In young children *acetone acidosis* (cyclic vomiting) may give difficulty. There may be severe vomiting with abdominal pain, and the cecum may be distended and tender. The smell of acetone on the breath and the urinary findings should distinguish. Acute *pyelitis* is recognized by the study of the urine. Inflammation of the ileocecal lymph nodes may be accompanied by pain and vomiting with tenderness and rigidity in the right iliac fossa. The diagnosis may be difficult.

The recognition of *chronic appendicitis* may be very difficult. Thorough study and observation for a period are essential. The X-ray study is specially important. Failure to visualize the appendix suggests that its lumen is obstructed. The distinction from gallbladder disease may be obscure, in fact the two often occur together, especially in older patients. Pelvic disease should be carefully excluded. A calculus in the kidney or ureter, pyelitis, and especially *stricture of the ureter* should be excluded. The slight results from medical treatment and the long duration of symptoms are points of importance. Tuberculosis of the cecum, actinomycosis and right inguinal hernia should be excluded. A tender movable cecum may be the cause of pain. Hysteria may simulate appendicitis very closely, and it may require keen judgment to make a diagnosis. Mucous colitis with enteralgia is sometimes mistaken for appendicitis. Ulceration or partial obstruction of the colon may suggest appendicitis. The referred pain of acute thoracic disease and the root pains of spondylitis have led to error, but this should not occur if a proper examination is made.

Perinephritic and pericecal abscess from perforation of ulcer, either simple or cancerous, and circumscribed peritonitis in this region from other causes, can rarely be differentiated until an exploratory incision is made.

Briefly stated, localized pain in the right iliac fossa, with or without induration or tumor, the existence of McBurney's tender point, fever, furred tongue, vomiting, with constipation or diarrhea, indicate appendicitis. The occurrence of general peritonitis is suggested by increase and diffusion of the abdominal pain, tympanites (as a rule), marked aggravation of the constitutional symptoms, particularly elevation of fever and increased rapidity of the pulse. Obliteration of hepatic dulness is rarely present, as the peritoneum in these cases does not often contain gas.

Appendicitis and Pregnancy.—The association is not uncommon. Of 103 perforative or gangrenous cases 89 were operated upon, with 36 deaths. Of 14 cases not operated upon, all died. Of the 103 cases 80 aborted before or after operation. Of 104 nonperforative cases 50 were operated upon with 1 death, of the remaining 54, 4 died; 13 of these patients aborted (Babler). Mild cases recover; in the severer form it is safer to operate at once.

Prognosis.—*There would be no percentage of deaths from appendicitis if every case commencing with acute pain and developing tenderness and rigidity of the abdomen and quickening of the pulse were operated upon within twelve hours* (Rutherford Morison).

While the majority of patients recover without operation it is never possible to predict the outcome at the onset of any attack. With early diagnosis and immediate operation the outlook is excellent. If peritonitis has set in the outcome is always uncertain. In the dangerous and perforative cases the outlook depends on the time of operation. *Purgation* adds enormously to the danger and active support should be given to the campaign of education of the public to the dangers of giving purgatives to a patient with abdominal pain. After recovery from an attack without operation there is a strong probability of recurrence. It would be interesting to know how many of the 18,100 fatal cases in 1930 in the United States had been operated upon and at what period.

Treatment.—Gradually the profession has learned to recognize that appendicitis is a surgical disease. In hospital practice the patients should be admitted directly to the surgical wards. Many lives are lost by temporizing. The general practitioner does well to remember—whether his leanings be toward conservative or radical methods of treatment—that the surgeon is often called too late, never too early.

There is no medicinal treatment of appendicitis. There are no remedies capable in any way of controlling the course of the disease. Rest in bed in the Fowler position, nothing by mouth, fluid by the drop method in the bowel, no purgation, the use of a small enema if necessary, gastric lavage if there is vomiting, are the wisest measures till a decision as to operation is reached. The practice of giving opium in some form in appendicitis and peritonitis is decreasing, but is still too common. The use of ice locally may relieve the pain. *Purgatives should not be given,* even if there is only a suspicion of appendicitis.

If the patient is seen within thirty-six hours of the onset, immediate operation is advisable as recovery is almost certain and more dangerous developments are prevented. If acute peritonitis has begun the best surgical judgment may have difficulty in deciding as to operation; each patient is a distinct problem. Operation is indicated in case of abscess.

In recurring appendicitis, when the attacks are of such severity and frequency as to disturb the patient, the mortality in capable hands is very small. It is best to operate between attacks. In the chronic variety operation should be done when the diagnosis is definite; it should not be done in a doubtful case on the chance of helping.

INTESTINAL OBSTRUCTION

Intestinal obstruction may be caused by strangulation, intussusception, twists and knots, strictures and tumors, by abnormal contents, and by paralysis of the muscular coat of the bowel. In a study of the statistics of 21 British Hospitals for five years Vick (1932) found 3625 cases of obstruction not due to hernia. The causes were: (1) Obstruction of the lumen, 71 (47 due to gallstones); (2) conditions in the wall, 971 (895 due to carcinoma); (3) external constriction, 1324 (505 due to adhesions and 790 to internal strangulation); (4) embolism and thrombosis, 49; (5) intussusception, 1034 (989 idiopathic); and (6) volvulus 176 cases. In the same period there were 3267 cases due to hernia, 1378 inguinal and 1348 femoral.

Etiology and Pathology.—(*a*) STRANGULATION.—This is a frequent cause of acute obstruction, and occurred in 34 per cent of 295 cases analyzed by Fitz, and in 35 per cent of 1,134 cases of Leichtenstern. Of the 101 cases of strangulation in Fitz's table, the following were the causes: Adhesions, 63; vitelline remains, 21; adherent appendix, 6; mesenteric and omental slits, 6; peritoneal pouches and openings, 3; adherent tube, 1; peduncular tumor, 1. The bands and adhesions result, in a majority of cases, from former peritonitis. A number of instances have followed pelvic operations in women. The strangulation may be recent and due to adhesion of the bowel to the abdominal wound or a coil may be caught between the pedicle of a tumor and the wall. Late occlusion is due to bands and adhesions.

The vitelline remains are represented by *Meckel's diverticulum*, which forms a finger-like projection from the ileum, usually within eighteen inches of the ileocecal valve. The coils of the intestine may be strangulated about the diverticulum when its end is attached to the abdominal wall, to the mesentery, or to another portion of the intestine, or a long diverticulum unattached may be twisted, or there may be inversion of the diverticulum into the lumen of the bowel causing obstruction or leading to intussusception.

Seventy per cent of the cases of obstruction from strangulation occur in males; 40 per cent of all the cases occur between the ages of fifteen and thirty years. In 90 per cent of the cases of obstruction from these causes the site is in the small bowel; the position of the strangulated portion was in the right iliac fossa in 67 per cent and in the lower abdomen in 83 per cent.

(*b*) INTUSSUSCEPTION.—In this condition one portion of the intestine slips into an adjacent portion, forming an invagination or intussusception. Irregular peristalsis is the essential cause. The two portions make a cylindrical tumor, which varies in length from a half inch to a foot or more. The condition is always a descending intussusception, and, as it proceeds, the middle and inner layers increase at the expense of the outer layer. An intussusception consists of three layers of bowel: the outermost, the intussuscipiens, or receiving layer; a middle or returning layer; and the innermost or entering layer. The student can obtain an idea of the arrangement by making the end of a glove-finger pass into the lower portion. The actual condition can be studied in the common postmortem invaginations in the small bowel of children. The cases are most common in early life; of 103 cases in children, nearly 50 per cent occurred in the fourth, fifth, and sixth months (Wiggin). No definite cause could be assigned in 42 cases; in the others diarrhea or habitual constipation had existed.

The site of the invagination varies. We may recognize (1) an *ileocecal*, when the ileocecal valve descends into the colon, probably favored by atony of the ileocecal valve. There are cases in which this is so extensive that the valve has been felt *per rectum*. This form occurred in 75 per cent. In the *ileocolic* the lower part of the ileum passes through the ileocecal valve. (2) The *ileal*, in which the ileum is alone involved. (3) The *colic*, in which it is confined to the large intestine. (4) *Colicorectal*, in which the colon and rectum are involved. (5) Intussusception of the appendix is rare, but there are cases, most of them in children.

In case of death from intussusception, the condition is very characteristic. Peritonitis or acute injection of the serous membrane may be present. When death occurs early, as it may from shock, there is little to be seen. The portion of bowel affected is large and thick, and forms an elongated tumor with a curved outline. The parts are swollen and congested, owing to the constriction of the mesentery between the layers. The entire mass may be of a deep livid-red color. In very recent processes there is only congestion, and perhaps a thin layer of lymph, and the intussusception can be reduced, but when it has lasted for a few days, lymph is thrown out, the layers are glued together, and the entering portion of the gut can not be withdrawn.

The anatomical condition accounts for the tumor present in two-thirds of all cases; and the engorgement, which results from the compression of the mesenteric vessels, explains the frequent occurrence of blood in the discharges, which has so important a diagnostic value. If the patient survives, necrosis and sloughing of the invaginated portion may occur, and, if union has taken place between the inner and outer layers, the calibre of the gut may be restored and a cure effected. Many cases are on record. In the museum of McGill University are 17 inches of small intestine, passed by a lad who had symptoms of internal strangulation, and who made a complete recovery.

(*c*) Volvulus.—This is most frequent between the ages of thirty and forty. In the great majority of cases the twist is axial and associated with an unusually long mesentery. In Vick's statistics, 85 were in the small bowel, 56 in the sigmoid and 35 in the cecum. Constipation is an important etiological factor. As a rule, in volvulus the loop of bowel is simply twisted upon its long axis, and the portions at the end of the loop cross each other and so cause strangulation. It occasionally happens that one portion of the bowel is twisted about another.

Traction kinks occur at three regions—the third portion of the duodenum, the last part of the ileum, and the sigmoid flexure. What is known as *gastromesenteric ileus* is caused by compression of the lower portion of the duodenum by the root of the mesentery with its contained blood-vessels. The condition has been described under acute dilatation of the stomach.

The *ileum kink* occurs within a few inches of the cecum. This portion has a short tight mesentery and a large loose cecum may sag over the brim of the pelvis and cause a definite kink of the ileum with constipation, pain in the right iliac fossa, and symptoms which simulate appendicitis. The recognition of this disturbance is usually difficult.

Traction of a very full sigmoid flexure may, without any special twist, compress and obstruct a neighboring coil of the colon.

(*d*) Strictures and Tumors.—These are less important causes of *acute* obstruction; there were only 15 instances out of 295 cases, in 14 of which the obstruction occurred in the large intestine (Fitz). They are common causes of *chronic* obstruction. Lipoma may occur, growing from the submucosa, and cause intussusception. In a number of cases the tumor has been passed *per rectum.*

The obstruction may result from: (1) *Congenital stricture.* These are rare. There may be faulty rotation of the bowel or more commonly the condition is that of complete occlusion, either an imperforate anus or the congenital defect by which the duodenum is not united to the pylorus. (2) *Simple cicatricial stenosis,* which results from ulceration, tuberculous or syphilitic and more rarely from dysentery. (3) *New growths.* The malignant structures are due chiefly to cylindrical epithelioma, which forms an annular tumor, most common in the colon, about the sigmoid flexure or the descending colon. Of benign growths, papillomata, adenomata, lipomata, and fibromata occasionally induce obstruction. (4) *Compression and traction.* Tumors of neighboring organs, particularly of the pelvic viscera, may cause obstruction by adhesion and traction. In the healing of tuberculous peritonitis the contraction of the thick exudate may cause compression and narrowing of the bowel.

(*e*) ABNORMAL CONTENTS.—Foreign bodies, such as fruit stones, coins, pins or false teeth, are occasionally swallowed. *Foods,* usually vegetable with much residue, such as figs or orange pulp, are sometimes responsible. The obstruction is usually in the ileum near the ileocecal junction. *Round worms* may become rolled into a tangled mass and cause obstruction. The majority of foreign bodies, such as coins and pins, cause no inconvenience, but in a day or two pass in the stools. Occasionally such a foreign body as a pin passes through the esophagus and lodges in some adjacent organ, as in the heart (Peabody), or a barley ear may reach the liver (Dock).

Drugs, such as magnesia or bismuth, have accumulated in the bowels and produced obstruction, but in the great majority of the cases the condition is caused by feces, gallstones or enteroliths. Of 44 cases, in 23 the obstruction was by gallstones, in 19 by feces, and in 2 by enteroliths. Obstruction by feces may happen at any period of life; it may occur in young children and persist for weeks. In fecal accumulation the large bowel may reach an enormous size and the contents become very hard. The retained masses may be channeled, and small quantities of fecal matter are passed until a mass too large enters the lumen and causes obstruction. There may be few symptoms, as the condition may be borne for weeks or even months.

Obstruction by *gall stones* is not very infrequent, as 23 cases were reported in the literature in eight years. The obstruction is usually in the ileocecal region, but it may be in the duodenum. These large gall stones ulcerate through the gallbladder, usually into the small intestine, occasionally into the colon. In the latter case they rarely cause obstruction. Courvoisier collected 131 cases in the literature.

Enteroliths may be formed of masses of hair, more commonly of the phosphates of lime and magnesia, with a nucleus formed of a foreign body or of hardened feces. Nearly every museum possesses specimens of this kind. They are very rare causes of obstruction.

(*f*) PARALYTIC ILEUS.—Without any obstruction in the lumen, in a localized area or in a wide section of the bowel, the muscular walls may be so paralyzed that no movement occurs, causing a condition which virtually amounts to obstruction. The best illustrations of local paralytic ileus are seen in the embolic and thrombotic processes in the mesenteric arteries, when the corresponding portions of the intestinal wall are in a state of infarction. This occurs in the verminous aneurism in a horse and is associated with intestinal colic. It is more common in the small than in the large bowel, but in one instance of paralytic ileus due to involvement of the transverse colon there was not, so far as one could discover, any affection of the blood vessels; the symptoms were those of acute obstruction.

Following operations, particularly on the abdomen, after injuries, following paracentesis in ascites, in pneumonia, pleurisy, and occasionally in heart disease, a paralytic state of the bowel may occur, with cessation of peristalsis, distention of the abdomen, vomiting and other signs of obstruction. There are remarkable cases of hysteria with symptoms of chronic obstruction of the bowels and fecal vomiting—the so-called ileus hystericus.

Symptoms.—(*a*) Acute Obstruction.—Pain, vomiting, constipation and collapse are the important features. *Pain* sets in early and may come on abruptly while the patient is walking, or, more commonly, during the performance of some action. It is at first colicky but subsequently becomes continuous and very intense. *Vomiting* follows quickly and is constant and most distressing. At first the contents of the stomach are voided, and then greenish, bile-stained material, and later the material vomited is a brownish-black liquid, with a distinctly fecal odor. This sequence of gastric, bilious, and, finally, stercoraceous vomiting is a most important diagnostic feature. The higher the obstruction is in the bowel, the more severe the vomiting. The *constipation* may be absolute, without the discharge of either feces or gas. Very often the contents of the bowel below the stricture are discharged. Distention of the abdomen usually occurs, and, when the large bowel is involved, it is extreme. On the other hand, if the obstruction is high up in the small intestine, there may be very slight tympany. Sounds of peristalsis are not heard—"deathly silence"—and the heart sounds may be heard very distinctly over the abdomen. At first the abdomen is not tender, but subsequently it may become acutely so. A tumor may be felt, especially in intussusception. If acute obstruction occurs secondary to chronic obstruction there may be marked peristalsis.

The constitutional symptoms from the outset are severe. The face is pallid and anxious, and *collapse* supervenes. The eyes become sunken, the features pinched, and the skin is covered with a cold, clammy sweat. The pulse becomes rapid and feeble; the blood pressure falls. There may be no fever. Toxemia is marked and is usually more acute the higher the seat of the obstruction. With intussusception there may be attacks of syncope and marked pallor. The tongue is dry and parched and the thirst is incessant. The urine is high-colored, scanty, and there may be suppression, particularly when the obstruction is high up in the bowel. This is probably due to the constant vomiting and the small amount of liquid absorbed. There is an increase in the nonprotein nitrogen of the blood, more rapid if the obstruction is high. The case terminates, as a rule, in from three to six days. In some instances the patient dies from shock or sinks into coma. A leukocytosis of 75,000 or 80,000 may be present.

(*b*) Chronic Obstruction.—When due to *fecal impaction*, there is a history of long-standing constipation. There may have been discharge of mucus, or, in some instances, the fecal masses have been channeled, and so have allowed the contents of the upper portion of the bowel to pass through. In elderly persons this is not infrequent; but examination, either *per rectum* or externally, in the course of the colon, will reveal the presence of hard scybalous masses. There may be retention of feces for weeks without serious symptoms. In other instances there are vomiting, pain in the abdomen, gradual distention, and finally the vomitus becomes fecal. The hardened masses may excite an intense colitis or even peritonitis.

Chronic intussusception is rare, occurs in adults and may be associated with tumors or polypi. The symptoms may be intermittent; attacks of colic occur with constipation and possibly the passage of mucus and blood. A tumor is palpable in some cases and may be more marked during acute exacerbations; occasionally it reaches the anus. There is always danger of acute obstruction or peritonitis.

In *stricture,* whether cicatricial or cancerous, the symptoms are very diverse. Constipation gradually comes on, is extremely variable, and it may be months or even years before there is complete obstruction. There are transient attacks, in which from some cause the feces accumulate above the stricture, the intestine becomes greatly distended, and in the swollen abdomen the coils can be seen in active peristalsis. In such attacks there may be vomiting, but it is very rarely fecal. In the majority of these cases the general health is seriously impaired; the patient becomes anemic and emaciated, and, finally, in an attack of complete obstruction, death occurs with the features of acute occlusion, or the course may be prolonged for ten or twelve days.

Diagnosis.—The diagnosis of obstruction does not offer great difficulty in the majority of cases but some conditions simulate it closely. In acute obstruction the X-ray study (without barium), especially of the gaseous distention and fluid levels, may be helpful. Acute *enteritis* with severe vomiting and pain may give difficulty, but the diarrhea makes the diagnosis clear. *Peritonitis* may cause confusion, but the local signs in the abdomen, the absence of peristalsis, and the general features should aid. In obstruction, peritonitis occurs in the later stages, and if the patient is seen then for the first time the recognition of the obstruction may be difficult. *Acute pancreatitis* may simulate obstruction very closely as also *mesenteric thrombosis* or *embolism.* The diagnosis may be in doubt until the abdomen is opened. *Lead poisoning* should not cause difficulty if a careful study is made; the blue line on the gums, the absence of vomiting, the milder pain and the general condition are important. *Hernia* must always be excluded, which is not easy in fat patients. The possibility of a small femoral or properitoneal hernia should be kept in mind. An obturator hernia can only be recognized after opening the abdomen. In some cases the necessary diagnosis is of a condition which demands exploration of the abdomen.

(*a*) Situation of the Obstruction.—A rectal and, in women, a vaginal examination gives information as to the condition of the pelvic and rectal contents, particularly in intussusception, in which the descending bowel can sometimes be felt. In obstruction high up the empty coils sink into the pelvis and can there be detected. In the inspection of the abdomen there are important indications, as the special prominence in certain regions, the occurrence of well-defined masses and hypertrophied coils in active peristalsis. John Wyllie called attention to the great value in diagnosis of the "patterns of abdominal tumidity." In obstruction of the lower end of the large intestine not only may the horseshoe of the colon stand out plainly, when the bowel is in rigid spasm, but even the pouches of the gut may be seen. When the cecum or lower end of the ileum is obstructed the tumidity is in the lower central region, and during spasm the coils of the small bowel may stand out prominently, one above the other, either obliquely or transversely placed—the so-called "ladder pattern." In obstruction of the duodenum or jejunum there may only be slight distention of the upper part of the abdomen, associated usually with rapid collapse and anuria. The acute toxemia may be due to proteose intoxication.

In the ileum and cecum the distention is more in the central portion of the abdomen; the vomiting is distinctly fecal and occurs early. In obstruction of the colon tympanites is much more extensive and general. Tenesmus is more common, with the passage of mucus and blood. The course is not so quick, the collapse does not supervene so rapidly, and the urinary secretion is not so much reduced.

In obstruction from stricture or tumor the situation can in some cases be accurately localized, but in others it is very uncertain. Examination of the rectum should first be made. The sigmoidoscope should be used cautiously. The quantity of fluid which can be passed into the large intestine should be estimated. The rectum may be inflated with air. In certain cases these measures give important indications as to the situation of an obstruction in the large bowel. An X-ray study should always be made.

(*b*) Nature of the Obstruction.—This is often difficult, not infrequently impossible, to determine. *Strangulation* is not common in very early life. In many instances there have been previous attacks of abdominal pain, or there are etiological factors which give a clue, such as old peritonitis or operation on the pelvic viscera. Neither the onset nor the character of the pain gives us any aid. In rare instances nausea and vomiting may be absent. The vomiting usually becomes fecal from the third to the fifth day. A tumor is not common in strangulation, and was present in only one-fifth of the cases. Fever is not of diagnostic value.

Intussusception is an affection of childhood, and is of all forms of internal obstruction the one most readily diagnosed. The onset is acute with pain and signs of shock after which the symptoms may decrease for a time. Vomiting is not constant. The presence of tumor, bloody stools and tenesmus are the important factors. The tumor is usually sausage-shaped and felt in the region of the transverse colon. It existed in 66 of 93 cases. It became evident the first day in more than one-third of the cases, on the second day in more than one-fourth, and on the third day in more than one-fifth. Blood in the stools occurs in at least three-fifths of the cases, spontaneously or following an enema. The blood may be mixed with mucus. Tenesmus is present in one-third of the cases. Fecal vomiting is not very common. *Henoch's purpura* may give difficulty; signs of purpura may be found elsewhere.

Volvulus can rarely be diagnosed. The frequency with which it involves the sigmoid flexure is to be borne in mind. The injection of fluid may give valuable indications.

In fecal obstruction the condition is usually clear, as the feces can be felt *per rectum* and also in the distended colon. Fecal vomiting, tympany, abdominal pain, nausea and vomiting are late and are not so constant. In obstruction by gall stone a few of the patients gave a previous history of gall-stone colic. Jaundice was present in only 2 of 23 cases. Pain and vomiting, as a rule, occur early and are severe, and fecal vomiting is present in two-thirds of the cases. A tumor is rarely evident.

Prognosis.—Recovery without operation results in a few cases, but as a rule death follows unless operation is done. Naturally the earlier the obstruction is relieved the better the outlook. The age, general condition and, in very acute cases, the degree of toxemia are important. Promptness in diagnosis and operative interference decide the outlook to a considerable extent.

Treatment.—In *acute* obstruction operation should be done at the earliest possible moment. In case of doubt or if operation is refused, nothing should be given by mouth, the stomach should be washed if there is vomiting or distention, nothing in the nature of a purgative should be given, and the colon may be irrigated very cautiously. Fluid can be given by the drop method by the bowel or subcutaneously. Morphia may be given to relieve the pain if operation is decided on or if the condition is hopeless. It should not be used while there is doubt, but hot or cold applications made to the abdomen.

In *chronic* obstruction the diet should be concentrated. Enemata of various kinds may be tried cautiously but purgatives should not be given. The use of mineral oil is sometimes helpful. Belladonna or atropine should be given to diminish spasm; opium or morphia should be used only after careful consideration.

CONSTIPATION

Definition.—Delay in the passage of the contents of the intestines.

Etiology.—General Causes.—(*a*) Constitutional peculiarities: Constipation may be a family complaint, possibly due to congenital muscular weakness of the colon. (*b*) Sedentary habits, particularly in persons who eat too much and neglect the calls of nature. (*c*) *Certain* diseases, such as anemia, hypothyroidism, neurasthenia, hysteria, chronic affections of the liver, stomach, and intestines, and the acute fevers. (*d*) Diet, either one which gives an irritating residue causing spasm of the colon or one which leaves too little. (*e*) That injurious habit, *drug taking*. The irritability produced by purgatives leads to disturbance of the mucous membrane and also of the sympathetic nervous system. (*f*) Disturbance in the act of defecation, frequently due to neglect. The feces are moved down to the pelvic colon and normally the impulse to defecate comes from the passage of this material into the rectum. Neglect of this impulse means that the sensation is gradually decreased, so that a stronger stimulus is required, or it is lost entirely. Atony and dilatation of the rectum result, with accumulation of feces in the colon which may result in spasmodic contraction or atony. The mental attitude is important; the individual thinks that his bowels will not move without help by drugs or enemata; the use of these in time renders normal function more difficult and so the vicious circle goes on.

Local Causes.—Weakness of the abdominal muscles in obesity or from overdistention in repeated pregnancies. Atony of the large bowel from chronic disease of the mucosa; the presence of tumors, physiological or pathological, pressing upon the bowel; enteritis; foreign bodies, large masses of scybala, and strictures of all kinds. A local cause is atony of the colon, particularly of the muscles of the sigmoid flexure by which the feces are propelled into the rectum. An obstinate form is that associated with a contracted state of the colon (spastic constipation). This is met with—first, as a sequence of chronic dysentery or ulcerative colitis; secondly, in cases of hysteria and neurasthenia, usually with vagotonia; and, thirdly, in very old persons often without any definite cause. This is common in those who have a nervous system easily disturbed. It may be that the sigmoid flexure and lower colon are in a spastic condition, while the transverse and ascending parts are in a state of atony and dilatation. The most characteristic sign of this variety is the presence of hard, globular masses, or small and sausage-like feces.

Radiography has taught us much of the conditions favoring intestinal stasis. The upward position in man favors viscerotopsis, with which we find associated many obstinate cases of constipation. There may be difficulty caused by a dropping of the cecum and the lower coil of the ileum. The obstruction may result in dilatation of the end of the ileum, with delay in the passage of the feces. Another point is the fixed splenic flexure of the colon. The sigmoid loop seems specially designed to promote stasis; the rectum may also present an elongated S-shaped loop, and, finally, there is the sharp pelvirectal flexure, above which the feces accumulate.

The rate of the passage of the feces through the bowel may be estimated accurately with the X-rays. After a barium meal the cecum is reached in about four hours, the hepatic flexure two hours later, the splenic flexure three hours after that, and the beginning of the pelvic colon twelve hours after the commencement of the meal. The feces do not pass beyond the pelvirectal flexure until just before defecation.

Hurst divides the causes into (1) delay in the passage through the colon with normal defecation (*colic constipation*); (2) normal passage through the colon with difficulty in evacuation from the pelvic colon (*dyschesia*); and (3) insufficient formation of feces.

Symptoms.—It is difficult to state exactly what symptoms are actually due to constipation. It occurs frequently in persons whose general and sympathetic nervous systems are disturbed. Many of the discomforts attributed to constipation are really due to sympathetic system disturbance and not to "intestinal auto-intoxication" about which so much nonsense has been talked and written. This is shown by the fact that relief often follows immediately after the bowels have moved. A "toxemia" could not disappear in such a short time. Persistent constipation may exist with good health, but regular and sufficient emptying of the bowel is the normal and should be attained. Whether this means two or three stools in the day, a daily movement, or one every two days depends on the individual.

Debility, lassitude, vertigo and mental depression are frequent symptoms in constipation, particularly in persons of a nervous temperament. Headache, loss of appetite, a furred tongue, foul breath and gastric disturbance may occur. In girls the skin is "muddy," acne is common, anemia may be associated, and there is a flabby state of the system generally.

When persistent, the accumulation of feces leads to unpleasant, sometimes serious, local conditions, such as piles, ulceration of the colon, distention of the sacculi, perforation, enteritis and occlusion. In women pressure may cause pain with menstruation and a sensation of fullness and distention. Neuralgia of the sacral nerves may be caused by an overloaded sigmoid flexure. The feces collect chiefly in the colon. Even in extreme grades of constipation it is rare to find dry feces in the cecum. The feces may form large tumors at the hepatic or splenic flexures, or a sausage-like, doughy mass above the navel, or an irregular tumor in the left inguinal region. In old persons the sacculi of the colon become distended and the scybala may remain and undergo calcification, forming enteroliths. In cases with prolonged retention the fecal masses become channeled and *diarrhea* may occur for days before the true condition is discovered. In women who have been habitually constipated attacks of diarrhea with nausea and vomiting should excite suspicion and lead to a thorough examination of the colon.

Captivated by the theories of Metchnikoff we have been on the crest of a colonic wave, and "intestinal toxemia" has been held responsible for many of the ills that flesh is heir to, particularly arteriosclerosis and old age. The seniles and preseniles of two continents have taken sour milk and lactobacillary compounds, to the great benefit of the manufacturing chemists! Some part of what is regarded as intestinal toxemia is really intestinal infection.

Constipation in infants is common and troublesome. The causes are congenital, dietetic and local. In some instances the child is constipated from birth, may not have a natural movement for years, and yet thrive and develop. There are cases of dilatation of the colon with persistent constipation which appears sometimes to be a congenital defect. In some patients there may be constricting bands or a congenital stricture.

Dietetic causes are more common. In sucklings it often arises from an unnatural dryness of the residue which passes into the colon, and it may be difficult to decide whether the fault is in the mother's milk or in the digestion of the child. Most probably it is in the latter, as some babies may be persistently costive on natural or artificial foods. Deficiency of fat in the milk is believed by some to be the cause. In children it is of the greatest importance that regular habits should be ensured. Carelessness on the part of the mother in this matter often lays the foundation of troublesome constipation in after life. Impairment of the contractility of the intestine in consequence of inflammation, disturbance in the intestinal secretions, and deficiency in the defecation reflex are the chief local causes.

Diagnosis.—Too often the statement of the patient is accepted without investigation. The diagnosis should include the cause of the constipation. It may be easy to overlook constipation. The patient may have a daily stool but of insufficient amount, or there may be marked retention of feces with several loose stools daily due to irritation or the passage of fluid contents through the mass. There may be retention with a daily stool which is very hard. Many have wrong ideas as to a normal stool and it is an advantage to inspect the movements. In the recognition of the exact condition, an X-ray study is of the greatest value.

Treatment.—Much may be done by systematic habits, particularly in the young. The patient should go to stool at a fixed hour every day, whether there is desire or not, and the desire should always be gratified. In adults the mental attitude is important. The need of the cultivation of regular habits is essential, but many patients are too careless and lazy to take sufficient trouble to insure this. Psychotherapy has a very definite place. Exercise in moderation is helpful, especially of the trunk and abdominal muscles. In stout persons and in women with pendulous abdomens the muscles should have the support of a bandage. Friction or massage is useful in the chronic cases. A good substitute is a metal ball weighing from four to six pounds, which may be rolled over the abdomen every morning for five or ten minutes. The function of the stomach should be thoroughly studied and any disturbance properly treated. The diet should be low in protein, with plenty of fruit and vegetables, particularly salads and tomatoes. It is often advisable to omit meat and substitute cereals, milk and milk foods. Oatmeal is usually laxative. A high fat diet (200 grams of fat per day) is helpful in some patients. Fluids should be taken freely. A tumblerful of hot or cold water on rising, taken slowly, is efficacious in many cases. A glass of hot water at night may also be tried. A pipe or a cigar after breakfast is an aid for many men.

When the condition is not very obstinate it is well to try to relieve it by hygienic and dietetic measures. If drugs must be used they should be the milder laxatives, such as mineral oil or one of its combinations, cascara or senna. Enemata are often necessary, and it is preferable to employ them early than constantly to use purgative pills. Glycerine in the form of suppository or as a small injection is valuable. Injections of tepid water, with or without soap, may be used with good effect. The patient should be in the dorsal position with the hips elevated, and it is best to let the fluid flow in slowly from a fountain syringe.

The usual remedies employed are often useless in *spastic constipation.* A very satisfactory measure is the olive or cotton seed oil injection; 6 to 10 ounces of oil are allowed to flow slowly (or are injected) into the bowel. The operation should take ten or fifteen minutes. This may be repeated every day until the intestine is cleared, and subsequently a smaller injection every few days will suffice. In the cases with a spastic colon the injection of oil at bedtime, which is retained during the night, is often effectual.

The ideal would be to manage constipation without the use of drugs but human nature being what it is we cannot hope for this. When drugs are used they should be as simple as possible. Mineral oil is often effectual, usually best taken about meal times. The combination with agar may be better and does not "leak" as often as the oil alone. Agar alone may be efficient. Castor oil is usually effectual (℥ ss-i, 15-30 cc.) and may be given in small doses (ʒ i, 4 cc.) each night with benefit. Cascara, phenolphthalein, senna and some of the combinations of milder laxatives often do well. Magnesia is often useful. The persistent use of strong saline purgatives is to be condemned but small doses of mild salines may be effectual.

In children the indications should be met, as far as possible, by hygienic and dietetic measures. In the constipation of sucklings a change in the diet of the mother may be tried, or from one to three teaspoonfuls of cream may be given before each nursing. In artificially fed children the top milk with the cream should be used. Drinking of water, barley water or oatmeal water will sometimes obviate the difficulty. If laxatives are required, simple syrup, manna, or olive oil may be sufficient. A conical piece of soap is sometimes efficacious. Massage along the colon may be tried. Small injections of cold water may be used but large injections should be avoided. If it is necessary to give a laxative, castor oil or fluid magnesia is the best. If there are signs of gastro-intestinal irritation, rhubarb and soda or gray powder may be given. In older children the diet should be carefully regulated.

VISCEROPTOSIS

(*Splanchnoptosis, Enteroptosis, Glénard's Disease*)

Definition.—"Dropping of the viscera" is not a disease, but a symptom group characterized by looseness of the mesenteric and peritoneal attachments, so that the stomach, intestines, particularly the transverse colon, liver, kidneys, and spleen occupy an abnormally low position.

Symptoms and Signs.—There are two varieties: in one, which may be called constitutional or *congenital*, it is an expression of an anomaly of development, a narrow upper abdominal opening, low diaphragm and elongated visceral ligaments, all of which combined lead to a greater or less degree of prolapse of the abdominal viscera. The second, or *acquired* visceroptosis, is largely due to relaxation of the abdominal wall. The support of the viscera is due to the integrity of the reflex arc and abdominal muscles, the tonic action of which, as shown by the studies of Keith and of Sherrington, is brought into play by a reflex, the afferent end organs of which are the peritoneal nerves and Pacinian bodies.

In the first group is embraced a somewhat motley series of cases, in which, with a pronounced nervous or neurasthenic basis, there are displacements of the viscera *with symptoms*. The patients are usually young, more frequently women than men, and of spare habit. The condition may follow an acute illness with wasting. They complain, as a rule, of dyspepsia, throbbing in the abdomen, and dragging pains or weakness in the back, and inability to perform the usual duties of life. A considerable proportion of the patients with neurasthenia present the local features of visceroptosis. One notices often an erythematous flushing of the skin; the scratch of the nail is followed by a line of hyperemia, less often of pallor. The pulsation of the abdominal aorta is readily seen.

In the second group inspection of the abdomen often shows a very relaxed abdominal wall. Peristalsis of the intestines may be seen, and in extreme cases the outlines of the stomach itself with its waves of peristalsis. On inflating the stomach the organ stands out with great prominence, and the lesser and greater curvatures are seen, the latter perhaps well below the navel. The waves of peristalsis are feeble and without the force of those seen in the stomach dilated from stricture of the pylorus. The condition of descensus ventriculi with atony is best studied in this group of cases. An important point to remember is that it may exist in an extreme grade without symptoms.

Radiography has given much information of the position of the viscera. The stomach may be vertically placed and reach far below the navel; its motility may be normal, but there may be stasis from associated pyloric spasm or from kinking of the duodenum. Clapotage or splashing is usually distinct.

There is usually much relaxation of the mesentery and of the peritoneal folds which support the intestines. The colon is displaced downward (coloptosis), with consequent kinking at the flexures. The descent may be so low that the transverse colon is at the brim of or even in the pelvis. It may indeed be fixed or bent in the form of a V. It is frequently to be felt as a firm cord crossing the abdomen at or below the level of the navel. This kinking may take place also at the pylorus, where the duodenum passes into the jejunum, and where the ileum enters the cecum.

The *cecum* may be very movable and with this there may be pain, attacks of colic and constipation. There may be fullness in the cecal region and on palpation the distended cecum is easily felt. The mass may be very movable. Incompetence of the ileocecal valve may exist. It is often difficult to know how much significance belongs to this condition. It is undoubtedly present in many healthy persons and frequently with an abnormally movable cecum. In others it seems to be associated with a variety of abdominal symptoms, often associated with intestinal stasis. The X-ray study is important in the diagnosis of the ileocecal incompetency and any associated conditions.

Nephroptosis, or displacement of the *kidney*, is one of the most constant phenomena in visceroptosis. It is well to distinguish between the kidney which one can just touch on deep inspiration—palpable kidney—one which is freely movable, and on deep inspiration descends so that one can put the fingers of the palpating hand above it and hold it down, and, thirdly, a floating kidney, which is easily grasped, readily moved to the middle line, and down toward the right iliac fossa. Some hold that the designation floating kidney should be restricted to the cases in which there is a mesonephron, but this is excessively rare, while extreme grades of renal mobility are common. Some of the more serious sequences, namely, Dietl's crises and intermittent hydronephrosis, will be considered with diseases of the kidney.

Displacement of the *liver* is very much less common. In thin women who have laced, the organ is often tilted forward, so that a large surface of the lobes comes in contact with the abdominal wall; it is a very common mistake under these circumstances to think that the organ is enlarged. Dislocation of the liver itself will be considered later.

Mobility of the *spleen* is sometimes very marked. In an extreme grade it may be found in almost any region of the abdomen and may be mistaken for a fibroid or ovarian tumor. A considerable proportion of the cases come first under the care of the gynecologist.

The explanation of the phenomena accompanying visceroptosis is by no means easy. It has been suggested that overfilling of the splanchnic vessels accounts for the exhaustion and nervousness. Many patients carry themselves badly, with resulting muscular strain, and this sometimes accounts for the pain in the back. In a large proportion of the cases no symptoms occur until after an illness or some protracted nervous strain.

Treatment.—In a majority of all cases four indications are present: To treat the existing neurasthenia, to relieve the nervous dyspepsia, to overcome the constipation, and to afford mechanical support to the organs. Three of these are considered under their appropriate sections. In cases in which enteroptosis has followed loss in weight after an acute illness or worries and cares an important indication is to fatten the patient.

A well-adapted abdominal support is one of the most important measures in enteroptosis. In many of the milder grades it alone suffices. There is no single simple measure which affords relief to distressing symptoms in so many cases as the abdominal support. It should fit the lower abdomen snugly, and be arranged with straps so that it can not ride up over the hips. A special form must be used for movable kidney. In some cases support may be given by the use of adhesive strapping. Exercises to strengthen the abdominal muscles and proper abdominal breathing are aids. General "setting-up" exercises are often helpful. The patients should rest and lie on the right side as much as possible; an hour's rest after meals is useful. Some are aided by having the foot of the bed elevated. Some of the more aggravated types of enteroptosis are combined with such features of neurasthenia that a rigid rest treatment is indicated. In a few very refractory cases surgical interference may be called for but it is rarely successful. With incompetency of the ileocecal valve general measures to relieve stasis are indicated and if not successful operation may be advisable.

And, lastly, the physician must be careful in dealing with the subjects of visceroptosis not to lay too much stress on the disorder. It is well never to tell the patient that a kidney is movable or the stomach and colon are low; the symptoms may date from a knowledge of the existence of the condition. A careful reticence is usually the part of wisdom.

NEOPLASM OF THE INTESTINE

New growth of the bowel occurs almost entirely in the colon; involvement of the small bowel is very rare. The majority of growths occur in the rectum or sigmoid. The age is usually between 40 and 60. The form is a columnar-celled carcinoma and a striking feature is the late occurrence of metastases.

Symptoms.—In the early stages these are generally indefinite and consist in abdominal discomfort, usually in the lower part, and constipation in one whose bowels have been regular or aggravation of existing constipation. Occasionally diarrhea occurs as an early feature, due to irritation from a growth which does not cause narrowing, or from retained feces. The constipation increases; ribbon-shaped or round small stools occur at times but are not distinctive. Sometimes acute obstruction occurs, perhaps after a period of indefinite symptoms or it may be the first manifestation. There is mucus in the stools and pus and blood (often occult) if ulceration results. The discomfort increases to pain which may be colicky and, if there is obstruction, visible peristalsis may be present. The features of obstruction gradually increase and at this stage a tumor may be felt by rectal or abdominal examination—occasionally a tumor is felt when there are no signs of obstruction. The tumor is usually hard, rarely painful and often movable. General features, emaciation, anemia, and cachexia, as a rule come on slowly and late in the course. Growths of the ascending colon are usually more acute in their course and show general features earlier. Peritonitis may result from perforation.

There are two forms of carcinoma of the *small bowel:* (1) *carcinoid* is not very malignant and causes metastasis very late if at all. It has been termed "rodent ulcer" of the intestine. (2) *Adenocarcinoma* which is more common, quite malignant and causes early metastasis. The most constant features are colicky pain, vomiting, and rapid loss in weight. There may be marked increase in peristalsis. The X-ray study is not of great help. Resection usually gives only temporary relief as in a large proportion of the cases metastasis is found at operation.

Diagnosis.—Disturbance of the bowels in a person over forty, without evident explanation, demands the consideration of new growth. The X-ray study is of great value. A study of the stools and a rectal examination with the finger and tube should always be made. *Diverticulitis,* especially in a single diverticulum, *ulcerative colitis* and *tuberculosis* of the cecum should be excluded. The *treatment* is surgical. The harm done by the careless giving of purgatives for constipation without a proper diagnosis of the cause is well illustrated in neoplasm of the bowel.

MISCELLANEOUS AFFECTIONS

MUCOUS COLITIS

Known by various names, such as *membranous enteritis, tubular diarrhea, mucous colic,* and *myxoneurosis intestinalis,* this disease has been recognized for several centuries. Spasticity of the colon is often associated with it; both represent disturbance of the sympathetic nervous system. The passage of mucus in large quantities from the bowel is met with, *first,* in catarrh of the intestine, due to various causes. It is not uncommon in children, and may be associated with disturbances of digestion and slight colic. *Secondly,* in local disease or irritation of the bowel, in cancer of the colon and rectum. In tubo-ovarian disease much mucus and slime may be passed. *Thirdly,* true mucous colitis, a *secretion neurosis* of the large intestine met with particularly in nervous and hysterical patients. It is more common in women. Some cases appear to be due to food allergy. There is an abnormal secretion of a tenacious mucus, which may be slimy and gelatinous, like frog-spawn, or it is passed in strings or strips, more rarely as a tubular membrane. The membrane *in situ* adheres closely to the mucosa, but is capable of separation without any lesion of the surface. Microscopically the casts are mucoid, of a uniform granular ground substance through which there are remnants of cells, some of which have undergone hyaline change. Triple phosphate, cholesterin, and fatty crystals are present, and occasionally fine, sandlike concretions. The epithelium of the mucosa seems to be intact.

Symptoms.—In a large proportion of all the cases the subjects are nervous in greater or less degree. Some cases have had hysterical outbreaks, and there may be hypochondriasis or melancholia. The patients are self-centred and often much worried about the mucous stools. Some of the cases are among the most distressing with which we have to deal, invalids of many years' standing, neurasthenic to an extreme degree, with recurring attacks of pain and the passage of large quantities of mucus or intestinal casts.

In many cases the attacks come on in paroxysms, associated with colicky pains, or occasionally crises of the greatest severity, so that appendicitis may be suspected. Emotional disturbances, worry of all sorts or an error in diet may bring on an attack. *Constipation* is a special feature in many cases. Sometimes there are attacks of *nervous diarrhea.* Some patients have a movement after each meal. This is due to an active gastrocolic reflex, so that feces reach the rectum after each meal.

While the disease is obstinate and distressing, it is rarely serious, though Herringham states that he knew of three cases of mucous colitis in which death occurred suddenly, in all with great pain in the left side of the abdomen. The abdomen itself is rarely distended. There is often a painful spot between the navel and the left costal border, tender on pressure, and sometimes the paroxysms of pain seem centred in this region. A spastic condition of the colon frequently exists and is easily recognized by palpation.

Diagnosis.—This is rarely doubtful, but it is important not to mistake the membranes for other substances; thus, the external cuticle of asparagus and undigested portions of meat or sausage skins sometimes assume forms not unlike mucous casts, but microscopic examination will quickly differentiate them. The presence of ulcers, polypi and neoplasm should be excluded. Mucous colitis with severe pain may be mistaken for appendicitis.

Treatment.—The mechanism of the condition should be carefully explained to the patient. An important point is to avoid fatigue, physical, emotional or nervous. The *diet* should be decided for each patient; it is usually best to avoid roughage. The psychical effect of a special diet should be considered. Many patients cut down the diet too much, one attack after another being blamed on some particular food when a nervous upset was responsible. Irrigations of the bowel should be used with great care. They may be given to empty the bowel when necessary but to many may be irritating. The injection of 6 ounces of oil at bedtime, to be retained through the night, is often useful. Every effort should be made to overcome constipation by general measures rather than by drugs. Mineral oil or its combinations may be used; strong salines should be avoided. Heat applied to the abdomen, dry or moist, is often helpful. Drugs are not of much value, but if there is marked spasm, bromide and belladonna or phenobarbital may be useful. It is quite useless to give bismuth and so-called intestinal remedies. First the basic neurasthenic state is to be dealt with, and this may suffice for a cure.

DILATATION OF THE COLON

There are four groups of cases. In the first the distention is entirely gaseous, and occurs not infrequently as a transient condition. In many cases it has an important influence, inasmuch as it may be extreme, pushing up the diaphragm and seriously impairing the action of the heart and lungs. It is an occasional cause of sudden heart failure. In pneumonia and other acute diseases this distention may be extreme.

In the second group are the cases in which the distention of the colon is caused by solid substances, as fecal matter. In institutions, particularly for the insane, it is not infrequent to find the aged with great distention. There may be small liquid movements which pass the solid material.

When, thirdly, the dilatation is due to an organic obstruction the colon may reach a very large size. These cases are common enough in malignant tumors and sometimes in volvulus. Dilatation of the sigmoid flexure occurs particularly when this portion of the bowel is congenitally very long. In such cases the bowel may be so distended that it occupies the greater part of the abdomen, pushing up the liver and the diaphragm. An acute condition is sometimes caused by a twist in the mesocolon. And, fourthly—

Idiopathic Dilatation.—Hirschprung's disease. This occurs in young children and a similar condition in adults is known as *megacolon.* In adult life it may be difficult to decide whether it existed from childhood in a mild form or developed recently. The sigmoid flexure alone or the entire colon is involved, and the size may be colossal. In Formad's case the circumference of the colon was from fifteen to thirty inches, and the weight of the contents forty-seven pounds. There is a congenital anomaly (muscular hyperplasia) with disturbance of the neuromuscular mechanism which involves a varying amount of the colon and may involve the rectum. The changes may be local. There may be a failure to relax at the pelvirectal or anal sphincter. The *features* are very definite—constipation, an enlarged abdomen, attacks of pain with increasing distention, and then diarrhea, either natural or induced, with relief. Such attacks may occur from birth and continue to the twentieth or thirtieth year. The abdominal picture is distinctive—the great enlargement of the upper half of the abdomen, the spreading of the costal arch, the remarkable length from the ensiform cartilage to the navel, and in the attacks the coils of the colon stand out prominently, and even the longitudinal bands may be seen.

The outlook is uncertain. Stretching of the pelvirectal sphincter may be useful. Every effort should be made to empty the bowel by irrigations. Mineral oil may be given freely. Lumbar sympathectomy has been successful. Parathormone, 10 to 30 units a day, has been used. Hurst, who terms it achalasia of the anal sphincter, holds that gradual dilatation of the anal sphincter is curative. After any treatment, the use of mineral oil and enemas should be continued as the hypertrophied colon is not likely to return to normal size.

INTESTINAL SAND

"Sable Intestinal."—There are two groups of cases in which sand-like material is passed with the stools. The *false,* in which it is made up of the remains of vegetable food and fruits which have resisted digestion or which have become encrusted with earthy salts. *True* intestinal sand of animal origin, gritty fine particles, usually gray, black or brown, is formed in the bowel and is made up largely of lime salts. In mucous colitis this material may be passed at intervals for months. In *treatment* the saturated fats, as in meat, cream and butter, should be left out of the diet; olive oil may be used instead. The usual management of mucous colitis is indicated.

DIVERTICULITIS—PERISIGMOIDITIS

Congenital diverticula, of which Meckel's is the type, may cause strangulation or obstruction.

Acquired diverticula, commonly hernial protrusion of the mucous and serous coats, occur anywhere in the intestinal tract. In the small bowel they rarely cause symptoms. They may occur throughout the colon but are most frequent in the sigmoid. They develop after the age of 40 and often in those who have used purgatives. This is termed *diverticulosis* and causes no symptoms. The diverticula may become the seat of inflammation—*diverticulitis.* There is usually constipation of long standing with discomfort or pain in the lower left abdomen. Telling and Gruner analyzed 324 cases; 68 per cent were males. The evaginations of the mucosa are usually the result of high intracolic pressure, associated with constipation.

The secondary pathological processes are *mechanical,* as torsion, formation of concretions and lodgment of foreign bodies; and *inflammatory,* acute diverticulitis, which may rapidly become gangrenous; chronic inflammation leading to thickening, and tumor formation and narrowing; perforation, causing local abscess, general peritonitis or fistula. Other changes are chronic local peritonitis with adhesions, metastatic suppuration, and in late stages cancer may develop. Adhesions may form with the bladder with a resulting vesicocolic fistula.

The *symptoms* may not permit of more than a tentative diagnosis. Pain in the left lower quadrant with tenderness, rigidity and a mass in a person over sixty, who has been constipated, should suggest diverticulitis as well as cancer. In acute exacerbations there may be fever, toxemia and leukocytosis.

The usual absence of blood in the stools, the long history of pain in the lower left quadrant, tumor formation and perhaps later disappearance, negative sigmoidoscopy, slight fever and good nutrition or even obesity are in favor of the former. Severe intestinal hemorrhage may occur. The X-ray study is of value.

In *treatment,* diverticulosis requires a diet without roughage or irritating substances and the prevention of constipation by the use of mineral oil and small oil enemas. In an acute attack of diverticulitis the patient should be at rest, on liquid diet and given mineral oil freely. Heat or cold may be applied to the abdomen. Otherwise keeping the feces soft and avoiding constipation are important. Operation may be required for acute conditions.

MELANOSIS OF THE COLON

In this there is pigmentation of the mucous membrane which varies from brown to black. It may involve the whole colon or be most marked in the upper or lower part. The rectum may show it also. The nature of the pigment is doubtful but it is usually regarded as melanin. Constipation is the rule in the patients and a free use of laxatives, especially cascara and also aloes, rhubarb and senna. These contain anthracene or emodin compounds. The condition is found on sigmoidoscopic examination. It does not seem to cause any symptoms. The pigmentation may disappear in a few months.

AFFECTIONS OF THE MESENTERY

Hemorrhage (*Hematoma*).—Instances in which the bleeding is confined to the mesenteric tissues are rare; more commonly the condition is associated with hemorrhagic infiltration of the pancreas and with retroperitoneal hemorrhage. It occurs in rupture of aneurisms, either of the abdominal aorta or the superior mesenteric artery, in malignant forms of infectious fevers, in smallpox, and sometimes when no predisposing conditions exist.

Affections of the Mesenteric Vessels.—(*a*) Aneurism (see page 879).

(*b*) Embolism and Thrombosis.—*Infarction of the Bowel.*—When the mesenteric vessels are blocked by emboli or thrombi, infarction follows in the territory supplied, which may pass on to gangrene or to perforation and peritonitis. If the superior mesenteric artery is blocked the result is fatal. In the veins the thrombosis may be primary, following infective processes in the intestines, particularly about the appendix, or in cachectic states. Secondary thrombosis is met with in cirrhosis of the liver, syphilis and pylephlebitis, or may result from the stasis caused by arterial emboli. There are two groups—acute and chronic. In the former the onset is sudden with violent paroxysmal abdominal pain, not specially localized, persistent vomiting which usually lessens after some hours, and bloody stools. The abdomen may be slightly full but there is no muscle spasm. There may be slight fever or the temperature is normal or subnormal. The signs of shock and collapse are usually marked. Signs of peritonitis may appear later. Death may occur in a few hours. In the *chronic* cases the onset is insidious; there may be vague abdominal discomfort without localized tenderness. The *diagnosis* is extremely difficult and the acute cases are usually regarded as obstruction. The occurrence of severe pain without rigidity of the abdominal walls is suggestive. Operation has been done with recovery in a few cases. In J. W. Elliot's successful case 48 inches of the bowel were resected.

Diseases of the Mesenteric Veins.—Dilatation and sclerosis occur in cirrhosis of the liver. In prolonged obstruction there may be large saccular dilatations with calcification of the intima, as in a case of obliteration of the venae portae described by the senior author. Suppuration of the mesenteric veins occurs usually with pylephlebitis. The mesentery may be much swollen and is like a bag of pus; only by careful dissection one sees that the pus is within channels representing dilated mesenteric veins.

Disorders of the Chyle Vessels.—Varicose, cavernous, and cystic chylangiomata are met with in the mucosa and submucosa of the small intestine, occasionally of the stomach. Extravasation of chyle into the mesenteric tissue is sometimes seen. Chylous cysts may occur at the root of the mesentery. There is an instance of a congenital malformation of the thoracic duct, in which the receptaculum formed a flattened cyst which discharged into the peritoneum, and a chylous ascitic fluid was withdrawn on several occasions. Homans reported the case of a girl who, from the third to the thirteenth year, had an enlarged abdomen. Laparotomy showed a series of cysts containing clear fluid, supposed to be dilated lymph vessels connected with the intestines. The diagnosis is hardly possible without opening the abdomen.

Cysts of the Mesentery.—They may be either dermoid, hydatid, serous, sanguineous, or chylous. They occur at any portion of the mesentery, and range from a few inches in diameter to large masses occupying the entire abdomen. They are frequently adherent to neighboring organs, the liver, spleen, uterus and sigmoid flexure.

The *clinical features* are variable. There may be vague abdominal pain, sometimes vomiting, occasionally signs of obstruction and a tumor. Sometimes a mass develops rapidly, particularly in the hemorrhagic forms. Colic and constipation or acute obstruction are present in some cases. The general health, as a rule, is well maintained in spite of the progressive enlargement of the abdomen, which is most prominent in the umbilical region. Mesenteric cysts may persist for many years.

The *diagnosis* is extremely uncertain and no single feature is in any way distinctive. The important signs are: the great mobility, the situation in the middle line and the zone of tympany in front of the tumor. Of these, the second is the only one which is at all constant, as when the tumors are large the mobility disappears, and at this stage the intestines are pushed to one side. It is most frequently mistaken for ovarian tumor. Movable kidney, hydronephrosis and cysts of the omentum have also been confused with it. The only treatment is surgical.

DIGESTIVE DISTURBANCE DUE TO FOOD ALLERGY

The disturbances are probably due to edema of the mucous membrane and spasm of smooth muscle. Reactions in the liver are also possible.

Etiology.—There is often a family history of allergy, found in 65 per cent of Rowe's cases. As to age, it is probably more common in children.

Clinical Features.—These are many and varied. In acute forms, paroxysmal attacks of abdominal pain with vomiting and diarrhea, lasting from 24 to 48 hours, occur. They may be frequent or occasional. In the intervals no evidence of abdominal disease can be found. In the *mouth*, there may be "canker sores," blisters, white patches and burning sensations. *Gastric* symptoms are belching, pyrosis, nausea and vomiting. Some cases of pylorospasm may be due to allergy. There may be abdominal pain, more in the upper right quadrant, suggesting hepatic disease or cholecystitis, or in the cecum and colon. There may be duodenal stasis with reversed peristalsis. Diarrhea is common and mucous colitis often occurs. In some attacks intestinal obstruction is suggested.

Diagnosis.—The history of allergy, familial or personal, is important. The relation of certain foods to attacks and dislike of certain foods are important. Skin tests are not very helpful in older patients; they are most useful in children. Eosinophilia with an attack is suggestive. The effect of epinephrine, (1-1000 solution) 5 to 10 minims hypodermically, is important if it gives relief. Rowe has emphasized the value of elimination food tests.

Treatment.—Any foods to which the patient is found to be sensitive, by skin tests or elimination tests, should be avoided. Ephedrine (gr. ½, 0.032 gm.) three times a day before meals may be useful. Epinephrine in the smallest dose found to be effective should be given hypodermically at the onset of an attack.

DISEASES OF THE LIVER

JAUNDICE

Definition.—Jaundice or icterus is a condition characterized by coloration of the skin, mucous membranes, and fluids of the body by bile pigment. It is a symptom, not a disease, and is met with in a variety of conditions. In *carotinemia* there is a yellow discoloration of the skin but the sclerotics are not involved. The blood serum and urine are colored owing to the presence of carotin, derived from foods rich in it (carrots, spinach, egg yolk, etc. but difficulty in diagnosis is not probable.

There is difference of opinion as to whether jaundice can occur without the action of the liver cells. Bilirubin may be formed in tissues or serous cavities from extravasated blood; this however is apparently not absorbed. Great importance attaches to the "reticulo-endothelial" system, the cells of which occur in various parts of the body. The chief interest with regard to jaundice belongs to those in the liver (cells of Kupffer), which lie along the venous capillaries, and those lining the sinuses of the spleen. There are also some in the bone marrow. It is suggested that these cells are concerned in the production of hemolytic jaundice and not the cells of the liver. The cells of the reticulo-endothelial system break down hemoglobin and manufacture bilirubin or its precursor and the liver cells pass it into the bile capillaries. The bile capillary begins with a blind end and is surrounded by the glandular cells. Between the glands are the capillaries passing from the portal system to the branch of the hepatic vein in the centre of the lobule. The Kupffer cells lie along the walls of the capillaries.

One theory of bilirubin formation is that the polygonal glandular cells of the liver are chiefly concerned in the transference of the bile pigment from the blood capillaries to the bile capillaries. In this passage the bilirubin is altered and so there are two varieties of bilirubin, one which has passed through the liver cells (giving the direct immediate reaction of van den Bergh) and one which has not done so and passes into the blood (indirect delayed reaction).

McNee suggests the following possibilities in the causation of jaundice: (1) Bile pigment passes through the polygonal cells to reach the bile capillaries but is obstructed and reabsorbed into the blood. (2) The polygonal cells are damaged; all or part of the bile pigment is unable to enter them and passes into the circulation by the hepatic veins. (3) With excessive blood destruction there may be too much bilirubin for the polygonal cells to handle. Some passes into the bile capillaries, coloring the stools, and the remainder into the circulation. (4) Damage of the polygonal cells and obstruction in the bile ducts.

By the van den Bergh test small amounts of bilirubin can be detected in the blood and measured quantitatively. Bilirubin may be present in the blood in increased amounts without clinical jaundice (*latent* jaundice). Normal serum contains bilirubin which gives the indirect or delayed reaction, sometimes called "functional bilirubin," in amounts of 0.2-0.5 of the van den Bergh unit (1-1,000,000 to 1-400,000). Of the two forms of bilirubin, one is found usually in obstructive jaundice and the other in hemolytic jaundice. These correspond to the two reactions given by the van den Bergh test. In obstructive jaundice the reaction is *direct* or *immediate;* the bilirubin has passed through the polygonal cells and then been absorbed. In hemolytic jaundice the reaction is *indirect* or *delayed;* the bilirubin has been formed independently of the liver cells and has not passed through them. In toxic and infective jaundice the reaction is *biphasic,* possibly due to both forms of bilirubin being present. In some cases two or three of the varieties of jaundice may be combined. The amount of bilirubin in the blood may be increased before jaundice is evident.

The *icterus index* is a quantitative estimation of the color of the blood serum.

The figures are 4 to 6 as normal; from 6 to 16 in latent jaundice; above 16 jaundice is usually evident.

Dissociated Jaundice.—In this the bile pigment and bile salts behave differently; one may be retained or reabsorbed while the other is excreted normally. Retention of pigment with excretion of bile salts is common in the late stages of catarrhal jaundice and the reverse in some cases of cirrhosis of the liver. Occasionally the kidneys excrete bile salts but not bile pigment.

OBSTRUCTIVE JAUNDICE

The chief causes of obstructive jaundice are: (1) Obstruction by foreign bodies within the ducts, as gall stones and parasites; (2) by inflammatory tumefaction of the duodenum or the lining membrane of the duct; (3) by stricture or obliteration of the duct; (4) by tumors closing the orifice of the duct or growing in its interior; (5) by pressure on the duct from without, as by tumors of the liver itself, of the stomach, pancreas, kidney, or omentum; by pressure of enlarged glands in the fissures of the liver, and, more rarely, of abdominal aneurism, fecal accumulation or the pregnant uterus. There are probably factors additional to the obstruction itself. There may be obstruction from cholangitis and also damage to the hepatic cells. Biliary thrombi in the bile capillaries are formed in some cases, possibly due to abnormal bile. Under obstructive jaundice may perhaps be placed the cases of jaundice from mental shock which "may conceivably cause spasm and reversed peristalsis of the bile-duct" (W. Hunter). In some of these cases the jaundice may appear with great rapidity.

Symptoms.—(*a*) *Icterus.*—The color ranges from a lemon-yellow to a deep olive-green or bronzed hue in permanent obstruction. In some instances the color of the skin is greenish-black, the so-called "black jaundice." The color of the skin is no certain indication of the amount of bilirubin in the blood. Except the central nervous system, all the tissues are stained.

(*b*) In the more chronic forms *pruritus* is a most distressing symptom. There may be a curious pre-icteric itching. Sweating is common, and may be localized to the abdomen or to the palms of the hands. Lichen, urticaria and boils may occur. *Xanthoma multiplex* is rare. Usually in the flat form, rarely nodular, they are most common in the eyelids and on the hands and feet but may be numerous over the body and occasionally they are found in the bile ducts. The patches contain cholesterol. After persisting for years they may disappear. In very chronic cases telangiectases develop in the skin, sometimes in large numbers over the body and face, occasionally on the tongue and lips, forming bright red patches from 1 to 2 cm. in breadth.

(*c*) The blood serum is tinged with bilirubin. With the van den Bergh test an *immediate direct* reaction is obtained. Figures of 50 units (1-4,000) have been found. At least four units (1-50,000) must be present before bile passes into the urine. This reaction is of aid in the diagnosis of obstructive from hemolytic jaundice.

(*d*) The *secretions* are colored with bile pigment. The sweat tinges the linen; the tears, saliva and milk are rarely stained. The expectoration is not often tinted except in pneumonia. The urine may contain the pigment before it is apparent in the conjunctiva. The color varies from light greenish yellow to a deep black-green. In jaundice of long standing or great intensity the urine usually contains albumin and always bile-stained casts.

(*e*) *Feces.*—The stools are of pale drab or slate-gray color, and usually fetid and pasty. The "clay-color" of the stools is also in part due to undigested fat which may be increased from the normal 7 to 10 per cent to 55 or 75 per cent. There may be constipation; in some instances, owing to decomposition, there is diarrhea.

(*f*) *Slow Pulse.*—The heart's action may fall to 40, 30, or even to 20 per minute. It is particularly noticeable in the cases of catarrhal and recent jaundice, and is not as a rule an unfavorable symptom. It occurs usually in the early stages of jaundice. The respirations may fall to 10 or even to 7 per minute. Xanthopsia, or yellow vision, may occur.

(*g*) *Hemorrhage.*—The tendency to bleeding in chronic icterus is a serious feature and the blood coagulation time may be much retarded. This is an important point as uncontrollable hemorrhage is a well-recognized accident in operating upon patients with chronic jaundice. Purpura, large subcutaneous extravasations, more rarely hemorrhages from the mucous membranes, occur in protracted jaundice and in the more severe forms.

(*h*) *Cerebral Symptoms.*—Irritability, great depression of spirits or even melancholia may be present. In any case of persistent jaundice special nervous phenomena may develop and rapidly prove fatal—such as sudden coma, acute delirium or convulsions. Usually the patient has a rapid pulse, slight fever, and a dry tongue, and passes into the "typhoid state." These features are not nearly so common in obstructive as in febrile jaundice, but they may terminate a chronic icterus in whatever way produced. The group of symptoms has been termed *cholemia.* In some cases the symptoms may be due to uremia.

TOXIC AND INFECTIVE JAUNDICE

This is the commonest form of jaundice and probably the mechanism varies in different cases depending on the relative extent of injury to the liver cells and obstruction. The latter is due to cholangitis with inflammatory changes in the bile capillaries and ducts. The results of the functional tests prove the presence of damage of the hepatic cells. There may be many grades of damage ranging from cloudy swelling (as in typhoid fever), to fatty degeneration (chloroform poisoning) or to marked necrosis (acute yellow atrophy). In the detoxicating function of the liver cells there is abundant opportunity for damage. The van den Bergh test is of little clinical value in this form, the reaction being *biphasic,* due possibly to the two varieties of bilirubin being present. The relative amounts may vary. "The absorbed bile in toxemic jaundice is usually rich in bile pigments which arise from the increased destruction of hemoglobin; it is deficient in bile salts owing to the impaired function of the liver cells" (Willcox). The mucous membrane of the duodenum may be swollen and show hemorrhages.

The main causes may be grouped as follows:

(1) *Infectious diseases,* as typhoid fever, pneumonia, yellow fever, etc.

(2) *Chemical poisons,* as chloroform, arsenobenzol derivatives, tetrachlorethane, inorganic arsenic compounds, phosphorus, etc.

(3) Certain *toxic conditions,* as acute yellow atrophy.

(4) In conditions termed infectious, febrile or malignant jaundice.

The *symptoms* are not so striking as in the obstructive variety. Bile is present in the stools and the skin has in many cases only a slight lemon tint. The urine may contain no bile pigment, but the urinary pigments are considerably increased. In severer forms, as acute yellow atrophy, the color may be more intense. The general disturbance may be profound, with high fever, delirium, convulsions, suppression of urine, black vomit and cutaneous hemorrhages. The toxemia may take the form of stupor or coma.

Certain special forms deserve notice.

Tetrachlorethane.—The inhaled vapor is a cause of illness. Headache, nausea, and abdominal discomfort may be present for a week or more before jaundice appears. If quickly removed from the influence of the vapor, recovery is prompt, but *icterus gravis* may occur with purpura, convulsions, suppression of urine and coma. Fever is absent and there is no anemia, and the jaundice is unusually deep. There is extensive degeneration of the liver cells, and if the disease lasts many weeks, a "replacement cirrhosis." Contraction of the liver with ascites may follow.

Trinitrotoluene.—Many munition workers suffered severely, some from the local effects, dermatitis or erythema, many more from inhalation of the dust or swallowing the powder. The toxic symptoms come on after a variable period of exposure from a few days to months. Nausea, weakness and pallor, with signs of irritation of the throat are early symptoms. Then jaundice begins, and if severe, there are the usual toxic features. The anemia resembles the pernicious type, with a high color index and leukopenia. At first enlarged, the liver may subsequently shrink, and some of the cases have the picture of acute yellow atrophy with purpura and hemorrhages. In both these forms when jaundice is severe, full alkaline treatment is helpful—sodium citrate and sodium bicarbonate, 30 grain (2 gm.) doses of each every two or three hours and intravenous injection of normal saline with two drams (8 gm.) of bicarbonate of soda to the pint (Willcox). Glucose should be given freely by mouth or intravenously. Dinitrophenol, dinitrobenzene and picric acid may cause toxic jaundice.

Arsenobenzol Derivatives.—Occasional fever with nausea, irritation of the skin and scattered purpura may follow a dose of arsphenamine. The severer symptoms usually come on in two or three days with fever, delirium, jaundice and death in coma or with convulsions. They are especially likely to occur if there is any hepatic disease. Purpura may be very extensive with hemorrhage from the mucous membranes. Death has followed within two days. The liver presents widespread necroses with fatty degeneration. In case of recovery the size of the liver may be greatly reduced.

HEMOLYTIC JAUNDICE

In this form the bilirubin is formed outside the liver, apart from the hepatic cells, and in this the reticulo-endothelial system, especially in the spleen, assumes great importance. With increased blood destruction the cells of the reticulo-endothelial system, especially of the spleen, become overactive with a resulting increased formation of bilirubin. The bilirubin formed in this way differs from that which has passed through the hepatic cells. The van den

Bergh test gives the *delayed indirect* reaction, the same as given by the bile pigment normally in the blood. The absence of bile pigment from the urine and its presence in the feces (acholuric jaundice) is important. The excretion of bilirubin by the kidney in hemolytic jaundice is different from that in obstructive jaundice and bile rarely, if ever, passes through the kidney in the hemolytic form. It may be excreted as urobilin. Biliary thrombi are often found in the bile capillaries. The importance of the spleen in hemolytic jaundice is proved by the cases of acholuric jaundice in which removal of the spleen results in the disappearance of the jaundice. In pernicious anemia the bilirubin content of the blood is always increased, usually to 3-5 units but this does not necessarily mean clinical jaundice.

The *diagnosis* of hemolytic jaundice is greatly aided by the van den Bergh reaction. Many cases of *latent jaundice* (in which there is retention of bile pigment without coloration of the skin or bile in the urine) belong here, and in these this reaction is essential in diagnosis.

HEREDITARY AND FAMILIAL JAUNDICE

A family form of icterus has long been known and there are several groups. First, *icterus neonatorum*, as in the remarkable instance described by Glaister (Lancet, March, 1879), in which a woman had eight children, six of whom died of jaundice shortly after birth; one had stenosis of the common duct, which, as John Thomson has shown, is, with angiocholitis, a common lesion in this affection. Still more remarkable is it that the mother of this woman had twelve children, all of whom were icteric after birth, but the jaundice gradually disappeared. A brother of the woman had several children who also were jaundiced at birth. Glaister states that all of the children of Morgagni, fifteen in number, had icterus neonatorum. In certain of these familial cases, it is stated that intramuscular injections of the mother's blood serum (10-15 cc.) daily for several days is curative (Hampson).

Secondly, the *acholuric* or chronic splenomegalic *hemolytic jaundice*, which may be hereditary or familial or sometimes acquired late in life. The red cells are fragile and easily hemolyzed with liberation of hemoglobin and an excess of bilirubin formed in the spleen. There is no obstruction. The jaundice is usually slight and varies from time to time. The feces are normal in color; the urine is free from bile. The red cells are very fragile and undergo hemolysis in 0.6 to 0.42 per cent sodium chloride solution (the normal is 0.42 to 0.34 per cent solution). Moderate secondary anemia is common. The spleen is usually enlarged but the liver is normal. In the acquired form the jaundice is less prominent but the anemia is more marked and may suggest the pernicious form. There may be a leukocytosis with myelocytes and an increase in eosinophiles. There is a positive indirect reaction with the van den Bergh test. In *diagnosis* the increased fragility of the red cells is characteristic with the other features. *Treatment* consists in removal of the spleen if possible and symptomatic measures.

Thirdly, cases with enlargement of the spleen and liver and marked constitutional disturbances, anemia, dwarfing of stature, infantilism, and slight jaundice. Cases described as Hanot's cirrhosis have occurred in several members of a family, and the jaundice has dated from childhood.

Diagnosis of Jaundice.—Clinical jaundice is usually easily recognized in daylight by the discoloration of the sclerotics; in artificial light slight grades are not seen. Yellow fat in the sclerotics and the pigmentation in negroes may give difficulty. If any doubt exists and in all cases of latent jaundice the van den Bergh test is positive. Amounts of 4 units are necessary in obstructive jaundice to cause surface pigmentation; in hemolytic jaundice larger amounts may be present without surface pigmentation. In the diagnosis of the form of jaundice the whole picture must be studied; the van den Bergh test is of value but is not infallible and there are puzzling exceptions to the general rules. The recognition of latent jaundice may suggest an early stage of carcinoma of the liver or myocardial failure.

Treatment.—This is essentially that of the causal condition but the irritation caused by the jaundice often demands relief. Warm alkaline baths, sponging the skin with a solution of sodium bicarbonate or phenol (1-2 per cent) or the application of 5 per cent menthol ointment may give relief. It is well to reduce the fats in the diet. The administration of calcium salts or blood transfusion is advisable before operation. Histamine (0.25 milligram) may be given hypodermically twice a day or ergotamine tartrate (gr. 1/60, 0.001 gm.) by mouth 3 times a day for 4 days.

ICTERUS NEONATORUM

Newborn infants are liable to jaundice, which in some instances rapidly proves fatal. A mild and severe form may be recognized.

The *mild or physiological icterus* of the new-born occurs in about 50 per cent of infants. The jaundice appears early, usually on the first or second day, and is of moderate intensity. The urine may be bile-stained and the feces colorless. The nutrition of the child is not usually disturbed, and in the majority the jaundice disappears within two weeks. This form is never fatal. The bilirubin content of the blood is increased and the van den Bergh reaction suggests that the jaundice is hemolytic and not obstructive.

The *severe form* of icterus in the new-born may depend upon (*a*) congenital absence of the common or hepatic duct, of which many instances are on record; (*b*) congenital syphilitic hepatitis; and (*c*) septic infection, associated with phlebitis of the umbilical vein. This is a severe and fatal form, in which hemorrhage from the cord may also occur.

Curiously enough, in contradistinction to other forms, the brain and cord may be stained yellow in icterus neonatorum, sometimes diffusely, more rarely in definite foci corresponding to the ganglion cells which have become deeply stained (Schmorl).

ACUTE YELLOW ATROPHY

(*Malignant Jaundice; Icterus gravis: Acute Necrosis*)

Definition.—An acute widespread autolytic necrosis of the liver cells, probably due to various causes, characterized by jaundice, toxemia and a reduction in the volume of the liver. It is a symptom-complex rather than a disease.

Etiology.—The first authentic account was given by the famous old Paris doctor—Ballonius—sometimes called the French Hippocrates (1538-1616). Bright gave a good description in 1836. It is a rare disease, as among 28,000 medical cases admitted to the Johns Hopkins Hospital in nearly twenty-three years there were only 3 cases. It varies in frequency in different countries, and seems to be rarer in the United States than in Germany and England. The majority of cases occur between the tenth and the fortieth year. Rolleston collected 42 cases occurring within the first ten years of life.

Acute necrosis of the liver occurs under many conditions: (*a*) In the infections, syphilis, typhoid fever, diphtheria and septicemia. (*b*) Nonbacterial poisons. The delayed chloroform poisoning is a hepatic necrosis resembling very closely acute yellow atrophy. Phosphorus produces a similar condition, and possibly mercury. Arsenobenzol compounds may cause it. (*c*) Autogenous poisons, produced in connection with pregnancy and parturition. The ordinary necrotic foci of the liver in pregnancy are the same kind but less in degree than those of acute yellow atrophy.

An exaggeration of any cause for toxic jaundice may lead to a clinical condition which we call acute yellow atrophy. Its association with pregnancy is remarkable. More than half of the cases occur in women, and in a large proportion of these during the middle or latter period of pregnancy. The disease has followed a profound shock or mental emotion. It may follow "catarrhal jaundice." It occurs occasionally in syphilis and other acute infections, and there are cases of cirrhosis of the liver associated with diffuse necrosis, intense jaundice and toxemia. We are ignorant of the conditions under which toxins cause this widespread necrosis.

Morbid Anatomy.—The liver is greatly reduced in size, looks thin and flattened, and may not have more than one-half or one-third of its normal weight. It is flabby and the capsule is wrinkled. Externally the organ has a greenish-yellow color. On section the color may be yellowish-brown, yellowish-red, or mottled, and the outlines of the lobules are indistinct. The yellow and dark-red portions represent different stages of the same process—the yellow an earlier, the red a more advanced stage. The organ may cut with considerable firmness. The liver cells are seen in all stages of necrosis, and in spots appear to have undergone complete destruction, leaving a fatty, granular *débris* with pigment grains and crystals of leucin and tyrosin. Hemorrhages occur between the liver cells. There is a cholangitis of the smaller bile ducts. Marchand, MacCallum, and others have described regenerative changes in the cases which do not run an acute course.

The other organs show extensive bile-staining, and there are numerous hemorrhages. The kidneys may show marked granular degeneration of the epithelium, and usually there is fatty degeneration of the heart. In a majority of the cases the spleen is enlarged.

Symptoms.—In the initial stage there may be gastroduodenal catarrh, and the jaundice is thought to be of a simple nature. In some instances this lasts only a few days, in others two or three weeks. Then severe symptoms set in—headache, delirium, trembling of the muscles, and, in some instances, convulsions. The picture may suggest meningitis. Vomiting is a constant symptom, and blood may be brought up. Hemorrhages occur into the skin or from the mucous surfaces; in pregnant women abortion may occur. The jaundice usually increases, coma sets in and gradually deepens until death. The temperature is variable; in a majority of the cases the disease runs an afebrile course, though sometimes just before death there is an elevation. In some instances there is marked pyrexia. The pulse is usually rapid, the tongue coated and dry, and the patient is in a toxic state. The liver may be enlarged at first but rapidly decreases in size and there may be complete obliteration of the liver dulness. There is marked disturbance of liver function. Ascites may occur.

The urine is bile-stained and often contains casts. Frequently albuminuria and occasionally albumosuria occur. Urea is markedly diminished. There is a corresponding increase in the percentage of nitrogen present as ammonia from the normal 2 to 5 per cent up to 20 per cent. The diminution in urea is probably partly due to the liver cells failing to manufacture urea from ammonia, but also to organic acids seizing on the ammonia and preventing the formation of urea. Leucin and tyrosin are not constantly present; of 23 cases collected by Hunter, in 9 neither was found; in 10 both were present; in 3 tyrosin only; in 1 leucin only. The leucin and tyrosin are probably derived from the liver cells as a result of their extensive destruction. In the majority of cases no bile enters the intestines, and the stools are clay-colored. The disease is almost invariably fatal but in a few instances recovery has occurred with a resulting cirrhosis.

The duration and the type of the disease depend upon the extent and the rapidity of progress of the necrosis. Cases have lasted as long as forty days, while death has occurred as early as the second day. A subacute form has been described with a slow necrosis lasting many months, associated with jaundice—a protracted stage from which recovery is possible by regeneration of liver tissue, but consecutive cirrhosis is the rule.

Diagnosis.—Jaundice with vomiting, dimunition of the liver volume, delirium, and the presence of leucin and tyrosin in the urine, are characteristic features. Leucin and tyrosin are not distinctive. They may be present in other forms of jaundice, some acute infections and leukemia.

It is not to be forgotten that any severe jaundice may be associated with intense cerebral symptoms. The clinical features in certain cases of *cirrhosis* are almost identical, but the history, the more constant occurrence of fever, and the absence of leucin and tyrosin are distinguishing signs. *Phosphorus* poisoning may closely simulate acute yellow atrophy, particularly in the hemorrhages, jaundice, and diminution in the liver volume, but the gastric symptoms are usually more marked, and leucin and tyrosin are stated not to occur in the urine.

Treatment.—Efforts should be made to eliminate toxins by free elimination, the giving of alkalies and the use of subcutaneous and intravenous saline injections. Gastric sedatives may be used to allay the vomiting. A milk diet with large amounts of sugar should be given with abundance of alkaline water. Dextrose should be given intravenously twice a day (250-500 cc. of a 25 per cent solution) and insulin (5 to 10 units).

AFFECTIONS OF THE BLOOD VESSELS OF THE LIVER

Anemia.—There are no symptoms indicative of this condition.

Hyperemia.—(*a*) Active Hyperemia.—After each meal the rapid absorption by the portal vessels induces transient congestion of the organ, which is entirely physiological: but it is quite possible that in persons who persistently eat and drink too much this active hyperemia may lead to functional disturbance and in the case of too much alcohol, to organic change. In the fevers an acute hyperemia may be present.

The *symptoms* are indefinite. Possibly the sense of distress or fullness in the right hypochondrium, so often mentioned by dyspeptics and by those who eat and drink freely, may be due to this cause. There are probably diurnal variations in the volume of the liver. In cirrhosis with enlargement the rapid reduction in volume after a copious hemorrhage indicates the important part which hyperemia plays even in organic troubles. Andrew H. Smith described a case of periodical enlargement of the liver.

(*b*) Passive Congestion.—This is much more common and results from an increase of pressure in the efferent vessels or sublobular branches of the hepatic veins. Every condition leading to stasis in the right heart affects these veins. In chronic valvular disease, myocardial insufficiency, fibrosis of the lung, and intrathoracic tumors, mechanical congestion occurs and leads to definite changes. The liver is enlarged, firm, and of a deep-red color; the hepatic vessels are greatly engorged, particularly the central vein in each lobule and its adjacent capillaries. On section the organ presents a peculiar mottled appearance, owing to the congested hepatic and anemic portal territories; hence the term *nutmeg* given to this condition. Gradually the distention of the central capillaries reaches such a grade that atrophy of the intervening liver cells is induced. Brown pigment is deposited about the centre of the lobules and the connective tissue is greatly increased. In the cardiac liver the organ is large in the early stage, but later it may become contracted. Occasionally the connective tissue is increased about the lobules as well, but the process usually extends from the sublobular and central veins.

The *symptoms* are not always to be separated from those of the associated conditions. Gastro-intestinal catarrh is usually present and hematemesis may occur. The portal obstruction in advanced cases leads to ascites, which may precede the development of general dropsy. There is often slight jaundice, the stools may be clay-colored, and the urine contains bile pigment. The liver is increased in size, may be a full hand's breadth below the costal margin and tender on pressure. There is pain if the enlargement has been rapid. It is in this condition particularly that we find pulsation of the liver. We must distinguish communicated pulsation from the heaving, diffuse impulse due to regurgitation into the hepatic veins, in which the whole liver dilates with each impulse.

The *diagnosis* is usually clear except when the myocardial weakness is not very evident. The results of cardiac treatment are of aid in the diagnosis from cirrhosis or syphilis. The indications for *treatment* are to restore the balance of the circulation and to unload the engorged portal vessels. The diet should be mostly milk and it may be well to keep down the amount of water for a few days. The bowels should be freely opened. An enema should be given followed by calomel, a compound cathartic pill or elaterin (gr. 1/10, 0.006 gm.) and Epsom salts repeated as necessary. Dry cups over the liver may be used. The causal condition should be treated.

Diseases of the Portal Vein.—(*a*) THROMBOSIS; ADHESIVE PYLEPHLEBITIS. —Coagulation of blood in the portal vein is met with in cirrhosis, in syphilis of the liver, invasion of the vein by cancer, proliferative peritonitis involving the gastrohepatic omentum, perforation of the vein by gall stones, and occasionally follows sclerosis of the walls of the portal vein or of its branches. In rare instances a complete collateral circulation is established, the thrombus undergoes the usual change, and ultimately the vein is represented by a fibrous cord, a condition which has been called *pylephlebitis adhesiva*. In a case of this kind the portal vein was represented by a narrow fibrous cord; the collateral circulation, which must have been established for years, ultimately failed, ascites and hematemesis supervened and rapidly proved fatal. The diagnosis can rarely be made. A suggestive combination is a *sudden* onset of intense engorgement of the branches of the portal system, leading to hematemesis, melena, ascites, and swelling of the spleen.

Infarcts (anemic or hemorrhagic) are not common in the liver. They occur in obstruction of the portal vessels, or of the portal and hepatic veins at the same time, occasionally in disease of the hepatic artery.

(*b*) SUPPURATIVE PYLEPHLEBITIS is considered in the section on abscess.

Affections of the hepatic vein are extremely rare. Dilatation occurs in cases of chronic enlargement of the right heart, from whatever cause. Emboli occasionally pass from the right auricle into the hepatic veins. *Obstruction* of the hepatic veins is rare. There are acute enlargement of the liver with a rounded edge, pain on pressure and ascites (transudate) which contains red cells and does not clot readily. The duration may be days to years.

Hepatic Artery.—Enlargement of this vessel is seen in cirrhosis of the liver. It may be the seat of extensive sclerosis. Aneurism of the hepatic artery is rare and will be referred to in the section on arteries.

DISEASES OF THE BILE PASSAGES AND GALLBLADDER

CATARRHAL JAUNDICE

Definition.—Jaundice due to hepatitis and cholangitis, and sometimes associated with obstruction of the terminal portion of the common duct. It is not always possible to decide accurately as to the exact condition and probably various lesions are responsible. The disease may occur in epidemics.

Etiology.—In one group the jaundice is due to an extension of an acute gastroduodenitis to the common duct, which is obstructed by swelling of the mucous membrane or by a plug of mucus completely obstructing the outflow of bile. In some cases evidence of infection is found in the duodenal contents and occasionally plugs of mucus are obtained by duodenal biliary drainage. In one case at postmortem the orifice was plugged with inspissated mucus, the common and hepatic ducts were slightly distended and contained a bile-tinged mucus, and there were no changes in the mucosa of the ducts. There is no sign of hepatitis in some cases. In other cases an infection of the finer ducts within the liver occurs which may be due to infection from the intestine. In another group there are no gastro-intestinal symptoms but jaundice with toxemia and hepatic insufficiency; at autopsy normal bile ducts and duodenum are found. The important lesion is the hepatitis and such cases possibly should be separated as infectious hepatitis or cholangitis. The van den Bergh test gives varying results so that probably there is a combination of obstructive and toxic and infective jaundice.

Symptoms.—There may be neither pain nor distress, and the patient's friends may first notice the yellow tint, or the patient may observe it in the looking-glass. In other instances there are dyspeptic symptoms and uneasy sensations in the hepatic region or pains in the back and limbs. In the epidemic form the onset may be more severe, with headache, chill, and vomiting. Fever is rarely present, though the temperature may reach 101° or 102°. All the signs of obstructive jaundice are present, the stools are clay-colored, and the urine contains bile pigment. The skin has a bright-yellow tint; the greenish, bronzed color is never seen in the simple form. Spider angiomata may occur on the face. They disappear in a few months. The pulse may be normal, but occasionally it is remarkably slow, and may fall to 40 or 30 beats in the minute, and the respirations to as low as 8 per minute. Sleepiness may be present and rarely a comatose state. The liver may be normal in size, but is usually slightly enlarged, and the edge can be felt below the costal margin. Occasionally the enlargement is more marked. As a rule the gallbladder can not be felt. The spleen may be increased in size. The duration is from four to eight weeks. There are mild cases in which the jaundice disappears within two weeks or it may persist for three months or even longer. Some cases go on to acute necrosis (acute yellow atrophy) with a fatal result. The stools should be carefully watched, for they give the first intimation of removal of the obstruction.

Diagnosis.—This is rarely difficult. The onset in young, comparatively healthy persons, the moderate icterus, the absence of pain and emaciation or evidences of cirrhosis or cancer usually make the diagnosis easy. Cases which persist for two or three months cause uneasiness, as the suspicion is aroused that it may be more than simple catarrh. There are instances in which time alone can determine the true nature of the case. The possibility of other forms must be borne in mind in anomalous types.

Treatment.—The patient should be in bed. The diet should be simple and the fats restricted. It is well to give carbohydrates freely. Measures should be used to allay gastric catarrh, if it is present. A dose of calomel may be given, and the bowels kept open subsequently by salines. The patient should not be violently purged. Daily lavage of the stomach with water at 95° is useful. Bismuth and bicarbonate of soda may be given, and the patient should drink freely of alkaline mineral waters. The method of drainage of the bile ducts devised by Lyon, in which a 25 per cent solution of magnesium sulphate is introduced into the duodenum, relaxing the sphincter of the common duct, is of great value and should be done as early as possible. If a plug of mucus can be dislodged, there may be an immediate flow of bile and rapid improvement. Daily duodenal biliary drainage should be done for some days. By the use of this method the duration is usually shortened, especially if it is done early. As there may be hepatitis and the possibility of permanent hepatic damage, the hepatic function should be carefully studied after the attack is over.

CHRONIC CHOLANGITIS

This may possibly occur as a sequel of an acute process but it is unusual to see a chronic, persistent jaundice due to this cause. A chronic catarrh always accompanies obstruction in the common duct, whether by gall stones, neoplasm, stricture, or external pressure. There are two groups of cases:

With Complete Obstruction of the Common Duct.—In this form the bile passages are greatly dilated, the common duct may reach the size of the thumb or larger, there is usually dilatation of the gallbladder and of the ducts within the liver. The contents of the ducts and of the gallbladder are a clear, colorless mucus. The mucosa may be everywhere smooth and not swollen. The clear mucus is usually sterile. The patients are the subjects of chronic jaundice, usually without fever.

With Incomplete Obstruction of the Duct.—There is pressure on the duct or there are gall stones, single or multiple, in the common duct or in the diverticulum of Vater. The bile passages are not so much dilated, and the contents are a bile-stained, turbid mucus. The gallbladder is rarely much dilated. In a majority of all cases stones are found in it.

The symptoms of this form are sometimes very distinctive. With it is associated most frequently the so-called hepatic intermittent fever, recurring attacks of chills, fever, and sweats. It is important to bear in mind that the chills, fever, and sweats do not necessarily mean suppuration.

SUPPURATIVE AND ULCERATIVE CHOLANGITIS

The condition is a diffuse, purulent cholangitis involving the larger and smaller ducts. In a large proportion of all cases there is associated suppurative disease of the gallbladder. In all forms of infection of the bile passages cultures of the duodenal contents may give information as to the infecting organism.

Etiology.—It is the most serious of the sequels of gall stones. Occasionally a diffuse suppurative angiocholitis follows the acute infectious cholecystitis; this, however, is rare, since fortunately in the latter condition the cystic duct is usually occluded. Cancer of the duct, or foreign bodies, such as lumbricoids or fish bones, are occasional causes. There may be extension from a suppurative pylephlebitis. In rare instances suppurative cholangitis occurs in acute infections, as pneumonia and influenza.

The common duct is greatly dilated and may reach the size of the index finger or the thumb; the walls are thickened, and there may be fistulous communications with the stomach, colon, or duodenum. The hepatic ducts and their extensions in the liver are dilated and contain pus mixed with bile. On section of the liver small abscesses are seen, which correspond to the dilated suppurating ducts. The gallbladder is usually distended, full of pus, and with adhesions to the neighboring parts, or it may have perforated.

Symptoms.—The symptoms of suppurative cholangitis are usually very severe. A previous history of gall stones, the development of a septic fever, the swelling and tenderness of the liver, the enlargement of the gallbladder, and the leukocytosis are suggestive features. Jaundice is always present but is variable. In some cases it is very intense, in others it is slight. There may be very little pain. There are progressive emaciation and loss of strength. In one case parotitis developed which subsided without suppuration.

Treatment.—With infection of the bile passage, the diet should be simple and water taken freely. Hexamine may be given in full dosage. Lyon's method of nonsurgical biliary drainage should always be tried. In some cases surgical drainage of the gallbladder has been of use. Vaccines prepared from duodenal cultures may be tried.

ACUTE CHOLECYSTITIS

Etiology.—Acute inflammation of the gallbladder is due to bacterial invasion, with or without the presence of gall stones. Three varieties or grades may be recognized: the catarrhal, the suppurative, and the phlegmonous. The condition is very serious, may be fatal, and may require prompt surgical intervention for its relief.

Acute noncalculous cholecystitis is a result of bacterial invasion, probably often from foci in the mouth and throat. The colon bacillus, the typhoid bacillus, staphylococci and streptococci are the organisms most often found. The frequency of gallbladder infection in the fevers, particularly in typhoid fever, has been mentioned. In many cases the organisms are found in the wall of the gallbladder when the contents are sterile.

The infection may be carried by the lymphatics, by the bile, by the blood, or by the bile ducts. With infection there are changes (1) in the mucous membrane, (2) in the wall, (3) in the peritoneal surface, tending to cause adhesions, and (4) in the bile in the gallbladder. The relative proportion of these varies greatly but they tend to be progressive.

Pathology.—The organ is usually distended and the walls tense. Adhesions may have formed with the bowel or omentum. In the acute stage the mucous membrane is swollen and the mucin increased. As the process continues the mucosa is thickened, the epithelium desquamates, there are areas of necrosis, and the villi may be hypertrophied and stand out, giving a strawberry appearance. With obstruction of the duct and pyogenic infection there may be acute necrotic cholecystitis, with rapid perforation, or a more chronic purulent cholecystitis—empyema of the gallbladder.

Symptoms.—Severe paroxysmal pain is, as a rule, the first indication, most commonly in the right side of the abdomen in the region of the liver. It may be in the epigastrium or low down in the region of the appendix. "Nausea, vomiting, rise of pulse and temperature, prostration, distention of the abdomen, rigidity, general tenderness becoming localized" usually follow (Richardson). In this form, without gall stones, jaundice is not often present. Signs at the base of the right lung are common in any form of acute biliary infection. Leukocytosis is common. The local tenderness is extreme, but it may be deceptive in its situation. Due probably to adhesions and inflammatory processes between the gallbladder and bowel are the intestinal symptoms; there may be complete stoppage of gas and feces; indeed, the operation for acute obstruction has been performed. The distended gallbladder may sometimes be felt. As a sequel there may be purulent distention. In the early stages, probably with catarrhal changes, the symptoms may be mainly gastric.

Diagnosis.—This is by no means easy and appendicitis or acute intestinal obstruction may be diagnosed. The history is often a valuable guide. Occurring during convalescence from typhoid fever or in a patient with previous cholecystitis, such a group of symptoms is highly suggestive. The differentiation of the variety of the cholecystitis is difficult. In the diagnosis of all infections of the bile tract the study by Lyon's method of the bile and its contents may be of great aid. For details his book on the subject should be consulted. In the acute suppurative and phlegmonous forms the symptoms are usually more severe, perforation is very apt to occur, with local or general peritonitis, and unless operative measures are undertaken death ensues.

There is an acute cholecystitis, probably an infective form, in which the patient has recurring attacks of pain in the region of the gallbladder. The diagnosis of gall stones is made, but an operation shows simply an enlarged gallbladder filled with mucus and bile, and the mucous membrane perhaps swollen and inflamed.

Treatment.—The patient should be at rest, given a simple fluid diet, and take water freely. The bowels are kept open by enemata and simple salines. An ice bag is applied over the gallbladder region. Sodium salicylate and hexamine may be given by mouth (of each gr. 15, 1 gm. t. i. d.). Lyon's method of bile duct drainage often gives excellent results. In the milder forms the inflammation subsides gradually; in severer form operation is indicated and the results are excellent. Increase in the local signs, an enlarged gallbladder, increasing leukocytosis and fever, are usually indications for operation. Foci of infection should be properly treated.

CHRONIC CHOLECYSTITIS

Etiology.—It often results from a previous attack of acute cholecystitis or may be associated with gall stones or chronic infection of the ducts. In some cases it is undoubtedly chronic from the onset, resulting from a persistent infection which is never acute enough to set up an active attack. The infection may be hematogenous from foci of infection, by the portal system or from the liver. Cholecystitis may occur at any age and probably begins frequently in early life with a slow development to the production of definite symptoms.

Pathology.—The gallbladder is usually distended and contains thick bile and mucus. The walls may be thickened. There may be destruction of the villi and a deposit of lipoid material in the mucous membrane—"strawberry gallbladder." Later small ulcers may result, fibrous changes occur and stones may form. The mucosa may be atrophic and sometimes the gallbladder is small and sclerotic; it may be surrounded by dense adhesions. The relationship between the lymphatics of the gallbladder and pancreas is important in explaining the association of infection in these organs.

Symptoms.—These are much the same as those from gall stones and a differential diagnosis may be impossible. Disturbance of the digestive tract is always marked. Flatulency after meals, complaint of fullness after a small meal, a sudden sensation of nausea sometimes with a feeling of faintness, a feeling of cold or slight chilly sensations, and sometimes regurgitation into the mouth are among the symptoms. The stomach contents are variable, achlorhydria is fairly common. The persistence of the symptoms and the lack of results from ordinary treatment are important. The X-ray study may show an enlarged gallbladder and cholecystography usually shows disturbance of function. Jaundice occurs in some cases, varying from time to time. The coexistence of ulcer, gastric or duodenal, and cholecystitis is not rare. There may be attacks of acute pain but tenderness on deep pressure over the gallbladder is much more common. There may be tenderness on pressure at the right costovertebral angle. In the intervals there may be an entire absence of any tenderness in the gallbladder region. Sometimes the gallbladder is palpable. W. J. Mayo called attention to a form of chronic cholecystitis without gall stones and accompanied with chronic interlobular pancreatitis in which the mucous membrane shows a strawberry-like appearance. The process is confined to the gallbladder; the glands along the ligament may be enlarged. The chief symptom is pain in the region of the gallbladder, but there is no distention and the chronic pancreatitis is not always expressed clinically.

Diagnosis.—The marked digestive disturbance, the variability and persistence of the symptoms, the local tenderness, the results of cholecystography and the study of the bile, especially from the gallbladder, obtained by duodenal drainage are important. In early stages, the diagnosis may be difficult as symptoms and signs are few and it must depend largely on the study of the bile.

Treatment.—The medical management is much the same as in gall stones; a simple diet, large amounts of water, keeping the bowels freely open and taking regular exercise. The *diet* must be chosen for each patient. Fats are useful to stimulate empyting of the gallbladder; butter, cream, eggs and olive oil are best. Fried foods should not be used. If cholesterol crystals are found in the bile or the blood cholesterol is high, a cholesterol-free diet should be given (no eggs, cream, cheese, liver, kidney, sausage, fat meat, and little butter). The administration of salicylate of sodium and hexamine seems sometimes to be of use; hexamine (methenamine) may be given in doses of 90 grains a day with enough alkali to make the urine alkaline and prevent urinary irritation. The taking of salines before breakfast is often helpful. In many cases nonsurgical drainage (Lyon) is advisable. It may relieve the symptoms materially and done at intervals keep the disturbance to a minimum. In many patients it is an excellent preparation for operation. The decision as to surgical interference must depend on the severity of the symptoms and the interference with health due to the condition. In some cases adhesions are present between the gallbladder and the colon, pylorus and duodenum and operation may be justified to correct them. If there is distinct evidence of a chronic suppurative process in the gallbladder, surgical measures should not be delayed. An important point in the decision as to operation in some cases rests with the condition of the heart. Myocardial disturbance is common with chronic gallbladder disease and this may be regarded as a contra-indication to operation when it is the treatment likely to help the myocardium. As a rule these patients stand operation surprisingly well. Proper preparation before operation is important.

CANCER OF THE BILE PASSAGES

Incidence.—Of 3,908 operations on the gallbladder and biliary passages, in 85 or 2.1 per cent cancer was found (Mayo). Cancer of the gallbladder is more common in women, 3 to 1 (Musser), and in three-fourths of the cases gall stones are or have been present. The fundus of the bladder is usually attacked first. Primary carcinoma of the bile ducts is rare.

Symptoms.—When the disease involves the gallbladder there is usually a history suggesting previous gallbladder disease. The first symptom is discomfort or pain in the gallbladder region, made worse by meals and by any jolting. Gastric disturbance is marked. A tumor is usually felt, variable in size, occasionally very large, due to distention of the gallbladder or involvement of contiguous parts. It is usually firm and hard. Jaundice may be due to involvement of the liver; it was present in 69 per cent of Musser's cases; pain is often of great severity and paroxysmal in character. The pain and tenderness on pressure persist in the intervals between the paroxysmal attacks. There is loss of weight, sometimes fever and sweats. When the liver is involved the picture is that of carcinoma of the organ.

Primary malignant disease in the *bile ducts* is less common, and rarely forms tumors that can be felt externally. The tumor is usually in the common duct, 72 of 90 cases collected by Rolleston. There is usually an early, intense, and persistent jaundice. Pain is variable. The gallbladder is usually enlarged in obstruction of the common duct by malignant disease. The dilated gallbladder may rupture. At best the *diagnosis* is doubtful, unless cleared up by an exploratory operation. A very interesting form of malignant disease of the ducts is that which involves the diverticulum of Vater of which Rolleston collected 23 cases.

Medical *treatment* is symptomatic. Removal has little chance of success unless operation is done early but except when there is evidence of metastases it is well to advise the attempt.

STENOSIS AND OBSTRUCTION OF THE BILE DUCTS

Stenosis.—Stenosis or complete occlusion very rarely follows ulceration, most commonly after the passage of a gallstone. In these instances the obstruction is usually low down in the common duct. Foreign bodies, such as the seeds of fruits, may enter the duct, and round worms may crawl into it. Liver flukes and echinococci are rare causes of obstruction in man.

Obstruction.—Obstruction by *pressure* from without may be due to cancer of the head of the pancreas, less often a chronic inflammation, compressing the terminal portion of the duct, and rarely, cancer of the pylorus. Secondary carcinomatous involvement of the lymph nodes of the liver is a common cause of occlusion of the duct. Rare causes are aneurism of a branch of the celiac axis and pressure of abdominal tumors. The most common cause is gall stones. Obstruction of the *cystic duct* may be due to infection.

SYMPTOMS.—The symptoms produced are those of chronic obstructive jaundice. At first, the liver is enlarged but in chronic cases it may be reduced in size, and of a deeply bronzed color. The hepatic intermittent fever is not often associated with complete occlusion of the duct from any cause, but it is most frequent in chronic obstruction by gall stones. Permanent occlusion of the duct terminates in death. In many cases the conditions which lead to the obstruction are in themselves fatal. The liver, which is not necessarily enlarged, presents a moderate grade of cirrhosis. Cases of cicatricial occlusion may last for years.

DIAGNOSIS.—A history of colic, jaundice of varying intensity, paroxysms of pain, and intermittent fever point to gall stones. In cancerous obstruction the tumor mass can sometimes be felt in the epigastric region. In cases in which the lymph nodes in the transverse fissure are cancerous the primary disease may be in the pelvic organs or the rectum, or there may be a gastric cancer, which has not given any symptoms. In these cases the examination of other lymphatic glands, as above the clavicle, may be of value. The gallbladder is usually enlarged in obstruction of the common duct, except in the cases of gall stones (*Courvoisier's law*). Great and progressive enlargement of the liver with jaundice and moderate continued fever is more commonly met with in cancer. A careful X-ray study should always be made.

Treatment.—This must depend on the diagnosis. If due to neoplasm little can be done. Drainage of the gallbladder or its junction to the bowel may give some relief. If caused by gall stones, operation by an experienced surgeon is indicated.

Congenital Obliteration of the Ducts.—John Thomson, in 1892, collected 49 cases and studied the condition thoroughly. Howard and Wolbach in 1911 brought the cases up to 76 and Holmes in 1919 found 108 cases. Thomson regards congenital malformation as the chief cause, but cholangitis and congenital cirrhosis of the liver are important factors. Jaundice sets in early, but may be delayed for ten or twelve days, and is progressive and deep. Hemorrhages in the skin, from the gastro-intestinal tract, and from the umbilical cord have occurred in fully 50 per cent. Nearly half of the patients die within the first month, a few live on for five or six months, but rarely as long as the tenth or twelfth. There is no treatment.

Mention may be made of *cystic dilatation* of the common duct which may be a congenital anomaly. It occurs more often in females. The symptoms usually date from childhood and may be intermittent. Pain in the upper abdomen, vomiting, jaundice, and a palpable tumor are present. The diagnosis is rarely made without exploration. The treatment is surgical.

CHOLELITHIASIS

No chapter in medicine is more interesting than that which deals with the question of gall stones. Few affections present so many points for study—chemical, bacteriological, pathological, and clinical.

Origin of Gall Stones.—There are three mechanisms specially concerned: (1) infection, (2) stasis, and (3) the cholesterol content of the blood.

(1) *Infection.*—The route may be (*a*) hematogenous, probably the most common, (*b*) by elimination through the liver, and (*c*) retrograde. Hematogenous infection may be from a focus of infection in any part of the body; disease of the appendix is sometimes responsible. The gallbladder is a peculiarly favorable habitat for organisms. Streptococci, staphylococci, pneu-

mococci, colon bacilli and typhoid bacilli have been found with varying conditions of the bile. Streptococcus infection is frequent. The typhoid bacillus may live indefinitely in the gallbladder and has been found in the interior of gall stones. The experimental production of gall stones has been accomplished by injecting organisms into the gallbladders of animals. The calculus associated with infection is composed largely of calcium salts.

(2) *Stasis.*—An inspissated condition of the bile occurs with this and precipitation is likely to occur. A nucleus is thus formed and other elements are deposited on it. Inspissation of the bile is favored by pregnancy and the acute infectious diseases. The views of Meltzer on disturbed contrary innervation of the gallbladder with retention of bile are of interest in this connection.

(3) *Cholesterol.*—In a number of cases of cholelithiasis there is an increase in the cholesterol content of the blood. In some cases this may be temporary and not present when the existence of gall stones is recognized. Cholesterol may be of exogenous or endogenous origin. There is often an increase in the blood cholesterol during typhoid fever, in diabetes and obesity and in pregnancy. It is evident that with a foreign body present there may be subsequent infection. A study of the cases in which cholesterol stones are found shows that a history of infection is generally lacking. The formation of a cholesterol stone may be favored by an increase in the cholesterol in the blood, by its increased excretion by the liver, or by deposit of material from inspissated bile.

Age.—The great majority of cases occur between thirty and sixty, forty to fifty being the most common decade. They are rare under twenty-five but cases have occurred in the newborn and in infants.

Sex.—Three-fourths of the cases occur in women. Pregnancy has an important influence. Some postmortem series show gall stones present in 25 per cent of women over 40 years of age.

All conditions which favor *stagnation of bile* predispose to the formation of stones. Among these may be mentioned corset-wearing, obesity, visceroptosis, and occupations requiring a "leaning forward" position. Lack of exercise, sedentary occupations, particularly when combined with overindulgence in food and constipation are also favoring circumstances.

Physical Characters of Gall Stones.—They may be single, in which case the stone is usually ovoid and may attain a very large size. Instances are on record of gall stones measuring more than 5 inches in length. They may be extremely numerous, ranging from a score to hundreds or even thousands, in which case the stones are very small. When moderately numerous, they show signs of mutual pressure and have a polygonal form, with smooth facets; occasionally, however, five or six gall stones of medium size are found which are round or ovoid and without facets. They are sometimes mulberry-shaped and very dark, consisting largely of bile-pigments. Again there are small, black calculi, rough and irregular in shape, and varying in size from grains of sand to small shot. These are sometimes known as gall-sand. The greater portion of the stone is made up of cholesterol, which may form the entire calculus, and is arranged in concentric laminae showing also radiating lines. Salts of lime and magnesia, bile acids, fatty acids, and traces of iron and copper are also found in them.

Seat of Formation.—Within the liver itself calculi are occasionally found, but are here usually small and few, and in the form of ovoid, greenish-black grains. A large majority of all calculi are formed in the gallbladder where the stones in the larger ducts have usually had their origin.

Symptoms.—In some cases gall stones may be latent or cause no symptoms directly referable to the gallbladder which may tolerate the presence of large numbers for an indefinite time. The most common symptoms are *digestive;* they are variable in time and character but always tend to be persistent. Discomfort, a sense of fullness, flatulency, nausea, and sometimes vomiting are frequent. These are caused by cholecystitis rather than by gall stones. There may be a sense of weight or oppression in the epigastrium perhaps with a feeling of faintness. Slight chilly sensations may occur at times. There may be attacks of more severe gastric disturbance in which pain is more marked with considerable vomiting. There is often the complaint of pain about the right shoulder or the angle of the right scapula which is described as "going straight through" or radiating from the front. There may be a curious feeling in the right side which the patient has difficulty in describing; it is like a "catch" or "stitch." Violent exercise or jolting, as in a motor trip, may increase the symptoms. Tenderness may be found on deep pressure in the region of the gallbladder or in the epigastrium, with varying resistance and muscle spasm. The pressure may have to be deep and is often done best by the thumb under the costal margin, the patient taking a deep inspiration. The "catch" in the breath may be characteristic.

Jaundice may occur and should be carefully looked for, especially after an increase in the symptoms. The stomach contents show nothing distinctive; hypo-acidity is probably most common. There is usually marked constipation. Obstinate attacks of urticaria may occur.

Certain important features are: (1) the mechanical accidents in consequence of migration of the stone or of obstruction, either in the ducts or intestines; (2) the septic, infectious accidents, either local (cholangitis and cholecystitis with empyema of the gallbladder, and the fistulae and abscess of the liver with infection of the neighboring parts) or general, fever and secondary visceral lesions.

Biliary Colic.—Gall stones may become engaged in the neck of the gallbladder or in the cystic or the common duct without producing severe symptoms. More commonly the violent symptoms known as biliary colic result. The attack sets in abruptly with agonizing pain in the right hypochondriac region, which radiates to the shoulder, or is very intense in the epigastric and lower thoracic regions. It is often associated with a rigor and fever from 102° to 103°. The pain is usually so intense that the patient rolls about in agony with vomiting, profuse sweating, and great depression of the circulation. There may be marked tenderness in the region of the liver, which may be enlarged, and the gallbladder may become palpable and very tender. In other cases the fever is more marked. The spleen may be enlarged. The symptoms of acute infectious cholecystitis and gall stone colic may be very similar. In a large number of cases jaundice occurs, but not always. It does not happen during the passage of the stone through the cystic duct but only when it becomes lodged in the common duct. The pain is due (*a*) to impaction of the stone about the orifice of the cystic duct or to slow progress in the duct, in which the stone takes a rotary course owing to the arrangement of the Heisterian valve; the cystic duct is poor in muscle fibres but rich in nerves and ganglia;

(*b*) to the acute inflammation which usually accompanies an attack; (*c*) to the stretching and distention of the gallbladder.

The attack varies in duration. It may last for a few hours, several days, or even a week or more. If the stone becomes impacted in the orifice of the common duct, the jaundice becomes intense; much more commonly it is a transient icterus.

Occasionally accidents occur, such as rupture of the duct with fatal peritonitis. Fatal syncope and convulsive seizures during an attack are rare events. Palpitation and distress about the heart may be present, and occasionally a mitral murmur occurs during the paroxysm, but the cardiac conditions described as coming on acutely in biliary colic are due to preexistent myocardial degeneration, not infrequent in patients with gall stones. In some cases attacks of angina pectoris occur secondary to gallbladder disease.

The *diagnosis* of acute hepatic colic is generally easy. The pain is in the upper abdominal and thoracic regions, whereas in nephritic colic it is in the lower abdomen. A history of previous attacks is an important guide, and the occurrence of jaundice, however slight, determines the diagnosis. To look for gall stones, the stools should be thoroughly mixed with water and carefully filtered through a narrow-meshed sieve. Concretions due to some fruits, *e. g.*, pears, or to olive oil should not be mistaken for gall stones. A remarkable xanthoma of the bile passages has been found in association with hepatic colic. In chronic gallbladder cases, with adhesions, the clinical picture may resemble closely that of ulcer. The presence of gall stones may be proved by X-ray examination in a considerable proportion of cases but not the pure cholesterol stones.

Obstruction of the Cystic Duct.—The effects may be thus enumerated: (*a*) *Dilatation* of the gallbladder. In acute obstruction the contents are bile mixed with much mucus or mucopurulent material. In chronic obstruction the bile is replaced by a clear fluid mucus due to absorption of the bile and other contents. By this time the lining is of fibrous tissue and the fluid is a transudate. This is an important point in diagnosis, as such a gallbladder may form a large tumor. A dilated gallbladder may reach an enormous size, and in such cases it has been mistaken for an ovarian tumor. In one case it was attached to the right broad ligament. The dilated gallbladder can usually be felt below the edge of the liver, and often has a characteristic outline like a gourd. An enlarged and relaxed organ may not be palpable, and in acute cases the distention may be upward toward the hilus of the liver. The dilated gallbladder usually projects directly downward, rarely to one side or the other, though occasionally towards the middle line. It may reach below the navel, and in persons with thin walls the outline can be accurately defined. Riedel called attention to a tongue-like *projection* of the anterior margin of the right lobe in connection with enlarged gallbladder. Distention of the gallbladder may occur without jaundice; indeed, the greatest enlargement has been met with in such cases.

Palpation.—There are two conditions in which gall stones may be felt; the large, loose, flaccid pouch with numerous stones in a person with a very relaxed abdominal wall—a well-known surgeon described the palpation of gall stones in himself—and the hard top of the single large ovoid stone about which the walls of the gallbladder have contracted.

(*b*) *Cholecystitis.*—The simple form is common, and to it are due probably many of the symptoms of the gall stone attack. Phlegmonous cholecystitis is rare. Perforation may occur with fatal peritonitis. Chronic cholecystitis in some grade is common and many of the symptoms are due to it. Adhesions may form to the stomach, duodenum or colon. With infection of the common duct, the pancreatic ducts may be involved and chronic pancreatitis result. *Suppurative cholecystitis* is much less common, and in the great majority of cases is associated with gall stones. There may be enormous dilatation, and over a litre of pus has been found. Perforation and the formation of abscesses in the neighborhood are not uncommon.

(*c*) *Calcification* of the gallbladder may be a termination of the previous condition. There are two forms: incrustration of the mucosa with lime salts and the true infiltration of the wall with lime, the so-called ossification.

(*d*) *Atrophy* of the gallbladder is not uncommon. It shrinks into a small fibroid mass, not larger, perhaps, than a walnut, or even has the form of a narrow fibrous string; more commonly it tightly embraces a stone. This condition is usually preceded by hydrops of the bladder.

(*e*) Occasionally the gallbladder presents *diverticula,* which may be cut off from the main portion, and usually contain calculi.

Obstruction of the Common Duct.—There may be a single stone tightly wedged in the duct in any part of its course, or a series of stones, sometimes extending into both hepatic and cystic ducts, or a stone lies in the diverticulum of Vater. There are three groups of cases: (*a*) In rare instances a stone tightly corks the common duct, causing *permanent occlusion;* or it may partly rest in the cystic duct, and may have caused thickening of the junction of the ducts; or a big stone may compress the hepatic or upper part of the common duct. The jaundice is deep and enduring, and there are no septic features. The pains, the previous attacks of colic, and the absence of enlarged gallbladder help to separate the condition from obstruction by new growths, although it cannot be differentiated with certainty. The ducts are usually much dilated and everywhere contain a clear mucoid fluid.

(*b*) *Incomplete Obstruction, with Infective Cholangitis.*—There may be a series of stones in the common duct, a single stone which is freely movable, or a stone (ball-valve stone) in the diverticulum of Vater. These conditions may be found at autopsy, without the subjects having had symptoms pointing to gall stones; but in a majority there are characteristic features. The common duct may be as large as the thumb; the hepatic duct and its branches through the liver may be greatly dilated, and the distention may be apparent beneath the liver capsule. Great enlargement of the gallbladder is rarer. The mucous membrane of the ducts is usually smooth and clear, and the contents consist of a thin, slightly turbid bile-stained mucus. Operation may be the only possible method by which a diagnosis can be made.

Naunyn gave as the distinguishing signs of stone in the common duct: "(1) The continuous or occasional presence of bile in the feces; (2) distinct variations in the intensity of the jaundice; (3) normal size or only slight enlargement of the liver; (4) absence of distention of the gallbladder; (5) enlargement of the spleen; (6) absence of ascites; (7) presence of febrile disturbance; and (8) duration of the jaundice for more than a year."

In connection with the ball-valve stone, most common in the diverticulum of Vater, though it may be in the common duct itself, there is a special symptom group: (*a*) Paroxysms with chills, fever, and sweating; the *hepatic intermittent fever* of Charcot; (*b*) jaundice of varying intensity, which persists for months or even years, and deepens after each paroxysm; (*c*) at the time of the paroxysm, pain in the region of the liver with gastric disturbance. These symptoms may continue on and off for years, without the development of suppurative cholangitis. The rigors are of intense severity, and the temperature rises to 103° or 105° F. The chills may recur daily for weeks and be attributed to malaria. The jaundice is variable, and deepens after each paroxysm. The itching may be most intense. Pain, which is sometimes severe and colicky, does not always occur. There may be marked vomiting and nausea. As a rule there is no progressive deterioration of health. In the intervals between the attacks the temperature is normal.

The history and postmortem examinations show conclusively that this condition may persist for years without suppuration within the ducts. It is probable that the toxic symptoms develop only when a certain grade of tension is reached. A valuable diagnostic point is the absence of dilatation of the gallbladder in cases of obstruction from stone—Courvoisier's rule.

(*c*) *Incomplete Obstruction with Suppurative Cholangitis.*—When suppurative cholangitis exists the mucosa is thickened, often eroded or ulcerated; there may be extensive suppuration in the ducts throughout the liver, and even empyema of the gallbladder. Occasionally the suppuration extends beyond the ducts, and there is localized liver abscess or perforation of the gallbladder with the formation of abscess between the liver and stomach. Clinically it is characterized by fever which may be intermittent, but more commonly is remittent and without prolonged intervals of apyrexia. The jaundice is rarely so intense, nor does it deepen after the paroxysms. There is usually greater enlargement of the liver with tenderness and definite signs of septicemia. The course is shorter and recovery never takes place.

THE MORE REMOTE EFFECTS OF GALL STONES.—(*a*) *Biliary Fistulae.*—(1) *Cutaneous.*—The external fistula is the most common, 184 out of 384 cases (Naunyn). A majority occur in the region of the navel, to which part the falciform ligament directs the suppuration. The number of stones discharged varies from one to hundreds. Of 184 cases in Courvoisier's statistics recovery took place in 78. In rare instances the fistula is in the right iliac fossa or even in the thigh.

(2) *Gastro-intestinal Fistulae.*—The duodenal is the most frequent, 108 of 384 cases (Naunyn). Usually the opening is between the fundus of the gallbladder and the first part of the duodenum. A big stone may ulcerate through, leaving little or no damage. In other instances the cicatrization leads to obstruction. Communication with the ileum and jejunum is rare.

Fistulae between the common duct and the duodenum occurred in 15 cases in Naunyn's series. Biliary gastric fistulae are rare. The vomiting of gall stones is not necessarily proof of perforation, as in the majority of such cases the stones probably pass up through the pylorus.

(3) *Bronchobiliary Fistulae.*—Of J. E. Graham's collected series of 35 cases, 19 were due to gall stones; 11 to hydatids; 2 to roundworms; and in 2 the cause was doubtful. The amebic liver abscess perforating into the lung may be followed by a permanent biliary fistula.

(4) Perforation may occur into the *portal vein*, of which a few cases are on record; one, according to tradition, was the famous Ignatius Loyola.

(5) Perforation into the *hepatic artery* or one of its branches is exceedingly rare. Either an erosion from the common duct or an hepatic aneurism may rupture into the gallbladder.

(6) Fistula into the *urinary passages* may be with the pelvis of the kidney, in which a gall stone has been found, or into the urinary bladder.

(7) Lastly, the communication between the *pericardium* and the biliary tract is referred to by Naunyn in a single case.

(*b*) *Perforation into the Peritoneum.*—Of 119 cases (Courvoisier) in 70 the rupture occurred directly into the peritoneal cavity; in 49 an encapsulated abscess formed. As a rule, the condition is due to an acute cholecystitis.

(*c*) *Intestinal Obstruction by Gall Stones.*—Of 295 cases of obstruction, analyzed by Fitz, 23 were by gall stones. Of Courvoisier's 131 cases, in 6 the calculi had a peculiar situation, as in a diverticulum or in the appendix. Of the remaining 125 cases, in 70 the stone was spontaneously passed, usually with severe symptoms. The postmortem reports show that in some of these cases very large stones have passed, as the gall duct has been enormously distended, its orifice admitting the finger freely. This, however, is extremely rare. The stones have been found most commonly in the ileum.

Diagnosis.—The frequency of gall stones in those over 40 years of age, especially women, should be remembered. With hepatic colic or lodgment of a stone in the common duct diagnosis is usually easy but in many cases the symptoms are digestive and do not suggest gall stones. The persistence and variability of the digestive symptoms with little result from symptomatic treatment are important. The X-ray study by a competent man gives positive results in many cases; pure cholesterol stones do not show in X-ray plates. A study of the material obtained by bile-duct drainage may be of aid. The exclusion of organic stomach disease is usually not difficult. In some cases the diagnosis has to be made of gallbladder disease, the presence of gall stones being in doubt. The diagnosis from *coronary artery occlusion* is important. Formerly the usual error consisted in mistaking coronary occlusion for gallbladder disease but now the reverse error is more common. Myocardial change is common with gallbladder disease and there may be considerable circulatory disturbance with an attack of biliary colic. A complete study should prevent a mistake. Of course the two conditions may be combined.

Prognosis.—The outlook is always uncertain. Many patients carry gall stones for years without any severe symptoms and with good general health, as postmortem studies prove. There is always the danger of colic, blocking of a duct, severe infection, or of carcinoma developing. The influence on the patient's comfort and general health may be marked. The presence of gall stones is always a danger and after long duration the outlook with operation may be serious owing to complicating conditions. Certain statistics suggest that in general the outlook is much better in women than in men.

Treatment.—GENERAL.—The decision for or against surgical treatment must first be made. There are patients in whom the symptoms are so slight that consent to surgery is almost out of the question or the general condition is such that operation involves great risk. As a general rule the condition should be regarded as a surgical one; regret for early operation is rare but common for delay. The patient is safer in the hands of a good surgeon than left to Nature with the assistance that we can give. With persistent symptoms, general ill-health, repeated attacks of colic, or evidence of infection or obstruction of the bile passages, there should be no delay in advising operation. In mild cases the problem should be frankly stated to the patient for decision. Delay to try the effects of careful medical treatment may be accepted but should not be urged. It is most justifiable if the symptoms are recent and mild, without evidence of infection, in elderly patients in whom symptoms have been slight and perhaps have grown less, and in those in whom operation involves great risk.

Foci of infection should be treated and special attention given to the mouth. The patient should take regular exercise. The diet should be simple and in some cases a cholesterol free diet seems useful. (No eggs, liver, kidney or sweetbread and as little fat as possible.) Water should be taken freely. The soda salts are believed to prevent the concentration of the bile; the sulphate or the phosphate may be taken in doses of 1 to 2 drams daily before breakfast. Some form of salicylate may be useful; acetylsalicylic acid (gr. 5, 0.3 gm.) may be given four or five times a day. Hexamine (gr. 15, 1 gm.) four times a day is useful. An alkali, as sodium bicarbonate or magnesia, is sometimes of value and belladonna may relieve discomfort. For the itching McCall Anderson's dusting powder may be used: starch, an ounce (30 gm.); camphor, a dram and a half (6 gm.), and oxide of zinc, half an ounce (15 gm.). Powdering with starch, strong alkaline baths (hot), histamine hypodermically (0.25 milligram) twice a day, ergotamine tartrate (gr. 1/60, 0.001 gm.) 3 times a day, and antipyrin (gr. v, 0.3 gm.), may be tried. Menthol ointment (5 per cent) sometimes gives relief.

In an attack of biliary *colic* the patient should be kept under morphia, given hypodermically, in quarter-grain (0.016 gm.) doses. In an agonizing paroxysm it is well to give a whiff or two of chloroform until the morphia has had time to act. Great relief is experienced from a hot bath and fomentations in the region of the liver. The patient should be given laxatives and drink copiously of alkaline mineral waters. Olive oil has proved useless in our hands. Since the days of Durande, whose mixture of ether with turpentine is still used in France, various remedies have been advised to dissolve the stones within the gallbladder, none of which is efficacious.

Surgical treatment, especially if undertaken early, is usually satisfactory. The possibility of re-formation of stones is very slight. It is probable that in the majority of instances the stones do not re-form, but were incompletely removed. Deaver reports an instance in which 200 stones were removed two years after the extraction of 120. After removal of the gallbladder stones may be formed in the hepatic ducts.

THE CIRRHOSES OF THE LIVER

General Considerations.—The many forms of cirrhoses of the liver have one feature in common—an increase in the connective tissue. We use the term cirrhosis (by which Laënnec characterized the tawny, yellow color of the common portal form) to indicate similar changes in other organs.

Etiology.—There are five types of primary lesion, any one of which may lead to cirrhosis.

(1) *Toxic Cirrhosis.*—This is the only acute type and it is seen post-partum, in chloroform narcosis and sometimes as a terminal lesion in any form of disease. There is a central necrosis about the hepatic vein which may be slight in amount, or in some cases an acute yellow atrophy, very extensive so that the liver is rapidly reduced in size. Into the necrotic areas leukocytes migrate, the dead liver cells are quickly removed and there is an apparent increase of the connective tissue. Great regeneration of the liver cells is possible. Clinically this type can scarcely be spoken of as cirrhosis.

(2) *Infectious Cirrhosis.*—Adami and his school hold that colon bacilli from the bowel pass to the liver and there gradually excite a slow proliferation of connective tissue, regarding it as a kind of subinfection. Mallory thinks that the only type of true infectious cirrhosis is through the bile ducts, usually when there is bile stasis or gall stones or other obstructions are present. Cases are described in which invasion occurs along apparently normal bile ducts, the organisms causing necrosis of the liver cells, proliferation of fibroblasts, and thickening of the walls of the smaller bile ducts which may be dilated and tortuous. Clinically this type is rare, and characterized by chronic jaundice and enlargement of the liver.

(3) *Pigment Cirrhosis.*—This may be an external pigment as in anthracosis in which the irritation of the coal particles reaching the liver through the lymphatics may excite a moderate grade of cirrhosis. The endogenous pigment is a transformation of hemoglobin as in malaria or hemochromatosis.

(4) *Syphilitic Cirrhosis.*—Whether congenital or acquired, the lesion is a diffuse proliferation of fibroblasts, or a more localized lesion, the gumma.

(5) *Alcoholic Cirrhosis.*—The liver cells, singly or in groups, undergo a slow necrosis, followed by a multiplication of the fibroblasts with hyalin degeneration of some cells and multiplication of others and increase in the smaller bile ducts. With fatty infiltration the organ may be enlarged.

Of these types the toxic and one form of the alcoholic are associated with contraction, the infectious, the pigmentary and the fatty cirrhosis with enlargement of the organ. Clinically we may consider four forms, the portal, the hypertrophic (of Hanot), the syphilitic, and the capsular.

PORTAL CIRRHOSIS

Etiology.—The disease occurs most frequently in middle-aged males who have been addicted to drink. Whisky, gin, and brandy are more potent to cause cirrhosis than beer. It is more common in countries in which strong spirits are used than in those in which malt liquors are taken. It is not always due to alcohol. Symmers believes that syphilis is an important factor in the etiology of the Laënnec cirrhosis. Among 1,000 autopsies in the Johns Hopkins Hospital there were 63 cases of small cirrhotic liver, and 8 cases of the fatty cirrhotic organ. The influence of chronic infection is probably an important factor. Any toxic agent which reaches the liver continuously or repeatedly tends to produce cirrhosis. Probably in many cases several factors combine to cause a chronic progressive hepatitis.

Cirrhosis of the liver in young children is not very rare. In a certain number of the cases there is an alcoholic history, in others syphilis has been present, while a third group, due to the infectious diseases, embraces a certain number of the cases of Hanot's hypertrophic cirrhosis.

Morbid Anatomy.—Portal cirrhosis occurs in two well-characterized forms: THE ATROPHIC CIRRHOSIS OF LAENNEC.—The organ is greatly reduced in size and may be deformed. The weight is sometimes not more than a pound or a pound and a half. It presents numerous granulations on the surface; is firm, hard, and cuts with great resistance. The substance is seen to be made up of greenish-yellow islands surrounded by grayish-white connective tissue. W. G. MacCallum has shown that regenerative changes in the cells are almost constantly present.

THE FATTY CIRRHOTIC LIVER.—Even in the contracted form the fat is increased, but in typical examples of this variety the organ is enlarged, smooth or very slightly granular, anemic, yellowish-white in color, and resembles an ordinary fatty liver. It is firm, cuts with resistance, and shows a great increase in the connective tissue. This form occurs most frequently in beer-drinkers.

The essential elements in cirrhosis are destruction of liver cells with fibrosis and obstruction to the portal circulation.

In a case of cirrhosis with contraction the peritoneum often contains a large quantity of fluid, the membrane is opaque, and there is chronic catarrh of the stomach and small intestines. The spleen is enlarged, in part, at least, from chronic congestion, possibly due in part to a toxic influence. The pancreas frequently shows interstitial changes. The kidneys are sometimes sclerotic, the bases of the lungs may be compressed by the ascitic fluid, the heart often shows marked degeneration, and arteriosclerosis is usually present. A remarkable feature is the association of acute *tuberculosis* with cirrhosis. Rolleston found that tuberculosis was present in 29 per cent of 706 fatal cases of cirrhosis. Peritoneal tuberculosis was found in 9 per cent of 584 cases.

The compensatory circulation is carried out by the following vessels: (1) The accessory portal system of Sappey, of which important branches pass in the round and suspensory ligaments and unite with the epigastric and mammary systems. These vessels are numerous and small. Occasionally a large single vein, which may attain the size of the little finger, passes from the hilus of the liver, follows the round ligament, and joins the epigastric veins at the navel. Although this has the position of the umbilical vein, it is usually a para-umbilical vein—that is, an enlarged vein by the side of the obliterated umbilical vessel. Rarely there is about the navel a bunch of varices, the so-called caput Medusae. Other branches of this system occur in the gastro-epiploic omentum, about the gallbladder, and, most important of all, in the suspensory ligament. These latter form large branches, which anastomose freely with the diaphragmatic veins, and so unite with the vena azygos. (2) By the anastomosis between the esophageal and gastric veins. The veins at the lower end of the esophagus may be enormously enlarged, producing varices. (3) The communications between the hemorrhoidal and the inferior mesenteric veins. The freedom of communication here is variable, and the hemorrhoidal veins may not be much enlarged. (4) The veins of Retzius, which unite the radicles of the portal branches in the intestines and mesentery with the inferior vena cava and its branches. To this system belongs the whole group of retroperitoneal veins, which are in most instances enormously enlarged, particularly about the kidneys, and which carry a considerable proportion of the portal blood.

Symptoms.—The most extreme grade of portal cirrhosis may exist without symptoms. *So long as the compensatory circulation is maintained* the patient may suffer little or no inconvenience. The remarkable efficiency of this collateral circulation is well seen in those rare instances of permanent obliteration of the portal vein. The symptoms may be divided into two groups—obstructive and toxic.

Obstructive.—The overfilling of the blood vessels of the stomach and intestine leads to chronic catarrh, and the patients suffer with nausea and vomiting, particularly in the morning; the tongue is furred and the bowels are irregular. Hematemesis may be an early feature; it is often profuse and liable to recur but seldom proves fatal. The amount vomited may be remarkable; one patient vomited ten pounds in seven days. Melena is common and hemorrhages from the bowels may occur for several years without hematemesis. The bleeding very often comes from esophageal varices. Epistaxis sometimes occurs. Enlargement of the *spleen* may be due to toxemia. The organ can usually be felt. Evidences of the establishment of the collateral circulation are seen in the enlarged epigastric and mammary veins, more rarely in the presence of the caput Medusae and the development of hemorrhoids. The distended venules in the lower thoracic zone along the line of attachment of the diaphragm are not specially marked in cirrhosis. The most striking feature of failure in the compensatory circulation is *ascites*, the effusion of serous fluid into the peritoneal cavity, which may appear suddenly. The conditions under which this occurs are obscure. In some cases it is due more to chronic peritonitis and perihepatitis than to the cirrhosis. The abdomen gradually distends, may reach a large size, and contain 15 to 20 litres. Edema of the feet may precede or develop with the ascites. The dropsy is rarely general.

Jaundice is usually slight and may be transient; it occurs in about one-third of the cases. The skin has frequently a sallow, slightly icteroid tint. The gastric secretions are usually reduced and there may be achlorhydria. The urine is often reduced in amount, contains urates in abundance, often a slight amount of albumin, and, if jaundice is intense, casts. The disease may be afebrile throughout, but in many cases there is slight fever. The liver functional tests may show marked decrease. The *blood* of some patients shows a rather high color index and the average size of the red cells may be greater than normal.

Examination at an early stage may show an enlarged and painful liver. In many of the cases of portal cirrhosis the organ is "enlarged at all stages of the disease, and, whether enlarged or contracted, the clinical symptoms and course are much the same" (Foxwell). A decrease in the size of the liver under observation may be a striking feature. The patient may first come under observation for dyspepsia, hematemesis, slight jaundice, or nervous symptoms. Later in the course the patient has an unmistakable hepatic facies; he is thin, the eyes are sunken, the conjunctivae watery, the nose and cheeks show distended venules, and the complexion is muddy or icteroid. On the enlarged abdomen the vessels are distended, and a bunch of dilated veins may surround the navel. A *venous hum*, sometimes accompanied by a thrill, may be heard in the epigastrium or over varicosities. *Nevi* of a remarkable character may appear on the skin, either localized stellate varices—spider angiomata—usually on the face, neck, and back, and also "mat" nevi—areas of skin of a reddish or purplish color due to the uniform distention of small venules. When much fluid is in the peritoneum it is impossible to make a satisfactory examination, but after withdrawal the area of liver dulness can be determined and on deep pressure the edge of the liver may be detected, and occasionally the hard, firm, and even granular surface. The spleen is palpable in about 75 per cent of the cases. Examination of the anus may show hemorrhoids.

Toxic Symptoms.—At any stage the patient may have cerebral symptoms, a noisy delirium, or stupor, coma, or even convulsions. The condition is not infrequently mistaken for uremia. The nature of the toxic agent is not settled. Without jaundice, and not attributable to cholemia, the symptoms may come on when the patient has not had alcohol for weeks.

The fatty cirrhotic liver may produce symptoms similar to those of the contracted form, but more frequently it is latent and is found accidentally in topers who have died from various diseases. A number of the cases clinically diagnosed as cirrhosis with enlargement come in this division.

Diagnosis.—In the early stages one can only be suspicious. With ascites, a well-marked history of alcoholism, the hepatic facies, and hemorrhage from the stomach or bowels, the diagnosis is rarely doubtful. If, after withdrawal of the fluid, the spleen is found to be enlarged and the liver either not palpable or, if it is enlarged, hard and regular, the probabilities in favor of cirrhosis are very great. In the early stages, when the liver is increased in size, it may be impossible to say whether it is a cirrhotic or a fatty liver. The differential diagnosis between common and syphilitic cirrhosis can usually be made. A history of syphilis or the existence of other syphilitic lesions, with irregularity on the surface or at the edge of the liver, and relatively greater enlargement of the left lobe, are in favor of the latter. Thrombosis or obliteration of the portal vein can rarely be differentiated. In a case of fibroid transformation of the portal vein, the collateral circulation had been established for years, and the symptoms were simply those of extreme portal obstruction, such as occur in cirrhosis. Thrombosis of the portal vein may occur in cirrhosis and be characterized by a rapidly developing ascites. The cardiac liver is usually easily recognized. Splenic anemia with cirrhosis may give difficulty, but the degree of splenomegaly, marked secondary anemia and leukopenia are usually distinctive.

Prognosis.—The outlook is bad. In alcoholic patients much depends on the ability to give up the use of alcohol. When the collateral circulation is fully established the patient may have no symptoms whatever. There are instances of enlargement of the liver, slight jaundice, cerebral symptoms, and even hematemesis, in which the liver becomes reduced in size, the symptoms disappear, and the patient may live in comparative comfort for years. There are cases, too, possibly syphilitic, in which, after one or two tappings, the symptoms disappear and the patients apparently recovered. The occurrence of fever and toxic symtoms, nephritis and acute tuberculous disease are ominous. Ascites is a serious event, especially if due to cirrhosis alone and not to an associated peritonitis. Of 34 cases with ascites 10 died before tapping was necessary; 14 were tapped, and the average duration of life after the swelling was first noticed was only eight weeks; of 10 cases the diagnosis was wrong in 4, and in the remaining 6, who were tapped oftener than once, chronic peritonitis and perihepatitis were present (Hale-White).

HYPERTROPHIC BILIARY CIRRHOSIS (*Hanot*)

This form was first described by Requin in 1846, but our accurate knowledge of it dates from the work of Hanot (1875), whose name it bears in France—*maladie de Hanot.* It is a rare disease.

Cirrhosis with enlargement occurs in portal cirrhosis; there is an enlarged fatty and cirrhotic liver of alcoholics, a pigmentary form occurs in hemochromatosis, and in syphilis the organ is often very large. The hypertrophic cirrhosis of Hanot is easily distinguished from these forms.

Etiology.—Males are more often affected than females—in 22 of Schachmann's 26 cases. The subjects are young; some of the cases in children probably belong to this form. Alcohol plays a minor part and not one of our patients had been a heavy drinker. The etiology is obscure; chronic infection may be responsible. Two of our patients were brothers.

Morbid Anatomy.—The organ is enlarged, weighing from 2,000 to 4,000 grams. The form is maintained, the surface is smooth, or presents small granulations; the color in advanced cases is of a dark olive green; the consistence is greatly increased. The section is uniform, greenish yellow in color, and the liver nodules may be seen separated by connective tissue. The bile-passages present nothing abnormal. The cirrhosis is mono- or multilobular, with a connective tissue rich in round cells. The bile vessels are the seat of cholangitis, catarrhal and productive, and there is an extraordinary development of new biliary canaliculi. The liver cells are neither fatty nor pigmented, and may be increased in size and show karyokinetic figures. From the supposed origin about the bile vessels it has been called biliary cirrhosis. The spleen is greatly enlarged and may weigh 600 or more grams.

Symptoms.—The cases occur in young persons; there is not, as a rule, an alcoholic history, and males are usually affected. The features are: (*a*) A remarkably *chronic course* of from four to six, or even ten years. (*b*) *Jaundice,* usually slight, often not more than a lemon tint, or a tinging of the conjunctivae. At any time during the course an *icterus gravis,* with high fever and delirium, may develop. There is bile in the urine; the stools are not clay colored as in obstructive jaundice but may be very dark. (*c*) Attacks of *pain* in the region of the liver, which may be severe and associated with nausea and vomiting. The pain may be slight and dragging, and in some cases is not prominent. The jaundice may deepen after attacks of pain. (*d*) *Enlarged liver.* A fullness in the upper abdominal zone may be the first complaint and the enlargement may be very marked. In one of our cases the left lobe was unusually prominent and stood out almost like a tumor. Exploration showed only an enlarged, smooth organ without adhesions. On palpation the hypertrophy is uniform, the consistence is increased, and the edge distinct and hard. The gallbladder is not enlarged. The flatness is much increased and may extend from the sixth rib to the level of the navel. (*e*) The spleen is enlarged, easily palpable, and very hard. (*f*) Certain negative features are of moment—the usual absence of ascites and of dilatation of the subcutaneous veins of the abdomen. Among other symptoms may be mentioned hemorrhages. One patient had bleeding at the gums for a year; another had had for years most remarkable attacks of purpura with urticaria. Pruritus, xanthoma, lichen, and telangiectasis may be present in the skin. The skin may become very bronzed, almost as deeply as in Addison's disease. Slight *fever* may be present, which increases during the crises of pain. There may be a marked leukocytosis. A curious attitude of the body has been seen, in which the right shoulder and right side appear dragged down. The patients die from icterus gravis, from hemorrhage, from an intercurrent infection, or in profound cachexia. Certain cases of cirrhosis of the liver in children are of this type; the enlargement of the spleen may be very pronounced.

Diagnosis.—The chronicity, the age, the jaundice with enlarged liver and spleen, and the absence of ascites aid in the distinction from portal cirrhosis with enlargement. Splenic anemia should not give difficulty, the blood findings, the absence of jaundice (except with a small liver), and the absence of marked hepatic enlargement should be distinctive. The marked smooth enlargement of syphilis may cause error if its possibility is not considered.

SYPHILITIC CIRRHOSIS

This is considered in the section on syphilis (p. 265). It is referred to again to emphasize (1) its frequency; (2) the great importance of its differentiation from the alcoholic form; (3) its curability in many cases; and (4) the tumor formations in connection with it.

CAPSULAR CIRRHOSIS—PERIHEPATITIS

Local capsulitis is common in many conditions of the liver. The form of disease here described is characterized by an enormous thickening of the entire capsule, with great contraction of the liver, but not necessarily with special increase in the connective tissue of the organ itself. Our chief knowledge of the disease we owe to Guy's Hospital physicians, particularly Hilton Fagge and Hale-White. The liver substance itself was "never markedly cirrhotic; its tissue was nearly always soft." Chronic capsulitis of the spleen and a chronic proliferative peritonitis are almost invariably present. In 19 of 22 cases the kidneys were granular; some regard it as a sequel of sclerotic nephritis. The symptoms are those of portal cirrhosis—*ascites,* often recurring and requiring many tappings. Jaundice is not often present. There are two groups of cases —the one in adults usually with ascites is regarded as ordinary cirrhosis and the diagnosis is rarely made. Signs of sclerotic nephritis, recurring ascites, and absence of jaundice are important diagnostic points. In the second group the perihepatitis, perisplenitis, and proliferative peritonitis are associated with adherent pericardium and chronic mediastinitis. In one such case the diagnosis of capsular hepatitis was very clear, as the liver could be grasped in the hand and formed a rounded, smooth organ resembling the spleen. The child was tapped 121 times.

Treatment of the Cirrhoses.—The portal function of the liver may be put out of action without much damage to the body. There may be an extreme grade of cirrhotic atrophy without symptoms; the portal vein may be obliterated, or, experimentally, the portal vein may be anastomosed with the cava. So long as there is an active compensatory circulation a patient with portal cirrhosis may remain well. In the biliary form toxemia is the special danger and we have no means of arresting the progress of the disease. In the alcoholic form it is too late, as a rule, to do much after symptoms have occurred. In a few cases an attack of jaundice or hematemesis may prove the salvation of the patient, who may afterward take to a temperate life. The *diet* should be very simple (largely milk and milk foods, simple carbohydrates and fruits). The amount of fluid must be decided for each patient. Some do best with moderate amounts. Others are better with the smallest quantity which is possible with comfort and a low or salt-free diet. A high carbohydrate diet with insulin may be helpful. Alcohol and highly spiced foods should be forbidden. The bowels should be kept open, for which the use of the salines is generally best; drastic purgation should be avoided. An occasional course of iodide may be given. With the advent of ascites the critical stage is reached. Restriction of fluid intake and free purgation may relieve a small exudate, rarely a large one, and it is best to tap early. In the syphilitic cirrhosis much more can be done, and a majority of the cases of cure after ascites are of this variety. Iodide in moderate doses, 5 to 10 drops of the saturated solution, and mercury save a number of cases. The diagnosis may be reached only after removal of the fluid, but in every case with a suspicion of syphilis, or with irregularity of the liver this treatment should be tried.

(*a*) *Tapping.*—When the ascites increases it is better to tap early. As Hale-White remarks, a patient with portal cirrhosis alone who is tapped rarely recovers, but there are instances in which early and repeated paracentesis is followed by cure. Accidents are rare; hemorrhage, acute peritonitis, or erysipelas at the point of puncture occasionally follow; collapse may occur during the operation, to guard against which Mead advised the use of the abdominal binder. Continuous drainage with Southey's tubes has no special advantages. (*b*) *Laparotomy*, with complete removal of the fluid, and freshening or rubbing the peritoneal surfaces, to stimulate the formation of adhesions. (*c*) *Omentopexy*, the stitching of the omentum to the abdominal wall, and the establishment of collateral circulation in this way between the portal and the systemic vessels. This operation is sometimes successful. In 224 cases there were 84 deaths and 129 recoveries; 11 cases doubtful. Among the 129 successful cases, in 25 the ascites recurred; 70 appeared to have completely recovered. (*d*) *Fistula of Eck.* The portocaval anastomosis has been performed in cirrhosis of the liver; one patient lived for three months. (*e*) *Autodrainage*, in which the fluid is drained into the subcutaneous tissues.

ABSCESS OF THE LIVER

Etiology.—Suppuration within the liver, either in the parenchyma or in the blood or bile passages, occurs under the following conditions:

(*a*) The *tropical abscess*, also called the *solitary*, commonly follows amebic dysentery. Cases may occur without a history of previous dysentery, and there have been fatal cases without any affection of the large bowel. In the

United States the large solitary abscess is not very infrequent. The relation of this form of abscess to amebic dysentery has been considered. The number of cases has been much reduced since the introduction of the emetine treatment.

(*b*) *Trauma* is an occasional cause. The injury is generally in the hepatic region. Injury to the head may be followed by liver abscess.

(*c*) *Embolic or pyemic abscesses* occur in pyemia or following foci of suppuration in the territory of the portal vessels. The infective agents may reach the liver through the hepatic artery, as when the original focus is in the area of the systemic circulation; though occasionally the infective agent, instead of passing through the lungs, reaches the liver through the inferior vena cava and the hepatic veins. A remarkable instance of multiple abscesses of arterial origin was shown in the case of aneurism of the hepatic artery reported by Ross and Osler. Infection through the portal vein is more common as from dysentery and other ulcerative affections of the bowels, appendicitis, occasionally with typhoid fever, in rectal affections, and in abscesses in the pelvis. In these cases the abscesses are multiple and, as a rule, within the branches of the portal vein—*suppurative pylephlebitis.*

(*d*) *Inflammation of the bile passages* may be caused by the infection with gall stones, more rarely by parasites—*suppurative cholangitis.* In some cases of tuberculosis of the liver the affection is chiefly of the bile ducts, with the formation of multiple tuberculous abscesses containing a bile-stained pus.

(*e*) *Foreign Bodies and Parasites.*—In rare instances foreign bodies, such as a needle, may pass from the stomach or gullet, lodge in the liver, and excite an abscess, or a foreign body, such as a needle or a fish-bone, has perforated a branch of the portal vein itself and induced pylephlebitis. Echinococcus cysts may cause suppuration, the penetration of round worms into the liver less commonly, and most rarely of all the liver fluke.

Morbid Anatomy.—(*a*) The Amebic Abscess.—This has been described under amebic dysentery.

(*b*) Of Septic and Pyemic Abscesses.—These are usually multiple, though occasionally, following injury, there may be a large solitary abscess.

In *suppurative pylephlebitis* the liver is uniformly enlarged. The capsule may be smooth and the external surface of normal appearance. On section there are isolated pockets of pus, either having a rounded outline or in some places distinctly dendritic, and from these the pus may be squeezed. The entire portal system within the liver may be involved; sometimes territories are cut off by thrombi. The suppuration may extend into the main branch or even into the mesenteric and gastric veins. In *suppurative cholangitis* there is usually obstruction by gall stones, the ducts are greatly distended, the gall-bladder enlarged and full of pus, and the branches within the liver are extremely distended, having an appearance not unlike that described in pylephlebitis. An abscess may have a sponge-like appearance due to the fusion of numerous points of suppuration. Suppuration about echinococcus cysts may be very extensive, forming enormous abscesses, the character of which is at once recognized by the remnants of the cysts.

Symptoms.—(*a*) Large Solitary Abscess.—This may be latent and without definite symptoms; death may occur suddenly from rupture. Fever, pain, enlargement of the liver, and a septic condition are the important symptoms.

The temperature is elevated at the outset and is of an intermittent or septic type. It is irregular, and may remain normal or even subnormal for a few days; then the patient has a rigor and the temperature rises to 103° F. or higher. Owing to this intermittent fever the disease may be mistaken for malaria. The fever may rise every afternoon without a chill. Profuse sweating is common, particularly when the patient falls asleep. In chronic cases there may be little or no fever. Patients with a liver abscess perforating the lung may cough up pus after the temperature has been normal for weeks. The *pain* is variable and usually referred to the back or shoulder; or there is a dull aching sensation in the right hypochondrium. When turned on the left side, the patient often complains of a heavy, dragging sensation, so that he usually prefers to lie on the right side. Pain on pressure over the liver is usually present, particularly on deep pressure at the costal margin in the nipple line.

The *enlargement* of the liver is most marked in the right lobe, and, as the abscess cavity is usually situated more toward the upper surface, the increase in volume is upward and to the right, not downward, as in cancer and other affections producing enlargement. Percussion in the midsternal and parasternal lines may show a normal limit. At the nipple-line the curve of liver dulness begins to rise, and in the midaxilla it may reach the fifth rib, while behind the dulness may be almost on a level with the angle of the scapula. The breath sounds at the right base are feeble, and with the fluoroscope the right side of the diaphragm is seen to be high. There are instances in which this characteristic feature is not present, as when the abscess occupies the left lobe. The enlargement of the liver may be so great as to cause bulging of the right side, and the edge may project a hand's-breadth or more below the costal margin. In such instances the surface is smooth. Palpation is painful, and there may be fremitus on deep inspiration. In some instances fluctuation may be detected. Adhesions may form to the abdominal wall and the abscess may point below the margin of the ribs, or even in the epigastric region.

In many cases the appearance of the patient is suggestive. The skin has a sallow, slightly icteroid tint, the face is pale, the complexion muddy, the conjunctivae are infiltrated, and often slightly bile-tinged. There is no internal affection associated with suppuration which gives just the same hue as certain instances of abscess of the liver. Marked jaundice is rare. Diarrhea may be present and give an important clue to the nature of the case, particularly if amebae are found in the stools. Constipation may occur. There is usually a polymorphonuclear leukocytosis.

Perforation of the lung may occur. The extension may be through the diaphragm, without actual rupture, and with the production of a purulent pleurisy and invasion of the lung. With cough of an aggravated and convulsive character, there are signs of involvement at the base of the right lung, defective resonance, feeble tubular breathing, and change in the tactile fremitus. There may be little to suggest the hepatic abscess.

The abscess may perforate externally or into the stomach or bowel; occasionally into the pericardium. The duration of this form is very variable. Some very acute cases occur; more often it proves fatal in six or eight weeks or may persist for several years.

The prognosis is always serious.

(*b*) Pyemic Abscess and Suppurative Pylephlebitis.—Clinically these conditions cannot be separated. Occurring in a general pyemia, no special features may be added. When there is suppuration within the portal vein the liver is uniformerly enlarged and tender, though pain may not be a marked feature. There is an irregular, septic fever, and the complexion is muddy, sometimes distinctly icteroid. The special features are those of pyemia, plus a slight icteroid tinge, and an enlarged and painful liver. The sweats, chills, prostration, and fever have nothing distinctive.

Diagnosis.—Abscess of the liver may be confounded with malarial fever but a proper study should prevent this. Practically an *intermittent fever* which resists quinine is not malarial. Exploratory aspiration is of value in case of extension of dulness upward, done in the axilla or back. A negative result does not exclude abscess. When the abscess bursts into the pleura a right-sided empyema is produced and perforation of the lung usually follows. When the liver abscess has been latent and dysenteric symptoms have not been marked, the condition may be considered as empyema or abscess of the lung. In such cases the anchovy-sauce color of the pus and the presence of amebae will enable one to make a definite diagnosis. Perforation externally is readily recognized, and yet in an abscess cavity in the epigastric region it may be difficult to say whether it has proceeded from the liver or is in the abdominal wall. When the abscess is large, and the adhesions are so firm that the liver does not descend during inspiration, the exploratory needle does not make an up-and-down movement. The diagnosis of suppurating echinococcus cyst is rarely possible, except in Australia and Iceland, where the hydatids are so common. Cases of *syphilis* of the liver have been regarded as abscess, as the fever may be high and intermittent. Knowledge of the possibility is the best safeguard.

Perhaps the most important affection which causes difficulty is the *intermittent fever* associated with gall stones. Postmortem examinations have shown conclusively that high fever and chills may recur at intervals for years without suppuration in the ducts. The distinctive features of this condition are paroxysms of fever with rigors and sweats—which may occur with great regularity, but which often are separated by long intervals—the deepening of the jaundice after the paroxysms, the entire apyrexia in the intervals, and the maintenance of the general nutrition. The time element is important, as in some cases the disease has lasted for several years. Finally, it is to be remembered that abscess of the liver, in temperate climates at least, is invariably secondary, and the primary source must be carefully sought for in dysentery, ulceration of the rectum, suppurating hemorrhoids, ulcer of the stomach, or in suppurative disease elsewhere, particularly within the skull or in the bones. Leukocytosis may be absent in amebic abscess of the liver; in septic cases it may be very high.

Treatment.—If there is evidence of amebic hepatitis or abscess, active treatment with emetine should be given, as the need for operation may be prevented. Pyemic abscess and suppurative pylephlebitis are invariably fatal. Treves reported a case of pyemic abscess following appendicitis in which the patient recovered after an exploratory operation. Surgical measures are not justified in these cases, unless an abscess shows signs of pointing. As the abscesses associated with dysentery are often single, they afford a reasonable hope of benefit from operation. If, however, the patient is expectorating the pus, if the general condition is good and the fever not marked, it is best to defer operation, as many recover spontaneously. The large single abscesses are the most favorable for operation. The general medical treatment is that of ordinary septicemia.

NEW GROWTHS IN THE LIVER

Etiology.—Cancer of the liver is third in order of frequency of internal cancer. It is rarely primary, usually secondary to cancer in other organs. It is a disease of late adult life. It occasionally occurs in children and there have been a few cases in infants. Women are attacked less frequently than men but secondary cancer is more common in women, owing to the frequency of cancer of the uterus and breast. In many cases trauma is an antecedent, and cancer of the gallbladder is associated in many instances with gallstones. Cancer is stated to be less common in the tropics.

Morbid Anatomy.—The following forms of new growths occur in the liver and have a clinical importance:

CANCER.—*Primary Cancer.*—This is rare; of 134 cases reported by Tull, in 99 the growth was of the liver cell (hepatoma) type and in 35 of the bile duct (cholangioma) type. There are nodular forms, in which there are scattered growths throughout the organ, and the massive form in which the solitary tumor occupies a large area, either a lobe or the greater part of it. A considerable number of the cases occur with cirrhosis—the so-called *cancer with cirrhosis.* The course is rapid, jaundice often occurs, splenic enlargement is not infrequent, ascites and edema are common and toxic features are frequent toward the close.

Secondary Cancer.—The organ may reach an enormous size, 30½ pounds (Osler), 33 pounds (Christian). The cancerous nodules project beneath the capsule, and can be felt during life or seen through thin abdominal walls. They are usually disseminated equally, though rarely they are confined to one lobe. The consistence of the nodule varies; in some cases they are firm and hard and those on the surface show a distinct umbilication, due to the shrinking of the fibrous tissue in the centre. These superficial masses are sometimes spoken of as "Farre's tubercles." More frequently the masses are on section grayish-white in color or hemorrhagic. Rupture of blood vessels is not uncommon; in one case there was an enormous clot beneath the capsule of the liver, with hemorrhage into the gallbladder and peritoneum. The secondary cancer shows the same structure as the initial lesion, and is usually an alveolar or cylindrical carcinoma. Degeneration is common in the secondary growths; thus hyaline transformation may convert large areas into a dense, dry, grayish-yellow mass. Extensive areas of fatty degeneration may occur, sclerosis is not uncommon, and hemorrhages are frequent. Suppuration sometimes follows.

PRIMARY ADENOMA.—Gordinier and Sawyer collected 44 cases, 28 of which were multiple, and of these 21 were associated with portal cirrhosis. In a majority of the cases the process appears to be secondary to a cirrhosis, a compensatory cell hypertrophy to offset the destruction of the liver cells. In some cases, however, it may be a primary affair. The clinical picture is that of cirrhosis, often of the Hanot type.

Sarcoma.—Of primary sarcoma few cases have been reported. Secondary sarcoma is more frequent, lymphosarcoma and myxosarcoma, less frequently gliosarcoma or the smooth or striped myoma. The most important form is the *melanosarcoma,* secondary to sarcoma of the eye or skin. Very rarely melanosarcoma occurs primarily in the liver. In this form the liver is greatly enlarged, is either uniformly infiltrated with the growth, which gives the cut surface the appearance of dark granite, or there are large nodular masses of a deep black or marbled color. There are usually extensive metastases and in some instances every organ of the body is involved. Nodules of melanosarcoma of the skin may give a clue to the diagnosis.

Other Forms of Liver Tumor.—Angioma occurs as a small, reddish body the size of a walnut, and consists simply of a series of dilated vessels. Occasionally angiomata grow and produce large tumors.

Cysts are occasionally found, either single, which is not very uncommon, or multiple, when they usually coexist with congenital cystic kidneys.

Symptoms.—It is often impossible to differentiate primary and secondary cancer of the liver unless the primary seat of the disease is evident. As a rule, cancer of the liver is associated with progressive enlargement; but in some cases of primary nodular cancer and in the cancer with cirrhosis the organ may not be enlarged. Gastric disturbance, loss of appetite, nausea and vomiting are frequent. Progressive loss of flesh and strength may be the first symptoms. *Pain* or a sensation of uneasiness in the right hypochondriac region may be present, but enormous enlargement of the liver may occur without any pain. *Jaundice,* which is present in at least half of the cases, is usually moderate, unless the common duct is occluded. *Ascites* is rare, except in the form of cancer with cirrhosis, in which the picture is that of cirrhosis with contraction. Pressure by nodules on the portal vein or extension of the cancer to the peritoneum may induce ascites.

Inspection shows the abdomen to be distended, particularly in the upper zone. In late stages, when emaciation is marked, the cancerous nodules can be plainly seen beneath the skin, and in rare instances even the umbilications. The superficial veins are enlarged. On palpation the liver is usually felt below the costal margin, descending with each inspiration. The surface is usually irregular, and may present large masses or smaller nodular bodies, either rounded or with central depressions. With diffuse infiltration the liver may be greatly enlarged and present a smooth surface. The growth is progressive, and the edge of the liver may ultimately extend below the level of the navel. Although generally uniform and producing enlargement of the whole organ, occasionally a tumor in the left lobe forms a mass occupying the epigastrium. By percussion the outline can be accurately limited and the progressive growth estimated. The spleen is rarely enlarged. *Fever* is present in many cases, usually continuous, ranging from 100° to 102° F.; it may be intermittent, with rigors. This may be associated with cancer alone or with suppuration. Edema of the feet, from anemia, usually supervenes. Cancer of the liver kills in from three to fifteen months. One of our patients lived for more than two years.

Diagnosis.—This is easy when the liver is greatly enlarged and the surface nodular. The smoother forms of diffuse carcinoma may be mistaken for fatty or amyloid liver, but jaundice, rapid enlargement, and more marked cachexia usually suffice to differentiate it. Perhaps the most puzzling conditions occur in the cases of enlarged syphilitic liver with irregular gummata. The large echinococcus liver may suggest carcinoma, but the nodules are usually softer, the disease lasts longer, and cachexia is not marked. Hydatid disease is usually localized and the general condition is better. With marked ascites the diagnosis from cirrhosis or syphilis may be difficult. The patient should be tapped and palpation done at once. The cirrhotic liver is less irregular and the spleen is often enlarged. If fever is marked an acute infection may be suspected. Careful search should always be made for primary growth.

Hypertrophic biliary cirrhosis may be mistaken for carcinoma, as the jaundice is usually deep and the liver large; but the absence of a marked cachexia and wasting and the painless, smooth character of the enlargement are against cancer. In large, rapidly growing secondary cancers the superficial rounded mass may almost fluctuate and these soft tumor-like projections may contain blood. The *cancer with cirrhosis* can scarcely be separated from cirrhosis itself. Perhaps the wasting is more extreme and more rapid, but the jaundice and ascites are identical. *Melanosarcoma* causes great enlargement and there are frequently symptoms of involvement of other viscera. Secondary tumors may occur in the skin. A very important symptom, not present in all cases, is the passage of a very dark-colored urine, which may, when first voided, be normal in color. A melanosarcoma of the eye, or the history of blindness in one eye, with subsequent extirpation, may indicate the true nature of the hepatic enlargement.

There are several conditions in which the liver itself, or portions of it, may be mistaken for cancer. (*a*) In syphilis the left lobe may increase out of all proportion to the right, and form a prominent mass in the epigastrium. (*b*) Riedel's tongue-like lobe in the neighborhood of the gallbladder, and often associated with distention of this organ. (*c*) The extreme left portion of the organ may be almost separated by a broad, flat band, containing little or no liver tissue. In a very thin person this may feel like a separate tumor mass. A small portion of the liver may rest directly upon the celiac axis, connected with the left lobe by a mesentery. Lastly, the contracted, deformed organ in perihepatitis may form a visible, freely movable tumor in the upper portion of the abdomen, without a semblance of the normal liver. Such an instance is figured in Osler's lectures on Abdominal Tumors.

Treatment.—Resection of tumors of the liver has been performed in some cases. Otherwise the treatment is symptomatic—any desired diet, keeping the bowels open, tapping if necessary and sufficient sedatives.

FATTY LIVER

Two different forms are recognized—fatty infiltration and fatty degeneration. Fatty *infiltration* occurs, to a certain extent, in normal livers, since the cells always contain minute globules of oil. In fatty *degeneration*, which is much less common, the protoplasm of the liver cells is destroyed and the fat takes its place, as in malignant jaundice and phosphorus poisoning.

Fatty liver occurs under the following conditions: (*a*) With general obesity, in which the liver appears to be one of the storehouses of the excessive fat. (*b*) In conditions in which oxidation processes are decreased, as in cachexia, profound anemia and pulmonary tuberculosis. The fatty infiltration of the liver in heavy drinkers is to be attributed to the excessive demand made by the alcohol upon the oxygen. (*c*) Certain poisons, such as phosphorus, produce an intense fatty degeneration with necrosis of the liver cells. The toxin of acute yellow atrophy, whatever its nature, acts in the same way.

The liver is uniformly increased in size. The edge may reach below the level of the navel. It is smooth, looks pale and bloodless; on section it is dry, and renders the surface of the knife greasy. The liver may weigh many pounds, but the specific gravity is so low that the organ floats in water.

The *symptoms* of fatty liver are not definite. Jaundice is never present; the stools may be light colored, but even in the most advanced grades the bile is still formed. Signs of portal obstruction are rare. The spleen is not enlarged. Hemorrhoids are not very infrequent. Altogether, the symptoms are chiefly those of the disease with which the degeneration is associated. In cases of great obesity the physical examination is uncertain; but in cachectic conditions the organ can be felt to be greatly enlarged, though smooth and painless. Fatty livers are among the largest met with at the bedside. In *treatment,* if the patient uses alcohol this should be stopped; the diet should be simple and the bowels kept open.

AMYLOID LIVER

The waxy, lardaceous, or amyloid liver occurs as part of a general degeneration, associated with cachexias, particularly when the result of long-standing suppuration. It is rare in the United States.

In practice, it is found oftenest in the prolonged suppuration of tuberculous disease, either of the lungs or bones. Next in frequency are the cases associated with syphilis. Here there may be ulceration of the rectum, with which it is often connected, or chronic bone disease, or it may be present without suppurative changes. It is found occasionally in rickets, in prolonged convalescence from the infectious fevers, and in the cachexia of cancer.

The amyloid liver is large, and may attain dimensions equalled only by those of the cancerous organ. Wilks speaks of a liver weighing fourteen pounds. It is solid, firm, resistant, on section anemic, and has a semitranslucent, infiltrated appearance. Stained with a dilute solution of iodine, the amyloid areas assume a rich mahogany-brown color.

There are no characteristic *symptoms.* Jaundice does not occur; the stools may be light-colored, but the secretion of bile persists. The physical examination shows the organ to be uniformly enlarged and painless, the surface smooth, the edge rounded, and the consistence greatly increased. Sometimes the edge, even in great enlargement, is sharp and hard. The spleen may be involved but there are no evidences of portal obstruction.

The *diagnosis* is, as a rule, easy. Progressive and great enlargement in connection with suppuration of long standing or with syphilis is almost always of this nature. In rare instances the amyloid liver is reduced in size. In *leukemia* the liver may attain considerable size and be smooth and uniform, resembling the fatty organ. The blood condition indicates the true nature of the case. Treatment is symptomatic and of the causal condition.

ANOMALIES IN FORM AND POSITION OF THE LIVER

In transposition of the viscera the right lobe of the organ may occupy the left side. A common and important anomaly is the tilting forward of the organ, so that the anteroposterior axis becomes vertical, not horizontal. Instead of the edge of the right lobe presenting just below the costal margin, a considerable portion of the surface of the lobe is in contact with the abdominal parietes, and the edge may be felt as low as the navel. This anteversion is apt to be mistaken for enlargement of the organ.

The "lacing" liver is met with in two chief types. In one the anterior portion, chiefly of the right lobe, is greatly prolonged, and may reach the transverse navel line, or even lower. A shallow transverse groove separates the thin extension from the main portion of the organ. The peritoneal coating of this groove may be fibroid, and in rare instances the deformed portion is connected with the organ by an almost tendinous membrane. The liver may be compressed laterally and have a pyramidal shape; the left border and the hinder margin of the left lobe may be much folded and incurved.

The projecting portion of the liver, extending low in the right flank, may be mistaken for a tumor, or more frequently for a movable right kidney. Its continuity with the liver itself may not be evident on palpation or on percussion, as coils of intestine may lie in front. It descends, however, with inspiration, and usually the margin can be traced continuously with that of the left lobe of the liver. The greatest difficulty arises when this anomalous lappet is naturally very thick and united to the liver by a very thin membrane, or when it is swollen in conditions of congestion.

The other principal type of lacing liver is quite different in shape. It is thick, broader above than below, and lies almost entirely above the transverse line of the cartilages. There is a narrow groove just above the anterior border, which is placed more transversely than normal.

Movable Liver.—This rare condition, usually found in women, has led in a considerable number to a mistaken diagnosis. A slight grade of mobility of the organ is found in the pendulous abdomen of enteroptosis and after repeated ascites.

The organ is so connected at its posterior margin with the inferior vena cava and diaphragm that any great mobility from this point is impossible, except on the theory of a mesohepar or congenital ligamentous union between these structures. The ligaments may show an extreme grade of relaxation (the suspensory 7.5 cm., and the triangular ligament 4 cm., in one of Leube's cases); and when the patient is in the erect posture the organ may drop down so far that its upper surface is entirely below the costal margin.

DISEASES OF THE PANCREAS

PANCREATIC INSUFFICIENCY

Failure of the internal secretion is followed by disturbance in the carbohydrate metabolism, of the external secretion by disturbances of digestion, or by the injurious effects of the retained secretion. Insufficiency of the external secretion is indicated by:

(*a*) Steatorrhea.—This consists in the presence of neutral unsplit fat in the stools. The proportion of fat in the feces varies; above 30 per cent of the dried weight suggests pancreatic insufficiency. The stools are either oily like butter, or gray like asbestos. The ability to digest fat differs greatly and there are healthy persons who constantly have a high percentage of fat in the stools. Steatorrhea may last for years without impairment of health. There is also a disturbance in the ratio between the neutral fats and the fatty acids. Cammidge gives the following average figures: Normal per cent, total fats 21, neutral fats 11, fatty acids 10; malignant disease, total fats 77, neutral fats 50, fatty acids 27; chronic pancreatitis, total fats 50, neutral fats 32, fatty acids 18.

(*b*) Azotorrhea, the presence of undigested protein materials in the stools. Normally only 5 or 6 per cent of the undigested proteins appears in the feces, but in pancreatic disease as much as 30 or 40 per cent may be recovered. Some claim that persistence of the nuclei of the meat fibres in the stools indicates defective tryptic digestion.

(*c*) Increase in *diastase* in the blood and urine.

Symptoms.—These are not striking and relate particularly to the digestive tract. In consequence of the lack of fat digestion there may be diarrhea with foul stools. The general condition suffers to a varying degree. Certain tests are of value: (1) Increased diastase in the blood and urine, (2) decreased sugar tolerance; the occurrence of hyperglycemia and glycosuria which may appear after taking 50 to 100 grams of dextrose, (3) the Loewi epinephrine mydriasis test (dilatation of the pupil in 20 to 60 minutes after instillation in the eye of one drop of 1-1000 solution of epinephrine, repeated in five minutes; the test may be positive in hyperthyroidism), (4) failure of the digestion of unboiled starch (boiled starch may be digested by saliva).

Treatment.—The amount of fat in the diet should be reduced and if there is evidence of disturbance from lack of protein digestion, the meats should be decreased. Pancreatic extract should be given in full dosage (15 grains, 1 gm.) three times a day. If there is lack of gastric secretion full doses of dilute HCl should be given.

There is a form of pancreatic insufficiency in children which may be congenital. In *congenital steatorrhea* the feces contain oil which solidifies on cooling. It appears to be a familial constitutional insufficiency of the pancreas. Associated with this is marked interference with development—*pancreatic infantilism.*

PANCREATIC NECROSIS

The entire series of pancreatic lesions, from hemorrhage to gangrene, and from fat necrosis to pancreatic cyst, may result from tryptic autodigestion (Chiari). This is met with under four conditions: (*a*) Trauma, as in gunshot wounds, blows, or perforation of a peptic ulcer. (*b*) Primary thrombosis in the venous radicles of the glands. (*c*) Obstruction of the free flow of secretion in the duct. (*d*) Entrance of bile into the ducts.

In the mildest forms there are only a few small hemorrhages or circumscribed areas of necrosis of the gland tissue with fat necrosis in the neighborhood; in severer forms groups of acini or the whole gland may be involved.

Fat necrosis occurs whenever the pancreatic juice, obstructed from any cause and dammed back on the gland, infiltrates its tissues, or escaping by the lymph spaces finds its way to structures at some distance from the gland. The necrosis is due to the fat-splitting ferment in the secretion (Opie).

Balser first called attention to this remarkable change which is found in the interlobular pancreatic tissue, in the mesentery, in the omentum, in the abdominal fatty tissue generally, and occasionally in the pericardial and subcutaneous fat. The necroses are most frequent in the acute and necrotic forms of pancreatitis, less common in the suppurative. In the pancreas the lobules are separated by a dead white necrotic tissue, which gives a remarkable appearance to the section. In the abdominal fat the areas are usually not larger than a pin's head; they at once attract attention, and may be mistaken, on superficial examination, for miliary tubercles or neoplasms. They may be larger; in some instances they are the size of a hen's egg. On section they have a soft tallowy consistence, and the substance is a combination of lime with certain fatty acids. The necroses may be crusted with lime.

HEMORRHAGE

Both Spiess (1866) and Zenker (1874) were acquainted with hemorrhage into the pancreas as a cause of sudden death, but its great medicolegal importance was first fully recognized by F. W. Draper, of Boston, whose townsmen, Harris, Fitz, Whitney, and others, contributed additional studies. In 4,000 autopsies Draper met with 19 cases of pancreatic hemorrhage, in 9 or 10 of which no other cause of death was found. When the bleeding is extensive the entire tissue of the gland is destroyed and the blood invades the retroperitoneal tissue. In other instances the peritoneal covering is broken and the blood fills the lesser peritoneum. The hemorrhage may be in connection with an acute pancreatitis or with necrotic inflammation of the gland.

The *symptoms* are those of *acute pancreatitis*. A well-marked tumor may sometimes be felt in the epigastrium. There may be tenderness and swelling in the course of the descending colon, with frequent stools, containing blood and mucus, and suggesting intussusception.

ACUTE PANCREATITIS

While for convenience a distinction is made between hemorrhagic, suppurative and gangrenous pancreatitis, yet they are practically different manifestations of the same process. The principal *etiological* factors are *stasis* and *infection* which may be by the ducts or metastatic from some focus which may be in the gallbladder, an ulcer, or in the bowel, more often the colon. The appendix does not seem to be responsible in many cases. It seems possible that infection may be carried to the pancreas by the lymphatics in the retroperitoneal tissues. Association with cholelithiasis is common, but the calculi are usually in the gallbladder and rarely in the ampulla, which suggests that direct regurgitation of bile into the pancreatic duct occurs rarely. Injection of bile into the pancreatic duct of dogs reproduces the lesion. Rupture of the pancreas from trauma is an occasional cause. Acute pancreatitis occurs occasionally in the acute infectious diseases, especially mumps, and in pyemia and infectious endocarditis. Otherwise it is found usually in adult life and more often in men. Streptococci and colon bacilli are the organisms most often present.

Pathology.—The fat necrosis is probably due to the action of the fat splitting ferment. It has been suggested that the hemorrhages may be due to trypsin digesting the walls of the vessels. The pancreatic juice is activated by calcium salts, by the action of bacteria or by the products of aseptic necrosis. The toxic features may be much the same as in acute intestinal obstruction.

The pancreas is enlarged and the interlobular tissues infiltrated with blood, and perhaps with clots. The anatomical appearances are very characteristic. The tissues about the gland are infiltrated with blood and there may be fluid in the lesser peritoneum. Areas of fat necrosis are seen in the retroperitoneal fat, the mesocolon and mesentery. The gland itself is swollen and in section the stroma has a mottled dark brown appearance and the outlines of the acini may be lost. Edema of the pancreas is found in some cases.

Symptoms.—In some cases there have been premonitory attacks of pain which may be general or in the upper part of the abdomen and suggest gastric ulcer or gall stones. The onset is very sudden with severe *pain* usually referred to the epigastrium and in some cases very severe in the lower dorsal region of the back. It is continuous but paroxysms of greater severity come at intervals. There may be tenderness in the left costovertebral angle. Vomiting soon begins and is frequent. There is constipation and no sounds of peristalsis can be heard. In the most acute cases there is a condition of *shock*. The symptoms of the attack are those of a very acute abdominal condition. There may be *cyanosis* especially of the neck and face. Examination shows fullness and tenderness in the upper abdomen and usually increasing distention. The tenderness may be specially marked across the epigastrium and there may be a distinct sense of resistance but marked rigidity is usually absent. Bluish discoloration about the navel and greenish discoloration in the loins have been noted (Turner). There is not likely to be any tumor mass felt until at least the third day. There may be marked leukocytosis. Glycosuria is rare; there is increase of diastase in the urine and blood. The temperature is rarely elevated and may be subnormal; the pulse is rapid. Morphia has little effect on the pain. The most acute cases, termed fulminating, show a very severe onset with marked shock and collapse. This has been explained as probably due to pressure on the celiac axis. In these cases there is profuse hemorrhage into the pancreas and death usually follows in two or three days.

In the acute cases of average severity, the onset is sudden, but less severe than in the preceding. Only part of the pancreas may be damaged and the most greatly damaged part may go on to necrosis and gangrene. Suppuration may follow, giving the picture of an *acute suppurative pancreatitis*. There may be a single abscess or numerous small ones. In one series of 38 cases, in 24 there was a single abscess. In some cases there is a diffuse purulent infiltration. Among the results are peripancreatic abscess with perforation into the stomach, duodenum or peritoneum and thrombosis of the portal vein. The course of the suppurative form is likely to be chronic. Jaundice, diarrhea and glycosuria have occurred but are rare. A tumor mass in the epigastrium may result. In less acute forms the process may be limited to a part of the pancreas, usually the head, and the hemorrhage is slight. The main symptoms are pain in the abdomen with nausea and vomiting, but the pulse and temperature may show no change and the condition may be overlooked, especially as it is often associated with cholecystitis.

In *gangrenous pancreatitis,* complete necrosis of the gland, or part of it, may follow hemorrhage or hemorrhagic inflammation, and in exceptional cases may occur after suppurative infiltration or after injury or perforation of an ulcer of the stomach. Symptoms of hemorrhagic pancreatitis may precede or be associated with it. Death usually follows in from ten to twenty days, with symptoms of collapse. The pancreas may present a dry necrotic appearance, but as a rule the organ is converted into a dark slate-colored mass lying nearly free in the omental cavity or attached by a few shreds. In other instances the totally or partially sequestrated organ may lie in a large abscess cavity, forming a palpable tumor in the epigastric region. The necrotic portion may be discharged *per rectum,* with recovery.

Diagnosis.—The sudden dramatic *onset* in the severe forms should always suggest the possibility of acute pancreatitis. Perforation of the stomach or bowel, mesenteric thrombosis and intestinal obstruction give features very similar, also the rupture of an aneurism. "Acute pancreatitis is to be suspected when a previously healthy person or a sufferer from occasional attacks of indigestion is suddenly seized with a violent pain in the epigastrium followed by vomiting and collapse, and in the course of twenty-four hours by a circumscribed epigastric swelling, tympanitic or resistant, with slight elevation of temperature. Circumscribed tenderness in the course of the pancreas and tender spots throughout the abdomen are valuable diagnostic signs" (Fitz). The mild forms are more difficult to recognize and are usually mistaken for cholecystitis. The presence of a tumor mass is of the greatest moment. Consideration of the possibility of acute pancreatitis is the best safeguard against error. Acute coronary artery occlusion should be kept in mind.

Treatment.—It is well to stop all intake by mouth and give fluid by rectum. Morphia should be given in full doses to control the pain. The decision as to exploration must depend on the condition; in the fulminant cases it may not be possible, in the less severe cases it is usually wise, in the mild cases it is not necessary. If gall stones are present they should be removed and the gallbladder drained. With signs of suppuration and abscess formation drainage is advisable. Otherwise symptomatic measures are indicated.

CHRONIC PANCREATITIS

Forms.—There is still a great deal of uncertainty about this condition. The truth is if operators regard an indurated or even nodular head of the pancreas as indicating a chronic pancreatitis they will find it frequently. Those who follow Virchow's postmortem technique and open the stomach and duodenum and press on the course of the bile duct know how common is this sensation over the head of the organ, which may be sliced with the conviction that there must be some special morbid change. W. J. Mayo remarks how frequently he has found the pancreas enlarged, indurated and nodulated in cases with no symptomatic evidence of pancreatic inflammation. Anatomically there are two forms:

(*a*) *Interlobular* pancreatitis follows occlusion of the duct or infection, such as occurs with calculi, biliary or pancreatic, with which colon bacilli, streptococci, or occasionally typhoid bacilli are associated. Even in advanced sclerosis of this type the islands of Langerhans are spared. It may occur as an independent affection. It is not uncommon in the bodies of adults to find the head of the pancreas extraordinarily hard and so dense that it feels like scirrhus. The condition is often present without symptoms of pancreatic disease during life. A special form is the chronic interstitial pancreatitis which accompanies hemochromatosis. Sclerosis of the head of the pancreas may cause obstruction of the duct.

(*b*) Chronic *interacinar* pancreatitis is characterized by a diffuse fibrosis penetrating between the acini, with little or no involvement of the interlobular tissues. It may follow infection but is more common with cirrhosis of the liver, chronic passive congestion and arteriosclerosis.

Etiology.—The main factor is *infection* of the ducts, which may be due to infection in the duodenum or of the bile ducts and gallbladder. The association of the duct of Wirsung with the common bile duct, which is surrounded by the head of the pancreas in the majority of cases, has an important influence. Infection of the bile ducts is common and the stasis which accompanies it, whether alone or with gall stones, is a contributing factor. Sclerosis of the pancreas occurs with cirrhosis of the liver, possibly due to alcohol in some cases, and with arteriosclerosis. The possibility of *syphilis* as an etiological factor should be kept in mind.

Symptoms.—The clinical picture is obscure. Cammidge describes four types: (*a*) The dyspeptic, in which the disease is due to morbid conditions of the bowels, and the symptoms are mainly referred to the digestive organs. (*b*) The cholelithic, associated with the presence of gall stones in the common duct; there is usually chronic jaundice and the dominant symptoms are hepatic. (*c*) A miscellaneous group in which the pancreatitis is secondary to malignant disease, etc. (*d*) The diabetic group with glycosuria, into which the preceding groups may merge in time. Certain cases of obscure abdominal pain may be due to chronic pancreatitis, possibly with mild acute exacerbations.

Symptoms of pancreatic insufficiency are generally present but cannot be regarded as distinctive, as biliary disease is so often present. Anorexia is common and occasional vomiting may be noted; there may be discomfort after meals but pain is not often present though colic may occur in the absence of gall stones. Jaundice may be found, due to obstruction of the common duct from stone or pressure from the pancreas if it surrounds the duct. Occasionally the pancreas can be felt; sometimes it is tender. Diarrhea is common with bulky fetid stools containing an excess of fat. There is marked loss of fat and nitrogen in the stools. There is a large amount of unsplit fat present. The extent of digestion of cell nuclei is of some value. Glycosuria occasionally results. The general health may suffer and emaciation result. Death may be due to exhaustion.

Diagnosis.—This is difficult. The absence or decrease of pancreatic secretion may be evident from the stools, but this may be due to obstruction preventing the pancreatic juice from reaching the intestine and not to pancreatic disease. Increased diastase in the blood and urine, Loewi's epinephrine mydriasis test and decreased carbohydrate tolerance are significant. With chronic jaundice of obscure causation chronic pancreatitis should be considered. Even at operation it may be difficult to tell whether new growth or pancreatitis is present; time decides.

Treatment.—Owing to the difficulty of diagnosis in the early stages it is impossible to speak positively in a great many cases, but in the forms which are associated with pain, jaundice, the presence of calculi, and infection of the ducts excellent results have followed free drainage of the bile passages. Removal of the gallbladder is sometimes more effectual than drainage alone. If obstruction is found this should be remedied if possible.

PANCREATIC CYSTS

As to *sex*, the total figures are about equal. As to *age*, the largest number are in the fourth decade; cases have occurred in infants.

Varieties.—TRAUMATIC CASES.—In one series of 33 cases 30 were men and only 3 in women. Blows on the abdomen or constantly repeated pressure are the most common forms of trauma. One case followed severe massage. Usually with the onset there are inflammatory symptoms, pain, and vomiting, sometimes suggestive of peritonitis. The contents of the cyst are usually bloody, though in 13 of the traumatic cases it was clear or yellowish.

CYSTS FOLLOWING INFLAMMATORY CONDITIONS.—In 51 cases the trouble began gradually after attacks of dyspepsia with colic, simulating somewhat that of gall stones. Occasionally the attack set in with very severe symptoms, suggestive of obstruction of the bowel. In this group the tumor appeared in 19 cases soon after the onset of the pain; in others it was delayed for a period of from a few weeks to two or three years. McPhedran reported a remarkable instance in which the tumor appeared in the epigastrium with signs of severe inflammation. It was opened and drained and believed to be a hydrops of the lesser peritoneal cavity. Three months later a second cyst developed, which appeared to spring directly from the pancreas.

CYSTS WITHOUT INFLAMMATORY OR TRAUMATIC ETIOLOGY.—Of 33 cases in this group 26 were in women. A remarkable feature is the duration—in one case for forty-seven years, in one between sixteen and twenty years, in others for sixteen and nine years, in the majority from two to four years.

Morbid Anatomy.—Körte recognizes (1) *retention cysts* due to plugging of the main duct; (2) *proliferation cysts* of the pancreatic tissue and cystoadenoma; (3) *retention cysts* arising from the alveoli of the gland and of the smaller ducts, which become cut off and dilate in consequence of chronic interstitial pancreatitis; (4) *pseudocysts* following inflammation or trauma of the pancreas, causing hemorrhage and hydrops of the lesser peritoneum.

Situation.—In its growth the cyst may (1) be in the lesser peritoneum, push the stomach upward, and reach the abdominal wall between the stomach and the transverse colon; (2) more rarely the cyst appears above the lesser curvature and pushes the stomach downward; in both of these the tumor is high in the abdomen; but (3) it may develop between the leaves of the transverse mesocolon and lie below both the colon and stomach. The relation of these two organs to the tumor is variable, but in the majority the stomach lies above and the transverse colon below the cyst. Occasionally the cyst may arise in the tail of the pancreas and project far over in the left hypochondrium in the position of the spleen or a renal tumor. In this situation the diagnosis is likely to be very difficult and may require exploration.

General Symptoms.—Apart from the features of onset already referred to, the patient may complain of no trouble unless the cyst reaches a large size. Painful colicky attacks, with nausea and vomiting and progressive enlargement of the abdomen, have frequently been noted. Fatty diarrhea from disturbance of the function of the pancreas is rare. Glycosuria has been present in a number of cases. Increased secretion of saliva, the so-called pancreatic salivation, is also rare. The symptoms are due largely to pressure, which may cause jaundice, disturbance of the stomach and intestines, or dyspnea. Very marked loss of weight has been present in a number of cases. Remarkable features are a sudden increase in size from hemorrhage or the transitory disappearance of the cyst. In one of Halsted's cases the girth of the abdomen decreased from 43 to 31 inches in ten days with profuse diarrhea. Sometimes the disappearance has followed blows.

Diagnosis.—The cyst occupies the upper abdomen, usually forming a semicircular bulging in the median line, rarely to either side. In 16 cases Körte states that the chief projection was below the navel. The tumor may occupy the greater part of the abdomen. The cyst is immobile, respiration having little or no influence on it. The stomach, as a rule, lies above it and the colon below. The relations of the cyst can be determined by an X-ray study. It may be impossible to distinguish between a true and a pseudocyst (lesser peritoneum). Mesenteric cysts are more movable.

In a majority of the cases the fluid is of a reddish or dark-brown color, and contains blood or blood coloring matter, cell detritus, fat granules, and sometimes cholesterin. The consistence of the fluid is usually mucoid, rarely thin. The reaction is alkaline, the specific gravity from 1.010 to 1.020.

Ferments may be present in the fluid or in the material from the fistula. In 20 of 54 cases only one ferment was present, in 20 cases two, and in 14 cases all three of the pancreatic ferments were found. In view of the wide occurrence of diastatic and fat-emulsifying ferments in various exudates, the only positive sign in the diagnosis of the pancreatic secretion is the digestion of fibrin and albumin.

Treatment.—This is surgical and the results are satisfactory. Of 160 cases of operation there were 150 recoveries. Removal may be possible or drainage alone may be advisable.

TUMORS OF THE PANCREAS

Of new growths in the organ carcinoma is the most frequent. Sarcoma, adenoma, and lymphoma are rare. *Adenoma* of the islands of Langerhans may cause hypoglycemia (hyperinsulinism).

Frequency.—In Vienna in 18,069 autopsies there were 22 cases of cancer of the pancreas (Biach). In 11,472 postmortems at Milan, Segré found 132 tumors of the pancreas, 127 of which were carcinomata, 2 sarcomata, 2 cysts, and 1 syphiloma. In 6,000 autopsies at Guy's Hospital there were only 20 cases of primary malignant disease of the organ (Hale-White). Among 42,000 admissions to the Johns Hopkins Hospital, Futcher reports 58 cases in which a clinical diagnosis was made; in 31 the diagnosis was verified by operation or autopsy. The head of the gland is most commonly involved, but the disease may be limited to the body or to the tail.

Symptoms.—The following are the most important features: (*a*) Epigastric *pain*, often early and persistent or occurring in paroxysms. (*b*) *Jaundice*, due to pressure of the tumor in the head of the pancreas on the bile duct. The jaundice is intense and permanent, and associated with dilatation of the gallbladder, which may reach a large size and is usually palpable. Jaundice does not occur if the tail of the pancreas is involved; in this event pain may radiate to the left back. (*c*) A *tumor* in the epigastrium. This is not common; in 137 cases Da Costa found a tumor in only 13 and Futcher in 12 of 31 cases. Palpation under anesthesia with the stomach empty would probably give a larger percentage. As the tumor rests directly upon the aorta there is usually a marked pulsation, sometimes with a bruit. There may be pressure on the portal vein, causing obstruction and its usual sequels. (*d*) Symptoms due to *loss of function* of the pancreas are less important. Fatty diarrhea is not very often present. In consequence of the absence of bile the stools are usually clay-colored and bulky with excess of neutral fat and fatty acid crystals. Glycosuria is not common. (*e*) Rapid wasting and cachexia. Of other symptoms nausea and vomiting are common. In some instances the pylorus is compressed and there is dilatation of the stomach. In a few cases there has been profuse salivation.

The points of greatest importance in the *diagnosis* are the intense and permanent jaundice, with dilatation of the gallbladder, rapid emaciation, and a tumor in the epigastric region. Of less importance are features pointing to disturbance of the functions of the gland. The diagnosis from primary carcinoma of the common bile duct or a gall stone plugging the duct completely may not be possible without operation. Chronic pancreatitis may give a similar picture if the common duct is compressed. Deformity of the duodenum may be found in the X-ray study.

The outlook in tumors of the pancreas is, as a rule, hopeless; but successful cases of operation have been reported. If there is doubt as to the diagnosis, operation should be done and if there is a growth of the pancreas an anastomosis should be made between the gallbladder and intestine to relieve the jaundice. Otherwise treatment is symptomatic.

PANCREATIC CALCULI

Pancreatic lithiasis is rare. Ackman and Ross (1932) found slightly over 100 cases reported. The majority of cases occur in males of middle age. In 1,500 autopsies at the Johns Hopkins Hospital there were 2 cases. Infection and stasis are the important factors.

The stones are usually numerous, either round in shape or rough, spinous and coral-like. The color is opaque white. They are composed chiefly of calcium carbonate and phosphate. The effects of the stones are: (1) A chronic interstitial inflammation of the gland substance with dilatation of the duct; sometimes cystic dilatation of the gland; (2) acute inflammation with suppuration; (3) the irritation of the stones may lead to carcinoma.

Symptoms.—Epigastric pain, sometimes colicky and worse after meals, attacks like gall stone colic (with the pain radiating to the left) and signs due to obstruction of the flow of pancreatic secretion are suggestive. A pancreatic stone may cause jaundice by pressing on the common duct or causing obstruction in the ampulla of Vater. The X-rays may aid in diagnosis. An analysis of calculi passed with the stools may alone serve to distinguish them from gall stones. Operation has given good results.

DISEASES OF THE PERITONEUM

ACUTE PERITONITIS

Definition.—Acute inflammation of the peritoneum due to infection.

Etiology.—The condition may be primary or secondary.

(*a*) Primary Peritonitis.—In this the organisms, usually the pneumococcus or streptococcus, reach the peritoneum by the blood or lymphatics. It is often a terminal infection, as seen in nephritis, gout and arteriosclerosis. Of 102 cases of peritonitis which came to autopsy at the Johns Hopkins Hospital, 12 were of this form.

(*b*) Secondary peritonitis is due to extension of inflammation from, or perforation of, one of the organs covered by the peritoneum. Peritonitis from extension may follow inflammation of the stomach or intestines, ulceration in these parts, cancer, acute suppurative inflammations of the spleen, liver, pancreas, retroperitoneal tissues and the pelvic viscera.

Perforative peritonitis is the most common, following external wounds, perforation of an ulcer of the stomach or bowels, perforation of the gall-bladder, abscess of the liver, spleen or kidneys. Two important causes are appendicitis and suppurating inflammation about the fallopian tubes and ovaries. There are instances in which peritonitis has followed rupture of an apparently normal Graafian follicle. Of the above 102 cases, 56 originated in an extension from some diseased abdominal viscus. The remaining 34 followed surgical operations upon the peritoneum or the contained organs.

The peritonitis of septicemia and pyemia is almost invariably the result of a local process. An exceedingly acute form of peritonitis may be caused by the development of tubercles on the membrane.

Morbid Anatomy.—In recent cases, on opening the abdomen the intestinal coils are distended and glued together with lymph, and the peritoneum presents a patchy, sometimes a uniform injection. The exudation may be: (*a*) *Fibrinous,* with little or no fluid, except a few pockets of clear serum between the coils. (*b*) *Serofibrinous.* The coils are covered with lymph, and there is a large amount of a yellowish, serofibrinous fluid. When the stomach or intestine is perforated this may be mixed with food or feces. (*c*) *Purulent,* in which the exudate is either thin and greenish yellow in color, or opaque white and creamy. (*d*) *Putrid.* Occasionally in puerperal and perforative peritonitis, particularly when the latter has been caused by cancer, the exudate is thin, grayish green in color, and has a gangrenous odor. (*e*) *Hemorrhagic.* This is sometimes found as an admixture in cases of acute peritonitis following wounds, and occurs in the cancerous and tuberculous forms. (*f*) A rare form occurs in which the injection is present, but almost all signs of exudation are wanting. Close inspection may be necessary to detect a slight dulling of the serous surfaces.

The amount of the effusion varies from half a litre to 20 or 30 litres. There are essential differences between the various kinds of peritonitis which depend often on the infecting organism.

Bacteriology.—A large number of organisms have been found. In 33 cases following operation the staphylococcus was present alone in 12, the streptococcus in 5, and the colon bacillus in 5. Other organisms were the penumococcus, *B. pyocyaneus,* and *B. aërogenes.* Of 56 cases of peritonitis following intestinal infections, the colon bacillus occurred in 43, usually with streptococci. The gonococcus is present in the form which arises from salpingitis and in the gonorrheal infections of children. Much attention has been paid to the *pneumococcus* in the causation of peritonitis; some cases are of the primary form without recognizable portal of entry; but there are many latent pneumococcic lesions, particularly of the middle ear and sinuses.

Symptoms.—In the perforative and septic cases the onset is marked by chilly feelings or an actual rigor with intense pain in the abdomen. The features of collapse may be marked. In typhoid fever, when the sensorium is benumbed, the onset may not be noticed. The *pain* is general, and is usually intense and aggravated by movements and pressure. It is usually a striking feature. A position is taken which relieves the tension of the abdominal muscles, so that the patient lies on the back with the thighs drawn up and the shoulders elevated. The greatest pain is usually below the umbilicus, but in peritonitis from perforation of the stomach pain may be referred to the back, chest, or shoulder. The respiration is superficial—costal in type—as it is painful to use the diaphragm. For the same reason the action of coughing is restrained and even the movements necessary for talking are limited. In this early stage the tenderness may be great and the abdominal muscles are often rigidly contracted. If the patient is at perfect rest the pain may be slight, and there are instances in which it is not at all marked, and may, indeed, be absent.

The abdomen gradually becomes distended and tense, is tympanitic and respiratory movement is absent. The pulse is rapid, small, and hard, and often has a peculiar wiry quality. It ranges from 110 to 150. The temperature may rise rapidly and reach 104° or 105° F., but the subsequent elevation is moderate. In some very severe cases there may be no fever throughout. The leukocyte count varies with the grade of infection. In the severe cases it may not be increased. The tongue at first is white and moist, but subsequently becomes dry and often red and fissured. *Vomiting* is an early and prominent feature and causes great pain. The contents of the stomach are first ejected, then a yellowish and bile-stained fluid, and finally a greenish and, in rare instances, a brownish black liquid with slight fecal odor. The bowels may be loose at the onset and constipation may follow. Frequent micturition may be present, less often retention. The urine is usually scanty and high-colored.

The appearance of the patient when *general peritonitis* has developed is very characteristic. The face is pinched, the eyes are sunken, and the expression is very anxious. The constant vomiting of fluids causes a wasted appearance, and the hands sometimes present the washer-woman's skin. Except in cholera, we see the Hippocratic facies more frequently in this than in any other disease—"*a sharp nose, hollow eyes, collapsed temples; the ears cold, contracted, and their lobes turned out; the skin about the forehead being rough, distended, and parched; the color of the whole face being brown, black, livid, or lead-colored.*" There are one or two additional points about the abdomen. The *tympanites* is usually excessive, owing to the great relaxation of the walls of the intestines by inflammation and exudation. There is absence of the sounds of peristalsis and the breath and heart sounds may be heard loudly. The diaphragm is pushed up and the apex beat of the heart may be dislocated to the fourth interspace. The liver dulness may be greatly reduced, or may, in the mammary line, be obliterated. This is not a distinctive feature of perforative peritonitis, as the liver dulness in the mammary line may be obliterated by tympanites alone. In the axillary line, the liver dulness, though diminished, may persist. Pneumoperitoneum following perforation more certainly obliterates hepatic dulness. In such cases the fluid effused produces a dulness in the lateral region; but with gas in the peritoneum, if the patient is turned on the left side, a clear note is heard beneath the seventh and eighth rib. Acute peritonitis may present a flat, rigid abdomen throughout its course.

Effusion of fluid is usually present except in some acute, rapidly fatal cases. The flanks are dull on percussion. The dulness may be movable, though this depends altogether upon the degree of adhesions. There may be considerable effusion without either movable dulness or fluctuation. A friction rub may be present, as first pointed out by Bright, but it is not nearly so common in acute as in chronic peritonitis.

There are modifications of the ordinary picture, due often to the special organism. In *pneumococcal peritonitis* children are more often affected than adults. There are two forms, diffuse and local. In the *diffuse* form the onset is acute followed by marked general features, severe pain, frequent vomiting, often severe diarrhea, with death within 36 or 48 hours. Some patients recover after a stormy course. In the more common *local* form the features are less severe. After an acute onset the condition improves but a few days later the symptoms become more severe and there is abscess formation usually in the lower abdomen. This may rupture internally or externally, often about the navel. The creamy, odorless, greenish pus is characteristic. General *gonococcal* peritonitis is more common in female children and may be much less severe than other forms. Local gonococcal pelvic peritonitis is common. *Streptococcal peritonitis* is usually very severe—the puerperal form especially so. In it the features of septicemia may be marked. *Local peritonitis* is common, especially secondary to appendicitis or pelvic infection. Local signs are evident, especially pain, tenderness and muscle spasm. There is always the danger of general peritonitis resulting if the process is acute; in other cases a local abscess may form. The term *spreading peritonitis* may be used to designate cases in which the process advances gradually from a local to a general involvement. The general features are less severe than in the acute general form and if not helped by operation the disease may last for some time, possibly with abscess formation.

Prognosis.—In the cases due to injury or perforation of an abdominal organ much depends on the interval between this and operation. Every hour of delay increases the risk. In the group due to extension from the pelvic organs the outlook is more favorable. The acute diffuse peritonitis usually terminates in death. The most intense forms may kill within thirty-six to forty-eight hours; more commonly death results in four or five days, or the attack may be prolonged to eight or ten days. The pulse becomes irregular, the heart-sounds weak, the breathing shallow; there are lividity with pallor, a cold skin with high rectal temperature. Death may occur with great suddenness. A low temperature, rapid pulse, marked distention, absence of leukocytosis and severe toxemia point to a fatal ending. The causal organism influences the outlook; cases due to the gonococcus and some forms of staphylococci are more favorable than those due to the streptococcus.

Diagnosis.—In typical cases the severe pain at onset, the distention of the abdomen, the tenderness, the fever, the gradual onset of effusion, collapse, and the vomiting give a characteristic picture. Careful inquiries should at once be made concerning the previous condition, from which a clue can often be had as to the starting-point of the trouble. In young adults a considerable proportion of all cases depends upon appendicitis, and there may be an account of previous attacks. In women the most frequent causes are suppurative processes in the pelvic viscera or acute puerperal infection. It is not always easy to determine the cause. Many patients come under observation with the abdomen distended and tender, and it is impossible to make a satisfactory examination. In such instances the pelvic organs should be examined with great care. Suggestive points in the *pneumococcus* form in children are the sudden onset, the severe toxemia, high fever, marked leukocytosis, vomiting, and diarrhea with less abdominal pain and tenderness as compared with other acute forms. The following conditions are most apt to be mistaken for acute peritonitis:

(*a*) *Acute Enterocolitis.*—Here the pain, distention and sensitiveness on pressure may be marked. The pain is more colicky in character and the diarrhea more frequent but muscle spasm is less marked.

(*b*) *So-called Hysterical Peritonitis.*—This has deceived the very elect, as almost every feature of genuine peritonitis may be simulated. The onset may be sudden, with severe pain in the abdomen, tenderness, vomiting, diarrhea, difficulty in micturition, and the characteristic decubitus. Even the temperature may be elevated. A case was reported by Bristowe with four attacks within a year, and it was not until special hysterical symptoms developed that the true nature of the trouble was suspected.

(*c*) *Obstruction* of the bowel may simulate peritonitis, both having pain, vomiting, tympanites, and constipation. They may both be present. It may be impossible to make a diagnosis before exploration.

(*d*) *Rupture of an abdominal aneurism or mesenteric thrombosis or embolism* may cause symptoms which simulate peritonitis. In the latter, a sudden onset with severe pain, collapse symptoms, frequent vomiting, and great distention of the abdomen may be present. A definite diagnosis may be possible only after the abdomen is opened.

(*e*) Acute pancreatitis, severe pyelitis in a child or a ruptured tubal pregnancy may be mistaken for peritonitis.

(*f*) Basal pneumonia or pleurisy should not cause difficulty if a careful examination is made. The same applies to lead colic and the crisis of tabes.

Treatment.—Something can be done in prevention by recognition and prompt treatment of conditions which may lead to general peritonitis, such as gastric ulcer, appendicitis, cholecystitis, etc. An early surgical consultation is important. With signs or suspicion of peritonitis, the patient should be at absolute rest and propped up in bed in a sitting position; nothing should be given by mouth; a solution of glucose (5 per cent) and sodium bicarbonate (2 per cent) should be given per rectum by the drop method and salt solution subcutaneously or intravenously. Purgatives should not be given. If there is shock from perforation, fluid may be given subcutaneously, and epinephrine (♏ xv, 1 cc.) as indicated. If there is much vomiting gastric lavage is indicated. If there is constant secretion into the stomach a small tube may be kept in position so that frequent lavage is possible without disturbing the patient. The rectal tube may be used to relieve tympanites. Turpentine stupes, an ice-bag or hot applications may be applied to the abdomen if they give comfort. Various serums have been used, especially the antigas gangrene serum. In a pneumococcus infection serum may be used for Types I and II. It is well to withhold morphia until a definite course of action is decided upon. If the condition is hopeless morphia should be given freely. In general, operation is indicated and as soon as possible, especially after perforation. In some cases delay may be advisable, for example until shock has passed, but this should be left to the judgment of the surgeon. In pneumococcus and gonococcus peritonitis delay is advisable unless an abscess forms.

PERITONITIS IN INFANTS AND CHILDREN

Peritonitis may occur in the fetus as a consequence of syphilis, and may lead to constriction of the bowel by fibrous adhesions.

In the newborn a septic peritonitis may extend from an inflamed cord. Distention of the abdomen, slight swelling and redness about the cord, and not infrequently jaundice are present. It is uncommon and existed in only 4 of 51 infants dying with inflammation of the cord and septicemia (Runge).

During childhood peritonitis arises from causes similar to those in the adult. Perforative appendicitis is common. Peritonitis following blows or kicks on the abdomen occurs more frequently at this period. In boys injury while playing football may be followed by diffuse peritonitis. A rare cause is extension through the diaphragm from an empyema. There are instances of peritonitis occurring in several children at the same school. It was in investigating an epidemic of this kind that Anstie received the postmortem wound of which he died. Peritonitis in children may follow the gonorrheal vulvitis so common in infant homes and hospitals.

LOCALIZED PERITONITIS

Subphrenic Peritonitis.—The peritoneum covering the right and left lobes of the liver may be involved in an extension from the pleura of suppurative, tuberculous, or cancerous processes. In various affections of the liver—cancer, abscess, hydatid disease, and in affections of the gallbladder—the inflammation may be localized to the peritoneum covering the upper surface of the organ. These forms of localized subphrenic peritonitis in the greater sac are not so important as those in the *lesser peritoneum.* The anatomical relations of this structure are as follows: It lies behind and below the stomach, the gastrohepatic omentum, and the anterior layer of the great omentum. Its lower limit forms the upper layer of the transverse mesocolon. On either side it reaches from the hepatic to the splenic flexure of the colon, and from the foramen of Winslow to the hilus of the spleen. Behind it covers and is tightly adherent to the front of the pancreas. Its upper limit is formed by the transverse fissure of the liver, and by that portion of the diaphragm which is covered by the lower layer of the right lateral ligament of the liver. The foramen of Winslow, through which the lesser communicates with the greater peritoneum, is readily closed by inflammation.

Inflammatory processes, exudates, and hemorrhages may be confined entirely to the *lesser peritoneum.* The exudate of tuberculous peritonitis may be localised in it. Perforation of certain parts of the stomach, of the duodenum, and of the colon may excite inflammation in it alone; and in various affections of the pancreas, particularly trauma and hemorrhage, the effusion into the sac has often been confounded with cyst of this organ.

There is a remarkable form of subphrenic abscesses containing air, which may simulate closely pneumothorax, and called by Leyden *pyopneumothorax subphrenicus.* In 142 of 170 recorded cases the cause was known. In a few instances, as in one reported by Meltzer, the subphrenic abscess seemed to have followed pneumonia. Pyothorax is an occasional cause. By far the most frequent condition is gastric ulcer, which occurred in 80 of the cases. Duodenal ulcer was the cause in 6 per cent. In about 10 per cent the appendix was the starting-point of the abscess. Cancer of the stomach is an occasional cause. Other rare causes are trauma, perforation of hepatic or renal abscess, lesions of the spleen, abscess and cysts of the pancreas. In a majority of the cases in which the stomach or duodenum is perforated—sometimes in the cases following trauma—the abscess contains air.

The *symptoms* of *subphrenic abscess* vary very considerably, depending a good deal upon the primary cause. The onset, as a rule, is abrupt, particularly when due to perforation of a gastric ulcer. There are severe pain, vomiting, often of bilious or of bloody material; respiration is embarrassed, owing to the involvement of the diaphragm; then the constitutional symptoms occur associated with suppuration, chills, irregular fever and emaciation. Subsequently perforation may take place into the pleura or into the lung, with severe cough and abundant purulent expectoration.

The *perihepatic abscess* beneath the arch of the diaphragm, whether to the right or left of the suspensory ligament, when it does not contain air, is almost invariably mistaken for empyema. Remarkable features are superadded when the abscess cavity contains air. On the right side, when the abscess is in the greater peritoneum, above the right lobe of the liver, the diaphragm may be pushed up to the level of the second or third rib, and the physical signs on percussion and auscultation are those of pneumothorax, particularly the tympanitic resonance and the movable dulness. The liver is usually greatly depressed and there is bulging on the right side. Still more obscure are the cases of air-containing abscesses due to perforation of the stomach or duodenum, in which the gas is contained in the lesser peritoneum. Here the diaphragm is pushed up and there are signs of pneumothorax on the left side. In a large majority of all the cases which follow perforation of a gastric ulcer the effusion lies between the diaphragm above, and the spleen, stomach, and the left lobe of the liver below. The X-ray is of value in diagnosis and on the left side the sign described by Fussell and Pancoast in perinephritic abscess may be helpful. This consists in a wave in the fluid seen with the fluoroscope when the patient's body is moved quickly from side to side. An exploratory puncture may find pus.

The prognosis in subphrenic abscess is not very hopeful. Of the cases on record about 20 per cent only have recovered.

Appendicular.—The most frequent cause of localized peritonitis in the male is appendicitis. The situation varies with the position of this extremely variable organ. The adhesion, perforation, and intraperitoneal abscess cavity may be within the pelvis, or to the left of the median line in the iliac region, in the lower right quadrant of the umbilical region—a not uncommon situation—or, most frequently in the right iliac fossa. In the most common situation the localized abscess lies upon the psoas muscle, bounded by the cecum on the right and the terminal portion of the ileum and its mesentery in front and to the left. In many of these cases the limitation is perfect, and postmortem records show that complete healing may take place with the obliteration of the appendix in a mass of firm scar tissue.

Pelvic Peritonitis.—The most frequent cause is inflammation about the uterus and Fallopian tubes. Puerperal septicemia, gonorrhea and tuberculosis are the usual causes. The tubes are the starting-point in a majority of the cases. The fimbriae become adherent and closely matted to the ovary, and a thickening of the parts, in which the individual organs are scarcely recognizable, is gradually produced. The tubes are dilated and filled with cheesy matter or pus, and there may be small abscess cavities in the broad ligaments. Rupture of one of these may cause general peritonitis, or the membrane may be involved by extension, as in tuberculosis of these parts.

The *treatment* of all these forms is surgical.

CHRONIC PERITONITIS

The following varieties may be recognized:

Local adhesive peritonitis, a very common condition, may occur wherever there has been inflammation, as about the appendix, gallbladder, colon, liver, spleen and pelvic organs. Points of thickening or puckering on the peritoneum occur sometimes with union of the coils or with fibrous bands. In a majority of such cases the condition is met accidentally postmortem. Two sets of *symptoms* may be caused by these adhesions. When a fibrous band is attached in such a way as to form a loop or snare, a coil of intestine may pass through it. Thus, of 295 cases of intestinal obstruction analyzed by Fitz, 63 were due to this cause. The second group is less serious and comprises cases with persistent abdominal pain of a colicky character, sometimes rendering life miserable. The symptoms depend largely on the area involved. Adhesions involving the pylorus or duodenum may suggest ulcer or about the colon they may cause marked stasis. A careful X-ray study is the greatest aid in determining the situation of and results from the adhesions.

Diffuse Adhesive Peritonitis.—This is a consequence of an acute inflammation, either simple or tuberculous. The peritoneum is obliterated. On cutting through the abdominal wall, the coils of intestines are uniformly matted together and can neither be separated from each other nor can the visceral and parietal layers be distinguished. There may be thickening of the layers, and the liver and spleen are usually involved in the adhesions.

Proliferative Peritonitis.—Apart from cancer and tubercle, which produce typical lesions of chronic peritonitis, the most characteristic form may be described under this heading. The essential feature is great thickening of the peritoneal layers, usually without much adhesion. The cases are sometimes seen with sclerosis of the stomach. It may occur in connection with a sclerotic condition of the cecum and the first part of the colon. It is not uncommon with cirrhosis of the liver in which event there is usually moderate effusion, rarely extensive ascites. The peritoneum is opaque white in color, and everywhere thickened, often in patches. The omentum is usually rolled and forms a thickened transverse mass between the stomach and the colon. The peritoneum over the stomach, intestines, and mesentery is sometimes greatly thickened. The liver and spleen may simply be adherent, or there is chronic perihepatitis or perisplenitis, so that a layer of firm, almost gristly connective tissue of from one-fourth to half an inch in thickness encircles these organs. Usually the volume of the liver is in consequence greatly reduced. The gastrohepatic omentum may be constricted by this new growth and the calibre of the portal vein much narrowed. A serous effusion may be present. On account of the adhesions which form, the peritoneum may be divided into three or four different sacs, as is described under tuberculous peritonitis. In these cases the intestines are usually free, though the mesentery is greatly shortened. There are instances in which the mesentery is so shortened by this proliferative change that the intestines form a ball not larger than a cocoanut situated in the middle line, and after the removal of the exudation can be felt as a solid tumor. The intestinal wall is greatly thickened and the mucous membrane of the ileum is thrown into folds like the valvulae conniventes. This proliferative peritonitis may be found in the subjects of chronic alcoholism. In long-continued ascites the serous surfaces generally become thickened and present an opaque, dead white color. This is observed especially in hepatic cirrhosis, but attends tumors, chronic passive congestion, etc. Syphilis may be responsible.

In all forms of chronic peritonitis a *friction* may be felt or heard usually in the upper abdomen. Polyorrhomenitis, *polyserositis*, generally chronic inflammation of the serous membranes, Concato's disease (as the Italians call it) may occur with this form as well as in the tuberculous variety. The pericardium and both pleurae may be involved. The *pericardial pseudocirrhosis* (Pick's disease) is an allied condition.

In some instances of chronic peritonitis the membrane presents numerous nodular thickenings, which may be mistaken for tubercles. Cases have been reported due to oat particles. J. F. Payne described a case with disseminated growths throughout the liver which were not cancerous. It has been suggested that some of the cases of tuberculous peritonitis cured by operation have been of this nature, but histological examination should determine. Miura, in Japan, reported a case in which these nodules contained the ova of a parasite. In one case the exciting cause was regarded as cholesterin plates, contained within the granulomatous nodules.

Chronic Hemorrhagic Peritonitis.—Blood-stained effusions in the peritoneum occur particularly in cancerous and tuberculous disease. A chronic inflammation analogous to the hemorrhagic pachymeningitis of the brain was described first by Virchow, and is localized most commonly in the pelvis. Layers of new connective tissue form on the surface of the peritoneum with large wide vessels from which hemorrhage occurs. This is repeated from time to time with the formation of regular layers of hemorrhagic effusion. It is rarely diffuse, more commonly circumscribed. Probably the spontaneous peritoneal hemorrhage with acute abdominal features (Churchman) may represent the primary form of this rare condition.

Treatment.—In cases with *adhesions* which are causing symptoms, great caution should be exercised in advising operation and a thorough X-ray study made to determine, if possible, the exact condition. For local adhesions of the pylorus, duodenum, and colon, causing obstruction, surgery may be beneficial. In the cases with extensive adhesions about the cecum and ascending colon, the chances are less favorable. Every effort should be made to help the action of the bowels by medical measures especially mineral oil and belladonna. An abdominal support may be of help. For *chronic proliferative peritonitis* very little can be done. If a primary cause is present such as renal and cardiac disease or syphilis, treatment should be directed to that. The treatment in general is practically that of ascites and tapping should be done whenever necessary. The injection of epinephrine (♏ xv, 1 cc.) into the peritoneal cavity after tapping has been of benefit. As a rule operation is not advisable and no benefit results from an attempt to produce additional adhesions.

NEW GROWTHS IN THE PERITONEUM

Tuberculous Peritonitis.—This has already been considered.

Cancer of the Peritoneum.—Although, as a rule, secondary to disease of the stomach, liver, or pelvic organs, cases of primary cancer occur. It is probable that the so-called primary cancers of the serous membranes are endotheliomata and not carcinomata. Secondary malignant peritonitis occurs in connection with all forms of cancer. It is usually characterized by a number of round tumors scattered over the entire peritoneum, sometimes small and miliary, at other times large and nodular, with puckered centres. The disease most commonly starts from the stomach or the ovaries. The omentum is indurated and, as in tuberculous peritonitis, forms a mass which lies transversely across the upper portion of the abdomen. Primary malignant disease of the peritoneum is extremely rare. *Colloid* sometimes occurs, forming enormous masses, which in one case weighed over 100 pounds. Peritoneal cancer spreads by the detachment of small particles which are carried in the lymph currents and by the movements to distant parts, or by contact of opposing surfaces. It occurs more frequently in women than in men, and more commonly at the later period of life than in the young.

The *diagnosis* is easy with a history of local malignant disease; as when it occurs with ovarian tumor or with gastric cancer. In cases in which there is no evidence of a primary lesion the diagnosis may be doubtful. The clinical picture is usually that of chronic *ascites* with progressive emaciation. There may be no fever. If there is much effusion nothing definite can be felt on examination. After tapping, irregular nodules or the curled omentum may be felt lying transversely across the upper abdomen. Multiple nodules, if large, indicate cancer, particularly in persons above middle life. Nodular tuberculous peritonitis is most frequent in children. The presence about the navel of secondary nodules and indurated masses is more common in cancer. Inflammation, suppuration, and the discharge of pus from the navel rarely occur except in tuberculous disease. Considerable enlargement of the inguinal glands may be present in cancer. The fluid in cancer and in tubercle may be much alike, hemorrhagic in both; more often in the latter. In cancer there may be large multinuclear cells or groups of cells—the sprouting cell-groups of Foulis—which are extremely suggestive. The *colloid cancer* may give a different picture; instead of ascitic fluid, the abdomen is occupied by semisolid gelatinous substance, and is firm, not fluctuating. Echinococci in the peritoneum may simulate cancer very closely.

Free solid tumors are sometimes met with, usually fibroid or calcareous, as in the case reported by Campbell and Ower, in which a man had had a movable tumor in his abdomen for more than twenty years. It had increased in size, and at his death was a rounded mass 8 by 9 cm.

ASCITES

Definition.—The accumulation of serous fluid in the peritoneal cavity.

Etiology.—Local Causes.—(*a*) Chronic inflammation of the peritoneum, either simple, cancerous, or tuberculous. (*b*) Portal obstruction in the terminal branches within the liver, as in cirrhosis, syphilis and chronic passive congestion, or by compression of the vein in the gastro-hepatic omentum, by proliferative peritonitis, gumma, new growths, or aneurism. (*c*) Thrombosis of the portal vein. (*d*) Tumors of the abdomen. The solid growths of the ovaries may cause ascites, which may completely mask the true condition. It is important to bear in mind this possibility in obscure ascites in women. An enlarged spleen may be associated with recurring ascites.

General Causes.—The ascites may be part of a general dropsy, the result of mechanical effects, as in heart disease. In cardiac lesions the effusion is sometimes confined to the peritoneum, in which case it is due to secondary changes in the liver, or it may be connected with a failure of the suction action of this organ by which the peritoneum is kept dry. Ascites occurs also in the dropsy of nephritis and severe anemia.

Signs.—A gradual uniform enlargement of the abdomen is the characteristic sign of ascites. (*a*) *Inspection.*—According to the amount of fluid the abdomen is protuberant and flattened at the sides. With large effusions, the skin is tense and may present lineae albicantes. Frequently the navel and the parts about it are very prominent. In many cases the superficial veins are enlarged and can be seen joining the thoracic vessels. Often it can be determined that the current is from below upward. In some instances, as in obliteration of the portal vein, these superficial abdominal vessels may be extensively varicose. About the navel in cases of cirrhosis there is occasionally a bunch of distended veins. The heart may be displaced upward.

(*b*) *Palpation.*—Fluctuation is obtained by placing one hand upon one side of the abdomen and giving a sharp tap on the opposite side with the other hand, when a wave is felt to strike as a definite shock against the applied hand. Even comparatively small quantities of fluid may give this fluctuation shock. When the abdominal walls are thick or very fat, an assistant may place the edge of the hand in front of the abdomen. In ascites Pitfield points out that if the patient is in a sitting position and percussion is done over the muscles of the lower back, the fluctuation wave can be felt in the lower front of the abdomen. In palpating for the solid organs in case of ascites the pads of the fingers are placed lightly upon the skin, and by a sudden depression of the fingers the fluid is displaced and the solid organ or tumor may be felt. By this method of "dipping" or displacement, the liver may be felt below the costal margin, or the spleen, or sometimes solid tumors of the omentum or intestine.

(*c*) *Percussion.*—In the dorsal position with a moderate quantity of fluid in the peritoneum the flanks are dull, while the umbilical and epigastric regions, in which the intestines float, are tympanitic. This area of clear resonance may have an oval outline. Having obtained the lateral limit of the dulness on one side, if the patient turns on the opposite side, the fluid gravitates to the dependent part and the uppermost flank is now tympanitic. In moderate effusions this movable dulness changes greatly in the different postures. Small amounts of fluid, probably under a litre, would scarcely give movable dulness, as the pelvis and the renal regions hold a considerable quantity. In such cases it is best to place the patient in the knee-elbow position, when a dull note will be determined at the most dependent portion. The diaphragm is pushed up, the liver dulness is high and the heart may be displaced. There may be dyspnea with thoracic signs of passive congestion or fluid.

Diagnosis.—The following are among the conditions which may be mistaken for ascites: *Ovarian tumor,* in which the sac develops, as a rule, unilaterally, though when large it is centrally placed. The dulness is anterior and the resonance is in the flanks, into which the intestines are pushed by the cyst. Examination *per vaginam* may give important indications. In those rare instances in which gas develops in the cyst the diagnosis may be very difficult. Succussion has been obtained in such cases. A *distended bladder* may reach above the umbilicus. In such instances some urine dribbles away, and suspicion of ascites or a cyst is occasionally entertained. A trocar may be thrust into a distended bladder, supposed to be an ovarian cyst, and it is stated that John Hunter tapped a bladder, thinking it to be ascites. Such a mistake is avoided by prior catheterization. Large pancreatic or hydatid cysts in the abdomen may simulate ascites.

The diagnosis of the *cause* is often impossible, before tapping is done, in the absence of a good history or previous observation. The cases due to cardiac disease, nephritis or anemia should be easily recognized. After tapping, the examination of the liver and spleen or finding a tumor may give the diagnosis. Careful search should be made for a primary growth; with secondary involvement of the peritoneum the general condition is usually suggestive. A rectal examination is important in all cases and a vaginal one in women. Cirrhosis of the liver, chronic and tuberculous peritonitis, and ascites due to solid tumors may give the greatest difficulty.

Ascitic Fluid.—Usually this is a clear serum, light yellow in the ascites of anemia and nephritis, often darker in color in cirrhosis of the liver. The specific gravity is low, seldom more than 1.010 or 1.015, whereas in the fluid of ovarian cysts or chronic peritonitis the specific gravity is over 1.015. It is albuminous and sometimes coagulates spontaneously. Dock has called attention to the importance of the study of the cells in the exudate. In cancer very characteristic forms, with nuclear figures, may be found. Hemorrhagic effusion usually occurs in cancer and tuberculosis, occasionally in cirrhosis and with ruptured tubal pregnancy.

CHYLOUS ASCITES.—Of the cases tabulated by McKenzie, Wallis, and Scholberg, 81 were in association with tumors, 46 with the infections, chiefly tuberculosis, 37 in association with affections of the thoracic duct and lymphatic system, and 78 in connection with diseases such as cirrhosis of the liver, cardiac disease, nephritis, amyloid disease, and thrombosis. In a certain number of cases the cause of the condition is unknown.

Quincke recognized two types, one in which there was a true milky or fatty fluid, the other in which the turbidity is due to fatty degeneration of cells or to chemical substances of a nonfatty nature. The fluid of the true *chylous* ascites is yellowish-white in color, contains fine fat globules, a creamy layer collects on standing, the specific gravity generally exceeds 1.012, and the fat content is high. As a rule, it tends to accumulate rapidly and large amounts may be removed. The fluid of *pseudochylous* ascites is milky white, the opacity may vary at different tappings. Microscopically there are many fine refractile granules, but they do not give reactions for fat, the cellular elements may be numerous, and a creamy layer rarely forms. The specific gravity is less than 1.012, and the total solids rarely exceed 2 per cent. The fat content is low. Lecithin combined with globulin appears to be the cause of the opalescence. Milky ascites is characteristic of no specific morbid lesion. The prognosis is usually grave.

Treatment.—This depends much on the nature of the cause. In cirrhosis early and repeated tapping may give time for the establishment of the collateral circulation, and temporary cures have followed this procedure. The injection of epinephrine (ʒ ss, 2 cc. of a 1-1000 solution) into the peritoneal cavity after tapping has been useful in some cases. Permanent drainage with Southey's tube, incision, and washing out the peritoneum have also been practised. Little is gained by restricting the amount of fluid. The intake of salt should be reduced to a minimum. The bowels should be kept open but excessive purging avoided. Diuretics are of little value in the presence of ascites owing to the pressure influencing the renal activity but may be useful early or after tapping. It is wise to give diuretics for a day or two before tapping so that they may act promptly. Diuretin (gr. 15, 1.0 gm.) or theocin gr. 5, 0.3 gm.) should be given three times a day. With heart disease the proper treatment should be given. In case of a solid tumor, as of the ovary, removal is curative. In the ascites of cardiac and renal disease cathartics are useful, particularly the bitartrate of potash, given alone or with jalap, and the large doses of salts given an hour before breakfast with as little water as possible. These sometimes cause rapid disappearance of the effusion. The ascites of the general anascara of nephritis will receive consideration under another section.

DISEASES OF THE OMENTUM

Torsion.—Though the first case was reported by Oberst in 1882, Bookman collected 131 cases in 1915. It is one of the causes of acute abdominal conditions. The torsion may occur with or without the presence of a hernial sac, with which fully 90 per cent of the cases have occurred. The twist is usually associated with adhesion of the free extremity to some structure. As the cases are usually in connection with hernia, the diagnosis of strangulation is made. Pain, muscular rigidity and vomiting are the usual features. The pain may be sudden in onset or recurrent for years. The bowels are usually open; there may be mucus and blood in the stools; sometimes there is constipation. The condition is mistaken for hernia, acute appendicitis, or intestinal obstruction. The existence of a hernia and the sudden appearance of an abodminal mass are suggestive. Early operation with removal of the strangulated portion is the only treatment.

SECTION VII

DISEASES OF THE RESPIRATORY SYSTEM

DISEASES OF THE NOSE

EPISTAXIS

Etiology.—Among *local* causes are trauma, small ulcers, picking or scratching the nose, new growths, and the presence of foreign bodies. In chronic nasal catarrh bleeding is not infrequent. The blood may come from one or both nostrils. The flow may be profuse after an injury.

Among *general* conditions the following are the most important: It occurs in growing children, particularly about the age of puberty; more frequently in the delicate than in the strong and vigorous. There is a family form in which many members in several generations are affected, a *hereditary multiple telangiectasis,* a special feature of which is recurring epistaxis. The disease has nothing to do with hemophilia, with which it has been confounded. The bleeding occurs from the telangiectasis in the nasal mucosa, and from those in the lips, tongue, and skin.

Epistaxis is common in persons of so-called plethoric habit. It is stated sometimes to precede, or to indicate a liability to, apoplexy. There may be a most extreme grade of cyanosis without its occurrence. It is frequent in hepatic cirrhosis. At high altitudes epistaxis is common. In hemophilia the nose ranks first of the mucous membranes from which bleeding arises. It occurs in all forms of chronic anemias and in conditions with hypertension. It occurs at the onset of certain fevers and is associated in some special way with typhoid fever. Vicarious epistaxis has been described in suppression of the menses. The blood comes from capillary oozing or diapedesis but may come from a small vessel or from capillary angiomata situated in the respiratory portion of the nostril and upon the cartilaginous septum.

Symptoms.—Slight hemorrhage is not associated with any special features. When the bleeding is protracted the patients have the more serious manifestations of loss of blood. In the slow dripping which takes place in some instances of hemophilia, a remarkable blood tumor projecting from one nostril and extending even below the mouth may be formed.

Death from ordinary epistaxis is very rare. The more blood that is lost the greater is the tendency to clotting with cessation of the bleeding.

Diagnosis.—This is usually easy. One point only need be mentioned; namely, that bleeding from the posterior nares occasionally occurs during sleep and the blood trickles into the pharynx and may be swallowed. If vomited, it may be regarded as hematemesis; or, if coughed up, as hemoptysis.

Treatment.—In a majority of the cases the bleeding ceases of itself. In the most frequent situation the introduction of absorbent cotton for about an inch, held in position by compressing the nostrils, will often control the bleeding. Astringents, such as zinc or alum may be used. If the bleeding comes from an ulcerated surface, an attempt should be made to apply the cautery. If the bleeding is at all severe and obstinate, the nares should be packed. A patient with epistaxis and spider angiomata of the skin and mucous membranes used a finger of a rubber glove with a small rubber tube and stopcock by which he could dilate the glove finger, inserted into the nostril, and so effectually control the bleeding. A solution of epinephrine or thromboplastine may be injected into the nostril. The injection of blood serum may be tried or transfusion done in severe cases.

DISEASES OF THE LARYNX

ACUTE LARYNGITIS

This may come on as an independent affection or in association with general inflammation of the upper respiratory passages.

Etiology.—Many cases are due to catching cold or to overuse of the voice; others come on in consequence of the inhalation of irritating gases. Very severe laryngitis is excited by traumatism, either injuries from without or the lodgment of foreign bodies. It may be caused by the action of very hot liquids or corrosive poisons. It may occur in the general catarrh of influenza and measles. The pneumococcus, streptococcus, influenza bacillus and *Micrococcus catarrhalis* are the organisms most commonly found.

Symptoms.—There is a sense of tickling referred to the larynx; cold air irritates and, owing to the increased sensibility of the mucous membrane, the act of inspiration may be painful. There is a dry cough and the voice is altered. At first it is simply husky, but soon phonation becomes painful, and finally the voice may be completely lost. In adults the respirations are not increased in frequency, but in children dyspnea is not uncommon and may occur in spasmodic attacks and become urgent if there is much edema with the inflammatory swelling.

The laryngoscope shows a swollen mucous membrane of the larynx, particularly the aryepiglottidean folds. The vocal cords have lost their smooth and shining appearance and are reddened and swollen. Their mobility also is greatly impaired, owing to the infiltration of the adjoining mucous membrane and of the muscles. A slight mucoid exudation may cover the parts. The constitutional symptoms are not severe. There is rarely much fever, and in many cases the patient is not seriously ill. Occasionally attacks come on with greater intensity, the cough is very distressing, deglutition is painful, and there may be urgent dyspnea.

Diagnosis.—There is rarely any difficulty in this if a satisfactory laryngoscopic examination can be made. The severer forms may simulate edema of the glottis. When the loss of voice is marked, the case may be mistaken for nervous aphonia, but the laryngoscope decides the question. Much more difficult is the diagnosis of acute laryngitis in children, particularly in the very young, in whom it is so hard to make a proper examination. From ordinary laryngismus it is to be distinguished by the presence of fever, the mode of onset, and particularly the coryza and the previous symptoms of hoarseness or loss of voice. Membranous laryngitis may at first be quite impossible to differentiate, but in a majority of cases of this affection there are patches on the pharynx and early swelling of the cervical glands. The symptoms, too, are much more severe.

Treatment.—Rest of the larynx should be enjoyed, so far as phonation is concerned; smoking should be forbidden. In cases of any severity the patient should be kept in bed. The room should be at an even temperature and the air saturated with moisture. Inhalations of benzoin, menthol and eucalyptus are helpful. Early in the disease, if there is much fever, aconite and citrate of potash may be given, and for the irritating cough a full dose of Dover's powder or codein at night. An ice-bag externally often gives great relief.

ACUTE FULMINATING LARYNGO-TRACHEO-BRONCHITIS

This usually occurs in young children and has severe general features with high fever and intense local inflammatory changes in the larynx, trachea and bronchi. There is a very tenacious exudate which may cause varying degrees of obstruction especially in the larynx, which rarely shows much edema. In some cases the obstruction is more in the trachea and bronchi. Cultures from the exudate usually show pneumococci and staphylococci. The frequency of streptococci is uncertain; there may be a terminal streptococcus infection. The signs of obstruction are marked with retraction on inspiration. The pulse and respiration rates are high. In the *diagnosis,* laryngeal diphtheria and foreign body have to be excluded. This is done best by direct laryngoscopy. In *treatment,* removal of the secretion is essential. This may require bronchoscopy if there is much secretion in the trachea or bronchi. As this may have to be repeated frequently, it is well to do a tracheotomy early so as to lessen irritation of the larynx. These patients require constant watching as obstruction may increase suddenly. Fluid should be given freely.

CHRONIC LARYNGITIS

Etiology.—The disease usually follows repeated acute attacks. The most common cause is overuse of the voice, particularly in persons whose occupation necessitates shouting. The constant inhalation of irritating substances, dusty occupations, smoking and nasal infection may also cause it.

Symptoms.—The voice is usually hoarse and rough and in severe cases may be almost lost. There is usually very little pain; only the unpleasant sense of tickling in the larynx, which causes a frequent desire to cough. With the laryngoscope the mucous membrane looks swollen, but much less red than in the acute condition. In association with the granular pharyngitis, the mucous glands of the epiglottis and of the ventricles may be involved.

Treatment.—Etiological factors should be corrected. The nostrils should be carefully examined, since chronic laryngitis may be dependent upon obstruction to the passage of air through the nose or rhinitis. Local applications can be made directly to the larynx. Among the remedies most recommended are solutions of nitrate of silver, perchloride of zinc, and tannic acid. Oily or saline sprays may be used. Among directions to be given are the avoidance of heated rooms and loud speaking, and abstinence from tobacco and alcohol. The throat should not be too much muffled, and morning and evening the neck should be sponged with cold water.

Hoarseness.—This results from many causes and an etiological diagnosis should be made as early as possible. Chronic laryngitis should only be diagnosed when every other cause is excluded, especially tuberculosis, syphilis and above all malignant disease. The conditions which the practitioner should especially have in mind are many; there are certain local causes which require the specialist for their recognition.

(1) *Local.*—Malignant disease, papilloma, tuberculosis, syphilis, leprosy, diphtheria, laryngismus stridulus, foreign body, vocal nodules, vocal abuse, and chronic laryngitis.

(2) *Secondary.*—Aneurism, goitre, thickened pleura, mitral stenosis, tabes, multiple sclerosis, syringomyelia, glossolabiopharyngeal paralysis and nephritis.

EDEMATOUS LARYNGITIS

It was described by Matthew Baillie (1812) and Pitcairn (one of the owners of the famous Gold-headed Cane) was one of the first cases.

Etiology.—Edema of the structures which form the glottis is met with (*a*) as a sequence of acute laryngitis and with acute streptococcal pharyngolaryngitis; (*b*) in chronic diseases of the larynx, as syphilis or tubercle; (*c*) in severe inflammatory diseases like diphtheria, in erysipelas of the neck, and in various forms of cellulitis; (*d*) occasionally in the acute infections—scarlet or typhoid fever; (*e*) from drinking very hot or irritating fluids; (*f*) from trauma due to a foreign body or instrumentation; and (*g*) from septic infection of ulcers. Noninflammatory causes are nephritis, angioneurotic edema and from the administration of iodide in a susceptible person.

Symptoms.—There is dyspnea, increasing in intensity, so that within an hour or two the condition may become very critical. There is sometimes marked stridor and the voice becomes husky and disappears. The laryngoscope shows enormous swelling of the epiglottis, which can sometimes be felt with the finger or even seen when the tongue is strongly depressed. The aryepiglottidean folds are the seat of the chief swelling and may almost meet in the middle line. Occasionally the edema is below the true cords. In acute septic *pharyngolaryngitis* the general and local symptoms are severe. Dundas-Grant has pointed out that in these cases the patient's voice suggests that he has quinsy but no evidence of this is found—"quinsy voice without quinsy." The *diagnosis* is rarely difficult, as even without the laryngoscope the swollen epiglottis can be seen or felt with the finger. The condition is often fatal.

Treatment.—An ice-bag should be placed on the larynx and the patient given ice to suck. The air of the room should be moist. If the symptoms are urgent, the throat should be sprayed with a strong solution of cocaine or epinephrine (1-1000) and the swollen epiglottis scarified. If relief does not follow, tracheotomy should immediately be performed. The high mortality is due to the fact that this operation is, as a rule, too long delayed. In angioneurotic edema, 15 minims (1 cc.) of epinephrine solution (1-1000) should be given hypodermically.

SPASMODIC LARYNGITIS

(*Laryngismus stridulus*)

Definition.—Spasmodic contraction of the intrinsic muscles of the larynx, usually in children, leading to closure of the glottis and dyspnea.

Etiology.—In children it may be a purely nervous affection, without any inflammatory condition of the larynx, and is most common with rickets and adenoids. The disease has close relations with tetany and may display many of the accessory phenomena of this disease. The attack may come on when the child has been scolded. It was supposed at one time that they were associated with enlargement of the thymus, and the condition received the name of *thymic asthma.*

In adults it may follow irritation of the pneumogastric nerves, as in aneurism or mediastinal tumor. The crises in tabes dorsalis are due to sudden spasm of the intrinsic muscles. It is occasionally seen in hysteria. There are attacks of spasmodic cough in adults with distressing spasm of the glottis, lasting for months and arousing the suspicion of aneurism or tumor.

During a paroxysm there is spasm of the adductors, but the precise nature of the influence causing it is not known, whether central or reflex from peripheral irritation. The disease is not so common in America as in England.

Symptoms.—The attacks may come on either in the night or in the day; often just as the child awakes. There is no cough or hoarseness, but the respiration is arrested and the child struggles for breath, the face gets congested, and then, with a sudden relaxation of the spasm, the air is drawn into the lungs with a high-pitched crowing sound, which has given to the affection the name of "child-crowing." Convulsions may occur or there may be carpopedal spasms. Death may, but rarely does, occur during the attack. With the cyanosis the spasm relaxes and respiration begins. The attacks may recur with great frequency throughout the day. The character of the attacks and the absence of symptoms in the intervals are important in diagnosis.

Treatment.—An open-air life, nourishing diet, cod-liver oil and tonic treatment are indicated. The bowels should be carefully regulated. Adenoids should be removed and any nasopharyngeal diseases treated. Hydrotherapy is often useful; two or three times a day the child should be placed in a warm bath, and the back and chest sponged for a minute or two with cold water. It may be employed when the child is in a paroxysm, though if the attack is severe it is better to dash cold water into the face. Sometimes placing the finger far back into the throat or pulling the tongue forward relieves the spasm. Amyl nitrite by inhalation may give relief. Small doses of sodium bromide, chloral hydrate or antipyrine are sometimes useful.

Spasmodic croup, believed to be a functional spasm of the muscles of the larynx, is most common between the ages of two and five years. The child goes to bed well, and about midnight or in the early morning hours awakes with oppressed breathing, harsh, croupy cough, and perhaps some huskiness of voice. The oppression and distress for a time are serious, the face is congested, and there are signs of cyanosis. The attack passes off abruptly, the child falls asleep and awakes the next morning feeling perfectly well. These attacks may be repeated for several nights in succession, and usually cause great alarm. There are instances in which the child is somewhat hoarse throughout the day, and has slight catarrhal symptoms and a croupy cough. There is probably slight catarrhal laryngitis with it. These cases are not infrequently mistaken for laryngeal diphtheria. To allay the spasm a whiff of chloroform or amyl nitrite may be administered, or the child may be placed in a hot bath. An emetic, such as wine of ipecac, will usually relieve the spasm, and is specially indicated if the child has overloaded the stomach.

TUBERCULOUS LARYNGITIS

Etiology.—Tubercles may arise primarily in the laryngeal mucosa, but in the great majority of cases the affection is secondary to pulmonary tuberculosis, in which it is met with in a proportion of from 18 to 30 per cent. Laryngitis may occur very early in pulmonary tuberculosis. There may be involvement of the larynx with very limited pulmonary signs.

Morbid Anatomy.—The mucosa is at first swollen and presents scattered tubercles, which seem to begin in the neighborhood of the blood vessels. By their fusion small tuberculous masses arise, which caseate and finally ulcerate. The ulcers are usually covered with a grayish exudate, and there is a general thickening of the mucosa about them, particularly marked upon the arytenoids. The ulcers may erode the true cords and destroy them, and passing deeply may cause perichondritis with necrosis and occasionally exfoliation of the cartilages. The disease may involve the pharynx and fauces. The epiglottis may be entirely destroyed. There are rare instances in which cicatricial changes go on to such a degree that stenosis of the larynx is induced.

Symptoms.—The first indication is slight huskiness of the voice, which finally deepens to hoarseness, and in advanced stages there may be complete loss of voice. There is something very suggestive in the early hoarseness of tuberculous laryngitis. The attention may be directed to the lungs simply by the quality of the voice.

The *cough* is in part due to involvement of the larynx. Early in the disease it is not very troublesome, but when the ulceration is extensive it becomes husky and ineffectual. Of the symptoms, none is more aggravating than the dysphagia, which is met with particularly when the epiglottis is involved, and when the ulceration has extended to the pharynx. In instances in which the epiglottis is in great part destroyed, with each attempt to take food there are distressing paroxysms of cough and even of suffocation with severe pain.

With the laryngoscope there is seen early a pallor of the mucous membrane, which looks thickened and infiltrated, particularly that covering the arytenoid cartilages. There may be congestion rather than pallor. The ulcers are very characteristic. They are broad and shallow, with gray bases and ill-defined outlines. The vocal cords are infiltrated and thickened, and ulceration is very common.

The *diagnosis* is rarely difficult, as it is usually associated with well-marked pulmonary disease. Simple laryngitis, syphilis and neoplasm have to be excluded. In case of doubt the secretion from the base of an ulcer should be examined for bacilli.

Treatment.—The voice should not be used. In the early stages no method of treatment is more effectual. Applications of lactic acid in glycerine and the electrocautery are the best local measures. The insufflation, three times a day, of a powder of iodoform with morphia, after cleansing the ulcers with a spray, relieves the pain in some cases. Cocaine (4-per-cent solution) applied with the atomizer will often enable the patient to swallow his food comfortably. There are, however, distressing cases of extensive ulceration in which even cocaine loses its good effects. Anesthesin (gr. v, 0.3 gm.) may be insufflated and give relief, or a combination of it and orthoform in equal parts. Injection of the laryngeal nerves with alcohol has relieved the pain. With loss of the glottis the difficulty in swallowing is less when the patient hangs the head over and sucks food through a tube. Heliotherapy has given good results.

SYPHILITIC LARYNGITIS

Syphilis attacks the larynx in congenital cases or as a secondary or tertiary manifestation of the acquired form.

Symptoms.—In *secondary* syphilis there is occasional erythema of the larynx, which may go on to definite catarrh, but has nothing characteristic. The process may proceed to the formation of superficial whitish ulcers, usually symmetrically placed on the cords or ventricular bands. Mucous patches and condylomata are rarely seen. The symptoms are practically those of slight loss of voice with laryngeal irritation, as in the simple catarrhal form.

The *tertiary* laryngeal lesions are numerous and serious. True gummata, varying in size from the head of a pin to a small nut, arise in the submucous tissue, most commonly at the base of the epiglottis. They go through the characteristic changes and may break down, producing extensive and deep ulceration, or—and this is more characteristic of syphilitic laryngitis—in their healing form a fibrous tissue which shrinks and produces stenosis. The ulceration may involve the cartilage, inducing necrosis and exfoliation, and even hemorrhage from erosion of the arteries. Edema may suddenly prove fatal. The cicatrices which follow the sclerosis of the gummata or the healing of the ulcers produce great deformity. The epiglottis may be tied down to the pharyngeal wall or to the epiglottic folds, or even to the tongue; and eventually a stenosis results, which may necessitate tracheotomy. The outlook for much improvement in these cases is unfavorable.

The laryngeal symptoms of *congenital* syphilis appear either early, within the first five or six months, or after puberty; most commonly in the former period. The gummatous infiltration leads to ulceration, most commonly of the epiglottis and in the ventricles, and the process may extend deeply and involve the cartilage. Cicatricial contraction may also occur.

The *diagnosis* of syphilis of the larynx is rarely difficult, since it occurs commonly with other features of the disease. The cough has a peculiar rough quality which is often suggestive.

Treatment.—The administration of antisyphilitic remedies is the most important, and under these the secondary lesions usually subside promptly. The tertiary laryngeal manifestations are always serious and difficult to treat. The deep ulceration is specially hard to combat, and the cicatrization may necessitate tracheotomy or gradual dilatation.

DISEASES OF THE BRONCHI

ACUTE TRACHEOBRONCHITIS

Acute inflammation of the trachea and larger bronchi is a very common disease, rarely serious in healthy adults, but which may be fatal in the old and in the young, owing to associated pulmonary complications. The trachea and bronchi are usually involved together but the process may be most marked in either of them. The bronchitis affects either the larger and medium sized tubes or the smaller bronchi, in which case it is known as capillary bronchitis. We shall speak here only of the former, as the latter is part and parcel of bronchopneumonia.

Etiology.—In a majority of cases it is an *acute infection* beginning as a simple coryza and extending to the air passages. It is very infectious, as noted by Benjamin Franklin, and prevails at times in epidemic form. It prevails in the cold changeable months. The association with cold is indicated in the popular expression "cold on the chest." It attacks persons of all ages, but more particularly the young and the old. Some individuals have a special predisposition and the slightest exposure may bring on an attack.

Acute bronchitis is associated with many infections, notably measles and typhoid fever. It is present also in asthma and whooping cough. The subjects of spinal curvature are specially liable to it. The bronchitis of nephritis, gout and heart disease is usually a chronic form. Inhalation of dust is a contributing factor in many cases. Irritating gases of all sorts may cause bronchitis. Ether inhalation is only too often followed by bronchitis. There is a spirochetal form which may be acute or chronic. Upper respiratory tract infection (tonsils, sinuses) may be responsible for repeated attacks.

Bacteriology.—The pneumococcus is responsible for many cases both in young and old. The infection may follow pneumonia, and bronchitis may recur winter after winter, with the sputum showing an almost pure culture of the pneumococcus. These germs may persist in the sputum for many years, with an almost daily cough, aggravated in the winter. The influenza bacillus is common and may be found alone or with streptococci. The *Micrococcus catarrhalis* is present in a number of cases, very often with other organisms. It is not possible to separate clinical groups of bronchitis to correspond with the chief infective agent. The pneumococcus carrier appears to be very liable to recurring attacks. The Vincent organism may cause ulcerative or membranous bronchitis with very severe features.

Morbid Anatomy.—The mucous membrane of the trachea and bronchi is reddened, congested, and covered with mucus and mucopus, which may be seen oozing from the smaller bronchi, some of which are dilated. The finer changes in the mucosa consist in desquamation of the ciliated epithelium, swelling and edema of the submucosa, and infiltration of the tissue with leukocytes. The mucous glands are much swollen.

Symptoms.—General.—The symptoms of an ordinary "cold" accompany the onset; the coryza extends to the larynx, producing hoarseness, and then to the trachea and bronchi, causing cough. A chill is rare, but there is a sense of oppression, with heaviness and pains in the bones and back. In mild cases there is scarcely any fever, but in severer forms the range is from 101° to 103° F. In *tracheitis* the sputum is often tough and tenacious, sometimes gelatinous, in a gray, mottled globular mass, often projected from the mouth in coughing. The amount is not large and it often accumulates on the cords, causing a desire to clear the throat. There may be severe discomfort or pain felt behind the sternum. The *bronchial* symptoms set in with a feeling of tightness and irritation beneath the sternum and a sensation of oppression in the chest. The cough is rough at first, and often of a ringing character. It comes on in paroxysms which rack and distress the patient extremely. The pain may be intense beneath the sternum and along the attachments of the diaphragm. At first the cough is dry and the expectoration scanty and viscid, but in a few days the secretion becomes mucopurulent and abundant, and finally purulent. With the loosening of the cough great relief is experienced. The sputum is made up largely of pus-cells, with a variable number of large round alveolar cells, many of which contain carbon grains, while others have undergone myelin degeneration.

Physical Signs.—The respiratory movements are not greatly increased in frequency unless the fever is high. There are instances, however, in which the breathing is rapid and when the smaller tubes are involved there is dyspnea. On palpation the bronchial fremitus can often be felt. On auscultation in the early stage, piping sibilant râles are everywhere to be heard. They are very changeable, and appear and disappear with coughing. With relaxation of the bronchial membranes and greater abundance of secretion, the râles change and become mucous and bubbling in quality. The bases of the lungs should be examined each day, particularly in children and the aged for signs of bronchopneumonia.

Course.—This depends on the conditions under which the disease arises. In healthy adults, by the end of a week the fever subsides and the cough loosens. In another week or ten days convalescence is fully established. In young children the chief risk is in the extension of the process downward. In measles and whooping cough the ordinary bronchitis is very apt to descend to the finer tubes, which become dilated and plugged with mucopus, inducing areas of collapse, and finally bronchopneumonia. This extension is indicated by changes in the physical signs. Usually at the base the râles are crackling and numerous and there may be areas of defective resonance and of feeble or distant tubular breathing. In the aged and debilitated there are similar dangers if the process extends to the smaller tubes. In old age the bronchial mucosa is less capable of expelling mucus, which is more apt to sag to the dependent parts with extension of the inflammation to the air-cells.

In *acute suppurative bronchitis,* there is very severe inflammation in the medium and small bronchi with purulent secretion. The onset is usually acute and followed by high fever, severe cough and extreme dyspnea. The sputum may be blood streaked at first but soon becomes purulent and profuse. Cyanosis may be very marked. There is marked toxemia. The lungs show many râles; there may be dulness at the bases. Death may occur in 2 or 3 days or the course be prolonged to death or recovery.

Diagnosis.—This is rarely difficult. Although the mode of onset may be brusque and perhaps simulate pneumonia, yet the absence of dulness and blowing breathing, and the general character of the bronchial inflammation, render the diagnosis easy. Bronchopneumonia is indicated by the greater severity of the symptoms, particularly the dyspnea, higher fever (except in the aged), the more paroxysmal and insistent cough, the changed color, and the physical signs. In tracheitis, direct inspection may be made.

Treatment.—We should do all in our power to lessen the risks of infection. The patient should sleep alone, the sputum should be carefully disinfected, and, when possible, there should be an abundance of sunlight and fresh air. Proper treatment of nasopharyngeal disease is important. In mild cases household measures suffice. A hot foot-bath, or a warm bath, a drink of hot lemonade, and a mustard plaster on the chest will often give relief. In severe cases the patient should be in bed. The diet should be simple and liquids taken freely. For the dry, racking cough, the symptom most complained of by the patient, Dover's powder is a useful remedy (gr. v-x, 0.03-0.06 gm.). It is a popular belief that quinine will check an oncoming cold but this is doubtful. It is a common custom when persons feel the approach of a cold to take a Turkish bath, and though the tightness and oppression may be relieved by it, there is risk in a majority of cases. Hydrotherapy is useful in the form of compresses to the thorax or a wet pack. Relief is obtained from the unpleasant sense of rawness by keeping the air of the room saturated with moisture and by counterirritation to the chest, especially in tracheitis. In this dry stage the old-fashioned mixture of the wines of antimony and ipecacuanha with liquor ammonii acetatis and nitrous ether is useful. If the pulse is very rapid, tincture of aconite may be given, particularly to children. The use of inhalations, such as the compound tincture of benzoin, often gives relief. For the cough, when dry and irritating, opium should be used in the form of Dover's powder or paregoric and ammonium chloride (gr. v, 0.03 gm.) given. In the very young and the aged care must be exercised in the use of opium, particularly if the secretions are free; but for the distressing, irritative cough, which keeps the patient awake, opium in some form gives the best relief. Codein is often helpful. As the cough loosens and the expectoration is more abundant, the patient becomes more comfortable. In this stage it is customary to ply him with expectorants of various sorts. Though useful occasionally, they should not be given as a routine. *Vaccine treatment* is very uncertain, even when a single organism has been recovered, but occasionally prompt and satisfactory results are seen, both in prophylaxis and treatment.

In the acute bronchitis of children, if the amount of secretion is large and difficult to expectorate, or if there is dyspnea and cyanosis, an emetic (a tablespoonful of ipecac wine) should be given and repeated if necessary.

In the acute forms due to chemical irritation from war or industrial gas the intratracheal instillation of a few cc. of equal parts guaiacol, camphor, and menthol, 5 per cent in olive oil *t.i.d.*, will be found very effective.

CHRONIC BRONCHITIS

Etiology.—This may follow repeated attacks of acute bronchitis and is common in chronic lung affections, heart disease, aneurism of the aorta, gout and renal disease. It is most frequent in the aged and in males. Climate and season have an important influence. It is the cause of the winter cough of the aged, which recurs with regularity as the weather gets cold and changeable. Owing to the more uniform heating of the houses, it is less common in Canada and in the United States than in England. The organisms are practically the same as in acute bronchitis, often in combination.

Morbid Anatomy.—The bronchial mucosa present a variety of changes, depending somewhat upon the disease with which chronic bronchitis is associated. In some cases the mucous membrane is very thin, so that the longitudinal bands of elastic tissue stand out prominently. There is often peribronchitis with fibrosis. The tubes are dilated, the muscular and glandular tissues atrophied, and the epithelium is in great part shed. In other instances the mucosa is thickened and infiltrated. There may be ulceration, particularly of the mucous follicles. Bronchiectasis is common and emphysema is a constant accompaniment.

Symptoms.—In the form in old persons, associated with emphysema, fibrosis or heart disease, the chief symptoms are as follows: Shortness of breath, which may not be noticeable except on exertion. The patients "puff and blow" on going up hill or up a flight of stairs. This is due not so much to chronic bronchitis as to associated emphysema or cardiac weakness. They complain of no pain. The cough is variable, changing with the weather and season. During the summer they may remain free, but each succeeding winter the cough comes on with severity and persists. There may be only a spell in the morning or the chief distress is at night. The sputum is very variable. In cases of so-called dry bronchitis there is no expectoration. Usually, however, it is abundant, mucopurulent or distinctly purulent. There are instances in which the patient for years coughs up a thin fluid sputum. There is rarely fever. The general health may be good and the disease may present no serious features apart from the liability to induce emphysema and bronchiectasis. In many cases it is incurable. Patients improve and the cough disappears in the summer only to return in the winter.

Physical Signs.—The chest is usually distended, the movements are limited, and the condition is often that which we see in emphysema. The percussion note is clear or hyperresonant. On ausculation, expiration is prolonged and wheezy, and râles of various sorts are heard—some high-pitched and piping, others deep and snoring. Crepitant râles are common at the bases. The association of fibrosis and bronchiectasis may give varied signs.

In children apart from chronic disease of the lungs, chronic bronchitis with cough, chiefly nocturnal, is a common accompaniment of enlarged tonsils and adenoids, of sinusitis and sometimes of enlarged bronchial glands. The child, a mouth breather, with the characteristic facies and chest, is often thin and underdeveloped, with slight evening fever. Diffuse râles are present at the apices or, more commonly, the bases. The cough, the fever and the chest signs may lead to the diagnosis of tuberculosis.

Clinical Varieties.—The description just given is of the ordinary chronic bronchitis which occurs with emphysema and heart disease and in many elderly men. There are certain forms which merit special description: (*a*) There is a form in young adults which may continue indefinitely without serious impairment of the health. In some cases it follows influenza and there may be slight bronchiectasis. It may be secondary to sinus infection.

(*b*) BRONCHORRHEA.—Excessive bronchial secretion is met with under several conditions. It must not be mistaken for the profuse expectoration of bronchiectasis. The secretion may be very liquid and watery—*bronchorrhoea serosa*—and in extraordinary amount. More commonly, it is purulent though thin, and with greenish or yellow-green masses. It may be thick and uniform. This profuse bronchial secretion is usually a manifestation of chronic bronchitis which may lead to dilatation of the tubes and ultimately to fetid bronchitis. In the young the condition may persist for years.

(*c*) PUTRID BRONCHITIS.—Fetid expectoration occurs with bronchiectasis, gangrene, abscess, or with decomposition of secretions within tuberculous cavities and in an empyema which has perforated the lung. There are instances in which, apart from any of these states, the expectoration has a fetid character. The sputum is abundant, usually thin, grayish-white in color, and separates into an upper fluid layer capped with frothy mucus and a thick sediment in which may sometimes be found dirty yellow masses the size of peas or beans—the so-called *Dittrich's* plugs. The affection is rare apart from the above-mentioned conditions. In severe cases it leads to changes in the bronchial walls and often to abscess or gangrene. Metastatic brain abscess has followed in a number of cases.

(*d*) DRY CATARRH.—The *catarrh sec* of Laënnec, a not uncommon form, is characterized by paroxysms of coughing of great intensity, with little or no expectoration. It is usually met with in elderly persons with emphysema, and is one of the most obstinate of all varieties of bronchitis.

The bronchitis with an unusual number of eosinophiles in the sputum is usually associated with asthma.

Diagnosis.—The recognition of chronic bronchitis is rarely difficult but associated conditions are frequently overlooked. Bronchiectasis, fibrosis or aneurism should be kept in mind. It is important to exclude pulmonary tuberculosis which may be difficult owing to the bronchitis and emphysema. The sputum should be thoroughly studied and the X-ray study is useful. Cough secondary to heart disease should be easily recognized; the signs are often more basal than apical and proper therapy has a marked effect.

Treatment.—Removal to a southern latitude may prevent the onset. In England the milder climate of Falmouth, Torquay, and Bournemouth is suitable for those who cannot go elsewhere. Egypt, southern France, southern California, and Florida furnish winter climates in which the subjects of chronic bronchitis live with the greatest comfort. With care chronic bronchitis may prove to be the slight ailment that, as Oliver Wendell Holmes remarked, promotes longevity.

The first endeavor is to ascertain, if possible, whether there are constitutional or local affections with which it is associated. In many instances there is arteriosclerosis or nephritis, with heart disease and emphysema. Careful search should be made for disease of the upper respiratory tract (throat, nose, sinuses) and proper treatment carried out. In the form occurring in the old prophylaxis is most important. There is no doubt that with prudence even in the most changeable weather much may be done to prevent bronchitis. Warm but light undergarments should be used and special care taken in the spring months not to change them for lighter ones before the warm weather is established. Respiratory exercises in the recumbent position to increase the expansion of the lower thorax and the action of the diaphragm are sometimes helpful. The use of autogenous vaccines as a preventive is sometimes successful and is worthy of trial.

Cure is seldom effected by medicinal remedies. There are instances in which iodide of potassium acts with remarkable benefit, and it should always be given a trial in cases of bronchitis of obscure origin. For the morning cough, bicarbonate of sodium (gr. xv, 1 gm.), chloride of sodium (gr. v, 0.3 gm.), spirit of chloroform (♏ v, 0.3 cc.) in anise water and taken with an equal amount of warm water will be found useful (Fowler). When there is much sense of tightness and fullness of the chest, the portable Turkish bath may be tried. When the secretion is excessive atropine is sometimes useful. When the heart is feeble, digitalis and strychnia are beneficial. Preparations of tar, creosote, and terebene are sometimes useful. The compound tincture of benzoin, menthol and eucalyptus are often useful in inhalations. If fetor be present, phenol in the form of spray (1 per cent solution) will lessen the odor, or thymol (1 to 1,000), but intratracheal medication is the most efficient. It is usually possible without much difficulty to inject with a suitable syringe about two drams (8 cc.) of olive oil, with gr. ½ (0.032 gm.) of iodoform, and gr. ⅛ (0.008 gm.) of morphia if there is irritating cough. For urgent dyspnea with cyanosis, venesection gives most relief. In the form in children, associated with adenoids, complete removal, followed by respiratory exercises, is indicated.

Bronchomoniliasis.—Infection with *Monilia* may occur alone or with other diseases, such as tuberculosis. The signs are of bronchitis or bronchopneumonia. In severe infections there may be emaciation and a picture like tuberculosis. The course may be prolonged with relapses. The *diagnosis* rests on the repeated finding of the fungus in the sputum. Agglutination and complement fixation tests may be useful. The persistent use of iodine, given as the tincture (♏ x-xx, 0.6-1.3 cc.), is the best treatment.

BRONCHIAL SPIROCHETOSIS

There is a form of bronchitis, acute or chronic, associated with infection with *Spirochœta bronchialis,* most common in some parts of the tropics but which has a wide distribution. This organism is often found in pulmonary abscess. It was described by Castellani in 1905.

Symptoms.—In the acute form the features are much as in ordinary bronchitis. The sputum is usually scanty and may contain small amounts of blood. The chronic form may follow an acute attack or come on gradually. The sputum is scanty and often blood-tinged; hemoptysis may occur. There may be fever. The lungs may show areas of dulness and various kinds of râles. Spirochetes in large numbers are found in the sputum. The mouth should be cleaned thoroughly to avoid the presence of mouth spirochetes. The outlook is good but the course may be very chronic.

Diagnosis.—The condition may be regarded as tuberculosis but careful study of the sputum should correct the error. The same applies to its distinction from other forms of bronchitis.

Treatment.—The same measures should be employed as in acute bronchitis. Arsenic in the form of Fowler's solution has given good results. The use of neo-arsphenamine seems advisable.

BRONCHIECTASIS

Definition.—Bronchiectasis is the condition of dilatation of one or more bronchi.

Etiology.—Dilatation follows various affections of the bronchi themselves, of the lungs and of the pleura. The condition may be unsuspected clinically and is much more common than indicated in the literature. Either the cases are now more often recognized or the disease has become more frequent. It occurs in from 2 to 4 per cent of the postmortems in general hospitals. A majority of the cases are recognized between the ages of 20 and 40 years but it is not uncommon in children, especially with sinus and tonsil infection. Males are more often affected. Following Fowler's classification, the causes are:

A. Intrinsic, *acting directly through the bronchi.*

(1) *Bronchitis.*—Chronic cough is a common antecedent, and the dilatation is a mechanical effect of constant forced expiration acting on bronchial walls weakened by disease. There are three groups: (*a*) The remarkable form of generalized dilatation of the smaller bronchi seen in children after the infections, particularly measles, bronchopneumonia and whooping cough. (*b*) Following an infective bronchitis, pneumococcal or influenzal, the cough persists and gradually the signs of diffuse bronchiectasis appear with fetid sputum. (*c*) The bronchitis following prolonged exposure to dust, as in miners and potters is often associated with bronchiectasis.

(2) *Stenosis* of a bronchus, either by compression from without by a tumor or aneurism, a growth in the wall or a foreign body within. The last is an important cause. As a result of the narrowing, the secretions accumulate, the walls are weakened and dilatation follows.

B. Extrinsic causes associated with changes in the lung tissue or pleura. (*a*) *Fibrosis* of the lung from whatever cause, syphilis, pneumonia, anthracosis and chronic fibroid pleurisy. (*b*) Acute *bronchopneumonia.* It is rare after delayed resolution in lobar pneumonia but may occur with bronchopneumonia. In a patient dead six weeks from the onset there were areas of bronchopneumonia, dilatation of the bronchi of both lower lobes, several spots of gangrene, and secondary abscess of the brain. (*c*) *Compression* of the lung. The tubes are rarely found dilated in the extreme compressed form of chronic empyema. Local compression by tumor or aneurism may be a cause without stenosis of the bronchus. The atelectatic bronchiectasis occurs in an area of lung which has not developed or not expanded after birth. The bronchial walls show an overgrowth of cartilage. (*d*) *Tuberculosis.* It is rare to dissect a lung in the chronic ulcerative form without finding somewhere a dilated bronchus. The more chronic the disease and the greater the fibrosis the more widespread the dilatation, and most often in the upper lobes.

C. Congenital.—This rare form occurs as a universal saccular distention of the bronchi, usually of one lung; or it may be confined to the bronchi of the third and fourth order in local areas of atelectasis.

Morbid Anatomy.—Three chief forms are recognized—*cylindrical, fusiform* and *saccular*—which may exist together in the same lung. The condition may be general or partial. Universal bronchiectasis occurs in rare congenital cases and occasionally as a sequence of interstitial pneumonia. The entire bronchial tree is represented by a series of sacculi. The walls are smooth and possibly without ulceration or erosion except in the dependent parts. The lining membrane of the sacculi is usually smooth and glistening. The dilatations may form large cysts immediately beneath the pleura. Intervening between the sacculi is dense fibrotic lung tissue. The partial dilatations are common in chronic tuberculosis, particularly at the apex, in chronic pleurisy at the base and in emphysema. Here the dilatation is more commonly cylindrical, sometimes fusiform. The bronchial mucous membrane is much involved and sometimes there is a narrowing of the lumen. Occasionally one meets with a single saccular bronchiectasis with chronic bronchitis or emphysema. Some of these look like simple cysts, with smooth walls and without fluid contents. An acute bronchiolectasis may follow the infectious diseases.

The essential factors are: (1) weakening of the bronchial walls, (2) increased pressure on the walls, especially from cough and secretion, and (3) pulling on the bronchial walls during inspiration by fibroid conditions. Any inflammatory process may damage the interstitial tissues with resulting fibrosis which may narrow or widen the bronchioles or bronchi. Bronchiolectasis or bronchiectasis results. Various organisms are found in the sputum; the influenza bacillus may predominate.

Symptoms.—There are *acute* cases, usually the bronchiolectasis of children which generally follows bronchopneumonia. In the limited dilatations of tuberculosis, emphysema and chronic bronchitis the symptoms are in great part those of the original disease, and often the condition is not suspected.

In extensive *saccular bronchiectasis* the characters of the cough and expectoration are distinctive. The patient will pass the greater part of the day without any cough and then in a severe paroxysm will bring up a large quantity of sputum. Of 23 cases the amount for twenty-four hours was in 2 less than 100 cc., in 11 from 100-300 cc., in 2 almost 500 cc., in 7 over 600 cc. In one case with over one litre per day the cavities were very small. Sometimes change of position will bring on a violent attack, probably due to the fact that some of the secretion flows from the dilatation to a normal tube. The daily spell of coughing is usually in the morning. The sputum is in many instances very characteristic, grayish or grayish brown in color, fluid, purulent, with a peculiar acid, sometimes fetid, odor. Placed in a conical glass, it separates into a thick granular layer below and a thin mucoid intervening layer above, which is capped by a brownish froth. Microscopically it shows pus cells and often large crystals of fatty acids, sometimes in enormous numbers and arranged in bunches. Hematoidin crystals are sometimes present. Elastic fibres are seldom found except when there is ulceration of the bronchial walls. In some cases the sputum is very fetid. Nummular expectoration, such as comes from tuberculous cavities, is not common. *Hemorrhage* occurs in the majority of cases and varies from slight bleeding to a hemorrhage which may be fatal. *Arthritis* may occur, and it is one of the conditions with which pulmonary osteo-arthropathy is commonly associated. Clubbing of the fingers and toes is common. There is a remarkable association of bronchiectasis with abscess of the brain. Among 13,700 autopsies at the London Hospital and the Brompton Hospital there were 19 cases of cerebral abscess with pulmonary disease, usually bronchiectasis (Schörstein). There is a *dry* form with a chronic dry cough, occasionally with blood-streaked sputum or hemoptysis and the signs of fibrosis. The diagnosis can be made only by bronchoscopy or the X-ray study with lipiodol.

Physical Signs.—The associated conditions are so various that the signs vary greatly. In deep-seated cases there may be no signs. The coexistence of tuberculosis, chronic bronchitis, emphysema or fibrosis gives a complicated picture. The signs are influenced by these factors. Dilatations near the surface yield a tympanitic note. In saccular bronchiectasis the signs vary as the cavity is empty or filled with secretion. On auscultation the breath sounds depend on associated changes unless the bronchiectasis is superficial, when cavernous breathing may be heard. Many varieties of râles are heard. In diffuse early cases they may have a very intense crackling quality which is sometimes suggestive of dilatation.

Certain points are worthy of emphasis. The disease begins in childhood probably in many cases but cough may be the only symptom for years. The cases with profuse sputum often represent a far advanced stage. The importance of upper respiratory tract infection in the etiology should be kept in mind. The disease is more frequent than is usually recognized. In children, a persistent cough, especially with indefinite signs at the bases, for which no evident cause is found, should suggest the need of excluding bronchiectasis. A careful search should be made for infection in the tonsils or sinuses. In cases secondary to these infections the process is usually bilateral.

The *course* is long with a tendency to slow progression. Exacerbation may follow an acute infection. The cases due to foreign body usually improve if removal is done. There may be pleurisy with marked thickening. Hemorrhage is common and may cause death. Septicemia may result. Many patients have a miserable existence from the persistent cough and general ill health.

Diagnosis.—In the extensive sacculated forms, unilateral and associated with interstitial pneumonia or chronic pleurisy, the diagnosis is easy. There is contraction of the side, which in some instances is not at all extreme. The cavernous signs may be chiefly at the base and may vary according to the condition of the cavity, whether full or empty. There may be marked amphoric phenomena and loud resonant râles. The patients frequently show signs of marked embarrassment of the circulation with dyspnea and cyanosis on exertion. A condition very difficult to distinguish from bronchiectasis is a limited pleural cavity communicating with a bronchus. After the introduction of lipiodol into the bronchi, the X-ray study is of the greatest value in showing the dilated bronchi. Bronchoscopy is also of aid especially in the recognition of stenosis. The intensity of the shadow in plates taken before and after evacuation of the contents may be suggestive.

The disease is often regarded as *tuberculosis,* which may coexist, but proper sputum examination should prevent this. The acuteness of abscess of the lung and the character of the sputum are usually distinctive. From chronic bronchitis the diagnosis is difficult but the sputum, the clubbing of the fingers and the X-ray study are aids. The possibility of a foreign body should be remembered.

Treatment.—Medical treatment is palliative only, since it is impossible to heal the cavities. Postural treatment is important, and the most favorable position should be studied for each patient. Sleeping with the head low favors "drainage." The reduction of the fluid intake to a minimum is sometimes useful. Codein may be given for cough. Intratracheal injections may be helpful; with a suitable syringe a dram may be injected of the following solution: Menthol 10 parts, guaiacol 2 parts, olive oil 88 parts; or when the odor is very offensive iodoform in olive oil. Creosote may be used in an inhaler or the vaporized fumes inhaled in a small room, the eyes being protected and the nostrils stuffed with absorbent cotton. Creosote may be taken internally in doses of ♏ v (0.3 cc.) with cod-liver oil. Careful search should be made for upper respiratory tract infection, especially in the sinuses, and proper treatment instituted. In some of these cases early diagnosis, especially in children, eradication of the focus of infection, and persistent bronchoscopic drainage may result in palliation if not effect a cure.

Surgical Treatment.—Thoracoplasty has been helpful in some cases. Lobectomy, if only one lobe is affected, is curative. Avulsion of the phrenic nerve causing relaxation of the diaphragm and partial collapse is useful in early cases, especially in children. Bronchoscopic drainage is very helpful and should be begun as early as possible. Artificial pneumothorax is usually ineffectual.

HAY FEVER AND BRONCHIAL ASTHMA

Definition.—Hay fever is an allergic coryza with a marked vasomotor reaction. Bronchial asthma is a reaction in the bronchi of allergic nature in sensitized persons with swelling of the mucous membrane and dyspnea. There are no essential differences between hay fever and asthma; in the one the nasal portion of the respiratory tract is affected, in the other the bronchial, in many instances both.

Etiology.—The word "asthma," which means a panting, was used by the older writers as we use the term dyspnea. Some still speak of "cardiac and renal asthma," but the term should be restricted to the independent disease, first separated in the seventeenth century by Van Helmont and by Willis. The latter speaks of the "tyranny and cruelty" of the disease, and suspected the cause to lurk in the "muscular coats of the pneumonic vessels," meaning the bronchi. Floyer (1698), who gives a good account of his own case in his *Treatise of the Asthma,* held the same views. With the introduction of accurate methods of diagnosis by Laënnec the independent disease was separated from a host of maladies with dyspnea as a prominent symptom.

Our modern conception of *hay fever* dates from the description by Bostock in 1819 and 1828 of the summer catarrh—Catarrhus aestivus. He recognized the periodicity, the disturbance of respiration as sometimes the only feature, and the association with the "effluvium from new hay." Elliotson (1831) first suggested that it was caused by the "effluvia of the grass and probably the pollen." Morrill Wyman (1854) separated the spring and autumn forms of hay fever. Blackley (1873) demonstrated that "pollen possesses the power of producing hay fever both in its asthmatic and catarrhal forms," and, as early as 1865, showed that skin reactions were present in sensitive persons. Then came many observations on the relation of nasal conditions to asthma and hay fever. Dunbar applied modern methods to the study of the pollen problem, separated the toxins, studied their reactions, cutaneous and serological, and introduced a specific therapy.

Finally Meltzer and his pupils Auer and Lewis (1910) brought the disease into the category of allergic phenomena. After an injection of horse serum a guinea-pig has no reaction, but ten days later if a second dose be given the animal will be found to have been "sensitized" by the first dose, and, in consequence, has alarming symptoms—sneezing, dyspnea at first, labored breathing and convulsions. Anatomically the lungs are voluminous, do not collapse, and the bronchi show marked congestion of the mucosa. An asthmatic subject, sensitive, say, to eggs, if injected with a small amount of egg albumen will have an attack with difficulty in expiring, not inspiring. The lungs become distended and the diaphragm does not move. The alveolar air has a low carbon dioxide content. An injection of epinephrine relieves the condition; just as, if given in time, it removes the anaphylactic symptoms in the guinea-pig. The part played by bronchial spasm is in question and its occurrence is not proved. There is in both forms marked swelling with increased secretion from the mucous membrane. The subjects of hay fever and asthma are sensitized to various "asthmogenic" agents, usually proteins, which may be inhaled, injected, or autogenous, the result of bacterial or other activity. The effect of pollen on the mucous membrane is direct by irritation and indirect by absorption of the protein. Sensitive individuals give skin reactions to some of the agents causing the asthma. The reaction may be immediate or delayed, or both; the former corresponds to the group giving a positive skin reaction and the latter to the group due to infection, rarely to food.

Many patients are sensitive to more than one protein (multiple sensitization). The same patient may be sensitive to plant, animal and bacterial proteins. In the nonsensitive group (usually due to infection) the disease appears later, after the fortieth year, and many of them have chronic bronchitis and cardiorenal changes. "As the age of onset increases the frequency of sensitization decreases." We may group the exciting agents into:

(1) Inspiratory.—*Vegetable,* the pollens of various grasses and flowers, the dust from certain cereals, moulds, etc. *Animal,* the emanations from horses, cats, birds and substances in dust.

(2) Ingested.—A host of vegetable and animal proteins, various grasses, wheat, oats; leguminous foods, peas, beans and lentils; fruits and nuts. Many animal substances, meat, milk and eggs, oysters, lobsters and crabs. Certain drugs, as acetylsalicylic acid, may be causal.

(3) Metabolic.—Abnormal products of primary digestion in stomach or bowels; faulty transmutation in the liver; lack of quantity or quality in the

internal secretions; imperfect metabolism in the tissues may be responsible for some obscure cases.

(4) Bacterial.—Many asthmatic and hay fever patients are sensitized to various organisms, varieties of streptococci being the most common. The exciting organism may exist in the sinuses or air passages.

Psychical Causes.—In some patients an anxiety neurosis or emotional disturbance plays some part and not infrequently this is an important factor in producing an attack in one who has had asthma.

Heredity.—This is present in a considerable proportion and the family history may show instances of other allergic phenomena in addition to asthma. Sensitization to a particular protein is not transmitted. When both parents have asthma or hay fever, all their children tend to have it. The tendency is transmitted.

Sympathetic Nervous System.—There is often disturbance of function in this. In some cases disturbance of the vagus plays a part and vagotonia is common. It has been suggested that the vagus nucleus may be hypersensitive to irritants carried by the blood or to peripheral or psychical stimuli.

Local Causes.—Conditions of the nose and pharynx, as swollen turbinates, deflected septum, polypi, sinusitis and diseased tonsils, play a part in some patients. They may supply extra irritation or infection associated with them may be responsible. Kern and Schenck (1934) showed that nasal polyps are usually associated with allergic states. The addition of some other factor to the special sensitization may be necessary to cause an attack. A person may be free in the city and suffer from an attack in the country or in one place. In these cases the individual becomes exposed to the special agent to which he is sensitized. Sleeping on a horsehair mattress or on a feather pillow may cause attacks in persons susceptible to these substances. There are children naturally sensitized to extraordinarily minute quantities of egg or meat. There is a morbid sensitiveness of the mucous membranes in many patients with hay fever. The subjects of asthma, particularly of horse asthma, are liable to serious attacks of serum sickness or anaphylactic shock after the administration of antitoxin. Inquiry should always be made as to previous asthma before giving either prophylactic or curative doses of serum.

On *bronchoscopic* examination the findings are: (1) changes in the mucosa of the trachea and bronchi, (2) abnormal secretions, tenacious or purulent, (3) collapse of the trachea and bronchi during cough and expiration, (4) absence of bronchial spasm, and (5) absence of mucosal erosion or ulceration (Clerf). The absence of spasm is to be noted. The presence of secretions and bronchial collapse are important factors.

Pathology.—Huber and Koessler, in reporting on four cases, point out a parallelism between the clinical picture and the structural changes. Of two cases of the form due to infection one had during life marked secretion and striking hypertrophy of the mucous glands of the bronchi was found; the other with unproductive cough and bronchospasm showed marked hypertrophy of the smooth muscle system. A case due to food sensitization showed hypertrophy of both glandular and muscular systems and one of horse asthma, death being due to acute anaphylaxis, showed acute emphysema and marked constriction of the bronchi and bronchioles. Irregular thickening of the pulmonary arteries was noted in three of the cases.

Symptoms.—Bostock's account of his attacks of *hay fever* (1819) may be abstracted. "A sensation of heat and fulness is experienced in the eyes with redness and a discharge of tears. There is much smarting and itching, the eyes become inflamed and discharge copiously. This state of the eyes recurs in paroxysms in June and July. There follow fulness in the head, particularly the fore part, irritation of the nose causing sneezing which may occur in fits of extreme violence. There is tightness in the chest, with difficulty in breathing and a feeling of want of air. The voice may be husky and to these symptoms may be added languor, loss of appetite, incapacity for exertion, restless nights often with profuse perspiration." In his second paper (1828) Bostock recognized that the eyes, the nose, the fauces and the lungs may be involved in varying degrees.

The *asthma* fit is thus described by Floyer (1698). "At first waking about one or two o'clock in the night the fit begins, the breath is very slow, but after a little time more strait, the diaphragm seems stiff and tied and is with difficulty moved downwards, but for enlarging the breast in inspiration the intercostal muscles, which serve for the raising of the ribs and the scapular muscles all join their force, and strain themselves for the enlarging of the cavity of the breast. He has to rise out of his bed and sit erect that the weight of the viscera may pull down the diaphragm. The muscles which serve for expiration cannot easily perform the contraction of the thorax, being hindered by the stiffness and inflation of the membranes. The expiration is slow, leisurely and wheezing, and the muscular fibres of the bronchi and the vesiculae of the lungs are contracted, and that produces the wheezing noise which is best heard in expiration." There is not much to add to this description.

The attack may last from a few minutes to several hours. When severe there are signs of defective aëration, cyanosis, with sweating, feeble pulse and cold extremities. Coughing is difficult, very tight and dry at first, and then more violent, with the expectoration of the distinctive sputum.

Physical Signs.—The chest looks full and fixed, and there is very little expansion. The breathing is costal, the diaphragm is low and the movement much restricted. Inspiration is short, expiration much prolonged, labored and accompanied by wheezing râles. Percussion may be hyperresonant—Biermer's "box tone"—the cardiac flatness is obliterated, and the liver dulness low. On auscultation inspiration is feeble, expiration prolonged and in both the normal characters are obscured by sibilant and sonorous râles. Towards the end the râles become moister. It is remarkable with what rapidity they may disappear. The *sputum* is distinctive. Early in the attack it is brought up with difficulty and consists of small round masses, gelatinous, like sago balls in a thin mucus, the so-called "perles" of Laënnec. Spread on glass with a black background, they can be unfolded and are seen to be moulds of the smaller tubes, many with a twisted appearance. A smaller number show the Curschmann spirals of which there are two forms, one a simple loose twist in which are entangled leukocytes, especially eosinophiles. The other, a form of spiral probably never met with except in true asthma, is a tightly coiled skein of mucus in which cells are entangled and through the centre of which runs a thread of clear translucent mucin. Curschmann's spirals are found in nearly all cases when looked for early and in the right way. In addition to the spirals and the eosinophiles, a third element is often present, the Charcot-

Leyden crystals, hexagonal, elongated pointed structures. They are found more often when the sputum changes to mucopurulent or if it is let stand for twenty-four hours. The character of the sputum in bronchial asthma points to a process which differs from the ordinary forms of bronchitis. The small size of many of the casts indicates involvement of the smaller tubes. In young children an attack may have an abrupt onset with slight fever, great distress, rapid pulse and respiration and cyanosis. The presence of a foreign body or laryngeal diphtheria may be suspected but the features due to a foreign body are more often regarded as asthma. In these cases the use of oxygen with atropine and epinephrine is indicated. Sedatives may be given later.

The *eosinophiles* in the blood are much increased, up to 53 per cent in one of our cases, and this may persist in moderate grade between attacks. In the secretion from the nose in hay fever and in the sputum of bronchial asthma, many eosinophiles may be found.

The *course* is variable. Hay fever usually recurs year by year, in spring or autumn, varying with the pollen to which the individual is sensitive. Forms of asthma due to protein are more variable. A child may recover completely after years of severe attacks. The results of treatment are important. The milder forms may persist through long life, and be, as Oliver Wendell Holmes said of his asthma, "the slight ailment that promotes longevity." In long-standing cases emphysema and chronic bronchitis complicate the disease and later hypertrophy of the heart. Even with these complications, in a suitable climate or with care, the patients may survive well into the seventh decade.

Diagnosis.—There is not any difficulty in recognizing hay fever but it is necessary to determine the particular pollen which is responsible if specific treatment is to be given. This is done by trying the skin reactions with extracts of various pollens. A positive result is shown by a local reaction. The picture of asthma is usually distinctive but to determine the particular protein (if any) responsible requires careful tests. Other forms of expiratory dyspnea rarely cause difficulty if a careful examination is made but it is common in hospital experience to have patients with marked cardiac or renal dyspnea sent in with a diagnosis of bronchial asthma. The use of the terms "cardiac and renal" asthma contributes to this error. The dyspnea of laryngeal or tracheal obstruction and that due to pressure, as from aneurism, is usually inspiratory. An occasional case of foreign body in a bronchus may simulate asthma particularly if the "asthmatoid wheeze" occurs. The X-ray study is of aid if doubt exists after thorough examination.

Prognosis.—In early life this depends largely on the possibility of an etiological diagnosis and the result of desensitization or removal of some source of irritation, as in the nose and throat. If the disease has existed for some time or begins after the age of thirty, the existence of emphysema and chronic bronchitis renders the outlook for complete recovery very doubtful. The "asthmatic constitution" is a permanent quality. Death occasionally occurs in young persons after a long period of severe attacks.

Treatment.—For *hay fever* change of locality during the pollen season may give freedom. Local treatment of the nose, if required, sometimes gives relief. The use of a cocaine spray is helpful but is a dangerous remedy. Epinephrine (1-1000 solution) may be applied or ephedrin sprays used to give temporary relief. Remedies which sometimes are of benefit are sodium bicarbonate internally in full dosage and locally as a spray, and calcium lactate which should be taken for a considerable period in doses of gr. xv (1 gm.) three times a day. Spraying the nose and throat with the specific pollen antigen may be useful, combined with immunization. Active immunization by pollen extracts is sometimes effective as a prophylactic. The particular pollen to which the patient is sensitive having been determined, an alcoholic solution of it is used, the first dose having a dilution insufficient to produce a skin reaction. Very small doses should be given to patients who are very sensitive as shown by skin tests. The strength of the injections is increased very gradually; they are repeated every four or five days until ten to twenty have been given. This should be done if possible before the usual time for the attacks. It is wise to repeat the treatment at least for two successive years. The prevention of recurrence offers difficulties, and each case should be studied in the light of recent investigations. In the nonsensitive forms cultures may show some dominant organism from which a vaccine may be prepared.

Careful study of each patient with *asthma* by modern methods is an essential preliminary. The tests are not very difficult, but the intelligent coöperation of the patient or of the parents of a child is essential. The reactions should first be studied. The nonsensitive group comprise as a rule older patients in whom the disease has come on late and who are subject to sinus infection or bronchitis or show cardiorenal changes. The treatment of these conditions may give relief and in some of these patients iodide is helpful. Vaccines may be prepared from the dominant organism in the sputum. The teeth and tonsils should be eliminated as factors of infection, and the condition of the intestines carefully studied. Nasal and sinus disease should be excluded or treated and there may be striking relief from local treatment.

In the *sensitive* groups—ingestion, inhalation and bacterial—separation from the exciting factor is important; this may be in occupation, environment, contact with animals or in diet. Desensitization for the responsible food protein may occur if it is totally abstained from for a long period. The best results are obtained by elimination of the etiological factor in this group. Special care has to be taken in the case of eggs as very minute quantities of the protein may cause attacks. Such articles as cakes, custards and puddings containing eggs must be excluded. The proteins of the cereals, wheat, barley, rice, rye, oat, buckwheat, may be the cause, and the hay fever patient sensitive to the pollen of the grasses may react to the proteins of wheat or rye. Protection may be obtained by giving small doses of the protein over long periods.

The horse asthmatics may be treated by beginning with the injection of a dilution of the hair protein 1:100,000 and this must be slowly and gradually increased. Injection of horse serum is of little or no value in the treatment of horse asthma (Walker). The prophylactic treatment is not without risks as in the case of an asthmatic of fifteen years' standing who received an injection on successive days of 0.01 and 0.02 mg. of an extract of horse hair; on the fourth day she had another of 0.03 mg. Within two minutes she complained of feeling hot, in three minutes the face was flushed, the eyes and nose "running" and the skin prickling. In five minutes asthma began with a choking sensation in the throat. Twelve minims of a 1:1000 epinephrine solution relieved the attack. Urticaria appeared and the attack was over in an hour and a half. In the bacterial cases the best results have been obtained by the use of vaccines prepared from cultures of the causal organism. The initial dose should be small and increased very gradually so that a reaction is not produced.

Nonspecific protein therapy has been used, as for example in the form of peptone, various methods of administration being employed. Thus a 5 per cent solution in normal saline may be given intravenously, beginning with 5 minims (0.3 cc.) and increasing each weekly dose by 2 minims. The method is not without danger and serious reactions sometimes result.

Treatment of the Attack.—Hypodermics of epinephrine (♏ xv, 1 cc. of a 1-1000 solution) or of atropine (gr. 1/100, 0.00065 gm.) may give prompt relief, but individual cases vary greatly. Smaller doses of epinephrine are sometimes efficient and some patients are helped by injections given once a week over a long period. Caution should be exercised in patients with sclerosis or high blood-pressure. Morphia (gr. ⅙-¼, 0.01-0.016 gm.) hypodermically is one of the best remedies. The inhalation of amyl nitrite may give prompt relief or a whiff of chloroform may relieve the spasm. Pilocarpine (gr. ⅛, 0.008 gm.) hypodermically may be tried. Iodide and belladonna taken for a long period may be helpful. Ephedrine is often useful as a spray (0.5-2 per cent solution), or by mouth (gr. ½-1, 0.03-0.06 gm.).

Usually a chronic asthmatic has some favorite substance to inhale or to smoke. Most of the cigarettes used for the purpose contain leaves of the Solanaceae, to which nitrate of potash is added. Stramonium leaves and potassium nitrate burnt together on a plate may be used. *Bronchoscopic treatment* is sometimes useful especially in the patients with chronic tracheobronchitis with increased secretion. Removal of the secretion is effective rather than any local applications. The duration of benefit varies greatly. X-ray therapy is of benefit to some patients.

FIBRINOUS BRONCHITIS

Definition.—An acute or chronic affection, characterized by the formation in the bronchial tubes of fibrinous casts, which are expelled in paroxysms of dyspnea and cough.

Fibrinous moulds of the bronchi are formed in diphtheria (with extension into the trachea and bronchi) in pneumonia, and occasionally in pulmonary tuberculosis, conditions which have nothing to do with true fibrinous bronchitis. As to tuberculosis Landis states that no instance occurred during thirteen years at the Phipps Institute, nor was it found in 662 autopsies on tuberculous subjects. Fibrinous casts are expectorated in chronic heart disease and in the albuminous expectoration following tapping of a pleural exudate. In hemoptysis blood casts may be expectorated, and they are not to be confounded with the casts of true fibrinous bronchitis which may be coughed up with profuse hemorrhage. In pneumonia small fibrinous plugs are not uncommon in the sputum, and in rare instances quite large moulds of the tubes may be coughed up. The mycelium of *Aspergillus fumigatus* may form membranous casts in the bronchi.

Pathology.—This is obscure. The membrane is identical with that to which the term croupous is applied, and the obscurity relates not so much to the mechanism of the production, which is probably the same as in other mucous surfaces, as to the curious limitation to certain bronchial territories and in the chronic form to the remarkable recurrence at stated or irregular intervals throughout a period of many years. In the fatal cases the bronchial mucous membrane may be found injected or pale. In Biermer's case the epithelial lining was intact beneath the cast, but in that of Kretschy the bronchi were denuded of their epithelium. Emphysema is almost invariably present. Sometimes a careful examination will reveal evidences of recent or antecedent pleurisy.

Clinical Description.—It is a rare affection and most common at the middle period of life. Of 27 cases, 15 were in males. The attacks may occur at definite intervals for months or years. The form and size of the casts may be identical at each attack as though each time precisely the same bronchial area was involved. The expectoration of the casts is associated with paroxysms of severe dyspnea and coughing, which occur at longer or shorter intervals. Fever and hemoptysis may be present during the attack. Physical signs usually indicate the portion of the lung affected, as there are suppressed breath sounds and numerous râles on coughing. A very dry râle, called the "*bruit de drapeau*," has been described, caused by the vibration of a loosened portion of the cast. There may be collapse of the lung from bronchial obstruction.

In five cases there were skin lesions. Tuberculosis is rarely present. The casts are usually rolled up and mixed with mucus and blood. When unrolled they are large white branching structures. The main stem may be as thick as the little finger. They have been described as fibrinous but they consist mainly of mucin. On section they show a concentrically stratified structure, with leukocytes and alveolar epithelium. Leyden's crystals and Curschmann's spirals are sometimes found. Death occurred in one case of the series.

The *acute form*, of which Bettman (1901) collected 15 cases, comes on most frequently during some fever, as typhoid, pneumonia, or the eruptive fevers. After a preliminary bronchitis the dyspnea increases, and then the casts are coughed up. Chills and fever have been present. Four of the 15 cases proved fatal, and the casts were found *in situ*. It is much more serious than the chronic form into which it may pass. Night after night distressing attacks of coughing may occur, with dyspnea and cyanosis, only relieved by the expectoration of large quantities of sputum with casts of all sizes, sometimes very small ones which "tail off" into true spirals. In a case of this type there were attacks of fever with toxemia and delirium. The casts may have an arborescent structure or come from a single tube or its bifurcation, in which case they show the characteristic structure.

Diagnosis.—Laryngeal or tracheal obstruction may be suggested by the dyspnea; sometimes the cast is caught in the larynx. Bronchial asthma and collapse of the lung should be excluded; the latter may be present from bronchial obstruction.

Treatment.—In the acute cases the treatment is that of acute bronchitis. We know of nothing which can prevent the recurrence of attacks in the chronic form. In the uncomplicated cases there is rarely any danger during the paroxysm, except from laryngeal obstruction. Inhalations of ether, vapor, or atomized lime water aid in the separation of the membranes. Intratracheal injections of olive oil with iodoform may be tried. The employment of emetics in some cases is effective in promoting the removal of the casts. Removal by the bronchoscope should be done. Infection in the upper respiratory tract should be eradicated.

TRACHEAL AND BRONCHIAL OBSTRUCTION AND STENOSIS

Etiology.—The causes *in* the *trachea* are: (1) stenosis due to the cicatrization of wounds, especially tracheotomy; (2) healing of an ulcer, as in syphilis; (3) tumor, usually papilloma; (4) a foreign body; and (5) diphtheritic membrane or tough tenacious secretion. The causes *outside* the *trachea* are: (1) strangulation; (2) pressure from an enlarged thyroid, rarely from enlarged lymph nodes; (3) pressure from an enlarged thymus; (4) enlargement of the mediastinal glands; and (5) intrathoracic tumor. *In* the *bronchi* the causes are: (1) a foreign body, or swelling of the mucous membrane due to a foreign body; (2) the healing of an ulcer; (3) new growth; (4) broncholithiasis; (5) the traction produced by fibrosis; (6) the presence of membrane in diphtheria or the casts of fibrinous bronchitis; (7) inspissated secretion; (8) congenital malformations, and (9) spasm or collapse of the bronchi. The influence of traction is seen especially in the small bronchi and bronchioles. The common causes *outside* the *bronchi* are: (1) enlargement of the mediastinal or bronchial glands; (2) aneurism; (3) neoplasm of the lung, pleura or esophagus; (4) mediastinal abscess; and (5) pericardial effusion.

Pathology.—This depends on the cause and degree of the changes. In the trachea the stenosis varies in extent. In the bronchi if the obstruction is sudden and complete, there is collapse of the portion of the lung supplied, the air is absorbed, and if the obstruction continues there will be fibrosis and dilatation of the bronchi. In partial obstruction the results depend on the degree of narrowing, the amount of air that can enter and of secretion that can escape. Abscess may follow. In cases of pressure or traction from without the effects are varied; fibrosis and bronchiectasis are probable results.

Symptoms.—In both trachea and bronchi much depends on the degree of obstruction and the rapidity of its occurrence. With obstruction in the *trachea,* dyspnea is the prominent symptom, usually with stridor and a form of respiration characteristic of tracheal obstruction. Cough occurs with a harsh metallic quality. If the obstruction is marked the dyspnea is extreme, the patient has to sit up or lean forward and cyanosis becomes marked. With extreme respiratory effort the larynx may move very slightly or not at all. The *signs* are not distinctive. The sounds over the trachea may be harsh and noisy; over the lungs the stridor may be heard with variable breath sounds, depending on the degree of obstruction.

When the obstruction is *bronchial,* cough is usual and may be paroxysmal but dyspnea is rarely as marked as in tracheal obstruction. The signs over the area of lung supplied vary with the conditions produced and there is no set picture. With complete blocking there is collapse; with a ball-valve action the lung will be emphysematous. Fibroid changes and bronchiectasis are common late results.

Diagnosis.—In the trachea this is aided by the laryngoscope and bronchoscope. The external causes of pressure may be evident at once. In the bronchial conditions a careful study of the signs with bronchoscopic and X-ray examination is usually sufficient.

Treatment.—This has to be governed by the causal conditions and in some cases can be palliative only. A prompt tracheotomy may be life saving in tracheal obstruction or bronchoscopy in bronchial obstruction.

FOREIGN BODIES IN THE BRONCHI[1]

Largely as a result of the splendid work of Chevalier Jackson of Philadelphia, we have learned that foreign bodies in the bronchi are not infrequent. A great variety of objects may gain entrance to the trachea, the majority of which (75 per cent) pass into the right bronchus. There are not necessarily any severe symptoms with this and the history may be quite negative. No age is exempt but the accident is particularly apt to occur in children. In the majority of cases there is a history of choking, cough, distress and dyspnea. Frequently after this there is a quiescent period before a return of symptoms. The objects that may be inhaled are many and some are of such a size that it does not seem possible that they can pass through the larynx. Many cases occur in children, often due to carelessness in allowing them to handle small objects which are promptly put in the mouth; in adults the pernicious habit of holding objects in the mouth, such as pins and tacks, is often responsible.

Pathology.—There is no one picture as the nature of the object, its size, the length of stay and the degree of obstruction have an influence. Vegetable substances, as a nut, often set up an intense tracheobronchitis in addition to the obstruction, while a pin may remain for years without causing any change. With complete obstruction there is collapse of the lung supplied; with partial obstruction varying grades of change. If the foreign body remains for some time, dilatation of the bronchus and fibrosis probably result. Drainage of the affected lung is interfered with and collection of secretions and infection result. Abscess or empyema may follow but are rare. Pneumonia in the true sense does not result; there may be pneumonitis.

Symptoms.—These are very varied, depending principally on the character of the foreign body. A very acute general process may result which ends fatally in a few days, as seen after the inhalation of vegetable substances particularly, or there may be an acute process which gradually subsides into a chronic condition. Cough is common and resulting conditions such as abscess or bronchiectasis give their usual symptoms. A foreign body in the trachea causes severe dyspnea with signs throughout both lungs on auscultation. A "slap" may be heard with coughing.

Physical Signs.—These are very varied and no set picture can be described. The most acute signs result from the inhalation of a nut, the peanut being most common in the United States. To this the name *Arachidic Bronchitis* has been given. The condition is an edematous, purulent, tracheobronchitis which may result in lung abscess. The cases are in children; the symptoms come on rapidly with high irregular fever, severe toxemia and the signs of an intense general bronchitis, with a great variety of râles mostly

[1] Fuller details are given in the Lumleian Lectures on "The Clinical Features of Foreign Bodies in the Bronchi," *Lancet*, 1924, i, 735, 787, 838.

coarse and bubbling. The "asthmatoid wheeze" is often present, the dyspnea is extreme, cyanosis is marked and there is tenacious purulent sputum. The condition is usually regarded as pneumonic but foreign bodies do not cause pneumonia. If a bronchus is plugged there is dulness with absence of breath and voice sounds. The lung supplied by the plugged bronchus contains much secretion and is described as "drowned" lung. If the foreign body acts as a ball-valve, letting air in but not out, the affected lung becomes distended but does not move with respiration. In general the signs are those of complete or partial obstruction of a bronchus and evidently will show much variation. If complete, the picture is that of collapse, often modified because the obstruction may not have been complete at first but becomes so later from swelling of the mucous membrane. With partial obstruction the signs may vary from hour to hour, often due to the amount of secretion which accumulates and then may be brought up. Diminished expansion, decreased vocal fremitus, varying grades of dulness (exceptions are an overdistended lung from ball-valve action and marked collapse) and breath sounds which may be distant or harsh and usually râles of many kinds are found.

The signs in the more chronic cases vary greatly depending on the character of the substance, the reaction set up, whether the bronchus is plugged and the changes in the supplied lung. In all cases there may be auscultation signs on the unaffected side due to extension of inflammation or secretions passing over. In cases of long duration, fibrosis, bronchiectasis and abscess may result with their usual features. Decreased expansion is always present on the affected side. Two special signs are important. One is the occurrence of very fine râles over a small area in the case of metallic bodies which do not plug the bronchus and the other the "*asthmatoid wheeze*" described by Jackson. This is a wheezing sound which varies in pitch and loudness and may be with inspiration or expiration or with both. It may be heard at a distance or with the bell of the stethoscope at the patient's mouth.

Diagnosis.—It is remarkable how often the diagnosis is missed because a proper history is not taken or the child's story is not believed. The acute features may lead to the diagnosis of pneumonia, which a careful examination should prevent. In the chronic cases tuberculosis is often diagnosed. The signs in a lobe which is completely shut off are often regarded as those of empyema. An exploratory puncture soon decides. The X-rays are of great aid but not all foreign bodies show in the plates. The changes in the involved lobe or lung are distinctive as a rule. The thought of the possibility of foreign body is the surest aid against error. A foreign body in the trachea may suggest diphtheria and edema of the glottis often occurs. A foreign body in the esophagus may give tracheobronchial symptoms due to overflow of secretion through the larynx or by pressure on or perforation into the trachea. It is easy to be misled in such cases.

Treatment.—This is removal by *bronchoscopy* done by skilled hands.

Broncholithiasis.—Calcified tracheabronchial lymph nodes may ulcerate into a bronchus; material, as from cavities, may become calcified, or enchondromas may become free. The calcified body may be smooth or rough. There may be no symptoms or signs. If inflammation is excited or obstruction caused it acts like a foreign body. There may be hemoptysis. In longstanding cases bronchiectasis or lung abscess may result. The diagnosis is usually made by expulsion of the substance, sometimes by the X-ray. Bronchoscopy should be done if there are signs of obstruction.

DISEASES OF THE LUNGS

CIRCULATORY DISTURBANCES IN THE LUNGS

Congestion.—There are two forms of hyperemia—active and passive.

1. ACTIVE CONGESTION.—About this much doubt and confusion exist. French writers regard it as an independent primary affection. English and American authors more correctly regard it as a symptomatic affection. Active fluxion to the lungs occurs with increased action of the heart, and when very hot air or irritating substances are inhaled. In diseases which interfere locally with the circulation the capillaries in the unaffected portions may be greatly distended. The importance of this collateral fluxion is probably exaggerated. In a series of pulmonary affections there is this associated congestion—in pneumonia, bronchitis, pleurisy and tuberculosis.

The *symptoms* of active hyperemia of the lungs as given by French writers are of an affection difficult to distinguish from anomalous or larval forms of pneumonia. The chief features are initial chill, pain, dyspnea, moderate cough, and temperature from 101° to 103° F. The physical signs are defective resonance, feeble breathing, sometimes bronchial, and fine râles. A majority of physicians would class such cases under pneumonia.

An intense and rapidly fatal congestion of the lung, following extreme heat or cold or sometimes violent exertion, is recognized by some authors. Renforth, the oarsman, is said to have died from this during a race near St. John, N. B. Leuf described cases in which, in association with drunkenness, exposure and cold, death occurred suddenly, the only lesion found being an extreme, almost hemorrhagic, congestion of the lungs. It is by no means certain that in these cases death really occurs from pulmonary congestion in the absence of specific statements as to the coronary arteries and heart.

2. PASSIVE CONGESTION.—Two forms of this may be recognized, the mechanical and the hypostatic.

(*a*) *Mechanical congestion* occurs whenever there is an obstacle to the return of the blood to the heart. It is common in affections of the left heart, particularly mitral stenosis. The lungs are voluminous, russet brown in color, cutting and tearing with great resistance. On section they show at first a brownish red tinge, and the cut surface becomes rapidly a vivid red color from oxidation of the abundant hemoglobin. This is known as *brown induration* of the lung. Occasionally this mechanical hyperemia follows pressure by tumors. So long as compensation is maintained the congestion of the lung in heart disease does not produce any symptoms, but with enfeebled heart action the engorgement becomes marked and there are dyspnea, cough, and expectoration with the characteristic alveolar cells.

(*b*) *Hypostatic Congestion.*—In fevers and adynamic states generally it is very common to find the bases of the lungs deeply congested, a condition induced partly by the effect of gravity, the patient lying recumbent in one posture for a long time, but chiefly by weakened heart action. That it is not an effect of gravity alone is shown by the fact that a healthy person may remain in bed an indefinite time without its occurrence. The posterior parts of the lung are dark in color and engorged with blood and serum; in some instances to such a degree that the alveoli no longer contain air and portions of the lung sink in water. The terms *splenization* and *hypostatic pneumonia* have been given to these advanced grades. It is common in long debilitating illness. With ascites, meteorism, and abdominal tumors the bases of the lungs may be compressed and congested. There is a form of passive congestion met with in injury to, and organic disease of, the brain. In cerebral apoplexy the bases of the lungs are deeply engorged, not quite airless, but heavy, and on section drip with blood and serum. This may occur in an extreme grade throughout the lungs in death from morphia poisoning. In some instances the lung tissue has a blackish, gelatinous, infiltrated appearance, almost like diffuse pulmonary infarction. Occasionally this is most marked in, and even confined to, the hemiplegic side. In prolonged coma the hypostatic congestion may be associated with patches of consolidation, due to the aspiration of food into the air passages.

The *symptoms* of hypostatic congestion are not characteristic. There are shortness of breath and cough with abundant sputum containing alveolar epithelium filled with yellow and black pigment—the so-called "heart-failure cells." On examination slight dulness, feeble, sometimes blowing, breathing and crackling or bubbling râles can be detected. Pulmonary infarction and edema may occur as complications.

Treatment.—The treatment is usually that of the condition with which the congestion is associated. In patients in whom passive congestion is probable, frequent change of position in bed is advisable and they should sit up in a chair occasionally if possible. Deep breathing for short periods is useful. The bowels should be kept open and freely moved if congestion is present. Active treatment for the heart is usually indicated. In the intense hyperemia, which may possibly occur primarily, and which is met with in heart disease and emphysema, bleeding should be done. From 20 to 30 ounces of blood should be taken.

Edema.—In all forms of intense congestion there is a transudation of serum from the engorged capillaries chiefly into the air cells, but also into the alveolar walls. Not only is it frequent in congestion, but also with inflammation, new growth, infarcts, and tubercles. When limited to the neighborhood of an affected part, the name collateral edema is applied to it.

Acute edema is met with: (1) in the infections, particularly pneumonia; (2) in nephritis especially with uremia; (3) in heart disease, particularly myocarditis and valve lesions; (4) in arteriosclerosis with high tension; (5) pregnancy; (6) angioneurotic edema; (7) as a complication of the epileptic fit, and (8) after thoracentesis. The theory most generally accepted is that of W. H. Welch, whose experiments indicate that pulmonary edema is due to a disproportionate weakness of the left ventricle, so that the blood accumulates in the lung capillaries until transudation occurs. Myocardial failure is the most important cause. Others regard it as due to disturbance in the vasomotor mechanism of the lungs with increased permeability of the capillaries. In some cases there are recurring attacks of acute edema without obvious cause. Anatomically the lung is anemic, heavy, sodden, pits on pressure, and on section a large quantity of clear or blood-tinged serum flows out. It may have in places a gelatinous aspect.

SYMPTOMS.—The onset is sudden with a feeling of oppression in the chest and rapid breathing which soon becomes dyspneic or orthopneic. There may be an incessant short cough and a copious frothy, sometimes blood-tinged, expectoration, which may be expelled in a gush from the mouth and nose. The face is pale and covered with a cold sweat; the pulse is feeble and the heart's action weak. The percussion note is usually impaired, especially over the lower parts; the breath sounds vary, at first they may be harsh but later become feeble and may be obscured by the râles. Early in the attack the râles are fine and crackling but soon become coarser and bubbling. The fine râles may be heard before there are any symptoms and give warning of an attack. Later, with fluid in the bronchi, they are very loud, coarse and bubbling. The attack may be fatal in less than an hour or may persist in some degree for twelve or twenty-four hours and then pass off. Lissaman reported a case with 72 attacks in two and a half years. There is no doubt of the *diagnosis* when the condition is fully developed but it is important to recognize the early stages when treatment is of more use. The dyspnea, the thin watery sputum and the character of the early râles are important. The outlook is always serious.

TREATMENT.—Venesection is often most helpful. Morphia (gr. ¼, 0.016 gm.) with atropine (gr. 1/50, 0.0012 gm.) should be given hypodermically and the atropine repeated in fifteen minutes if there is no change. Aromatic spirit of ammonia (ʒ i, 4 cc.) may be given by mouth. One of the digitalis preparations should be given intramuscularly and repeated every three hours if indicated. If hypertension is present nitroglycerine (gr. 1/100, 0.0006 gm.) is to be given under the tongue and repeated until an effect is produced. Inhalation of chloroform, artificial respiration, dry cupping and the use of oxygen may be helpful. Patients who have repeated attacks should be warned against overexertion and with the first symptoms of an attack should be given ammonia with morphia and atropine hypodermically.

Pulmonary Hemorrhage.—This occurs in two forms—*bronchopulmonary hemorrhage*, in which the blood is poured into the bronchi and expectorated, and *pulmonary infarction*, in which the hemorrhage takes place into the air cells and lung tissue.

1. BRONCHOPULMONARY HEMORRHAGE; HEMOPTYSIS.—The term hemoptysis should be restricted to the spitting of blood from hemorrhage below the vocal cords. It results from a variety of conditions, among which the following are the most important: (*a*) In young persons hemoptysis may occur without warning, and after continuing for a few days disappear and leave no ill traces. There may be at the time of the attack no physical signs indicating pulmonary disease. In such cases good health may be preserved and no further trouble occur, but tuberculosis should be suspected. In Ware's contribution, of 386 cases of hemoptysis in private practice 62 recovered and pulmonary disease did not subsequently develop. (*b*) *Hemoptysis in pulmonary tuberculosis,* which is considered on page 186. (*c*) With certain diseases of a bronchus or lung, as pneumonia (in the initial stage), infarction, and cancer, occasionally in syphilis, the spirochetal bronchitis, gangrene, abscess, and bronchiectasis. (*d*) In heart affections, particularly mitral lesions. It may

be profuse and recur at intervals for years. (*e*) *In ulcerative affections of the larynx, trachea, or bronchi.* Sometimes the hemorrhage is profuse and rapidly fatal, as when the ulcer erodes a large branch of the pulmonary artery. (*f*) *Aneurism.* It may be sudden and rapidly fatal when the sac bursts into the air passages. Slight bleeding may continue for weeks or months, due to pressure on the mucous membrane or erosion of the lung; or in some cases the sac "weeps" through the laminae of fibrin. (*g*) *Vicarious hemorrhage* occurs in rare instances in cases of interrupted menstruation. The instances are well authenticated. Flint mentions a case under observation for four years, and Hippocrates refers to it in the aphorism, "Hemoptysis in a woman is removed by an eruption of the menses." Periodical hemoptysis has been met with after the removal of both ovaries. Fatal hemorrhage has occurred from the lung during menstruation when no lesion was found to account for it. In tuberculous women the tendency to hemoptysis is increased at the menstrual period. (*h*) *Permanent high arterial tension.* Hemoptysis, sometimes profuse, may occur at intervals. (*i*) Hemoptysis occurs sometimes in *malignant fevers* and in *purpura hemorrhagica, hemophilia* and *leukemia.* (*j*) Due to trauma. (*k*) There is endemic hemoptysis, due to the bronchial fluke, seen in China and Japan.

Symptoms.—Hemoptysis sets in, as a rule, suddenly. Often without warning the patient experiences a warm, saltish taste as the mouth fills with blood. Coughing is usually induced. There may be only an ounce or so brought up before the hemorrhage stops, or the bleeding may continue for days, the patient bringing up small quantities. In other instances, particularly when a large vessel is eroded or an aneurism bursts, the amount is large, and the patient, after a few attempts at coughing, shows signs of suffocation and death is produced by inundation of the bronchial system. Fatal hemorrhage may occur into a large cavity without hemoptysis. The blood from the lungs generally has characters which distinguish it readily from vomited blood. It is alkaline, frothy, mixed with mucus, and air-bubbles are present in the clot. Blood-moulds of the smaller bronchi are sometimes seen. Patients can usually tell whether the blood has been brought up by coughing or vomiting, and in a majority of cases the history gives important indications. In hemoptysis connected with menstrual disturbances the practitioner should see that the blood is actually coughed up, since deception may be practised. The spurious hemoptysis of hysteria is considered with that disease. Naturally, the patient is alarmed by the bleeding, but, unless very profuse, as when due to rupture of an aneurism in a pulmonary cavity, the danger is rarely immediate. The ultimate prognosis depends on the cause. The attacks are apt to recur for a few days and the sputum may remain blood-tinged for a longer period. In the great majority of cases the hemorrhage ceases spontaneously. Blood may be swallowed and produce vomiting, and, after a day or two, the stools may be dark in color. It is not advisable to percuss the chest during an attack of hemoptysis; auscultation may show widespread râles.

Treatment of Pulmonary Hemorrhage.—The pressure within the pulmonary artery is considerably less than that in the aortic system. The system is under vasomotor control, but our knowledge of the mutual relations of pressure in the aorta and in the pulmonary artery, under varying conditions, is imperfect. There may be an influence on the systemic blood pressure without any on the pulmonary, and the pressure in the one may rise while it falls in the other, or it may rise and fall in both together. The researches of Brodie and Dixon indicate that drugs which raise the peripheral blood pressure by vasoconstriction increase the total blood in the lung. Thus ergot, a remedy commonly used, causes a rise in the pulmonary blood-pressure, while aconite produces a fall.

The anatomical condition in hemoptysis is either hyperemia of the bronchial mucosa (or the lung tissue) or a perforated vessel. In the latter case the patient may pass rapidly beyond treatment, though there are instances of the most profuse hemorrhage which must have come from a perforated artery or a ruptured aneurism, in which recovery has occurred. When the blood is brought up in large quantities, it is almost certain that an aneurism has ruptured or a vessel has been eroded. In the instances in which the sputum is blood tinged or when the blood is in smaller quantities, bleeding comes by diapedesis from hyperemic vessels. In such cases the hemorrhage may be beneficial in relieving congestion.

The truth, *Das Blut ist ein ganz besonderer Saft*, is strikingly emphasized by the frightened state of the patient. Rest of the body and peace of the mind—"*quies, securitas, silentium*" of Celsus—should be secured. If there is marked restlessness, morphine hypodermically (gr. 1/6, 0.011 gm.) is advisable. Turn the patient on the affected side, if known, as regurgitation is less apt to occur into the bronchi of the sound lung. As Aretaeus remarks, in hemoptysis the patient despairs from the first and needs to be strongly reassured. Death is rarely due directly to hemoptysis; patients die after, not of it (S. West). In the majority of cases of mild hemoptysis this is sufficient. Even when the patient insists upon going about, the bleeding may stop spontaneously. The diet should be liquid. Alcohol should not be used. The patient may, if he wishes, have ice to suck. For cough, which is always present and disturbing, codein can be given freely. Digitalis should not be used. Aconite may be used when there is much vascular excitement. Ergot, tannic acid, and lead have no influence in hemoptysis; ergot probably does harm. In Europe the intravenous injection of 10 cc. of a 1 per cent solution of Congo red has been used. It is important that the Congo red should be absolutely pure, and fresh solutions only should be used. One of the most satisfactory means of lowering blood-pressure is purgation, and when the bleeding is protracted salts may be freely given. In profuse hemoptysis, as from erosion of an artery or rupture of an aneurism, a fatal result is common, and yet postmortem evidence shows that thrombosis may occur with healing in a rupture of considerable size. The fainting induced by loss of blood probably promotes thrombosis, and it was on this principle that formerly patients were bled from the arm, or from both arms, as in the case of Laurence Sterne. The ice-bag is of doubtful utility. In protracted cases artificial *pneumothorax* is very useful, especially in tuberculous patients. *Blood transfusion* may be required if the bleeding is severe.

2. Pulmonary Infarction.—The blood is effused into the air cells and interstitial tissue. It is usually diffuse, the parenchyma not being broken, as is the brain tissue in cerebral apoplexy. Sometimes, in disease of the brain, in septic conditions, and in malignant fevers, the lung tissue is uniformly infiltrated with blood and has a black, gelatinous appearance.

Etiology.—This results from the blocking of a branch of the pulmonary artery by an embolus or thrombus. (1) *Embolism.* The embolus may originate: (*a*) in the systemic venous system. This follows *phlebitis* with thrombosis, most common in the femoral or pelvic veins, but not rare in smaller veins. It happens after operations, particularly in the pelvis or on the appendix; (*b*) in the *right heart,* especially in the auricle with myocardial failure. Vegetations from the valves of the right heart (rarely from the left heart through an open septum) may be detached; (*c*) in the *pulmonary artery;* (*d*) *fat* embolism usually follows operations or fracture, especially in fat persons; (*e*) in portions of *new growth* which gain entrance into veins; (*f*) *hydatid* embolism; and (*g*) *air* embolism. (2) *Thrombosis.* This occurs secondary to embolism but may be primary in the pulmonary vessels, either with atheroma or disease of the lung.

Blocking of the pulmonary arteries is not always followed by infarction; partly because the wide capillaries furnish sufficient anastomosis, and partly because the bronchial vessels may keep up the circulation. The infarctions are chiefly at the periphery of the lung, usually wedge-shaped, with the base of the wedge toward the surface. When recent, they are dark in color, hard and firm, and look on section like an ordinary blood-clot. Gradual changes go on and the color becomes a reddish brown. The pleura over an infarct is inflamed. A section shows the air cells to be distended with red blood cells, which may also be in the alveolar walls. The infarcts may be multiple and vary in size from a walnut to an orange. Very large ones may involve the greater part of a lobe. In the artery passing to the affected territory a thrombus or an embolus is found. In many cases the source of the embolus can not be discovered. It is not infrequent to find total obstruction of a large branch of a pulmonary artery without hemorrhage into the corresponding lung area. The further history of an infarction is variable. It is possible that in some instances the circulation is reestablished and the blood removed. More commonly, if the patient lives, the usual changes go on in the extravasated blood and ultimately a pigmented, puckered, fibroid patch results. Abscess and empyema result if the embolus is infective. Occasionally gangrene results. A gangrenous infarct may rupture and produce fatal pneumothorax.

Symptoms.—The clinical features vary widely, much depending on the size of the infarct and whether the embolus is infective or not. In the case of a large embolus blocking a main branch of the pulmonary artery death may be almost instantaneous, perhaps after a cry. In other cases there are sudden severe dyspnea, thoracic pain, distress and cyanosis, followed by unconsciousness and death. In cases of moderate severity, there is sudden thoracic *pain* with dyspnea, cough and *hemoptysis* of varying amounts. The symptoms occur with varying degrees of severity and in the milder forms only slight pain, moderate distress and cough are seen. The *signs* are not distinctive; there is decreased expansion, if the infarct is single, with diminished vocal fremitus as a rule; the percussion note is dull; the breath sounds are decreased or absent, but blowing breathing and a friction rub may be heard. There may be râles in the adjoining areas. The signs persist for some time and a dull area may remain, partly due to pleural thickening. If the embolus is infective, suppuration and its results follow. A lower lobe is usually involved. The X-ray plate may show the affected area.

Postoperative Embolism.—This may occur in the first few days after operation and is often regarded as pneumonia, from which the diagnosis may be difficult, but as a rule the breathing is not tubular and characteristic râles are absent. The mortality is high. The infarction may occur in the second or third week after operation, usually after an ordinary convalescence or there may have been slight fever (probably from phlebitis). The onset is sudden with sharp thoracic pain, dyspnea, increase in the respiration and pulse rate, and often high fever, which rises for two or three days. Cough may not appear for a day; with it there may be bloody sputum or a frank hemoptysis. The signs are as given before, a friction rub usually being prominent.

Fat Embolism.—The symptoms may be pulmonary and cerebral. The pulmonary features are dyspnea, increased respiration rate, cyanosis and cough, sometimes with hemoptysis. There is fever with increased pulse rate and a drop in blood pressure. The sputum and urine may contain fat droplets. There may be petechiae in the skin. The signs in the lungs are most marked at the bases. Death may be rapid and occur on the operating table. The majority of deaths occur within two or three days.

Diagnosis.—The dramatic onset and death in severe cases should make the diagnosis clear but such instances are sometimes mistaken for cerebral hemorrhage. The moderately severe cases may be regarded as pneumonia or pleurisy. The mild cases are easily overlooked and regarded as pleurisy or "intercostal neuralgia." They explain many puzzling thoracic conditions in acute infections and after operation. Collapse of the lung should always be considered.

Prognosis.—This depends largely on the size of the occluded vessel. With severe features the outlook is always serious; in moderate or mild forms there is little danger. Recurrence is evidently more likely if the embolus comes from the heart than from a thrombophlebitis.

Treatment.—Care should be taken to ensure rest in all cases of phlebitis and peripheral thrombosis until the clot is organized. Sodium citrate (gr. 5-10, 0.3-0.6 gm. three times a day) is useful in an illness in which thrombosis may occur, especially if the patient is taking large amounts of milk. In an attack, the giving of morphine (gr. ¼, 0.016 gm.) and atropine (gr. 1/100, 0.0006 gm.) is wise with cardiac stimulation if required. Venesection is useful if there is much venous fullness. The pain should be relieved when necessary and other symptomatic measures used as indicated.

PULMONARY FIBROSIS

This condition, known also as fibroid disease and cirrhosis of the lung or chronic interstitial pneumonia, is not a disease but represents the result of many inflammatory and irritative processes. Fibroid change may start in the tissue about the bronchi and blood vessels, the interlobular septa, the alveolar walls or in the pleura. So diverse are the forms and so varied the conditions under which it occurs that a classification is difficult. We recognize two chief forms—*local,* involving a limited area of the lung, and *diffuse,* invading both lungs or an entire organ.

Etiology.—(*a*) LOCAL fibroid change is common. It is a constant accompaniment of tubercle, in the evolution of which interstitial changes play a very important rôle. In tumors, abscess, gummata, hydatids and emphysema it also occurs. Fibroid processes are frequent at the apices of the lungs and may be due to a limited healed tuberculosis, to fibroid induration or result from thickening of the pleura.

(*b*) DIFFUSE FIBROSIS is met with :(1) As a sequence of *acute lobar pneumonia.* Although extremely rare, this is a possible termination. From unknown causes resolution fails to take place. Organization goes on in the fibrinous plugs within the air cells and the alveolar walls become greatly thickened by a growth, first of nuclear and subsequently of fibrillated connective tissue. Macroscopically a smooth, grayish, homogeneous tissue which has the peculiar translucency of all newly-formed connective tissue is produced. This has been called gray induration.

(2) *Bronchopneumonia.*—These cases are relatively common especially after influenzal pneumonia. The process may be specially marked about the hilum and spread outward and downward. The lower lobes are most often involved. Compensatory emphysema is frequent. The fibrosis may extend from the bronchi, which are usually dilated.

(3) *Bronchiectasis* may be followed by fibrosis of the lung. The alveolar walls are thickened and the lobules converted into firm grayish masses, in which there is no trace of normal lung tissue. This may go on and involve a lobe or the whole lung. Many of these cases are tuberculous from the outset.

(4) *Chronic fibrosis,* due to inhalation of dust or irritating fumes.

(5) *Syphilis* of the lung may present the features of a chronic fibrosis.

(6) Fibroid changes may follow the compression by aneurism or new growth, any local bronchial or pulmonary process or any condition causing obstruction or stenosis, as a foreign body.

(7) Repeated mild *bronchial infections* or persistent low grade infection as from infected sinuses.

(8) *Pleurogenous Interstitial Fibrosis.*—This term is applied to that form which follows invasion from the pleura. Doubt has been expressed whether this really occurs. While Wilson Fox was probably correct in questioning whether an entire lung can become cirrhosed by a gradual invasion from the pleura, there can be no doubt that there are instances of primitive dry pleurisy, which gradually compress the lung and lead to interstitial fibrosis. This may be due in part to the fibroid change which follows prolonged compression. In some cases there is a distinct connection between the thickened pleura and the dense strands of fibrous tissue passing from it into the lung substance. Instances occur in which one lobe or the greater part of it presents, on section, a mottled appearance, owing to the increased thickness of the interlobar septa—a condition which may exist without involvement of the pleura. In many other cases, however, the extension seems to be so definitely associated with pleurisy that there is no doubt as to the causal connection between the two processes. In these instances the lung is removed with great difficulty, owing to the close adhesion of the pleura to the chest wall.

Morbid Anatomy.—There are two chief forms, the massive or lobar and the localized form. In the *massive* form the disease is unilateral; the chest of the affected side is sunken, deformed, and the shoulder much depressed. The heart is drawn over to the affected side. The unaffected lung is emphysematous and covers the greater portion of the mediastinum. It is scarcely credible in how small a space, close to the spine, the fibrosed lung may lie. The adhesions between the pleural membranes may be extremely dense and thick, particularly in the pleurogenous cases; but when the disease has originated in the lung there may be little thickening of the pleura. The organ is airless, firm, and hard. It strongly resists cutting, and on section shows a grayish fibroid tissue of variable amount, through which pass the blood vessels and bronchi. The latter may be slightly or enormously dilated. There are instances in which the entire lung is converted into a series of bronchiectatic cavities and the fibrosis is apparent only in certain areas or at the root. The tuberculous cases can usually be differentiated by the presence of an apical cavity, not bronchiectatic, often large, and the other lung almost invariably shows tuberculous lesions. Aneurisms are not infrequent in the cavities. The heart is hypertrophied, particularly the right ventricle, and there may be marked atheromatous changes in the vessels. An amyloid condition of the viscera is found in some cases.

In the *localized* form the areas are smaller, often centrally placed, and most frequently in the lower lobes. They are pigmented, show dilated bronchi, and when multiple are separated by emphysematous lung tissue.

A *reticular form* has been described in which the lungs are intersected by grayish fibroid strands following the lines of the interlobular septa. *Peribronchial fibrosis* is very common, figures largely in X-ray reports on the thorax, and results from many infections, possibly also from the irritation produced by gas. It is not necessarily tuberculous.

Symptoms and Course.—The disease is essentially chronic, extending over many years, and the general health may be fairly good. In a well-marked case the patient complains of chronic cough and perhaps shortness of breath. In other respects he is well and is usually able to do light work. The patients are often regarded as tuberculous, though there may be scarcely a symptom of that disease except the cough. There are instances, however, of fibroid tuberculosis which can not be distinguished from ordinary fibrosis except by the presence of tubercle bacilli in the sputum. As the bronchi are usually dilated, the symptoms and signs may be those of *bronchiectasis.* The cough is paroxysmal and the sputum generally copious and mucopurulent or seropurulent. It is sometimes fetid. *Hemorrhage* is not infrequent, and occurred in more than one-half of the cases analyzed by Bastian. Walking on the level and in the ordinary affairs of life, the patient may show no shortness of breath, but in the ascent of stairs and on exertion there may be dyspnea. Cyanosis and clubbing of the fingers are common.

Physical Signs.—*Inspection.*—If unilateral the affected side is immobile, retracted, and shrunken, and contrasts in a striking way with the voluminous healthy one. The intercostal spaces are obliterated and the ribs may even overlap. The shoulder is drawn down and the spine is bowed. The muscles of the shoulder girdle are wasted. The heart is greatly displaced, being drawn over by the shrinkage of the lung to the affected side. When the left lung is affected there may be a large area of visible impulse in the second, third, and fourth interspaces. Mensuration shows a great diminution in the affected side, and with the saddle-tape the expansion may be seen to be negative. The *percussion* note varies with the degree of emphysema and fibrosis, and the condition of the bronchi. It may be flat, particularly at the base or apex.

In the axilla there may be flat tympany or an amphoric note over a large sacculated bronchus. On the opposite side the percussion note is usually hyper-resonant. The *breath sounds* vary greatly, depending on the amount of fibrosis, the extent of bronchiectasis and especially on the degree of pleural thickening. They may be amphoric over cavities; râles of many kinds are frequent. The voice sounds are usually exaggerated. Cardiac murmurs are not uncommon, particularly when the right heart fails. The physical signs vary considerably, according to the stage of the process. The disease is essentially chronic, and may persist for fifteen or twenty years. Death occurs sometimes from hemorrhage, more commonly from gradual failure of the right heart, and occasionally from amyloid degeneration.

In the *diffuse general* forms the symptoms are the same but the signs are less definite. There is usually marked emphysema with signs of bronchitis. Only an X-ray study may give definite information as to the extent of fibrosis.

Diagnosis.—This is never difficult but it may be impossible to say, without a clear history, whether the origin is pleuritic or pneumonic. Between cases of this kind and fibroid tuberculous it is not always easy to discriminate, as the conditions may be almost identical. When tuberculosis is present, however, bacilli are present in the sputum, and there may be signs of disease in the other lung. The X-ray study is of great aid.

Treatment.—It is usually for an intercurrent affection or an aggravation of the cough that the patient seeks relief. Nothing can be done for the condition itself. When possible the patient should live in a mild climate and avoid exposure to cold and damp. A distressing feature in some cases is putrefaction of the contents of the dilated tubes, for which the same measures may be used as in fetid bronchitis.

PNEUMOCONIOSIS—SILICOSIS

Definition.—Under this term are embraced those forms of fibrosis of the lung due to the inhalation of dust. They have received various names, according to the nature of the inhaled particles—*anthracosis, siderosis, chalicosis, silicosis* and *asbestosis*. However, the most important constituent in all the inorganic dusts is *silica*. The significance of sericite is not decided. Cases due to dust from organic material such as cotton, shoddy, tobacco, etc., are rare and less serious.

Etiology.—This is entirely a question of exposure to dust and so occupation plays an important part. Hygienic conditions, such as ventilation, have an influence. The disease occurs almost entirely in males. Probably about half a million workers in the United States are exposed to silica dust. The danger is in proportion to the amount of dust which is inhaled, the size of the particles and the silica content. Another factor is exposure to alkaline silica mixtures as in the manufacture of scouring soaps and powders. The length of time required for definite changes to result varies greatly in different trades; an average may be put at 8 to 10 years. There are *acute* cases, usually in workers with alkaline silica mixtures, in which the exposure is less than a year. In coal miners it may be 20 years before symptoms appear; the amount of silica in the dust of coal mines is usually small. While it seems probable that coal dust itself causes some changes, these do not seem to be marked and silica is the essential factor. *Tuberculosis* is often associated and some hold that the combination is really a new condition and not one disease superimposed on the other. The tuberculosis may have existed before the silicosis, possibly latent, or contracted after it. In the majority of acute fatal cases of silicosis, tuberculosis is found. It is suggested that workers with syphilis develop silicosis rapidly and that the disease runs a rapid course.

The results are due to three factors: (1) mechanical, (2) chemical and (3) infection. The chemical changes seem to be the most important. If free silica is inhaled it is probably converted to silicates in the tissues. The silica content of the lung varies; if more than 1 per cent of the dried lung it has played an important part. An amount of over 3 per cent has been found.

Organic dust is not so serious, and it has been questioned if pneumoconiosis is ever produced by it alone. The workers in cotton and woolen mills have a high death rate from tuberculosis, but the dust is probably not a serious factor. In the grinding of rags, new workers may have attacks of catarrh and fever with shivering ("Shoddy fever," Oliver). The dust of *grain* in threshing may cause irritation of the bronchi, headache and sometimes fever.

The dust particles inhaled into the lungs are dealt with by the ciliated epithelium and the phagocytes. The ordinary mucous corpuscles take in a large number of the particles which fall upon the trachea and main bronchi. The cilia sweep the mucus out to a point from which it can be expelled by coughing. In dwellers in the country, where the air is pure, they are able to prevent the access of dust particles to the lung tissue, so that even in adults these organs present a rosy tint, very different from the dark appearance of the lungs of dwellers in cities.

In the development of the condition an important part is played by the mononuclear phagocytic cells which ingest the dust particles and carry them into the tissues. They pass into the lymphatics, where they cause irritation with resulting changes. The process has been divided into three stages. (1) There is inflammation of the lymphatics with localization in areas, sometimes forming nodules ("pseudotubercle"), and changes in the lymph nodes at the roots of the lungs. Fibrosis accompanies these changes. (2) The fibrosis increases often in local areas so that the nodules are more prominent. (3) The areas are larger and the general fibrosis is more marked with increased involvement of the lymph nodes at the hilum. Emphysema gradually becomes more marked and there may be thickening of the pleura.

In *asbestosis* irregular structures with a yellow color ("asbestosis bodies") are found in the lungs and sputum. Asbestos contains various silicates, principally magnesium silicate.

Morbid Anatomy.—It is not uncommon to find in persons whose lungs are only moderately involved the bronchial glands sclerosed and hard. The fibroid changes usually begin in the peribronchial lymph tissue, and in early stages the sclerosis may be largely confined to these regions. In later stages there is general fibrosis. A Nova Scotian miner, aged thirty-six, died in the Montreal General Hospital, of small-pox, after an illness of a few days. In his lungs (externally coal-black) there were round and linear patches ranging in size from a pea to a hazelnut, of an intensely black color, airless and firm, and surrounded by a crepitant tissue, slate gray in color. In the centre of each of these areas was a small bronchus. Many were situated just beneath the pleura, and formed typical examples of limited fibroid bronchopneumonia. There is usually thickening of the alveolar walls, particularly in certain areas. By the gradual coalescence of these fibroid patches large portions of the lung are converted into firm areas of fibrosis, grayish black in the coal miner, steel gray in the stone worker.

A second important factor is *chronic bronchitis,* which is present in a large proportion and really causes the chief symptoms. A third is the occurrence of *emphysema,* which is almost invariably associated with long-standing cases. With the changes so far described, unless the sclerotic area is unusually extensive, the case may present the features of chronic bronchitis with emphysema, but finally another element may come into play. In the fibroid areas softening may occur, probably a process of necrosis similar to that by which softening is produced in fibromyomata of the uterus. At first these are small and contain a dark liquid. They rarely attain a large size unless a communication is formed with the bronchus, in which case they may become converted into suppurating cavities.

Tuberculosis.—As mentioned, this occurs in a large percentage of those with silicosis. Apparently this is least marked in workers in coal mines and the mortality from tuberculosis among them seems to be less than in the general population.

Symptoms.—Except in the acute cases the symptoms do not come on until the patient has worked for a variable number of years in the dusty atmosphere. As a rule there are cough and failing health for a prolonged period of time before complete disability. The coincident emphysema is responsible in great part for the shortness of breath and wheezy condition of these patients. The sputum is usually mucopurulent, often profuse, and in anthracosis very dark in color—the so-called "black spit," while in silicosis there may be seen under the microscope the bright angular particles of silica. In asbestosis the "asbestosis bodies" are found in the sputum. The *signs* are those of chronic bronchitis and emphysema, to which are added later those of fibrosis of the lung and often those of myocardial failure.

Prognosis.—This is very variable and depends greatly on the kind of dust, the amount of change produced and whether tuberculosis is added. The disease may progress after the exposure to dust has ceased as the reaction of the tissues to the contained silica continues. Symptoms may appear years after exposure, due to continued action of the silica in the tissues. The presence of tuberculosis or myocardial change is serious.

Diagnosis.—This is rarely difficult; the history of exposure to dust is important. It must be borne in mind that chronic bronchitis and emphysema form essential parts of the process and that in late stages there may be tuberculous infection. The X-ray study is the most important means of diagnosis. The picture in the early stages shows increase in the normal shadows especially about the hilum, and as the disease advances there are circumscribed dense areas. Miliary tuberculosis may be suggested. The diaphragm shows limitation of motion in the later stages. The diagnosis of tuberculosis may be difficult; sputum examinations may decide.

Prophylaxis.—Much has been done to reduce the prevalence of the disease by proper ventilation of works and the protection of the men. The conversion of dry into wet mining prevents the distribution of injurious dust.

Treatment.—This is practically that of chronic bronchitis and emphysema. The patient should change his occupation.

EMPHYSEMA

Definition.—The condition in which the infundibular passages and the alveoli are dilated and the alveolar walls atrophied.

Floyer of Litchfield first described the anatomical condition and spoke of the disease as "flatulent asthma" (1698), meaning a disorder in which the lungs were blown up with air. A practical division may be made into compensatory, hypertrophic, and atrophic forms, the acute vesicular emphysema, and the interstitial forms. The last two do not in reality come under the above definition, but for convenience they may be considered here. *Obstructive* emphysema occurs with a foreign body in a bronchus which has a ball-valve action, allowing air to enter but not to escape.

COMPENSATORY EMPHYSEMA

Whenever a region of the lung does not expand fully in inspiration, either another portion of the lung must expand or the chest wall sink in order to occupy the space. The former almost invariably occurs. In bronchopneumonia there is distention of the air-vesicles in the adjacent healthy lobules, and the same happens in the neighborhood of tuberculous areas and cicatrices. With general pleural adhesions there is often compensatory emphysema, particularly at the anterior margins of the lung. The most advanced example of this form is seen in fibrosis, when the unaffected lung or portions of lung increase greatly in size, owing to distention of the air vesicles. A similar though less marked condition is seen in extensive pleurisy with effusion and in pneumothorax.

At first, this distention is a simple physiological process and the alveolar walls are stretched but not atrophied. Ultimately, however, in many cases they waste and the contiguous air cells fuse, producing true emphysema.

HYPERTROPHIC EMPHYSEMA

The large-lunged emphysema of Jenner, also termed substantive or idiopathic, is a well-marked affection, characterized by enlargement of the lungs, due to distention of the air cells and atrophy of their walls, and clinically by imperfect aëration of the blood and more or less marked dyspnea.

Etiology.—Emphysema is the result of persistently high intra-alveolar tension acting upon a congenitally weak lung tissue. Strongly in favor of the view that the nutritive change in the air cells is the primary factor are the markedly *hereditary* character of the disease and the frequency with which it starts early in life. To James Jackson, Jr., of Boston, we owe the first observations on its hereditary character. Working under Louis' direction, he found that in 18 out of 28 cases one or both parents were affected.

In childhood it may follow recurring asthmatic attacks or bronchitis with adenoids or tonsillar disease. It may occur in several members of the same family. We are ignorant as to the nature of this congenital pulmonary weakness. Cohnheim thought it probably due to a defect in the development of the elastic-tissue fibres, which is borne out by Eppinger's observations.

Heightened pressure within the air cells may be due to forcible inspiration or expiration. Much discussion has taken place as to the part played by these two acts in the production of the disease. The *inspiratory* theory was advanced by Laënnec and subsequently modified by Gairdner, who held that in chronic bronchitis areas of collapse were induced, and compensatory distention took place in the adjacent lobules. This unquestionably does occur in compensatory emphysema, but probably is not a factor of much moment in this form. The *expiratory* theory, supported by Mendelssohn and Jenner, accounts for the condition in a more satisfactory way. In all straining efforts and violent attacks of coughing the glottis is closed and the chest walls strongly compressed by muscular effort, so that the strain is thrown upon those parts of the lung least protected, as the apices and the anterior margins, where we find the emphysema most advanced. The sternum and costal cartilages gradually yield to the heightened intrathoracic pressure and, in advanced cases, give the characteristic rotundity to the thorax.

Freund's Theory.—A primary disease of the costal cartilages, a chronic hyperplasia with premature ossification, brings about a state of rigid dilatation of the chest in the inspiratory position, to which the emphysema is secondary. It is probable that there is a group of cases in which such changes occur in young persons, particularly in the cartilages of the first three ribs. For such a condition Freund's operation (of resection) would be indicated.

Of other etiological factors *occupation* is the most important. The disease is met with in players on wind instruments and in glass blowers, but by no means invariably, and in occupations necessitating heavy lifting or straining. Whooping cough and bronchitis play a rôle, not so much from changes induced in the bronchi as from the prolonged attacks of coughing.

Morbid Anatomy.—The thorax is capacious, usually barrel-shaped, and the cartilages are calcified. On removal of the sternum, the anterior mediastinum is completely occupied by the margins of the lungs, and the pericardial sac may not be visible. The organs are very large and have lost their elasticity, so that they do not collapse in the thorax or on the table. The pleura is pale and there is often an absence of pigment, sometimes in patches, termed by Virchow *albinism* of the lung. To the touch they have a peculiar, downy, feathery feel, and pit readily on pressure. This is one of the most marked features. Beneath the pleura greatly enlarged air vesicles may be readily seen. They vary in size from .5 to 3 mm., and irregular bullae, the size of a walnut or larger, may project from the free margins. The best idea of the extreme rarefaction of the tissue is obtained from sections of a lung distended and dried. At the anterior margins the structure may form an irregular series of air chambers, resembling the frog's lung. On careful inspection, remnants of the interlobular septa or the alveoli may be seen on these emphysematous vesicles. Though general, the distention is more marked, as a rule, at the anterior margins, and is often specially marked at the inner surface of the lobe near the root, where in extreme cases air-spaces as large as a hen's egg may sometimes be found. Microscopically there is atrophy of the alveolar walls, with a coalescence of neighboring air cells. In this process the capillary network disappears before the walls are completely atrophied. The loss of the elastic tissue is a special feature. In certain cases there may be a congenital defect in this tissue. The epithelium of the air cells undergoes a fatty change, but the distended air-spaces retain a pavement layer.

The *bronchi* show important changes. In the larger tubes the mucous membrane may be rough and thickened from chronic bronchitis; often the longitudinal lines of submucous elastic tissue stand out prominently. In the advanced cases many of the smaller tubes are dilated, particularly when, in addition to emphysema, there are peribronchial fibroid changes. Bronchiectasis is not an invariable accompaniment of emphysema, but, as Laënnec remarks, it is difficult to understand why it is not more common. Of associated morbid changes the most important are found in the *heart.* The right chambers may be dilated and hypertrophied, the tricuspid orifice large, and the valve segments are often thickened at the edges. In advanced cases the cardiac hypertrophy is general. The pulmonary artery and its branches may be wide and show marked atheromatous changes. *Pneumothorax* may follow the rupture of an emphysematous bleb.

Symptoms.—The disease may be tolerably advanced before any special symptoms occur. A child may be somewhat short of breath on going upstairs or be unable to run and play as other children without great discomfort; or, perhaps, has attacks of slight lividity. Doubtless much depends upon the completeness of cardiac compensation. When this is perfect, there may be no special interruption of the pulmonary circulation and, except with violent exertion, there is no interference with the aëration of the blood. In well-marked cases the following are the most important symptoms: *Dyspnea,* which may be felt only on slight exertion, or may be persistent, and aggravated by intercurrent attacks of bronchitis. The respirations are often harsh and wheezy, and expiration is distinctly prolonged. The vital capacity is usually greatly reduced. The dyspnea may be marked with very slight exertion or even on speaking, especially rapidly.

Cyanosis of an extreme grade is more common in emphysema than in other affections with the exception of congenital heart disease. It is one of the few diseases in which a patient may be able to go about with a lividity of startling intensity. The contrast between the extreme cyanosis and the comparative comfort of the patient is very striking. In other affections of the heart and lungs with a similar degree of cyanosis the patient is invariably in bed and usually in a state of orthopnea. One condition must be referred to, viz., the extraordinary cyanosis in cases of poisoning by aniline products, which is in most part due to the conversion of the hemoglobin into methemoglobin.

Bronchitis with associated cough is frequent and often the direct cause of the distress. The contrast between emphysematous patients in the winter and summer is marked in this respect. In the latter they may be comfortable and able to keep at work, but with the cold and changeable weather they are laid up with bronchitis. Finally the two conditions become inseparable and the patient has persistently more or less cough. The acute bronchitis may produce attacks not unlike asthma. In some instances this is true asthma, with which emphysema is frequently associated.

As age advances, and with successive attacks of bronchitis, the condition grows slowly worse. In old persons the dyspnea may begin at once on exertion and subside as quickly with rest. The dyspnea in such cases is often regarded as due to cardiac disease. The affection can generally be told at a glance—the rounded shoulders, barrel chest, the thin yet oftentimes muscular form, and sometimes a characteristic facial expression. There is another group of patients from twenty-five to forty years of age who, winter after winter, have attacks of intense cyanosis in consequence of an aggravated bronchitis. These patients may have been subject to dyspnea from infancy, due probably to a primary defect of structure in the lung tissue.

PHYSICAL SIGNS.—*Inspection.*—The thorax is markedly altered in shape; the anteroposterior diameter is increased and may be even greater than the lateral, so that the chest is barrel-shaped. The appearance is somewhat as if the chest was in a permanent inspiratory position. The sternum and costal cartilages are prominent. The lower zone of the thorax looks large and the intercostal spaces are much widened, particularly in the hypochondriac regions. The sternal fossa is deep, the clavicles stand out with great prominence, and the neck looks shortened from the elevation of the thorax and the sternum. A zone of dilated venules may be seen along the line of attachment of the diaphragm. Though this is common in emphysema, it is by no means peculiar to it or indeed to any special affection.

The curve of the spine is increased and the back is rounded, so that the scapulae seem to be almost horizontal. Mensuration shows the rounded form of the chest and the very slight expansion on deep inspiration. The respiratory movements, which may look energetic and forcible, exercise little or no influence. The chest does not expand but there is a general elevation. The inspiratory effort is short and quick; the expiratory movement is prolonged. There may be retraction instead of distention in the upper abdominal region during inspiration, and a transverse curve crossing the abdomen at the level of the twelfth rib is sometimes seen. The apex beat of the heart is not visible, and there is usually marked pulsation in the epigastric region. The cervical veins stand out prominently and may pulsate.

Palpation.—The vocal fremitus is somewhat enfeebled but not lost. The apex beat can rarely be felt. *Percussion* gives greatly increased resonance, full and drum-like—hyperresonance. The note may have a tympanitic quality. There may be marked variations in the note in local areas at different times especially in the lower backs. The area of resonance is greatly extended, the heart dulness may be obliterated, the upper limit of liver dulness is lowered, and the resonance may extend to the costal margin. Behind, a clear percussion note extends to a much lower level than normal. The level of splenic dulness may be lowered.

On *auscultation* the breath sounds are usually enfeebled; with bronchitis they may be harsh or masked by bronchitic râles. There may be prolongation of expiration, and the normal ratio may be reversed. It is often wheezy and harsh and associated with coarse and sibilant râles. It is said that in interstitial emphysema there may be a friction sound heard, not unlike that of pleurisy. The heart sounds are usually feeble but clear; in advanced cases, when there is marked cyanosis, a tricuspid regurgitant murmur may be heard. Accentuation of the pulmonary second sound may be present.

Course.—This is slow but progressive, the recurring attacks of bronchitis aggravating the condition. Death may occur from intercurrent pneumonia and dropsy may supervene from cardiac failure. Occasionally death results from cardiac failure, with extreme cyanosis. Pneumothorax may occur. Duckworth called attention to occasional fatal hemorrhage in emphysema.

Treatment.—The measures mentioned in connection with bronchitis should be employed. In children with asthma and emphysema the nose should be carefully examined. No remedy has any influence over the progress of the condition itself. Bronchitis is the great danger for these patients, and therefore when possible they should live in an equable climate. They do well in southern California and in Egypt. In consequence of the venous engorgement they are subject to gastric and intestinal disturbance, and it is particularly important to keep the bowels regulated and avoid flatulency, which often seriously aggravates the dyspnea. Patients who come into the hospital in a state of urgent dyspnea and lividity, with great engorgement of the veins, should be bled. Inhalation of oxygen may be used. Epinephrine hypodermically (♏ xv, 1 cc.) may give relief. Strychnine will be found useful. In children, with insufficiency of expiration and the lower edge of the lungs below the usual level, pressure on the lower ribs may correct this. Breathing exercises to aid expiration are helpful. Breathing of compressed air in a pneumatic cabinet gives temporary relief. Resection of the first costal cartilage or of the first three cartilages has been practised (Freund's operation). It is not likely to be of benefit in the aged in whom the condition is established, but in a special group in the young in which the primary trouble appears to be in the cartilages good results may follow.

ATROPHIC EMPHYSEMA

A senile change, called by Sir William Jenner small-lunged emphysema, is really a primary atrophy of the lung, coming on in advanced life, and scarcely constitutes a special affection. It occurs in old persons who may have had a winter cough and shortness of breath for years. In contrast to the essential hypertrophic emphysema, the chest is small and the ribs obliquely placed. The thoracic muscles are usually atrophied. The lung is converted into a series of large vesicles, on the walls of which the remnants of air cells may be seen. The *treatment* is largely of associated bronchitis or heart disease.

ACUTE VESICULAR EMPHYSEMA

When death occurs from bronchitis of the smaller tubes or diffuse bronchopneumonia, when strong inspiratory efforts have been made, the lungs are large in volume and the air cells much distended. Clinically, this condition may occur rapidly in cardiac dyspnea. The area of pulmonary resonance is much increased; piping râles and prolonged expiration are heard everywhere. A similar condition may follow pressure on the vagi.

INTERSTITIAL EMPHYSEMA

This may result from trauma, penetrating wounds, and violent coughing as in pneumonia or influenza. Beads of air are seen in the interlobular and subpleural tissue, sometimes forming large bullae beneath the pleura. If rupture occurs close to the root of the lung, the air passes along the trachea into the subcutaneous tissues of the neck. The *diagnosis* is made by the finding of subcutaneous air in the neck. It is usually quickly absorbed. Sedatives should be given if necessary. After tracheotomy the reverse may occur and the air may pass from the tracheotomy wound along the windpipe and bronchi and appear beneath the surface of the pleura. From interstitial emphysema spontaneous pneumothorax may arise in healthy persons.

COLLAPSE OF THE LUNG

Congenital.—This occurs in stillborn and weak infants, due to weakness of the muscles, obstruction of the trachea and bronchi, or syphilis. The lungs are unexpanded and solid if the condition is total; if partial there are areas containing air. The condition is chiefly of pathological interest.

Acquired.—Collapse of an air-containing lung may be of two kinds: (1) active, in which some disturbance of the respiratory mechanism occurs, and (2) passive, in which pressure from without, as from pleural effusion, pneumothorax, or obstruction of a bronchus is responsible.

Active collapse (massive collapse) occurs after operations, especially on the abdomen, injuries to the chest, trunk and pelvis, gunshot wounds of the chest (not necessarily on the injured side), with occlusion of a bronchus, allergic reactions (?) and after some acute infections, as diphtheria, in which paralysis of the diaphragm occurs. The explanation is not always evident. Paralysis of the diaphragm is suggested; also that the costal part of the diaphragm does not contract, with a tendency to lack of expansion of the lower lobes. Bronchial spasm due to reflex irritation from other parts is suggested. The cough reflex may be inhibited. In marked cases the heart is displaced to the affected side and the other lung is voluminous. The collapse may involve one lobe (usually a lower one), a portion of a lobe, or the whole lung. A plug of mucus or secretion, or a foreign body, completely closing a bronchus is one cause, the mechanism of which is clear but not all cases are due to this.

The *symptoms* appear usually within 24 hours of the operation or injury, but may be delayed for some days. The onset is sudden with severe dyspnea, cyanosis and prostration. There may be pain, usually in the lower thorax. There is cough which depends somewhat on associated bronchitis or pneumonia. There is usually fever with increase in the pulse and respiration rate. In milder attacks the symptoms may not be marked. There is decreased expansion on the affected side, to which the trachea and heart are displaced, and increased movement on the sound side. The costal movement is absent or reversed on the affected side. Vocal fremitus is variable; the percussion note may be dull but is often tympanitic; the breath sounds are usually bronchial or tubular but may be distant; râles are not constant but are numerous as the lung expands. The voice sounds are usually exaggerated but may be absent. The X-ray shows a dense shadow over the affected area with the diaphragm high and immobile and the trachea and heart displaced. Bronchitis, pneumonia or pleurisy may follow and influence the signs.

The *diagnosis* may be difficult, especially from lobar pneumonia; the displacement of the heart *toward* the affected side in collapse is most important.

In pneumothorax and pleural effusion the heart is displaced *away* from the affected side. The distention of the sound side may suggest pneumothorax at first but a thorough study should prevent error. From pulmonary embolism, the bloody sputum and absence of marked cardiac displacement should aid. The presence of a foreign body should be excluded. Bronchoscopy should be done to exclude bronchial obstruction due to secretion.

In *treatment,* change in position after operation or injury and collapse, and encouraging the patient to take deep breaths help in prevention. When collapse has occurred the patient should be turned on the normal side and encouraged to cough. Morphine and atropine should be given to control pain and distress. Strychnine in full doses hypodermically is useful (gr. 1/20, 0.003 gm., every 2 or 3 hours). Active stimulation should be given if there is collapse (digitalis, caffeine). Inhalation of oxygen may be of great value. In cases in which the signs suggest obstruction of a bronchus, bronchoscopy should be done. The removal of a plug of mucus in a bronchus results in prompt improvement.

Passive collapse may be general or local and in mild forms is very common. Pleural effusion, pneumothorax, pressure of an aneurism or a foreign body in a bronchus may cause collapse of a large area. Dorsal decubitus and abdominal distention cause collapse at the bases. Small areas of collapse occur with severe bronchitis, bronchopneumonia, etc.

The symptoms are so mixed with those of the causal condition that a definite description is not possible. Tympany may be marked, as above a pleural effusion. In the cases due to outside pressure, as aneurism, or a foreign body the vocal fremitus and breath sounds are decreased and the percussion note is dull. With incomplete collapse, dulness and many crackling râles are found. The course depends on the causal condition; a collapsed lung may expand again after a long period of collapse but there is always danger of fibroid change. The diagnosis rarely offers difficulty; the X-ray study is of great help.

The *treatment* is that of the original condition. Much may be done to prevent lower lobe collapse in a long illness by change in position and encouragement of deep breathing.

GANGRENE OF THE LUNG

Etiology.—Gangrene of the lung is not an affection *per se,* but occurs in a variety of conditions when necrotic areas undergo putrefaction. It is not easy to say why gangrene should occur in one case and not in another, as the germs of putrefaction are always in the air passages, and yet necrotic territories rarely become gangrenous. Total obstruction of a pulmonary artery, as a rule, causes infarction, and the area shut off does not often, though it may, slough. Another factor seems to be necessary—probably a lowered tissue resistance, the result of general or local causes. Spirochetes and fusiform bacilli from the mouth or pharyngeal infection may be responsible. It is met with (1) as a sequence of lobar pneumonia. This rarely occurs in a previously healthy person—more commonly in the debilitated or diabetic subject. (2) Gangrene is very prone to follow aspiration pneumonia, since the foreign particles rapidly undergo putrefactive changes. Of a similar nature are the cases of gangrene due to perforation of cancer of the esophagus into the lung or into a bronchus. (3) The putrid contents of a bronchiectatic, more commonly of a tuberculous, cavity may excite gangrene in the neighboring tissues. The pressure bronchiectasis following aneurism or tumor may lead to extensive sloughing. (4) Gangrene may follow simple embolism of the pulmonary artery. More commonly, the embolus is derived from a part which is mortified or comes from a focus of bone disease. (5) Gangrene may occur in conditions of debility during convalescence from protracted fever—occasionally without our being able to assign any reasonable cause.

Morbid Anatomy.—Laënnec, who first accurately described pulmonary gangrene, recognized a diffuse and a circumscribed form. The former, though rare, is sometimes seen with pneumonia, more rarely after obliteration of a large branch of the pulmonary artery. It may involve the greater part of a lobe, and the lung tissue is converted into a horribly offensive greenish-black mass, torn and ragged in the centre. In the *circumscribed* form there is well-marked limitation between the gangrenous area and the surrounding tissue. The focus may be single or multiple. The lower lobe is more commonly affected than the upper, and the peripheral more than the central portion of the lung. A gangrenous area is at first uniformly greenish brown in color; but softening rapidly takes place with the formation of a cavity with shreddy, irregular walls and a greenish, offensive fluid. The lung tissue in the immediate neighborhood shows a zone of deep congestion, often consolidation, and outside this an intense edema. In the embolic cases the plugged artery can sometimes be found. When rapidly extending, vessels may be opened and a copious hemorrhage ensue. Perforation of the pleura is not uncommon. The decomposing material usually excites an intense bronchitis. Embolic processes are not infrequent. There is a remarkable association in some cases between gangrene of the lung and abscess of the brain.

Symptoms and Course.—Usually definite symptoms of local pulmonary disease precede the characteristic features of gangrene. These are very varied, depending on the primary disease. The sputum is very characteristic. It is intensely fetid—usually profuse—and, if expectorated into a conical glass, separates into three layers—a greenish brown, heavy sediment; an intervening thin liquid, which sometimes has a greenish or a brownish tint; and, on top, a thick, frothy layer. Spread on a glass plate, the shreddy *débris* of lung tissue can readily be picked out. Even large fragments of lung may be coughed up. Robertson, of Onancock, Va., sent one several centimetres in length, which had been expectorated by a lad of eighteen, who had severe gangrene and recovered. Elastic fibres are usually found with granular matter, pigment grains, fatty crystals, bacteria, and leptothrix. The peculiar plugs of sputum which occur in bronchiectasis are not found. Blood is often present, and, as a rule, is much altered. The sputum has, in a majority of the cases, an intensely fetid odor, which may permeate the entire room. It is much more offensive than in fetid bronchitis or abscess of the lung. The fetor is particularly marked when there is free communication between the gangrenous cavities and the bronchi. Localized gangrene, unsuspected during life and without fetor of the breath, may be found postmortem.

The physical signs, when extensive destruction has occurred, are those of cavity, but the limited circumscribed areas may be difficult to detect. Bronchitis is always present. The X-ray examination aids in diagnosis.

Among the general symptoms may be mentioned fever, usually of moderate grade; the pulse is rapid, and very often the constitutional depression is severe. But the only special features indicative of gangrene are the sputum and the fetor of the breath. The patient generally sinks from exhaustion. Fatal hemorrhage may ensue.

Treatment.—This is very unsatisfactory. Postural drainage should be tried if possible. An antiseptic spray of weak phenol solution may be employed. If the patient's condition is good and the gangrenous region can be localized, surgical interference is indicated. With the possibility that spirochetal infection may be important etiologically, the use of neoarsphenamine (0.3-0.5 gm.) intravenously is advisable.

ABSCESS OF THE LUNG

Etiology.—Suppuration occurs in the lung under the following conditions: (1) As a sequence of inflammation, either lobar or lobular. In lobar pneumonia the abscesses are of small size and usually involve, as Addison remarked, several points at the same time. Abscess formation is frequent in the deglutition and aspiration forms of bronchopneumonia. (2) After wounds of the neck or operations upon the throat, particularly the tonsils, and tooth extraction; in suppurative disease of the nose or larynx, occasionally of the ear, infective particles reach the bronchi and excite inflammation which may end in abscess. Abscess of the lung after *tonsillectomy* occurs with alarming frequency. Moore, as the result of a careful study, estimates its occurrence as one in 2500-3000 tonsillectomies, which is probably conservative. The abscess may follow inspiration or embolism; emboli lodge in the right lung more often than in the left. (3) Cancer of a bronchus or of the esophagus, perforating the root of the lung or the bronchi, may produce suppuration. (4) Embolic abscesses, the result of infective emboli, may be numerous and present very definite characters. As a rule they are superficial, beneath the pleura, and often wedge-shaped. The pleura is usually covered with greenish lymph, and perforation may occur with the production of pyopneumothorax. (5) Perforation of the lung from without, foreign bodies, and, in the right lung, perforation from subphrenic or liver abscess or a suppurating echinococcus cyst are occasional causes. (6) Suppurative processes play an important part in pulmonary tuberculosis. A study of 172 cases from various causes proved bronchoscopically at the Jefferson Hospital (Flick *et al.*, 1929) showed that the upper were involved more often than the lower lobes. In the pus a variety of organisms is found; anaerobic forms are frequent. Spirochetes and fungi (especially monilia) are common.

Pathology.—The abscess is usually single, except in the embolic cases, and is surrounded by an area of congested and edematous lung tissue. As rupture into a bronchus usually occurs early there is rarely much fibrosis about the abscess. The abscess increases in size by extension.

Symptoms.—If abscess occurs in the course of another disease, the symptoms are increased, with higher fever, perhaps chills, toxemia and cough. If the abscess forms, as after tonsillectomy, in a patient previously well, pain and cough are frequent with fever, sometimes chills, and perhaps dyspnea. Leukocytosis is the rule. The signs are often slight, depending on the size of the abscess and its relation to the surface. There are decreased expansion, dulness which may be slight, decreased vocal fremitus and breath sounds, without râles over the area but a few may be heard in adjoining areas. Often the first characteristic sign is the appearance of a large amount of foul pus when the abscess ruptures into a bronchus. If the patient is first seen after rupture the signs of cavity may be found and the sputum is of great aid in diagnosis. The odor is offensive, yet it rarely has the horrible fetor of gangrene or putrid bronchitis. Hemoptysis occurs fairly often. Fragments of lung tissue and elastic tissue with alveolar arrangement may be found. The presence of this with the physical signs and the X-ray study rarely leave any question as to the diagnosis. Embolic cases usually run a fatal course. Recovery occasionally occurs after pneumonia. In abscess following *tonsillectomy,* the symptoms usually appear within a week after operation but may be much later (five weeks). Pain, chills or chilly sensations, fever, cough and purulent sputum are the early features.

Diagnosis.—Before rupture, suspicion only may be possible unless the X-ray report is definite. After rupture, an *interlobar empyema* may be distinguished only by the absence of elastic fibres. In gangrene the odor of the breath and sputum is usually distinctive. In bronchiectasis, tuberculous cavity and fetid bronchitis, a thorough study of the sputum is important. In the diagnosis of a bronchial new growth with an abscess secondary to it, bronchoscopy is essential.

Treatment.—The patient should be in bed and nourished as well as possible. The essential point is to secure thorough drainage. Postural drainage should be carried out; the best method depends somewhat on the situation of the abscess and should be found for each patient. The X-ray picture is sometimes a guide as to the best position to favor drainage. With abscess of the lower lobe, if possible, the foot of the bed should be elevated and the patient lie without a pillow. The head should be lowered over the side of the bed during coughing. After the abscess has ruptured, bronchoscopic drainage with the injection of antiseptics, done by *skilful hands,* is most satisfactory. The earlier it is begun the better. Whenever possible this should be done; a general anesthetic is not required. When the abscess is well defined and superficial, an attempt may be made to open and drain it. Operation is not advisable early and is most useful in chronic cases. Artificial pneumothorax is not advised as it often interferes with drainage. Thoracoplasty may be done for a chronic abscess if other measures fail. As many abscesses contain spirochetes, neoarsphenamine may be given intravenously. It is difficult to judge as to the value of this.

NEW GROWTHS OF THE LUNGS AND BRONCHI

Primary tumors of the bronchi and lungs appear to be increasing in frequency. In perhaps 85 per cent of cases the primary growth is in a bronchus; later it may involve the lung tissue. Secondary neoplasm in the lung is common, especially from neoplasm of the kidney.

Etiology.—There is no clear explanation of the increase in these or of reasons for it. Irritation of the bronchial mucous membrane by gases or tar is suggested. In the workers in the Schneeberg and Joachimstal mines there is a high incidence, perhaps due to radioactive material in these mines. As to age it is well to recognize that it may occur in young adults.

Pathology.—Sarcoma is very rare. Benign tumors, as adenoma, occur in the bronchi. Carcinoma usually begins in the wall of a bronchus, as a rule of some size. There has been much discussion as to the histological characters of the tumors. Those from the mucous glands may show the same character in the metastases, as in the brain. The tumors tend to extend by continuity and metastases are common, most often to the pleura.

Symptoms.—The *onset* is usually insidious and in a surprisingly large number of cases the patient comes on account of symptoms due to a *metastasis.* This is often in the nervous system or spinal cord and metastatic brain tumors have been operated upon. The early symptoms are usually *pain* and *cough* with little sputum, which may be blood stained. Dyspnea and hemoptysis may follow. These features are usually persistent. Loss of weight and strength with anemia follow later; fever occurs in some cases. There may be a pleural effusion or, if the growth causes much obstruction, infection below it with purulent sputum. The *physical signs* in the early stages are those of obstruction and evidently vary with the degree of this, as with a foreign body in a bronchus. There can be no set picture but as a rule the signs of obstruction increase steadily. As the growth increases, invades the lung and involves the lymph glands, the local signs are more marked. There may be marked dulness. With definite obstruction, the signs in the lung supplied are marked and vary with the amount of drainage. In the later stages fever is usually present. The supraclavicular and axillary glands may be enlarged.

The *benign tumors* (fibromata and adenomata) are rare. They cause bronchial obstruction, often with bronchiectasis, and in some cases can be removed through the bronchoscope.

Diagnosis.—The only hope for these patients lies in early diagnosis. As cough is an important early symptom, we should endeavor to be much more persevering and alert in making an exact diagnosis of the cause of persistent cough. Careful study soon excludes any general cause, such as bronchitis, and a short period of observation and study should exclude tuberculosis, the diagnosis often made in bronchial neoplasms. The possibility of neoplasm should be kept in mind. The symptoms and signs ought to excite suspicion. The *bronchoscopic* study is essential and should be done early. By it the presence of a growth is proved and a portion of tissue can usually be removed for examination. The X-ray study may show bronchial obstruction and also extension of the growth. It is evident that many pulmonary and bronchial conditions may give difficulty. Consideration of the possibility of neoplasm is a great safeguard. With a pleural effusion or signs of metastases most prominent, the diagnosis may be very difficult.

Treatment.—In a few cases the growth has been removed through the bronchoscope. With early diagnosis and the advances in lung surgery we may hope that some may be saved by operation. Otherwise intensive X-ray treatment is indicated; it often prolongs life and lessens discomfort. Radium therapy does not seem to be as effective.

New Growths of the Lung Parenchyma.—Primary growths are rare; extension may occur from a bronchial neoplasm. The early symptoms are not distinctive and definite signs may be late. With increase in size, diminished expansion, dulness and altered breath sounds are found. The X-ray study is the most important aid in diagnosis. In *treatment*, early diagnosis and surgical removal offer the only chance. X-ray therapy should be used otherwise.

Mediastinum.—Quite early the glands become involved, increase rapidly, compress the adjoining structure and the picture is that of a mediastinal tumor with its dominant pressure symptoms.

CYSTS OF THE LUNG

Dermoid Cyst.—This may give no symptoms or gradually increase in size and cause symptoms by pressure. They may become infected. Rupture into a bronchus may occur. The symptoms are variable depending on the size and situation of the cyst. The *diagnosis* is usually difficult and made by the X-ray study. If treatment is required this must be surgical.

Congenital Air Cyst.—In 1934, Wood found 122 cases reported. The etiology is obscure. There are two forms. (1) The *solitary cyst* (or multiple large cyst). This is usually large, and may give severe symptoms in early life. There are attacks of dyspnea and cyanosis without any evident cause. Signs suggesting pneumothorax may be found. The X-ray study shows a large air sac which may replace a lobe or the whole lung, and simulate pneumothorax. Studies after the injection of iodized oil may be useful. Progressive dyspnea in adults without evident cause is suggestive. The heart is displaced away from the lesion. (2) *Multiple small cysts* of the lung, honeycomb type. The number varies and the symptoms are not marked unless they largely replace the lung tissue. They are not recognized as a rule until late childhood or adult life. In *diagnosis*, the bronchoscopic and X-ray study is important. In *treatment* of a large cyst, puncture may be done. The injection of iodized oil has been useful. With increased pressure, aspiration or permanent drainage may be done.

DISEASES OF THE PLEURA

ACUTE PLEURISY

Anatomically, the cases may be divided into dry or adhesive pleurisy and pleurisy with effusion. Another classification is into primary or secondary forms. According to the course, a division may be made into *acute* and *chronic pleurisy*, and this is perhaps the most satisfactory.

FIBRINOUS OR PLASTIC PLEURISY

In this the pleural membrane is covered by a sheeting of lymph of variable thickness, which gives it a turbid, granular appearance, or the fibrin may exist in distinct layers. It occurs (1) as an apparently primary affection, following cold or exposure but there is always infection from some source. It may be secondary to acute throat infection; tuberculosis has always to be considered unless another cause is evident. Cases occur in which the disease sets in with the usual symptoms of pain in the side and slight fever with the physical signs of fibrinous pleurisy. After a few days, the friction rub disappears and no exudation occurs. Union takes place between the membranes and possibly the pleuritic adhesions found so often postmortem originate in these slight fibrinous pleurisies.

(2) Fibrinous pleurisy occurs as a *secondary* process in acute diseases of the lung, such as pneumonia, which is always accompanied by a certain amount of pleurisy, usually of this form. Cancer, abscess, infarction and gangrene also cause plastic pleurisy when the surface of the lung becomes involved. It is especially associated in a large number of cases with tuberculosis.

Symptoms.—The onset is usually sudden but may be preceded by malaise. There is *pain* which may be severe and aggravated by cough or a deep breath. It is generally in the lower thorax. Cough occurs and is without sputum. There is usually slight fever but occasionally it is high. There is less expansion on the affected side; vocal fremitus shows little change; the friction may be felt; there may be slight dulness. On auscultation, the breath sounds are usually less well heard than normally, probably due largely to the diminished movement, and a friction rub is heard which varies greatly in character and loudness. There may be very fine crackling râles heard at the end of inspiration and it is often difficult to decide whether they are produced in the lung or pleura. The typical rub is a creaking, rough sound heard with inspiration and sometimes with expiration. It may be heard over a small or large area. A deep breath or a change in position may increase the rub. If on the left side there may be also a pleuropericardial friction rub. Pleurisy in the interlobar areas and of the mediastinal pleura does not give definite signs. The X-ray study may aid in their recognition.

The *course* is variable. The rub and the fever may disappear in a few days or the process may go on to effusion. Slight adhesions probably form in most cases and there may be discomfort or slight pain for some months.

Diagnosis.—This may be very easy or difficult. The general appearance with the "catch" on taking a deep breath is significant. There is no doubt if a definite rub is heard. In some cases with very fine râles the diagnosis lies between a lung condition and pleurisy. The X-ray study may aid in this. That convenient diagnosis, "intercostal neuralgia" should be made with great hesitation. It is probably a very rare condition. The root pains of spondylitis should not cause error, nor those due to aneurism or tumor. An effort should always be made to decide the cause of the pleurisy and tuberculosis should be proved or excluded.

SEROFIBRINOUS PLEURISY

In a majority of cases there is, with the fibrin, a variable amount of fluid exudate, which produces the condition known as pleurisy with effusion.

Etiology.—Of 194 cases in fifteen years in the Hopkins Hospital, there were 161 males and 33 females. Under twenty years of age there were 20 patients; 18 were over sixty years of age. The greatest number (59) was in the fifth decade. Cold acts as a predisposing agent, which permits the action of various micro-organisms. A majority of the cases are tuberculous. This view is based upon: (1) *Postmortem evidence.* Tubercles have been found in acute cases, thought to have been "rheumatic" or due to cold. (2) The not infrequent presence of *tuberculous lesions,* often latent, in the lung or elsewhere. (3) The character of the *exudate.* If coagulated and the coagulum digested and centrifugalized, tubercle bacilli may be found. Injected into a guinea-pig, in amounts of 15 cc. or more, tuberculosis followed in a large percentage. Cultures from the fluid may be positive for tubercle bacilli. The cytodiagnosis shows that as in other tuberculous exudates the mononuclear leukocytes predominate. (4) The *tuberculin* reaction is positive in a considerable percentage of the cases. (5) The subsequent history. Of 90 cases of acute pleurisy under the observation of H. I. Bowditch between 1849 and 1879, 32 died of or had pulmonary tuberculosis. Hamman collected 562 cases in which the subsequent history was sought; of these 167, 29.7 per cent became tuberculous. Serous effusion may occur with infectious diseases, *e.g.* typhoid fever, lobar pneumonia, septicemia and scarlet fever. Other conditions are new growth of a bronchus, lung or pleura, pulmonary infarcts and trauma of the thorax.

Bacteriology.—The tubercle bacillus is present in a large proportion of all cases of primary or so-called idiopathic pleurisy. A large amount of the exudate must be taken to make the test of animal inoculation complete. Eichhorst found that 62 per cent were demonstrated as tuberculous when 15 cc. of the exudate were inoculated into test animals, while less than 10 per cent showed tuberculosis when only 1 cc. of the exudate was used. The newer methods make the results of cultures for the tubercle bacillus much more often positive.

The *pneumococcus* pleurisy is almost always secondary to a focus of inflammation in the lung but may be primary. The exudate is usually purulent and the outlook is favorable. The *streptococcus* pleurisy may occur from direct infection of the pleura through the lung in streptococcus pneumonia; in other instances it follows infection of more distant parts. Acute streptococcus pleurisy is the most serious of all forms. Among other bacteria are the staphylococcus, Friedländer's bacillus, the typhoid bacillus, and the diphtheria bacillus.

Morbid Anatomy.—The serous exudate is abundant and fibrin is found on the pleural surfaces and scattered through the fluid in the form of flocculi. The proportions of these constituents vary a great deal. In some instances there is very little membranous fibrin; in others it forms thick, creamy layers and exists in the dependent part of the fluid as whitish, curd-like masses. The fluid is of a lemon color, either clear or slightly turbid, depending on the number of formed elements. In some instances it has a dark brown color. The microscopic examination shows leukocytes, occasional swollen cells, which may be derived from the pleural endothelium, shreds of fibrillated fibrin, and a variable number of red blood cells. Some exudates contain large numbers of eosinophiles. A large number of cells undergoing mitotic division is diagnostic of malignant disease. The fluid is rich in albumin and sometimes coagulates spontaneously. Its composition closely resembles that of blood serum. Cholesterin, uric acid, and sugar are occasionally found. The amount of the effusion varies from ½ to 5 litres. Enormous amounts are sometimes removed, 188 ounces in one case (E. C. Carter). The *lung* is more or less compressed. If the exudation is limited the lower lobe alone is collapsed; but in an extensive effusion the entire lung is close to the spine, dark and airless, or even bloodless—*i. e.*, carnified.

In large exudations the adjacent organs are displaced; the liver is depressed and the heart dislocated. With reference to the position of the heart, the following statements may be made: (1) Even in the most extensive left sided exudation there is no rotation of the apex of the heart, which in no case was to the right of the midsternal line; (2) the relative position of the apex and base is usually maintained; in some instances the apex is lifted, in others the whole heart lies more transversely; (3) the right chambers of the heart occupy the greater portion of the front, so that the displacement is rather a definite dislocation of the mediastinum, with the pericardium, to the right, than any special twisting of the heart itself; (4) the kink or twist in the inferior vena cava described by Bartels may be present.

Symptoms.—Prodromes are not uncommon, but the disease may set in abruptly with a chill, followed by fever and a severe pain in the side. In very many cases, however, the onset is insidious, particularly in children and in elderly persons. Slight dyspnea on exertion and an increasing pallor may be the only features. Washbourn called attention to the frequency with which the pneumococcus pleurisy sets in with the features of pneumonia. The *pain* is the most distressing symptom, and is usually referred to the nipple or axillary regions. It must be remembered that pleuritic pain may be felt in the abdomen or low down in the back, particularly when the diaphragmatic surface of the pleura is involved. It is lancinating, sharp, and severe, and is aggravated by cough. At this early stage, on auscultation, sometimes indeed on palpation, a dry friction rub can be detected. The fever rarely rises so rapidly as in pneumonia, and does not reach the same grade. A temperature of from 102° to 103° F. is an average pyrexia. It may drop to normal at the end of a week or ten days without any definite change in the physical signs, or may persist for several weeks. *Cough* is an early symptom but is rarely so distressing or frequent as in pneumonia. There are instances in which it is absent. The expectoration is usually slight in amount, mucoid, and occasionally streaked with blood.

At the outset there may be *dyspnea,* due partly to the fever and partly to the pain. Later it results from the compression of the lung, particularly if the exudation has taken place rapidly and in cases with very rapid effusion the dyspnea may be marked. When, however, the fluid is effused slowly, one lung may be entirely compressed without inducing shortness of breath, except on exertion, and the patient will lie quietly in bed without evincing the slightest respiratory distress. When the effusion is large the patient usually prefers to lie upon the affected side.

Physical Signs.—Inspection shows some degree of immobility on the affected side, depending upon the amount of exudation and in large effusions an increase in volume, which may appear to be much more than it really is as determined by mensuration. The intercostal depressions are obliterated. In right sided effusions the apex beat may be lifted to the fourth interspace, be pushed beyond the left nipple, or even seen in the axilla. When the exudation is on the left side, the heart impulse may not be visible; but if the effusion is large it is seen in the third and fourth spaces on the right side, and sometimes as far out as the nipple, or even beyond it. In massive effusion on the left side there may be a prominence below the left costal margin.

Palpation enables us to determine the deficient movements on the affected side, the obliteration of the intercostal spaces, and the position of the heart's impulse. In simple serofibrinous effusion there is rarely any edema of the chest walls. It is scarcely ever possible to obtain fluctuation. Tactile fremitus is greatly diminished or abolished. If the effusion is slight there may be only enfeeblement. The absence of the voice vibrations in effusions of any size is a valuable sign. In children and occasionally in adults there may be much effusion with retention of fremitus. In very rare cases the vibrations may be communicated through localized pleural adhesions. Pitfield has described a useful sign which consists in the transmission of vibrations, when percussion is done over the fluid, to the lumbar muscles on the same side. It is present even with small amounts of fluid.

Mensuration.—A difference of half an inch to an inch, or even, in large effusions, an inch and a half, may be found between the two sides.

Percussion.—Early there may be no alteration, but with the accumulation of fluid the resonance becomes defective, and finally gives place to flatness. From day to day the gradual increase in height of the fluid may be studied. In a pleuritic effusion rising to the fourth rib in front the percussion signs are usually very suggestive. Above the fluid the note is often tympanitic (Skodaic resonance), most marked in front. It shades into a flat note in the lower mammary and axillary regions. The dulness has a peculiar wooden quality and the *resistance* is marked, especially on direct percussion, differing from that of pneumonia and readily recognized by skilled fingers. When the patient is in the erect posture the upper line of dulness is not horizontal, but is higher behind than in front. The curve marking the intersection of the plane of contact of lung and fluid with the chest wall is known as "Ellis's line" which Garland verified clinically and by animal experiments. With medium-sized effusions this line begins lowest behind, advances upward and forward in a letter-S curve to the axillary region, whence it proceeds in a straight decline to the sternum. This curve is demonstrable only when the patient is in the erect position. Grocco, in 1902, called attention to the existence of a triangular area of relative dulness, along the spine, on the side opposite to the pleurisy, in width from 2 to 5 cm., and with the apex upward. It can be demonstrated in a large majority of all cases, particularly in young and thin persons. It is probably due to bulging of the mediastinum, by the fluid, across the middle line.

On the right side the dulness passes without change into that of the liver. On the left side it may obliterate Traube's semilunar space. If the effusion is moderate, *movable dulness* may be obtained by marking carefully, in the sitting posture, the upper limit in the mammary region, and then in the recumbent position, noting the change in the height of dulness. This sign can not always be obtained. In very copious exudation the dulness may reach the clavicle and even extend beyond the sternal margin of the opposite side.

Auscultation.—A friction rub may be heard early, which disappears as the fluid accumulates. With even a slight exudation there is weakened or distant breathing. Often the breath sounds are audible, though distant, and have a tubular quality. Sometimes only a puffing tubular expiration is heard, which may have a metallic or amphoric quality. Loud resonant râles accompanying this may suggest a cavity. These pseudocavernous signs are most frequent in children and lead to error. Above the dulness the breath sounds are usually harsh and exaggerated, and may have a tubular quality with variable râles. The vocal resonance is usually diminished or absent. The whispered voice is said to be transmitted through a serous and not through a purulent exudate (Baccelli's sign), but this is not always true. There may be bronchophony. The voice sometimes has a curious nasal, squeaking character, termed by Laënnec *egophony*, especially about the upper level of the fluid. In typical form this is not common, but there may be a curious twang-like quality of the voice, particularly at the outer angle of the scapula.

When the apex of the heart lies beneath the sternum there may be no impulse. The determination of the situation of the organ may rest with the position of maximum loudness of the sounds. A systolic murmur may be heard. There may be a pleuropericardial friction rub.

Blood Count.—Emerson studied 89 cases of acute pleurisy with effusion in which blood counts were made before the temperature reached normal and only 26 had a leukocytosis between 10,000 and 15,000; only one was above 15,000. In 12 cases the count was below 5,000.

The X-ray pictures are of much value in diagnosis. They show that the effusion is not always in the lower portion of the chest with the patient in the upright position, but that it may represent a vertical column in the lateral aspect of the chest, compressing the lung toward the spine. The effusion is not always mobile, but may be fixed by adhesions. In this event shifting dulness is not likely to be demonstrated.

Course.—This is very variable. After a week or ten days the fever subsides, the cough and pain disappear, and a slight effusion may be quickly absorbed. When the effusion reaches as high as the fourth rib recovery is usually slower. Many patients come under observation, after some weeks' illness, with the fluid up to the clavicle. The fever may last from ten to twenty days without exciting anxiety, though, as a rule, in ordinary pleurisy, the temperature in cases of moderate severity is normal within eight or ten days. Left to itself, the natural tendency is to resorption; but this may take place very slowly. With the absorption of the fluid there is a redux-friction crepitus, either leathery and creaking or crackling and râle-like, and for months, or even longer, defective resonance and feeble breathing are found at the base. Rare modes of termination are perforation and discharge through the lung, and externally through the chest wall.

The immediate *prognosis* in pleurisy with effusion is good. Of 320 cases at St. Bartholomew's Hospital, only 6.1 per cent died before leaving the hospital (Hedges). A serofibrinous exudate may persist for months, particularly in tuberculous cases, and sometimes reaccumulates after aspiration and resists all treatment. After persistence for more than twelve months, in spite of repeated tapping, a serous effusion was cured by incision without deformity of the chest (S. West). When one pleura is full and the heart is greatly dislocated, the condition, although in a majority of cases producing remarkably little disturbance, is not without risk. The ultimate outlook depends much on the cause.

PURULENT PLEURISY: EMPYEMA

Etiology.—Empyema is rarely primary and if so is usually due to the pneumococcus. It may be due to involvement from without, as in fracture of a rib, a penetrating wound or disease of the esophagus. It occurs with acute infectious diseases, especially pneumonia. In the majority it is due to infection from the lung, pneumonia especially, infarction, particularly infective, abscess, gangrene, tuberculosis, etc. It is common in children below the age of ten years. The pneumococcus is the most common organism, then the ordinary pus organisms and tubercle bacilli; in rare cases the influenza bacillus, spirochetes and streptothrix organisms have been found.

Morbid Anatomy.—On opening an empyema postmortem we usually find that the effusion has separated into a clear, greenish yellow serum above and thick, cream-like pus below. The fluid may be scarcely more than turbid, with flocculi of fibrin through it. In the pneumococcus empyema the pus is usually thick and creamy. It usually has a heavy, sweetish odor, but in some instances—particularly following wounds—it is fetid. In cases of gangrene the pus has a horribly stinking odor. The pleural membranes are greatly thickened. On the costal pleura there may be erosions, and in old cases fistulous communications are common. The lung may be compressed to a small area and the visceral pleura may show perforations.

Symptoms.—Purulent pleurisy may begin abruptly, with the symptoms already described. More frequently it comes on insidiously in the course of other diseases or follows a serofibrinous pleurisy. There may be no pain in the chest, very little cough, and no dyspnea, unless the amount is large. Symptoms of septic infection are rarely wanting. If in a child, there is gradually developing pallor and weakness; sweats occur with irregular fever. A cough is by no means constant. The leukocytes are usually much increased; in one fatal case they numbered 115,000.

Physical Signs.—Practically they are those of pleurisy with effusion but there are additional points to be mentioned. In empyema, particularly in children, the disproportion between the sides may be extreme. The intercostal spaces may not only be obliterated but may bulge. There may be edema of the chest walls. The subcutaneous veins may be very distinct. It must not be forgotten that in children the breath sounds may be *loud and tubular* over a purulent effusion of considerable size. The displacement of the heart and liver are more marked in empyema than in serous effusion.

A curious phenomenon associated generally with empyema, but sometimes occurring in the serofibrinous exudate, is *pulsating pleurisy*, first described by MacDonnell, Sr., of Montreal. In 95 cases collected by Sailer it was much more frequent in males than in females. In 38 there was a tumor; that is, *empyema necessitatis*. In all but one case the fluid was purulent. Pneumothorax may be present. There are two groups of cases, the intrapleural pulsating pleurisy and the pulsating *empyema necessitatis*, in which there is an external pulsating tumor. No satisfactory explanation has been offered how the heart impulse is thus forcibly communicated through the effusion.

Empyema is a chronic affection, which in a few instances terminates naturally in recovery, but a majority of cases, if left alone, ends in death. The following are some modes of natural cure: (*a*) By *absorption* of the fluid.

In small effusions this may take place gradually. The chest wall sinks. The pleural layers become greatly thickened and enclose between them the inspissated pus, in which lime salts are gradually deposited. (*b*) By *perforation* of the lung. Although in this event death may take place rapidly, by suffocation, as Aretaeus says, yet if it occurs gradually recovery may follow. Empyema may discharge by opening into the bronchus and forming a fistula, or by producing necrosis of the pulmonary pleura, sufficient to allow soaking of the pus through the spongy lung tissue into the bronchi. In the first way pneumothorax usually, though not always, develops. In the second way the pus is discharged, without formation of pneumothorax. Even with a bronchial fistula recovery is possible. (*c*) By *perforation* of the chest wall—*empyema necessitatis.* This is by no means unfavorable, as many cases recover. The perforation may occur anywhere in the chest wall, but is more common in front. It may be from the third to the sixth interspace, usually, according to Marshall, in the fifth. It may perforate in more than one place, and there may be a fistulous communication which opens into the pleura at some distance from the external orifice. The tumor, when near the heart, may pulsate. The discharge may persist for years. In Copeland's Dictionary is mention of a physician who had a pleural fistula for thirteen years and enjoyed fair health.

An empyema may perforate neighboring organs, the esophagus, peritoneum, pericardium, or the stomach. A remarkable sequel is a pleuro-esophageal fistula; in one case there was a fistulous communication through the chest wall. Some remarkable cases pass down the spine and along the psoas into the iliac fossa, and simulate a psoas or lumbar abscess.

Encapsulated Empyema.—In lobar or bronchopneumonia, pockets of pus from the size of an egg to an orange may form. A good many cases are with streptococcus empyema, and H. M. Thomas, Jr., called attention to the frequency of abdominal pain and meteorism, the early prostration, the high leukocytosis, and the danger of rupture into the pleura. The condition may be revealed only by the X-ray study.

OTHER VARIETIES OF PLEURISY

Hemorrhagic Pleurisy.—A bloody effusion is met with under the following conditions: (*a*) In the pleurisy of *asthenic states,* such as cancer, nephritis, and occasionally in the malignant fevers. It is interesting to note the frequency with which hemorrhagic pleurisy is found in cirrhosis of the liver. It occurred in the patient in whom Laënnec first accurately described this disease. While this may be a simple hemorrhagic pleursy, in a majority of the cases it is tuberculous. (*b*) *Tuberculous pleurisy,* in which the bloody effusion may result from the rupture of newly formed vessels in the soft exudate with the eruption of miliary tubercles, or it may come from more slowly formed tubercles in a pleurisy secondary to pulmonary disease. (*c*) *Cancerous pleurisy,* whether primary or secondary, is frequently hemorrhagic. (*d*) Occasionally hemorrhagic exudation is found in healthy individuals, with no sign of tuberculosis or cancer. In one such case, the patient was healthy eight years afterward. (*e*) During aspiration the lung may be wounded and blood be mixed with the serofibrinous exudate. The condition of hemorrhagic pleurisy is to be distinguished from hemothorax.

In *eosinophilic pleural effusion* a large percentage of eosinophiles is found in the fluid. The cause is obscure; it occurs with various conditions but tuberculosis is not common.

Cholesterol Pleurisy.—In this the pleural fluid is rich in cholesterol in crystalline form. Stein (1932) found 21 cases reported. Many of the patients have pulmonary tuberculosis or had previous pleural effusion. The diagnosis is made by finding the cholesterol crystals in the fluid.

Diaphragmatic Pleurisy.—The inflammation may be limited partly or chiefly to the diaphragmatic surface. A distressing cough is common but *pain* is usually the most prominent symptom, increased by cough or any movement; it may be referred to the shoulder or abdomen. The pleurisy is often dry but there may be effusion, either serofibrinous or purulent, which is circumscribed on the diaphragmatic surface. In these cases the pain may simulate that of acute abdominal disease. It may be intensified by pressure over the lower ribs, especially the tenth. A friction rub is often heard; if present it may be evident over a small area only. The lower lobe may show signs of collapse or congestion and fine râles may be heard over it which are difficult to distinguish from a friction rub. The diaphragm is fixed and the respiration is thoracic and short. Hiccough is common. Andral noted severe dyspnea and attacks simulating angina in some cases. The effusion is usually plastic, not serous. Serous or purulent effusions of any size limited to the diaphragmatic surface are extremely rare. Intense subjective with relatively less objective features are suggestive of diaphragmatic pleurisy. There may be marked hyperesthesia over the lower thorax and upper abdomen, with tenderness along the edge of the trapezius of the affected side. The X-ray study is of aid.

Encysted Pleurisy.—The effusion may be circumscribed by adhesions or separated into pockets or loculi, which communicate with each other. This is most common in empyema. In these cases there have usually been, at different parts of the pleura, multiple adhesions by which the fluid is limited. In other instances the recent membranes may encapsulate the exudation on the diaphragmatic surface or on the pleura posterior to the midaxillary line. In some cases the tactile fremitus is retained along lines of adhesion. The condition may be very puzzling and present difficulties in diagnosis. The exploratory needle should be freely used and the X-rays employed.

Interlobar pleurisy forms an interesting and not uncommon variety. In many instances of acute pleurisy the interlobar serous surfaces are involved and closely adherent; sometimes the fluid is encysted between them. These collections may perforate the bronchi, and the cases present special difficulties in diagnosis. The X-ray study is of great value.

Chylothorax.—This is a rare condition first described by Bartolet in 1633. E. H. Funk found only 54 cases of chylous effusion reported in 1918. Three forms of milk-like effusion occur; (1) chylous, (2) chyliform, and (3) pseudochylous. The cause of the *chylous* effusion is trauma, in which the thoracic duct is ruptured, or pressure, as by malignant growth, causing a backward flow along the pulmonary and pleural lymphatics. The fluid accumulates rapidly. The signs are those of an effusion and the diagnosis is made only by aspiration. The fluid is milky in appearance and contains fat in minute globules. The fat may be as high as 4 per cent. The specific gravity exceeds 1.012. The *chyliform* effusion is usually associated with tuberculosis or neoplasm and accumulates slowly. The milky appearance is regarded as due to fat liberated by the breaking down of leukocytes and endothelial cells which have undergone fatty degeneration. The *pseudochylous* fluid has a specific gravity below 1.012 and is poor in solids. It occurs in heart disease, amyloid disease, tuberculosis, neoplasm, and nephritis (syphilitic?). The appearance is due to calcium phosphate, cholesterol or a lecithin globulin compound.

Treatment.—Injury to the thoracic duct during operation may require ligation. For the effusion tapping is indicated if pressure symptoms are marked but a large amount should not be removed at one time. Any underlying condition should receive proper treatment.

Diagnosis of Pleurisy

Acute plastic pleurisy is readily recognized. In the diagnosis of pleuritic effusion the first question is, Does a fluid exudate exist? the second, What is its nature? In large effusions the increase in size of the affected side, the immobility, the absence of tactile fremitus, the resistance, with the displacement of organs, give indications of the presence of fluid. The chief difficulty arises in effusions of moderate extent, when the dulness, the presence of bronchophony, and, perhaps, tubular breathing may simulate *pneumonia.* The chief points to be borne in mind are: (*a*) Differences in the onset and in the general characters of the two affections, more particularly the initial chill, the higher fever, more urgent dyspnea, and the rusty expectoration of pneumonia. Some cases of pneumococcus pleurisy set in like pneumonia. (*b*) Certain physical signs—the more wooden dulness, the greater resistance, and the marked diminution or the absence of tactile fremitus in pleurisy. The auscultatory signs may be deceptive. It is usually, indeed, the persistence of tubular breathing, particularly high-pitched, even amphoric expiration, heard in some cases of pleurisy, which has raised the doubt. The intercostal spaces are more commonly obliterated in pleuritic effusion than in pneumonia. The displacement of organs is a valuable sign. With an exploring needle the question is usually easily settled. Pus is sometimes not obtained if too small a needle is used. Pneumothorax is an occasional sequence of puncture. The needle is especially useful in the diagnosis from collapse of the lung and thickened pleura. In massive pneumonia, in which the bronchi are plugged, if the patient has not been seen from the outset, the diagnosis may be impossible without it.

On the left side it may be difficult to differentiate a large *pericardial* from a pleural effusion. The retention of resonance at the base, the presence of tympany toward the axilla, the absence of dislocation of the heart to the right, the feebleness of the pulse and the heart-sounds, and the urgency of the dyspnea, out of proportion to the extent of the effusion, are the chief points to be considered. *Hydrothorax* presents signs identical with those of serofibrinous effusion. Certain *tumors* within the chest may simulate pleural effusion. It should be remembered that many intrathoracic growths are accompanied by exudation. Malignant disease of the lung and pleura and hydatids of the pleura produce extensive dulness, with suppression of the breath sounds, closely simulating effusion.

On the right side, abscess of the liver, subdiaphragmatic abscess, and hydatid cysts may press upward and produce dulness and enfeebled breathing. Often in these cases there is a friction sound, which should excite suspicion, and the upper outline of the dulness is sometimes plainly convex. In a case of cancer of the kidney the growth involved the diaphragm very early, and for months there were signs of pleurisy before our attention was directed to the kidney. In case of doubt the X-ray study is a great aid; exploratory puncture should be done without hesitation.

The second question, as to the *nature of the fluid,* is quickly decided by the use of the needle. Persistent fever, sweats, a leukocytosis, and increase in the pallor suggest the presence of pus. In children the complexion is often sallow and earthy. In protracted cases, even in children, when the general symptoms and the appearance have been strongly suggestive of pus, the syringe has withdrawn clear fluid. On the other hand, effusions of short duration may be purulent, even when the general symptoms do not suggest it. In pneumonia, the possibility of empyema should always be in mind during the course, and suspected if the crisis is delayed or fever continues, if chills and sweats follow, or if the cough changes to one of paroxysmal type of great intensity. There are three groups: (*a*) The presence of the empyema is readily detected. (*b*) It is suspected, but it is not possible to locate pus by the ordinary physical signs. The exploratory needle should be freely used. (*c*) In a few instances small interlobar collections, small mural abscesses, and the diaphragmatic form may escape detection until an exploratory operation is performed. The *prognostic* import of the causal organism is as follows: The pneumococcus is of favorable significance, as such cases usually get well rapidly, sometimes with a single aspiration. The streptococcus empyema is the most serious form, and even after a free drainage the patient may succumb to septicemia. A sterile fluid indicates in a majority of instances a tuberculous origin. In the distinction between an exudate (pleurisy) and a transudate (hydrothorax) from the fluid, the points are: Specific gravity above 1.018 in exudate, below 1.015 in transudate; albumin 30 to 65 gms. per litre and fibrinogen 1 in exudate, and 10 to 30 gms. albumin and fibrinogen 0.1 gm. in transudate.

Treatment

Acute Fibrinous Pleurisy.—The patient should be in bed. At the outset the severe pain may be relieved by hot or cold applications or counterirritation but a hypodermic of morphia is more effective. It is well to administer a mercurial and saline purge. Fixing the side by strapping with adhesive plaster, which should pass well over the middle line, applied tightly and evenly at full expiration, gives great relief. Dry cupping may be employed. Artificial pneumothorax may be done if the pain is severe and not relieved by other measures. The ice-bag may be used as in pneumonia. Codein may be required for cough. The open-air treatment should be begun early, as a majority of the cases are tuberculous.

When *effusion* has taken place, mustard plasters or iodine, producing slight counterirritation, appear useful, particularly in the later stages. Iodide of potassium is of doubtful benefit. By some the salicylates are believed to be of special efficacy but drug treatment is unsatisfactory. A dry diet and saline purges (in concentrated form before breakfast) may be tried and a salt-free diet has been advised, but these measures are disappointing.

Early and if necessary repeated *aspiration* is the most satisfactory treatment. Effusion of sufficient extent to give definite signs is the indication for aspiration; early tapping usually shortens the course materially and repetition may not be necessary. The results obtained by Delafield in 200 cases treated by early aspiration have never been equalled. The credit of introducing aspiration in pleuritic effusions is due to Morrill Wyman, of Cambridge, Mass., and Henry I. Bowditch, of Boston. Years prior to Dieulafoy's work, aspiration was in constant use at the Massachusetts General Hospital and advocated repeatedly by Bowditch. As the question is of historical interest, we give Bowditch's conclusions concerning aspiration, which practically represent the opinion of to-day: "(1) The operation is perfectly simple, but slightly painful, and can be done with ease upon any patient in however advanced a stage of the disease. (2) It should be performed forthwith in *all* cases in which there is complete filling up of one side of the chest. (3) He had determined to use it in *any* case of even *moderate* effusion lasting more than a few weeks and in which there should seem to be a disposition to resist ordinary modes of treatment. (4) He urged this practice upon the profession as a very important measure in practical medicine; believing that by this method death may frequently be prevented from ensuing either by sudden attack of dyspnea or subsequent phthisis, and, finally, from the gradual wearing out of the powers of life or inability to absorb the fluid." When the fluid reaches to the clavicle the indication for aspiration is imperative. Fever is not a contra-indication; indeed, often with serous exudates the temperature falls after aspiration. In cases with tuberculosis of the lung on the affected side it may be wiser to delay aspiration as the fluid keeps the lung at rest.

The operation is simple and practically without risk. The spot selected for puncture should be in the sixth intercostal space in the midaxilla or at the outer angle of the scapula in the eighth space. The axilla is usually preferable as the patient does not have to sit up. If he has to be in a sitting position, he should be supported in front. The arm of the patient should be brought forward with the hand on the opposite shoulder, so as to widen the spaces. The area should be painted with iodine and the skin and deeper tissues anesthetized by novocaine. The needle should be thrust in close to the upper margin of the rib, so as to avoid the intercostal artery, the wounding of which, however, is exceedingly rare. The fluid should be withdrawn slowly. The amount will depend on the size of the exudate but it is safer not to exceed 1500 cc. As the fluid is withdrawn it may be replaced by oxygen or air and if this is done, larger amounts of fluid may be removed. In chronic cases of serous pleurisy after the failure of repeated tappings S. West showed the value of free incision and drainage. He reported cases of recovery after effusions of fifteen and eighteen months' standing.

Repeated tapping may be required in some cases. In the chronic cases the injection of epinephrine (20 to 30 drops of a 1-1,000 solution) into the pleural cavity after aspiration has proved of value.

Symptoms and Accidents During Paracentesis.—*Pain* is usually complained of after a certain amount of fluid has been withdrawn; it is sharp and cutting in character. *Coughing* occurs toward the close, and may be severe and paroxysmal. Pain, cough or distress may compel withdrawal of the needle.

Pneumothorax of slight extent often follows an exploratory puncture or aspiration. *Subcutaneous emphysema* may develop from the point of puncture, without the production of pneumothorax. *Faintness* is not uncommon and convulsions may occur during the withdrawal or while irrigating the pleura. These symptoms are of reflex origin from the pleura. Hemiplegia may follow. And lastly *sudden death* may occur from syncope or from the pleural reflex.

These serious events may follow exploratory puncture of the lung. Such accidents are explained by the studies of Capps and Lewis, who have shown that a sudden and sometimes fatal fall in blood pressure may follow the experimental irrigation of the pleura in dogs. Occasionally toxic symptoms arise resembling those of "serum illness"—pains in the joints, albumin in the urine, and edema—suggestive of the absorption of toxins that act like a foreign protein. Expectoration of a large quantity of *albuminous fluid* may occur suddenly after the tapping, associated with dyspnea. Some cases have proved rapidly fatal, with the features of an acute edema of the lungs. It occurs usually after large amounts are removed.

The after-treatment of pleurisy is important and the patients should be handled exactly as if they had an early tuberculous lung lesion unless the effusion is proved to be due to some other cause.

Empyema.—A majority of the cases get well, provided that free drainage is obtained. In some cases recovery follows aspiration, especially if done early in the empyema of pneumonia. The good results in any method depend upon the thoroughness with which the cavity is drained. In the subsequent treatment a point of great importance in facilitating the closure of the cavity is the distention of the lung on the affected side. This may be accomplished by the method advised by Ralston James, especially in children. The patient daily, for a certain time, increasing gradually with the increase of his strength, transfers water from one bottle to another by air-pressure. The bottles should be large, holding at least a gallon each, and by the arrangement of tubes, as in the Wolff's bottle, an expiratory effort of the patient forces the water from one bottle into the other. Equally efficacious is the plan advised by Naunyn. The patient sits in an arm-chair grasping strongly one of the rungs with the hand and forcibly compressing the sound side against the back of the chair; then forcible inspiratory efforts are made which act chiefly on the compressed lung, as the sound side is fixed. The cavity is gradually closed, partly by the falling in of the chest wall and partly by the expansion of the lung. The cavity may fail to close after operation and a chronic empyema remains with a sinus. In such cases the lung is collapsed, often fibroid, and there is great thickening of the pleura. In some instances thoracoplasty is indicated.

The physician is often asked, in cases of empyema with emaciation, fever and feeble, rapid pulse, whether the patient can stand the operation. Even in the most desperate cases one should never hesitate to secure drainage.

CHRONIC PLEURISY

This affection occurs in two forms:

Chronic pleurisy with effusion in which the disease may set in insidiously or follow an acute serofibrinous pleurisy. The fluid may persist for months or even years without undergoing any special alteration and without becoming purulent.

Chronic Dry Pleurisy.—The cases are met with (*a*) *as a sequence of ordinary pleural effusion.* When the exudate is absorbed and the layers of the pleura come together there is between them a variable amount of fibrinous material which undergoes organization, and is converted into a layer of firm connective tissue. This process goes on at the base, and is represented by slight flattening, deficient expansion, defective resonance on percussion and enfeebled breathing. After recovery from empyema the flattening and retraction may be more marked. In both cases the condition can be greatly benefited by pulmonary gymnastics. In these firm, fibrinous membranes calcification may occur, particularly after empyema. It is not very uncommon to find between the false membranes a small pocket of fluid forming a sort of pleural cyst. In the great majority of these cases the condition need not cause anxiety. There may be an occasional dragging pain at the base of the lung or a stitch in the side, but patients may remain in perfectly good health. The most advanced grade of this secondary dry pleurisy is seen in cases of empyema which have perforated and ultimately healed by a gradual absorption or discharge of the pus, with retraction of the chest and fibrosis of the lung. Traumatic lesions, such as gunshot wounds, may be followed by an identical condition. Postmortem, it is impossible to separate the layers of the pleura, which are greatly thickened, particularly at the base, and surround a compressed airless, fibroid lung. Bronchiectasis may follow, sometimes not only on the affected side, but also in the lower lobe of the other lung.

(*b*) *Primitive Dry Pleurisy.*—This condition may follow directly the acute plastic pleurisy or it may set in without any acute symptoms and the patient's attention is called to it by feeling the pleural friction. A constant effect of this primitive dry pleurisy is the adhesion of the layers. This is probably an invariable result, whether the pleurisy is primary or secondary. The organization of the thin layer of exudation in pneumonia unites the two surfaces by delicate bands. *Pleural adhesions* are extremely common and may be limited in extent or universal. Thin fibrous adhesions do not produce any alteration in the percussion note and, if limited, there is no special change on auscultation. When, however, there is general adhesion the expansion of the lung is considerably impaired. We should naturally think that universal adhesions would interfere materially with the function of the lungs, but practically we see many instances in which there has not been the slightest disturbance. The physical *signs* of thickened pleura are by no means constant. There is diminished expansion, absence of Litten's sign, decreased vocal fremitus, various degrees of dulness and diminished breath sounds. The extent of thickening influences the signs which may vary considerably. The amount of fibrosis in the lungs also has an influence.

It is probable that a primitive dry pleurisy may lead to great thickening of the membranes, and ultimate invasion of the lung, causing fibrosis.

(*c*) There is a primitive dry pleurisy of *tuberculous* origin. In it both parietal and costal layers are greatly thickened—perhaps from 2 to 3 mm. each—and present firm fibroid, caseous masses and small tubercles, while uniting the two thickened layers is a reddish-gray fibroid tissue, sometimes infiltrated with serum. This may be a local process confined to one pleura, or it may be in both. These cases are sometimes associated with a similar condition in the pericardium and peritoneum.

Occasionally remarkable vasomotor phenomena occur in chronic pleurisy, whether simple or in connection with tuberculosis of an apex. Flushing or sweating of one cheek or dilatation of the pupil are the common manifestations. They appear to be due to involvement of the first thoracic ganglion at the top of the pleural cavity.

Treatment.—It is well to carry out the general treatment for tuberculosis. In some cases the use of exercises may be of value, but the chances of helping the local condition materially by any treatment are not good.

HYDROTHORAX

Hydrothorax is a transudation of simple noninflammatory fluid into the pleural cavities and occurs as a secondary process in many affections. The fluid is pale yellow with a specfic gravity below 1.015; it does not clot; the cells are scanty and the amount of albumin is small. It occurs with cardiac disease, in acute or chronic nephritis, in severe anemia, from pressure due to new growth and obstruction of the azygos veins. It occurs more often on the right side and if on both sides, there is more fluid on the right side. In renal disease hydrothorax is almost always bilateral, but in heart affections the right side is more commonly involved. The physical *signs* are those of pleural effusion but the exudation is rarely excessive. In kidney and heart disease, even when there is no general dropsy, the occurrence of dyspnea should at once direct attention to the pleura. In chronic myocardial disease the effusion is usually on the right side, and may recur for months. The greater frequency of the dextral effusion has been attributed to compression of the azygos vein, but compression of the pulmonary veins by the dilated right auricle seems more probable. Postmortem records show the frequency with which this condition is overlooked. The primary condition should be treated. Saline purges will in many cases rapidly reduce the fluid but, if necessary, aspiration should be practised repeatedly.

HEMOTHORAX

This results from trauma to or disease of the vessels of the chest wall, pleura, lung and mediastinum especially tuberculosis and neoplasm. It is a common sequence of wounds of the chest. A high velocity bullet may pass through the chest and lung without causing serious damage and the man may be about within a week. The blood usually comes from the lung. The amount varies from a few ounces to several pints. When withdrawn the blood forms a scanty clot because much of the fibrin has been deposited on the pleura. The fluid is not all blood, but mixed with serous exudate with many leukocytes, endothelial and eosinophile cells. Even when large amounts are present there may be no signs of anemia. The pleural surfaces are covered with a thin film of fibrin. The lower lobe is often collapsed. Pneumothorax and pneumohemothorax are rare, 8 cases of the latter and 4 of the former in 328 cases of gunshot wounds of the chest (Bradford and Elliott).

Symptoms.—Shock, cough, dyspnea and hemoptysis are present in a majority of the cases. Slight fever is frequent and the pulse is quickened. If not infected the progress is uneventful. The cough lessens, slight fever persists, but with moderate exudates the absorption is rapid. A slight icteric tinge of the skin may be present. With massive hemorrhage, as from an aneurism, there is collapse and sudden death.

The *signs* vary with the amount of fluid. With a massive exudate there is a flat note on percussion, absence of fremitus, and distant or feeble tubular breathing. The signs are often less distinctive than with simple effusion. With the fluoroscope the diaphragm is seen to be high. A phenomenon, not seen in ordinary effusion, is the early flattening and immobility of the side, which with the high level of the diaphragm speaks for massive *collapse* of the lung, with displacement of the heart to the affected side. This may take place with moderate effusion and may disappear rapidly. Contralateral collapse of the unaffected lung occurs not infrequently, with flatness at the opposite base, tubular breathing and increased fremitus.

Complications.—Septic infection is indicated by increasing fever and pulse rate, persistence of cough, increase of the exudate, sweats, etc. Secondary hemorrhage is rare. Pneumonia, pericarditis, purulent bronchitis, abscess and gangrene, and general streptococcus infection may occur.

Treatment.—Without infection a majority of the cases get well with rest in bed, but increase of the dyspnea may demand aspiration. Oxygen replacement is useful in large effusions. Infection calls for free drainage.

PNEUMOTHORAX

(*Hydropneumothorax and Pyopneumothorax*)

Air alone in the pleural cavity, to which the term pneumothorax is strictly applicable, is a rare condition. It is often associated with a serous fluid—hydropneumothorax, or with pus—pyopneumothorax.

Etiology.—There exists normally within the pleural cavity of an adult a negative pressure of several (3 to 5) millimetres of mercury, due to the recoil of the distended, perfectly elastic lung. Hence, through any opening connecting the pleural cavity with the external air we should expect air to rush in until this negative pressure is relieved. To explain the absence of pneumothorax in a few cases of injury laying the pleura bare, in which it would be expected, S. West assumed the existence of a cohesion between the plurae, but this force has not been satisfactorily demonstrated.

If the opening causing the pneumothorax remains patent, as in some external wounds and in perforations through consolidated areas of the lung, the intrathoracic pressure is that of the atmosphere. The lung will collapse as much as possible by virtue of its own elastic tension, the intercostal grooves are obliterated, the heart is displaced, and the diaphragm depressed, because the negative pressure by which these organs are partly retained in their ordinary position has been relieved. If the opening becomes closed the intrathoracic pressure may rise above the atmospheric and the displacements be much increased. But most perforations through the lungs are valvular, a property of lung tissue, and the intrapleural pressure is soon about 7 mm. of mercury. If there be a fluid exudate the pressure may be higher, but the high pressures supposed are more apparent than real, and that measured at the autopsy table is probably not that during life. It is more a question of the amount of distention than the actual pressure which determines the discomfort.

Pneumothorax arises: (1) In perforating wounds of the chest, sometimes associated with extensive cutaneous emphysema. It may follow exploratory puncture with a small needle. Pneumothorax rarely follows fracture of a rib, even though the lung may be torn. (2) In perforation of the pleura through the diaphragm, usually by malignant disease of the stomach or colon, or abscess of the liver. The pleura may also be perforated in cancer of the esophagus. (3) When the lung is perforated, by far the most common cause: (*a*) In the normal lung from rupture of air vesicles or an emphysematous bleb—*spontaneous* form. The air may be absorbed and no ill effect follow. It does not necessary excite pleurisy, as pointed out many years ago by Gairdner, but inflammation and effusion are the usual result. (*b*) From perforation due to local disease of the lung, either the softening of a caseous focus or the breaking of a tuberculous cavity. Probably 90 per cent of all cases are due to this cause. Less common are the cases due to septic bronchopneumonia, abscess, infarct and gangrene. (*c*) Perforation of the lung from the pleura, which arises in certain cases of empyema and produces a pleurobronchial fistula. (4) Spontaneously, by the development in pleural exudates of the gas bacillus. *Hemopneumothorax* may be spontaneous, the blood coming from the torn lung, from torn adhesions or from a cavity which has ruptured into the pleura.

Among 918 cases collected by Black the causal factors were: tuberculosis 715, pulmonary gangrene 65, empyema 45, trauma 32, bronchiectasis 10, pulmonary abscess 10, emphysema 7, pulmonary infarction 4, thoracentesis 3, and many rare causes with one or two examples.

Pneumothorax occurs chiefly in adults, is rare in young children and more frequent in males than in females.

A remarkable recurrent variety has been described; in Goodhart's case the pneumothorax developed first in one side and then in the other.

Morbid Anatomy.—If a trocar is inserted between the ribs there may be a jet of air of sufficient strength to blow out a lighted match. On opening the thorax the mediastinum and pericardium are seen to be displaced to the opposite side; but the heart is not rotated, and the relation of its parts is maintained much as in the normal condition. A serous or purulent fluid is usually present and the membranes are inflamed. The cause of the pneumothorax can usually be found without difficulty. In the great majority of instances it is the perforation of a tuberculous cavity or a breaking of a superficial caseous focus. The orifice of rupture may be extremely small. In chronic cases there may be a fistula of considerable size communicating with the bronchus. The lung is usually compressed and fibrosed.

Symptoms.—The rupture may be felt or even heard by the patient. In some cases there may be discomfort or pain, with mild dyspnea but not enough to compel him to go to bed. The condition may be found on a routine examination. This is often the case with a localized pneumothorax. In others the *onset* may be sudden with severe pain, marked dyspnea and cyanosis, and signs of shock. The respirations are rapid and shallow with increased heart rate and a small pulse. In severe cases the color becomes livid, the pulse feeble and rapid, there is sweating with great respiratory distress—the pneumothorax acutissimus of Unverricht. The patient may become unconscious and die within twenty-four hours. In 23 per cent of 385 cases the onset was *insidious* (O. H. P. Pepper). The "splash" may be the first indication to the patient of any change.

Physical Signs.—*Inspection* shows marked enlargement of the affected side with immobility. The patient usually lies on the affected side and is propped up. The heart impulse is usually much displaced. On *palpation* the fremitus is greatly diminished or more commonly abolished. It may be increased in front due possibly to adhesions or a lung pressed against the chest wall. On *percussion* the resonance has a tympanitic or amphoric quality but this is not always the case. It may be a dull tympany. In some instances there is a full, hyperresonant note, like emphysema; while in others there is dulness. These extreme variations depend doubtless upon the degree of intrapleural tension. Error in diagnosis may result from ignorance of the fact that the percussion note may be "muffled, toneless, almost dull" (Walshe). There is usually dulness at the base from fluid and shifting dulness may be marked. When recumbent the tympanitic note on the right side may reach the costal border, when erect the dulness may be at the third rib. The liver flatness may be obliterated. On *auscultation* the breath sounds are suppressed. Sometimes there is a distant feeble inspiratory sound of marked amphoric quality or hollow cavernous sounds. The contrast between the loud exaggerated breath sounds on the normal side and the feeble or absent breath sounds on the other is very suggestive. The râles have a peculiar metallic quality, and on coughing or deep inspiration there may be what Laënnec termed the metallic tinkle. This sound, like striking a glass vessel with a pin, may be heard some distance from the patient or in all parts of the room (Allbutt). A gurgling sound may be heard during inspiration, the so-called "water whistle noise." The voice has a curious metallic echo. The *coin-sound* is very characteristic. To obtain it the auscultator should place one ear on the back of the chest while the assistant taps one coin on another on the front of the chest. The metallic echoing sound produced is one of the most characteristic signs of pneumothorax. The Hippocratic *succussion splash* may be obtained when the auscultator's head is placed upon the chest while the patient's body is shaken. A splashing sound is produced, which may be audible at a distance. A patient may himself notice it in making abrupt movements. The splash depends on fluid and air. Of other signs displacement of organs is most constant. The heart may be "drawn over" to the opposite side, and the liver greatly displaced.

Gas Analysis.—Emerson determined experimentally that of the air introduced, the oxygen rapidly diminishes, but the nitrogen remains very constant. An increasing amount of oxygen suggests an open fistula. Air is absorbed rapidly from the normal pleura and in spontaneous cases the signs may disappear within a week; in other instances weeks or months may elapse.

Diagnosis.—When the percussion note is dull the condition may be mistaken for effusion. Massive collapse of the lung simulates it closely.

Diaphragmatic or congenital hernia following a crush or other accident may closely simulate it. Pneumothorax in a patient with emphysema may cause difficulty. Percussion of the lower border of the lung on the affected side shows that the resonance in pneumothorax extends to the lowest part of the pleural cavity and is fixed, not changing with in- and expiration. Very large cavities with tympanitic percussion and râles of an amphoric, metallic quality, may simulate pneumothorax. In total excavation of one lung the amphoric and metallic phenomena may be intense, but the absence of dislocation of the organs, of the succussion splash, and of the coin-sound differentiates this condition. While this is true in the great majority of cases, the coin-sound may be heard over a large cavity in the right upper lobe. Pyopneumothorax subphrenicus may simulate true pneumothorax closely. The recognition of cystic disease of the lung and localized pneumothorax may depend on the X-ray study.

X-ray Examination.—The characteristic features are an abnormally clear zone without the normal lung markings, the shadow of the collapsed lung, not always easy to see, and the visceral displacements. The fluid shows as an opaque shadow and with the fluoroscope a wavy outline of the fluid may be seen in shaking the patient. An aneurism pressing on a bronchus may cause inflation of the lung and features suggestive of pneumothorax.

Prognosis.—This depends largely upon the cause but it is usually serious. The tuberculous cases may die within a few weeks. Of 22 tuberculosis cases 20 died (J. H. H. Series). There are tuberculous cases in which pneumothorax, if occurring early, seems to arrest the progress of the tuberculosis. There is a chronic pneumothorax which may last several years. The outlook in spontaneous pneumothorax is good. It may recur or appear later in the other side. Though usually not tuberculous and due to a ruptured bleb or a tear, it may be followed years later by tuberculosis of the lung (Hamman).

Treatment.—The patient should be kept as quiet as possible and morphia given to secure this if necessary. He should be encouraged to suppress cough and avoid deep respirations. Strapping the affected side and the giving of sedatives, such as codein and heroin, may lessen cough. With fluid present it may be necessary to remove some if there are pressure symptoms, but it is better left alone if possible for two weeks or until the fistula is closed. There are three groups of cases: First, in severe cases with urgent dyspnea, great displacement of the heart, cyanosis, and low blood pressure, a needle should be inserted into the pleura to allow air to escape. Immediate aspiration has saved life. The degree of intrapleural pressure is a guide to the need of removing air. Secondly, the spontaneous cases which usually do well, as the air is quickly absorbed; so also with the traumatic variety. Very many of the tuberculous cases are best let alone, if the patient is doing well, or if the disease in the other lung is advanced. Thirdly, when there is pus, and the patient is not doing well aspiration should be done. In the tuberculous variety with pyopneumothorax it is usually best not to interfere. In some cases resection of one or two ribs may be done. Of nine cases in our series two recovered. Repeated aspiration may result in improvement.

When the pneumothorax follows carcinoma, gangrene or abscess of the lung, the course is rapidly fatal. When an empyema has preceded the pneumothorax, recovery may follow surgical drainage.

NEW GROWTHS OF THE PLEURA

Primary neoplasm of the pleura is rare and may be endothelioma, carcinoma or sarcoma. Secondary involvement is more common and may be due to direct extension from growth in the lung or mediastinum, or metastases from other parts. It is not infrequently secondary to cancer of the breast.

Symptoms.—These are not characteristic and may be those of pleural effusion. Dyspnea, cough and pain are usual. In some cases the pleura is thickened and a coarse friction rub is heard. The pleural fluid is usually hemorrhagic and may contain cells which suggest the diagnosis. The glands in the neck or axilla may be enlarged. Progressive weakness, anemia and emaciation may be the main features. Nodules may appear on the ribs. Cachexia may be late and the course may be prolonged for one or two years.

Diagnosis.—The occurrence of pleural effusion, especially if chronic and hemorrhagic, without evident cause should excite suspicion. A careful study should be made of the cells in the fluid. The X-ray study is important.

Treatment.—This is palliative and repeated tapping may be necessary. Sometimes replacement of the fluid by oxygen or air is an advantage. Sedatives should be used as required. X-ray therapy may give relief.

AFFECTIONS OF THE MEDIASTINUM

Lymphadenitis.—The greater number of glands is on the right side, and the right bronchus passes off at a higher level (fifth dorsal vertebra) than the left. The glands are enlarged in inflammatory affections of the lungs and in pneumoconiosis. In the acute affections of childhood, including throat and sinus infections, they are swollen. They are almost constantly involved in tuberculosis of the lungs and may be the only organs found tuberculous. Often in children the glands at the lung root become enlarged and caseous and penetrate deeply into the hilus and into the lung itself.

SYMPTOMS.—These are not very definite in the simple and tuberculous forms and depend greatly on the extent of enlargement, the degree of infection or caseation and whether the glands exert pressure. *Cough* is frequent and may be irritative, paroxysmal and nonproductive. Sometimes there may be considerable dyspnea, so that asthma is suspected. There may be a special susceptibility to bronchitis. *Fever* of slight grade is common and may persist for months. In children there are often malnutrition, weakness, anemia and loss of weight. The *signs* are indefinite and vary with the amount of enlargement. There may be dulness in the interscapular regions or beside the sternum from the clavicle to the third rib. The breath sounds may be harsh over these areas but they are often so normally. If there is pressure on a bronchus to a lower lobe the note may show impairment and the breath sounds be feeble. The sign described by d'Espine is not of much value. Other signs of pressure may be found. If suppuration occurs the general features may be more marked, and rupture into a bronchus may suggest abscess. Invasion of the mediastinum, lung, pleura or pericardium may occur. The *diagnosis* may be difficult and even the X-ray study may not be positive although sometimes of the greatest value. Enlargement of the glands is common and may represent an old healed process of no present significance. Comparison on successive studies may be helpful. The use of tuberculin aids in the recognition of the tuberculous cases.

Treatment.—This must be of the causal condition. In children in whom enlargement of the glands is found it is wise to regard the adenitis as tuberculous until proved otherwise.

Suppurative Lymphadenitis.—Occasionally abscess in the bronchial or tracheal lymph nodes is found. It may follow simple adenitis but is most frequently associated with tubercle. The liquid portion may gradually be absorbed and the inspissated contents undergo calcification. Long continued *fever* may be present and the diagnosis may be difficult. Perforation may occur into the esophagus or into a bronchus, or in rare instances, as in the case reported by Sidney Phillips, perforation of the aorta, as well as a bronchus, which did not prove fatal rapidly, but caused repeated attacks of hemoptysis during a period of sixteen months.

Tumors.—*Sarcoma* is by far the most frequent tumor. Ross, in a study of 60 cases, found 44 cases of sarcoma and 10 of carcinoma. The lung was usually involved. In nearly 70 per cent the anterior glands were affected. There are three chief points of origin, the thymus, the lymph glands, and the pleura and lung. The enlarged glands of Hodgkin's disease and leukemia, and intrathoracic goitre may be added. Males are more frequently affected than females. The age is most commonly between thirty and fifty.

Symptoms.—The signs of mediastinal tumor are those of *intrathoracic pressure.* In some cases almost the entire chest is filled with the masses. The heart and lungs are displaced and it is marvelous how life can be maintained with such dislocation and compression of the organs. *Pain* is an important feature, usually fairly constant and often with exacerbations. It may be felt beneath the sternum or round the thorax. Pressure on the trachea may cause stridor, sometimes with wheezing. The patient may have to lean forward. *Dyspnea* is one of the earliest and most constant symptoms, and may be due to pressure on the trachea or the recurrent laryngeal nerves. It may also be due to pressure upon the heart or vessels. In a few cases it results from the pleural effusion which so frequently accompanies intrathoracic growths. Associated with the dyspnea is *cough,* often severe and paroxysmal, with the quality of the so-called aneurismal cough when a recurrent nerve is involved. The voice may be affected from a similar cause. Hemoptysis may occur and suggest pulmonary tuberculosis. Pressure on the vessels is common, and on the subclavian artery may cause inequality of the radial pulses. The superior vena cava may be compressed and obliterated, and when the process goes on slowly the collateral circulation may be completely established. Less commonly the inferior vena cava or one or other of the subclavian veins is compressed. The arteries are much more rarely obstructed. There may be *dysphagia,* due to compression of the esophagus. There may be pupillary changes, usually contraction. Expectoration of blood, pus, and hair is characteristic of the dermoid cyst.

Physical Signs.—On inspection there may be orthopnea and marked cyanosis of the upper part of the body possibly with edema. In such instances, if of long duration, there are signs of collateral circulation and the superficial mammary and epigastric veins are enlarged. In cases of chronic obstruction the fingers may be clubbed. There may be bulging of the sternum or the tumor may erode the bone and form a prominence. The rapidly growing lymphoid tumors more commonly than others perforate the chest wall. In Hodgkin's disease the sternum may be eroded and perforated. The perforation may be on one side of the breast-bone. The projecting tumor may pulsate; the heart may be dislocated and its impulse much out of place. Contraction of one side of the thorax has been noted in a few instances. The larynx may be fixed. On palpation the fremitus is absent wherever the tumor reaches the chest wall. If pulsating, it rarely has the forcible, heaving impulse of an aneurism. On *percussion* the results are variable. There may be dulness over the manubrium and sometimes in the back. With compression of a bronchus, extension to a lung or pleural effusion many variations are found. The same applies to auscultation but there is usually silence over a dull area. The heart sounds are not transmitted and the respiratory murmur is feeble or inaudible, rarely bronchial. Vocal resonance is, as a rule, absent. Pleural effusion occurs in many instances of mediastinal growth.

Tumors of the *anterior mediastinum* originate usually in the thymus, or its remnants, or in the connective tissue; the sternum is pushed forward and often eroded. The growth may be felt in the suprasternal fossa; the cervical glands are usually involved. Pressure is chiefly upon the venous trunks. Dyspnea is prominent. A retrosternal goitre may give similar signs.

Intrathoracic tumors in the *middle* and *posterior mediastinum* originate most commonly in the lymph nodes. The symptoms are out of all proportion to the signs; there is urgent dyspnea and cough, which is sometimes loud and ringing. The pressure is chiefly upon the gullet, the recurrent laryngeal nerve and sometimes upon the azygos vein.

In a third group, tumors originating in the *pleura* and the *lung*, the pressure symptoms are not so marked. Pleural exudate is very much more common; the patient becomes anemic and emaciation is rapid. There may be secondary involvement of the lymph nodes in the neck.

Diagnosis.—Given the signs of increased intrathoracic pressure various conditions have to be considered. The results of the X-ray study are of great importance and may be decisive. The general features, enlarged cervical or axillary glands, and a hemorrhagic pleural fluid are important. The diagnosis from a new growth of the lung may be impossible and the diagnosis of mediastinal tumor from aneurism is sometimes extremely difficult. An interesting case reported by Sokolosski, in Bd. 19 of the *Deutsches Archiv für klinische Medicin,* in which Oppolzer diagnosed aneurism and Skoda mediastinal tumor, illustrates how the most skillful observers may be unable to agree. Scarcely a sign is found in aneurism which may not be duplicated in mediastinal tumor. This is not strange, since the features in both are largely due to pressure. The cyanosis, venous engorgement, and collateral circulation are as a rule, more marked in tumor. The time element is important. If the condition has persisted for more than eighteen months the disease is probably aneurism but there are exceptions. The diastolic shock so often felt over an aneurism is rarely, if ever, present in mediastinal growths, even when they perforate the sternum and have communicated pulsation. Tracheal tugging rarely occurs with tumor. Another point of importance is that a tumor from the mediastinum, eroding the sternum, and appearing externally, if aneurismal, has forcible, heaving, and distinctly expansile pulsations. Radiating pain in the back, arms and neck is rather in favor of aneurism, as is also improvement from iodide. The traumatic cyanosis of the upper half of the body which follows compression injuries of the thorax could scarcely be mistaken for the effect of tumor. The X-ray study is rarely at fault in differentiating aneurism and tumor. The frequency of *pleural effusion* with mediastinal tumor is to be remembered. It may give curiously complex characters to the physical signs which are profoundly modified after aspiration.

The *treatment* is largely symptomatic and palliative but in some cases deep X-ray or radium therapy gives relief and prolongs life. With early diagnosis there may be a possibility of removal, especially in the anterior mediastinum. Occasionally a tumor of the mediastinum is operable. Intrathoracic goitre can be removed.

Abscess of the Mediastinum.—Hare collected 115 cases of mediastinal abscess, in 77 of which there were details sufficient for analysis. The great majority occurred in males; 44 were instances of acute abscess. The anterior mediastinum is most commonly the seat of the suppuration. The cases are most frequent after trauma; some have followed erysipelas or occurred with eruptive fevers. Injury or disease of the esophagus, trachea or bronchi, and extension of infection from the lung, pleura, pericardium, spine or sternum may be responsible. Many cases, particularly the chronic abscesses, are tuberculous. Of *symptoms, pain* behind the sternum is the most common. It may be throbbing, and in the acute cases is associated with fever, sometimes with chills and sweats. If the abscess is large there may be dyspnea and features due to increased intrathoracic pressure. The pus may burrow into the abdomen, perforate through an intercostal space, erode the sternum or discharge into the trachea or esophagus. In chronic abscess the pus may become inspissated. The *physical signs* are indefinite. A pulsating and fluctuating tumor may appear at the border of the sternum or at the sternal notch. The *diagnosis* is first of some condition causing mediastinal pressure. The X-ray study gives valuable aid. Fever, perhaps with chills, leukocytosis and any evidence of "pointing" suggest abscess. The *prognosis* is serious unless it is possible to drain the abscess early. The *treatment* is surgical.

Mediastinitis, Acute and Indurative.—The *acute* form occurs with pericarditis and pleurisy, with the infections, particularly pneumonia and syphilis, and may follow trauma, especially penetrating wounds. The *symptoms* are indefinite and it is rarely recognized clinically. Pain behind the sternum and pressure signs may be present and a well-marked creaking friction with dulling of the percussion note on the sternum (C. P. Howard). It may pass on to abscess formation or more commonly to the *indurative form,* in which there is great increase in the fibrous tissues in the mediastinum, usually with adherent pericarditis. The process may extend and seriously compress or obliterate the vessels. Certain cases of fibroid obliteration of the superior vena cava originate in this way. It is sometimes associated with chronic polyserositis. The process may begin about the aorta and is then usually syphilitic. Cyanosis, dyspnea and cough are the prominent symptoms. The superficial veins are enlarged, the sternal note is flat, the X-ray picture shows a broad mediastinal shadow, and sometimes a loud creaking friction is heard. Swelling of the feet and ascites may be present, and when the thoracic duct is involved the ascitic fluid may be chylous. The heart may be enlarged, with adherent pericardium and the picture at the end may be that of cardiac dropsy. The *treatment* is that of the original condition in acute cases; in the chronic forms due to syphilis iodide should be given freely.

Suppurative mediastinitis (abscess) may follow the acute simple form or arise from trauma or perforation of the esophagus, trachea or bronchi. The general features are usually severe fever, chills and leukocytosis. Dyspnea and cyanosis with signs of mediastinal pressure are present. The course is usually downward unless relieved by operation or external pointing. The abscess may rupture into adjacent organs. Surgical drainage is the only treatment.

Miscellaneous Affections.—In Hare's 520 cases there were 7 of fibroma, 11 of dermoid cyst, 8 of hydatid cyst, and cases of lipoma and gumma.

Cysts of the Mediastinum.—*Simple* cysts are usually small and rarely cause symptoms. *Dermoid* cysts are rare and the symptoms begin in early adult lift, often before the age of twenty. Their size varies from a walnut to a child's head. The symptoms are thoracic pain, cough and profuse expectoration which may contain hair, cartilage, bones and teeth. Hemoptysis may occur; the sputum is often foul and may contain fat droplets. The diagnosis may be made by the presence of hair in the sputum or by a tooth being seen in an X-ray plate. The symptoms of *teratomata* usually begin about puberty. The tumors consist of masses of tissue containing small cysts. *Hydatid cyst* is rare in this situation. The diagnosis of cysts depends largely on the X-ray study and occasionally on tapping. The serological reaction is useful in hydatid cyst. Surgical *treatment* is indicated.

Emphysema of the Mediastinum.—Air in the tissues of the mediastinum is met with in cases of trauma, and occasionally in fatal cases of diphtheria and whooping cough. It may extend to the subcutaneous tissues. Champneys called attention to its frequency after tracheotomy, in which the conditions favoring its production are division of the deep fascia, obstruction in the air passages and inspiratory efforts. It is often associated with pneumothorax, and more often with rupture of the lung without pneumothorax, the pleura remaining intact and the air dissecting its way into the mediastinum and neck. The *symptoms* and *signs* are indefinite. Crackling sounds may be heard over the sternum, often influenced by respiration and the heart movements. Subcutaneous emphysema may be found in the neck. There is no treatment for the condition itself, only for the causal lesion.

DISEASES OF THE DIAPHRAGM

From its importance in respiration any disturbance of the function of the diaphragm may result in marked symptoms, especially in respiration. With inflammation of either surface the proper contraction is affected. *Diaphragmatic hernia* is usually congenital, rare, and best recognized by an X-ray study. *Acquired hernia* or *evisceration* usually results from injuries or wounds, especially stab wounds, sometimes from severe vomiting, and is nearly always on the left side. There are likely to be shock, vomiting, dyspnea, and the features resulting from peritonitis and pleuritis. There will be flattening of the side of the abdomen with absence of thoracic motion and of breath sounds on the affected side. Hiccough, cough and gastric symptoms are common. The X-ray picture is definite. The *diagnosis* has to be made from pneumothorax and eventration of the diaphragm. *Eventration* of the diaphragm is rare. In this the abdominal viscera are displaced upward on account of thinning of half the diaphragm. The condition is usually congenital and recognized accidentally in an X-ray examination.

Various grades of "*para-esophageal*" *hernia* occur and are not uncommon. Usually a portion of the stomach is involved but sometimes the colon. The hernia enters into the posterior mediastinum, not into the pleural cavity. There is often a hiatus between the esophagus and diaphragm. The *symptoms* are largely gastric, discomfort, pain which may radiate to the back, and belching. The severity tends to increase as the condition becomes more marked. Later there may be pressure on the lungs and heart. The *treatment* of hernia is in general surgical. In some cases phrenicotomy with paralysis of the diaphragm results in improvement.

Paralysis may occur with central lesions or injury or disease of the phrenic nerves. It is seen with diphtheria, epidemic encephalitis and acute poliomyelitis. The arch of the diaphragm is high and there may be collapse of the lower lobe on the affected side. Bilateral paralysis is always serious. There is severe dyspnea, the movements of the epigastrium and hypochondria are reversed, the lower thorax expands horizontally to a marked extent and with the fluoroscope the high position of the arches and absence of movement can be seen. Clonic *spasm* is present with hiccough, which, in acute illness, is a sign of gravity. Tonic spasm is sometimes seen in patients with emphysema and severe bronchitis. It occurs in tetanus, rabies and strychnine poisoning. *Postencephalitic tic* of the diaphragm has occurred with a rate of 60 to 90 per minute. Blocking of the phrenic nerves by the injection of alcohol or exposing them and freezing with ethyl chloride spray may relieve the condition.

Inflammation is common and usually secondary to some process in the thorax or abdomen. Primary involvement occurs in trichiniasis and some cases of severe scurvy. The lymphatic supply favors infection. The best example of an acute process is seen in diaphragmatic pleurisy. The most important causes of more chronic inflammation are pleuritis and tuberculosis. With irritation of the diaphragm or its serous covering, pain may be felt in the shoulder, due to stimulation of the sensory terminals of the phrenic nerve. As a result of an acute process changes in the muscle and adhesions are common with resulting restriction of motion. This causes dyspnea and possibly the pain and soreness in the lower thorax so common after pleurisy. Diminished expansion of the lower thorax, absence of Litten's sign, dulness and feeble breath sounds are found, due in part to thickened pleura. The X-ray study confirms the diagnosis and by it the exact condition can be determined. The extent of deformity of the diaphragm and restriction of motion are often striking. In pulmonary tuberculosis there may be decreased movement of the diaphragm even when the lung lesion is apical. In pneumoconiosis, in some cases of emphysema and fibroid change, the deformity of the diaphragm and its restricted function are marked. In advanced stages of all these diseases this plays a considerable part in causing the symptoms, especially dyspnea. There may be rapid and extensive changes in the diaphragm with acute peritonitis as from a perforated gastric ulcer. Collapse of the lung may follow.

SECTION VIII

DISEASES OF THE KIDNEYS

MALFORMATIONS

Newman classifies them as follows: A. Displacements without mobility—(1) congenital displacement without deformity; (2) congenital displacement with deformity; (3) acquired displacements. B. Malformations of the kidney. (1) Variations in number—(*a*) supernumerary kidney; (*b*) single kidney, congenital absence of one kidney, atrophy of one kidney; (*c*) absence of both kidneys. (2) Variations in form and size—(*a*) general variations in form, lobulation, etc.; (*b*) hypertrophy of one kidney; (*c*) fusion of two kidneys—horseshoe kidney, sigmoid kidney, disk-shaped kidney. In the *horseshoe* kidney, the commonest form of fusion, the lower poles are usually joined. It may be recognized during life by palpation, pyelography or in the X-ray plate. C. Variations in pelvis, ureters, and blood vessels.

The *fused* kidneys may form a large mass, which is often displaced, being in an iliac fossa, in the mid line of the abdomen, or even in the pelvis. Under these circumstances it may be mistaken for a new growth. The organ has been removed under the belief that it was a floating kidney. One patient lived eleven days with complete anuria.

Congenital Hydro-Ureter and Hydronephrosis.—In this rare condition one kidney may be involved or one kidney with the ureters. A man aged 21 under the care of Halsted had from his second year severe attacks of abdominal pain in which a swelling would appear between the hip and costal margin and subside with the passage of a large amount of urine; a huge hydronephrotic sac was drained. Of the bilateral congenital form there are two varieties:

(1) A remarkable hypertrophy and dilatation of the bladder and ureters, with congenital defect of the abdominal muscles. The bladder may form a large tumor, and the ureters may be visible through the thin abdominal walls as coils resembling the small intestine.

(2) There is a form of dilatation of the bladder, enlargement of the ureters and pelvis, with a clinical picture of chronic pyelonephritis and retention of urine, resembling obstruction, but in which, postmortem, there is no demonstrable organic obstruction. There appears to be a congenital maldevelopment of the musculature of the pelvis, ureters and bladder wall, or "an acquired vesical paresis, so that efforts of micturition become weaker and weaker as time goes on." The bladder distends, the ureteral meatuses become insufficient, secondary infection follows, and the child from three to six years of age comes under observation with the signs of an extensive pyelonephritis. The prognosis in such cases is extremely grave.

MOVABLE KIDNEY

(*Floating Kidney; Palpable Kidney; Ren mobilis; Nephroptosis*)

This was known to Riolan in the seventeenth century and to Matthew Baillie and to Rayer in the first half of the nineteenth century.

The kidney is held in position by its fatty capsule, by the peritoneum which passes in front of it, and by the blood vessels. Usually fixed, under certain circumstances one or the other organ, more rarely both, becomes movable. In very rare cases the kidney is surrounded, to some extent, by the peritoneum, and is anchored at the hilus by a mesonephron. Some would limit the term floating kidney to this condition.

Movable kidney is almost always acquired. It is more common in women. Of 667 cases collected by Kuttner, 584 were in women and only 83 in men. It is more common on the right than on the left side. Of 727 cases analyzed by this author, it occurred on the right in 553 cases, on the left in 81, and on both sides in 93. The greater frequency in women is partly due to compression of the lower thoracic zone by tight lacing (now rare), and to the relaxation of the abdominal walls which follows repeated pregnancies. Movable kidney, however, is by no means uncommon in nulliparae. There may be a congenitally relaxed condition of the peritoneal attachments as the condition has been met with in infants and children. Wasting of the fat about the kidney, trauma and the lifting of heavy weights are occasional factors. The kidney is sometimes dragged down by tumors. The greater frequency on the right side is probably associated with the position of the kidney just beneath the liver, and the depression to which the organ is subjected with descent of the diaphragm in inspiration.

Many cases present that combination of neurasthenia with gastro-intestinal disturbance which was described by Glénard as *enteroptosis*.

To determine the presence of a movable kidney the patient should be in the dorsal position, with the head moderately low and the abdominal walls relaxed. The left hand is placed in the lumbar region behind the eleventh and twelfth ribs; the right hand in the hypochondriac region, in the nipple line, just under the edge of the liver. Bimanual palpation may detect the presence of a firm, rounded body. If nothing is felt, the patient should be asked to draw a deep breath, when, if the organ is palpable, it is touched by the fingers of the right hand. Various grades of mobility may be recognized. It may be possible barely to feel the lower edge on deep palpation—*palpable kidney*—or the organ may be so far displaced that on drawing the deepest breath the fingers of the right hand may be, in a thin person, slipped above the upper end of the organ, which can be readily held down—*movable kidney*. In a third group the organ is freely movable, and may even be felt just above Poupart's ligament or in the midline, or it can be pushed over beyond this point. To this the term *floating kidney* is appropriate.

The movable kidney may be tender on pressure, especially when it is grasped very firmly, when there is a dull pain or sometimes a sickening sensation. Examination of the patient from behind may show a distinct flattening in the lumbar region on the side in which the kidney is mobile.

Symptoms.—In a large majority of cases there are no symptoms, and if detected accidentally it is well not to let the patient know of its presence. Too much stress may be laid upon the condition. Pain in the lumbar region or a sense of dragging and discomfort may be present. In a large group the symptoms are those of neurasthenia with dyspepsia. In women the nervous symptoms may be marked, and in men various grades of hypochondriasis. Dilatation of the stomach has been observed, due to pressure of the dislocated kidney upon the duodenum. Constipation is not infrequent. Some writers have described pressure upon the gall ducts, with jaundice, but this is very rare. Fecal accumulation and even obstruction may be associated with the displaced organ.

Dietl's Crises.—In connection with movable kidney, nearly always in women, and on the right side, there are remarkable attacks characterized by pain, chill, nausea, vomiting, fever and collapse. They were described first by Dietl, in 1864, and attributed to twist or kink of the renal vessels or of the ureter. In the subject of movable kidney they may recur at intervals for months or years. A sudden exertion, an error in diet, or standing for a long time may bring on an attack. The pain is in the renal region, of great intensity, simulating colic, and radiates down to the ureter and through to the back. The patient feels nauseated and cold, or there may be a severe chill; vomiting is common. The urine is scanty and contains an excess of urate and oxalates; sometimes it is bloody. The affected side is tender, the muscular tension increases, and the kidney may be enlarged, sensitive to pressure and less movable; but there is no positive tumor. In other cases a *tumor* rapidly forms from dilatation of the pelvis of the kidney. Appearing at the edge of the epigastric region, it may gradually reach the size of a large orange or a cocoanut and fills the entire renal region. This may happen within thirty-six or forty-eight hours. The nausea persists, there is fever, the patient looks ill, and the urine may be scanty or bloody. The general symptoms abate, the local tenderness lessens, the amount of urine may increase rapidly, and in ten or twelve hours the tumor may disappear. With a return of the symptoms the tumor reappears, and again subsides. This is *intermittent hydronephrosis* which may progress to permanent hydronephrosis.

Diagnosis.—The diagnosis of movable kidney is rarely doubtful. Tumors of the gallbladder, ovarian growth, cysts and tumors of the bowels and carcinoma of the pylorus may in rare instances be confounded with it.

Treatment.—In many instances great relief is experienced from some form of abdominal support which is often better than special pads. It should be applied in the morning, with the patient in the dorsal position. In some cases a support in the lower abdominal zone is sufficient. In the attacks of severe colic morphia may be required. The intermittent hydronephrosis may be relieved by a support but if not operation is advisable. The kidney may have to be fixed in position. This is a suitable procedure for severe cases, and relief is afforded in many instances by the operation, though not in all. Increase in weight often helps to hold the kidney in place. Attention should always be given to the state of the nervous system and in some cases a prolonged rest treatment is indicated.

CIRCULATORY DISTURBANCES

The secretion of urine is accomplished by the maintenance of a certain blood pressure within the glomeruli and by the activity of the renal epithelium. The watery elements are filtered from the glomeruli, the amount depending on the rapidity and the pressure of the blood current; the quality whether normal or abnormal, depending upon the condition of the capillary and glomerular epithelium. The integrity of the epithelium covering the capillary tufts within Bowman's capsule is essential to the production of a normal urine. If under any circumstances their nutrition fails, as when, for example, the rapidity of the blood current is lowered, so that they are deprived of the necessary amount of oxygen, the material which filters through is no longer normal, but contains serum albumin. The renal epithelium is extremely sensitive to circulatory changes, and compression of the renal artery for only a few minutes causes serious disturbance.

The circulation of the kidney is influenced by reflex stimuli coming from the skin. Exposure to cold causes heightened blood pressure within the kidneys and increased secretion of urine. Bradford has shown that after excision of portions of the kidney, to as much as one-third of the total weight, there is a remarkable increase in the flow of urine.

Congestion.—(1) Active Hyperemia.—The most typical congestion is that in the early stage of acute nephritis, when the organ may be large, soft, of a dark color, and on section blood drips from it freely. Turpentine, cantharides and copaiba cause extreme hyperemia of the organ.

It has been held that in all the acute fevers the kidneys are congested, and that this explained the scanty, high-colored and often albuminous urine. On the other hand, the kidney in acute fever may be small, pale and bloodless; this anemia, increasing with the pyrexia and interfering with the nutrition of the epithelium, may account for the scanty urine and the presence of albumin. In prolonged fevers it is probable that relaxation of the arteries again takes place. Certainly it is rare to find marked anemia postmortem; the kidney of fever is commonly swollen, the blood vessels are congested, and the cortex frequently shows traces of cloudy swelling. The circulatory disturbances in acute fevers are probably less important than the effects of the specific agents of the disease, their toxins or the altered metabolism.

(2) Passive Congestion; Mechanical Hyperemia.—This is found in chronic disease of the heart or lung, with impeded circulation, and as a result of pressure upon the renal veins by tumors, the pregnant uterus or ascitic fluid. In the passive congestion of chronic heart disease, the organs are enlarged and firm, the capsule strips off readily, as a rule, the cortex is of a deep red color, and the pyramids of a purple red. The section is coarse looking, the substance is very firm, and resists cutting and tearing. The interstitial tissue is increased, and there is a small-celled infiltration between the tubules. Here and there the Malpighian tufts have become sclerosed. The blood vessels are usually thickened, and there may be more or less granular, fatty, or hyaline changes in the epithelium of the tubules. The condition is indeed a diffuse nephritis. The urine is usually reduced, is of high specific

gravity, and contains albumin. Hyaline casts and blood corpuscles are not uncommon. In some cases (over half) with macroscopically no signs of chronic or acute nephritis the urinary features lead to the diagnosis of acute nephritis (Emerson). In uncomplicated cases uremia is rare. In the cardiac cases with extensive arteriosclerosis, the kidneys are more involved and the renal function is likely to be disturbed.

ANOMALIES OF THE URINARY SECRETION

ANURIA

Total suppression of urine occurs under the following conditions:

(*a*) As an event in the intense congestion of *acute nephritis*. For a time no urine may be formed; more often the amount is greatly reduced.

(*b*) Complete *anuria* is seen when renal stones block both ureters; or a calculus blocks the active kidney, the other being represented by a shell of tissue. In this "obstructive suppression," there is a condition which has been called "latent uremia." There may be very little discomfort, and the symptoms are unlike those of ordinary uremia. Convulsions occurred in only 5 of 41 cases (Herter); headache in only 6; vomiting in only 12. Consciousness is retained; the pupils are usually contracted; the temperature may be low; there are twitchings and perhaps occasional vomiting. Of 41 cases, 35 occurred in males. Of 36 cases with absolute anuria, in 11 the condition lasted more than four days, in 18 from seven to fourteen days, and in 7 cases longer than fourteen days (Herter). Obstructive suppression occurs when cancer compresses both ureters and involves their orifices in the bladder. Both ureters may be accidentally tied in an operation.

(*c*) Cases occur from *prerenal* causes. The following are among the more important: Fevers and inflammation; acute poisoning by phosphorus, mercury, lead and turpentine; aortic thrombosis involving the renal arteries; in the collapse after severe injuries or after operations, or, indeed, after the passing of a catheter; in the collapse stage of cholera and yellow fever; and, lastly, there is a hysterical anuria, of which Charcot reported a case in which anuria lasted for eleven days, but one must be very suspicious of deception.

A patient may live for ten to twenty-three days with complete suppression. Weakness, vertigo, nausea, dulness and drowsiness passing into coma are the usual features. The blood contains larger amounts of nitrogen and urea than is usual in uremia. Myers notes a case of recovery after twenty-three days of anuria.

Treatment.—In the obstructive cases surgical interference should be resorted to. In the nonobstructive cases, cupping over the loins, hot applications, free purging, and sweating with pilocarpine and sweat baths are indicated. Potassium citrate and sodium bicarbonate, 20 grains (1.3 gm.) of each, may be given every two hours by mouth, or a 2 per cent solution of each by rectum. Alkalosis should be kept in mind. When the secretion is once started diuretin often acts well. Large hot bowel irrigations with normal salt solution may stimulate the activity of the kidneys.

HEMATURIA

Etiology.—(1) Essential Hematuria.—How much basis there is for this group is a question and it is doubtful if the term should be retained. To make this diagnosis is to confess our inability to find any positive cause. Some are due to varicosity of vessels in the papillae. The bleeding is spontaneous, often associated with pain, though some attacks are painless. The X-ray picture is negative, the hemorrhage ceases of itself, and rarely do the attacks recur with such frequency that the patient becomes anemic. The condition was referred to under Gull's name of "renal epistaxis" in previous editions. It is rarely serious, and many cases recover spontaneously; in others nephrotomy stops the bleeding. Purpura should always be considered.

(2) General Diseases.—In the specific fevers, purpura, scurvy, the anemias, hemophilia and leukemia. It may be caused by malaria.

(3) Renal Causes.—Acute congestion and inflammation, as in nephritis, pyelitis, or pyelonephritis, or due to toxic agents, such as turpentine, carbolic acid and cantharides. Renal infarction, as in ulcerative endocarditis. New growths, in which the bleeding is usually profuse. In tuberculosis at the onset, when the papillae are involved, there may be bleeding. Stone in the kidney is a frequent cause. Parasites: The *Filaria bancrofti* and *Bilharzia* cause a form of hematuria met with in the tropics. The echinococcus is rarely associated with hemorrhage. It sometimes occurs in floating kidney and hydronephrosis. An unusual cause is the painful, villous tumor of the renal pelvis. It is difficult to distinguish the condition from stone. Angioma, papilloma and capillary nevi of the papillae may cause bleeding.

(4) Affections of the Urinary Passages.—Stone in and stricture of the ureter, tumors, polypi, tuberculosis, diverticula, or ulceration of the bladder, cystitis, calculus, parasites, and, very rarely, ruptured veins in the bladder. Bleeding from the urethra occasionally occurs in gonorrhea and as a result of the lodgment of a calculus. In females it may be due to prolapse or tumor of the urethra. Hematuria may be an early symptom in malignant disease or from an enlarged prostate.

(5) Trauma.—Injuries may produce bleeding from any part of the urinary passages. By a fall or blow on the back the kidney may be injured, and this may be followed by free bleeding; less commonly the blood comes from injury of the bladder or prostate. Blood from the urethra may be due to injury by the passage of a catheter or sound, or sometimes to falls. Transient hematuria follows all operations on the kidney.

(6) Exercise.—After strenuous exercise or exposure to cold temporary hematuria may occur with blood casts, followed by transient albuminuria, in individuals who show no signs of nephritis.

Diagnosis.—This is usually easy. The color of the urine varies from a light smoky to a bright red, or it may have a dark color. The blood cells are readily recognized microscopically, either plainly visible and retaining their color, in which case they are usually crenated, or simply as shadows. In ammoniacal urine or urines of low specific gravity the hemoglobin is rapidly dissolved from the corpuscles.

It is important to distinguish between blood coming from the bladder and from the kidneys. From the bladder the blood may be found only with the last portions of urine, or at the termination of micturition. In hemorrhage from the kidneys the blood and urine are intimately mixed. Clots are more commonly found with blood from the kidneys, and may form moulds of the pelvis or ureter. When the seat of the bleeding is in the bladder, on washing out this organ, the water is more or less blood-tinged; but if the source of the bleeding is higher, the water comes away clear. In many instances it is difficult to settle the question by the urine alone, and the symptoms and the physical signs must be taken into account. Cystoscopic examination of the bladder and catheterization of the ureters are aids in the diagnosis of doubtful cases. The recognition of the cause may be difficult. New growth, tuberculosis and calculus should always be considered.

Treatment.—The essential treatment must depend on the cause. In all forms of hematuria rest is essential. In that produced by renal calculi the recumbent posture may suffice to check the bleeding. It is doubtful if drugs have any influence. Cold may be applied to the loins or dry cups in the lumbar region. Incision of the kidney has cured the so-called essential hematuria.

HEMOGLOBINURIA

This is characterized by the presence of blood pigment in the urine. The blood cells are absent or in small numbers. The coloring matter is not always hemoglobin, but not infrequently methemoglobin. The urine has a red or brownish-red, sometimes quite black, color, and usually deposits a very heavy brownish sediment. When the hemoglobin is in small quantities, it may give a smoky color to the urine. Microscopic examination shows the presence of granular pigment, sometimes fragments of blood disks, epithelium, and often darkly pigmented urates. The urine is also albuminous. The number of red blood cells bears no proportion to the intensity of the color of the urine. Examined spectroscopically, there are either the two absorption bands of oxyhemoglobin or the three absorption bands of methemoglobin, of which the one in the red near *C* is characteristic. There are two clinical groups.

Toxic Hemoglobinuria.—This is caused by poisons which produce rapid dissolution of the blood corpuscles, such as potassium chlorate in large doses, pyrogallic acid, carbolic acid, arseniuretted hydrogen, carbon monoxide, naphthol, and muscarine; it also occurs in scarlet fever, yellow fever, typhoid fever, malaria, favism and syphilis. It has followed severe burns. Exposure to excessive cold and violent muscular exertion are stated to produce hemoglobinuria. A remarkable toxic form occurs in horses, coming on with great suddenness and associated with paresis of the hind legs. Death may occur in a few hours or a few days. The animals are attacked only after being stalled for some days and then taken out and driven, particularly in cold weather. The form of hemoglobinuria from cold and exertion is extremely rare. No instance of it, even in association with frost-bites, came under our observation in Canada. Blood transfused from one mammal into another causes dissolution of the corpuscles with the production of hemoglobinuria; and, lastly, there is the *epidemic hemoglobinuria* of the newborn, associated with jaundice, cyanosis and nervous symptoms.

Paroxysmal Hemoglobinuria.—This is characterized by the occasional passage of bloody urine, in which the coloring matter only is present. It is more frequent in males and occurs chiefly in adults. It seems specially associated with cold and exertion, and has been brought on, in a susceptible person, by the use of a cold foot-bath. It occurs in persons subject to Raynaud's disease, and the relation between these two affections is extremely close. Druitt, the author of the well-known *Surgical Vade-mecum,* gave a graphic description of his sufferings, which lasted for many years, and were accompanied with local asphyxia and local syncope. The connection, however, is not very common. The relation of hemoglobinuria to malaria has been considered. *Syphilis* is present in some cases and should always be considered. In one case after fifteen injections of arsphenamine, the hemoglobinuria disappeared (Brem).

Symptoms.—The attacks may come on suddenly after exposure to cold or as a result of mental or bodily exhaustion. They may be preceded by chills and pyrexia or the temperature is subnormal. There may be vomiting and diarrhea. Pain in the lumbar region is not uncommon. The hemoglobinuria rarely persists for more than a day or two—sometimes not for a day. There are instances in which, even in a single day, there are two or three paroxysms, and in the intervals clear urine is passed. Jaundice has been present in a number of cases. The disease is rarely if ever fatal.

The blood serum of these patients contains a complex hemolysin, a potential toxin, capable of dissolving the patient's own corpuscles and those of other individuals. It is an amboceptor component of the hemolysin, not the complement, that is peculiar, and this amboceptor differs "from other known hemolytic amboceptors in that it will unite with the red blood corpuscles only at a low temperature in the presence of complement, and furthermore in that it is capable of bringing about the solution of the patient's own cells (autohemolytic action), and those of other members of the group to which the patient belongs, as well as the cells of members of other groups" (Moss). Atmospheric cold and congestion of the peripheral vessels will reduce the temperature of the blood sufficiently to permit the union of the amboceptor and corpuscles, and hemolysis occurs.

The *treatment* of paroxysmal hemoglobinuria is unsatisfactory. Amyl nitrite will sometimes cut short or prevent an attack (Chvostek). During the paroxysm the patient should be kept warm and given hot drinks. If there is a syphilitic history active treatment should be given. In a warm climate the attacks are much less frequent. It is possible that an antitoxin may be obtained to neutralize the hemolytic amboceptor of the disease.

ALBUMINURIA: PROTEINURIA

"Reasons drawn from the urine are as brittle as the urinal" is a dictum of Thomas Fuller peculiarly appropriate in connection with this subject.

Blood serum contains two proteins, albumin and globulin, either of which or both may appear in the urine. The relative amounts vary in different conditions. The term proteinuria is more comprehensive than albuminuria. Crystalline proteins occur rarely. The presence of protein in the urine, formerly regarded as indicative of nephritis, is now recognized as occurring under many circumstances without serious organic change in the kidney. Two groups may be recognized—one in which the kidneys show no coarse lesions, and one in which there are evident anatomical changes.

Albuminuria without Coarse Renal Lesions.—(*a*) Functional or Orthostatic Albuminuria.—When protein substances transude there is probably disturbance in the nutrition of the epithelium of the capillaries of the tuft or of the cells surrounding the glomerulus. This is still in dispute, and many hold that there is a physiological albuminuria which may follow muscular work, the ingestion of food rich in albumin, violent exertion or cold bathing. On one point all agree, that the cause must be something unusual and excessive, as severe exertion in a football match or a race, etc. The presence of protein in the urine is usually indicative of some change in the renal or glomerular epithelium, which may be transient and unimportant, depending on variations in the circulation or the irritating effects of substances taken with the food or temporarily present, as in febrile states. It is possible that altered protein in the blood serum may be at fault.

Albuminuria of adolescence and cyclic albuminuria, in which the albumin is present only at certain times during the day—*orthostatic albuminuria*—are interesting forms. A majority of the cases occur in young persons—males more commonly—and the condition is often discovered accidentally. These are often the children of neurotic parents, and show asthenia and vasomotor instability with an irritable heart and varying blood pressure. Renal stasis may be responsible, caused by compression of the left renal vein between the aorta and mesenteric artery. This is favored by the aorta being pushed forward by lordosis or the mesenteric artery pulled on by visceroptosis. In such cases with a proper abdominal support the albuminuria disappears. Some cases last only during puberty, some throughout life. The condition is common, particularly in young men in training—the athletic albuminuria to which Collier called attention. Of 156 men in training 130 had albumin in the urine. Erlanger and Hooker have shown that the protein is excreted only during periods with low pulse pressure. The urine, as a rule, contains only a small amount of protein, but in some instances large quantities are present. The ratio of albumin to globulin is 2 to 1 (in nephritis it may be 6 to 1). The most striking feature is the variability. It may be absent in the morning and present only after exertion; or it may be greatly increased after taking food, particularly proteins. Even the change to the upright position (orthostatic) may suffice to cause it. Support of a movable kidney may stop it. The quantity of urine may be but little, if at all, increased, the specific gravity is usually normal, and the color may be high. Occasionally hyaline casts are found, and in some instances there has been transient glycosuria. As a rule, the pulse is not of high tension and the second aortic sound is not accentuated. Calcium lactate (gr. xv, 1 gm., three times a day) may cause a disappearance of the albumin.

Goodhart, from a study of the after history of more than 250 cases, holds that albuminuria of the adolescent has no sinister effect on health or the duration of life, and that with due circumspection such patients ought not to be excluded from the advantages of life insurance.

(*b*) Febrile Albuminuria.—Pyrexia, by whatever cause produced, may cause slight albuminuria, due to slight changes in the glomeruli induced by the fever, such as cloudy swelling, which can not be regarded as an organic lesion. It is extremely common, occurring in pneumonia (in about 70 per cent of our cases), diphtheria, typhoid fever (about 60 per cent of our cases), malaria, especially the estivo-autumnal type, and in acute tonsillitis. The amount is slight, and it usually disappears with the cessation of the fever. Hyaline and even epithelial casts accompany the condition.

(*c*) Hemic Changes.—Purpura, scurvy, chronic poisoning by lead or mercury, syphilis, leukemia and profound anemia may be associated with albuminuria. Abnormal ingredients in the blood, such as bile pigment, may cause the passage of small amounts of albumin.

The transient albuminuria of pregnancy may belong to this hemic group, although in a majority of such cases there are changes in the renal tissue. Albumin may be found sometimes after the inhalation of ether or chloroform.

(*d*) Nervous System.—In many morbid conditions of the nervous system, albumin may be present in the urine, and there are instances in young nervous persons not easy to separate from the orthostatic forms. In brain tumors, following epileptic attacks, in various types of meningitis, it has been present. In meningeal hemorrhage, as pointed out by Guillain, the albumin may be very abundant, 5 to 20 grams in the litre.

Albuminuria with Lesions of the Urinary Organs.—(*a*) *Congestion* of the kidney, either active, such as follows exposure to cold and is associated with the early stages of nephritis, or passive, due to passive congestion, or to pressure on the renal veins by the pregnant uterus or tumors.

(*b*) *Organic disease* of the kidneys—acute and chronic nephritis, infarction, amyloid degeneration, suppurative nephritis, nephrosis and tumors.

(*c*) Affections of the pelvis, ureters, bladder and prostate, when associated with the formation of pus or hematuria.

(*d*) Hereditary familial albuminuria and hemorrhagic nephritis. Families have been described in which through two and three generations members have had albuminuria, high blood pressure, occasional hematuria or sometimes only microscopic blood, from early childhood. Some of the patients died early from uremia; others lived to adult life. Hypertension and cardiovascular features have been present in some cases.

Prognosis.—Febrile albuminuria is transient, and in a majority of the cases depending upon hemic causes it disappears and leaves the kidneys intact. A trace of albumin in a man over forty, with or without a few hyaline casts, is not of much significance, except as an indication that his kidneys, like his hair, are beginning to turn "gray" with age. In many instances the discovery is a positive advantage, as the man is made to realize, perhaps for the first time, that he has been living carelessly. The question was discussed from this standpoint in a paper with the paradoxical title "On the Advantages of a Trace of Albumin and a Few Tube-casts in the Urine of Men over Fifty Years of Age" (*N. Y. Med. Jour.*, vol. lxxiv). The persistence of a slight amount of albumin in young men without increased arterial tension is less serious, as even after continuing for years it may disappear. Practically in all cases the presence of albumin indicates a change of some sort, the nature, extent, and gravity of which it is difficult to estimate; so that other considerations, such as the presence of casts, renal function, nitrogenous retention, increased tension, and the general condition must be carefully considered.

The physician is often consulted as to the relation of albuminuria and life insurance. Naturally, companies lay great stress upon the presence of albumin, but in chronic interstitial nephritis it is often absent or transient, even when the disease is well developed. After the fortieth year, from a standpoint of life insurance, the state of the arteries and the blood pressure are usually more important than the condition of the urine.

Albumosuria.—Albumose (proteose) and peptone are occasionally found in the urine, but are of slight clinical significance. They are found in many febrile diseases, in chronic suppuration, and whenever protein materials are undergoing autolysis, as in pneumonia, acute yellow atrophy of the liver and during the involution of the uterus.

Myelopathic albumosuria, "*Kahler's disease,*" is characterized by multiple myelomata with excretion of the *Bence-Jones body,* discovered by him in 1848. Some believe that it is not a proteose but a higher protein of endogenous origin derived from the tumor cells of a myeloma or from the abnormal synthesis of a body protein. Males above forty years of age are usually affected. The Bence-Jones body appears rarely with other tumors of the bones. The myeloma is a true tumor, the cells of which resemble the plasma rather than the myelocytes of the bone marrow (Christian). In *multiple myelomata* there is involvement of the spine, ribs or sternum, with protuberances or deformity of the spine. Pain, often intermittent, is common, sometimes due to pressure on the cord or nerves. The average duration is from one to two years. The Bence-Jones body is found in the urine in about 80 per cent and has been found in the blood serum. The disease runs a fatal course. The simplest reaction is the white precipitate formed on adding nitric acid to the urine; when boiled it disappears, to reappear on cooling. The urine may be of a milky white color when passed.

BACTERIURIA

Described first by Roberts in 1881, much attention has been paid to it and its importance recognized both as a secondary and a primary affection. The secondary form is best illustrated by the bacilluria of typhoid fever. In the cases in which there is no recognizable cause or primary focus, the colon bacillus and streptococci are the commonest organisms. The bacilli may come directly from the blood, as in typhoid fever, and probably multiply in the urinary passages, or they may come from a focus of infection anywhere from Bowman's capsule to the prostate.

Clinically there are two groups of cases, bacilluria pure and simple and bacilluric cystitis or pyelitis. In the former there may be no symptoms; the urine may have a slight haziness due to the enormous number of organisms but there is no pus. In the other there are signs of inflammatory reaction in the urinary passages with pus. Usually with the *B. coli* infection the urine is acid, with the staphylococcus alkaline and often with marked phosphaturia. The cases are often very intractable. Without cystitis or pyelitis there may be no symptoms, but in many instances there are all the phenomena of these affections. Many cases clear up rapidly with hexamine (methenamine). Vaccine therapy has been used but not with very good results.

PYURIA

Causes.—(*a*) Pyelitis and Pyelonephritis.—In large abscesses of the kidney the pus may be intermittent, while in calculus and tuberculous pyelitis the pyuria is usually continuous, though varying in intensity. In cases due to the colon or tubercle bacillus the urine is acid, in those due to the proteus bacillus alkaline, while in staphylococcus cases the urine is either less acid than normal or alkaline. In pyelitis and pyelonephritis following cystitis the urine is alkaline or acid, depending upon the infecting organism; more mucus, frequent micturition, and a previous bladder history are aids in diagnosis. H. Cabot points out that if the fresh urine shows cocci in abundance, with a small amount of albumin, few red blood cells, many leukocytes or a little pus, and the renal function near normal, it is probably a coccus infection and mostly in the cortex. If there are many bacilli, little albumin, much pus and greatly decreased renal function it is probably a colon bacillus infection with the first effect on the convoluted tubes and the lesion of the pelvis secondary.

(*b*) CYSTITIS.—The urine is usually acid, especially in women, since the colon bacillus is a very common cause of these infections. The pus and mucus are more ropy, and triple phosphate crystals are found in the freshly passed urine in the alkaline infections. Pus may come from the prostate.

(*c*) URETHRITIS, particularly gonorrhea. The pus appears first, is in small quantities, and there are signs of local inflammation.

(*d*) In LEUKORRHEA the quantity of pus is usually small, and large flakes of vaginal epithelium are numerous. In doubtful cases, when leukorrhea is present, the urine should be withdrawn through a catheter.

(*e*) RUPTURE OF ABSCESSES INTO THE URINARY PASSAGES.—In such cases as pelvic or perityphlitic abscess there have been previous symptoms of pus formation. A large amount is passed within a short time, then the discharge stops abruptly or rapidly diminishes within a few days.

Pus gives to the urine a white or yellowish-white appearance. On settling, the sediment is sometimes ropy, the supernatant fluid usually turbid. In cases due to urea-decomposing microbes (proteus bacillus, various staphylococci) the odor may be ammoniacal even in fresh urine. The pus cells are usually well formed when the pus comes from the bladder; the protoplasm is granular, and often shows many translucent processes.

The only sediment likely to be confounded with pus is that of the phosphates; but it is whiter and less dense, and is distinguished immediately by microscopic examination or by the addition of acid. With the pus there is always more or less epithelium from the bladder and pelves of the kidneys, but since in these situations the forms of cells are practically identical, they afford no information as to the locality from which the pus has come.

The treatment is considered under the conditions in which pyuria occurs.

CHYLURIA—NONPARASITIC

This is a rare affection, occurring in temperate regions and unassociated with *Filaria*. The urine is of an opaque white color; it resembles milk, is occasionally mixed with blood (hematochyluria), and sometimes coagulates into a jelly-like mass. In other instances there is at the bottom of the vessel a loose clot which may be distinctly blood tinged. The turbidity seems to be caused by numerous minute granules—more rarely oil droplets similar to those of milk. The urine may be much more milky shortly after taking food, and the recumbent posture increases the milkiness. In one case the urine became chylous in the bladder, and Hertz found obstruction of the thoracic duct and a communicating ruptured lymphatic vessel in the bladder.

LITHURIA

The general relations of uric acid have been considered under gout.

Occurrence in the Urine.—The uric acid occurs in combination chiefly with ammonium and sodium, forming the acid urates. In smaller quantities are the potassium, calcium and lithium salts. The uric acid may be separated from its bases and crystallize in rhombs or prisms, usually of a deep red color, owing to the staining of the urinary pigments. The sediment is granular and the crystals look like grains of Cayenne pepper. It is important not to mistake a deposit of uric acid for an excess. The deposition of uric acid in the urine is due to conditions which diminish the solvent power rather than to increase in the quantity. Of the conditions which cause precipitation of uric acid Roberts gives the following: "(1) High acidity; (2) poverty in mineral salts; (3) low pigmentation; and (4) high percentage of uric acid." The acidity is probably the most important.

In health the amount of uric acid excreted bears a fairly constant ratio to the urea eliminated. The average ratio is 1 to 50, while the average ratio of the nitrogen of uric acid to the total nitrogen in the urine is 1 to 70. In several cases of gout Futcher found that in the intervals between acute attacks the uric acid was reduced to a much greater extent than the urea, so that the ratio of the former to the latter often varied between 1 to 300 up to (in one case) 1 to 1,500, a return to about the normal proportions occurring during the acute attacks.

More common is the precipitation of amorphous urates, forming the so-called brick-dust deposit, which has a pinkish color, due to urinary pigment. It is composed chiefly of the acid sodium urates. It occurs particularly in very acid urine of a high specific gravity. As the urates are more soluble in warm solutions, they often deposit as the urine cools. This usually does not mean excessive excretion, but conditions favoring the deposit.

Treatment.—Meat, fish, tea and coffee should be excluded from the diet and the patient drink water freely. Alkalies and salicylic acid may be given.

OXALURIA

The discovery of calcium oxalate crystals in the urine by Donné in 1838 led to the description of the so-called oxalic acid diathesis. It is claimed that all the oxalic acid in the urine enters the body with the food (Dunlop). In health none, or only a trace, is formed in the body. The amount fluctuates with the food taken, and is usually below 10 milligrams daily (H. Baldwin). It seems to be formed in the body when there is an absence of free hydrochloric acid in the gastric juice, and in connection with excessive fermentation in the intestines. It never forms a heavy deposit.

When in excess and present for any considerable time, the condition is known as *oxaluria*, the chief interest of which is in the fact that the crystals may be deposited before the urine is voided, and form a *calculus*. Some hold that there is a special diathesis associated with its presence in excess and manifested by dyspepsia, irritability, depression, lassitude, and sometimes marked hypochondriasis. There may be in addition neuralgic pains and general nervous symptoms. These symptoms are probably dependent upon some disturbance of metabolism of which the oxaluria is a manifestation. It is a feature in many gouty persons and in the condition called lithemia.

Treatment.—Water should be taken freely. In the diet the following should be avoided: spinach, rhubarb, strawberries, cranberries, asparagus, radish, horse-radish, grapes and currants.

CYSTINURIA

This rare condition, an "inborn error of metabolism" (Garrod), is of clinical importance because cystin is very sparingly soluble and calculi may be formed, renal or vesical. It is strongly hereditary and has been traced through three generations. The quantity excreted is 0.3 to 0.5 gram per diem, and the excretion persists for years, or even for life. Cystin is an aminoderivative of thiolactic acid in which two molecules are linked together by their sulphur atoms. In the urinary sediment the colorless hexagonal crystals of cystin are readily detected. In some cases there is also the excretion of diamines (cadaverin and putrescin) in the urine and feces.

Treatment.—This involves a decreased production of cystin by reducing the amount of protein in the diet and an increased solubility in the urine by giving sodium bicarbonate (90 to 150 grains, 6 to 10 gms. a day).

PHOSPHATURIA

Phosphoric acid is excreted from the body in combination with potassium, sodium, calcium and magnesium, forming two classes, the alkaline phosphates of sodium and potassium and the earthy phosphates of lime and magnesia. The amount of phosphoric acid (P_2O_5) excreted in the twenty-four hours varies between 1 and 5 grams, with an average of 2.5 grams. It is derived mainly from phosphoric acid in the food, but also as a decomposition product from nuclein, protagon and lecithin. Of the alkaline phosphates, those in combination with sodium are the most abundant. The alkaline phosphates are more abundant than the earthy phosphates.

Of the *earthy phosphates,* those of lime are abundant, of magnesium scanty. In urine which has undergone ammoniacal fermentation, either in- or outside the body, there is in addition the ammonio-magnesium or triple phosphate. The earthy phosphates occur as a sediment when the alkalinity is due to a fixed alkali, or under certain circumstances the deposit may take place within the bladder, and then the phosphates are passed at the end of micturition as a whitish fluid, popularly confounded with spermatorrhea. Study of patients with symptoms of neurasthenia and a phosphate sediment in the fresh urine indicates an abnormality in the calcium metabolism, an absolute increase of this with a decrease of the phosphoric acid. The calcium phosphate may be precipitated by heat and produce a cloudiness which may be mistaken for albumin, but is dissolved upon making the urine acid. This is frequent in persons suffering from dyspepsia or debility. The phosphates may be deposited in urine which has undergone decomposition, in which the carbonate of ammonia from the urea combines with the magnesium phosphates. This is seen in *cystitis,* due to a urea decomposing microbe.

The clinical significance of an excess of phosphates, to which the term *phosphaturia* is applied, has been much discussed. A deposit does not necessarily mean an excess, to determine which a careful analysis of the twenty-four hours' urine should be made. The amount is increased in wasting diseases, such as tuberculosis, acute yellow atrophy of the liver, leukemia and severe anemia and diminished in acute diseases and during pregnancy.

Teisser, of Lyons, in 1876, described a condition to which he gave the name of "essential phosphaturia," also called "phosphatic diabetes," the symptoms of which are polyuria, thirst, emaciation, and a great increase in the excretion of phosphates, which may rise to 7 to 9 grams a day. The condition sometimes simulates diabetes very closely, even to the pruritus and dry skin. In a case of this kind, Barker found the metabolism normal for carbohydrates, but the organic phosphorus percentage was high; the chief abnormality was an abnormally large amount of organic acids.

INDICANURIA

Indican is the indoxyl-sulphate of potassium, in which form it appears in the urine and is colorless. When concentrated acids or strong oxidizing agents are added to the urine, this substance is decomposed and the indigo set free. It is derived from indol, formed in the intestine by the decomposition of protein under the influence of bacteria. When absorbed, this is oxidized in the tissues to indoxyl, which combines with potassium sulphate, forming indican.

It is often found in persons of good health or with slight digestive complaints. It is not specially associated with constipation (Allen Jones). In gall stone attacks, hyperchlorhydria, wasting diseases, peritonitis and empyema it is usually present. In a few cases it is constantly present and in excess. Barr found only 32 such cases among 2,092 patients, and in these the symptoms did not suggest "intestinal auto-intoxication," nor did lactobacillary treatment have the slightest influence on the condition.

Indican has occasionally been found in calculi. Though, as a rule, the urine is colorless when passed, there are instances in which decomposition has taken place within the body, and a blue color is noticed immediately after the urine is voided. Sometimes in alkaline urine on exposure there is a bluish film on the surface. Methylene blue must be excluded.

MELANURIA

"Black urine" may be dark when passed or may become so later. In the following conditions melanuria may occur: (1) *Jaundice.* Only in very chronic cases of deeply bronzed icterus is the urine quite dark. (2) *Hematuria* and *hemoglobinuria.* Here it is an exaggeration of the smoky tint due to the presence of blood. (3) *Hematoporphyrinuria.* (4) Melanuria, in which the urine has, as a rule, the normal color when passed, and on standing becomes black as ink. In some instances it is black when passed. Melanuria of this type only occurs with the presence of melanotic tumors. (5) *Alkaptonuria.* (6) *Indicanuria.* When rich in indoxyl sulphate the urine is brown or becomes so after standing, due to the oxidation products of indol. In any disease leading to an abundant secretion of indican, as intestinal obstruction, black urine may be passed. As Garrod suggests, it is probable that black urine in tuberculosis is of an allied nature. (7) After certain articles of *diet* and *drugs.* Some dark colored pigments, as in black cherries, plums and bilberries, cause darkening of the urine. Resorcin may do the same. Carboluria has been ascribed to hydrochinone formed from phenol. Naphthalene, creosote and the salicylates may cause darkening of the urine, or even blackness.

ALKAPTONURIA

"Alkaptonuria is not the manifestation of a disease, but is rather of the nature of an alternative course of metabolism, harmless and usually congenital and lifelong" (Garrod). It is an anomaly which may be regarded as "a rare recessive character in the Mendelian sense." The tyrosin in the protein molecule is not completely broken down and the intermediate product, homogentisic acid, is found in the urine. There are two points of clinical interest. The alkapton urine reduces Fehling's solution, and diabetes may be suggested, but it does not ferment, and is optically inactive. The linen may be stained by the urine, which in some cases is dark when passed. In 1866 Virchow described blackening of the cartilages and ligaments—*ochronosis.*

PNEUMATURIA

Gas may be passed with the urine: (1) After mechanical introduction of air in vesical irrigation or cystoscopic examination. (2) As a result of infection with gas forming organisms. Glycosuria has been present in a majority of the cases. The yeast fungus, the colon bacillus and the gas bacillus have been found. (3) In cases of vesico-enteric fistula.

In gas production within the bladder the symptoms are those of a mild cystitis, with the passage of gas at the end of micturition, sometimes with a loud sound. The diagnosis is readily made by causing the patient to urinate in a bath or by plunging the end of the catherer under water.

OTHER SUBSTANCES

Lipuria.—Fat in the urine, or lipuria, occurs, first, without disease of the kidneys, as in excess of fat in the food, after administration of cod-liver oil, in fat embolism occurring after fractures, in the fatty degeneration in phosphorus poisoning, in prolonged suppuration, as in tuberculosis and pyemia, in the lipemia of diabetes mellitus; secondly, with disease of the kidneys, as in nephrosis; and thirdly, in chyluria. The urine is usually turbid but there may be fat drops as well, and fatty crystals have been found. In a few instances calculi form composed of fat and coated with phosphates.

Pentosuria.—This may be a familial anomaly or follow the eating of certain fruits or drinking of fruit juices. The subjects are usually regarded as diabetics, an error avoided by the special tests for the pentoses.

Lipaciduria is applied to the condition in which there are volatile fatty acids in the urine, such as acetic, butyric, formic, and propionic acid.

Ketonuria.—The occurrence of *acetone, diacetic acid,* and *β-oxybutyric acid* has been considered under Diabetes.

Hematoporphyria.—The porphyrins are colored compounds, close to hematin and bilirubin, which may be the parent substances. Porphyrin may be an intermediate product in the conversion of hemoglobin to bilirubin. They occur in traces in normal urine (uroporphyrin and coproporphyrin), feces and bile, and in larger amounts in pulmonary tuberculosis, pleurisy with effusion, lead poisoning, etc. The *congenital* form is very rare. It is a family disease and occurs most often in males. The urine is red or sometimes brown. There may be brown pigmentation of the bones and a pink color of the enamel of the milk teeth. The spleen may be enlarged. A serious feature is the occurrence of hydroa vacciniforme which recurs year after year. Bullae may form on the conjunctivae and blindness result. In some cases the disease occurs in acute forms (acute toxic and acute idiopathic) with toxic symptoms, severe abdominal pain, and an ascending paralysis (much like Landry's paralysis) which may prove fatal.

Hematoporphyrinuria.—This usually results in females from the taking of sulphonal, more rarely trional, over long periods as a rule. The urine has a color like port wine. The outlook is serious. The drug should be stopped and sodium bicarbonate and calcium given in full doses.

Tyrosinosis.—Under this term, Medes (1932) describes an error in the metabolism of tyrosine. The substance excreted is p-hydroxyphenylpyruvic acid. It does not cause pigmentation, as ochronosis, but reduces copper solutions.

UREMIA

Definition.—A symptom-complex due to toxemia from renal insufficiency developing in the course of nephritis. The nature of the toxin is in doubt.

Etiology.—This has been and is the subject of much investigation. It seems probable that the factors are not the same in all cases; there may be several toxins concerned and such factors as acidosis and vascular disease, especially of the cerebral vessels, are not constant. The general metabolism is disturbed with results which we can estimate only partially. Some of the theories are as follows:

(1) Historically the view that retention of *urea* is responsible came first as the name implies. The picture seen in anuria, which causes extreme nitrogen retention, is not that of uremia. But it is difficult to exclude urea retention as having no part. Quite marked symptoms were experienced by Hewlett and his coworkers following the ingestion of large amounts of urea. Canti found the amount of urea to be uniform in the various body fluids, including edema fluid. In the cerebrospinal fluid an increase of urea is always found and Canti considered that increase in the nonprotein nitrogen above 0.2 per cent in this fluid means uremia. If it was 0.3 per cent or over, death followed. It is evident that because increase in urea is found it is not necessarily the cause of uremia. (2) That it is due to disturbance of an internal secretion of the kidney; of this there is no evidence. (3) That it is due to *nephrolysins;* for this evidence is lacking. (4) The view put forward by Traube that the important factor is *edema* of the brain. This is found but may be part of a general edema

due to failure of the circulation with myocardial insufficiency—a passive edema. It may play a part, as edema of the brain is found in the form of uremia in which coma is a marked feature. The improvement in such cases which may result from lumbar puncture is to be noted. (5) *Acidosis* is often associated and undoubtedly is responsible for some of the symptoms but can not be regarded as the cause. There is evidence that the toxins are in colloid combinations and so influenced by hydrogen ion concentration. (6) Disturbance of metabolism may result in the production of toxins. It has been stated that trimethylamine is found in the blood in increased amounts; it is responsible for the curious odor usually associated with uremia. (7) Foster isolated from the blood of patients with uremia of the convulsive form a toxic base of undetermined chemical structure, which causes convulsions and death in animals. Probably several factors are concerned in many cases.

Foster described three forms of uremia, but the majority of cases are not uncomplicated. (1) *Retention* form. In this there is a simple retention of urinary nitrogenous waste—a urinary poisoning. (2) *Cerebral edema* form. In this there is defective water and salt excretion with a resulting cerebral edema. (3) *Toxic* or *epileptiform* form. In this toxemia is marked, the result of abnormal metabolism. The first two represent a failure of excretion of water, salt and nitrogenous material. The third may show these but also a toxic base which causes convulsive seizures in animals. Hewlett showed that urea in the blood in amounts over 150 mg. per 100 cc. produces symptoms like some of those in uremia.

It seems best with our present knowledge to regard the essential cause to be toxins, due to retention and probably to disturbed metabolism, with added factors such as acidosis, cerebral edema and vascular disease. To which perhaps should be added in some cases, the influence of terminal infections. The only form in which complete recovery may result is that manifested especially by convulsions and amaurosis. Certain manifestations often regarded as uremic evidently are due to cardiovascular disease and hypertension ("hypertensive encephalopathy") and some designate them as "false uremia." Both varieties of disturbance may be present in the patient.

Pathology.—There are no findings characteristic of uremia. The renal lesions are not peculiar. There may be ulceration of the lower bowel. The degree of cerebral edema is variable and it is not always present. In some cases of uremia with convulsions hyperemia of the brain with minute hemorrhages through the substance has been found.

Symptoms.—These are shown in remarkable variety and many combinations are seen; some are more or less constant while others are rarer. The cerebral, respiratory and gastro-intestinal manifestations are the most important. In general certain forms can be recognized: (1) In that with convulsions, often acute, headache, amaurosis and coma occur and recovery may follow. (2) Coma of slow onset is the most striking feature, perhaps with dyspnea, Cheyne-Stokes breathing and acidosis. (3) Marked psychical disturbance, hallucinations, delusions, mental dullness, gastro-intestinal disturbances are the features with coma as a terminal event. A division into acute and chronic forms is convenient but, in all, disturbance in the nervous system is prominent.

Among the CEREBRAL symptoms are: (*a*) *Maniacal.*—These may come on abruptly in an individual who has shown no indications of mental trouble, and who may not be known to have nephritis. In one such case the patient became suddenly maniacal and died in six days. More commonly the delirium is less violent, but the patient is noisy, talkative, restless and sleepless.

(*b*) *Delusional Psychosis.*—Cases are by no means uncommon, and excellent clinical reports have been issued on the subject. Delusions of persecution are common and the patients may commit suicide. The condition is of interest medicolegally because of its bearing on testamentary capacity. Profound melancholia may also supervene.

(*c*) *Convulsions.*—These may come on unexpectedly or be preceded by headache, muscular twitching and restlessness. The attacks may be general and identical with those of epilepsy, though the initial cry may not be present. The fits may recur rapidly, and in the interval the patient is usually unconscious. Sometimes the temperature is elevated, but more frequently it is low and may sink rapidly after the attack. Local convulsions may occur in most characteristic form. A remarkable sequence of the convulsions is blindness—*uremic amaurosis*—which may persist for several days. This may occur apart from the convulsions and usually passes off in a day or two. There are, as a rule, no ophthalmoscopic changes. Sometimes uremic deafness supervenes and is probably also a cerebral manifestation. It may also occur with persistent headache, nausea and other gastric symptoms.

(*d*) *Coma.*—Unconsciousness invariably accompanies the general convulsions but coma may develop gradually without any convulsive seizures. Frequently it is preceded by headache, and the patient gradually becomes dull and apathetic. In these cases there may have been no previous indications of renal disease, and unless the urine is examined the nature of the case may be overlooked. Twitchings of the muscles occur, particularly in the face and hands, but there are many cases of coma in which the muscles are not involved. In some cases a condition of torpor persists for weeks or even months. The tongue is usually furred and the breath foul and heavy.

(*e*) *Local Palsies.*—In the course of chronic nephritis, hemiplegia, aphasia or monoplegia may come on spontaneously or follow a convulsion, and postmortem no gross lesions of the brain be found, but only a localized or diffuse edema. These cases may simulate almost every form of organic paralysis of cerebral origin. They are probably due to vascular changes but, in view of the temporary character, their nature is not easy to determine.

(*f*) Of other cerebral symptoms, HEADACHE is important. It is often occipital and extends to the neck. It may be an early feature and associated with giddiness. Other nervous symptoms are intense itching of the skin, numbness and tingling in the fingers, and cramps in the muscles of the calves, particularly at night. An erythema may be present.

UREMIC DYSPNEA was classified by Palmer Howard as follows: (*a*) Continuous dyspnea; (*b*) paroxysmal dyspnea; (*c*) both types alternating; and (*d*) Cheyne-Stokes breathing. The alkalinity of the blood is diminished. The acidosis is due to a nonvolatile acid and to the failure of the kidney to excrete acid sodium phosphate. The paroxysmal attacks of dyspnea are most commonly nocturnal; the patient may gasp for breath and show great distress. Occasionally the breathing is noisy and stridulous and sometimes has a hissing character. The Cheyne-Stokes type may persist for weeks or months. One patient, up and about, could feed himself only in the apnea period. Though usually serious and occurring with coma and other symptoms, recovery may follow even after persistence for a long period.

The relationship of *edema* is important. In some cases of nephritis with edema in which diuresis occurs, uremia follows the disappearance of the edema. It may also result from restriction of the fluid intake, suggesting in both cases a greater concentration of toxins in the blood and tissues.

The GASTRO-INTESTINAL manifestations often set in with abruptness. Uncontrollable vomiting may come on and its cause be quite unrecognized. The vomitus contains considerable amounts of urea. The attacks may be preceded by nausea and associated with diarrhea. The *diarrhea* may come on without the vomiting; sometimes it is profuse and associated with inflammation of the colon. Ulceration and intestinal hemorrhage may result.

A special UREMIC STOMATITIS has been described in which the mucosa of the lips, gums, and tongue is swollen and erythematous. The saliva may be decreased, and there is difficulty in swallowing and in mastication. The tongue is usually very foul and the breath heavy and fetid. There may be a tenacious coating in the mouth, pharynx and trachea. A cutaneous erythema may occur and a remarkable urea "frost" on the skin.

FEVER is not uncommon in uremic states, and may occur with the acute nephritis, with the complications, and as a manifestation of uremia itself.

Very many patients with chronic uremia succumb to terminal infections—acute peritonitis, pericarditis, pleurisy, meningitis or endocarditis.

Diagnosis.—Blood analyses are of great value, both for diagnosis and prognosis. Nonprotein nitrogen above 120 mg., urea nitrogen above 80 mg., uric acid above 6 mg., and creatinine above 4 mg. per 100 cc. of blood are significant. The estimation of the urea in the saliva is useful as its urea content increases with that of the blood. The maximum normal urea and ammonia nitrogen in the saliva is 16 mg. per 100 cc. corresponding to 20 mg. of *urea nitrogen* per 100 cc. of blood. In the "edema form" there may not be any increase. The test of renal function by phenolsulphonephthalein is of value both in diagnosis and in giving warning of impending uremia. In uremia the elimination of phthalein is nil or only a faint trace in two hours. In patients with chronic nephritis in whom the elimination in two hours is below 10 per cent there is danger of uremia.

Uremia may be confounded with:

(*a*) *Cerebral* lesions, such as hemorrhage, embolism, thrombosis, encephalitis, meningitis or tumor. In hemorrhage, so common in nephritis with hypertension, the sudden loss of consciousness, particularly if with convulsions, may simulate uremia; but the mode of onset, the complete hemiplegia, and conjugate deviation of the eyes, suggest hemorrhage. There are cases of uremic hemiplegia or monoplegia which can not be separated from those of organic lesion and which postmortem show no trace of coarse disease of the brain. In some cases it is impossible to distinguish between the two conditions. Lumbar puncture is of great aid, as it may show blood in the fluid in hemorrhage; the presence of urea in large amounts (over 0.2 per cent) suggests uremia. Cases of meningitis, in deep coma, with slight fever, furred tongue, but no localizing symptoms, may be regarded as uremia.

(*b*) Certain *infectious* diseases. Uremia may persist for weeks or months and the patient lies in a condition of torpor or coma, with a heavily coated, perhaps dry, tongue, muscular twitchings, a rapid feeble pulse, with slight fever. This naturally suggests one of the infectious diseases. Cases of this kind have been mistaken for typhoid fever and miliary tuberculosis.

(*c*) Uremic *coma* may be confounded with poisoning by alcohol or opium. In opium poisoning the respiration is slow and the pupils contracted; in alcoholism they are more commonly dilated. In uremia they are not constant; they may be widely dilated or of medium size. The examination of the eye grounds determines the presence of albuminuric retinitis. The urine should be examined. The odor of the breath sometimes gives an important hint. The condition of the heart and arteries should also be taken into account. Sudden uremic coma is more common in chronic interstitial nephritis. The character of the delirium in alcoholism is sometimes important, and the coma is not so deep as in uremia or opium poisoning. It may for a time be impossible to determine whether the condition is due to uremia, profound alcoholism or hemorrhage. In sudden coma, it is to be remembered that insensibility may occur after prolonged muscular exertion, as in a long race, with stertorous breathing and dilated pupils. Cases have occurred when sunstroke could be excluded; the condition may be due to the too rapid accumulation of waste products with hyperpyrexia from suspension of sweating.

(*d*) In patients with *myocardial failure* the features of this may lead to the missing of the signs of uremia. With marked dyspnea the absence of sufficient causal circulatory factors should excite suspicion. With vomiting or diarrhea as the prominent feature only a thorough study may give the correct diagnosis.

(*e*) *Vascular Disease.*—It may be difficult to decide how much this is responsible for the symptoms. The examination of the eye grounds may be of aid. In many cases the causes are multiple.

(*f*) The coma of diabetes mellitus and hypoglycemia should not give difficulty.

The treatment will be considered under Chronic Nephritis (page 703).

ACUTE NEPHRITIS

Definition.—Acute diffuse nephritis, due to infection or to the action of toxic agents upon the kidneys. In all instances changes exist in the epithelial, vascular and intertubular tissues, which vary in intensity in different forms: hence tubular, glomerular and acute interstitial forms are described. As the most striking changes are in the glomeruli, the term glomerulonephritis is commonly used.

When we employ the term "acute nephritis," it is well to keep in mind that we are discussing the first stages of a process which may pass on to subacute and chronic stages. In some cases the condition may clear and the patient recovers or the early acute stages may be overlooked and the disease is recognized first in a subacute or chronic stage. While we use certain designations for nephritis it is well to realize that all cases can not be put in definite categories. It is more important to recognize and understand the conditions in a given patient than to place his malady under some particular part of a classification.

There are two main forms of acute nephritis which may be described as (1) edematous and (2) hemorrhagic. A third form, less important, termed focal embolic glomerulonephritis, occurs with subacute bacterial endocarditis.

Etiology.—The following are the principal causes of acute nephritis:

(1) *Cold.*—Exposure to cold and wet is given as a common cause and determines, possibly in a few cases, an acute attack but more often this represents an exacerbation of existing disease.

(2) The organisms or toxins of the acute infections, particularly scarlet fever. In young children pneumococcus infection may be responsible. Many cases are due to streptococcus infection, as in the tonsils. An acute hematogenous infection may cause a severe nephritis and all grades of severity may occur. Syphilis is a factor in some cases. In exudative erythema and purpuric affections acute nephritis is not uncommon.

(3) *Epidemic Nephritis.*—Described first during the American Civil War and noted by Italian observers, it prevailed widely during the Great War (trench nephritis). This was generally the hemorrhagic variety.

(4) *Toxic agents,* such as turpentine, potassium chlorate and phenol may cause an acute congestion which sometimes terminates in nephritis. Alcohol probably never excites an acute nephritis.

(5) Acute nephritis occurs occasionally in connection with extensive lesions of the skin, as in burns or in chronic skin diseases, and also after trauma. It may follow operations on the kidney.

There is often a latent period in the occurrence of acute diffuse nephritis. In scarlet fever nephritis occurs usually about the third week and when secondary to throat infection after an interval of 10 to 20 days. It is suggested that allergy may play a part in this. The views as to the process involved are: (1) Toxic. The kidney lesion is regarded as due to the effect of toxins. (2) Ischemia. This may be due to active constriction or swelling of the endothelium of the capillaries. (3) Capillary damage. This may be part of widespread injury to the capillaries, the glomerulus showing marked damage. It may be that more than one process is concerned.

Morbid Anatomy.—The kidneys may present in mild cases no evident gross alterations. When seen early in more severe forms the organs are congested, swollen, dark, and on section may drip blood. In other instances the surface is pale and mottled, the capsule strips off readily, and the cortex is swollen, turbid, and of a grayish red color, while the pyramids have an intense beefy red tint. The glomeruli may stand out plainly, being deeply swollen and congested; in other instances they are pale.

The histology may be thus summarized: (*a*) *Glomerular changes.* The tufts suffer first, and there is either an acute intracapillary glomerulitis, in which the capillaries become filled with cells and thrombi, or involvement of the epithelium of the tuft and of Bowman's capsule, the cavity of which contains leukocytes and red blood corpuscles.

(*b*) *The alterations in the tubular epithelium consist* in cloudy swelling, fatty change and hyaline degeneration. In the convoluted tubules, the accumulation of altered cells with leukocytes and red blood corpuscles causes the enlargement and swelling of the organ.

(*c*) *Interstitial changes.* In the milder forms a simple inflammatory exudate —serum mixed with leukocytes and red blood corpuscles—exists between the tubules. In severer cases areas of small celled infiltration occur about the capsules and between the convoluted tubes.

Symptoms.—*Acute Diffuse Glomerulonephritis.*—The *onset* is usually sudden, and when the nephritis follows cold, edema may be noticed within twenty-four hours. After fevers the onset is less abrupt, but the patient gradually becomes pale and a puffiness of the face or swelling of the ankles is first noticed. In children there may be convulsions at the outset. Chilliness or rigors initiate the attack in a limited number of cases. The onset may be insidious with headache, nausea, vomiting and general malaise. The fever is variable. In young children with nephritis from cold or scarlet fever the temperature may, for a few days, range from 101° to 103°.

The most characteristic features are the *urinary changes.* There may at first be suppression; more commonly the urine is scanty, highly colored, and contains blood, albumin and casts. The quantity is reduced and only 4 or 5 ounces may be passed in twenty-four hours; the specific gravity is high—1.025, or more; the color varies from a smoky to a deep porter color, but is seldom bright red. On standing there is a heavy deposit; microscopically there are blood corpuscles, epithelium from the urinary passages, and hyaline, blood and epithelial casts. The albumin is abundant, forming a curdy, thick precipitate. Large amounts are seen in the acute nephritis of syphilis. The excretion of urea is reduced, though the percentage is high.

Edema is an early and often a marked feature. In cases of extensive dropsy effusion may take place into the plurae and peritoneum. There are cases of scarlatinal nephritis in which the edema of the extremities is trivial and effusion into the plurae extensive. The lungs may become edematous. In rare cases there is edema of the glottis. Epistaxis may occur or cutaneous ecchymoses may develop in the course of the disease.

The pulse may be hard, the tension increased, and the second sound in the aortic area accentuated. The blood pressure is variable but often increased. Occasionally dilatation of the heart comes on rapidly and may cause sudden death. The skin is dry and it may be difficult to induce sweating.

Uremic symptoms occur in a limited number of cases, either at the onset with suppression, more commonly later in the disease. Ocular changes are not so common in acute as in chronic nephritis, but hemorrhagic retinitis may occur and occasionally papillitis.

The *course* varies considerably. The description just given is of the form which most commonly follows scarlet fever. In many of the febrile cases dropsy is not prominent, and the diagnosis rests rather with the examination of the urine. Moreover, the condition may be transient and less serious. In other cases there may be hematuria and pronounced interference with the renal function. The most intense acute nephritis may exist without anasarca. In *scarlatinal* nephritis, in which the glomeruli are most seriously affected, suppression of urine may be an early symptom, the edema is apt to be extreme, and uremic manifestations are common. Acute nephritis in children may set in very insidiously with transient or slight edema, and the symptoms may point rather to the digestive system or to brain disease.

Hemorrhagic Nephritis.—This occurs especially with streptococcus infections, particularly of the upper respiratory tract. The pathology is described by Fahr as "a diffuse capillaritis of the glomerular loops." Small punctate hemorrhages may be seen on the cut surface of the kidney. The *symptoms* may be slight; fatigue, anorexia and headache may be the complaints. Edema is slight or absent. There may be slight fever, increased pulse rate and a mild leukocytosis. In the early stages the urinary findings may not be distinctive but show only an acute process. The predominance of red blood cells and their persistence are suggestive. The amount of urine may not be greatly decreased. The renal function is altered but slightly. The edema is usually of short duration and the albuminuria lessens but the red blood cells persist in the urine. Many patients recover after several weeks but in others the red cells may be found for a long time representing a subacute stage. It rarely becomes chronic. In some patients a focus of infection may be responsible for a recurrence and in many instances this is in the tonsils.

Embolic Focal Nephritis.—This occurs with subacute bacterial endocarditis due to *Streptococcus viridans* infection. Vegetations from the valves block the artery to a glomerulus or some of the glomerular loops. The occurrence of red blood cells in the urine is the main manifestation. Albuminuria is usual. There is no edema or change in renal function.

Diagnosis.—It is very important to bear in mind that the most serious involvement of the kidneys may be manifested only by slight edema of the feet or puffiness of the eyelids, without impairment of the general health. On the other hand, from the urine alone a diagnosis can not be made with certainty, since simple cloudy swelling and circulatory changes may cause a similar condition of urine. The first indication may be a uremic convulsion, particularly in the acute nephritis of pregnancy, and the practitioner should examine the urine regularly during pregnancy.

In nephritis in scarlet fever the symptoms are usually marked and the diagnosis is rarely in doubt. Every case in which albumin is present should not be called acute nephritis, not even if casts be present. The common febrile albuminuria, although it represents the first link in the chain of events leading to acute nephritis, should not be placed in the same category. The most frequent error is to regard *acute exacerbations* in chronic nephritis as primary acute attacks. The history, the condition of the heart and vessels, the blood pressure and the eyegrounds are important points in recognizing the existence of former nephritis. However there are cases in which it is very difficult to decide this point; they should be treated as acute nephritis.

There are occasional cases of acute nephritis with anasarca, in which albumin is absent or present only as a trace, but these are rare. Casts are usually found, and the absence of albumin is rarely permanent. The urine may be reduced in amount.

The character of the casts is of use in the diagnosis of the form of nephritis, but scarcely of such value as has been stated. The hyaline and granular casts are common to all varieties. The blood and epithelial casts, particularly leukocyte casts, are most common in acute cases.

The *hemorrhagic* form may not be recognized unless a careful urinary study is made. The persistence of red blood cells in the urine after the acute features of the attack are over is suggestive. *Pyelitis* may give difficulty at the onset but there is rarely edema with it and the urinary findings are helpful.

Prognosis.—The outlook varies somewhat with the cause. Recoveries in the form following exposure to cold are much more frequent than after scarlatinal nephritis. In younger children the mortality is high. Serious features are low arterial tension, uremia, and effusion into the serous sacs. The persistence of edema after the first month, pallor, and a large amount of albumin indicate the possibility of the disease becoming chronic. For some months after the disappearance of edema there may be traces of albumin and a few casts. If the nephritis is due to a focus of infection which can be removed the outlook is naturally better. The blood chemistry is of value as indicating the degree of retention, and the functional tests aid in estimating improvement in the working of the kidney.

In scarlatinal nephritis, if the progress is favorable, the edema diminishes in a week or ten days, the urine increases, the albumin lessens, and by the end of a month the dropsy has disappeared and the urine is nearly free. In very young children the course may be rapid, and the urine may be free from albumin in the fourth week. Other cases are more insidious, and though the dropsy may disappear, the albumin persists in the urine, the anemia is marked, and the condition becomes chronic, or, after several recurrences of the dropsy, improves and complete recovery takes place.

Prophylaxis.—Care is important in the infectious diseases which may be complicated by nephritis. Proper treatment of foci of infection, especially the tonsils, is of value. Care should be taken not to give any drugs which may irritate the kidney.

Treatment.—The indications are: (1) To remove the cause if possible; (2) to lessen the work of the kidney; (3) to aid elimination by the bowels; and (4) to meet symptoms as they arise. The patient should be in bed and remain there until all traces of the disease have disappeared or until there is no hope of complete recovery. A period of three months should be allowed for this. The presence of red blood cells in the urine is an indication for absolute rest. The patient should be clad in flannel. Any focus of infection should be removed.

Diet.—It is well to restrict the diet for some days to fruit juices, sugar and water. Barley water, lactose and cream may be added later. For children some form of candy made of sugar, butter and perhaps a small amount of cream is a welcome addition. Whey is useful and later milk may be given in small amounts. Broths and beef tea should not be given. As convalescence is established, bread and butter, lettuce and green vegetables, grapes, oranges and other fruit may be given. Meats should not be given for some time. As there is marked retention of the chlorides, which bear a relation to the edema, salt should be withheld. With vomiting, glucose solution (10 per cent) may be given intravenously twice a day (300 cc.) or by bowel (5 per cent solution).

The *fluid* intake must be governed by the condition. With edema it is well to restrict the total intake to 700 to 1000 cc. Otherwise the patient may drink freely of alkaline waters, ordinary water or lemonade. A useful drink is a dram of cream of tartar in a pint of boiling water with the juice of half a lemon and a little sugar. Taken cold, this is a pleasant drink. Alkaline drinks are useful if there is acidosis. Fluid may be given by the bowel or subcutaneously if it is not well taken by mouth.

No remedies control directly the changes in the kidneys, unless in syphilis.

At the onset, when there is pain in the back or hematuria, the use of dry cups is advisable and hot poultices are often useful. In cases which set in with suppression of urine these measures should be adopted, and in addition a hot bath or hot pack and a free purge. Sweat baths are to be used with caution and not given if there is weakness of the circulation. They are often of no value but occasionally their use is followed by marked improvement. In children the hot pack is usually satisfactory. It is applied by wringing a blanket out of hot water, wrapping the child in it, covering this with a dry blanket, and then with a rubber cloth. In this the child may remain for an hour. It may be repeated daily.

The *bowels* should be kept open by a morning saline purge; in children fluid magnesia is readily taken; in adults the sulphate of magnesia or Rochelle salts may be given in the morning, before anything is taken into the stomach. The compound jalap powder (gr. xx, 1.3 gm.) or, if necessary elaterin (gr. 1/20, 0.003 gm.) may be used. If the edema is not extreme, the urine not very concentrated, and uremic symptoms are not present, the bowels should be kept loose without active purgation. If these measures fail to reduce the edema and it has become extreme, the skin may be punctured or drained by a fine aspirator needle and the fluid allowed to flow through rubber tubing. If dyspnea is marked, owing to hydrothorax, aspiration should be performed. In some instances ascites may require paracentesis. If uremic convulsions occur, the intensity of the paroxysms may be limited by the use of chloroform; to an adult morphia hypodermically should be given at once and from a robust adult 20 ounces of blood may be withdrawn. In children the loins may be dry cupped, the hot pack used and a brisk purgative given. Bromide of potassium and chloral sometimes prove useful. Gastric lavage is useful for vomiting. Lumbar puncture with the withdrawal of fluid up to 30 cc. may be helpful.

As to the use of *diuretics* in acute nephritis, it is well to avoid them in the early stages; later potassium citrate may be given. Digitalis should be given only when the myocardial condition requires it. For the persistent *albuminuria*, we have no remedy of the slightest value.

For *anemia* iron should be employed but not until the acute symptoms have subsided. In children, the syrup of the iodide of iron is useful. In convalescence care should be taken to guard the patient against cold. The diet should still consist chiefly of milk, fruit juices and sugars with a gradual return to mixed food. A change to a warm climate is often beneficial.

In *hemorrhagic nephritis*, the same treatment applies but the dietary restrictions may be less strict and water can usually be given freely. Careful search must be made for a focus of infection and this should be removed as soon as possible. The patient should be in bed as long as red blood cells are found in the urine.

NEPHROSIS.—This term is applied to conditions, rather than a disease entity, in which there are degenerative, not inflammatory, changes which affect particularly the tubules; the glomeruli are only affected secondarily. There is much confusion in the use of this term and to apply it to cases of nephritis because there is marked edema does not add to the clarity of our views of nephritis. True nephrosis is a rare disease. The term should not be employed to include glomerulonephritis with edema. The conditions in which tubular degeneration predominates are: (1) febrile albuminuria, (2) metallic poisoning (mercury and bismuth), (3) the nephrosis of pregnancy, and (4) lipoid nephrosis. True lipoid nephrosis is a rare condition.

Lipoid Nephrosis.—The cause is usually obscure and infection does not seem to be responsible. Metabolic disturbance may be the primary factor with the renal changes secondary. Syphilis has been suggested but this is not proved and syphilitic treatment is not helpful. The onset is gradual. *Edema* is a striking feature and the anasarca may be extreme, with effusion into the serous cavities. The edema is marked in dependent parts. The amount of urine is diminished, it has a high specific gravity and contains large amounts of serum albumin with many casts which may be fatty or hyaline with fat droplets. Sometimes doubly refractive fat globules are found. The blood pressure is not increased, there is no hypertrophy of the heart and no marked nitrogen retention. There is a reduction in the total amount of protein in the blood serum with relative increase in globulin and an increase in the cholesterol content (lipoidema, hypercholesteremia), and a high chloride content in the blood. There may be a moderate secondary anemia. The disease is usually in a chronic stage when recognized. There is "a disturbance of the chemical balance of the body colloids with an increase of osmotic pressure in the body fluids and cells so that water is held in these cells in an abnormal way." (O'Hare).

The *diagnosis* depends largely on a knowledge of the condition and has to be made from subacute or chronic nephritis with edema. The general features, the absence of hypertension and eyeground changes, the few cellular elements in the urine, and the high cholesterol and globulin content of the blood are important. The *course* is usually prolonged and the condition is essentially chronic but recovery may occur, especially in children; an intercurrent infection is often responsible for death. In *treatment*, the diet should be rich in protein, owing to the great protein loss, and amounts of 2 or 3 grams per kilo of body weight may be given. The salt intake should be as small as possible. Milk should not be given. The fat in the diet should be reduced to a minimum. The usual measures for edema should be employed but drastic purgation and sweating are inadvisable. Theocin in 5 grain (0.3 gm.) doses three times a day or calcium chloride in 30 grains (2 gm.) doses every four hours may be given. Novasurol (merbaphen) in doses of 0.5 to 2 cc. of the 10 per cent solution intramuscularly every four days may be used with or without ammonium chloride (10 gr., 0.6 gm. three times a day). The use of novasurol is not without danger. Thyroid gland extract may be useful, the dose being determined by giving gr. i (0.06 gm.) three times a day and gradually increasing the amount.

CHRONIC NEPHRITIS

In nephritis there are two principal departures from normal in the renal function: (1) The kidney lets out material which should be kept in (*e.g.* albumin) and (2) keeps in material which should be passed out. The first represents the significant urinary findings, the second the changes in the blood and body fluids. In addition the metabolism of the body is altered and cardiovascular changes are common. Much of the confusion relates to the part played by the circulation; in certain forms the renal changes are secondary to vascular disease; in other cases one cause may be responsible both for renal and general sclerotic vascular changes. The student will do well to recognize that the estimation of the conditions present in a given patient is more important than placing him in some particular classification.

A clinical classification of chronic nephritis offers many difficulties. In all forms we deal with a diffuse process, involving epithelial, interstitial and glomerular tissue. A functional diagnosis is of great value but the function of the kidney may be influenced by factors outside the kidney itself. As regards an etiological classification there is more opportunity for this in acute nephritis than in the chronic forms.

Two main forms may be recognized: (1) The sclerotic or chronic interstitial—the "dry" form, in which there is hypertension, a retention of nitrogenous products in the blood, often ending in uremia, and (2) the chronic parenchymatous—the "wet" form, in which there is retention of water and salt with resulting edema. There are many intermediate forms and the terms mentioned may be regarded as describing the cases at each end of a series with every grade of variation between. The tendency is to consider the occurrence of hypertension and edema with the result of the functional tests as designating a symptom-complex rather than a distinct disease. The most useful tests in estimating the kidney function are: (1) The phthalein test. (2) The determination of the total nonprotein nitrogen, urea nitrogen, uric acid and creatinine content of the blood. (3) The two-hour test in which the patient is given full diet with fluid at mealtime only. The urine is collected every two hours from 8 a. m. to 10 p. m. and from 10 p. m. to 8 a. m. The important points are the lowering of the maximum specific gravity, the fixation of specific gravity and an increase in the night urine. (4) The urea concentration test in which the patient empties the bladder and takes 15 grams of urea in 100 cc. of water. The urine is passed one and two hours later and the urea content determined. If the urea is over 2 per cent the kidneys are fairly efficient. The second specimen is the more reliable as diuresis may dilute the first; not more than 125 cc. should be passed in the second hour. (5) The urea clearance test. (6) The response to the action of a diuretic.

The *amyloid* kidney may be spoken of as a variety of nephrosis, but in reality it is a degeneration which may accompany any form of nephritis.

CHRONIC NEPHRITIS WITH EDEMA

This form—nephritis with edema, "chronic parenchymatous"—is often rather a subacute than a chronic affection. If the patient lives sufficiently long, interstitial changes develop with finally a secondary contracted kidney.

Etiology.—In many cases the disease follows an acute nephritis, but more frequently than is usually stated the onset is insidious and independent of any recognized acute attack. Continued bacterial septicemia, secondary to a focal infection, is an important cause. The fevers may play a rôle in certain cases and some have laid stress upon malaria as a cause. The use of alcohol is believed by some to lead to this form of nephritis. In chronic suppuration, syphilis and tuberculosis a diffuse nephritis is not uncommon, sometimes with amyloid disease. Males are rather more subject to the affection than females. It is met with most commonly in young adults, and is not infrequent in children as a sequence of the nephritis of scarlet fever.

Morbid Anatomy.—Several varieties are recognized. In the *large white kidney* of Wilks, the organ is enlarged, the capsule is thin, and the surface white with the stellate veins injected; it is not common in America. On section the cortex is swollen, yellowish white, and often presents opaque areas. The pyramids may be deeply congested. On microscopic examination the epithelium is granular and fatty, and the tubules of the cortex are distended, and contain casts. Hyaline changes are present in the epithelial cells. The glomeruli are large, the capsules thickened, the capillaries show hyaline changes, and the epithelium of the tuft and of the capsule is extensively altered. The interstitial tissue is increased but not to an extreme degree.

The second variety results from gradual increase in the connective tissue and subsequent shrinkage, forming what is called the *small white kidney* or pale granular kidney. It is doubtful whether this is always preceded by the large white kidney. Some hold that it may be a primary independent form. The capsule is thickened and the surface rough and granular. On section the resistance is greatly increased, the cortex is reduced and presents numerous opaque white or whitish yellow foci, consisting of accumulations of fatty epithelium in the convoluted tubules. This combination of contracted kidney with areas of marked fatty degeneration has been given the name of small granular fatty kidney. The interstitial changes are marked, many glomeruli are destroyed, the degeneration of epithelium in the convoluted tubules is widespread, and the arteries are greatly thickened.

There is a variety known as *chronic hemorrhagic nephritis*, in which the organs are enlarged, yellowish white in color, and in the cortex are many brownish red areas, due to hemorrhage into and about the tubes. In other respects the changes are identical with those in the large white kidney.

Edema.—This is an important feature; two main factors are (1) intracapillary pressure and (2) colloid osmotic pressure of the plasma proteins. The intracapillary pressure is easily affected by a rise in the venous pressure from back pressure. Loss of serum albumin from the blood favors edema more than a loss of globulin and the loss of albumin is marked, not that of globulin, in nephritis. With alteration of the osmotic properties of the blood there is absorption and retention of fluid by the tissues. The influence of sodium chloride is from the sodium ion. Other factors may be concerned, myocardial insufficiency, poor nutrition and anemia. There may be salt retention without edema. There may be high lipoid content of the blood and pseudochylous ascites may occur. Salt retention and loss of protein, to a relative variable extent, are probably the important factors.

Symptoms.—Following an acute nephritis, the disease may present, in a modified way, the symptoms of that affection. In many cases it sets in insidiously, and after an attack of dyspepsia or a period of failing health and loss of strength the patient becomes pale, and puffiness of the eyelids or swollen feet are noticed in the morning. It is surprising for how long some of these patients may delay seeking advice and come under observation with a serious condition.

The *urine* is, as a rule, diminished in quantity, averaging 500 cc. It has a dirty yellow, sometimes smoky, color, and is turbid from the presence of urates. On standing, a heavy sediment falls, in which are numerous casts, hyaline, both large and small, epithelial, granular and fatty casts. Leukocytes are abundant; red blood cells and epithelium are frequently met with. The protein is abundant and the ratio of albumin to globulin is about 6 to 1. It is more abundant in the urine passed during the day. The specific gravity may be high in the early stages—from 1.020 to 1.025, even 1.040—though in the later stages it is lower. The urea is reduced in quantity. As the patient improves larger amounts of urine are voided.

Edema is a marked and obstinate feature. The face is pale and puffy, and in the morning the eyelids are edematous. The anasarca is general and there may be involvement of the serous sacs. There is often a distinctive appearance of the face; the complexion is pasty, the pallor marked, and the eyelids edematous. The dropsy is peculiarly obstinate. Uremic symptoms are common, though convulsions are less frequent than in sclerotic nephritis.

The blood pressure may be increased; the vessels ultimately become stiff and the heart hypertrophied, though there are instances in which the heart is not enlarged. The aortic second sound may be accentuated. *Anemia* is a marked feature and may be partly responsible for the weakness and dyspnea. Retinal changes, though less frequent than in sclerotic nephritis, occur in a number of cases.

Gastro-intestinal symptoms are common. Vomiting is frequently distressing and serious, and diarrhea may be profuse. Ulceration of the colon may prove fatal.

The *functional* tests may show great variations. In many cases the greatest change is in the ability to secrete water and salt, in others the reduction in function is more general and the phthalein excretion may be much reduced. In some cases there is hyperpermeability.

In some patients after a year or more there is a change in the picture. The edema lessens and the amount of urine increases. This is probably secondary to hypertrophy of the heart with higher blood pressure, with changes in the kidney. The disease has progressed to the form termed *secondary contracted kidney*. In this the quantity of urine is fairly large; the amount of protein is variable and there are many kinds of casts. The picture approaches that of chronic sclerotic nephritis and after some years it may be difficult, in the absence of a good history, to make a distinction.

Diagnosis.—This is not difficult in the average case with edema, anemia and urinary changes. In the absence of edema and without a good history there may be doubt. There is a group of cases in which the kidneys have been damaged but the condition is not progressive. There is proteinuria but the function is good and there are no cardiovascular lesions. Such a kidney may be able to do its work perfectly well but may be more susceptible to damage from infection. The term "leaky" kidney is sometimes applied to this condition. The good general health, the absence of symptoms and the functional tests aid its diagnosis. There are cases between the two principal forms of chronic nephritis which one has difficulty in classifying and the diagnosis of chronic nephritis is enough.

Prognosis.—This is extremely grave. Death is caused either by great effusion with edema of the lungs, by uremia, or by secondary inflammation of the serous membranes. Occasionally in children, even when the disease has persisted for some time, the symptoms disappear and recovery takes place. The frequency of acute exacerbations adds to the uncertainty of prognosis. A marked decrease in the kidney function is of grave omen.

Treatment.—This in many ways is similar to that of acute nephritis, with the exception of diet. The patient should be at rest if conditions demand it, otherwise exertion short of fatigue is advisable. Any foci of infection should be corrected and special care taken against chilling. Iron should be given if there is marked anemia; Basham's mixture is a favorite prescription. If the patient can live in a warm equable climate it is an advantage. Care should be taken to avoid exposure and chilling.

Diet.—This must be decided for each patient but we have erred in reducing the amount of protein, from a lack of which many nephritic patients suffer. From 60 to 70 grams a day can be given and larger amounts if the tests show good function and there is no increase in the nitrogen content of the blood. The amount of protein lost in the urine should be made up. Liver, kidney, sweetbread and meat extracts should be excluded. The effect of various amounts of protein should be observed and the most suitable amount chosen. There is no reason for excluding eggs and these patients should not be given an exclusive milk diet except for short periods and for special indications. If there is marked lipoidemia the fat in the diet should be reduced. *Salt* should be restricted; it is rarely necessary to give an absolutely salt-free diet and some patients seem to be injured by it. *Alcohol* should not be taken in any form. The effect of *tea* and *coffee* should be studied. The amount of fluid has to be decided for each patient; an average is 1200-1500 cc. per day. If larger amounts increase the quantity of urine proportionally they may be given. The Karrell diet consists in giving 200 cc. of milk at 8 a. m., 12 noon, and 4 and 8 p. m., and nothing more. After a week, a soft egg with bread may be added and the diet gradually increased, but the intake of fluid should be kept at 800 cc. a day for some time. Some patients with marked edema do well with this, but in others more fluid is advisable.

Edema.—With fluid in the serous sacs causing distress, tapping should be done. The use of punctures of the legs and scrotum has the danger of infection. The insertion of needles in the legs is the best method. They are inserted subcutaneously, as nearly parallel as possible to the surface, and held by strapping. Rubber tubing is attached. This is better than making incisions.

Diuretics.—These should be used cautiously and some may do harm; they should be stopped unless there is a prompt response. The combination of calcium lactate in large doses (ʒ i, 4 gm.) with theocin (gr. v, 0.3 gm.) three times a day is sometimes effectual. Digitalis should only be used if there is myocardial failure. The alkaline diuretics are usually safe but do not have much effect. Urea has been given (15-30 gm. daily) and some explain the diuresis which may follow increased protein in the diet as due to the increased production and diuretic effect of urea. Its use is only advisable if kidney function is good and there is no urea retention. The care of the bowels is important; salines are best and mercurials should be avoided owing to the danger of salivation. Novasurol (merbaphen) may be tried cautiously. Salyrgan in 10 per cent solution (0.5 cc. intravenously increased to 1 or 2 cc. once or twice a week) may be effective.

Decapsulation.—In patients with persistent edema, but no signs of cardiovascular changes, in whom treatment is not effective, this is worth consideration. The results in some cases have been excellent.

RENAL SCLEROSIS: CHRONIC INTERSTITIAL NEPHRITIS

(*Contracted Kidney; Arteriosclerotic Kidney; Senile Kidney*)

There is difficulty in deciding as to the sequence of events which cause the changes included under this heading. The disease, or symptom-complex, represents much more than a renal lesion alone; the vascular system and metabolic changes are involved with it. In some cases the process begins in the kidney and in others the vascular disease (hypertension, arteriosclerosis) is primary with the renal changes secondary. The final clinical picture may be the same but there are differences in the pathological findings. It is not always possible —to put it mildly—to predict the pathological findings from the clinical study.

Etiology and Morbid Anatomy.—Sclerosis of the kidney is met with (*a*) as a sequence of parenchymatous nephritis, forming the secondary contracted kidney (*b*) as a primary independent affection; (*c*) as a sequence of arteriosclerosis and hypertension; and (*d*) as a senile change.

(*a*) SECONDARY FORM.—The changes, especially in the glomeruli, suggest that the fibrosis has followed a previous acute inflammatory condition. The kidneys are contracted and granular; the cortex is narrowed. The glomeruli show marked changes, which are general but show variation in different tufts. The tubules are damaged, either destroyed or showing marked changes. Interstitial tissue is increased. The vessels show extensive changes.

(*b*) In the PRIMARY FORM the organ is smaller than in the secondary form, the capsule is very adherent, the granulations small, the organ of a reddish brown color, the cysts numerous, the arteries very sclerotic, and the cortex greatly reduced in volume. The chief reason for calling this primary is that one can find no history of previous renal disease. Some families show the disease in many members for several generations but probably these are usually cases of primary hypertension. Lead is a rare cause in America but a more common cause in England. It is not always easy to differentiate between the secondary and primary forms. As a rule, the former is paler and not so small. Of 174 cases, in 79 the combined weight of the kidneys was about 300 grams, in 57 cases 200 to 300 grams, in 30 cases 150 to 200 grams, and below 150 grams in 8 cases (Emerson). Unilateral nephritis is extremely rare, not occurring once in the series.

(*c*) With HYPERTENSION and ARTERIOSCLEROSIS. The organ is hard, red, and not necessarily greatly contracted. The small renal vessels (arterioles) are especially involved in the group beginning with hypertension. The changes in the glomeruli vary greatly and the tubules show extensive degeneration. In the *arteriosclerotic* form the surface may be smooth or the capsule only slightly thickened and adherent, tearing the substance very little as it is stripped off. In other cases the atrophy is in spots, affecting certain vascular districts, so that there is a sunken, deep red patch on the surface, or one pole of the kidney is shrunken, or the process is general in both kidneys, but the resulting contraction gives a warty rather than a granular surface.

(*d*) In the SENILE FORM, the organs are reduced in size, the capsules thickened and adherent, the pelvic fat increased, cortical and pyramidal portions uniformly wasted, and the arteries of the kidney substance prominent.

Almost invariably associated with chronic sclerotic nephritis are general arteriosclerosis and hypertrophy of the left ventricle. The changes in the arteries will be described elsewhere. In some cases the disease is latent, and the patients die of apoplexy or of acute uremia. In the arteriosclerotic form death is more commonly cardiac, and the condition of the kidneys may be entirely overlooked.

The disease is really one which involves the *cardiovascular-renal system.* Much discussion has taken place as to the association of hypertrophy of the heart and sclerosis of the blood vessels with the renal changes. A complete solution of the problems has scarcely yet been offered. The process may begin as hypertension with resulting vascular and renal changes. The essential cause of the hypertension is not known. Dating from the time of Bright it was thought that the heart had greater difficulty in driving the blood through the capillary system. Traube held that the obliteration of a large number of capillary territories in the kidney raised the arterial pressure and led to hypertrophy of the heart. In explanation of the muscular hypertrophy of the walls of the smaller arteries George Johnson introduced the view of a stop-cock action of these vessels under the influence of irritating ingredients in the blood. The mechanical view was thus put by Cohnheim. The activity of the circulation through the kidneys at any moment does not depend upon the need of these organs for blood, but upon the amount of material for the urinary secretion existing in the blood. When parts of both kidneys have undergone atrophy, the blood flow in the parts remaining must be as great as it would have been to the whole of the organs, had they been intact; but in order that such a quantity of blood should pass through the restricted capillary area now open to it an excessive pressure is necessary. This can result only by increased force on the part of the left ventricle. In this way both hypertension and the cardiovascular changes are explained.

The chemical view supposes the production (*a*) by the kidneys, (*b*) by the adrenal glands, of pressor substances but proof of this is lacking. The results from the removal of certain adrenal tumors and division of the sympathetic nerves to these glands speak for some influence.

Symptoms.—Many cases are latent, and are not recognized until the occurrence of one of the serious or fatal complications. Even an advanced grade of contracted kidney may be compatible with great mental and bodily activity. There may have been no symptoms to suggest to the patient the existence of a serious malady. In other cases the general health is disturbed. The patient complains of lassitude, is sleepless, has to get up at night to micturate; the digestion is disordered, the tongue is furred; there are complaints of headache, failing vision, vertigo and dyspnea.

So complex and varied is the clinical picture that it will be best to consider the symptoms under the various systems.

Urinary System.—In the *small contracted kidney* polyuria is common. Frequently the patient has to get up two or three times during the night to void and there is increased thirst. It is for these symptoms occasionally that relief is sought but in many cases this feature is not present. A careful study of the urine and the anatomical condition showed that no close parallelism could be made between the weight of the kidney, its appearance, and the urine it secreted before death. Of 174 cases with autopsy, in almost a third the renal changes were so slight that the nephritis was not mentioned as a part of the clinical diagnosis (Emerson). The color of the urine is a light yellow, and the specific gravity ranges from 1.005 to 1.012. Persistent *low specific gravity* is one of the most constant and important features. Traces of albumin are found, but may be absent at times, particularly in the early morning urine. It may be apparent only with the more delicate tests. The sediment is scanty, and in it a few hyaline or granular casts are found. The quantity of the solid constituents of the urine is, as a rule, diminished, though in some instances the urea may be excreted in full amount. In attacks of dyspepsia or bronchitis, or in the later stages when the heart fails, the albumin may be greatly increased and the urine diminished. Occasionally blood occurs in the urine, and there may be hematuria. Slight leakage, represented by the presence of a few red cells, may be present early and persist for years. In the *arteriosclerotic form* the quantity of urine is normal, or reduced rather than increased; the specific gravity is normal or high, the color of the urine is good, and there are hyaline and finely granular casts. The amount of albumin varies with the food and exercise, is usually in excess of that with the contracted kidneys, and does not show often albumin free intervals, also it is more common to find albumin without casts, while in the contracted kidney casts may occur without albumin.

The functional findings are very variable in different stages. They are of value in determining the approach of uremia. As Janeway showed, in the majority of cases death is not from renal insufficiency but from cardiac failure or cerebral vascular disease. Functional tests aid in deciding whether myocardial or renal insufficiency is the more important factor.

Circulatory System.—The pulse is hard, the pressure increased, and the vessel wall, as a rule, thickened. A distinction must be made between increased tension and thickening of the arterial wall. The tension may be plus in a normal vessel, but in chronic nephritis it is more common to have increased tension in a stiff artery.

A pulse of increased tension has the following characters: It is hard and incompressible, requiring a good deal of force to overcome it; it is persistent, and in the intervals between the beats the vessel feels full and can be rolled beneath the finger. These characters may be present in a vessel the walls of which are little, if at all, increased in thickness. To estimate the latter the pulse wave should be obliterated in the radial in two places and the vessel wall felt between them. In a normal vessel the arterial wall, under these circumstances, can not be differentiated from the surrounding tissue; whereas, if thickened, the vessel can be rolled beneath the finger. Palpation should not be limited to the radial artery; the femoral, brachial, temporal and posterior tibial should be examined. Persistent *high blood pressure* is a most important feature. It may rise to 250 mm. or 300 mm. With edema and cardiac dilatation the pressure may fall, but not necessarily. The *cardiac* features are equally important, though often less obvious. Hypertrophy of the left ventricle occurs to overcome the resistance and the enlargement of the heart ultimately becomes more general. The apex is displaced downward and to the left; the impulse is forcible and may be heaving. In elderly persons with emphysema the displacement of the apex may not be evident. The first sound at the apex may be duplicated; more commonly the second sound at the aortic cartilage is accentuated. In many cases a systolic murmur develops at the apex, as a result of relative mitral insufficiency. It may be loud and transmitted to the axilla. Finally the hypertrophy fails, the heart becomes dilated, gallop rhythm is present, and the general condition is that of chronic myocardial failure. In the arteriosclerotic form the picture may be cardiac from beginning to close—dyspnea and signs of dilated heart.

BLOOD.—The estimation of the nonprotein N, urea N, uric acid and creatinin is particularly important, an increase meaning retention. The urea N (normal 12-15 mg. per 100 cc.) is increased to 15-50 mgs. in chronic nephritis and 80-300 in uremia. Creatinin (normal 1-2.5) may be increased as high as 20 in chronic nephritis and in uremia. These findings are important in diagnosis and prognosis. It is a question which is most useful. Persistent low urea content in the blood, in the absence of edema, is evidence against renal disease. Increase in the uric acid content alone is not significant. In the immediate prognosis the creatinin estimation is important. Amounts from 3 to 5 mg. per 100 cc. of blood are unfavorable and if above 5 mg. an early termination may be expected. Severe *anemia* may occur, apparently due to disturbance of the function of the bone marrow. It suggests primary renal disease. It is not due to excessive hemolysis. It does not usually respond to treatment and is of unfavorable prognosis.

RESPIRATORY SYSTEM.—Sudden edema of the glottis may occur. Effusion into the plurae or sudden edema of the lungs may prove fatal. Acute pleurisy and pneumonia are not uncommon. Bronchitis is frequent, particularly in the winter. Sudden attacks of *dyspnea,* particularly at night, are not infrequent. This may be a uremic symptom or due to acidosis but is often cardiac. Cheyne-Stokes breathing may be present, most commonly toward the close, but the patient may be walking about and even attending to his occupation.

ACIDOSIS.—The majority of advanced cases show some degree of acidosis, which is often severe and hastens a fatal issue.

DIGESTIVE SYSTEM.—Dyspepsia and loss of appetite are common. Hematemesis and hemorrhage from the bowel may occur. Severe and uncontrollable vomiting may be the first symptom. This is usually regarded as a manifestation of uremia, but it may occur without any other indications, and prove fatal without any suspicion of nephritis. Severe and even fatal diarrhea may develop. The tongue may be coated and the breath heavy and urinous.

NERVOUS SYSTEM.—Various cerebral manifestations have been mentioned under uremia. Headache, sometimes of the migraine type, may be an early and persistent feature of chronic nephritis. A morning headache which wakes the patient early and lasts until midday is not uncommon. In hypertension mental work often causes headache. Cerebral hemorrhage often occurs with hypertension and sclerotic nephritis and may take place into the meninges or the cerebrum. It is usually associated with marked changes in the vessels. Neuralgias, in various regions, are not uncommon.

SPECIAL SENSES.—Troubles in vision may be the first symptom and in many cases the condition is diagnosed first by the ophthalmic surgeon. The retinal arteries show various grades of sclerosis. The flame-shaped retinal hemorrhages are common. Less frequent is diffuse retinitis. Sudden blindness may supervene without retinal changes—uremic amaurosis. Diplopia is a rare event. Recurring conjunctival and palpebral hemorrhages are fairly common, particularly in the arteriosclerotic form. Auditory troubles are by no means infrequent and ringing in the ears, with dizziness, is not uncommon. Various forms of deafness may occur.

SKIN.—Edema is not common; slight puffiness of the ankles may be present, but in a majority of the cases dropsy does not supervene. When extensive, it is almost always the result of myocardial failure. The skin is often dry and pale, and sweats are not common. In some instances the sweat may deposit a white frost of urea on the surface of the skin. Eczema is a common accompaniment. Tingling of the fingers or numbness and pallor—dead fingers—are not in any way peculiar to nephritis. Intolerable itching of the skin may be present, and cramps in the muscles are not rare.

Hemorrhages are not infrequent, particularly epistaxis. Severe and widespread purpura is a not uncommon terminal event and the primary disease may not be recognized. Bronchopulmonary hemorrhages may occur. Ascites is rare except in association with cirrhosis of the liver.

Diagnosis.—The autopsy often discloses the true nature of the disease, one of the many intercurrent affections of which may have proved fatal. The early stages of sclerotic nephritis are difficult to recognize. In a patient with hypertension (particularly if the vessel's wall is sclerotic), with the apex beat of the heart dislocated to the left, the second aortic sound ringing and accentuated, the urine abundant and of low specific gravity, with a trace of albumin and an occasional hyaline or granular cast, the diagnosis may be safely made. Of all the indications, that offered by the pulse is the most important. Persistent high tension with thickening of the arterial wall in a man under fifty means that serious mischief has taken place, that cardiovascular are certainly, and renal changes most probably, present. In the *arteriosclerotic* cases the history is of the "strenuous life"—work, alcohol, tobacco, Venus—and not of an infection or of lead or gout. The urine is not of persistently low specific gravity, there may be little or no albumin except in intercurrent attacks; the symptoms are cardiac rather than renal or cerebral; the ocular changes are hemorrhagic, not the true albuminuric retinitis. Primary hypertension should be distinguished and in this the functional tests are of value but in some cases it may be difficult to decide whether the condition was primarily essential hypertension or nephritis. As a rule the distinction is not important when this stage is reached.

Prognosis.—Chronic nephritis is an incurable affection, and the anatomical conditions on which it depends are as much beyond the reach of medicine as wrinkled skin or gray hair. However, it is compatible with the enjoyment of life for many years, and increased tension, thickening of the arterial walls, and polyuria with a small quantity of albumin, neither doom a man to death within a short time nor necessarily interfere with an active life so long as proper care be taken. Patients with high tension and a little albumin in the urine with hyaline casts may live for ten, twelve, or even fifteen years. Serious indications are the occurrence of uremic symptoms, dilatation of the heart, serous effusions, Cheyne-Stokes breathing, marked acidosis, persistent vomiting, and diarrhea. The functional tests and blood analysis give valuable information and are material aids in prognosis. Severe anemia is of grave significance and treatment usually has little effect on it.

Treatment.—Patients without local indications or in whom the condition has been accidentally discovered should so regulate their lives as to throw the least possible strain upon heart, arteries and kidneys. A quiet life without mental worry, with gentle but not excessive exercise, and residence in an equable climate, should be recommended. In addition they should be told to keep the bowels open, the skin active by a daily tepid bath with friction, and the urinary secretion free by drinking daily a definite amount of water. Alcohol should be strictly prohibited. Tea and coffee are allowable. If the patient is overweight this should be remedied.

The *diet* should be light and nourishing, and the patient should be warned not to eat excessively, and to take meat in moderate amount only once a day. Care in food and drink is probably the most important element in the treatment of early cases. One day a week with a diet of milk or green vegetables and fruit is useful. The salt intake should be small. A patient in good circumstances may be urged to go away during the winter months. There is no doubt of the value of avoiding changeable winter weather.

At this period medicines are not required unless for certain special symptoms. Patients derive much benefit from an annual visit to certain mineral springs, such as Poland, Bedford, Saratoga, in America, and Vichy and others in Europe. Mineral waters have no curative influence upon nephritis; they simply help the circulation and keep the drains flushed. When the patient's condition is good, medicines are not indicated, since no drugs are known to have any influence upon the progress of the disease. Sooner or later conditions arise which demand treatment. Of these the most important are:

(*a*) *Hypertension.*—It is to be remembered that a certain increase of tension is not only necessary but unavoidable in chronic nephritis, and a serious danger is too great lowering of the tension. In many cases the hypertension has been primary and the nephritis secondary. The happy medium must be sought between such heightened tension as throws a serious strain upon the heart and risks rupture of the vessels and lower tension which is liable to be associated with serous effusions. In cases with persistent high tension the diet should be light, an occasional saline purge should be given, and sweating promoted by hot baths. A few days in bed on milk diet is sometimes useful. An occasional venesection helps some patients.

(*b*) *Anemia* is best met by the use of iron.

(*c*) *Myocardial Insufficiency.*—The patient should be allowed to assume the nost comfortable position but rest should be as complete as possible. The diet should be greatly restricted and it is often wise to give no food for a day. Then milk (750 to 1000 cc. a day) may be allowed. Later it is well to give food in small amounts with frequent feedings. The total intake of fluids must depend somewhat on the presence of edema. With this the amount of fluid should not be over 1500 cc. and salt withheld as far as possible. Free purgation is indicated, for which calomel or elaterin (gr. 1/20, 0.003 gm.) and salines may be used. With marked dilatation of the heart, venesection is advisable unless the patient is anemic. Digitalis in the usual dosage is indicated and a high blood pressure is not a contra-indication to its use. Theobromine (gr. v, 0.3 gm.), diuretin (gr. xv, 1 gm.), and theocin (gr. iii, 0.2 gm.) may be tried, if there is much edema.

(*d*) *Vasodilators.*—The giving of these is not indicated for the purpose of reducing pressure but they may be of service in relieving symptoms, especially headache, dizziness and dyspnea. Nitroglycerine may be given beginning with gr. 1/100 (0.00065 gm.) and increasing till an effect is produced. Sodium nitrite is often more useful in doses of gr. ½-ii (0.03-0.12 gm.). Erythrol tetranitrate has a more prolonged effect. The dose of the vasodilator should be that which produces an effect.

(*e*) *Uremic Symptoms.*—Even before marked manifestations are present there may be extreme restlessness, mental wandering, a heavy, foul breath, and a coated tongue. Headache is not often complained of, though intense frontal headache may be an early symptom of uremia. The patient may complain of palpitation, feelings of numbness, and sometimes nocturnal cramps. For these symptoms the saline purgatives should be ordered, and hot baths, so as to induce copious sweating. Water should be given freely, by mouth, by the drop method by the bowel, and by subcutaneous injection if necessary. Irrigation of the bowel with hot water is useful. If signs of acidosis are present, sodium bicarbonate (ʒ i, 4 gm., a day) should be given. For the uremic convulsions, if severe, inhalations of chloroform may be used. If the patient is robust and full-blooded, from 12 to 20 ounces of blood should be removed. *Lumbar puncture* is often useful and can be done without hesitation; it sometimes relieves dyspnea. The patient should be freely sweated and if the convulsions recur chloral may be given, either by the mouth or per rectum, or, better still, morphia. For the restlessness and delirium morphia is indispensable. Since its recommendation in uremic states by Stephen MacKenzie, it has been used extensively and is of great value in these cases. It is of special value in the dyspnea and Cheyne-Stokes breathing of advanced arteriosclerosis with chronic uremia.

AMYLOID DISEASE

Amyloid (lardaceous or waxy) degeneration of the kidneys is an event in the process of chronic nephritis, most commonly in the chronic nephritis following fevers or of cachectic states. It has no claim to be regarded as a variety of nephritis. The affection of the kidneys is generally part of a widespread amyloid degeneration occurring in prolonged suppuration, as in bone disease, syphilis, tuberculosis, and occasionally leukemia, lead poisoning and gout. It varies curiously in frequency in different localities.

The amyloid kidney is large and pale, the surface smooth, and the venae stellatae well marked. On section the cortex is large and may show a peculiar glistening, infiltrated appearance with the glomeruli distinct. The pyramids, in striking contrast to the cortex, are of a deep red color. A section soaked in dilute tincture of iodine shows spots of a walnut or mahogany brown color. The Malpighian tufts and the straight vessels may be most affected. In lardaceous disease the kidneys are not always enlarged but may be normal in size or small, pale, and granular. The amyloid change is first seen in the Malpighian tufts, and then involves the afferent and efferent vessels and the straight vessels. In later stages the tubules are affected, chiefly the membrane, rarely, if ever, the cells themselves.

Symptoms.—The renal features alone may not indicate amyloid disease. Usually the associated condition gives a hint of the nature of the process. The urine, as a rule, shows important changes; the quantity is increased, and it is pale, clear and of low specific gravity. Albumin is usually abundant but may be scanty, and in rare instances absent. Possibly the variations in the situation of the amyloid changes may account for this, since the albumin is less likely to be present when the change is confined to the vasa recta. In addition to ordinary albumin, globulin may be present. The casts are variable, usually hyaline, often fatty or finely granular. Occasionally the amyloid reaction can be detected in the hyaline casts. Edema is present in many instances, particularly when there is much anemia or profound cachexia, but it is not invariable. Diarrhea is common.

Increased blood pressure and cardiac hypertrophy are not usually present, except in those cases in which amyloid degeneration occurs with chronic nephritis; under which circumstances there may be uremia and retinal changes, which, as a rule, are not met with in other forms.

Diagnosis.—By the urine alone it is not possible to recognize amyloid changes in the kidney. Usually, however, there is no difficulty, since the disease comes on in association with syphilis, prolonged suppuration, bone disease or tuberculosis, and there is enlargement of the liver and spleen. A suspicious circumstance is polyuria with a large amount of albumin and few casts, or when, in these constitutional affections, a large quantity of clear, pale urine is passed, even without albumin.

The *prognosis* depends rather on the causal condition. As a rule it is grave. The *treatment* is that of the causal condition.

PYELITIS

Definition.—Inflammation of the pelvis of the kidney and the conditions which result from it.

Etiology.—Pyelitis in almost all cases is induced by infection, rarely by the irritation of substances such as turpentine. Normally the kidney can eliminate without harm to itself, apparently, various bacteria carried to it by the blood; it probably becomes infected only when its resistance is lowered, as a result of some general cause, as anemia or an acute infection, or of some local cause, as nephritis, displacement, congestion due to pressure upon the ureter, ureteral stricture, twisted ureter (Dietl's crisis), or of operation, or when the number or virulence of the organisms is increased. These same factors probably play an important rôle in other causes of pyelitis, ascending infection from an infected bladder and tuberculous infection. Other causes described are various fevers, foci of infection, cancer, hydatids, the ova of certain parasites, cold and overexertion. Calculus seems not to be a common cause. It is not uncommon in pregnancy. It is more common in females, especially in childhood. The colon bacillus is the most frequent organism.

Morbid Anatomy.—In the early stages the mucous membrane is turbid, somewhat swollen, and may show ecchymoses or a grayish pseudomembrane. The urine in the pelvis is cloudy and contains numbers of epithelial cells.

In the calculous pyelitis there may be only slight turbidity of the membrane, which has been called catarrhal pyelitis. More commonly the mucosa is roughened, grayish in color, and thick. Under these circumstances there is almost always some dilatation of the calyces and flattening of the papillae. Following this condition there may be (*a*) extension of the suppurative processes to the kidney itself, *pyelonephritis;* (*b*) a gradual dilatation of the calyces with atrophy of the kidney substance, and finally the production of *pyonephrosis,* in which the kidney is represented by a sac of pus with or without a thin shell of renal tissue. (*c*) After the kidney structure has been destroyed by suppuration, if the obstruction at the orifice of the pelvis persists, the fluid portions may be absorbed and the pus become inspissated, so that the organ is represented by a series of sacculi containing grayish, putty-like masses, which may become impregnated with lime salts.

Tuberculous pyelitis usually starts upon the apices of the pyramids, and may at first be limited but ultimately the condition produced may be similar to that of calculous pyelitis. Pyonephrosis is quite as frequent a sequence, while the transformation of the pus into a putty-like material impregnated with salts is even commoner. The pyelitis consecutive to *cystitis* is generally bilateral, and the kidneys are sometimes involved, forming the so-called *surgical kidneys*—acute suppurative nephritis.

Symptoms.—There is great variation in the severity of pyelitis. In mild grades there is pain in the back or side, and usually tenderness on pressure over the kidney. The urine, turbid and containing pus cells, some mucus, and occasional red blood cells, is acid or alkaline, depending on the infecting organism; usually the albuminuria is of higher grade comparatively than the pyuria. Before pyuria is established there may be attacks of pain on the affected side (not reaching the severity of renal colic), rigors, high fever and sweats. Under these circumstances the urine, which may have been clear, becomes turbid or smoky from the presence of blood, and may contain large numbers of mucous cells and transitional epithelium. The statement is made that the epithelium in the urine in pyelitis is characteristic. This is erroneous, as may be demonstrated by comparing scrapings of the mucosa of the renal pelvis and the bladder.

In *severe* attacks the patient may be acutely ill for some days with high fever and chills, rapid pulse, toxemia, vomiting and prostration. The picture may suggest septicemia or some acute abdominal condition may be suspected on account of the pain, tenderness, vomiting and leukocytosis. Frequent micturition is common. As a rule these subside gradually so that in a week or ten days the patient is convalescent. In less acute cases the fever is less but there may be anemia with leukocytosis, loss of weight and strength, and occasional exacerbations. In young *children,* usually girls, the general features may be severe with slight local manifestations and few pus cells in the urine, which is acid and often contains colon bacilli.

When the pyelitis has become *chronic* the features are:

(*a*) *Pyuria.*—The pus is in variable amount, and may be intermittent. Thus, when only one kidney is involved, the ureter may be temporarily blocked, and normal urine is passed for a time; then there is a sudden outflow of the pent-up pus and the urine becomes purulent. Coincident with this retention, a mass may be felt on the side affected. Occasionally, in rapidly advancing pyelonephritis, portions of the kidney tissue, particularly of the apices of the pyramids, may slough away and appear in the urine; or solid cheesy moulds of the calyces are passed. Casts from the kidney tubules are sometimes present. The reaction of the urine depends upon the organism and whether the bladder is infected, when vesical irritability and frequent micturition may be present. Polyuria is usually present in chronic cases.

(*b*) Intermittent *fever* with chills is usually in suppurative pyelitis. The chills may recur regularly and the cases mistaken for malaria.

(*c*) The general condition often indicates prolonged suppuration. There is more or less wasting with anemia and a progressive failure of health. Secondary abscesses may develop and the clinical picture becomes that of pyemia. In some instances, particularly of tuberculous pyelitis, the clinical course may resemble that of typhoid fever. There are instances of pyuria recurring, at intervals, for many years without impairment of the bodily vigor. Some of these patients have practically no discomfort.

(*d*) Physical examination usually reveals tenderness or a definite swelling on the affected side, which may vary much in size and attain large dimensions if the kidney becomes enormously distended, as in pyonephrosis.

(*e*) Occasionally nervous symptoms, which may be associated with dyspnea, supervene, or the termination may be in a curious toxemia or by coma, not unlike that of diabetes. These have been attributed to the absorption of the decomposing materials in the urine. A form of paraplegia has been described with some cases of abscess of the kidney, but whether due to myelitis or to a peripheral neuritis has not been determined.

In suppurative nephritis following cystitis, the patient complains of pain in the back, the fever becomes high, irregular, and associated with chills, and in acute cases a typhoid state may precede the fatal event.

Diagnosis.—The local symptoms usually direct attention to the kidney and the tenderness and the urinary findings give the diagnosis. In cases without marked local symptoms it may be difficult to determine whether the pyelitis is primary or secondary to a general infection. Cultures from the urine give the causal organism. The possibility of *ureteral stricture* being responsible for the symptoms must be kept in mind. Between the tuberculous and the calculous forms of pyelitis the detection of tubercle bacilli or an X-ray study showing stone may decide. The examination for bacilli should be made systematically, and in suspicious cases injections of guinea-pigs should be made. From *perinephric abscess* pyonephrosis is distinguished by the more definite character of the tumor, the absence of edematous swelling in the lumbar region, and, most important of all, the history. The urine in perinephric abscess may be free from pus. There are cases, however, in which it is difficult to make a satisfactory diagnosis.

Suppurative pyelitis and *cystitis* are apt to be confounded. The two conditions may coexist and prove puzzling, but the history, the higher relative grade of albuminuria in pyelitis, the polyuria, the mode of development, the local signs in one lumbar region, and the absence of pain in the bladder should be sufficient. By the cystoscope, it may be definitely determined whether the pus comes from the kidneys or from the bladder.

In the diagnosis of pyelitis from pyelonephritis, the functional test is important; this is normal in pyelitis and reduced in pyelonephritis. The X-ray study gives much information as to the condition of the pelves of the kidneys.

Prognosis.—In attacks coming on during the fevers the outlook is good but there is always a tendency to relapse. In very acute or chronic cases severe toxemia is of grave omen. Tuberculous pyelitis may terminate favorably by inspissation of the pus and conversion into a putty-like substance with deposition of lime salts. With pyonephrosis the dangers are increased. Perforation may occur into the peritoneum, the patient may be worn out by the infection, or amyloid disease may develop.

Treatment.—In acute attacks the patient should be in bed, the diet of fluids only, especially milk and fruit juices, and the bowels kept open. Water should be given freely, by bowel or subcutaneously if there is vomiting. The reaction of the urine should be changed as soon as possible. If it is acid, as is usual in acute attacks, potassium citrate or acetate (gr. 15, 1 gm. every 2 or 3 hours) with sodium bicarbonate (gr. 30, 2 gm. three times a day) may be given at first and the dosage reduced later. When the fever drops or after the urine is alkaline for a few days, acid sodium phosphate (gr. xv, 1 gm.) can be given and as soon as the urine is acid hexamine (methenamine) in full dosage (gr. 10, 0.6 gm. three times a day and gradually increasing, if no irritation results, to 90 to 120 grains a day). When the urine is alkaline water should be given as freely as possible but when acid and antiseptics are being taken smaller amounts are advisable so that the antiseptic is not diluted too much. Sodium benzoate (gr. 10, 0.6 gm. three times a day) is sometimes useful with hexamine. Hexylresorcinol may be effective in doses of 0.15 to 0.6 gm. (gr. ii-x) three times a day. If the infection continues it is well to change the reaction every 7 to 10 days. *Ketogenic Diet.* By this the pH of the urine may be reduced to 5.5 or less and the concentration of beta-oxy-butyric acid be 0.5 per cent or more. The ratio of ketogenic to antiketogenic elements may be begun as 3 to 1. The protein in the diet may be kept at one gram per kilo of weight in children and 0.6 gram in adults. The main part of the diet otherwise is fat and there may be difficulty in giving this. Butter, cream and olive oil are used freely. The total fluid intake should be kept low. Usually after several days the pH falls; the diet should be given for three weeks. This treatment seems to be most effective in children.

Washing out the kidney pelvis may be done. The use of an autogenous vaccine is sometimes helpful. In the chronic cases much the same treatment should be given but the diet can be more liberal. When a tumor has formed the kidney should be explored, and, if necessary, nephrotomy or nephrectomy performed, if the other kidney functions sufficiently.

HYDRONEPHROSIS

Definition.—Dilatation of the pelvis and calyx of the kidney with atrophy of its substance, caused by the accumulation of nonpurulent fluids, the result of obstruction.

Etiology.—The condition may be *congenital,* owing to some abnormality in the ureter or urethra. The tumor produced may be large enough to retard labor. Sometimes it is associated with other malformations. There is a condition of moderate dilatation, apparently congenital, which is not connected with any obstruction in the ducts. In some instances there has been contraction or twisting of the ureter, or it is inserted into the kidney at an acute angle or at a high level. In adult life the condition may be due to lodgment of a *calculus* or to *ureteral stricture.* Hunner has demonstrated the frequency of this latter condition and that it is often secondary to a focus of infection elsewhere, as in the tonsils.

New growths may induce hydronephrosis; more commonly by pressure upon the ureter from without, particularly tumors of the ovaries and uterus. Occasionally cicatricial bands compress the ureter. Displacement of a movable kidney may be responsible. Obstruction within the bladder may result from cancer, hypertrophy of the prostate, and in the urethra from stricture. It is stated that slight grades of hydronephrosis have been found in patients with excessive polyuria.

Pathology.—When the ureter is blocked the secretion accumulates in the pelvis and infundibula. Sometimes acute inflammation follows, but more commonly the gradual pressure causes atrophy of the papillae with gradual distention and wasting of the organ. In acquired cases from pressure, even when dilatation is extreme, there is usually a thin layer of renal structure. In the most extreme stages the kidney is represented by a large cyst, which may show on its inner surface imperfect septa. The fluid is thin and yellowish and contains traces of urinary salts and sometimes albumin. The secretion may be turbid from small quantities of pus.

Total occlusion does not always lead to a hydronephrosis, but may be followed by atrophy of the kidney. It appears that when the obstruction is intermittent or not complete the greatest dilatation is apt to follow. The sac may be enormous, and cause a large abdominal tumor. It has even been mistaken for ascites. Enlargement of the other kidney may compensate for the defect. Hypertrophy of the left side of the heart usually follows.

Symptoms.—When small, it may not be noticed. The congenital cases when bilateral usually prove fatal within a few days; when unilateral, the tumor may not be noticed for some time. It increases progressively and has all the characters of a renal tumor. In adult life many cases, due to pressure by tumors, give rise to no symptoms.

In *intermittent* hydronephrosis the tumor suddenly disappears with the discharge of a large quantity of clear fluid; the sac gradually refills, and the process may be repeated for years. In these cases the obstruction is unilateral; a cicatricial stricture exists, or a valve is present in the ureter, or the ureter enters the upper part of the pelvis. Many of the cases are in women and associated with movable kidney.

The examination shows, in *unilateral hydronephrosis,* a tumor occupying the renal region. When of moderate size it is readily recognized, but when large it may be confounded with ovarian or other tumors. In young children it may be mistaken for sarcoma of the kidney or of the retroperitoneal glands, the common cause of abdominal tumor in early life. The large hydronephrotic sac may be mistaken for ovarian tumor. The latter is, as a rule, more mobile, and rarely fills the deeper portion of the lumbar region so thoroughly. The ascending colon may be found passing over the renal tumor, and vaginal examination gives important indications. The fluid of the renal cyst is clear, or turbid from the presence of cell elements, rarely colloid; the specific gravity is low; albumin and traces of urea and uric acid are usually present; and the epithelial elements in it may be similar to those found in the pelvis of the kidney. In old sacs the fluid may not be characteristic, since the urinary salts disappear, but in one case of several years' duration oxalates of lime and urea were found.

Diagnosis.—Perhaps the greatest difficulty is given by hydronephrosis in a movable kidney. Here, the history of sudden disappearance of the tumor with the passage of a large quantity of fluid is of great importance. In those rare instances of an enormous sac filling the entire abdomen, and sometimes mistaken for ascites, the character of the fluid might be the only point of difference. The tumor of *pyonephrosis* may be practically the same in physical characteristics. Fever is usually present, and pus is often found in the urine. In these cases, when in doubt, an exploratory operation should be done.

The *outlook* depends much upon the cause. When single, the condition may never produce serious trouble, and the intermittent cases may persist for years, and finally disappear. Occasionally the cyst ruptures into the peritoneum, more rarely through the diaphragm into the lung. The sac may discharge spontaneously through the ureter and the fluid never reaccumulate. In *bilateral* hydronephrosis there is danger of uremia and blocking of the ureter on the sound side by calculus has been followed by uremia. And, lastly, the sac may suppurate, and the condition change to pyonephrosis.

Treatment.—Cases of intermittent hydronephrosis which do not cause serious symptoms should be let alone. In cases due to ureteral stricture this should be treated. When the sac reaches a large size aspiration may be performed and repeated if necessary, but as a rule operation is to be preferred. It should not be delayed in cases due to calculus. When the sac is large, it may be incised and drained, or, as a last resort, the kidney may be removed. A carefully adapted abdominal support will sometimes prevent the recurrence of an intermittent hydronephrosis. In bilateral cases the cause should be treated if this is possible and every effort made to prevent urinary tract infection.

PYONEPHROSIS

Distention of the pelvis of the kidney with pus may result from pyelitis or hydronephrosis and occurs particularly with calculus and tuberculosis. The amount of pus may be so large that a tumor of considerable size results. The *symptoms* are local, especially discomfort or pain, and general due to the infection, chills and fever being common. There may be a marked toxemia. The enlarged kidney is palpable and tender. The urine contains pus unless the ureter is plugged. The *diagnosis* from hydronephrosis is made by the symptoms of infection and pus in the urine. In *treatment* if the infection is bilateral, large amounts of water with urinary antiseptics should be given. If one kidney is involved and the other is normal, removal of the kidney is indicated.

NEPHROLITHIASIS (Renal Calculus)

Definition.—The formation in the kidney or in its pelvis of concretions, by the deposition of certain of the solid constituents of the urine.

Etiology.—In the kidney substance itself the separation of the urinary salts produces a condition to which, unfortunately, the term "infarct" has been applied. Three varieties may be recognized: (1) The uric acid infarct, usually met with at the apices of the pyramids in newborn children and during the first weeks of life. Priapism and attacks of crying in the newborn have been attributed to the passage of these infarcts; (2) the sodium urate infarct, sometimes associated with ammonium urate, which forms whitish lines at the apices of the pyramids and is met with chiefly, but not always, in gouty persons; and (3) the lime infarcts, forming very opaque white lines in the pyramids, usually in old people.

In the pelvis and calyces concretions of the following forms occur: (*a*) Small gritty particles, *renal sand,* ranging in size from the individual grains of the uric acid sediment to bodies 1 or 2 mm. in diameter. These may be passed in the urine for long periods without producing any symptoms, since they are too fine to be arrested in their downward passage. They may cause symptoms in children, especially if the urine is highly acid.

(*b*) Larger concretions, ranging in size from a small pea to a bean, and either solitary or multiple in the calyces and pelvis. It is the smaller of these calculi which, in their passage, produce attacks of renal colic. They may be rounded and smooth, or present numerous irregular projections.

(*c*) The dendritic form of calculus. The orifice of the ureter may be blocked by a Y-shaped stone. The pelvis itself may be occupied by the concretion, which forms a more or less distinct mould. These are the remarkable *coral calculi,* which form complete moulds of infundibula and calyces, the latter even presenting cup-like depressions corresponding to the apices of the papillae. Some of these casts in stone of the renal pelvis are as beautifully moulded as Hyrtl's corrosion preparations.

Chemically, the varieties of calculi are: (1) *Uric acid* and *urates,* forming the renal sand, the small solitary, or the large dendritic stones. They are very hard, the surface is smooth, and the color reddish. The larger stones are usually stratified and very dense. Usually uric acid and urates are mixed, but in children stones composed of urates alone may occur. Uric acid calculi are rare.

(2) *Calcium oxalate,* which forms mulberry-shaped calculi, studded with points and spines. They are often very dark, intensely hard, and are a mixture of oxalate of lime and uric acid. These comprise the great majority of renal calculi. A high blood calcium, as in hyperparathyroidism or due to excess of vitamin D, favors their production.

(3) *Phosphatic calculi* contain calcium phosphate and ammoniomagnesium phosphate, sometimes with a small amount of calcium carbonate. They occur in alkaline urine. The phosphatic salts may be deposited about the uric acid or calcium oxalate stones.

(4) Rare forms of calculi are made up of cystin, xanthine, carbonate of lime, indigo and urostealith.

Calculi may be produced by an excess of a sparingly soluble abnormal ingredient, such as cystin or xanthine. Albumin, mucus, blood and epithelial threads may be the starting point of stone. *Infection* plays an important part, probably often from a distant focus. The demonstration of organisms in the centre of renal calculi suggests that in some cases the nucleus of the stone is an agglutinated mass of bacteria. Ureteral stricture may favor their formation.

Renal calculi are most common in the early and later period of life. They are moderately frequent in the United States, but there do not appear to be special districts, corresponding to the "stone counties" in England. Men are more often affected than women. Sedentary occupations may predispose to stone. There may be an association with certain bone lesions, injuries of the vertebrae, infected compound fractures, osteomyelitis, bone tuberculosis and osteitis fibrosa (these with hypercalcemia). In some of these there is urinary tract infection.

Pathology.—It is not uncommon to find stones of various sizes in the calyces without any destruction of the mucous membrane or dilatation of the pelvis. A turbid urine fills the pelvis, in which there are cells from the epithelial lining. There are cases in which, apparently, the stones may go on forming and are passed for years without seriously impairing the health and without inconvenience, except the attacks of renal colic. More remarkable are the cases of coral-like calculi, which may occupy the entire pelvis and calyces without causing pyelitis, but which gradually lead to more or less induration of the kidney. The most serious effects are when the stone excites a suppurative pyelitis and pyonephrosis. Of 140 kidneys containing stones removed at the Mayo clinic, 9 were cancerous (Correll).

Symptoms.—The effects of renal calculi are mechanical and due to the results of infection. Patients may pass gravel for years without having an attack of renal colic, and a stone may never lodge in the ureter. In other instances, the formation of calculi goes on year by year and the patient has recurring attacks such as were so graphically described by Montaigne in his own case. A patient may pass numbers of calculi or a single calculus and never be troubled again. The large coral calculi may excite no symptoms. In a remarkable specimen in the McGill Medical Museum, the patient, a middle-aged woman, died suddenly with uremic symptoms. There was no pyelitis, but the kidneys were sclerotic.

Renal colic ensues when a stone enters the ureter or follows an acute pyelitis. An attack may set in abruptly without apparent cause, or may follow a strain or jolting. It is characterized by agonizing pain, which starts in the flank of the affected side, passes down the ureter and is felt in the testicle and along the inner side of the thigh. The pain may also radiate through the abdomen and chest and be very intense in the back. In severe attacks nausea and vomiting follow and the patient is collapsed. Perspiration breaks out and the pulse is feeble and quick. A chill may precede the outbreak, and the temperature rise as high as 103°. No one has more graphically described an attack of "the stone" than Montaigne, who was a sufferer for many years: "Thou art seen to sweat with pain, to look pale and red, to tremble, to vomit well-nigh to blood, to suffer strange contortions and convulsions, by starts to let tears drop from thine eyes, to urine thick, black, and frightful water, or to have it suppressed by some sharp and craggy stone, that cruelly pricks and tears thee." From personal experience the senior author described three sorts of pain in an attack of renal colic: (*a*) A constant localized, dull pain, the area of which could be covered on the skin of the back in the renal region by a penny piece, and which could be imitated exactly by deep firm pressure on a superficial bone. (*b*) Paroxysms of pain radiating in the course of the ureter or into the flank, and as they increase accompanied by sweating, weakness and nausea. (*c*) Flushes or rushes of hot pain at intervals, often momentary, usually passing to the back, less often toward the groin. Dozens of these flushes relieved the monotony of *b*.

The symptoms persist for a variable period. In short attacks they do not last longer than an hour; in other instances they continue for a day or more, with temporary relief. Micturition is frequent, occasionally painful, and the urine, as a rule, is bloody. The red blood cells may only be found by the microscope. There are instances in which a large amount of clear urine is passed, probably from the other kidney. In rare cases the secretion of urine is completely suppressed, even when the opposite kidney is normal, and death may follow. This most frequently happens when the second kidney is diseased, or when only a single kidney exists. Orchitis may follow an attack.

After the attack of colic has passed there is more or less aching on the affected side, and the patient can usually tell from which kidney the stone has come. Examination during the attack is usually negative. Very rarely the kidney is palpable. Tenderness on the affected side is common. In very thin persons it may be possible to feel the stone in the ureter; or the patient may complain of a grating sensation.

When the calculi remain in the kidney they may produce very definite and characteristic symptoms, of which the following are the most important:

(*a*) *Pain*, usually in the back, which is often no more than a dull soreness, but which may be severe and come on in paroxysms. It is usually on the side affected, but may be referred to the *opposite kidney*, and there are instances in which the pain has been confined to the sound side. It radiates in the direction of the ureter and may be felt in the scrotum or penis. Vesical irritability is common. Pains of a similar nature may occur in movable kidney or be referred in prostatic disease, and surgeons have incised the kidney for stone and found none. In an instance in which pain was present for a couple of years the exploration revealed only a contracted kidney.

(*b*) *Hematuria.*—Although this occurs most frequently when the stone becomes engaged in the ureter, it may also come on when the stones are in the pelvis. The bleeding is seldom profuse but may persist for a long time. It is aggravated by exertion and lessened by rest. Frequently the red blood cells are only evident microscopically. The urine may be free for days, and then a sudden exertion or a rough ride may cause hematuria.

(*c*) *Pyelitis.*—(1) There may be attacks of severe pain in the back, not amounting to actual colic, which are initiated by a heavy chill followed by fever, in which the temperature may reach 104° or 105°, followed by profuse sweating. The urine, which has been clear, may become turbid and contain blood and epithelium from the pelvis. Such attacks may recur at intervals for months or years. This renal intermittent fever, due to the presence of calculi, is analogous to the hepatic intermittent fever, due to gall stones, and in both severe paroxysms may occur without any evidence of suppuration.

(2) More frequently the symptoms of purulent pyelitis are present; pain in the renal region, recurring chills, and pus in the urine, with or without indications of pyonephrosis.

(*d*) *Pyuria.*—There are instances of stone in the kidney in which pus occurs continuously or intermittently in the urine for many years.

Patients with stone in the kidney are often robust, high livers, and gouty. Attacks of dyspepsia are not uncommon, or they may have severe headaches.

Diagnosis.—The X-ray picture is rarely at fault; calculi do not show in 5 to 10 per cent of cases (cystin, xanthine and uric acid stones). Calcification of the intrarenal arteries may simulate stone. The use of the cystoscope with ureteral catheterization is of great value. Renal may be mistaken for intestinal colic, particularly if distention of the bowels is marked, or for biliary colic. The situation and direction of the pain, the retraction and tenderness of the testicle, hematuria, vesical irritability and changes in the urine are distinctive features. Attention may again be called to the fact that attacks simulating renal colic are associated with movable kidney, stricture of the ureter and disease of the prostate or even, possibly, with the accumulation of oxalates or uric acid in the pelvis of the kidney. In carcinoma of the ureter the pain is felt in many areas and is not typical. Hemorrhage may follow catheterization of the ureter. The diagnosis between a stone in the kidney and stone in the bladder rarely gives difficulty with the X-rays and cystoscope. It is stated that differences occur in the symptoms produced by different sorts of calculi. The large uric acid calculus less frequently produces severe symptoms but as the oxalate of lime is rougher, it is apt to produce more pain (often of a radiating character) and to cause hemorrhage. In both these forms the urine is acid. The phosphatic calculi are stated to produce the most intense pain and the urine is commonly alkaline. *Infarction* of the kidney may suggest stone, especially if there is pain and hematuria. There is practically always marked cardiac disease in these cases and infarction elsewhere is common.

Treatment.—In the attacks of renal colic great relief is experienced by a hot bath, which is sometimes sufficient to relax the spasm. When the pain is very intense morphia (gr. ¼, 0.016 gm.) and atropine (gr. 1/100, 0.006 gm.) should be given hypodermically and inhalations of chloroform may be necessary. Hot local applications are sometimes grateful. The patient may drink freely of hot lemonade or alkaline water. Occasionally change in posture or inversion gives great relief. In milder attacks it is wise to give tincture of belladonna (♏. 10, 0.6 cc.) with potassium acetate (gr. 15, 1 gm.) every 3 hours with large amounts of water. Surgical interference should be considered in all cases, especially when the stone is large or the associated pyelitis severe. Removal of a stone in the ureter by approach from the bladder or by operation should not be postponed. The function of the kidneys should be studied carefully before operation and especially with a stone in each kidney.

The patient should, as far as possible, live a quiet life, avoiding sudden exertion and jolting. An essential feature is to keep the urine abundant and, in the uric acid or uratic cases, alkaline. The patient should drink a large quantity of mineral water [1] or distilled water, which is just as satisfactory. The pains in the back are often greatly relieved by this treatment. Many patients find benefit from a stay at Saratoga, Bedford, Poland or other springs in the United States, or at Vichy or Ems in Europe.

If a stone has been passed its composition should be determined so that treatment can be carried out to prevent the further formation of stones if possible. For the rare uric acid stones, an alkaline urine is advisable, but for oxalate and phosphatic stones an acid reaction should be maintained. For oxalate calculi foods containing oxalic acid should be avoided. The most important are tea, coffee, cocoa, pepper, rhubarb, spinach, beetroot, beans, currants and figs. For uric acid calculi the diet is that indicated in gout.

[1] Some of these, if we judge by the laudatory reports, are as potent as the waters of Corsena, declared by Montaigne to be "powerful enough to break stones."

TUMORS OF THE KIDNEY

These are benign and malignant. Of the *benign* tumors, the most common are the small nodular *fibromata* which occur frequently in the pyramids, and occasionally *lipoma, angioma,* or *lymphadenoma.* The *adenomata* may be congenital; small nodules of aberrant adrenal tissue are not uncommon.

Malignant growths may be primary or secondary. The *sarcomata* are alveolar sarcoma or the remarkable form containing striped muscular fibres—rhabdomyoma. They usually occur in young children, grow rapidly and reach a large size. The most common and important renal tumor is the *hypernephroma,* the exact nature of which is doubtful. It often has metastases in the lungs which may give the first symptoms. Of 163 cases only 6 were extrarenal (Ellis). They may be small and in the renal cortex or form large tumors with extensive metastases. Most so-called carcinomas and sarcomas of the kidney are really hypernephromata. About 6 per cent of cases of new growth are associated with calculi.

The tumors attain a very large size and in children they may be enormous. They grow rapidly, are often soft, and hemorrhage frequently takes place into them. In the sarcomata, invasion of the pelvis or of the renal vein is common. The rhabdomyomata rarely form very large tumors, and death occurs shortly after birth. A child aged three years and a half died suddenly of embolism of the pulmonary artery and tricuspid orifice by a fragment of the tumor, which had grown into the renal vein. In association with new growth of the *adrenal cortex* precocious development of the external genitals has been noted, with overgrowth of the body, growth of hair on the face, and development of the breasts with menstruation in girls.

Symptoms.—The following are the most important: (*a*) *Hematuria* in more than half the cases may be the first indication. Its occurrence may be variable and intermittent. The blood is fluid or clotted, and there may be moulds of the pelvis of the kidney and of the ureter, which are rare except in cancer. Cancer cells are sometimes recognized in the urine.

(*b*) *Pain* is an uncertain symptom. In several of the largest tumors which have come under our observation there has been no discomfort from beginning to close. When present, it is of a dragging, dull character, situated in the flank and radiating down the thigh. The passage of the clots may cause great pain. In one case the growth was at first upward, and the symptoms for some months were those of pleurisy.

(*c*) Progressive *emaciation.* This may be marked and advance rapidly or there may be a large tumor without emaciation.

Physical Signs.—In almost all instances *tumor* is present. When small and on the right side, it may be very movable; in some instances, occupying a position in the iliac fossa, it has been mistaken for ovarian tumor. The large growths fill the flank and gradually extend toward the middle line, occupying the right or left half of the abdomen. Inspection may show two or three hemispherical projections corresponding to distended sections of the organ. In children the abdomen may reach an enormous size and the veins are prominent. On palpation the tumor is felt to occupy the lumbar region and can usually be lifted slightly; in some cases it is very movable, even when large;

in others it is fixed, firm, and solid. The respiratory movements have slight influence upon it. Rapidly growing renal tumors are soft and may give a sense of fluctuation. A point of importance is the fact that the colon crosses the tumor, and can usually be detected without difficulty. *Metastases* may give the first symptoms, especially in the lungs, brain or bones.

Prognosis.—Unless an early diagnosis is made so that removal is possible, the outlook is hopeless. The course may be prolonged in some cases for several years.

Diagnosis.—With hematuria, cystoscopy will show the affected kidney and the X-ray study and urinary examination should exclude calculus and tuberculosis. The diagnosis from *adrenal tumors* is difficult. The form described by Hutchison, usually in children and showing metastases in the skull, swelling of the eyelids, choked disk and severe anemia should be kept in mind. In children very large abdominal tumors are either renal or retroperitoneal. The retroperitoneal sarcoma (Lobstein's cancer) is more central, but may attain as large a size. If the case is seen only toward the end, a differential diagnosis may be impossible; but, as a rule, the sarcoma is less movable. It is to be remembered that these tumors may invade the kidney. On the left side an enlarged spleen is readily distinguished, as the edge is distinct and the notch or notches well marked; it descends during respiration, and the colon lies behind, not in front of it. On the right side growths of the liver are occasionally confounded with renal tumors: but such instances are rare, and there can usually be detected a zone of resonance between the upper margin of the renal tumor and the ribs. Late in the disease this is not possible, for the renal tumor is close to the liver. *Metastases* should be searched for, especially in the lungs.

A malignant growth in a movable kidney may be deceptive and simulate cancer of the ovary or myoma of the uterus. The great mobility upward of the renal growth and the negative pelvic examination are important.

Treatment.—When the growth is small, metastases excluded, and the patient in good condition removal of the organ may be undertaken, but the percentage of cases of recovery is very small, only 5.4 per cent (G. Walker). Otherwise the treatment is symptomatic.

CYSTIC DISEASE OF THE KIDNEY

Small Cysts.—These occur with chronic nephritis, and result from dilatation of obstructed tubules or Bowman's capsules. There are cases in elderly persons difficult to classify, in which the kidneys are greatly enlarged, very cystic, and yet not so large as in the congenital form.

Solitary Cysts.—Solitary cysts, ranging in size from a marble to an orange, or even larger, are occasionally found in kidneys which present no other changes. In exceptional cases they may form tumors of considerable size. Newman operated on one which contained 25 ounces of blood. They too, in all probability, result from obstruction.

Polycystic Kidneys.—In this condition, the greatly enlarged organs, weighing even as much as six pounds, are represented by a conglomeration of cysts, varying in size from a pea to a marble. Little or no renal tissue may be noticeable, although in sections it is seen that a certain amount remains in the interspaces. The cysts contain a clear or turbid fluid, sometimes reddish brown or even blackish, and may be of a colloidal consistence. Albumin, blood crystals, cholesterin, with triple phosphates and fat drops, are found in the contents. Urea and uric acid are rarely present. The cysts are lined by flattened epithelium. They occur in the fetus and sometimes are of such a size as to obstruct labor. In the adult they are usually bilateral, and there is every reason to believe that they begin in early life and increase gradually. A progressive growth has been noticed. They may be found with cystic disease of the liver and other organs. It is difficult to account for the origin of this remarkable condition, which some regard as a defect of development rather than a pathological change, and point to the association in the fetal cases of other anomalies, as imperforate anus. Others believe the condition to be a new growth—a sort of mucoid endothelioma. Several members of a family may be affected. In one instance mother and son were subjects of the disease. The average *age* at recognition is about 40 years.

SYMPTOMS.—Of a series of cases seen in adults the condition was recognized during life in the majority. The features are characteristic.

(*a*) *Bilateral renal tumors,* which may increase in size under observation. They may cause great enlargement of the upper zone of the abdomen. The colon and stomach are in front of the tumors, on the surface of which in thin subjects the cysts may be palpable or visible. While both kidneys are, as a rule, involved, one may be much smaller than the other.

(*b*) *Hematuria,* which may recur at intervals for years.

(*c*) The signs of a *chronic nephritis:* (1) pallor or muddy complexion; in rare instances a bronzing of the skin; (2) arteriosclerosis; (3) cardiac hypertrophy with accentuated second sound; (4) urine abundant, a low specific gravity, with albumin, and hyaline and granular casts, and in one case cholesterin crystals. Death occurs from uremia or the cardiovascular complications of chronic nephritis. A rare event is rupture of a cyst with perinephric abscess and peritonitis. The skin may be much pigmented.

Diagnosis.—If both enlarged kidneys can be felt and there are the signs of chronic nephritis, there is no difficulty. If only one kidney is felt, with hematuria the diagnosis of neoplasm may be made. Urographic studies should be made of both kidneys.

TREATMENT.—Operation, by exposing the kidney and draining the cysts, has been successful. When the condition is unilateral the kidney has been removed and the patients have remained well for years. Otherwise the treatment is that of chronic nephritis.

Other Varieties.—Occasionally the kidneys and liver present numerous small cysts scattered through the substance. The spleen and thyroid may be involved, and there may be congenital malformation of the heart. The cysts in the kidney are small, and neither so numerous nor so thickly set as in the conglomerate form, though the condition is probably the result of some congenital defect. There are cases, however, in which the kidneys are very large. It is more common in the lower animals than in man.

Echinococcus cysts are noted in the section on parasites. Paranephric cysts (external to the capsule) are rare; they may reach a large size.

PERINEPHRITIS AND PERINEPHRIC ABSCESS

Perinephritis.—This occurs in various forms. There may be *fibrosis* of the capsule of the kidney, a chronic fibrotic process with sclerosis of the perirenal fat and a *fibrolipomatous* process. The fatty capsule of the kidney is firm, with numerous bands of fibrous tissue, and is stripped off from the proper capsule with great difficulty. The main *symptom* is pain which is usually persistent. Mathé (1933) has emphasized the lack of mobility of the kidney, shown by a pyelogram taken in the upright position.

Perinephric Abscess.—Suppuration in the connective tissue about the kidney may follow (1) blows and injuries; (2) extension of inflammation from the pelvis of the kidney, the kidney itself, or the ureters; (3) rupture of a septic infarct in the kidney; (4) perforation of the bowel, most commonly the appendix, in some instances the colon; (5) extension of suppuration from the spine, as in caries, or from the pleura, as in empyema; (6) as a sequel of the fevers, particularly in children; and (7) from a distant focus of infection. In many instances the organism is a staphylococcus.

Postmortem the kidney is surrounded by pus, particularly at the posterior part, though the pus may lie altogether in front, between the kidney and the peritoneum. Usually the abscess cavity is extensive. The pus is often offensive and may have a distinctly fecal odor from contact with the large bowel. It may burrow in various directions and burst into the pleura and be discharged through the lungs. A more frequent direction is down the psoas muscle, when it appears in the groin, or it may pass along the iliacus fascia and appear at Poupart's ligament. It may perforate the bowel or rupture into the peritoneum; sometimes it penetrates the bladder or vagina.

Symptoms.—There may be intense *pain,* aggravated by pressure, in the lumbar region. In other instances the onset is insidious, without pain in the renal region; signs of deep seated suppuration may be detected. The pain may be referred to the neighborhood of the hip joint or to the joint itself, or radiate down the thigh and be associated with retraction of the testis. The patient lies with the thigh flexed, so as to relax the psoas muscle, and in walking throws, as far as possible, the weight on the opposite leg. He keeps the spine immobile, walks stooped and can voluntarily adduct the thigh only with difficulty.

There may be pus in the urine if the disease has extended from the pelvis or the kidney, but in other forms the urine is clear. When pus has formed there are usually chills with irregular fever and sweats. There may be swelling in the back or deep seated induration is felt between the last rib and the crest of the ilium. Bimanual palpation may reveal a distinct tumor mass. Edema or puffiness of the skin is frequently present. Leukocytosis is common.

Diagnosis.—This is usually easy except in the early stages; when doubt exists the aspirator needle should be used. With the X-ray, a lateral curvature of the spine with the concavity toward the affected side may be found. The kidney may be fixed and its shadow somewhat obscured. It is usually possible, especially by the X-ray, to exclude disease of the vertebra. In children hip-joint disease may be suspected, but the pain is higher, and there is no fullness or tenderness over the hip-joint itself. In left-sided abscess, with the fluoroscope, on quickly moving the patient, a wave can be seen in the fluid.

Treatment.—The treatment is clear—early, free, and permanent drainage.

SECTION IX

DISEASES OF THE BLOOD-FORMING ORGANS

ANEMIA

Anemia, a reduction of the amount of blood as a whole or of its corpuscles, or of certain of its constituents, may be due to failure in the manufacture, to increase in the consumption, or to a loss, sudden or gradual, as in hemorrhage. Anemia may be local in certain parts, or general.

Local Anemia.—Tissue irrigation with blood is primarily from the heart, but provision is made for variations in the supply, according to the needs of a part. The sluices are worked by the stop-cock action of the arteries, which contract or expand under vasomotor influence, central and peripheral. If the sluices of one large district are too widely open, so much blood may enter that other important regions have not a sufficient supply. Local anemia of the brain, causing syncope, ensues when the mesenteric channels, capable of holding all the blood, are wide open. Emotional stimuli, reflex from pain, etc., removal of pressure, as after tapping in ascites, may cause this. Possibly many symptoms in enteroptosis are due to relative anemia of the nervous system, owing to the persistent overfilling of the mesenteric reservoir. We know little of local anemia of the various organs, but functional disturbance in the kidneys, heart, etc., may result from a permanently low pressure in the local blood "mains." Anemia from arterial spasm is seen in Raynaud's disease, which usually affects the peripheral vessels, causing local syncope of the fingers, but may occur in the visceral vessels, particularly of the brain, and cause temporary hemiplegia, aphasia, etc.

Pseudo-anemia is common. Pallor may exist with a normal or even a plus blood count and color index. The transient pallor in nausea and after a drinking bout is a vasomotor affair. In aortic insufficiency, in lead-workers, in the morphia habitué, the skin may be permanently pale. The skin of the face may be unusually thick or the capillaries poorly developed, as in sedentary workers in contrast to the ruddy complexion of country people. The Latin races are paler than the Anglo-Saxons. There are healthy and strong individuals with a permanent pallor and normal blood.

General Anemia—Classification.—This offers many difficulties, as shown by the number of classifications suggested. The division into primary and secondary anemias is no longer suitable. One method is by etiology, another by the changes in the red blood cells or by their size. It is probable that any classification made at present will require revision in the future. Ottenberg (1933) suggests three main groups: (1) Due to some deficiency, (2) Due to direct injury to the blood forming organs, and (3) Due to blood destruction. Under the first heading are the anemias due to a lack of the "anti-anemic" principle, as in pernicious anemia, nutritional anemias and those due to hemorrhage. Under the second heading come aplastic anemia, that due to radio-active substances, and the anemia with certain bone diseases. In the third group, due to hemolysis, are the anemias secondary to many infections, as malaria, and to those with conditions such as sickle cell anemia. While in the majority of cases with a careful study the classification of a given case may be made with accuracy we must acknowledge that there are anomalous cases in which an exact designation is difficult or impossible. It appears at times that there are more such cases to-day than twenty-five years ago. This may be due to more elaborate methods of study and more complicated classifications. The terminology has become a special language.

Acute Anemia from Hemorrhage

Etiology.—In rupture of a large vessel or an aneurism, in peptic ulcer, or in injury to blood vessels the loss of three or four pounds of blood may prove fatal. Seven and a half pounds may be shed into one cavity (rupture of an aneurism into the pleura). A patient with hematemesis lost ten pounds of blood in one week, and yet recovered from the immediate effects. Even after the severest traumatic hemorrhage the blood count is rarely so low as in severe cases of pernicious anemia.

Symptoms.—Dyspnea, rapid action of the heart, and faintness are the prominent symptoms of an acutely produced anemia. There is marked pallor of the skin and mucous membranes, the pulse is jerking, the vessels throb, particularly the abdominal aorta, and the pistol shot sound is heard over them, the temperature is low, the patient feels giddy and faint and has noises in the ears. The blood pressure is low. If the bleeding continues there may be nausea, vomiting, and, with the rapid loss of large quantities of blood, convulsions. There is a great diminution of the red blood cells, often below 2,000,000 per c.mm. The hemoglobin is proportionately lower. Irregularity in the red blood cells is seen; nucleated cells, usually normoblasts, may appear early; the leukocytes are increased, usually the multinuclear neutrophiles. The process of regeneration goes on with great rapidity; the watery and saline constituents are readily restored; the albuminous elements are quickly renewed, but it may take weeks or months for the red blood corpuscles to reach normal. In a case of purpura the red cells fell between the 20th and 30th of April to below 2,000,000. It was not until July that the red blood corpuscles reached 4,000,000, and the blood was not normal until September. The hemoglobin is restored more slowly than the corpuscles.

In repeated hemorrhages the picture depends upon the interval between the losses of blood. If long enough to allow of complete regeneration each time the total amount of blood lost may be very great. Ehrlich mentions a patient with hemoptysis who lost 20 kilograms of blood in 6½ months. If the intervals are short, so that complete recovery from each loss is not possible, a chronic anemia is induced with a low color index.

Treatment.—In severe cases blood transfusion should be done as soon as possible. Normal saline solution may be given subcutaneously or intravenously but only if shock is marked in cases in which the bleeding may occur again, as in peptic ulcer. The patient should be at rest and given as nutritious a diet as possible with abundance of vitamins. Iron is to be given freely as Blaud's mass, 60 to 90 grains a day (4-6 gm.) or as iron and ammonium citrate 90 grains (6 gm.) a day. There is no gain in giving iron hypodermically.

Chronic Secondary Hypochromic or Microcytic Anemia

Synonyms.—Chronic *secondary* or *symptomatic* anemia. In this group the anemia occurs with another disease to which it is secondary. The color index is low and usually a large number of the red cells are below the normal size.

Etiology.—There are many causes, the most important of which are:

(*a*) *Inanition.*—This may be brought about by defective food supply or by conditions which interfere with the proper reception, digestion and absorption of the food. Lack of vitamins may be a factor.

(*b*) *Infections.*—In many acute fevers anemia is produced, which may persist after the infection has subsided. We see this particularly in typhoid fever, rheumatic fever, sepsis and malaria. Certain animal parasites, as the hookworm and diphyllobothrium, cause a profound anemia.

(*c*) *Intoxications.*—Inorganic poisons, such as lead, mercury, arsenic; organic poisons, as the toxins of various fevers; and certain autogenous poisons occurring in chronic affections, such as nephritis and jaundice.

An interesting type of toxic anemia is caused by arseniuretted hydrogen gas in submarines due to the slow action of gas evolved from the metallic portion of the battery plates. Of thirty cases studied by Dudley, the chief symptoms were dyspnea, albuminuria, puffiness of the face, conjunctivitis, jaundice and mild neuritic symptoms. The anemia was never extreme, the color index was, as a rule, high, with numerous megaloblasts.

(*d*) *Hemorrhage.*—This, if repeated, may cause severe anemia. This is particularly shown in cases of persistent bleeding from hemorrhoids.

(*e*) Long continued drain upon the system, as in chronic suppuration, prolonged lactation, and malignant disease.

Symptoms.—Loss of bodily and mental vigor with loss of weight and obvious anemia are the important features. The patient tires easily, the appetite is poor, digestion often faulty, palpitation is complained of, and there may be feelings of faintness, and, as the anemia progresses, swelling of the feet. There is not infrequently slight fever. Petechiae on the skin are not uncommon and retinal hemorrhages may occur. The blood picture is distinctive. The red blood cells are reduced, but rarely below two millions per c.mm. The hemoglobin is relatively lower than the red cells, thus with 70 per cent of red cells there may be only 40 per cent of hemoglobin, a low color index. The red blood corpuscles are irregular in shape, nucleated forms may be present, and the leukocytes are sometimes increased in number.

The *diagnosis* of secondary anemia rarely gives difficulty except in cases in which the blood picture may suggest the pernicious form. There are cases of very severe anemia in hookworm infection or cancer of the stomach but the other features of pernicious anemia are lacking. The diagnosis of the *cause* of secondary anemia may be difficult. There are patients with a persistent tendency to anemia, perhaps lasting for years, in whom no cause can be found. A congenitally inefficient bone marrow may be responsible. Some are probably cases of idiopathic hypochromic anemia.

Treatment.—The cause of the anemia should be sought and the necessary indications met. The large group depending on the drain on the albuminous materials of the blood, as in nephritis and suppuration, is difficult to treat successfully, and so long as the cause keeps up it is impossible to restore the normal blood condition. The anemia of inanition requires plenty of nourishing food, especially meat, and abundant vitamins. When dependent on organic changes in the gastro-intestinal mucosa not much can be expected from either food or medicine. In toxic cases due to mercury and lead the poison must be eliminated and a nutritious diet given with full doses of iron. In a great majority of the cases there is deficient blood formation, and the indications are briefly three: plenty of food, an open-air life and iron. As a rule, it makes but little difference what form of the drug is administered except that the inorganic preparations are best. The important point is to give *enough* and too often patients suffer from insufficient dosage. The best forms are Blaud's mass, 60 to 90 grains a day (4-6 gm.), making sure, if in pill form, that the pills are soft; iron and ammonium citrate 90 grains (6 gm.) a day in a 25 per cent solution, and ferrous sulphate (gr. x, 0.6 gm.) a day. Small doses of arsenic may be added with advantage; copper does not require to be given. There does not seem to be any advantage in giving iron hypodermically. Intravenous administration is to be condemned. In some severe forms secondary to chronic hemorrhages, liver therapy may be successful. In the majority of cases of secondary anemia it is not of value. In severe forms the patient should be at rest in bed and in the open air, if possible.

Idiopathic Hypochromic Anemia

Synonyms.—Idiopathic microcytic anemia; simple achlorhydric anemia.

Definition.—An anemia occurring especially but not exclusively in women, usually between the ages of 30 or 50 years, with an insidious onset, a chronic anemia, achlorhydria usually and a response to iron therapy.

Etiology.—A deficiency of iron possibly associated with achlorhydria, which is not always found, and disturbance of absorption from the intestine are suggested. Defective diet may be a factor. Pregnancy, lactation and excessive menstruation probably have an influence. The cases in males are few.

Pathology.—The bone marrow shows hyperplasia and an increase in the number of normoblasts.

Symptoms.—The onset is insidious but as there is often a history of symptoms for a long time it is difficult to know the time of onset. The main complaints are those due to anemia, asthenia, pallor, dyspnea, etc., and a group of digestive disturbances, glossitis, stomatitis, dysphagia and indigestion with constipation usually and diarrhea in some cases. There may be functional nervous disturbances as paresthesia, pruritus, and instability. Changes in the nails are common; they may be tender and brittle. The hair is often dry and may turn gray at an early age. There is marked *pallor*, often with undernutrition. The *blood* shows a low hemoglobin and a reduction in the red cells, much less relatively than in the hemoglobin. An average count is Hb. 40 per cent and red cells 3,500,000. The color index is low, often 0.5 or 0.6. There may be leukopenia. An occasional normoblast may be seen. The average size of the red cells is decreased. The icterus index is below normal. The *tongue* often shows changes; it may be smooth and red without papillæ. There may be marked *glossitis.* The gastric analysis shows absence of free hydrochloric acid but this is not invariable and the acid may appear after histamine is given. The achlorhydria may precede the anemia and remain after it is corrected. The spleen is enlarged in some instances. The *Plummer-Vinson syndrome* occurs with this anemia. The *course* is chronic without treatment and there is a strong tendency to recurrence.

Diagnosis.—This has to be made from chronic hypochromic anemia. The absence of the causal factors of the latter and the special features of this form usually suffice but in some cases the distinction may be difficult. The blood study distinguishes it from pernicious anemia. If the spleen is enlarged, splenic anemia is suggested; the result of therapy is important.

Treatment.—Good general hygiene, a varied diet with sufficient vitamins and iron in large dosage, as in chronic hypochromic anemia, are indicated. Maintenance doses should be given after the blood returns to normal to prevent recurrence. Dilute hydrochloric acid should be given if there is achlorhydria.

Plummer-Vinson Syndrome.—This shows a combination of glossitis, anemia and dysphagia and there is doubt as to its essential nature. The *cause* is in dispute but the local changes in the mucous membrane seem important. The anemia may be due to insufficient food due to the difficulty in swallowing. Some regard the anemia as the essential feature. It occurs usually in middle aged women with dysphagia, at first intermittent and later more constant, with severe choking attacks. The difficulty seems to be at the junction of the pharynx and esophagus and may be due to failure to relax rather than to spasm. The mucous membrane of the mouth and tongue has a smooth glossy appearance, is dry and easily injured. These changes extend to the pharynx and occasionally to the esophagus. In some cases the entrance to the esophagus is small and spasm is regarded as important. Other features are anemia, which is usually of a hypochromic form, enlargement of the spleen, and disturbance of the general health. In *treatment* every effort should be made to give sufficient food and a diet high in vitamins. Iron and ammonium citrate gr. 90 (6 gm.) per day should be given. Local sedatives, such as vaseline, may be applied to the pharynx.

Chlorosis

Definition.—An anemia of unknown cause, in young girls, characterized by a marked diminution of the hemoglobin with cardiovascular and sometimes nervous symptoms.

Occurrence.—Chlorosis has practically disappeared in America. This is one of the unexplained changes in the occurrence of disease. Forty years ago it was common; now it is extinct.

Etiology.—It is a disease of girls and it is doubtful if males are ever affected. The age of onset is between the fourteenth and seventeenth years;

recurrences, which are common, may extend into the third decade. The disease is most common among ill-fed, overworked girls confined in close, badly lighted rooms. Cases occur, however, under the most favorable conditions, but not often in countrybred girls, as Maudlin sings in the *Compleat Angler*. Lack of proper exercise and fresh air with improper food are factors. Emotional and nervous disturbances may be prominent. Menstrual disturbances are common but are probably a sequence. Constipation has been assigned as a cause.

Symptoms.—(*a*) General.—The subcutaneous fat is well retained or even increased. The complexion is peculiar, a curious yellow green tinge, which has given the disease its name, and its popular designation, the green sickness. Occasionally the skin shows pigmentation, particularly about the joints. The color may be deceptive, as the cheeks may have a reddish tint, particularly on exertion. The subjects complain of breathlessness and palpitation, and syncope is frequent, which often lead to the suspicion of heart or lung disease. Puffiness of the face and swelling of the ankles may suggest nephritis. The eyes have a peculiar brilliancy and the sclerotics are of a bluish color.

(*b*) Special Features.—*Blood*.—The drop looks pale. The essential feature is not a reduction in the number of cells but in the hemoglobin. The corpuscles look pale. There may be all the features of a profound anemia with the number of red cells nearly normal. No other form of anemia presents this feature, at least with the same constancy and in the same degree. In severe cases the red cells may be irregular in size and shape. Nucleated red cells (normoblasts) may be found in severe cases. The leukocytes may show a slight increase; the blood plates may be increased.

(*c*) Gastro-intestinal Symptoms.—The appetite is capricious, and patients may have a longing for unusual articles, particularly acids, and all sorts of indigestible things, such as chalk or even earth. Gastric distress is frequent. Constipation is common and usually obstinate.

(*d*) Circulatory Symptoms.—Palpitation of the heart may be the most distressing symptom. The transverse dulness may be increased. A systolic murmur is heard at the apex or at the base; more commonly at the latter, but in extreme cases at both. A diastolic murmur is rare. Over the jugular vein a continuous murmur may be heard. The pulse is usually full and soft. Pulsation in the peripheral veins is sometimes seen.

Thrombosis in the veins may occur, most commonly in the femoral and in the cerebral sinuses. In 86 cases the veins of the legs were affected in 48, the cerebral sinuses in 29 (Lichtenstern). The danger in femoral thrombosis is pulmonary embolism—in 13 of 52 cases (Welch).

Fever is not uncommon. Dermatographia is common. Hysterical manifestations are not infrequent. Menstrual disturbances are common and with improvement in the blood this function is usually restored.

Diagnosis.—Chlorosis is often recognized at a glance. The well-nourished condition, the peculiar complexion, most marked in brunettes, and the white or bluish sclerotics are characteristic. A special danger exists of mistaking the early stage of pulmonary tuberculosis for chlorosis. The palpitation of the heart and shortness of breath suggest heart disease, and the edema of the feet and pallor cause the cases to be mistaken for nephritis. The characters of the blood separate chlorosis from other forms of anemia.

Treatment.—This affords one of the most brilliant instances—of which we have but three or four—of the specific action of a remedy. Iron should be given in large doses as in other hypochromic anemias. An important point is to persist in the use of iron for at least three months, and it is wise to resume it in smaller doses, as recurrences are common. The diet should consist of good, easily digested food. Special care should be taken to prevent constipation. For the dyspeptic symptoms dilute hydrochloric acid is often useful. Rest in bed is important in severe cases.

Pernicious or Addisonian Anemia

Definition.—A severe and usually characteristic megalocytic anemia of unknown etiology and characterized by an embryonic type of hematopoiesis. It is to be noted that not all megalocytic anemias come under pernicious anemia.

History.—Addison, after whom the disease should be called, gave the first accurate account (1855). Channing described cases of severe anemia in the puerperal state. The writings of Gusserow and Biermer did much to awaken interest in the disease. The studies of Pepper (Secundus), H. C. Wood, and Palmer Howard made the disease familiar to American and Canadian physicians. Minot and Murphy introduced liver therapy in 1926 and Sturgis and Isaacs, in 1929, the use of desiccated defatted hog stomach.

Distribution.—It is a widespread disease, the incidence of which in any community is a good deal a matter of keenness on the part of the practitioners (Cabot). It appears to be increasing.

Etiology.—The figures quoted are from Cabot's analysis of some 1,200 cases in his article in our *System of Medicine.* It is a disease of middle life; a great majority—922—occurred over the age of 36. The youngest patient we have seen was a boy of ten years. Two or three cases may occur in one family and other relatives may show allied conditions such as achlorhydria.

The discovery by Minot and his coworkers that in liver and kidney there is a substance which profoundly influences the disease suggests several possibilities as to its nature. There is a lack of some substance, not identified, which is normally formed in the stomach, absorbed from the intestine and stored in the liver and probably in other organs. The individual is unable to obtain or form this substance from the protein ingested. Some modification of this in the body, probably in the liver, may be lacking. Is a hormone concerned? A predisposing constitutional factor is suggested, especially in the occurrence of achlorhydria, which may long precede the occurrence of the anemia, and be found in other members of the family. The work of Castle, which shows that meat previously digested in a normal human stomach and then fed to a pernicious anemia patient is effectual in treatment, is important. Infection of the gastro-intestinal tract can not be disregarded but has it any causal effect (as by influence on the liver) or is it a result largely of the achlorhydria? How many patients have the anti-anemic principle in the liver but not utilised?

Sex.—It is more common in males, but under the age of 30 women are more often affected.

Among other factors in cases *resembling* Addisonian anemia are:

Pregnancy and Parturition.—The anemia may (1) come on during pregnancy or (2) follow delivery, without any special loss of blood, or (3) be an acute septic anemia. There were 18 in Cabot's series of 1,200 cases. As a rule, cases in this group are readily recognized.

Intestinal Parasites.—Anemia of a severe and even pernicious type may be associated with diphyllobothrium or hookworm.

Hemorrhage.—Anemia after hemorrhage is usually of the hypochromic type, but in every series of cases of Addison's anemia will be found a few with a history of bleeding piles, epistaxis or loss of blood from other sources.

Certain *nutritional* anemias, and that of *sprue* and some forms of *fatty diarrhea.*

We have not got much beyond the position of Addison, who characterized the disease which he was describing as "a general anemia occurring without any discoverable cause whatever; cases in which there had been no previous loss of blood, no existing diarrhea, no chlorosis, no purpura, no renal, splenic, myasmatic, glandular, strumous or malignant disease."

Pathology.—The body is rarely emaciated. A lemon tint of the skin is present in a majority of the cases. The muscles may be intensely red, like horseflesh, while the fat is light yellow. Hemorrhages are common on the skin and serous surfaces. The heart is usually large, flabby, and empty. The myocardium is intensely fatty, and of a pale, light yellow color. In no affection do we see more extreme fatty degeneration. The lungs show no special changes. The stomach in many instances is normal, but in some cases the mucosa is extensively atrophied. The liver may be enlarged and fatty. The iron is in excess, a striking contrast to the cases of hypochromic anemia. It is deposited in the outer and middle zones of the lobules.

The spleen shows no important changes. The iron pigment is usually in excess. The lymph nodes may be of a deep red color. The amount of iron pigment is increased in the kidneys, chiefly in the convoluted tubules. The bone marrow is usually red, lymphoid in character, showing great numbers of nucleated red corpuscles, especially megaloblasts. There are cases in which the bone marrow shows no signs of activity—*aplastic anemia.*

Spinal cord lesions were present in 84 per cent of the postmortems collected by Cabot, a sclerosis chiefly of the posterior and lateral columns. Foci of a similar nature occur in the brain in the gray and white matter (Woltman).

Symptoms.—The description given by Addison is masterly: "It makes its approach in so slow and insidious a manner that the patient can hardly fix a date to the earliest feeling of that languor which is shortly to become so extreme. The countenance gets pale, the whites of the eyes become pearly, the general frame flabby rather than wasted, the pulse perhaps large, but remarkably soft and compressible, and occasionally with a slight jerk, especially under the slightest excitement. There is an increasing indisposition to exertion, with an uncomfortable feeling of faintness or breathlessness in attempting it; the heart is readily made to palpitate; the whole surface of the body presents a blanched, smooth, and waxy appearance; the lips, gums, and tongue seem bloodless, the flabbiness of the solids increases, the appetite fails, extreme languor and faintness supervene, breathlessness and palpitation are produced by the most trifling exertion or emotion; some slight edema is probably perceived about the ankles; the debility becomes extreme—the patient can no longer rise from bed; the mind occasionally wanders; he falls into a prostrate and half-torpid state, and at length expires; nevertheless, to the very last, and after a sickness of several months' duration, the bulkiness of the general frame and the amount of obesity often present a most striking contrast to the failure and exhaustion observable in every other respect."

A surprising fact is that there are patients with extreme anemia who are remarkably vigorous. One may see patients with a count of about two million red cells who insist that they are able to do everything as usual except for a little shortness of breath.

The appearance of the patient is usually very characteristic. The combination of a lemon-yellow tint of the skin with retention of the fat gives a very suggestive picture. Sometimes the tint is icteroid. In rare cases there is a white, anemic pallor, and in a third group a brownish tinge of the skin (sometimes associated with leukoderma) deep enough to suggest Addison's disease. Muscular weakness, palpitation, headache, dyspnea, vertigo and edema of the feet are common. *Fever* is usually present if the anemia is severe. Hunter emphasizes the seasonal character of the onset and relapses, usually from July to September, and the importance of *glossitis.* This latter occurs early, may be sudden in onset and occurs periodically. It may be least marked when the anemia is severe.

Gastro-intestinal symptoms are common. Paroxysms of abdominal pain with or without diarrhea may occur in crises. In fully one-half of the cases diarrhea occurs at some time during the course. Hydrochloric acid is practically always absent and this has been noted in some cases long before the onset of the anemia. The acid does not return when the blood count becomes normal. There may be marked glossitis and ulceration. The tongue is often smooth and glistening with atrophy of the papillae. Pyorrhea alveolaris is present in many cases and the teeth are often very bad.

Complaint of palpitation and disturbance of the *heart* is common. Slight dilatation is common; murmurs are rarely missed, generally hemic and basic. Apex diastolic murmurs may occur without valve lesions. Extraordinary throbbing of the arteries may be seen; the pulse may be collapsing. Anginal attacks may occur. Edema is common, usually in the feet, sometimes in the hands. The urine is usually of low specific gravity and pale. Sometimes it is of a deep sherry color, due to excess of urobilin. Increase of *urobilin* and urobilinogen in the stools, duodenal contents and urine is a constant finding, and the presence of these substances in the absence of biliary or hepatic disease is suggestive of pernicious anemia.

Nervous System.—The more carefully the patients are studied, the greater the frequency of nervous lesions. Numbness and tingling are common and sometimes there are marked neuritic pains. Multiple neuritis may be a feature of the disease. There are three groups of cases:

(*a*) The patient may have had no special symptoms pointing to involvement of the nervous system, but postmortem lesions of the cord are found.

(*b*) With the anemia there are signs of spinal cord lesions, a posterolateral sclerosis, with spastic features and increased reflexes, or the picture may be rather of the tabetic type—lightning pains, girdle sensation, areas of anesthesia and loss of the reflexes.

(*c*) There is a group (Russell, Batten, and Collier) in which the nervous changes, usually posterolateral sclerosis, precede the anemia.

As the disease progresses there may be great depression, sometimes delusions, but mental symptoms, as a rule, are not marked.

Hemorrhages are not uncommon, chiefly in the form of small petechiae. Retinal hemorrhages are frequent. Optic neuritis is rare.

Blood.—The drop may look of fair color but it is abnormally fluid. The *red cells* are greatly diminished; the average count in 81 patients, when they came under observation, was 1,575,000 per c.mm. There is no other disease which so often reduces the red blood corpuscles below 2,000,000. In 12 per cent of our cases the count was under 1,000,000. The count in a patient of Quincke's was 143,000 per c.mm. Capillary red cell counts average nearly 20 per cent higher than counts of the venous blood and more macrocytes are found in the capillary blood, probably due to the movement of the larger cells being slowed in the narrow capillaries (Duke and Stofer). This may explain the good color of the skin with a severe anemia. The *hemoglobin,* though quantitatively reduced, is relatively high. The color index is 1 or over.

Marked irregularity in size and shape of the red cells with many large forms is a special feature. Megalocytosis is a most essential feature. On the other hand, there are small red corpuscles—microcytes, from 2 to 6 μ in diameter, and of a deep red color. The large volume of the average red cell is a constant feature. The determination of the volume index is significant. The *Price-Jones curve* is determined by measuring the diameter of 500 red blood cells and charting the results with the number of cells as ordinates and the cell diameters as abscissæ, so that a red cell diameter distribution curve is obtained. If the variation in the size of the red cells is greater than normal the base of the curve is widened. The irregularity in shape is remarkable. Some are elongated, rod-like, others pyriform; one end of the corpuscle may be of normal shape, while the other is extended like the neck of a bottle. The reticulocytes are normal except in remissions. The bilirubin in the blood serum is greatly increased and varies inversely with the degree of anemia. The icterus index may be 20 or 25 (normal 4 to 6) and the van den Bergh reaction gives 1 to 2 mg. per 100 cc. (normal maximum 0.6). The serum in other anemias is much paler. The cholestral figures are low in the whole blood (Gibson and Howard).

Nucleated red cells are present at some time, varying in numbers from day to day. There are two main types—normoblasts of the average size and the megaloblasts, which are much larger. There are frequently intermediate forms between these two groups. The nucleated red cells vary extraordinarily and in the blood crises, a large number of nucleated reds appear. In one such crisis there were 14,388 normoblasts, 460 intermediates, and 138 megaloblasts per c.mm.

The *leukocytes* are generally diminished in number (2,000-4,000). There is often a marked increase in the small mononuclear forms. Levine and Ladd found that in a series nearly 40 per cent had eosinophiles of 5 per cent or over; 30 per cent had from 6 to 28 per cent. Myelocytes are frequently present, even up to 8 and 10 per cent. The blood plates are usually low; counts of 100,000 and less are not uncommon (Pratt).

The *metabolism* has been the subject of many studies. A pathological destruction of proteins is usually present but a positive nitrogen balance may be maintained by forced feeding (Mosenthal).

Prognosis and Course.—The disease may run a very acute course. In a patient of Finley's in Montreal the fatal termination occurred within ten days of the onset of symptoms. The introduction of liver therapy has completely altered the prognosis and gives the hope that the majority of patients can look forward to a great prolongation of life. It is essential that liver or ventriculin therapy be continued permanently in the necessary amount. The spinal

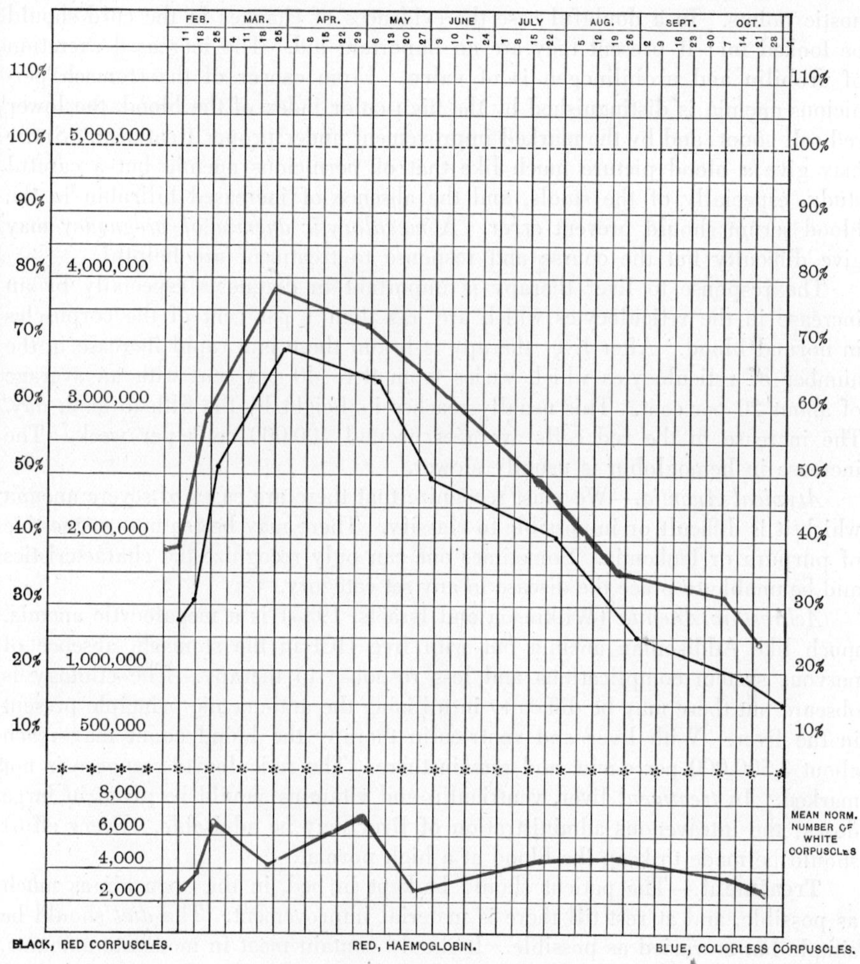

Chart XVI.—Pernicious Anemia

cord symptoms may improve but not necessarily even when the anemia is overcome.

The ultimate prognosis before the introduction of liver treatment was bad; only one patient in our series appeared to have recovered completely, another was alive and in good health six years after the last attack, and a third four years after. In Cabot's series there were ten cases which had lasted seven years or more, but there were only 6 out of 1,200 cases which he regarded as having completely recovered.

Diagnosis.—There is something very characteristic about the general appearance of a patient with Addisonian anemia. The lemon colored tint of the skin may suggest jaundice; the anemia, puffy face, swollen ankles, and albumin in the urine, nephritis; the pigmentation, Addison's disease; the shortness of breath and palpitation, heart disease; the pallor and gastric symptoms, cancer of the stomach. The usual retention of fat, the insidious onset, the absence of signs of local disease and the blood features are the important diagnostic points. In a doubtful case the evidences of changes in the cord should be looked for; if present they are an important aid. The increased excretion of urobilin and urobilinogen is of value. From cancer of the stomach pernicious anemia is distinguished by the high color index of the blood, the lower red cell count, and by the marked improvement under proper treatment. *Sprue* may give a blood picture much like that of pernicious anemia but a careful study, especially of the stools, and the absence of increased bilirubin in the blood serum should prevent error. A *megalocytic anemia of pregnancy* may give difficulty but the course and response to treatment are helpful.

The response to liver therapy is important in diagnosis especially by an increase in the reticulocytes which are less than 1 per cent of the corpuscles in normal blood. After liver therapy is begun there is a rapid increase in the number of reticulocytes which varies from 8 to 40 per cent with an average of about 20 per cent. This usually reaches its height by the fifth to tenth day. The increase in the red cells averages around 400,000 cells per week. The increase in hemoglobin is usually slower.

Atypical Anemia.—We must recognize that there are cases of severe anemia which it is difficult or impossible to classify. There may be features suggestive of purpura or leukemia. Sometimes one can only recognize the characteristics and be unable to place the disease in any set category.

Achresthic Anemia (Wilkinson and Israëls, 1935) is a megalocytic anemia, much like Addisonian anemia but with free HCl in the stomach, absence of nervous system complications and less response to therapy. The etiology is obscure but there may be difficulty in utilizing the anti-anemic principle present in the liver. With liver and ventriculin therapy the blood count may reach about 3,500,000 per c.mm. and remain there. The reticulocyte response is not marked. In *treatment* liver, ventriculin and vitamins should be given in large doses; the intravenous administration of liver may be advisable. Every effort should be made to keep the blood at a high normal.

Treatment.—The patient should be kept in bed, in the open air as much as possible, and at rest till there is material improvement. The *diet* should be simple but as varied as possible. It should contain meat in moderate amounts, fresh vegetables and fruits, and foods rich in vitamins. Liver and kidney are protein foods of special, one might say, specific value. *Liver* should be taken in amounts of one-half to one pound a day. If liver extract is used an amount (which contains a nonprotein fraction) representing one-half pound should be given each day, usually divided into three doses. The most satisfactory method is to give the liver extract intramuscularly, 2 cc. daily or every other day. This may be kept up until the blood count is normal. Intravenous administration is not advised except in an emergency. *Ventriculin* (desiccated defatted hog stomach) is given in daily doses of 10 grams for each million deficit in the blood count. The liver extract and ventriculin can be given by mouth in water, orange juice or tomato juice. In some reported cases in which the blood could not be brought to normal by liver therapy, the addition of iron in large doses was beneficial. In the treatment of the spinal cord lesions the blood should be brought to normal as soon as possible and kept at a high normal. Massage and measures to improve the condition by reeducation should be carried on steadily. In some cases, reports suggest that very large doses of iron (150 grains daily of Blaud's mass) for two or three months have been useful. If *hypothyroidism* is present, thyroid gland extract should be given until the basal metabolism is about normal.

Watch should be kept for any digestive disturbance, especially diarrhea, and the diet reduced. If there is constipation enemata may be used. It is well to give dilute hydrochloric acid in full doses (ʒ i, 4 cc.), during and after each meal or twice after the meal (15 and 30 minutes). Care should be taken of the mouth and teeth, and mouth infection thoroughly treated. Focal infection anywhere should receive proper treatment. Other measures which have been advocated include ultraviolet radiation and the use of insulin. Some give this in small doses, as 5 to 10 units, twice a day, others in larger amounts. After improvement the patient should be carefully watched and a blood count made each month. The patient must continue to take liver, liver extract or ventriculin in sufficient amount: an average is half a pound of liver, 3 vials of liver extract or 10 grams of ventriculin, on 4 or 5 days each week.

Transfusion is required only in cases in which the patient's condition is very grave when he comes under observation. It may tide him over until liver therapy can be effective.

Aplastic Anemia

In this the bone marrow ceases to function. Usually all three elements are concerned with decrease in red cells, leukocytes and platelets. In rare cases there is alteration of one only or one may be particularly involved. In aplastic anemia the red cell formation is specially concerned; in agranulocytosis the leukopoietic tissues; and in malignant thrombocytopenia the megakaryocytes.

Etiology.—The disease occurs in both sexes and usually in young adult life. There are two groups, *primary* in which no cause is evident and *secondary* to a variety of influences among which are radioactive substances, benzol, arsenobenzol, sepsis, acute infectious diseases (especially in children) and extreme malnutrition.

Pathology.—There is aplasia of the bone marrow which is fatty and atrophic. There are extensive hemorrhages.

Symptoms.—The onset is usually insidious. There is anemia, which increases rapidly, with hemorrhages from the mucous membranes and into the skin. Fever is common. The *blood* shows a marked anemia, the red cells usually falling to one million with a color index about normal. The leukocytes fall to low figures, even below 1000, and the platelets are few. The red cells show little change other than the decrease in number. The *course* is usually rapidly fatal and recovery very rare, occurring sometimes in the secondary form. In *treatment,* repeated transfusions may be given and measures used for the causal condition in the secondary form.

Sickle Cell Anemia

This is a familial and hereditary disease, probably congenital, occurring almost exclusively in negroes or mulattoes, characterized by the presence of sickle shaped red cells in the blood. It seems to exist from birth and has periods of activity and remission. It occurs in two forms, (1) active and (2) latent, the latter being more common. The main features are dyspnea, weakness, nausea, vomiting and abdominal pain, pallor, adenitis, enlargement of the liver and sometimes of the spleen, edema of the ankles with leg ulcers which suggest syphilis, and in some patients a curious green color of the sclerotics. Fever is common and may occur for two or three weeks at intervals. The blood shows a marked anemia with the red cells between one and a half and three millions, a color index near 1 and a leukocytosis of 10,000 to 25,000. Many of the red cells have a crescent or sickle shape: in sealed fresh wet preparations the number of sickle cells increases markedly. Myelocytes and nucleated red cells of all varieties are found. There is no increased fragility of the red cells and the coagulation time is normal. The blood serum is very yellow and contains large amounts of bilirubin. The *prognosis* in severe forms is grave by reason of increased susceptibility to acute infections and myocardial failure. The *treatment* is that of a secondary anemia. Splenectomy has not proved to be of definite value.

There is a condition in which the red cells are *elliptical* in shape. It is hereditary, transmitted by both sexes and not limited to any race. Studies of the bone marrow do not show any abnormality. There does not seem to be any tendency to anemia. It may be confused with sickle cell anemia.

Miscellaneous Anemias

Acute Hemolytic Anemia.—This is also termed acute febrile anemia. It occurs at any age but most often in youth. Possibly different conditions are included under this term. The picture is that of an acute general infection, often with high fever, but cultures are negative. There is a rapidly progressive anemia and the red cells may fall below one million. The color index is about normal. There is a high percentage of reticulocytes and there may be many normoblasts and megaloblasts. There may be a marked leukocytosis with many immature cells so that leukemia is suggested. The platelets are diminished and there may be extensive hemorrhages. There may be enlargement of the liver, spleen and lymph nodes. There may be cardiac dilatation and pericarditis has been described. The duration is variable; some cases become subacute and progress for some time. Hemolysis persists as long as there is fever. In *treatment,* one measure appears to have been useful—transfusion.

Acute Hemolytic Anemia of Pregnancy.—The common forms of anemia may occur in pregnancy or this form may appear in a patient who already has anemia. A true pernicious anemia may appear during pregnancy and disappear after delivery but this is very rare. There is a form which comes on in women previously healthy and disappears after delivery if she survives it. The features are those given for acute hemolytic anemia. There is fever and the blood shows a severe anemia of a megalocytic form. There is evidence of marked regeneration of the red cells. Myelocytes are often present. The platelets are diminished. Purpura and hemorrhages may occur. There may be mouth lesions and digestive disturbance is frequent but achlorhydria is rare. The condition continues until the uterus is emptied. In *treatment*, blood transfusions are essential. Liver should be given freely even if the results do not seem to be uniform. The weight of opinion is against interference to terminate the pregnancy as this may be dangerous.

Chronic Hemolytic Anemia.—This occurs most often in young adults and the etiology is obscure. There is anemia of various degrees, which may be severe, with a color index about normal and a permanent increase in the reticulocytes and megaloblasts. Leukocytosis is not common. Exacerbations of hemolysis occur with jaundice and sometimes hemoglobinuria. The spleen may be enlarged. The picture is much like congenital acholuric jaundice but without the family history and the red cells do not show the changes of that disease. The course is slow and death occurs after some years. In *treatment*, removal of the spleen may be helpful if it is enlarged. The usual remedies for anemia have no effect and transfusion appears to be harmful.

Anemia in Childhood.—This is complicated by the responses which the blood-forming organs make as they are different and more varied than in adults. In general one may say that the same forms occur as in adult life with the exception of pernicious anemia which does not occur below the age of 10 years. The factors of improper or insufficient diet and digestive disturbance are important. Aplastic and acute hemolytic anemia are more common than in the adult. If infection occurs very curious blood pictures may result. In many of the nutritional anemias of children there is marked iron deficiency.

Von Jaksch's Anemia.—This probably represents the reaction of a young blood system to various agents, infectious or nutritional. It may be a subchronic hemolytic anemia. It usually begins between the ages of six months to two years and often in children with rickets. There are slight fever, digestive disturbances, anemia and an enlarged spleen. The liver may be enlarged. There is a marked anemia, usually of secondary type, with leukocytosis and a relative lymphocytosis; nucleated red cells are present, sometimes in large numbers. Many patients recover. In *treatment* every effort should be made to aid nutrition with sunlight and fresh air. Vitamins should be given in sufficient amounts, especially vitamin C. Liver and iron are useful. Transfusion should be done if the anemia is severe.

LEUKEMIA

Definition.—A disease characterized by a permanent increase in the leukocytes of the blood, associated with hyperplasia of the leukopoietic tissues and the occurrence of abnormal white cells in the blood.

History.—In October, 1845, Hughes Bennett recorded a case of "suppuration of the blood with enlargement of the spleen and liver," and named the disease "leukocythemia." A month later Virchow described a similar condition of "white blood" to which he gave the name "leukemia." In 1870 Neumann determined the importance of changes in the bone marrow.

Classification.—The most common forms are those which involve the neutrophile cells (myeloid or myelogenous) and those which involve the lymphocytes (lymphoid or lymphatic leukemia). Eosinophilic and monocytic forms occur. Confusion in classification may occur on account of the difficulty in deciding as to the nature of immature cells. This is especially the case in acute leukemia but the clinical features are practically the same.

Etiology.—This is obscure. In the acute forms the picture suggests an infection but the chronic forms suggest neoplasm involving a system. Certain of the lesions are much like tumor formations. The acute forms occur more often at a younger age than the chronic, and chronic lymphatic at an older age than chronic myeloid leukemia.

The relation to *pregnancy* is interesting. Conception is rare during the course. The disease may begin during pregnancy and progress rapidly. In Cameron's case (Montreal) the grandmother, mother and brother had symptoms suggestive of leukemia. The disease was first noticed when her sixth child was three months old and he died of leukemia at the sixth month. She was leukemic through her seventh pregnancy and delivered with a red cell count of one million and the white blood count 1:10. The child had purpura and died on the fourth day with the red cell count normal and leukocytes about 35,000. Another child aged 8 had leukemia.

Pathology.—Dropsy is sometimes present. The heart and veins are distended with large blood-cots. In one case the weight of blood in the heart chambers was 620 grams. There may be remarkable distention of the portal, cerebral, pulmonary and subcutaneous veins. The blood is usually clotted, and the enormous increase in the leukocytes gives a pus like appearance to the coagula, so that it has happened more than once, as in Virchow's memorable case, that on opening the right auricle the observer at first thought he had cut into an abscess. The coagula have a peculiar greenish color, so intense as to suggest the color of chloroma. The fibrin is increased.

In the *myeloid* form the spleen is greatly enlarged, the capsule may be thickened, and the vessels at the hilus enlarged. The weight may range from 2 to 18 pounds. The organ shows chronic hyperplasia. It cuts with resistance, has a reddish brown color, and the Malpighian bodies are invisible. Grayish white, circumscribed, lymphoid tumors may occur throughout the organ, contrasting strongly with the reddish-brown matrix. The medulla of the long bones may resemble the matter which forms the core of an abscess, or may be dark brown in color. There may be hemorrhagic infarctions. There may be much expansion of the shell of bone with localized swellings.

In the *lymphatic* form there is enlargement of the lymph nodes and other lymphoid tissues. Leukemic enlargements may occur in the stomach, intestine, kidney, omentum and peritoneum. The thymus may be enlarged in the acute cases. The liver may be greatly enlarged, due to a diffuse leukemic infiltration or to definite growths. Tumors of the skin are rare.

I. Chronic Myeloid Leukemia.—This form is rather more common in males than in females, and between the 30th and 50th years. The youngest of our patients was a child of eight months. It has followed trauma. The disease usually appears in healthy persons without any recognizable cause.

Symptoms.—Anemia is not a necessary accompaniment of all stages of the disease; the subjects may look very healthy and well. The *onset* is insidious, and, as a rule, the patient seeks advice for progressive enlargement of the abdomen and shortness of breath, or for pallor, palpitation, and other symptoms of anemia. Epistaxis is common. Gastro-intestinal symptoms may precede the onset. Occasionally the first symptoms are of a very serious nature. In one case a boy played lacrosse two days before the onset of the final hematemesis; and in another case a girl, who had, it was supposed, only a slight chlorosis, died of fatal hemorrhage from the stomach before any suspicion had been aroused as to the true condition.

The increase in the size of the *spleen* is the most prominent feature in a majority of the cases. Pain and tenderness are common, though the progressive enlargement may be painless. A creaking fremitus may be felt on palpation. The enlarged organ extends downward to the right, and may be felt just at the costal edge, or when large it may extend as far over as the navel. In some cases it occupies fully one-half of the abdomen, reaching to the pubes below and extending beyond the middle line. As a rule, the edge, in some the notch or notches, can be felt distinctly. Its size varies greatly from time to time and it may be perceptibly larger after meals. A hemorrhage or free diarrhea may reduce the size. The pressure of the enlarged organ may cause distress after eating; in one case it caused fatal obstruction of the bowels. On auscultation a murmur may sometimes be heard over the spleen and Gerhardt described a pulsation in it.

The long bones are tender; leukemic tumors are rare but there may be tender localized swellings, particularly on the ribs, which yield to pressure. There may be marked tenderness over the lower sternum.

The *pulse* is usually rapid, soft, compressible, but often full in volume. The veins may be large and full, and pulsation in those of the hand and arm is common. Toward the close edema in the feet or general anasarca may occur. *Hemorrhage* is common. There may be extensive purpura, or a hemorrhagic exudate into the pleura or peritoneum. Epistaxis is the most frequent form. Hemoptysis, hematuria and intestinal hemorrhage are rare. Bleeding from the gums may be present. Hematemesis proved fatal in two of our cases, and in a third a large cerebral hemorrhage rapidly killed.

Local *gangrene* may develop, with signs of intense infection and high fever. There are very few pulmonary symptoms. The shortness of breath is due, as a rule, to the anemia. Toward the end there may be edema of the lungs or pneumonia. Gastro-intestinal symptoms are rarely absent; nausea and vomiting are early features in some cases, and diarrhea may be troublesome, even fatal. There may be a dysenteric process in the colon. Jaundice rarely occurs. Ascites may be prominent, probably due to the splenic tumor. A leukemic peritonitis may occur.

The *nervous system* is not often involved. Facial paralysis has been noted. Headache, dizziness, and fainting spells are due to anemia. Paraplegia may be due to pressure of a leukemic tumor on the cord. There is a peculiar *retinitis,* due chiefly to the extravasation of blood, but there may be aggregations of leukocytes, forming small leukemic growths. Optic neuritis is rare. *Deafness* is frequent; it may appear early and possibly is due to hemorrhage. Features like Ménière's disease may come on suddenly, due to leukemic infiltration or hemorrhage into the semicircular canal.

The urine presents no constant changes; uric acid is always in excess. *Priapism* may occur sometimes at the onset, and may persist for weeks. The cause is thrombosis of the veins in some cases.

Fever was present in two-thirds of our series. Periods of pyrexia may alternate with prolonged intervals of freedom. The *basal metabolic rate* is nearly always elevated and often corresponds to the severity of the leukemia. The increase may be as high as 40.

Blood.—In all forms of the disease the diagnosis must be made by the examination of the blood, as it alone offers distinctive features.

The striking change is an increase in the *leukocytes.* The average in our series was 298,700 per c.mm., and the average ratio to the red cells was 1 to 10. Counts above 500,000 are common, and they may rise above 1,000,000. The proportion of white to red cells may be 1 to 5, or even reach 1 to 1. There are instances in which the number of leukocytes exceeded that of the red corpuscles. The increase is in all the forms. The polynuclear neutrophiles make up from 30 to 50 per cent; both the small and the large lymphocytes are increased; the eosinophiles and the mast cells show both a percentage and absolute increase. The abnormal cells, the myelocytes, range up to 50 per cent. The great majority are neutrophilic but eosinophilic and basophilic myelocytes are present in small numbers. A variable number of myeloblasts occur. The tendency is for the percentage of immature cells to increase. Normoblasts and megaloblasts are common. At first the red cell count may be normal, but sooner or later anemia comes on, and the count may fall to 2,000,000. The color index is usually low. The blood plates vary in number and decrease in the later stages. Charcot-Leyden crystals may separate from the clots and the hemoglobin shows a remarkable tendency to crystallize.

Aleukemic Intervals.—The white cells may fall to normal or even below. In one of our patients the leukocytes diminished from 500,000 on Jan. 26 to 6,000 on Feb. 16, and throughout the greater part of March were as low as 2,000. This followed the use of arsenic. With this the spleen may or may not reduce. The same may occur spontaneously, but has been frequently seen following benzol, radium and X-ray treatment, and intercurrent infections. These aleukemic phases are only transitory. In some cases there may be no increase in the leukocytes but abnormal forms are present.

II. Chronic Lymphatic Leukemia.—This is less common. Cases of three to thirteen years' duration have been reported. A patient of W. H. Draper of New York seen ten years after the onset had a sheaf of blood counts from every clinician of note in Europe and the United States. There was no anemia, the leukocytes were 242,000 per c.mm., the superficial lymph nodes were enlarged and the spleen of moderate size.

It occurs in older persons, rarely, if ever, in children; the general health may be very good and the only inconvenience felt is from the enlarged glands. The spleen is rarely very large; the mesenteric and retroperitoneal glands may form big tumors. After lasting two or more years acute symptoms may come on—fever, hemorrhages, stomatitis, tonsillitis. Pigmentation of the skin, itching with urticaria and lymphomas may be present, giving a skin picture very like that of Hodgkin's disease. The blood shows at first little or no anemia. The leukocytes are usually above 100,000 per c.mm. and very high counts are not as common as in myeloid leukemia. The small lymphocytes predominate up to 90-95 per cent. The large forms are rare until the late stages when anemia supervenes. The granulocytes are diminished but sometimes the eosinophiles are increased.

III. Acute leukemia is the most terrible of all blood diseases. It occurs both in the myeloid and lymphatic forms and the relative frequency is difficult to state. The former is more common than we formerly thought. It occurs in younger persons and more frequently in males. In onset and course the disease resembles an acute infection. Swelling of the tonsils, ulcerative angina, stomatitis, fever, hemorrhages and a rapid anemia are the dominant features. Dyspnea, nausea, vomiting and diarrhea are not uncommon. Some cases resemble fulminant purpura and cutaneous hemorrhages may be present before the patient feels ill. The glands of the neck enlarge and usually other groups, but death may occur without marked adenitis. The spleen is usually palpable, rarely very large. Hemorrhages from the mucous membranes and into the serous sacs are common. Subperiosteal leukemic infiltration may occur and cause pain so that *arthritis* or *bone disease* is suspected. The course is rapid, and death may occur within a week of onset; more often in from three to six weeks. Remissions may occur and a case beginning acutely may linger for three or four months or occasionally pass into the chronic form.

Leukemia cutis is characterized by nodular tumors in the skin, which may break down rapidly, hemorrhages, pigmentation of the skin and fever. The spleen and lymph nodes may be little, if at all, enlarged.

The *blood picture* in the acute form may give the only data for diagnosis. The anemia is rapid with the usual changes in the blood cells. The leukocytes are increased but less as a rule than in the chronic forms. Counts of 20,000 to 30,000 are found early but may be much higher before death. In rare cases the leukocytes are low and necrosis then seems more severe. The majority of the cells are immature and it may not be possible to decide whether they are myeloblasts or lymphoblasts. If variations of one type of cell can be distinguished it is possible to diagnose the myeloid or lymphatic form. Clinically they are much alike and the outlook is the same.

Enlargement of the spleen and lymph nodes is less marked than in the chronic forms. Lymphoid swellings in the mouth, throat and intestines are common, and small tumors may be widely scattered on the serous membranes, skin, in the lungs, and even in the nervous system. The bone marrow is deep red, but the changes depend much on the duration of the disease.

Acute monocytic leukemia.—This is a rare form and has the features of acute leukemia. The predominant cell is the monocyte about which there is much controversy among hematologists.

IV. Atypical Leukemias.—(1) *Mixed* leukemias are probably rare if they actually occur.

(2) *Cases with atypical blood changes,* such as a very high percentage of eosinophiles. Atypical cells are common in acute forms.

(3) *Chloroma* is an atypical form of leukemia in which the leukemic tumors have a greenish color. It is more common in children. Exophthalmos is frequent owing to tumor formation in the orbit. The tumor growths occur chiefly in the skull, orbit, long bones, and throughout the viscera. The typical picture of this distribution may be present without the green tint of chloroma. The nature of the pigment is unknown. The meninges may be involved with pressure on the cord or nerve roots. The blood picture is that of leukemia, usually with acute or subacute features. The blood picture may be atypical in the early stages.

(4) *Subacute Leukemia.*—There is an insidious onset with a course of several months characterized by necrotic processes in the mouth or throat, fever and a progressive anemia. The leukocytes may not be greatly increased but there are immature forms, lymphoblastic or myeloblastic in origin.

Diagnosis.—The recognition of the acute forms may be difficult, particularly those which begin with marked angina and cutaneous hemorrhages. It may not be until a blood examination is made or the glands enlarge that suspicion is aroused. The chronic forms are easily recognized. In the myeloid form the enlarged spleen at once suggests a blood count, upon which the diagnosis rests. The diagnosis may be made by the ophthalmic surgeon. In the lymphatic form, too, the diagnosis rests with the blood examination. There are certain cases of *sepsis* with marked lymphocytosis, in which the leukocytes may reach 30,000 or 40,000 per c.mm. When the regional lymph nodes are involved this may raise a doubt. *Infectious mononucleosis* may give difficulty; the absence of anemia is important. Under treatment with arsenic, radium or X-rays the increase of leukocytes in leukemia may disappear but the differential count still be characteristic.

Prognosis.—Recovery is practically unknown. The acute cases die within three months; the chronic forms last from six months to four or five years, or longer. The chronic lymphatic form is the most protracted.

Association with Other Diseases.—Tuberculosis is not uncommon. Dock collected 27 cases, in none of which did the tuberculosis show any special influence. Intercurrent infections as influenza, erysipelas or sepsis may have a remarkable effect in reducing the number of leukocytes.

Treatment.—Fresh air, good diet, and abstention from mental worry and care are important general indications. The *indicatio morbi* can not be met. No treatment seems to influence the acute forms; blood transfusion may be tried. There are certain remedies which have an influence upon the chronic forms. *Arsenic* should always be given. Fowler's solution can be begun in doses of three drops and increased to the limit of tolerance or sodium cacodylate given by injection. *Benzol* has been used but should be given with caution and discontinued if there is a drop in the red cell count. If the number of leukocytes decreases steadily, the drug should be discontinued when they fall to 25,000. The dose is ʒ i (4 cc.) per day given in capsules with olive oil. The *X-rays* and *radium*, while not curative, add materially to the duration of life. They should not be used in the acute forms. The exposure should be over the spleen and long bones and care taken to watch for signs of toxemia. They usually cause a marked drop in the leukocytes. Either may be used with arsenic. X-ray or radium treatment should not be given if there is marked anemia or thrombopenia, or when there are many immature lymphocytes in the blood. Removal of the spleen has been done after radium treatment but the value of this is doubtful. Recurrence is to be expected after any treatment. The patient should be kept under observation with frequent blood counts and X-ray treatment resumed as soon as the leukocytes increase.

AGRANULOCYTOSIS

Synonyms.—Granulopenia; Granulocytopenia; Malignant neutropenia; Neutropenic State.

Definition.—This is a condition which may occur with a number of diseases and is not a distinct entity. There is a marked leukopenia, due to altered function of the leukopoietic tissues, most marked in the granulocytes. In one form, agranulocytic angina, the agranulocytosis is apparently primary and the other features secondary. In certain other forms the blood condition appears to be secondary.

A classification may be made as follows: (1) Agranulocytic angina; (2) cases secondary to infection as pneumonia, influenza, osteomyelitis, sepsis, etc.; (3) cases due to toxic influence, as radioactive substances, and benzol. Certain drugs are important causes, arsphenamine, hydroquinone, amidopyrine and certain barbituric acid derivatives. A common factor is the presence of the benzene ring. Particular interest belongs to the number of cases in those who have taken amidopyrine. Idiosyncrasy seems to be important when we consider the number of persons who take these drugs.

Etiology.—The condition may occur at any age and in either sex, but is more common in females. Agranulocytic angina is most common in middle aged women. The essential cause varies and the variety of causal agents suggests that the leukopoietic part of the bone marrow is easily disturbed. It may be a primary aplasia or some interference with the development of the leukocytes. The bone marrow may show granulocytic aplasia.

Clinical Features.—Disturbance of the leukopoietic tissues of the bone marrow may occur in varying grades of severity, especially in the secondary forms. There may be individuals who have a persistent low leukocyte count with good health. Such may be more likely to show severe features if a possible causal disturbance occurs. In women it sometimes has an association with menstruation. A definite disease picture is shown by:

Agranulocytic Angina.—This shows fever, toxemia, an ulcerative angina and marked granulocytopenia. The onset is sudden with fever, chills, marked prostration, and necrotic lesions in the tonsils and pharynx, and sometimes on the larynx, gums and tongue; occasionally they occur in the vagina and rectum. The fever may be high and toxemia marked. The necrotic, ulcerative lesions in the mouth and throat are usually marked and the cervical lymph nodes may be enlarged. The local lesions show an absence of reaction. The necrotic process may involve the esophagus, stomach and bowel. The liver and spleen may be enlarged. Jaundice occurs in some cases. The blood shows no changes in the red cells except anemia in prolonged attacks. The leukocytes are greatly reduced in number, sometimes below 1000. There is marked reduction in the granular cells which may be entirely absent both in the blood and bone marrow. The toxemia may be very marked. The *course* varies from acute cases which are fatal in a few days to chronic cases which may last for months. Relapse may occur after a period of good health, suggesting a susceptibility in the bone marrow. The mortality is high, up to 75 per cent, in untreated cases.

The *diagnosis* must depend chiefly on the blood examination which gives distinctive results. There may be difficulty with acute leukemia, if leukopenia is present, but the absence of immature leukocytes is significant. In *treatment,* every effort should be made to give nourishment and fluids as freely as possible. The ordinary measures for an acute infection should be used. Treatment of the lesions in the mouth by mild antiseptic solutions may be used. Blood transfusion is not indicated unless there is marked anemia, but some patients without anemia seem to have been helped by it. Benefit has been reported from mild X-ray therapy over the long bones. The best results have followed the use of Nucleotide K-96, given intramuscularly. Improvement is not seen until at least the third and more often the fifth day. Adenine sulphate may be given in doses of 0.5 gram, intravenously, in 20-30 cc. of water, twice in twenty-four hours. Leukocytic extracts may be used or a leukocytic cream (Strumia, 1934).

HODGKIN'S DISEASE

Definition.—A general disease of a malignant character with specific changes in the lymph nodes and lymphoid tissue. Anatomically there is a specific hyperplasia of the reticulo-endothelial cells, proliferation of endothelial cells, formation of mononuclear and multinuclear giant cells and the presence of eosinophiles. Degenerative changes and fibrosis follow.

History.—In 1832 Hodgkin recorded a series of cases with enlarged lymph nodes and spleen. From the group that Hodgkin described, Wilks picked out the disease and called it *anemia lymphatica.* Other names given to it are *adénie, pseudoleukemia, lymphadenoma and malignant lymphoma.*

Etiology.—A widely spread disease, a majority of the cases occur in young adults, and more frequently in males than in females. Twins and sisters have been attacked. The cause is unknown. Certain features suggest an infection: the rapid couse of some cases, the association with local irritation in the mouth and tonsils, the frequency with which the disease starts in the cervical glands, the gradual extension from one gland group to another, and the recurring exacerbations of fever. The work of M. H. Gordon suggests a specific infective agent, possibly a virus. When suspensions of the tissue are inoculated into the brains of rabbits, a specific encephalitis is produced. Material from acute cases of Hodgkin's disease give more acute symptoms in the animals than from chronic cases. The production of this "encephalitic syndrome" is useful in diagnosis as inoculation of material from lymphosarcoma, tuberculosis or leukemia does not cause it. Sternberg suggested that the disease was a special form of tuberculosis but when present tuberculosis appears to be a terminal infection. In many ways the disease suggests a form of "malignant growth" of the lymphatic system.

Morbid Anatomy.—The superficial lymph nodes are extensively involved, and from the cervical groups they may form continuous chains to the mediastinal and axillary glands. The masses may pass beneath the pectoral muscles and even beneath the scapulae. Of the internal glands, those of the thorax are most often affected, and the tracheal and bronchial groups may form large masses. The trachea and the aorta with its branches may be completely surrounded; the veins may be compressed, rarely the aorta itself. The masses perforate the sternum and invade the lung deeply. The retroperitoneal glands may form a continuous chain from the diaphragm to the inguinal canals. They may compress the ureters, the lumbar and sacral nerves, and the iliac veins. They may adhere to the broad ligament and the uterus and simulate fibroids. At an early stage the glands are soft; later they may become firm and hard. Fusion of contiguous glands does not often occur, and they tend to remain discrete. The capsule may be infiltrated and adjacent tissues invaded. On section the gland presents a grayish white semitranslucent appearance, broken by intersecting strands of fibrous tissue; there is no caseation or necrosis unless secondary infection has occurred.

The *spleen* is enlarged in 75 per cent of the cases; in young children the enlargement may be great, but the organ rarely reaches the size of the spleen in leukemia. In more than half of the cases lymphoid growths are present. The marrow of the long bones may be converted into a rich lymphoid tissue. The lymphatic structures of the tonsillar ring and of the intestines may show marked hyperplasia. The liver is often enlarged, and may present scattered nodular tumors, which may also occur in the kidneys.

Histology.—The studies of Andrewes and of Dorothy Reed show a very characteristic microscopic picture—proliferation of the endothelial and reticular cells, with the formation of lymphoid cells of uniform size and shape, and characteristic giant cells, the so-called lymphadenoma cells, containing four or more nuclei. Eosinophiles are always present, and proliferation of the stroma leads to fibrosis of the gland. The difference between the soft and hard forms depends largely upon the stage. When tuberculosis occurs as a secondary infection the two processes may be readily distinguished.

Symptoms.—A tonsillitis may precede the onset. Enlargement of the cervical glands is usually an initial feature; it is rare to find other superficial groups or the deeper glands attacked first. Months or several years may elapse before the glands in the axillae and groin become involved. During what may be called the first stage the patient's general condition is good; then anemia comes on, not marked at first, but usually progressive. In the majority of cases the *spleen* is enlarged. There may be very little pain until the internal glands become involved. The lymph nodes of the thorax and abdomen are frequently affected. The thymus gland may be involved. With swelling of the *mediastinal glands* there are cough, dyspnea, and often intense cyanosis, with all the signs of intrathoracic tumor. Involvement of the lung may be followed by necrosis with cavity formation and occasionally pyopneumothorax. There may be moderate *fever*. Bronzing of the skin may occur, apart from the use of arsenic. Pruritus may be present and boils and echthymatous blebs may occur. The blood shows a *secondary anemia* sometimes with a moderate leukocytosis. The leukocytes show no characteristic changes. There may be a moderate eosinophilia and, as the anemia progresses, nucleated red cells appear, and toward the end there may be a great increase in the lymphocytes. As the disease progresses there is marked emaciation with asthenia, and sometimes anasarca. This represents the common course, but there are many variations, among which are the following:

(*a*) An ACUTE FORM has been described. In one case beginning, like so many cases of lymphatic leukemia, with angina, the whole course was less than ten weeks. Ziegler mentioned two cases of death within a month.

(*b*) LOCALIZED FORM.—The enlargement may be localized to certain groups, in the neck, groin, retroperitoneum or thorax. Some of these cases present great difficulty in diagnosis, particularly if there are febrile paroxysms with slight involvement of the external groups. The disease may be confined to one region for a year or more before there is any extension. The localized mediastinal group often presents a remarkable picture—pressure signs, pain, orthopnea—and, unless there are other groups involved, or enlargement of the spleen, it may be difficult to make the diagnosis during life.

(*c*) WITH RELAPSING PYREXIA.—First recorded by Murchison in 1870, this form was studied by Pel and Ebstein. MacNalty made a careful study of this remarkable syndrome. Relapsing pyrexia may occur in cases with involvement of the internal glands alone, or, more frequently, with a general involvement. "Following on a period of low pyrexia, or of normal or subnormal temperature, there is a steady rise occupying two or four days to a maximum, which may reach 105°. For about three days the temperature remains at a high level, and then there is a gradual fall by lysis occupying about three days, and the temperature then becomes subnormal" (MacNalty). An afebrile period of ten days or two weeks then occurs, followed by another bout of fever. This may be repeated for many months. In one case the fever lasted exactly fourteen days for many successive paroxysms. During the fever the glands swell and may become tender. This febrile form may occur with involvement of the internal glands alone. In one patient whose cervical glands had been thoroughly removed there were typical Pel-Ebstein paroxysms, and we could find no enlarged glands, internal or external.

(*d*) LATENT TYPE.—Ziegler called attention to the importance of this form, in which anemia, fever, and constitutional symptoms may be present with enlargement of the internal glands.

(*e*) SPLENOMEGALIC FORM.—Enlargement of the spleen is present in a large proportion of cases. Whether or not there is a type involving the spleen without the lymph nodes is still a question. It is not improbable that the disease may originate in the lymphoid tissue of the spleen, and such cases have been reported. It is very difficult to distinguish them clinically from the early stages of splenic anemia.

(*f*) LYMPHOGRANULOMATOSIS.—The *skin lesions* may be in the rare form of a true lymphogranulomatosis or show a wide variety of changes. Among these are: pruritus, urticaria, edema, petechiae and marked pigmentation. The occasional occurrence of herpes zoster should be noted.

(*g*) BONE LESIONS may suggest osteomyelitis or bone tumor. There may be a granulomatous periostitis with osteophytes or rarefaction of the bone and synovitis may occur. The *vertebrae* are often involved with a resulting pressure *myelitis* or pressure on the *nerve roots.* These cases may show very puzzling nervous system manifestations early in the course.

Diagnosis.—(*a*) TUBERCULOSIS.—With enlargement of the glands on one side of the neck in a young person, it is often not easy to determine whether the disease is tuberculosis or Hodgkin's disease. Two points should be decided. First, one of the enlarged glands should be excised and carefully studied. The histological changes in Hodgkin's disease differ markedly from those in tuberculosis. Secondly, tuberculin should be used if the patient is afebrile. In early tuberculous adenitis the reaction is prompt and decisive.

Other points are the tendency in tuberculous adenitis to coalescence of the glands, adhesion to the skin, with suppuration, etc., and the liability to tuberculosis of the lung or pleura. There is a form of generalized tuberculous adenitis which occurs particularly in negroes and simulates Hodgkin's disease with enlargement of the gland groups in the neck, arms and axilla, never perhaps so much as in Hodgkin's disease, but with firm, elastic masses. There is irregular fever, not with periods of apyrexia; the course may be protracted, and at autopsy only the lymph nodes found involved.

(*b*) LEUKEMIA.—The blood examination gives the diagnosis and difficulty arises only in the cases of leukemia in which the leukocytes decrease or for a time become normal. Histologically there are striking differences between the structure of the glands in the two conditions.

(*c*) LYMPHOSARCOMA.—Clinically the case may resemble Hodgkin's disease very closely, and in the literature the two diseases have been confounded. The glands, as a rule, form larger masses, the capsules are involved, and adjacent structures are attacked, but this may be the case in Hodgkin's disease. Pressure signs in the chest and abdomen are more common in sarcoma. The most satisfactory mode of diagnosis is by examination of a gland.

Course.—There are acute cases in which the disease advances rapidly and death follows in a few months but, as a rule, it lasts for two to four years. In rare cases the duration may be ten or twelve years. Remarkable periods of quiescence may occur, in which the glands diminish in size, the fever disappears, and the general condition improves. Even a large group of glands may almost completely disappear, or a tumor mass in the neck may subside while the inguinal glands are enlarging. Usually cachexia with anemia and edema precedes death. A fatal event may occur early from great enlargement of the mediastinal glands.

Treatment.—Every effort should be made to aid the general nutrition and iron should be given for anemia. Removal of the glands seems to have gone out of fashion but it may delay the course. Radium and the X-rays do good if begun early before fibrosis and degenerative changes have occurred. The glands are often temporarily reduced in size but there is no proof of a complete cure. The use of Coley's fluid at the same time appears to be helpful. Other local treatment of the glands seems to do but little good.

Arsenic is the only drug which has a positive value and in some cases the effects are striking. It may be given in the form of Fowler's solution in increasing doses or as sodium cacodylate (gr. i-ii, 0.06-0.12 gm.) intramuscularly daily or every second day. Ill effects from the larger doses are rare. For the pressure pains morphia should be given.

PURPURA

Strictly speaking, purpura is not a disease; but under this term are conveniently arranged a number of affections characterized by extravasations of blood into the skin or mucous membranes. The basis of modern classification is the number of blood platelets but it must be recognized that there are borderline cases. This gives two main groups: (1) Nonthrombopenic Purpura and (2) Thrombopenic Purpura.

The purpuric spots vary from 1 to 3 or 4 mm. in diameter. When small and pinpoint-like they are called petechiae; when large, they are known as ecchymoses. At first bright red in color, they become darker, and gradually fade to brownish stains. They do not disappear on pressure.

The following is a provisional grouping of the cases:

Symptomatic Purpura.—(*a*) INFECTIOUS.—In pyemia, septicemia and malignant endocarditis (particularly in the last) ecchymoses may be very abundant. In typhus fever the rash is always purpuric. Measles, scarlet fever, and more particularly smallpox and cerebrospinal fever may have an extensive purpuric rash.

(*b*) TOXIC.—The venom of snakes produces extravasation of blood with great rapidity—a condition carefully studied by Weir Mitchell. Certain medicines, particularly copaiba, quinine, belladonna, mercury, ergot and the iodides may be followed by a petechial rash. Purpura may follow the use of small doses of iodide of potassium and death may be caused by a small amount, as in a case reported by Stephen Mackenzie of a child who died after a dose of 2½ grains. An erythema may precede the hemorrhage. It is not always a simple purpura but may be an acute febrile eruption of great intensity. Workers with benzol, used as a solvent for rubber, may have severe purpura. Cases such as those reported by Selling have been in connection with the coating of tin cans, while the Swedish cases occurred with the manufacture of bicycle tires. Under this division comes the purpura often associated with jaundice.

(*c*) CACHECTIC.—Under this heading are best described the instances of purpura which occur in cancer, tuberculosis, Hodgkin's disease, nephritis, scurvy and in the debility of old age. In these cases the spots are usually confined to the extremities. They may be very abundant on the lower limbs and about the wrists and hands. This constitutes the commonest variety and many examples can be seen in the wards of any large hospital.

(*d*) NEURITIC.—One variety is met with in cases of organic disease, the so-called myelopathic purpura, seen occasionally in tabes dorsalis, particularly following attacks of the lightning pains and, as a rule, involving the area of the skin in which the pains are most intense. Cases occur in acute myelitis, and occasionally in severe neuralgia. Another form is the remarkable hysterical condition in which stigmata, or bleeding points, appear upon the skin.

(*e*) WITH ANEMIA.—This is marked in conditions with changes in the bone-marrow, as aplastic anemia.

(*f*) MECHANICAL.—This is most frequent with venous stasis, as in the paroxysms of whooping cough, in epilepsy and about tight bandages.

Arthritic Purpura.—This form is characterized by involvement of the joints. It is often known, therefore, as "rheumatic," though in reality the evidence for this is not conclusive. It seems more satisfactory to use the designation arthritic. Three groups may be recognized:

(*a*) PURPURA SIMPLEX.—A mild form, often known as *purpura simplex*, is most common in children, in whom, with or without articular pain, purpuric spots appear upon the legs, less commonly upon the trunk and arms. As pointed out by Graves, this form may be associated with diarrhea. The disease is seldom severe. There may be loss of appetite and slight anemia. Fever is not, as a rule, present, and the patients get well in a week or ten days.

Usually regarded as rheumatic, and associated, in some instances, with arthritic manifestations, yet in a majority the arthritis is slighter than in rheumatic fever and no other manifestations are present. The average duration is two to four weeks, but there are chronic cases lasting a year or more.

(*b*) Anaphylactoid Purpura (*Schönlein-Henoch Disease; Hemorrhagic Capillary Toxicosis*).—In this form the cause is not in any change in the blood. The *skin lesions* are various; erythema, urticaria, edema and purpura occur. The erythematous exudate rather than purpura is the important lesion. There may be arthritis (Schönlein's disease) and abdominal colic, with or without bleeding from a mucous membrane (Henoch's Purpura). The blood platelets show little alteration. The cases in this group may show great variation in the clinical features so that their recognition is difficult.

In the *etiology* the influence of a histamine-like substance on the capillaries is suggested with the activation of a latent capillary toxicosis. It occurs especially in early life and more often in males. The nature of the disease is obscure. Its resemblance to serum sickness suggested the term *anaphylactoid* purpura. It appears to be a disease of the capillaries, not of the blood. In some cases there may be an acute throat infection. Sensitization to some food is found occasionally. The onset of *symptoms* may be with headache and malaise. Fever is common but is rarely high. The arthritis may precede the skin manifestations or occur after them. The *arthritis* is rarely severe, usually multiple, and may shift from joint to joint. The skin lesions are very varied, erythema, urticaria, edema and purpura. The *purpura* is the hemorrhagic form of an exudative process. The purpuric spots are of small size, occur especially on the legs, and appear in successive crops. Edema is fairly common and may be marked. The *abdominal* symptoms may be prominent. The *pain* is colicky, often very severe and may continue for days. The abdominal wall is rigid and there may be considerable tenderness. As constipation is common and vomiting may occur, the diagnosis of intestinal obstruction may be made. Blood may be passed from the stools or vomited. The acute features last for a few days and frequently recur. *Acute nephritis* occurs with the abdominal form. It is of the hemorrhagic form and may be so severe that death results. It rarely progresses to a chronic form but red blood cells in the urine may persist for some time. There is an intense reaction to tuberculin in some cases. Cerebral hemorrhage has proved fatal. In *diagnosis,* a careful search for the skin lesions is important; the purpuric spots may be very few. The blood shows a normal bleeding and coagulation time. There may be a leukocytosis. The blood platelets are usually normal in number. The acute abdominal features may suggest the need of exploration, an error which is not uncommon. In *prognosis,* the chief dangers are acute nephritis and cerebral hemorrhage.

Visceral Lesions in Purpura.—In any form of purpura, in the erythemas, and in urticaria *visceral* lesions may occur. (*a*) *Gastro-intestinal crises,* pain, vomiting, melena and diarrhea. The attacks have often been mistaken for appendicitis or intussusception, and at operation the condition has been found to be an acute serohemorrhagic infiltration of a limited area of the stomach or bowel. Identical attacks occur in angioneurotic edema. Intussusception has occurred with purpura. These crises may occur for years in children before an outbreak of purpura or urticaria gives a clue to their nature. (*b*) Enlargement of the *spleen* is usually present in these cases. (*c*) *Acute nephritis* may occur and form the most serious complication, of which seven cases in the series died (*Am. J. Med. Sc.*, Jan., 1904).

Chronic Purpura.—For years patients may have outbreaks of purpura without serious symptoms. One patient was practically never free from spots somewhere on the skin for thirty-three years, during which time she had had several severe attacks of nose-bleed, during which the purpura increased greatly. Another patient had recurring purpura on the legs for many years, with great pigmentation and thickening of the skin. There is a form of intermittent purpura with attacks over long series of years, as long as twenty, sometimes only on the skin, at other times with involvement of the mucous membranes (Elsner).

Essential Thrombopenic Purpura (*Purpura Haemorrhagica*).—In this disease (*morbus maculosus* of Werlhof) there is severe purpura, with reduction in the number of blood platelets and changes in the cells of the capillaries. Hemorrhage occurs into the skin and from the nose, mouth, lungs, digestive tract, urinary tract and uterus. It may occur in the brain and adrenal glands. There is apparently alteration in the capillaries, which renders them more permeable, with change in the platelets which some regard as secondary. The skin hemorrhages may be very extensive. Inflammatory phenomena do not occur. The disease is most common in children but may occur at any age. There are acute and chronic forms. In the former the attack may last from two weeks to three months. The chronic form is more frequent and may continue for years or occur intermittently with intervals of years between attacks. The *features* of the disease consist in the hemorrhages with the results from them and the changes in the blood. The *platelets* are greatly reduced and may fall to very low figures. The number may fall before a hemorrhage and in the intermittent forms the number may be normal between attacks. In the chronic form the count is permanently low. The *bleeding* time is increased. The *clot* is firm but it does not retract and there is no extrusion of serum. The *coagulation* time is normal. The blood has the character of a secondary anemia and nucleated red cells and myelocytes may be found. There is often a leukocytosis. The *capillary resistance test* is positive. This is done by placing the cuff of the blood pressure apparatus well above the elbow and maintaining a pressure between the systolic and diastolic pressure for about five minutes. A few minutes later hemorrhages are found in the skin of the forearm. Flicking the skin brings them out or increases them. Striking the skin over the sternum with a percussion hammer causes a local hemorrhage.

As regards the *course*, the frequency of spontaneous remissions should be remembered. Special attention should be given to the bleeding time as an indication for treatment. The symptoms may be mild and clear rapidly or in fulminant forms death may occur in a short time.

Diagnosis.—Purpura with bleeding from the mucous membranes is the characteristic point. Erythema and urticaria do not occur. A complete blood examination is essential and serves to distinguish this disease from scurvy and hemophilia. The diagnosis from *scurvy* may be made by the previous history, the circumstances under which the disease occurs and the absence of swelling of the gums. The malignant forms of the fevers, particularly smallpox and measles, are distinguished by the prodromes and the higher temperature. The special points in the diagnosis from *hemophilia* are considered under that disease. The possibility of mistaking the acute forms of *leukemia* for purpura should be kept in mind.

Treatment.—In *symptomatic purpura* attention should be paid to the conditions under which it occurs, and measures should be employed to increase the strength and to restore a normal blood condition. Tonics, good food and fresh air meet these indications. The patient should always be at rest in bed. In the simple purpura of children, or that associated with articular trouble, arsenic in full doses should be given. No good is obtained from small doses, but Fowler's solution should be given freely. In *anaphylactoid purpura* treatment is not very satisfactory. The patient should be kept in bed. In the arthritic form salicylates and local applications may relieve the pain. Alkalies may be given until the urine is alkaline. Calcium lactate (gr. xv, i gm.) by mouth three times a day or calcium chloride intravenously (25 cc. of a 10 per cent solution) in severe cases, should be given.

In *purpura hemorrhagica* the calcium salts, preferably the lactate, may be given in doses of 15 grains (1 gm.) three or four times a day for a few days. In bleeding from the mouth and nose the inhalation of carbon dioxide, irrigations with 2 per cent gelatin solution, and epinephrine should be tried. The last remedy has often acted promptly. Repeated *blood transfusions* (300 cc.) are the best means to control the bleeding time. The intramuscular injection of 20-40 cc. of citrated blood is a useful measure in severe cases. In *chronic* cases any focal infection should be treated and protein sensitization searched for. The *diet* should have a high protein and vitamin content, especially vitamin C. The use of ultraviolet light therapy seems useful. Ligation of the splenic artery appears to be as successful as splenectomy and entails less risk. Splenectomy has been successful and good results have been reported from liver therapy, as in pernicious anemia.

Miscellaneous Forms.—*Purpura fulminans* shows remarkable ecchymoses over the greater part of the skin. Hemorrhages from the mucous membranes may occur. All the typical cases have been in children and all have been fatal. The cause is obscure but some infection is suggested. Malignant forms of purpura occur in certain acute diseases, such as smallpox. Purpura of *endocrine* and *nervous origin* has been described. It may occur with menstruation. It has been described after severe fright and with organic nervous system disease. A segmental distribution has been noted. The so-called senile *purpura* is probably due to capillary weakness.

Other forms of hemorrhagic diseases may be mentioned. *Hereditary pseudohemophilia* shows normal coagulation time. The clinical features are much like purpura hemorrhagica. There is an increase in the bleeding time. The platelets may be normal in number or somewhat reduced but abnormal in morphology. The condition may improve in adult life. In treatment, arsenic may be useful; splenectomy should not be done. *Hereditary thrombopenia* is described with a positive capillary resistance test, reduced number of platelets, normal coagulation time and increased bleeding time. *Fibropenia* has a complete lack of fibrinogen in the blood, apparently due to constitutional deficiency. *Bernuth's pseudohemophilia* can only be distinguished from hemophilia by a study of the living capillaries which remain open after injury.

In hemophilia they close normally. The condition termed "*hereditary hemorrhagic thrombo-asthenia*" is a family disease with epistaxis and ecchymoses. There may be an intermittent prolongation of the bleeding time.

HEMORRHAGIC DISEASES OF THE NEWBORN

Syphilis Haemorrhagica Neonatorum.—The child may be born healthy or there may be signs of hemorrhage at birth. Then in a few days there are extensive cutaneous extravasations and bleeding from the mucous surfaces and the navel. There may be deep jaundice. Extravasations in the organs and syphilitic changes in the liver and other organs are found.

Epidemic Hemoglobinuria (*Winckel's Disease*).—Hemoglobinuria in the newborn is a fatal affection, which sets in usually about the fourth day after birth. It may follow infection of the umbilicus. The child becomes jaundiced, and there are marked gastro-intestinal symptoms, with fever, jaundice, rapid respiration and sometimes cyanosis. The urine contains albumin and methemoglobin. The disease has to be distinguished from simple icterus neonatorum, with which there may sometimes be blood or blood pigment in the urine. The spleen is swollen, and there are punctiform hemorrhages in different parts. Some cases have shown marked acute fatty degeneration of the internal organs—the so-called *Buhl's disease*.

Morbus Masculosus Neonatorum (Hemorrhagic Disease of the New Born). Apart from visceral hemorrhages, the result of injuries at birth, bleeding from one or more of the surfaces is not uncommon in the newborn; 50 cases occurred in 6,700 deliveries (C. W. Townsend). Of Townsend's cases, in 20 the blood came from the bowels, in 14 from the stomach, in 14 from the mouth, in 12 from the nose, in 18 from the navel, in 3 from the navel alone. The bleeding begins within the first week, but in rare instances is delayed to the second or third. Thirty-one of the patients died and 19 recovered. The disease is usually of brief duration, death occurring in from one to seven days unless treatment is given. The temperature is often elevated. The nature of the disease is unknown. As a rule, nothing abnormal is found postmortem. The general nature of the affection, its self-limited character, the presence of fever, and the greater prevalence in hospitals suggest an infectious origin (Townsend). The bleeding may be associated with intense hematogenous jaundice. Not every case of bleeding from the stomach or bowels belongs in this category. Ulcers of the esophagus, stomach and duodenum have been found in the newborn. The child may draw blood from the breast and subsequently vomit it.

Treatment.—The most useful measure is the intramuscular injection of fresh or citrated human blood in amounts of 20-40 cc. This should be repeated every four to eight hours if the hemorrhage continues.

HEMOPHILIA

Definition.—A disease characterized by deficiency in the thromboplastic substances, thereby rendering the individual liable to severe and recurring hemorrhages. The defect is hereditary, confined to the male sex but transmitted by the female alone.

History.—Our knowledge of this remarkable condition dates from 1803, when John C. Otto, a Philadelphia physician, published "an account of an hemorrhagic disposition occurring in certain families," and first used the word "bleeder." The works of Grandidier and of Wickham Legg give full clinical details, and the monograph of Bulloch and Fildes (Dulan & Co., London, 1911) presents in extraordinary detail every aspect of the disease.

Distribution.—A majority of the cases have been reported from Germany, Switzerland and the United States. Jews are supposed to be more prone to the disease, but this Bulloch doubts, and he discredits the negro cases.

SEX.—Bulloch and Fildes claim to have established the fact of immunity in females, denying the authenticity of all the published cases. "In none of the families of bleeders . . . do we find any unequivocal evidence of abnormality in the women, that is to say, any abnormality beyond what might be expected in any collection of females taken at random."

INHERITANCE.—Otto pointed out in his original paper that while the females do not themselves bleed they alone transmit the tendency. Of 171 recorded instances of transmission, 160 conform to the "law of Nasse" that the disease is transmitted by the unaffected female—"the conductor" (Bulloch and Fildes). They explain the 11 exceptions, and conclude that the disease is not propagated through a male. Hemophilia without demonstrable inheritance is very rare. It is the best illustration in man of sex-limited inheritance, the mechanism of which has been worked out so beautifully by Morgan and his pupils in Drosophilia.

Pathogenesis.—The blood looks normal. Delay in the coagulation time, 30 or 40 minutes up to some hours and imperfect clot formation are the outstanding features. In contrast to purpura haemorrhagica the platelets are normal. The essential defect is a congenital inability to produce a proper thrombin, through the agency of which the fibrinogen is converted into fibrin. Sahli suggested that the disease was due to a deficiency in the thrombokinase. "It may be classed as one of the ferment-deficiency diseases, with a strong hereditary association similar to other ferment-deficiency diseases such as cystinuria, alkaptonuria, etc." (Vines). The deficiency is relative, not absolute, and is on the organic side of the clotting mechanism, and not in the inorganic side, *e. g.*, due to lack of calcium salts. One of the difficulties in explaining the bleeding in hemophilia is the fact that the hemorrhage continues in spite of the presence of clots in and about the wound. Addis believes that a higher amount of thrombokinase is required to produce rapid clotting in hemophilic than in normal blood. In a wound, coagulation may occur only in those parts, as at the side, where the concentration of this material is highest; but the clot itself prevents the addition of further quantities of the thrombokinase from the tissues, and when the quantity of thrombin set free from the primary clot is insufficient completely to coagulate the blood in the centre of the wound, the bleeding may continue indefinitely.

Symptoms.—"The cardinal symptoms are three in number . . . an *inherited* tendency in *males* to *bleed*" (Bulloch and Fildes). A trifling injury, of no moment in a normal person, determines a hemorrhage, which has no tendency to stop, but the blood trickles or oozes until death follows or there is arrest. The bleeding may be external, internal or into joints. A majority of the attacks may be traced to trauma but spontaneous bleeding may occur. The liability is first noticed in early childhood, perhaps with circumcision, and persists to adult life, gradually diminishing and eventually disappearing, sometimes about puberty. Tooth extraction is a common cause. Epistaxis is frequent, heading the list in Grandidier's series of 334 cases. Other localities were: mouth 43, stomach 15, bowels 36, urethra 16, lungs 17, and a few instances of bleeding from the tongue, finger tips, tear papilla, eyelids, external ear, vulva, navel and scrotum. Trivial operations have been followed by fatal hemorrhage. Blows may cause large ecchymoses. Abdominal colic, due to bleeding into the intestinal wall, may occur as in anaphylactoid purpura. The diagnosis of appendicitis may be made. The capillary resistance test is negative.

Hemarthrosis, due to bleeding from the synovial membrane, and periarticular bleedings occur. The onset is rapid with marked swelling and a variable amount of pain. The knee or elbow is most often attacked, and the affection has been mistaken for tuberculosis or an acute septic infection. König makes three stages—hemarthrosis, panarthritis and deformity.

Prevention.—The women of bleeder families should not marry or marrying, they should not bear children. Males may marry safely.

Diagnosis.—The monograph by Bulloch and Fildes should be read by all who value accuracy of observation and investigation. Forms of bleeding are so common that it is a simple matter to construct a pedigree showing an inherited "hemorrhagic diathesis." It is essential for the diagnosis that the individual should have been more or less subject to bleeding from various parts throughout his life. "No solitary hemorrhage, however inexplicable, should, in our opinion, be regarded as hemophilia; it is necessary to show that the individual has been repeatedly attacked, if not from birth, from infancy" (Bulloch and Fildes). There is no method by which we can determine the deficiency of the process on which the bleeding depends. There may be great variability in the tendency to bleed.

In the diagnosis from *thrombopenic purpura* the following points are important. In hemophilia puncture of the skin rarely causes hemorrhage, in purpura it usually does; the number of blood plates is normal in hemophilia, much reduced in purpura; the coagulation time is prolonged in hemophilia (but not constantly so; it may be normal between attacks), normal or nearly so in purpura; the "bleeding time" is not prolonged in hemophilia, much prolonged in purpura; in hemophilia the blood clot retracts normally but not in purpura; the application of a tourniquet to the upper arm is without result in hemophilia but in purpura results in the formation of petechiae on the forearm. As regards heredity, it is well to remember that there are cases of hereditary purpura, some being found in hemophiliac families.

In *prevention* every effort should be made to avoid trauma and active games are forbidden. Operations should be avoided if possible. The giving of calcium lactate and thymus gland extract at intervals has been advised but it is not well to expect much from these measures.

Treatment.—This consists in an attempt to supply the missing substance by the injection of serum or transfusion. A useful measure is the subcutaneous or intramuscular injection of fresh or citrated human blood in doses of 20 to 40 cc. Previous testing is not necessary. Fresh blood or serum from animals, such as the horse or rabbit, is also effective given subcutaneously in the same dosage. The injection should be repeated every twelve hours while necessary. The use of fresh antidiphtheritic serum may be effectual. With obstinate bleeding and severe anemia repeated transfusions should be done. For surface hemorrhage, compression should be employed combined with the application of various substances, as epinephrine (1 to 1000), normal human blood or serum. The last has been injected into or around the wound with advantage. The feeding of liver (not liver extract) has been suggested. In arthritic hemorrhage, operation is contra-indicated but aspiration may be done for excessive effusion. The joint should be kept at rest in the acute stage and passive motion begun as soon as this is over. The use of ovarian extract has been suggested and large amounts are given by mouth (120 grains) or estrin or theelin by injection. The reports on this treatment are contradictory. Protein shock by the use of typhoid vaccine, peptone or horse serum apparently has an effect in some cases. The use of snake venom is being investigated but as yet it is not possible to decide as to its value.

POLYCYTHEMIA VERA, ERYTHREMIA

(*Vaquez' Disease, Osler's Disease*)

Definition.—A symptom-complex characterized by cyanosis, polycythemia and splenic enlargement. It is possible that it is not a specific disease but a syndrome with a varied etiology and pathology. Lucas (1912) pointed out the difficulty of distinguishing between primary and secondary polycythemia.

Etiology.—The cause is unknown. There is overactivity of the erythropoietic tissue of the bone marrow. This may be due to overactivity of the factor which is lacking in pernicious anemia or the bone marrow may be specially susceptible to it. Another view is that it represents a change in the blood forming tissues comparable to leukemia. In a few cases the blood shows features of both diseases; either may be primary. Cholesterol has been suggested as a factor. Disturbance of the pulmonary diffusion of oxygen with resulting lack in the tissues and stimulation of the bone marrow have been suggested. The disease occurs in both sexes and is most common between 40 and 50 years of age.

Pathology.—We see polycythemia as a *secondary* condition in high altitudes, in congenital heart disease, in Ayerza's disease, with marked loss of fluid and in emphysema of the lungs. The high altitude form is compensatory to lack of oxygen and there is increased activity of the bone marrow. In erythremia proper an increased activity of the bone marrow is present. The *blood* has a high uric acid content (probably endogenous); the iron content is high; the resistance of the corpuscles is increased; the viscosity is high; and the coagulation time is prolonged. The splenic enlargement is a result of increased blood formation and destruction. In the cases with pulmonary arteriosclerosis there is marked right heart hypertrophy.

Symptoms.—The three cardinal features are a change in the appearance of the patient, enlargement of the spleen and polycythemia. The superficial blood vessels, capillaries, and veins look full, so that the skin is always congested, in warm weather of a brick red color, in cold weather cyanosed. The engorgement of the face may be extreme, extending to the conjunctivae, and in cold weather the cyanosis of the face and hands may be marked as any that is ever seen. There is often marked vasomotor instability, the hand becoming engorged when held down, and rapidly anemic when held up.

The *spleen* is usually enlarged and may vary in size. It is hard, firm and painless. Cirrhosis of the liver is sometimes found.

The total bulk of *blood* is enormously increased, and the ratio of corpuscles to plasma is high. The polycythemia ranges from 7 to 12 or even 13 millions of red cells per cmm. As a rule, they are normal in appearance and shape; nucleated red cells may be present; the hemoglobin ranges up to 150 per cent, but the color index rarely reaches one. Moderate leukocytosis is the rule with a varying percentage of the different forms; a few myelocytes may be present. The specific gravity is high.

Of other symptoms the most common are inacapacity for work, headache, flushing and giddiness. Constipation is common, and albuminuria is usually present. The blood pressure may be high; occasionally there are hemorrhages into the skin and from the mucous membranes. Hematemesis and hematuria may occur. Recurring ascites, probably in association with the splenic tumor or secondary to hepatic cirrhosis, is present in some cases. There may be syncope and extreme prostration. Digestive disturbances may occur with pain of such severity that the abdomen has been explored. The cyanosis is intermittent in some cases. Vascular changes are common, vasomotor disturbance, arteriosclerosis, thromboangiitis obliterans and acute myocardial insufficiency.

Christian emphasized the frequency of nervous symptoms, among which are headache, dizziness, paresthesias, paresis and paralysis. Disturbances of vision are common. In some cases the symptoms suggest brain tumor. In early stages circulatory disturbance is probably responsible; later cerebral hemorrhage or thrombosis occurs.

A form is described as *benign familial polycythemia* in which there is polycythemia and splenomegaly without the typical picture of polycythemia vera. Geisböck described a variety, *polycythemia hypertonica,* with increased tension, arteriosclerosis and nephritis. In the condition called "Ayerza's Disease" or "cardiacos negros," associated with syphilitic disease of the pulmonary arteries, there is headache, vertigo, somnolence, cyanosis, dyspnea, cough, hemoptysis and polycythemia. There is a pulmonary stage lasting for some years followed by the "cardiacos negros" stage lasting for two to five years, with marked enlargement of the right heart. The X-ray shows the dilated pulmonary artery.

Diagnosis.—The features above referred to are sufficient in the absence of congenital heart disease, emphysema, and forms of cyanosis associated with poisoning by coal tar products. There is a *splenomegalic polycythemia* which occurs with tuberculosis of the spleen and with obstruction of the portal system.

Prognosis.—The prognosis is bad for cure, but the condition may persist for years with reasonably good health. Cardiac failure, vascular accidents, hemorrhage, and recurring ascites have been the usual modes of death.

Treatment.—The *diet* should be low in protein, especially the purin bases, and iron. When there is much fullness of the head and vertigo, venesection gives temporary relief. Inhalations of oxygen may be tried when the cyanosis is extreme. Good results are reported from the use of arsenic. Fowler's solution is begun in doses of three drops and increased to 15 to 20 drops three times a day. The dose then may be reduced and further dosage guided by the results. The use of phenylhydrazin hydrochloride in doses of gr. 1½ (0.1 gm.) once daily, with a careful watch of the blood count, has proved useful. It should not be used if there is hepatic cirrhosis. Acetylphenylhydrazin is said to be less toxic and is given in the same dosage. Benzol is of value in some cases in doses of ℳ xv (1 cc.) three times a day. The blood count is a guide for the proper dose. If syphilis is suspected, active treatment should be given. Radium and X-ray treatment over the long bones has apparently been useful in some cases; it should not be given over the spleen. The number of leukocytes is a guide in any treatment; leukcopenia should be avoided. Splenectomy should not be performed.

ENTEROGENOUS CYANOSIS

(*Methemoglobinemia and Sulphemoglobinemia*)

Definition.—A form of permanent cyanosis due to changes in the composition of the hemoglobin of the blood.

Etiology.—Certain drugs, such as potassium chlorate, phenacetine, acetanilide, trional, sulphonal and nitrites induce changes in the hemoglobin. Carbon monoxide and sulphuretted hydrogen may cause a chronic cyanosis. Stokvis brought evidence to show that certain cases of chronic cyanosis are associated with intestinal disturbances, and he gives this form the name "enterogenous." Some are associated with methemoglobinemia, others with sulphemoglobinemia. Nitrite-producing organisms give a reducing substance which acts on hemoglobin. In a doubtful case, with absence of lesions of the heart or lungs, a spectroscopic examination of the blood will determine if the cyanosis is of this nature, and which of the two derivatives of hemoglobin is causing it.

Gibson and Douglas obtained from the blood of one patient a pure culture of a colon organism and suggested the name "microbic cyanosis." Methemoglobinemia has been met with in Winckel's disease. Boycott discovered an infective methemoglobinemia in rats, caused by Gaertner's bacillus, which gives a remarkable bluish tint to the skin of white rats.

Symptoms.—These are emotional disturbances, headache, vertigo, asthenia, palpitation of the heart and syncope. The cyanosis varies in degree and may be extreme. There may be some polycythemia. In methemoglobinemia there is direct action of the drug on the hemoglobin; in sulphemoglobinemia, the hemoglobin combines with hydrogen sulphide absorbed from the bowel, so that constipation is usual in these cases.

In *sulphemoglobinemia* the appearance of the patients is much the same. They look badly, even death-like, but feel comfortable, and there is no shortness of breath. The main complaints are cyanosis, constipation, weakness and headache. A nitrite-producing bacillus has been found in the saliva.

Treatment.—The use of any causal drug should be discontinued. In some cases of methemoglobinemia a milk diet has proved useful; meat and eggs should be excluded. Irrigation of the colon should be done systematically. In sulphemoglobinemia every effort should be made to keep the bowels moving freely. The use of a vaccine made from the nitrite-producing organism has proved successful. Foci of infection should be treated, especially in the mouth.

If the causal drug is stopped, methemoglobinemia clears rapidly but weeks or months are required for sulphemoglobinemia to disappear.

DISEASES OF THE SPLEEN

GENERAL REMARKS

Though a ductless gland, the spleen is not known to have an internal secretion, and its functions are ill understood. It is not an organ essential to life. In the fetus it takes part in the formation of red and white blood corpuscles, and as it contains hematoblasts, it is possible that in the adult this function may be exercised to some extent, particularly in cases of severe anemia. The reticulo-endothelial system is specially concerned in this. The relation to the blood platelets is obscure.

Hemolysis is generally believed to be its special function, based upon the presence of a large percentage of organic compounds of iron, the deposit in the organ of blood pigments in various diseases, the presence of many macrophages containing red blood corpuscles, and upon the evidence, after removal of the spleen, of compensatory hemolysis in many newly formed hemolymph glands (Warthin). An important function is *contraction* which adds red blood cells to the circulating blood and probably is important in a single hemorrhage rather than in repeated bleeding. Contraction may be stimulated by epinephrine and, it is suggested, by central nervous control.

Removal of the spleen, an operation practised by the ancients in the belief that it improved the wind of runners, is not, as a rule, followed by serious effects. There may be slight eosinophilia and anemia, which may persist for some time and later there is usually slight leukocytosis, with relative increase of the lymphocytes. After removal, an accessory spleen may increase greatly in size. There are cases of congenital absence of the spleen.

In infections the organ enlarges and micro-organisms are present in large numbers. It has been supposed to play some part in the processes of immunity and phagocytosis goes on actively in the organ. In experimental anemia caused by various hemolytic agents the spleen enlarges, and in these conditions Bunting and Norris found evidence of vicarious blood formation. Chronic splenomegaly may be present with little disturbance of health.

MOVABLE SPLEEN

Movable or wandering spleen is seen most frequently in women the subjects of enteroptosis. It may be present without signs of displacement of other organs. It may be found accidentally in individuals who present no symptoms. In other cases there are dragging, uneasy feelings in the back and side. All grades are met with, from a spleen that can be felt completely below the margin of the ribs to a condition in which the tumor impinges upon the pelvis; indeed the organ has been found in an inguinal hernia! In the large majority of cases the spleen is enlarged. Sometimes it appears that the enlargement has caused relaxation of the ligaments; in other instances the relaxation seems congenital, as movable spleens have been found in members of the same family. Possibly trauma may account for some of the cases.

Apart from the dragging, uneasy sensations and the worry in nervous patients, a movable spleen causes few serious symptoms. *Torsion* of the pedicle may produce a serious condition, leading to great swelling of the organ, high fever or necrosis. The diagnostic features are a sudden onset with intense pain and symptoms of peritonitis; a splenic tumor appears in a few hours with absence of the normal splenic dulness. There is absence of rigidity of the abdominal wall at first.

The *diagnosis* of a movable spleen is usually easy unless the organ becomes fixed and is deformed by adhesions and perisplenitis. The shape and the sharp margin with the notches are points to be specially noted.

The *treatment* is important. The organ may be kept in position by a properly adapted belt and pad. Removal of the organ has been done, but is unnecessary as a rule. Splenectomy is indicated for torsion.

RUPTURE OF THE SPLEEN

Special interest attaches to the rupture which may occur spontaneously or from trauma in typhoid fever or malaria. Rupture of a malarial spleen may follow a blow, a fall, or exploratory puncture. Fatal hemorrhage may follow puncture of a swollen spleen with a hypodermic needle. There may be delayed hemorrhage following trauma. After an injury the patient may not seem ill and the latent period may be as long as three weeks. During this time there may be pain in the splenic region with some muscular rigidity, leukocytosis, diminished expansion on the left side and left basal pleurisy. With the final rupture there is severe pain and collapse. Occasionally rupture results from the breaking of an infarct or abscess. The symptoms are those of hemorrhage into the peritoneum, and the condition demands immediate operation.

INFARCT, ABSCESS, CYSTS AND TUBERCULOSIS OF THE SPLEEN

Emboli causing *infarcts* may be infective or simple and are most frequent in ulcerative endocarditis and septic conditions. Infarcts may follow the formation of thrombi in the branches of the splenic artery in acute fevers. In a few instances the infarcts have followed thrombosis in the splenic veins. They are chiefly of pathological interest. Infarct may be suspected in endocarditis, septicemia or pyemia when there are pain in the splenic region, tenderness on pressure, and swelling of the organ; a friction rub is often heard. Sometimes with infective infarcts large *abscesses* are formed, and in rare instances the whole organ may be converted into a sac of pus. Operation is indicated for abscess.

Tumors of the spleen, hydatid and other *cysts,* abscess and *gummata* are rare conditions of anatomical interest. Sarcoma is the most important primary tumor. *Abscess* may result from extension but is usually due to hemotogenous infection. With the general features of infection there is a large tender spleen, often adherent to the abdominal wall. In *Hodgkin's* disease the organ may be enlarged and smooth, or irregular from the presence of nodular tumors.

Cysts are rare (dermoid, hydatid and serous or hemorrhagic); the senior author saw but two, one an echinococcus, and the other a double cyst of the hilus. The latter probably arose from a hematoma, subcapsular or in the hilus.

Very small cysts occur in connection with polycystic disease of the liver and kidneys. The diagnosis of cysts is not often made; the mass is usually irregular in the region of the spleen, but the splenic outlines are marked. In the case with two cysts at the hilus, the tumor was very movable and irregular. Operation is usually successful.

Primary tuberculosis is rare. In some cases the symptoms resemble those of an acute infection, with pain in the splenic region and enlargement of the organ. In the chronic cases there is progressive enlargement of the spleen, often with cyanosis and sometimes with polycythemia. Splenectomy has been successful in some cases.

PRIMARY SPLENOMEGALY WITH ANEMIA

(*Splenic Anemia, Banti's Disease*)

Definition.—A primary disease of the spleen of unknown origin, characterized by progressive enlargement, anemia, a tendency to hemorrhage, and in some cases a secondary cirrhosis of the liver, with jaundice and ascites. That the spleen itself is essentially concerned is shown by the fact that complete recovery may follow its removal.

History.—The name "splenic anemia" was applied to a group of cases by Griesinger in 1866. H. C. Wood, in 1871, described cases as the splenic form of pseudoleukemia. The real study of the disease was initiated by Banti in 1883. In France the condition was called "primitive splenomegaly," and different types have been described. There is unfortunately a confusion in terminology; some use the term Banti's disease as synonymous with splenic anemia, while others restrict it to the cases of splenic anemia in which cirrhosis of the liver develops; not all cases of splenic anemia progress to the stage of Banti's disease. The latter usage is to be preferred.

Etiology.—In the majority of cases the enlargement of the spleen comes on without any recognizable cause. Obstruction of the venous outflow may be important. In a few cases malaria has been present, but in the greater number the first thing noticed has been the mechanical inconvenience of the big spleen. Males are more frequently attacked than females. It is a disease of young and middle life, the majority of cases occurring before the fortieth year. Gibson found a streptothrix (possibly Nocardia) in some cases.

Morbid Anatomy.—The spleen is greatly enlarged, very firm, the capsule thickened, the texture very tough and firm, and in a state of advanced fibrosis. Banti described a proliferation of the endothelial cells of the venous sinuses of the pulp. The blood-vessels in the neighborhood of the spleen may be very large, particularly the vasa brevia; the splenic vein and the portal vein may be enormously dilated, and show atheroma and calcification. The lymphatic glands are not involved. Hyperplasia of the bone marrow has been found, but no other changes of special importance.

Symptoms.—The disease is extraordinarily chronic; eight of our cases had a longer duration than ten years. Usually the first feature is:

Splenomegaly.—The enlargement is uniform, smooth, painless and usually reaches to the navel. It may exist for years without any symptoms other than the inconvenience caused by the distention and weight. Following an infarct pain may be present. Enlargement of the spleen may persist for many years without any consecutive change in the liver.

Anemia.—Sooner or later the patients become anemic. This may develop with rapidity but more commonly the process is gradual and the patient may come under observation for the first time with swelling of the feet, shortness of breath and advanced anemia. The blood picture is that of a secondary anemia with a low color index and a marked leukopenia. The red blood cells may fall as low as two million and in a series of uncomplicated cases the average leukocyte count was under 3,500 per c.mm. There are no special changes in the differential count. Some divide the cases into two groups depending on the number of platelets and suggest that in the thrombocytopenic group the splenomegaly is primary and so splenectomy more likely to be useful. Some patients have permanent slight anemia of the secondary type; others show recurring attacks of severe anemia, which may be independent of hemorrhage.

Hemorrhages.—Bleeding, usually hematemesis, may be a special feature and occur at intervals for many years. One of our patients had recurring attacks for twelve years, and one at the London Hospital for fifteen years (Hutchison). In such cases the diagnosis of peptic ulcer may be made. The bleeding may be of great severity. On several occasions one of our patients was brought into the hospital completely exsanguine; in three the hemorrhage proved directly fatal. The bleeding comes, as a rule, from esophageal varices. Melena, hematuria and purpura may occur.

Cirrhosis of the Liver.—This develops in a large number of the cases. The liver may be enlarged for a time, but not extremely so, and goes on to contraction with subsequent ascites. The cirrhosis is progressive. *Jaundice,* usually slight, may be present and persist for a long period. *Ascites* may be due to the enlarged spleen itself or to secondary cirrhosis of the liver.

Course.—It is extraordinarily chronic. Some cases never progress to the stage of Banti's disease. A patient may for years have a large spleen causing no inconvenience, then anemia may occur, from which recovery gradually takes place; or the first symptom may be ascites or a severe hemorrhage from the stomach. As a rule, the anemia becomes chronic.

Diagnosis.—Here may be mentioned other forms of splenomegaly.

SPLENOMEGALY WITH CHRONIC ACHOLURIC HEMOLYTIC JAUNDICE.—The form, first described by Minkowski, is usually a familial form, often hereditary. There are congenital (more common) and acquired forms. It is consistent with good health throughout life, and there may be no symptoms. Characteristic features are: (*a*) its familial form; (*b*) chronic enlargement of the spleen; (*c*) chronic slight jaundice; (*d*) presence of urobilin in the urine, but absence of bile pigment. The red blood corpuscles have an increased fragility. They show hemolysis in a 0.6 per cent solution of sodium chloride and this is complete at 0.4 per cent, the normal figures being 0.44 per cent to 0.3 per cent solution. There may be large numbers of reticulocytes. There is usually a moderate anemia. There may be acute attacks with fever, vomiting, abdominal pain, increase in the jaundice and in the anemia. Some of these attacks are due to gall stones. There is a tendency to chronic indolent leg ulcers. The *diagnosis* depends largely on the recognition of the fragility of the red cells. In *treatment* the patient should avoid chilling and exposure. If the condition is severe splenectomy should be done. Gall stones may require operation.

Splenomegaly of the Gaucher Type (see page 769).

Splenomegaly with Eosinophilia.—This is a rare condition with marked enlargement of the spleen and leukocytosis. In one case the leukocytes were 34,000 with 70 to 80 per cent of eosinophiles. Nucleated red cells are present in moderate numbers, both normoblasts and megaloblasts. The spleen shows a large number of eosinophiles. Following splenectomy there was a great increase in the number of leukocytes in two of the reported cases, to 138,000 and 211,000. The eosinophilia also increased to 90 per cent in Giffin's case. There may be hyperplasia of certain elements in the bone marrow. Splenectomy seems to have resulted in benefit in the general condition but the eosinophilia became more marked. This may be due to the loss of the phagocytic influence of the spleen. The condition may represent an unusual form of leukemia.

Thrombophlebitic Splenomegaly.—This is due to thrombosis in the splenic or in the portal vein or its branches. The thrombosis is usually of long duration and the thrombus is calcified; there may be channels through it. The thrombosis is probably secondary to phlebitis. The spleen is often enormously enlarged and perisplenitis with dense adhesions is common.

Hepatic Splenomegaly.—Three varieties of cirrhosis of the liver may lead to great enlargement of the spleen with anemia and a symptom-complex resembling that of splenic anemia.

(*a*) *Portal Cirrhosis.*—With recurring hemorrhages, a consecutive anemia, ascites, and an unusually large spleen, the condition may simulate closely the last stage of splenic anemia. The history, particularly the late appearance of the hepatic changes, may be the most important point. In the cases in which we have been in doubt the difficulty has arisen from an imperfect history and from the presence of recurring hemorrhages.

(*b*) *Syphilitic Cirrhosis.*—Great enlargement of the spleen may occur with hepatic syphilis, congenital or acquired and the picture may be similar to splenic anemia—slight jaundice, ascites, big spleen, recurring hemorrhages, and anemia. A search for the features of hepatic syphilis, the Wassermann test and the effect of syphilitic treatment are important. Syphilis may cause marked enlargement of the spleen without involvement of the liver. In some cases, there is little change in the spleen from specific treatment.

(*c*) In a few cases of hypertrophic cirrhosis, as in Hanot's form and in hemochromatosis, the spleen may be greatly enlarged.

Myelophthisic Splenomegaly.—In this the blood is of a fetal type with moderate anemia and many nucleated red cells. There is no evidence of hemolysis or increased red cell fragility.

Pernicious Anemia.—Sometimes the spleen is greatly enlarged but the blood findings give the diagnosis. In some cases of *Hodgkin's disease* the spleen may be markedly enlarged.

Tropical Splenomegaly.—Kala-azar can be distinguished by finding the Leishman-Donovan bodies. There are big spleens with anemia in the Tropics which are not kala-azar, and some of these are of the splenic anemia type.

Subleukemic Splenic Reticulo-endotheliosis is probably a subleukemic form of monocytic leukemia with marked splenomegaly. Leukemic reticulo-endotheliosis may show "generalized involvement of the entire reticulo-endothelial system, with or without localized tumors, with predominant involvement of the bone marrow, of lymphatic structures or of the liver or spleen" (Giffin and Watkins, 1934). The primitive free reticulo-endothelial cell may be found in the blood. The *diagnosis* is made by finding the reticular cells and reticular monocytes in the blood. The percentage of these cells increases as the disease progresses. Removal of the spleen is not indicated.

The cause of the enlarged spleen in malaria, leukemia, and erythremia is determined by the blood examination; in Hodgkin's disease, carcinoma, amyloid disease and endocarditis, other features usually prevent error.

Treatment.—This consists in splenectomy or ligation of the splenic artery, done as early as possible; with severe anemia the usual treatment should be given and especially blood transfusion. When marked hepatic changes have occurred, operation is usually contra-indicated. In the cases too far advanced for operation the treatment is that of any severe anemia and with cirrhosis of the liver and ascites the usual measures should be adopted. If there is any evidence of syphilis active treatment should be given.

XANTHOMATOSES

The term "xanthomatosis" is not a very satisfactory one but it seems to be firmly established. Probably the term "lipoidosis" would be more satisfactory.

The cases fall into two main groups: (1) Generalized. (a) Symptomatic in other diseases in which there are disturbances of lipoid metabolism, for example, in diabetes mellitus and jaundice, and (b) essential or primary forms which show a constitutional anomaly of lipoid metabolism.

(2) Localized. This may be described as "essential" or "primary" xanthomatosis. Under this heading come (1) Gaucher's disease, (2) Niemann-Pick disease, (3) Hand-Schüller-Christian disease, and (4) Primary cases which occur in the skin and internal organs. The forms on the eyelids belong here.

In the first group of generalized cases the lipoid is in the cells of the connective tissue and the endothelium of the lymph vessels. The material consists of a cholesterin fatty acid ester. The same material may be deposited in certain organs, for example, in the meninges, the spleen, the adrenal glands, etc.

In the group of essential or primary forms, there is a difference in the character of the deposited lipoids. This can be made out by microchemical methods. The condition is closely associated with the reticulo-endothelial system.

A rare form may be mentioned—"*Pseudoxanthoma elasticum*" (Sugg and Stetson, 1934). In this there is a curious loose and wrinkled appearance of the skin of the neck and axillae, and small subcutaneous nodules. There may be striae of varying widths and lengths. The same condition occurs in the mucous membrane of the mouth and nose, and occasionally on the back, arms and legs. The elastic fibres in the deeper parts of the skin show marked degeneration. There are also curious streaks in the retina with ultimate disturbance of vision. Possibly there may be an hereditary element in the disease. There is no definite treatment, but it is stated that X-ray therapy has given good results in some cases.

Gaucher's Disease.—This rare familial disease was described by Gaucher in 1882. It usually begins in childhood before the 12th year and is more frequent in girls. There are characteristic large foam cells which are found in the spleen, liver, bone marrow, lymph nodes and the reticulo-endothelial system generally. The diagnosis may be made by study of material obtained by splenic puncture. The special contained subtance is kerasin which does not give the stains for fat but does for iron. The main features are a progressive enlargement of the spleen often to an enormous size, with the general health remaining good, followed by enlargement of the liver without jaundice and rarely with ascites. There is a brownish yellow pigmentation of the skin, sometimes with wedge-shaped yellowish thickened areas on the conjunctiva on each side of the cornea. Anemia usually appears late and is moderate; leukopenia is usual. The disease is chronic and may persist for twenty years or more without much disturbance of the general health. There may be changes in the bones and joints. The diagnosis is suggested by the general features and is made beyond doubt by examination of the spleen, after puncture or removal. Splenectomy is advisable but not always curative.

Niemann-Pick Disease: Lipoid Histiocytosis.—This is a very rare disease of infants described by Niemann in 1914, apparently due to a lipoid metabolic disturbance in the reticulo-endothelial system. The spleen is much like that in Gaucher's splenomegaly but the material in the large cells is lipoid in character and probably belongs to the phosphatid group. Enlarged liver and spleen with ascites and edema, and leukocytosis, occur without jaundice. There are digestive disturbances, slow growth, and anemia. The course is usually fairly acute with death generally before the end of the second year. There is no known treatment of value.

Hand-Schüller-Christian Disease.—This is a congenital familial disease and occurs predominantly in males. The essential *etiology* is in doubt. There is a disturbance in lipoid metabolism and the lesions contain considerable cholesterol. The bones, particularly of the skull, show numerous defects, sometimes with cyst formation. So-called "foam cells" may almost completely replace the bone marrow and the subsequent formation of granulomatous tissue is the cause of the defects. Granulomatous masses may invade the orbit. Changes about the base of the skull, involving the pituitary gland, are apparently responsible for the diabetes insipidus and disturbance of growth. The pituitary gland may be infiltrated with the foam cells.

The *symptoms* usually begin in the second year; the main features being (1) defects of bones, particularly of the skull; (2) exophthalmos, and (3) diabetes insipidus. There are other features: Interference with growth, pigmentation of the skin, cyanosis and dyspnea, enlargement of the spleen, liver and lymph nodes. There may be jaundice in some cases. In some cases gingivitis and stomatitis are marked early in the disease. Anemia may be marked. In the *diagnosis,* the general features are suggestive and the bony changes are characteristic. Spontaneous remissions apparently occur.

In *treatment* a low fat diet is suggested. The giving of thyroid and pituitary gland extract has been done. The diabetes insipidus can possibly be aided by pituitary gland extract subcutaneously or by nasal spray. Small doses of insulin have been useful in thin and anemic patients. X-ray therapy has been employed and seems to have a beneficial effect on the bone lesions. It should not be used in patients who are very anemic or show hemorrhagic features.

SECTION X

DISEASES OF THE CIRCULATORY SYSTEM

DISEASES OF THE PERICARDIUM

PERICARDITIS

—Pericarditis is the result of infective processes or arises by extension of inflammation from contiguous organs. The pus cocci, the pneumococcus and the tubercle bacillus are the chief causal organisms.

Etiology.—PRIMARY, so-called idiopathic, inflammation is rare; but it has occurred in children without any evidence of rheumatic fever or of other disease. Tonsillitis should be looked for and certain cases are tuberculous.

Pericarditis from *injury* usually comes under the care of the surgeon in connection with the primary wound. The trauma may be from within, due to the passage of a foreign body—a needle, a pin or a bone—through the esophagus—a variety exceedingly common in cows and horses.

SECONDARY.—(*a*) This occurs most frequently with *rheumatic fever*. In our 330 cases of rheumatic fever (Johns Hopkins Hospital) pericarditis occurred in twenty—practically 6 per cent. The disease may be associated with acute tonsillitis in rheumatic subjects. The pericarditis may precede the arthritis. (*b*) In septic processes; in acute bone necrosis and puerperal fever it is not uncommon. (*c*) In *tuberculosis,* in which the disease may be primary or part of a general involvement of the serous sacs or with extensive pulmonary disease. (*d*) In the *fevers.* Not infrequent after scarlet fever, it is rare in measles, smallpox, typhoid fever and diphtheria. In *pneumonia* it is not uncommon, occurring in 31 among 665 cases (Chatard). In 184 postmortems there were 29 instances of pericarditis. It is most frequent in double pneumonia, and in our series with disease of the right side, if only one lung was involved. Pericarditis sometimes complicates *chorea;* it was present in 19 of 73 autopsies; in only 8 of these was arthritis present. (*e*) *Terminal* pericarditis. In gout, chronic nephritis, arteriosclerosis, diabetes and chronic illness of all sorts pericarditis is common and often overlooked. (*f*) *By Extension.* This occurs in pneumonia but with simple pleurisy it is rare. In ulcerative endocarditis, purulent myocarditis, and in aneurism of the aorta pericarditis may occur. It may follow extension of infection from the mediastinal glands, the ribs, sternum, vertebrae, and even from the abdominal viscera. (*g*) With *coronary artery occlusion* or myocardial infarction.

Pericarditis occurs at all ages. Cases have been reported in the fetus. In the newborn it may result from septic infection through the navel. Throughout childhood the incidence of rheumatic fever and scarlet fever makes it a frequent affection, whereas late in life it is most often associated with tuberculosis, nephritis and gout. Males are somewhat more frequently attacked than females. The so-called epidemics of pericarditis have been outbreaks of pneumonia with this as a frequent complication.

ACUTE FIBRINOUS PERICARDITIS

This, the most common and benign form, has a small amount of exudate which coats the surface in a thin layer and may be partial or general. In the mildest grades the membrane looks lustreless and roughened, due to a thin fibrinous sheeting, which can be lifted, showing beneath an injected or ecchymotic serosa. As the fibrinous sheeting increases in thickness the constant movement of the adjacent surfaces gives to it sometimes a ridge-like, at others a honeycombed appearance. With more abundant fibrinous exudation the membranes present an appearance like buttered surfaces which have been drawn apart. The fibrin is in shreds and the heart presents a curious shaggy appearance—the hairy heart of old writers, *cor villosum.*

In mild grades the subadjacent muscle looks normal, but in the more prolonged and severe cases there is *myocarditis,* and for 2 or 3 mm. beneath the visceral layer the muscle presents a pale, turbid appearance. Some of these acute cases are tuberculous and the granulations are easily overlooked.

There is usually a slight amount of fluid entangled in the meshes of fibrin, but there may be a very thick exudate without much serous effusion.

Symptoms.—Unless sought for there may be no objective signs and for this reason it is often overlooked, and in hospitals the disease is relatively more common in the postmortem room than in the wards.

Pain is a variable symptom, not usually intense, and in this form rarely excited by pressure. It is more marked in the early stage, and may be referred to the precordia, to the left shoulder, to the region of the xiphoid cartilage or to the abdomen. The last may be so marked that the abdomen has been opened. There may be pain on swallowing. In some instances the pain is of an aggravated character resembling angina. Cough and dyspnea may occur. *Fever* is usually present, but it is not always easy to say how much depends upon the primary disease, and how much upon the pericarditis. It is as a rule not high, rarely exceeding 103.5° F. In rheumatic cases hyperpyrexia has been observed.

Physical Signs.—*Inspection* is negative; *palpation* may reveal a distinct fremitus caused by rubbing of the roughened pericardial surfaces. This is usually best marked over the right ventricle. It is not always felt, even when the friction sound on auscultation is loud and clear.

Auscultation.—The *friction* sound is one of the most distinctive of physical signs. It is double, corresponding to the systole and diastole; but the synchronism with the heart sounds is not accurate, and the to and fro murmur usually outlasts the time occupied by the first and second sounds. In rare instances the friction is single; sometimes it appears to be triple—a sort of canter rhythm. The sounds have a peculiar rubbing, grating quality, characteristic when once recognized, and rarely simulated by endocardial murmurs. Sometimes instead of grating there is a creaking quality—the *bruit de cuir neuf*—the new leather murmur of the French. The pericardial friction appears superficial, very close to the ear, and is usually intensified by pressure with the stethoscope. It is best heard over the right ventricle, the part of the heart most closely in contact with the front of the chest—that is, in the fourth and fifth interspaces and adjacent portions of the sternum. There are instances in which the friction is most marked at the base, over the aorta, and at the superior reflection of the pericardium. Occasionally it is best heard at the apex. It may be limited to a narrow area, or transmitted up and down the sternum. There are no definite lines of transmission as in endocardial murmurs. An important point is the variability of the sounds, both in position and quality; they may be heard at one visit and not at another. The maximum of intensity will be found to vary with position, change of which may increase or decrease the rub. Friction may be present with a thin layer of exudate; on the other hand it may not be present with a thick, buttery layer. The rub may be entirely obscured by the loud râles in pneumonia, in which disease pericarditis is recognized clinically in about half the cases.

Diagnosis.—There is rarely any difficulty in determining the presence of a dry pericarditis, for the friction sounds are distinctive. The double murmur of aortic disease may simulate a pericardial rub. The constant character of the aortic murmur, the transmission, the phenomena in the arteries, the blood pressure and associated conditions should prevent this error.

Pleuropericardial friction is common, and may be associated with endo-pericarditis, particularly in pneumonia. It is frequent, too, in tuberculosis. It is best heard over the left border of the heart, and is much affected by the respiratory movement. Holding the breath or taking a deep inspiration may abolish it. The rhythm is not the simple to and fro diastolic and systolic, but the respiratory rhythm is superadded, usually intensifying the murmur during expiration and lessening it on inspiration. In tuberculosis of the lungs there are instances in which, with the friction, a loud systolic click is heard, due to the compression of a thin layer of lung and the expulsion of air from a softening focus or from a bronchus.

And, lastly, it is not very uncommon, in the region of the apex beat, to hear a series of fine crepitant sounds, systolic in time, often very distinct, suggestive of pericardial adhesions, but heard too frequently for this cause.

Course.—Simple fibrinous pericarditis never kills, but it occurs so often with serious affections that we have frequent opportunities to see all stages of its progress. In the majority of cases the inflammation subsides and the thin fibrinous laminae gradually become converted into connective tissue, which unites the pericardial surfaces firmly together. A very thin layer may "clear" without leaving adhesions. In other instances the inflammation progresses, with increase of the exudation, and the condition is changed to pericarditis with effusion. In some instances the simple plastic pericarditis becomes chronic, and great thickening of both layers gradually results.

PERICARDITIS WITH EFFUSION

Etiology.—Commonly a direct sequence of the dry or plastic pericarditis of which it is sometimes called the second stage, this form is found most frequently with rheumatic fever, tuberculosis and septicemia, and sets in usually with precordial pain, slight fever or a distinct chill. In children the disease may, like pleurisy, come on without local symptoms, and, after a week or two of failing health, slight fever, shortness of breath, and increasing pallor, the physician may find, to his astonishment, signs of extensive pericardial effusion. These latent cases are often tuberculous. W. Ewart called special attention to latent and ephemeral pericardial effusions, which he thought to be often of short duration and of moderate size, with an absence of the painful features of pericarditis. These are by no means rare but careful observation is required for their recognition.

Morbid Anatomy.—The effusion may be serofibrinous, hemorrhagic or purulent. The amount varies from 200 to 300 cc. to 2 litres. In serofibrinous exudation the pericardial membranes are covered with thick, creamy fibrin, which may be in ridges or honeycombed, or present long, villous extensions. The parietal layer may be several millimetres in thickness and form a firm, leathery membrane. The hemorrhagic exudation is usually associated with tuberculous or cancerous pericarditis, or in the aged. The lymph is less abundant, but both surfaces are injected and often show numerous hemorrhages. Thick, curdy masses of lymph are usually found in the dependent part of the sac. In many cases the effusion is really seropurulent, a thin, turbid exudation containing flocculi of fibrin.

The pericardial layers are greatly thickened and covered with fibrin. When the fluid is pus, they present a grayish, rough, granular surface. Sometimes there are distinct erosions on the visceral membrane. The heart muscle becomes involved to a greater or less extent and, on section, the tissue, for a depth of from 2 to 3 mm., is pale and turbid, and shows evidence of fatty and granular change. Endocarditis coexists frequently, but rarely results from the extension of the inflammation through the wall of the heart.

Symptoms.—Even with copious effusion the onset and course may be so insidious that no suspicion of the true nature of the disease is aroused.

As in the simple pericarditis, *pain* may be present, either sharp and stabbing or as a sense of distress and discomfort in the cardiac region. It is more frequent with effusion than in the plastic form. Pressure at the lower end of the sternum usually aggravates it. *Dyspnea* is a common and important symptom, one which, perhaps, more than any other, excites suspicion and leads to a careful examination. The patient is restless, lies upon the left side or, as the effusion increases, sits up in bed. Associated with the dyspnea is in many cases a peculiarly dusky, anxious countenance. The pulse is rapid, small, sometimes irregular, and may present the *pulsus paradoxus,* in which during each inspiration the pulse beat becomes very weak or is lost. These are due, in great part, to the direct mechanical effect of the pericardial fluid which embarrasses the heart's action. Other pressure effects are distention of the veins of the neck, *dysphagia,* which may be marked, and irritative cough from compression of the trachea. Aphonia is not uncommon, owing to compression or irritation of the recurrent laryngeal nerve. In massive effusion the pericardial sac occupies a large portion of the anterolateral region of the left side and the condition may be mistaken for pneumonia or pleurisy. Even in moderate grades the left lung is somewhat compressed, an additional element in the production of the dyspnea. Great restlessness, insomnia, and in the later stages low delirium and coma occur in the more severe cases. Delirium and marked cerebral symptoms are associated with the hyperpyrexia of rheumatic cases, but in addition there may be peculiar mental symptoms. The patient may become melancholic and show suicidal tendencies or the condition resembles closely delirium tremens. Sibson, who specially described the condition, states that the majority of such cases recover. Chorea may also occur, as pointed out by Bright. Convulsions are rare but have occurred during paracentesis.

Physical Signs.—*Inspection.*—In children the precordia bulges and with copious exudation the anterolateral region of the left chest becomes enlarged. A wavy impulse may be seen in the third and fourth interspaces, or there may be no impulse visible. The intercostal spaces bulge somewhat and there may be edema of the wall. Owing to compression of the lung, the expansion of the left side is greatly diminished. The diaphragm and left lobe of the liver may be pushed down and produce a prominence in the epigastric region. There may be marked distention of the veins of the neck and arms.

Palpation.—A gradual diminution and final obliteration of the cardiac impulse is a striking feature in progressive effusion. The position of the apex beat is not constant. In large effusions it is usually not felt. In children as the fluid collects the pulsation may be best seen in the fourth space, but this may not be the apex itself. The pericardial friction may lessen with the effusion, though it often persists with considerable fluid or it may be felt in the erect and not in the recumbent posture.

Percussion gives most important indications. The gradual distention of the pericardial sac pushes aside the margins of the lungs so that a large area comes in contact with the chest wall and gives a greatly increased area of dulness. The form of this dulness is irregularly pear-shaped; the base or broad surface directed downward and the stem or apex directed upward. The rapid transition from lung resonance to pericardial flatness is striking. Shifting dulness at the base, that is a change in the width of the dull area with the patient recumbent and sitting, wider when recumbent, is an important sign. There is a disproportionate extension of dulness upward, and to the right, with dulness in the right fifth interspace, extending one or two inches to the right of the sternum (Rotch's sign). Williamson could not verify this in an experimental study. In large effusions there may be altered resonance in the left axilla, and an area of dulness near the angle of the scapula with bronchial breathing, which may alter when the patient leans forward. It may extend to the base of the lung and have a rectangular shape.

Auscultation.—The friction sound heard in the early stages may disappear when the effusion is copious, but often persists at the base or over a limited area. It may be audible in the erect and not in the recumbent posture. With the absorption of the fluid the friction returns. An important sign is the gradual weakening of the heart sounds, which with the increase in the effusion may become so muffled and indistinct as to be scarcely audible. Occasionally a systolic endocardial murmur is heard. Early and persistent accentuation of the pulmonary second sound may be present.

Important accessory signs in large effusion are due to pressure on the left lung. The anterolateral margin of the lower lobe is pushed aside and in some instances compressed, so that percussion in the axillary region gives a modified note, usually a dull tympany. Variations in the position of the patient may change the note in this area, over which on auscultation there is either feeble or tubular breathing. The left lobe of the liver is pushed down. There may be changes in the electrocardiographic tracings.

Course.—Cases vary extremely in the rapidity with which the effusion forms. In every instance, when a pericardial friction murmur has been detected, the practitioner should outline with care the upper and lateral limits of cardiac dulness, mark the position of the apex beat, and note the intensity of the heart sounds. In many instances the exudation is slight in amount, reaches a maximum within forty-eight hours, and then gradually subsides. In other instances the accumulation is more gradual and progressive, increasing for several weeks. To such cases the term *chronic* has been applied. The rapidity with which a serofibrinous effusion may be absorbed is surprising. The possibility of the absorption of a purulent exudate is shown by the cases in which the pericardium contains semi-solid grayish masses in all stages of calcification. With serofibrinous effusion, if moderate in amount, recovery is the rule, with inevitable union of the pericardial layers. In some septic cases there is a rapid formation of pus and a fatal result may follow in three or four days. More commonly, when death occurs with large effusion, it is due to gradual asthenia or to pressure on the great veins. If the pressure in the pericardium exceeds that in the venae cavae, the circulation stops. The signs of danger may appear very rapidly so that constant watch is important.

Prognosis.—In the serofibrinous effusions the outlook is good and a large majority of the rheumatic cases recover but with a damaged myocardium. The purulent effusions are more dangerous; the septic cases are usually fatal, and recovery is rare in the slow, insidious tuberculous forms. In nephritis, gout, acute infectious diseases and in old age the outlook is always grave.

Diagnosis.—Probably no serious disease is so frequently overlooked. Post-mortem experience shows how often pericarditis is not recognized, or goes on to resolution and adhesion without attracting notice. In a case of rheumatic fever, watched from the outset, with the attention directed daily to the heart, it is one of the simplest of diseases to diagnose; but when one is called to a case for the first time and finds perhaps an increased area of precordial dulness, it is often very hard to determine with certainty whether or not effusion is present. The difficulty usually lies in distinguishing between dilatation of the heart and pericardial effusion. Although the differential signs are simple on paper, it is notoriously difficult in certain cases, particularly in stout persons, to say which condition exists. The special points are:

(*a*) The character of the impulse, which in dilatation, particularly in thin-chested people, is commonly visible and wavy. (*b*) The shock of the cardiac sounds is more distinctly palpable in dilatation. (*c*) The area of dulness in dilatation rarely has a triangular form; nor does it, except in mitral stenosis, reach so high along the left sternal margin or so low in the fifth and sixth interspaces *without visible or palpable impulse.* An upper limit of dulness shifting with change of position speaks strongly for effusion. (*d*) In dilatation the heart sounds are clearer, often sharp or fetal in character; gallop rhythm is common, whereas in effusion the sounds are distant and muffled. (*e*) Rarely in dilatation is the distention sufficient to compress the lung and produce a tympanitic note in the axillary region, or dulness behind. (*f*) The X-ray picture may be very definite.

The number of excellent observers who have failed to discriminate between these two conditions, and who have performed paracentesis *cordis* instead of paracentesis *pericardii,* is perhaps the best comment on the difficulties to be encountered in the diagnosis.

Massive (1½ to 2-litre) exudations have been confounded with a pleural effusion and the pericardium has been tapped under the impression that the exudate was pleuritic. The dull tympany in the infrascapular region or axilla, the absence of well-defined movable dulness, and the feeble, muffled sounds are indicative points. Followed from day to day there is rarely much difficulty, but it is different when a patient seen for the first time presents a large area of dulness in the left chest, and there is no pericardial friction murmur. Some cases have been regarded as encapsulated pleural effusions.

A special difficulty exists in recognizing the large exudate in pneumonia. The effusion may be much larger than the signs indicate, and the involvement of the adjacent lung and pleura is confusing. An encapsulated pericardial effusion may give a local area of dulness or show in the X-ray plate.

The nature of the fluid can not be determined positively without aspiration; but a fairly accurate opinion can be formed from the primary disease and the general condition. In rheumatic cases the exudation is usually sero-fibrinous; in septic and tuberculous cases it is often purulent from the outset; in senile, nephritic and tuberculous cases it may be hemorrhagic.

Treatment.—The patient should have absolute quiet, mentally and bodily. A support in front of the patient on which he can rest often gives comfort. Drugs such as aconite or digitalis are of doubtful utility. The diet should be simple and liquids are usually best. The ice bag is of great value. It may be applied to the precordia at first for an hour at a time, and then continuously. It reduces the frequency of the heart's action and seems to retard the progress of an effusion. Blisters are not indicated in the early stage but simple counter-irritation may give relief. Morphia should be given for pain or severe distress.

When *effusion* is present, the following measures may be adopted: Blisters to the precordia, a practice not so much in vogue now as formerly. It is surprising in some instances, how quickly an effusion subsides on their application. Purges and iodide of potassium are of doubtful utility. The action of the kidneys may be promoted by alkaline diuretics.

When serious signs occur, as dyspnea, sudden marked drop in blood-pressure, small rapid pulse and a dusky anxious countenance, paracentesis or incision of the pericardium should be performed. With a serofibrinous exudate, aspiration is sufficient; but when the exudate is purulent, the pericardium should be freely incised and drained. The puncture may be made in the fifth or sixth interspace, outside the left nipple line. In large effusions the pericardium can be readily reached by thrusting the needle upward and backward close to the costal margin in the left costoxiphoid angle. With an earlier operation in many instances and a more radical one in others—incision and free drainage, when the fluid is purulent—the percentage of recoveries will be increased. Repeated tapping may be needed. One patient with tuberculous effusion, tapped three times, recovered and was alive three years afterward. In convalescence, the patient should be quiet for some time; the condition of the myocardium is the best indication as to the duration of rest.

CHRONIC ADHESIVE PERICARDITIS

(Adherent Pericardium, Indurative Mediastino-pericarditis)

The remote prognosis in pericarditis is very variable. Some patients get well and have no further trouble, but in young persons serious results sometimes follow adhesions and thickening of the layers. As Sequira pointed out, the danger is directly in proportion to the amount of dilatation and weakening of the pericardium in consequence of the inflammation. The loss of the support afforded to the heart by the fibrous bag in which it is inclosed is an important factor. There are two forms of adherent pericardium.

(*a*) Simple adhesion of the peri- and epicardial layers, a common sequence of pericarditis, met with postmortem as an accidental finding. It is not necessarily associated with disturbance in the function of the heart, which in a large proportion of the cases is neither dilated nor hypertrophied.

(*b*) Adherent pericardium with chronic mediastinitis and union of the outer layer of the pericardium to the pleura and chest wall. This constitutes a most serious form of cardiac disease, particularly in early life, and may lead to an extreme grade of hypertrophy and dilatation. The peritoneum may be involved with perihepatitis, cirrhosis, and ascites (*Pick's disease*).

Symptoms.—The symptoms of adherent pericardium are those of hypertrophy and dilatation of the heart, and later of cardiac insufficiency. G. D. Head in a study of 59 cases divides them into (1) a small group with no symptoms, (2) a larger group with all the features of cardiac disease, and (3) a group comprising 11 cases in his series in which the features were hepatic. To this last group much attention has been paid since Pick's description. The adhesions compress the great veins. The *hepatic* features dominate the picture and the diagnosis of cirrhosis of the liver is usually made. Recurring ascites is the special feature and one patient was tapped 121 times. There is chronic peritonitis, with great thickening of the capsule of the liver and consequent contraction of the organ.

Diagnosis.—The following are important points. *Inspection.* A majority of the signs of value come under this heading. (*a*) The precordia is prominent and there may be marked asymmetry, owing to the enormous enlargement of the heart. (*b*) The extent of the cardiac impulse is greatly increased, and may sometimes be seen from the third to the sixth interspaces, and in extreme cases from the right parasternal line to outside the left nipple. (*c*) The character of the cardiac impulse. It is undulatory, wavy, and in the apex region there is marked systolic retraction. (*d*) Diaphragm phenomena (*Broadbent's sign*). When the heart is adherent over a large area of the diaphragm there is a systolic tug, which may be communicated through the diaphragm to the points of its attachment on the wall, causing a visible retraction. This had long been recognized in the region of the apex but John Broadbent called attention to the fact that it was frequently best seen on the left side behind, between the eleventh and twelfth ribs. This sign may be very localized. One difficulty is that, as A. W. Tallant pointed out, it may occur in thin chested persons with great hypertrophy of the heart. Sir William Broadbent called attention to the fact that owing to the attachment of the heart to the central tendon of the diaphragm this part does not descend with inspiration, during which act there is not the visible movement in the epigastrium. The respiratory movement of the left thorax is decreased. (*e*) Diastolic collapse of the cervical veins, Friedreich's sign, is not of much moment. (*f*) Distention of the cervical veins may be marked and increased during inspiration.

Palpation.—The apex beat is fixed, and turning the patient on his side does not alter its position. On palpation a *diastolic shock* or rebound is felt, which some regard as the most reliable sign of adherent pericardium.

Percussion.—The area of cardiac dulness is usually much increased. In many instances there are adhesions between the pleura and pericardium, and the cardiac dulness above and to the left may be fixed and uninfluenced by deep inspiration. This is an uncertain sign.

Auscultation.—The phenomena are variable and uncertain. In children, following rheumatic fever, endocarditis is usually present. Even in the absence of endocarditis, when the dilatation reaches a certain grade, there are murmurs of relative insufficiency, which may be present at the mitral and also at the tricuspid and pulmonary orifices. Theodore Fisher pointed out that there may be a well-marked presystolic murmur with adherent pericardium. Occasionally the layers of the pericardium are united in places by strong fibrous bands. In one such case Drasche heard a remarkable whirring, systolic murmur with a twanging quality. There may be crepitant sounds at the borders of the heart with a cardiorespiratory rhythm.

The *pulsus paradoxus,* in which during inspiration the pulse wave is small and feeble, is sometimes present, but it is not a diagnostic sign of either simple pericardial adhesion or of the cicatricial mediastino-pericarditis. It is probably due to varying intrathoracic pressure. The X-ray study may show irregularity of the borders of the heart, diminished movement of the diaphragm or it may be pulled upward with systole. Calcium deposits may be observed.

The *prognosis* depends largely on the extent of the adhesions but especially on the state of the myocardium. Adhesions sufficient to give marked signs usually mean a seriously impaired heart. *Treatment* has to be directed to the heart muscle and is largely that of myocarditis. *Cardiolysis,* Brauer's operation, has been helpful in some cases. Portions of the fourth, fifth, and sixth left ribs with the corresponding cartilages are resected, by which the heart's action is less embarrassed. It is a justifiable procedure in selected cases when the myocardium is in fair condition.

OTHER AFFECTIONS OF THE PERICARDIUM

Hydropericardium.—The pericardial sac contains postmortem a few cubic centimetres of clear, citron colored fluid. With general dropsy, due to kidney or heart disease, more commonly the former, the effusion may be excessive, adding to the embarrassment of the heart and the lungs, particularly when the pleural cavities contain fluid. There are rare instances in which effusion into the pericardium occurs after scarlet fever with few, if any, other dropsical symptoms. Hydropericardium is frequently overlooked. The features are much as in pericarditis with effusion except for the absence of pericardial friction. The treatment is that of the original condition with tapping if the symptoms demand it.

In rare cases the serum has a milky character—chylopericardium.

Hemopericardium.—This is met with in aneurism of the first part of the aorta, of the cardiac wall, or of the coronary arteries, and in rupture and wounds of the heart. Death usually follows before there is time for the production of symptoms other than those of rapid collapse. In rupture of the heart the patient may live for hours or even days with signs of progressive heart failure, dyspnea and effusion. In the pericarditis of tuberculosis, cancer and nephritis, and in old people the exudate is often blood stained.

Pneumopericardium.—This is an excessively rare condition, of which we have seen but one instance, from rupture of a cancer of the stomach. In James' series of 38 cases, perforation of the sac occurred in all but 5, in which the gas bacillus was the possible cause. Seven cases were due to perforation of the esophagus and eight to penetrating wounds from without. The physical signs are most characteristic. Tympany replaces the normal pericardial flatness. On auscultation there is a splashing, gurgling, churning sound, called by the French *bruit de moulin.* This was described in 19 of the cases collected by James. Of the 38 cases, 26 died.

Calcified Pericardium.—This may follow pericarditis, particularly the suppurative and tuberculous forms; occasionally it extends from calcified valves. The majority of the cases are instances of polyserositis and tuberculous in origin. A few cases follow rheumatic fever. It may be partial or complete. Of 59 cases collected by A. E. Jones, in 38 there were no cardiac symptoms. It is usually found at autopsy. There may be the signs of adherent pericardium. The X-ray study may give the diagnosis by the dense or mottled shadow of the heart. Studies should be made from different angles. The right heart is usually more involved than the left. There may be calcified thrombi in the heart

DISEASES OF THE HEART

SYMPTOMATIC AND MECHANICAL DISORDERS

SYMPTOMATIC DISORDERS

Introduction.—There are a number of disturbances referred to the heart which can not be termed diseases—symptom-complex is a better designation. They may occur without any sign of organic cardiac disease but frequently cause extreme distress to the individual. It is not possible to group them in any systematic way. In some there are only subjective sensations, in others these occur with objective findings. We should remember that back of subjective disorders there is some cause and the effort should always be made to find it. Disturbances in the nervous system, especially psychical, and in the internal secretions, infection in some form, unrecognized myocardial disease and the effects of toxic agents are particularly important.

(1) **Heart Consciousness.**—In health we are unconscious of the action of the heart. A not infrequent indication of debility or overwork is the consciousness of the cardiac pulsations which may be regular or irregular. This may be most evident when the patient is lying down. It is usually due to nervous fatigue, some form of debility or anemia, or flatulence. It may be present with organic disease and hypertrophy.

(2) **Precordial Pain.**—This may be referred to the whole precordia or to local areas, most often about the apex or outside it. The area corresponds to the distribution of the eighth cervical to the fourth dorsal segments. A distinction should be made between *aortic* pain (aortitis, acute and chronic, many cases of angina pectoris, and aneurism) and *cardiac* pain. The former is usually felt over the upper part of the sternum and may be referred to the arms. It is important to secure an exact statement of the seat of pain. The influence of exertion, emotion, fear and excitement in causation is important. Many serious forms of heart disease are unaccompanied by pain. There are many causes for more or less persistent precordial pain: (1) Myocardial, in which the pain is prolonged and usually most marked at the left border of the heart. It may amount only to a feeling of deep-seated discomfort or pressure, or a sense of weight or oppression. (2) Dilatation. (3) Pericarditis. (4) Valvular disease, especially aortic. (5) Disease of the coronary arteries. (6) Certain toxic influences, especially tobacco. (7) With the "Effort Syndrome." (8) Angina pectoris (some cases). (9) With digestive disturbances, especially distention and heart-burn. (10) In a large group in which no evidence of cardiac disease can be found and often termed "cardiac neurosis," which means little. This is common in women and especially marked in those who are "neurotic." Two forms are common: in one there is a dull more or less continuous pain and in the other sharp stabbing pains of short duration. Emotion is a frequent exciting cause. In some definite disturbances of sensation can be found, usually near the apex. (11) From involvement of the posterior nerve roots, as in spondylitis, and spinal cord lesions. (12) Referred pain as in some cases of gallbladder disease.

The term "pseudo-angina pectoris" should be dropped. Some use it as synonymous with "vasomotor angina pectoris." The group includes cases in neurotic persons or in those who have used too much tobacco. The attacks have no necessary relation to exertion and may come on at night or when the patient is at rest; they are commoner in women and may occur at any age; and are not associated with demonstrable organic disease of the heart or aorta. The attacks may last for an hour or longer. There is often a feeling of distention and the patients are usually restless, complaining of a number of symptoms. It must be remembered that there are cases of mild angina pectoris. It is safer to regard doubtful cases as examples of this or of coronary artery disease than to label them "pseudo-angina."

The *diagnosis* of pain is based on the patient's statement; the estimation of its severity is made by observation; the recognition of its cause demands thorough study. Careful search should be made for organic disease; always suspect this until its absence is proved. Special attention should be given to the nervous system. The cause of pain mistakenly regarded as cardiac but due to disease elsewhere is usually recognized by a thorough examination.

The *treatment* must be based on accurate diagnosis. In the "nervous group," the meaning of the symptom should be explained and every effort made to correct the causal factors. The use of sedatives is indicated until there is improvement in the general condition. A dose of aromatic spirit of ammonia with valerian or Hoffman's anodyne is often helpful in an attack.

(3) **"Effort Syndrome," "Neurocirculatory Asthenia," "Disordered Action of the Heart," "Irritable Heart."**—The condition to which these

terms are applied does not represent a specific disease but a combination of symptoms in which shortness of breath, fatigue and vasomotor disturbances are the principal features. The condition is not confined to soldiers; it occurs in civil life, and in females and children as well as in men. The subjects are usually of a subnormal type physically and unable to do heavy physical work. The majority lead a sedentary life. The etiological factors are many. The general "makeup" is largely responsible. Infection may play a part, especially rheumatic fever, tonsillitis, influenza, focal infection, etc.; syphilis plays a very small part. Hyperthyroidism is a factor in a small percentage only. Disturbance of the central nervous system is important. Certain of the patients are of the visceroptotic build, with long thin bodies and poor muscular development, and cardioptosis ("dropped heart") is relatively common. Stress and strain which they are unfitted to endure is a frequent determining factor.

Symptoms.—Shortness of breath, rarely at rest, but on exertion, is the most frequent complaint, and is increased by effort, especially if hurried. With this are severe fatigue and exhaustion, sometimes with tremor. *Pain* is common, usually precordial or in the lower left costal region, and increased by exercise. Precordial tenderness and disturbance of sensation may accompany it. Palpitation of the heart on exertion and excitement often occurs. Syncope is not uncommon, some attacks being of the vasovagal form. Giddiness is frequent and may occur with change in position or on exertion. *Vasomotor* phenomena are common; the hands and feet are blue, there is profuse sweating and dermographia is marked. The patients show nervous instability and are easily upset. The pulse rate is increased and responds quickly to exertion. The return to normal after exercise is slow. The blood pressure tends to be low. The heart shows absence of signs of myocardial disease. Cardiorespiratory murmurs are common. Care must be taken to recognize the condition in which an overacting "nervous" heart simulates mitral stenosis.

Diagnosis.—These patients should be carefully studied to exclude organic disease. Tuberculosis, thyroid dysfunction and focal infection are among the possibilities which should be kept in mind. The *prognosis* should be guarded until the progress can be observed. Many of them improve temporarily and relapse. Some do not seem to have it in them to make any sustained effort to help themselves.

In *treatment* any suggestion of "heart disease" should be avoided and every effort made to explain the condition. Search should be made for the etiology and a causal factor treated if possible, especially a focus of infection or an anxiety neurosis. Tobacco and alcohol should be forbidden. The whole method of life should be reviewed and every effort made to improve the general health by proper exercise, bathing and good hygiene. Cardiac drugs are not needed but general tonics or sedatives should be given if indicated.

(4) **Cardiac Asthenia in Children.**—This may occur at any age in children but especially about puberty. The complaints are of dizziness, weakness, discomfort about the heart and sometimes of syncope. The children are often pale and flabby with little endurance, and show vasomotor instability. The heart rate is increased and there may be sinus irregularity or extra systoles. The heart may be centrally placed and occasionally is slightly enlarged. A systolic murmur at the apex is common. Care should be taken to exclude myocardial disease or a focus of infection. These children should have long

hours of rest and take regular exercise, carefully supervised and increased gradually. Anemia should be treated.

(5) **Vasovagal Attacks.**—These are characterized by a loss of consciousness and may occur in a variety of circumstances. Many disturbing occurrences may initiate them, as nervous upsets, some unpleasant happening, fatigue, a close atmosphere, etc. They happen in both sexes and at any age, but more often in youth.

The loss of consciousness may come on suddenly or gradually. In the former event the patient may fall. If there is warning this is usually in the form of severe weakness, perhaps nausea and sometimes dizziness with a sensation of falling. There is usually marked pallor. The heart rate drops, often to about 40, and the blood pressure falls rapidly. In one attack which occurred while the blood pressure was being taken with the patient standing, the diastolic pressure was very low—about 10—just as the patient fell. He did not have aortic insufficiency. The radial pulse may not be felt. Profuse sweating usually occurs. The unconsciousness is usually of short duration; the patient is confused for a few minutes and weak for some time afterwards.

There is apparently marked vasodilatation and the slow heart rate is due to increased action of the vagus. It is probably due to nervous system disturbance in which the carotid sinus plays a part. Overaction of the depressor nerve may also be responsible. The attacks are not dangerous but are unpleasant and if frequent cause nervous worry which probably favors more attacks.

Treatment.—If any cause can be determined this should be corrected or avoided as the case may be. Atropine will control or lessen the overaction of the vagus. In an attack the patient should be kept with the head low and the clothing made loose around the neck. A dose of aromatic spirit of ammonia or whisky—best taken neat—is helpful. If an attack is prolonged 10 minims of epinephrine solution (1 to 1000) should be given hypodermically.

(6) **Palpitation.**—In health we are unconscious of the action of the heart. One indication of cardiac failure or stress is the consciousness of the cardiac pulsations, which may, however, be perfectly regular and orderly. This is not palpitation. The term is properly limited to irregular, rapid or forcible action of the heart perceptible to the individual. Extra systoles, auricular fibrillation and paroxysmal tachycardia are present in some cases.

Etiology.—The expression "perceptible to the individual" covers the essential element in palpitation of the heart. The most extreme disturbance of rhythm may be unattended with subjective sensations and there may be no consciousness of disturbed action. On the other hand, there are cases in which complaint is made of distressing palpitation and sensations of throbbing, in which examination reveals a regular heart, the sensations being entirely subjective. This occurs in a large group in which there is increased nervous excitability. Palpitation may be marked at puberty, at the climacteric, and occasionally during menstruation. It is common in anemia, hysteria and neurasthenia, and particularly with dyspepsia. Emotions, such as fright, are common causes of palpitation. It may occur as a sequence of the acute fevers. Females are more liable to the affection than males. Disturbance of the general health from many conditions may be responsible.

In a second group the palpitation results from the action of tobacco, coffee, tea and alcohol. Palpitation may be associated with organic disease of the heart, either of the myocardium or valves. As a rule it is a purely nervous phenomenon, seldom associated with organic disease in which the most violent action and extreme irregularity may exist without subjective consciousness of the disturbance. It often occurs with hyperthyroidism.

Symptoms.—In the mildest form, such as occurs during a dyspeptic attack, there are slight fluttering of the heart and a sense of what patients sometimes call "goneness." In more severe attacks the heart beats violently, its pulsations are visible, the rate is much increased, the arteries throb forcibly, and there is a sense of distress. In some instances the heart's action is not quickened. The most striking cases are in neurasthenic women, in whom the entrance of a person into the room may cause violent action of the heart and throbbing of the arteries. The pulse may be increased to 150 or 160. A diffuse flushing of the skin may appear at the same time. After such attacks a large quantity of pale urine may be passed. In many cases of palpitation, particularly in young men, the condition is relieved by exertion.

The examination usually shows a heart of normal size. The second sound at the base may be accentuated. A murmur may be heard over the pulmonary artery or at the apex in cases of rapid action in neurasthenia or severe anemia. The attacks may be transient, lasting only a few minutes, or may persist for an hour or more. In some instances any attempt at exertion renews the attack. Sometimes in vigorous young adults who are upset nervously, especially after exertion or during excitement, the signs of mitral stenosis are simulated. There is a systolic shock preceded by a suggestion of a thrill. On auscultation it may be difficult to decide whether or not there is a short presystolic murmur. A short period of observation usually removes the uncertainty and the administration of amyl nitrite, which increases the murmur of mitral stenosis, is an aid. Organic murmurs are sometimes increased by pressure on the eyeballs.

The *diagnosis* should always include the conditions which are responsible. Nervous states (especially anxiety neuroses and those due to disturbance in the sexual sphere), anemia, gastro-intestinal disorders, and particularly disease of the thyroid gland should be considered. In the condition termed *phrenocardia* there are palpitation, pain in the cardiac region or to the left of the apex, and respiratory disorder shown by attempts to take a deep breath. There may be spasm of the diaphragm with cardioptosis. The *prognosis* is that of the underlying condition, which it may be difficult to remedy.

Treatment.—An important element is to get the patient's mind quieted and assure him that there is no actual danger. The mental element is often very strong. If an underlying cause can be found this should receive attention. Before using drugs, it is well to try the effect of hygienic measures. As a rule, moderate exercise may be taken with advantage. Regular hours should be kept, and at least ten hours of the twenty-four should be spent in the recumbent posture. A tepid bath may be taken in the morning, or, if the patient is weak and nervous, in the evening, followed by a thorough rubbing. Hot baths and the Turkish bath should be avoided. It is best to prohibit alcohol, tea and coffee. The diet should be light and the patient should avoid taking large meals. Articles of food known to cause flatulency should not be used. Tobacco should be forbidden. Sexual excitement is particularly pernicious, and the patient should be warned on this point. The cases of palpitation due to excesses or to errors in diet and dyspepsia are usually remedied by hygienic measures.

A course of iron is often useful. Strychnia is valuable and best administered as the tincture of nux vomica which should be given freely, 20 minims (1.3 cc.) three times a day. If there is great rapidity of action, aconite may be tried. There are patients with sleeplessness and restlessness who are greatly benefited by sedatives or a hypnotic. Digitalis is rarely indicated but in obstinate cases it may be tried.

MECHANICAL DISORDERS OF THE HEART BEAT

Normal Mechanism.—The normal heart beat is initiated by a stimulus which originates in highly specialized tissue situated at the junction of the superior vena cava and the right auricle (sino-auricular node). This node under normal conditions determines the rate and rhythm of the heart, and is designated the "pacemaker." The excitation wave, immediately followed by muscular contraction, first sweeps over the walls of the auricles and then passes to the ventricles by a special conduction system, having its beginning in the node of Tawara, situated low down on the right side of the interauricular septum, and continued forward and downward as a narrow neuromuscular band (bundle of His), which upon reaching the intraventricular septum divides into a right and left branch supplying the respective ventricles; after further multiple subdivisions, the end branches terminate as the fibres of Purkinje, bringing the conduction system into intimate relation with the ventricular musculature. The efficiency of the heart depends in considerable degree upon the integrity of these structures and the orderly exercise of their functions. In health, under ordinary circumstances, stimuli are rhythmically generated in the sino-auricular node at the rate of 72 per minute and reach the ventricular walls after a lapse of approximately 0.2 second, causing contraction of auricles and ventricles as a result of the stimulus. An epitome of the myocardial functions is as follows: "The muscular fibres of the heart possess the power of rhythmically creating a stimulus, of being able to receive a stimulus, of responding to a stimulus by contracting, of conveying the stimulus from muscle fibre to muscle fibre, and of maintaining a certain ill-defined condition called tone" (Gaskell). Disturbance, impairment or loss of these functions occasion mechanical disorders of the heart beat.

The stimulus and contraction normally proceed in a regular way but if the excitability of any other part is sufficiently increased, a stimulus may originate there, giving rise to irregular contractions. After contraction has occurred, for a time the muscle can not be stimulated to contract again (refractory period). The muscle either contracts with its full power or does not contract at all in response to stimulation, "all or none." The longer the interval since the previous contraction, the weaker the stimulus which produces contraction. Also the longer the period of rest (diastole) the better prepared the muscle is to contract. Increase in rate is largely at the expense of diastole, so that with rapid rates the rest period of the heart is markedly shortened. The normal times are auricular systole .1 second, ventricular systole .3 second, and diastole .4 second. While the heart has the inherent power of originating stimuli and contracting, yet nervous control plays a part. This can influence all the functions of the heart muscle. The vagus depresses excitability, contractility, conductivity and tonicity. Inhibition of the heart may result from excessive stimulus of the vagus. The sympathetic supply increases contractility and conductivity. Much of the importance of the heart action pertains to systole and diastole is less regarded. It might be well to give more attention to diastole, which is the rest period and specially associated with tonicity, in the maintenance of which the vagus influences probably play a large part.

DISTURBANCES OF RATE

(1) **Tachycardia** (with Normal Mechanism).—The rapid action may be perfectly natural. There are individuals whose normal heart rate is 100 or even more per minute. Emotional causes, violent exercise and fevers all produce increase in the rapidity of the heart's action. The extremely rapid action which follows fright may persist for days or even weeks. It is not uncommon at the menopause.

There are cases in which it depends upon changes in the pneumogastrics or in the medulla. A tumor or clot in or about the medulla or pressure upon the vagi may be associated with rapid heart. Tachycardia occurs under many conditions, such as hyperthyroidism, mitral stenosis (apart from fibrillation), interference with the vagus (mediastinal tumor, etc.), postfebrile conditions, anemia, the effect of certain drugs (belladonna, thyroid extract), nervous disturbance, "effort syndrome," toxic states (tobacco), etc. The tachycardia may persist for months or indefinitely, and interfere with the amount of exertion such persons can make; in addition there is weakness and sometimes syncope. The diagnosis of the cause is essential and on this the treatment must be based.

(2) **Bradycardia** (True).—Slow action of the heart is sometimes normal and may be a family peculiarity. Napoleon is stated to have had a pulse of only 40 per minute. In any cases of slow pulse rate it is important to make sure that the number of heart and arterial beats correspond. The heart contractions, not the pulse waves, should be taken into account.

Physiological Bradycardia.—As age advances the pulse rate becomes slower. In the puerperal state the pulse may beat from 40 to 60 per minute. It is seen in premature labor as well as at term but the explanation is not clear. Slowness of the pulse is associated with hunger. Bradycardia depending on individual peculiarity is rare.

Pathological bradycardia is met with under the following conditions: (*a*) In convalescence from acute fevers. This is common, particularly after pneumonia, typhoid fever, influenza and diphtheria. It is most frequent in young persons and in cases which have run a normal course. (*b*) In diseases of the digestive system, such as chronic dyspepsia, ulcer or cancer of the stomach, and jaundice. (*c*) In diseases of the respiratory system. Here it is by no means so common, but is not infrequent in emphysema. (*d*) In diseases of the circulatory system. Bradycardia is not common in diseases of the valves. It is most frequent in fatty and fibroid changes in the heart, but is not constant in them. Sino-auricular block is a rare cause. (*e*) It occurs occasionally in nephritis and may be a feature of uremia. (*f*) From the action of toxic agents as in uremia, poisoning by lead and alcohol; it may follow the use of tobacco, coffee and digitalis. (*g*) In constitutional disorders, such as anemia and diabetes. (*h*) In diseases of the nervous system. Apoplexy, epilepsy, one stage of tuberculous meningitis, cerebral tumors, affections of the medulla, and diseases and injuries of the cervical cord may be associated with a slow pulse. In general paresis, dementia praecox, mania, and melancholia it is not infrequent. (*i*) It occurs occasionally in affections of the skin and sexual organs, and in sunstroke, or in prolonged exhaustion from any cause. (*j*) In hypothyroidism. (*k*) In heart block and in the Stokes-Adams syndrome.

Treatment.—For the bradycardia itself little can be done. The cause should receive attention.

DISTURBANCES OF RHYTHM AND FORCE

1. **Sinus Arrhythmia.**—This depends on changes in the control of the sino-auricular node in which the effect of vagus influence is important. It is frequently seen in connection with respiration, especially in deep breathing. The rate increases with inspiration and slows with expiration. This is common in young children and about the time of puberty, and is seen occasionally in adults. In some cases it may be responsible for attacks of faintness or syncope, sometimes with a slow rate and a low blood pressure. The occurrence

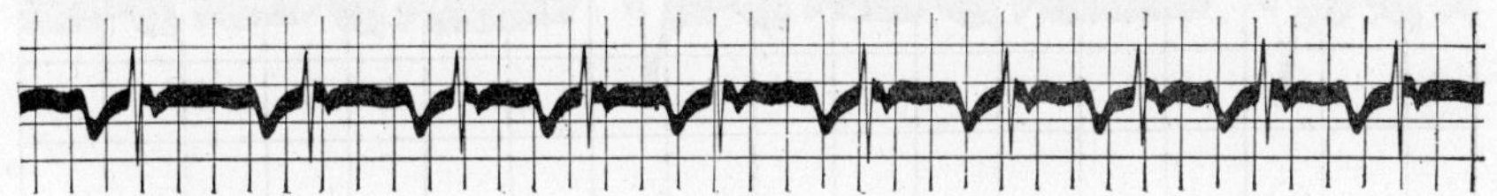

FIG. 1.—SINUS ARRHYTHMIA.

This exhibits a variation occasioned by a difference in length of diastoles. The systoles are the product of a normal mechanism and are unevenly spaced but show no variation.

of irregularity, also with slow pulse rate, and which has no order in its occurrence, is sometimes seen. This may occur after the administration of digitalis, in rheumatic myocarditis or with the bradycardia so common after pneumonia. The condition is not serious in any way.

Diagnosis.—This is usually clear. The irregularity is of the whole beat and the pulse and apex beat correspond. The occurrence with respiration is significant. Exercise, fever and atropine usually abolish this irregularity.

Treatment.—None is required and this condition should not be regarded as an indication for rest or lessened activity.

2. **Extra Systole (Premature Contraction).**—This is a common form of irregularity, to understand which it must be remembered that to a stimulus strong enough to set up a contraction the heart answers with all the contractility of which it is capable at the moment (Bowditch's law of maximal contraction). A second property of the heart muscle is that it possesses a "refractory phase" in which normally it is not excitable or answers only to very strong stimuli. The auricle, the auriculoventricular node or the ventricle may originate an abnormal stimulus for contraction, the sinus rhythm not being altered. Extra systoles may occur regularly or irregularly and often or seldom. Auricular and ventricular extra systoles are more common than the nodal form. (*a*) *Auricular extra systole.* The premature stimulus and contraction

of the auricle usually cause a premature contraction of the ventricle, but the stimulus may travel slowly, so that the auricular *contraction* interval is prolonged, or it may not reach the ventricle—it is blocked. (*b*) *Nodal* or *auriculoventricular extra systole.* The stimulus arises in the auriculoventricular junctional tissue and passes both to the auricle and ventricle. The two may contract together or either may be first. (*c*) *Ventricular extra systole.* The extra impulse arising in the ventricle and causing it to contract anticipates the next regular impulse from the auricle which arrives when the ventricle is in the "refractory phase" and hence it does not contract, so that the auricular impulse is wasted. The interval which follows the premature contraction will therefore be longer than normal (compensatory pause). In consequence of this prolonged interval of rest the next contraction is likely to be more forcible than normal. If the ventricular extra systole occurs early enough to permit the next regular auricular stimulus to arrive when the ventricle can contract,

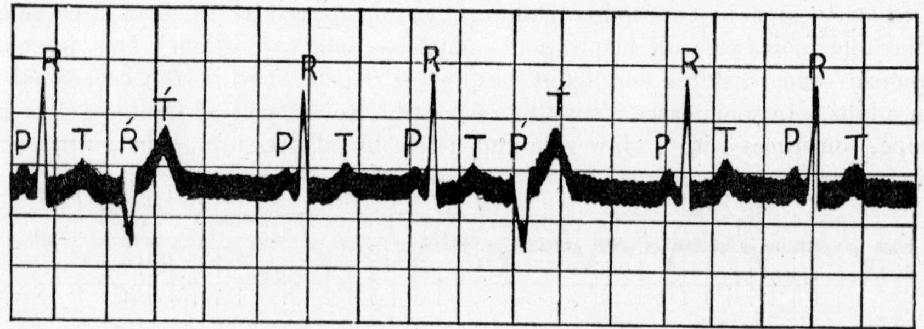

FIG. 2.—VENTRICULAR PREMATURE CONTRACTIONS.

Ventricular extra systoles or premature contractions shown by R′—T′ complexes which differ in their appearance from the normal R—T complex that in the R′—T′ complex the R′ is inverted and the T′ is wider and of greater amplitude.

there is a premature contraction between two normal beats. The premature contraction is not as strong as a normal one and hence the pulse wave resulting is smaller. If the contraction is very feeble (and the earlier it occurs in diastole the weaker it is) the aortic valves may not be opened or the wave may not reach the wrist. This results in a dropped beat. If an extra systole occurs regularly after each normal beat, then the apex impulse and the pulse wave occur in pairs—*pulsus bigeminus;* or if the extra systole occurs after two normal beats, the impulse and pulse occur in threes—*pulsus trigeminus,* and so on.

On auscultation two sounds are heard with the extra systole, if the aortic valves are opened, otherwise only a first sound. Evidently there can be many variations in the sounds and character of the pulse. Graphic records are usually necessary to distinguish between the auricular, nodal and ventricular forms of premature contractions. If a murmur is present it may be absent or less loudly heard with the premature beat. Fever, exercise, a change in posture, and a rapid heart rate may cause the temporary disappearance of extra systoles. They tend to be more frequent with a slowing heart, as after exercise, on taking the recumbent posture or after fever.

Symptoms.—The irregularity, inequality and intermission of the pulse in every day experience are largely due to extra systoles, which may present all sorts of combinations. There may be no actual pathological change, and so far as the maintenance of the circulation is concerned the heart may be acting in a satisfactory manner. The *subjective sensations* vary greatly. In some the extra systoles are not noticed but many complain of a variety of symptoms and especially of the pause with the succeeding strong contraction. Some patients are greatly disturbed by them and they are a common cause of palpitation.

Extra systoles occur at all ages and under the most varied conditions but are most common in persons over fifty. There are several classes of cases. The irregularity may be a life-long condition, without any recognizable disease and without any impairment of the function of the heart. This may be a peculiarity of the heart muscle of the individual, who has extra systole for the same reason—physiological but not well understood—as the dog and horse, in which animals it is common. The late Chancellor Ferrier, of McGill University, who died at the age of eighty-seven, had an extremely irregular heart action for the last fifty years of his life. In debilitated and neurasthenic persons there may be an irritable weakness of the heart with extra systoles and distressing palpitation. In a second group tobacco, tea, coffee or toxins of the infectious diseases are responsible. Digitalis may be a cause. Reflexly, as in flatulent dyspepsia, extra systoles may arise. Thirdly, high blood pressure can set up extra systoles; also change in posture. And, lastly, organic disease of the heart itself, especially myocardial.

The *significance* of extra systoles is not always easy to determine. They are often temporary, especially in young persons, but should not be regarded lightly. It is wiser to regard them as meaning some pathological change until the contrary is proved than to make light of them and recognize the error later. Nervous strain seems to be often responsible. In those over fifty years of age they may be the warning of myocardial damage. The patient seen to-day with extra systoles may return with auricular fibrillation in two or three years. The *diagnosis* is usually easy. The occurrence of an extra systole is felt at the apex and wrist and heard on auscultation. In the cases in which the contractions do not send a pulse wave to the wrist, the impulse may be felt at the apex or the sound heard. Tracings are rarely necessary.

Treatment.—This must depend on the other conditions found and not on the extra systoles themselves. The nature of the process should be explained. In nervous patients, sedatives are indicated. Quinine sulphate (gr. v-x, 0.3-0.6 gm.) with strychnine (gr. 1/30, 0.002 gm.) or quinidine gr. iii (0.2 gm.) sometimes lessen or stop extra systoles. Digitalis may have some effect but probably only if there is myocardial change.

(3) **Simple Paroxysmal Tachycardia.**—This is characterized by paroxysmal attacks, beginning and ending abruptly, in which the heart rate increases to between 100 and 200 a minute (the common rate is 140 to 190) and is regular. The abnormal impulses arise from a new focus which may be in the auricle or ventricle, usually in the auricle, and rarely in the junctional tissue. They represent "essentially a regular series of extra systoles" (Lewis).

It may occur at any age but is most frequent in young adults, and more often in males. There may be cardiac disease but most patients show no sign of any lesion. Naturally one is suspicious of some underlying factor (myocardial). Exertion, emotion or digestive disturbance may initiate an attack but usually no cause can be given. The duration of an attack varies from a few seconds to ten or more days.

The *symptoms* vary greatly with the duration and severity of the attack. A striking feature is the abrupt onset. In very short attacks the patient may not be conscious of any disturbance or make any complaint. In more marked attacks there may be discomfort and palpitation, with weakness, sweating and gastric disturbance. Thoracic *pain* of varying distribution is common, sometimes with disturbance of sensation. If dilatation of the heart follows there are the symptoms associated with it. In the examination there may be little except the rapid heart and the general condition is often good. There may be marked pulsation in the veins of the neck. The heart rate should be determined by auscultation. The sounds are short and sharp, like the fetal heart sounds. A previous murmur may have disappeared. Enlargement of the heart, passive congestion of the lungs, sometimes with bloody sputum, cyanosis, edema, and enlargement of the liver with tenderness may be found. These disappear rapidly when normal rhythm is restored.

In *diagnosis* the history of previous attacks with an abrupt onset and a sudden termination is important. The cases of tachycardia of other etiology rarely cause doubt. The rapid rate with loss of compensation should not cause difficulty. Change in posture and exertion do not alter the rate in paroxysmal tachycardia. In cases of doubt a tracing is diagnostic.

The *outlook* is good but always has an element of uncertainty. In prolonged attacks with marked disturbance of the circulation there is always some danger. The condition of the heart between attacks and the behavior of the muscle during the attack are important points. As to the patient becoming free of the attacks, it is difficult to speak with any certainty. The condition is compatible with long life.

Attacks of paroxysmal tachycardia (not simple) may be due to auricular fibrillation or auricular flutter. The usual features of these irregularities are present; in case of doubt, tracings give the diagnosis. *Ventricular paroxysmal tachycardia* is rare and usually occurs in patients with coronary artery disease and myocardial failure and especially with coronary artery occlusion. Overdosage of digitalis may be a cause. It may be suspected if there is a very rapid rate in a patient with chronic cardiac disease, with slight irregularity. The diagnosis can be made only by electrocardiographic study giving evidence that the impulses arise in the ventricle and that the auricular rate is slower than that of the ventricle.

Treatment.—The patient should be quiet and in the position which gives him the greatest comfort. The diet should be liquid. If there is gastric disturbance, the giving of sedatives and alkalies may be useful. An ice bag over the precordia often gives relief, if it does not stop the attack. The most diverse procedures may stop an attack, such as placing the head between the knees, being suspended with the head down, pressure on the right carotid artery, or on the eye-balls, any sustained respiratory effort, the production of vomiting, the application of a tight abdominal binder, etc. Quinidine (gr. v, 0.3 gm.) may be given every 2 or 3 hours for several doses in an attack. Smaller doses may be given steadily in the hope of preventing an attack. The use of epinephrine (♏ x, 0.6 cc. of a 1-10,000 solution) intravenously may be effectual. Chloral hydrate or morphia may be given to secure sleep. Any indicated symptomatic treatment should be given. Between attacks, any exciting cause should be avoided, the general health improved if possible, and attention paid to any gastro-intestinal disturbance. The wearing of an abdominal binder is sometimes useful.

(4) **Auricular Flutter.**—In this condition the impulses arise in the auricle, probably from a circular wave of contraction, which cause it to beat rhythmically at a rate of 200 to 350 per minute. As Lewis says, this may not be readily distinguished from paroxysmal tachycardia but when the rate is over 200 special characteristics appear. Lewis regards the circus movement as important in auricular flutter. The difference between it and fibrillation is largely one of degree. Heart block is almost always present with it, the ventricular rate being half that of the auricle; 2 :1 block is common but other ratios occur. There may be a change from one ratio to another. The rate of the auricle is regular; the ventricle is usually regular but sometimes irregular. It is most frequent in advanced years, more common in males and usually associated

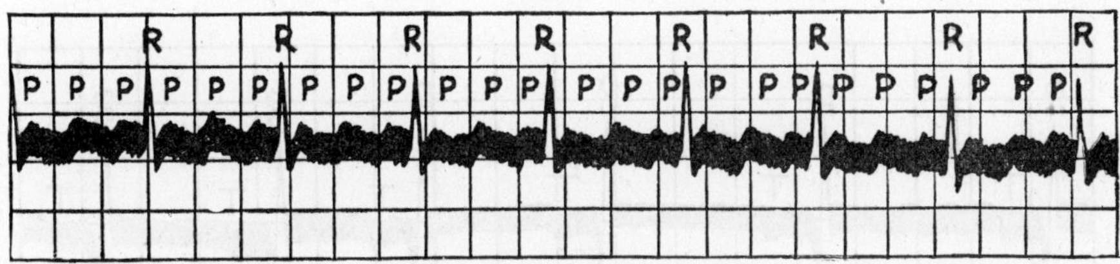

FIG. 3.—AURICULAR FLUTTER.

Auricular flutter shown by the occurrence of three auricular contractions (P waves) to one contraction of the ventricles as indicated by the R wave. The auricular rate is 300 per minute and the ventricular rate is 100 per minute.

with arteriosclerosis and myocarditis but may occur with acute infections, after an operation or with cardiac failure.

The *symptoms* are fewer than might be expected and depend on the state of the myocardium. There may be a complaint of palpitation and attacks of syncope. Occasionally the ventricle takes the auricular rate, with which the condition is grave, but such attacks are usually of short duration. The duration is variable; it may last a very short time or persist for months or years. The heart may return to normal rhythm or pass into auricular fibrillation abruptly. The attacks begin and end abruptly. The effect on the heart depends greatly on the condition of the myocardium, but the duration and ventricular rate also have an influence. There is always a probability of a return of the condition. The *diagnosis* may be possible by electrocardiographic study only. A persistent regular ventricular rate of 125 to 160 suggests flutter, especially in a patient over 50 years of age. There is no change of the rate with exercise or rest. Pressure over the carotid artery may slow the ventricle for a brief period. Digitalis usually slows the ventricle and makes it irregular. The *treatment* consists in the use of digitalis in full doses until a definite effect is produced. This may be a change to auricular fibrillation. As a rule the administration of digitalis should be continued in amounts sufficient to control the rate of the ventricle. Quinidine has been useful in some cases and full dosage may be required.

(5) **Auricular Filbrillation.**—This common form of cardiac irregularity is exceedingly important to recognize clinically. Transient and recurring forms are observed as a result of acute infections, as pneumonia, and preceding the permanent form. A study of its features in this condition gave Mackenzie the clue to its explanation. He found that in certain cases the transition from regular to irregular pulse of this type occurred with suddenness, and that, whereas before the irregularity supervened the jugular pulse showed the normal features, with a marked presystolic murmur and thrill at the apex, after the irregularity was established, the auricular wave disappeared from the jugular pulse and the presystolic murmur from the apex. The inference drawn was that the right auricle was so dilated as to prevent a normal auricular contraction. Complete proof of the cause was supplied by Lewis, who found that patients with this irregularity showed in tracings from the auricle numerous small and continuous waves, similar to those obtained in the dog after fibrillation of the auricle has been induced by faradic stimulation, or by ligation of the right coronary artery. The auricles do not contract but are in diastole

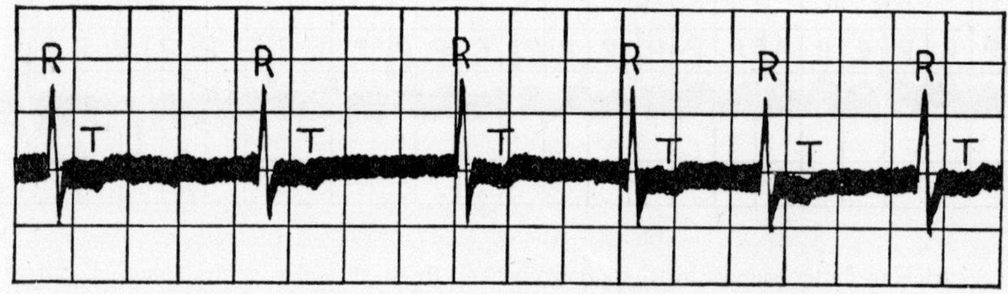

Fig. 4.—Auricular Fibrillation.

Auricular fibrillation shown by the absence of the P wave and the total irregularity of the occurrence of the R—T complex, which represents the contraction of the ventricle.

with many fibrillary twitchings. Numerous impulses come to the auriculoventricular bundle but only some are able to pass and these reach the ventricle irregularly. Hence the contractions of the ventricle are disturbed and irregular. The state of the bundle determines how many impulses pass and hence the ventricular rate shows great variation. Lewis regards auricular fibrillation as due to a *circus movement* in the auricle, "a single wave is propagated and revolves perpetually upon a re-entrant path." This is repeated as an average 450 times per minute. The relation of the refractory period to the speed at which the wave moves is important. If the advancing wave of contraction reaches muscle in the refractory period, evidently the contraction will stop. Quinidine acts by lengthening the refractory period so that the head of the circulating wave catches up with its tail, so to speak. When this happens the circus movement ceases. But quinidine also slows conduction which favors the circus movement. One effect tends to shorten the gap between "the crest of the movement and its wake," the other to lengthen it. Only if the first predominates will the abnormal movement terminate.

Auricular fibrillation forms a large proportion of the cases showing myocardial failure with an irregular pulse. Many of the contractions fail to reach the wrist (*pulse deficit*). It is a sign of marked myocardial disease, as seen in the late stages of mitral stenosis, toxic thyroid disease and myocardial failure with arteriosclerosis. It occurs occasionally in acute infectious diseases. The average age of onset in those with a previous history of rheumatic fever is 20 to 40; in the nonrheumatic group between 50 and 60.

The *symptoms* depend largely on the associated conditions and are often those of marked myocardial failure. The ventricular rate has some influence, as when it is very rapid (120-160), the distress and general symptoms of dilatation are more marked. The *pulse* is extremely irregular in every way and an irregular pulse with a rate over 120 is usually due to fibrillation. The more rapid the rate, the greater the irregularity. The *diagnosis* is clear with a very rapid heart, as all irregular hearts with a rate of 120 or more have auricular fibrillation, but when the rate is below 100 there may be slight difficulty until a careful study is made. With very many extra systoles there may be difficulty. The marked irregularity in every way—force, rhythm and rate—is usually sufficient. Tracings remove any doubt. In some cases fibrillation is present without marked rapidity of rate. This may be in patients who are taking digitalis but not always.

In *prognosis* the occurrence of fibrillation is of grave omen. The condition is compatible with life for years but means serious myocardial damage. The ventricular rate is of value, a persistent rate of 120 or over means a grave outlook and each increase in rate above this is more serious. The paroxysmal attacks, as in pneumonia or after operation, are usually temporary. They, and the more permanent fibrillation, are more serious with thyroid disease but often disappear after correction of the thyroid condition. The influence of treatment is of value in estimating the outlook.

Treatment.—For the general condition of the heart the problem is that of myocardial insufficiency, and for this and for the fibrillation the remedy is *digitalis,* which acts by blocking the passage of many of the impulses from auricle to ventricle. The dosage is that which keeps the heart at the best possible rate and must be decided for each patient. It depends somewhat on the severity of the condition; the present tendency is to give larger doses than formerly. In any case the object is to produce the desired effect, whatever dose is required. Most of the patients should continue the use of digitalis permanently in the dosage found to be most suitable.

The use of *quinidine* has been successful in a considerable number of cases, especially in paroxysmal auricular fibrillation and in connection with thyrotoxicosis. It probably depresses conduction. As a rule the patients should first have the advantage of digitalis, but this should be stopped for several days before quinidine is given. The patients should be carefully chosen; those in whom the fibrillation is recent (within six months); those without marked evidence of myocardial degeneration or arteriosclerosis are the most favorable. In patients with cardiac disease of long duration with decompensation, especially if the liver is enlarged, acute or subacute endocarditis, multiple valve lesions, coronary artery disease, heart block or angina pectoris, quinidine is not likely to be of use. It is well to give two doses of 3 grains (0.2 gm.) on the first day. The next day it is given in doses of 6 grains (0.4 gm.) three times and continued for three or four days. If there is an effect the drug should be given in smaller doses (0.2 gm. once or twice a day) for some time. The duration of this has to be settled for each patient. Some prefer to give larger doses, especially if the usual dosage is without effect. The risk of embolism is comparatively slight. Various disturbances may occur, such as dizziness, weakness, palpitation, dyspnea, diarrhea, etc. Sudden collapse or additional disturbance of rhythm may result. The drug should be stopped if any of these appear. If quinidine has an influence on the fibrillation, it is of value in determining how much part fibrillation plays in the myocardial failure. Sometimes it is well to give it permanently in doses of gr. v-x (0.3—0.6 gm.) a day.

Quinidine is useful in postoperative paroxysmal auricular fibrillation and in auricular fibrillation with thyroid disease. A dose of 3 grains (0.2 gm.) may be given to see if there is any idiosyncrasy, which usually shows in two or three hours. If this does not appear 5 grains (0.3 gm.) may be given every 2 hours until the pulse is regular or a total amount of 30 grains (2 gm.) has been given.

(6) **Heart block.**—In the adult heart the auriculoventricular bundle of His is 18 mm. long, 2.5 mm. broad, and 1.5 mm. thick; it arises in the septum of the auricles below the foramen ovale and passes downward and forward through the trigonum fibrosum of auriculoventricular junction, where it comes into close relation with the mesial leaflet of the tricuspid valve. Passing along the upper edge of the muscular septum, just where it joins with the posterior edge of the membranous septum, it radiates throughout the ventricles. If the function of the auriculoventricular bundle is impaired there may be a delay in the conduction of the impulse or it may be blocked completely. This may occur only with certain impulses (*partial heart block*) or with all (*complete heart-block*). Intermittent and variable forms have been observed. In complete block the ventricles assume their own rhythm (usually about 30 to 40 a minute).

Etiology.—Auriculoventricular heart block may occur at any age depending on the cause and may be congenital. It is more common in males. It is not infrequent, but usually temporary, in infectious diseases, especially rheumatic fever, influenza, diphtheria and pneumonia, but occurs in many others.

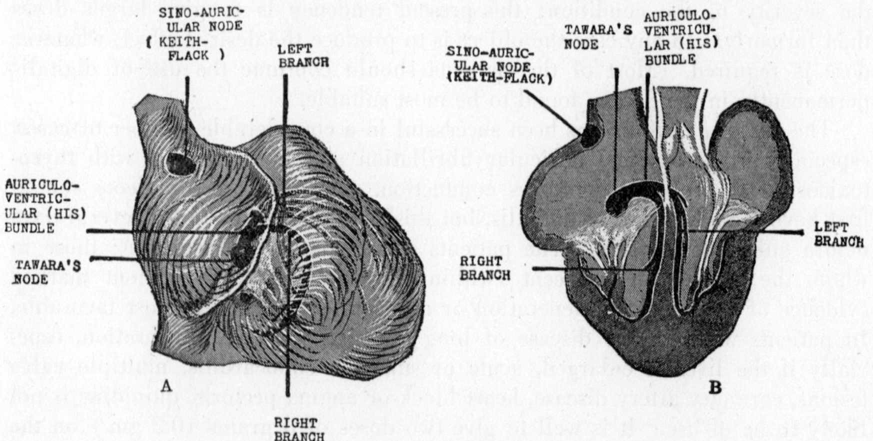

FIGS. 5 AND 6.—DIAGRAM SHOWING THE SINO-AURICULAR NODE AND THE AURICULO-VENTRICULAR BUNDLE.

A, viewed from the right; B, cross section of the heart, viewed from the front. (Kindness of A. D. Hirschfelder.)

In this group acute inflammatory changes or the influence of toxins may be responsible. Syphilis is a cause by the auriculoventricular bundle being affected in myocardial involvement or by a gumma. Any form of myocarditis, acute or chronic, may be responsible. The action of digitalis in auricular fibrillation depends largely on its action on the impulses passing from auricle to ventricle and hence it is one of the causes of heart block. The lesion in the bundle may be acute, usually in infections, or chronic, with fibrosis, gumma, etc. Heart block usually occurs with marked myocardial degeneration, involving both the muscle and the conduction system. Varying grades of *delayed conduction* with increase in the P-R interval are common and may go on to definite block.

The *symptoms* are variable, and depend to a considerable extent on the associated conditions. Some patients make little complaint, but dizziness, weakness and fainting attacks are not uncommon. In the more severe forms the syncopal attacks are more frequent. One variety is described under the

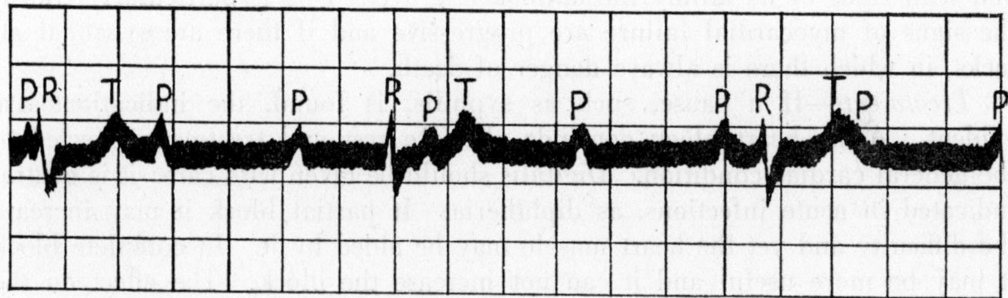

Fig. 7.—Complete Heart Block.

Complete heart-block or complete A-V dissociation shown by the auricle beating at a rate of 82 per minute in response to stimuli from the normal pacemaker, the sino-auricular node; the ventricle at a rate of 28 per minute in response to stimuli originating in the junctional tissue.

Stokes-Adams syndrome. Heart block occurs without the Stokes-Adams syndrome and the syndrome may be due to other causes. The *signs* vary with the grade of block. An early manifestation may be reduplication of the first or second sound due to lengthening of the A-V interval which represents a delay in conduction. A dropped beat is easily recognized and if the ventricle is beating regularly at half the rate of the auricle (2:1 block) the pulse may be 40 to 50 a minute. Halving of the ventricular rate under digitalis therapy is always suggestive. It may be that the auricular rate can be counted by the pulsations in the veins of the neck. In *complete* block the ventricle beats at about 35 and independently of the auricle. While the diagnosis can often be made from the physical signs, tracings render it certain. The more frequent contractions of the auricle may be seen with the fluoroscope.

Stokes-Adams Syndrome.—This may occur with heart block, more often partial than complete, or in conditions in which the rate is low from other causes. Clinically this presents three features: (*a*) *Slow pulse,* usually permanent, but sometimes paroxysmal, falling to 40, 20, or even 6 per minute; (*b*) *cerebral attacks*—vertigo of a transient character, syncope, pseudo-apoplectiform attacks or epileptiform seizures; (c) *visible auricular impulses* in the veins of the neck, as noted by Stokes—the beats varying greatly; a 2:1 or 3:1 rhythm is the most common. There are several groups of cases. It is usually a senile manifestation associated with arteriosclerosis. The cases in young adults and middle age may be of syphilitic origin. In some cases of slow pulse in this group the auricular as well as the ventricular rate may be slow and equal, the normal sequence of events being preserved; the origin of the condition is probably vagal. The outlook in this class of cases is good; in the others it is a serious disease and usually fatal, though it may last for years. The cerebral attacks are due to anemia of the brain or of the medulla. Syncopal attacks in patients with heart block may be due to transient ventricular fibrillation, the pulse rate rising with the attack and not slowing.

The *prognosis* in the cases of auriculoventricular heart block with acute infectious disease is usually good, with the exception of diphtheria and some cases of rheumatic fever. In the chronic forms the outlook is grave and sudden death is always possible. The syncopal and convulsive attacks are always serious. In some of the cases due to syphilis proper treatment may result in great improvement. In every case the state of the myocardium is important and with signs of its failure the outlook is grave. This is particularly true if the signs of myocardial failure are progressive and if there are syncopal attacks, in which there is always danger of death.

Treatment.—If a cause, such as syphilis, is found, the indications are evident. Acute heart block demands absolute rest and treatment directed to the general cardiac condition. Digitalis should be given with care; it is contraindicated in acute infections, as diphtheria. It partial block it may increase the difficulty and yet the heart muscle may be aided by it. In complete block it may be more useful and it can not increase the block. The effect on the myocardium must decide. In partial heart block the giving of atropine may be useful but rather in the cases due to acute infections than those with sclerotic processes. In the Stokes-Adams syndrome the injection of epinephrine (♏ 5-10, 0.3-0.6 cc. of 1-1000 solution) subcutaneously (not intravenously) may have a marked effect which lasts for ten or twelve hours. Barium chloride (gr. ½, 0.03 gm.) has not proved to be of value. Ephedrine sulphate (gr. ⅜) is of value and may be given twice a day to prevent attacks.

Sino-auricular Block.—This is not common and may occur in healthy persons. Either the sino-auricular node does not function at intervals or the stimulus is not transmitted to the auricle. In consequence the auricle and ventricle fail to contract and there is a pause, usually less than the length of two cardiac cycles. A whole beat fails to occur. It may be associated with auriculoventricular block and over-action of the vagus or digitalis may be a cause in some cases. It may occur in children after various infections and sometimes after exertion or excitement in apparently healthy persons. The rate may vary from 40 to 80. The electrocardiogram shows normal findings. If the interval between the sino-auricular impulses is great, the ventricles may contract from an ectopic focus ("ventricular escape"). Treatment is not required.

Bundle Branch or Intraventricular Block.—In this there is delay or block in the conduction system below the bifurcation of the bundle of His. It is evidence of myocardial degeneration and is often found in patients who have marked symptoms and signs of this, especially with coronary artery disease. The grade of block varies. King has shown that the diagnosis may be made clinically by (1) a visible and palpable bifid apex thrust and (2) feeble heart sounds with a sound as of an asynchronous murmur accompanying the two elements of the systolic thrust. There is usually evidence of myocardial disease. The *diagnosis* can be made with certainty only by the electrocardiogram. It always demands a serious prognosis and the majority of the patients showing it do not live two years, but there are striking exceptions. In some

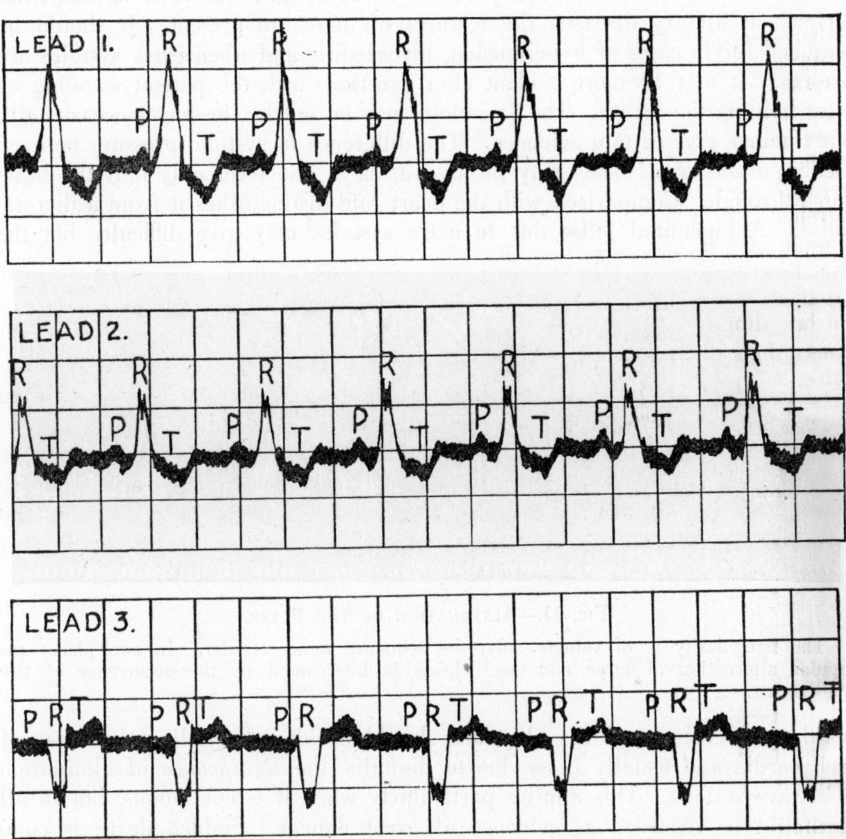

Figs. 8, 9, 10.—Bundle Branch Block.

Left Bundle Branch Block shown by tall wide R wave notched and directed upward in Lead I and downward in Lead III followed by a large T wave opposite in direction to the R wave. Right Bundle Branch Block is recognized by the R wave extending downward in Lead I and upward in Lead III with the T wave in Lead III directed downward.

cases it is a temporary condition. *Treatment* must be decided by the myocardial condition.

(7) **Pulsus Alternans.**—In this there is disturbance of the ventricular systole, so that larger and smaller amounts of blood are expelled by alternate contractions and consequently the pulse shows alternate large and small beats. It may occur with a very rapid heart rate, especially paroxysmal tachycardia and auricular flutter. Its occurrence when the heart rate is normal or nearly so has a very different and more serious meaning. It is observed in a variety of conditions in which marked circulatory disease is present, in severe infec-

tions, especially pneumonia, in uremia and in patients under the influence of digitalis. It occurs most often in advanced life in males with myocardial degeneration. It is essentially due to a partial failure of contractility, the most important of the myocardial functions, and is associated with conditions which cause heart failure. It is comparatively common but frequently overlooked.

The condition itself probably causes no *symptoms* but as it accompanies serious circulatory diseases, the features of these are present. It should be searched for in cases of hypertension, myocarditis and when extra systoles are present. It may be more evident after exertion, with the patient standing or after holding the breath. The variations may be felt by the finger occasionally but tracings give certain evidence. The difference in systolic pressure between the large and small beats may be an aid, as at one level only half the beats come through. Comparison with the heart rate distinguishes it from a dicrotic pulse. A bigeminal pulse due to extra systoles may give difficulty but the

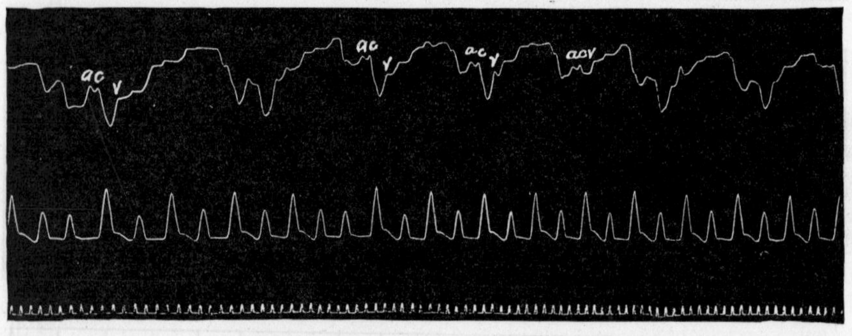

Fig. 11.—Alternation of the Pulse.

The irregularity is of volume only, the sequence being regular. In two places the regular alternation of large and small beats is interrupted by the occurrence of two small beats.

regular intervals in pulsus alternans should decide. Excluding the cases of tachycardia and usually those due to digitalis, the *significance* of alternation is always serious. This applies particularly when it is continuous, but in all it should be regarded as evidence of great danger. Sudden death is comparatively common. The *treatment* is that of the underlying condition and special emphasis should be placed on rest, thorough and prolonged.

(8) **Gallop Rhythm.**—A disturbance of rhythm in which three heart sounds are heard. At rapid rates the sounds suggest the gallop of a horse; at slower rates a canter (canter rhythm). The third sound may originate in various ways. If it comes after the second sound the term *protodiastolic* is applied (much the most common form); if just before the first sound it is termed *presystolic* (next in frequency); if between the two sounds, *mesodiastolic;* and last and rarest, during systole, *systolic.* In the *protodiastolic* form the extra sound corresponds in time with the normal third sound, much accentuated. Gallop rhythm is found most often with myocardial weakness and dilatation and usually is of grave prognosis. Certain cases, such as those with neurocirculatory asthenia, mitral stenosis and partial heart block are not as serious. The condition of the myocardium is the important point and treatment should be directed to it.

Comment.—While the study of cardiac arrhythmias by tracings has added greatly to our understanding of their mechanism, the student should remember that nearly all of them can be recognized by careful clinical observation. A diagnosis of an arrhythmia is not sufficient in itself; the attempt should be made to decide what is responsible. Too often the diagnosis of an arrhythmia by instrumental means is regarded as sufficient and little attention is paid to the cause. This consists in myocardial change in the great majority of cases and it should always be in mind. The efficiency of the myocardium is the essential point to determine and its function is to carry on the mass movement of blood. To pay the principal attention to an arrhythmia is often to miss the essential lesion.

AFFECTIONS OF THE MYOCARDIUM

HYPERTROPHY

Varieties.—The heart enlarges to meet a demand for extra work, either general, as in the hypertrophy of work, or special to combat a deficiency of cardiac structure, such as a damaged valve. There are two forms, one in which the cavity or cavities are of normal size, and the other in which the cavities are enlarged and the walls increased in thickness. The so-called concentric hypertrophy in which there is diminution of the size of the cavity with thickening of the walls is, as a rule, a postmortem change. The enlargement may affect the entire organ, or one side, or only one chamber. Naturally, as the left ventricle does the chief work the change is most frequently found here. Eyster believes that the most important factor is not increased work in itself but the muscle injury and reaction to injury that result from abnormal stretching of the muscle (when the fibres show hydropic degeneration) in the initial period of the overload.

Hypertrophy of the left ventricle alone, or with general enlargement of the heart, is brought about by—

Conditions affecting the heart itself: (*a*) Disease of the aortic valve; (*b*) mitral insufficiency; (*c*) pericardial adhesions; (*d*) sclerotic myocarditis; (*e*) disturbed innervation with overaction, as in exophthalmic goitre, and as a result of the action of alcohol, in the "beer heart." In all of these the work of the heart is increased. With the valve lesions the increase is due to increased intraventricular pressure with more blood to handle; in the case of the adherent pericardium and myocarditis, to direct interference with the proper contraction of the chambers.

Conditions acting upon the blood vessels: (*a*) Hypertension, with or without renal disease, especially capillary sclerosis of the renal arteries and the splanchnic vessels; (*b*) all states of increased arterial tension induced by contraction of the arterioles under the influence of spasm or toxic substances, which, as Bright suggested, "by affecting the minute capillary circulation, render great action necessary to send the blood through the distant subdivisions of the vascular system"; (*c*) narrowing of the aorta, as in congenital stenosis.

Right ventricle hypertrophy occurs with the following conditions: (*a*) *Lesions of the mitral valve,* either incompetence or stenosis, which increase the resistance in the pulmonary vessels. (*b*) *Pulmonary lesions* with atheroma or obliteration of any number of vessels within the lungs, as in emphysema or fibrosis. (*c*) *Valvular lesions* on the right side occasionally cause hypertrophy in the adult, not infrequently in the fetus. (*d*) *Chronic valvular disease of the left heart* and *pericardial adhesions* are sooner or later associated with hypertrophy of the right ventricle.

In the auricles simple hypertrophy is never seen; there is always dilatation with hypertrophy. In the left auricle this develops in lesions of the mitral orifice, particularly stenosis. The right auricle hypertrophies when there is increased pressure in the lesser circulation. Narrowing of the tricuspid orifice is a rare cause.

Symptoms.—There may be no complaint due to the hypertrophy and if associated with renal disease or hypertension there may be a sense of well-being. If the cardiac defect is not fully compensated, there are the usual features of myocardial insufficiency.

In hypertrophy of the *right auricle* the venous pulsation in the neck may be more evident, and an increase in dulness to the right of the sternum in the third and fourth interspaces may be detected. Hypertrophy of the *right ventricle* causes a slight bulging of the costal angle with a positive instead of a negative pulsation at this spot. There may be a heaving impulse of the lower sternum and costal cartilages. The venous pulsation in the neck is usually marked, and the first sound over the tricuspid area louder than normal. Hypertrophy of the *left auricle,* which is never unassociated with dilatation, may be detected occasionally by dulness toward the base of the left lung behind; it is diagnosed by the extension backward of the cardiac shadow in oblique illumination by the X-rays. Hypertrophy of the *left ventricle* is usually easy to diagnose. There is a forcible apex impulse, both visible and palpable, which may cause a movement of a large area of the chest wall. The apex beat, if there be only slight enlargement is usually displaced downward, and is in the 6th or 7th spaces; but if the enlargement be marked, the apex beat is well outside the nipple line. The first sound is usually marked and sometimes has a distinct booming quality. The second sound at the base is accentuated. The pulse is full and the blood pressure is usually raised.

DILATATION

As with other hollow muscular organs, the size of the chambers of the heart varies greatly within normal limits. Dilatation may be acute and quite transitory, as after severe muscular effort, or it may be chronic, in which case it is associated with hypertrophy. Not always, however; there is an extraordinary heart in the McGill University Museum with a parchment like thinning of the walls and uniform dilatation of all the chambers; in places in the right auricle and ventricle only the epicardium remains. Dilatation is pathological only when excessive or permanent. Increase in capacity means increased work and resulting hypertrophy to meet the demand.

Etiology.—Two important causes combine to produce dilatation—increased pressure within the cavities and impaired resistance, due to weakening of the muscular wall—which may act singly but are often combined. A weakened wall due either to structural change in the muscle or to a diminution of its natural tonus may yield to a normal distending force.

(*a*) Heightened endocardiac pressure results from an increased amount of blood to be moved or an obstacle to be overcome. It does not necessarily cause dilatation; simple hypertrophy may follow, as in the early period of aortic stenosis and the left ventricle hypertrophy in nephritis.

The size of the cardiac chambers varies in health. With slow action of the heart the dilatation is complete and fuller than it is with rapid action. Moderate exertion in a normal heart, or even prolonged exertion in a well-trained heart, lessens the heart size, but in conditions of ill health dilatation occurs. Physiologically, the limits of dilatation are reached when the chamber does not empty during systole. This occurs as an acute transient condition in severe exertion in an untrained or feeble condition.

There may be great dilatation of the *right heart,* as shown by the increased epigastric pulsation and increase in the cardiac dulness. The *safety valve* action of the tricuspid valves may come into play, relieving the lungs by permitting regurgitation into the auricle. With rest the condition is removed, but, if it has been extreme, the heart may suffer a strain from which it may recover slowly, or the individual may never be able again to undertake severe exertion. In the process of training the getting wind, as it is called, is largely a gradual increase in the capability of the heart, particularly of the right chambers. A degree of exertion can be safely maintained in full training which is impossible under other circumstances, because, by a gradual process the heart has strengthened its reserve force—widened enormously its limit of physiological work.

Endurance in prolonged contests is measured by the capabilities of the heart, which by increasing its tonus has increased its resistance to dilatation. We have no positive knowledge of the nature of the changes in the heart in this process, but it must be in the direction of increased muscular and nervous energy. Evidence is lacking to prove that prolonged athletic training causes hypertrophy of itself, but no man becomes a great runner or oarsman who has not naturally a capable if not a large heart. Master McGrath, the celebrated greyhound, and Eclipse, the race horse, both famous for endurance rather than speed, had very large hearts.

Excessive dilatation during severe muscular effort results in *heart strain.* A man, perhaps in poor condition, calls upon his heart for extra work during the ascent of a mountain, and has precordial discomfort and distress in the epigastrium. He breathes rapidly for some time, is "puffed," as we say, but the symptoms pass off after a night's rest. An attempt to repeat the exercise is followed by another attack or dyspnea may come on while at rest. For months such a man may be unfitted for severe exertion or he may be permanently incapacitated. In some way he has overstrained his heart. In such cases there was probably previous myocardial change. The "heart-shock" of Latham includes cases of this nature—sudden cardiac breakdown during exertion, not due to rupture of a valve.

Acute dilatation may occur in infectious diseases, especially pneumonia, diphtheria and rheumatic fever, with chronic myocardial disease from exertion, with the establishment of a new rhythm, as auricular fibrillation, in paroxysmal tachycardia, in Graves' disease and in coronary artery occlusion.

Dilatation occurs in all forms of *valve lesions.* In *aortic insufficiency* blood enters the left ventricle during diastole from the unguarded aorta and from the left auricle, and the quantity of blood at the termination of diastole subjects the walls to increased pressure, under which they yield. In time they augment in thickness and present the typical eccentric hypertrophy which is usually so marked in this condition.

In *mitral insufficiency* blood which should have been driven into the aorta is forced into and dilates the auricle from which it came, and then in the diastole of the ventricle a large amount is returned from the auricle and with increased force. In *mitral stenosis* the left auricle is the seat of greatly increased tension during diastole, and dilates as well as hypertrophies; the distention may be enormous. Dilatation of the *right ventricle* is produced by a number of conditions, which were considered under hypertrophy. All circumstances which permanently increase the tension in the pulmonary vessels causes its dilatation. Occlusion of the right coronary arter, may cause right heart failure.

(*b*) Impaired nutrition of the myocardium may lead to a diminution of the resisting power so that dilatation readily occurs.

The loss of tone due to parenchymatous degeneration or myocarditis in fevers may lead to a fatal condition of acute dilatation. The changes in the heart muscle which accompany acute endocarditis or pericarditis may lead to dilatation, especially in the latter disease. In anemia and leukemia the dilatation may be considerable. In fibrosis of the walls the yielding is always where this process is most advanced, as at the left apex. Under any of these circumstances the walls may yield with normal blood pressure.

Pericardial adhesions are a cause of dilatation, and we generally find in cases with extensive and firm union considerable hypertrophy and dilatation. There is usually here some impairment of the superficial layers of muscle. Dilatation is a common sequence of hypertrophy, usually after a long period. In many cases this occurs with the appearance of auricular fibrillation.

ACUTE MYOCARDITIS

Etiology.—Acute myocarditis occurs most often with infectious diseases among which rheumatic fever takes first place. Of other infections, scarlet fever, diphtheria, pneumonia, septicemia and influenza should be mentioned. The results of electrocardiographic studies in patients with acute infectious diseases show that disturbances of rhythm are common. This speaks for myocardial change which may represent an inflammatory or degenerative process. Myocarditis of some extent occurs with acute pericarditis and endocarditis.

Pathology.—While parenchymatous and interstitial forms are distinguished, in most cases both are present. Acute degenerative changes are often found. In rheumatic myocarditis, the Aschoff nodes are regarded as characteristic. Suppurative myocarditis occurs with malignant endocarditis and septicopyemia.

Symptoms.—As myocarditis occurs usually with a general infection and often with endocarditis and pericarditis it is difficult to separate the features due to it alone. There is dyspnea or increase in it if already present; there may be complaint of precordial discomfort or pain; vomiting may occur; and the general condition is worse. The *pulse* becomes more rapid as a rule—an exception is in diphtheria with bradycardia—and is feeble. There may be irregularity. The *heart* shows a widespread feeble impulse with a wavy character and the dulness is increased both right and left. The first sound may be short and sharp or blurred. Systolic murmurs are common both at the apex and base. There may be evidence of passive congestion at the bases of the lungs; enlargement of the liver is not marked as a rule.

Diagnosis.—The occurrence of severe myocardial failure in an acute infection is usually evident. Disturbances of rhythm, especially heart block, are significant. The increase in cardiac dulness is important, especially in children. To distinguish acute endocarditis from acute myocarditis may be impossible for some time.

Prognosis.—This depends somewhat on the original disease but with severe myocarditis is grave. Vomiting, restlessness, delirium, syncopal attacks, a very rapid heart, cyanosis and severe dyspnea are ominous signs.

Treatment.—The patient should be in the most comfortable position. The diet, during the acute infection, will probably have to be liquid, but soft foods may be given if the patient can take them. Carbohydrates should be given freely and in some cases glucose solution is given intravenously with advantage but only small quantities at a time. An ice-bag should be kept over the precordium. Rest should be secured for which sedatives, such as phenobarbital or bromide, may be used, but morphia hypodermically is often best. Digitalis is not indicated as a rule, except if auricular fibrillation appears when it may be of benefit. Caffeine may be tried but the results are doubtful. The *convalescence* should be prolonged and the patient kept at rest for weeks or months. Exertion should be resumed very gradually. Anemia should be treated by iron.

CHRONIC MYOCARDITIS—MYOCARDIAL INSUFFICIENCY

The term *chronic myocarditis* suggests a chronic inflammatory condition of the myocardium, but by custom its use includes various changes, especially chronic fibrosis, which may follow an acute inflammation or develop gradually from a variety of causes. Fibrous myocarditis, chronic interstitial myocarditis, cardiosclerosis, myocardosis and myocardial degeneration are some of the terms employed to designate these changes in the myocardium. In the consideration of cardiac disease in general, the myocardium must always be considered. The work of the heart is to move the blood and the myocardium supplies the power. A decrease in the efficiency of the myocardium is the usual cause of symptoms and hence it is difficult clinically to separate chronic myocarditis and myocardial insufficiency. However, we are able in some cases to recognize myocardial change before there are symptoms. The electrocardiographic study is of great value in this regard, but the interpretation should take the patient into account as well as his tracings.

With lessening of the muscular power of the heart the rapidity with which the blood circulates is diminished, and the tissues fail to receive their proper supply of oxygen and food, and to be relieved of their waste products—this is myocardial failure. The same effect may be produced in another way. The amount of blood in the body is much less than the total capacity of the vascular bed, and an adequate blood supply is only kept up by a general constriction of arterioles which dam the blood in the arterial system, but if there is a general vasodilatation of the arterioles, especially those in the splanchnic area, the heart does not receive an amount of blood sufficient to supply the bodily needs, with the same effect on the organs as in certain forms of cardiac failure. This condition does not concern us here, but is mentioned to avoid the impression that all failure of the circulation means failure of the heart.

The failure in muscular power may affect any cavity singly or the whole heart. Weakness of the *left ventricle* fails to give proper filling of the aterial system and general anemia of the tissues results. Failure of the *left auricle* means stasis in the lung vessels with deficient aëration of the blood, and a tendency to edema of the lung or to effusion into the pleural cavities. Failure of the *right heart* gives cyanosis of the organs, dyspnea at rest and on slight exertion, with stasis in the abdominal organs and edema.

The *reserve* power of the myocardium disappears in heart failure. This reserve, greatest in youth, is increased by adequate nutrition, certain congenital endowments, and, apart from other defects, by hypertrophy. It is lessened by defects in the cardiac structure, gross or minute, by defective nutrition, by bacterial and other poisons, and with advancing years. We have at present no means of gauging this reserve power of the organ.

The failure may be sudden or slow, according to the kind and rapidity of the lesion which causes it. When the left ventricle fails the effect may vary from immediate death, through all forms of fainting, giddiness, sense of dissolution, to a mild sense of bodily or mental fatigue; when the right ventricle fails the effect varies from a sudden dyspnea to a dyspnea which comes on with slight exertion.

As to the actual condition in myocardial failure generally, it is by no means easy in all cases to say what has been the cause. The lesions to which the myocardium is liable are described further on, yet there is a proportion of cases in which neither by postmortem examination nor microscopic search can the cause of the failure be suggested. Disturbances in conduction, ventricular fibrillation, or other changes may be responsible. One or more of the functions of the heart muscle may be affected.

Acute Myocardial Insufficiency.—Causes: (*a*) Wounds of the heart, (*b*) spontaneous rupture or rupture of valves, (*c*) rapid pericardial effusion, (*d*) access of air to the chambers of the heart, as from operations on the neck or after exposure to a high atmospheric pressure, (*e*) large thrombi quickly formed in a heart cavity, (*f*) sudden interference with the coronary circulation, (*g*) mechanical interference from pressure on the trachea or larynx, as in strangulation, (*h*) acute infections, such as diphtheria or pericarditis, (*i*) certain poisons, such as cocaine, phosphorus, etc., (*j*) stimulation of the vagus nerve, its centre in the medulla, or its termination in the heart.

Chronic Myocardial Insufficiency.—Causes: (*a*) Lesions of the heart muscle. *All cardiac failure is muscular.* The myocardium may be insufficiently nourished, as in coronary artery sclerosis. One or more of the functions of the cardiac muscle may be interfered with without producing any changes that can be detected by the microscope. (*b*) Lesions of the valves. (*c*) Lesions affecting the vascular fields of the efferent arteries. Emphysema, chronic bronchitis, asthma, fibrosis of the lungs, chest deformities, and mitral disease produce an embarrassment of the right heart; conditions causing hypertension and capillary fibrosis, especially of the splanchnic and renal area, produce failure of the left heart. (*d*) Overexertion. (*e*) Certain poisons, such as alcohol (especially beer) and phosphorus. (*f*) Other causes, such as adherent pericardium and exophthalmic goitre.

Anatomical Basis of Myocardial Insufficiency.—I. Lesions of the Coronary Arteries.—A knowledge of the changes produced in the myocardium by disease of the coronary vessels aids in the understanding of many problems in cardiac pathology. Anastomoses exist between the right and left coronary arteries and between the branches of each coronary artery. These become larger with increase in age. The vessels of Thebesius aid in supplying the myocardium when the coronary arteries are occluded as do also the "myocardial sinusoids." Coronary occlusion results in infarction with resulting permanent changes in the affected area.

An important effect of coronary artery disease is seen in the production of *fibrous myocarditis.* This may result from the gradual transformation of areas of anemic necrosis. More commonly it is caused by the narrowing of a coronary branch in a process of obliterative endarteritis. The sclerosis is most frequent at the apex of the left ventricle and in the septum, but may occur in any portion. In the septum and walls there are often streaks and patches seen only in carefully made serial sections. Hypertrophy of the heart is commonly associated with this degeneration.

Septic Infarcts.—In pyemia the smaller branches of the coronary arteries may be blocked with emboli which give rise to infectious or septic infarcts in the myocardium in the form of abscesses, varying in size from a pea to a pin's head. These may not cause any disturbance, but when large they may perforate into the ventricle or into the pericardium.

II. Acute Interstitial Myocarditis.—In some infectious diseases and in acute pericarditis the intermuscular connective tissue may be swollen and infiltrated with small round cells and leukocytes, the blood vessels dilated, and the muscle fibres the seat of granular, fatty, and hyaline degeneration. Occasionally, in pyemia the infiltration with pus cells is diffuse and chiefly in the interstitial tissue. Councilman described this condition in gonorrhea, and demonstrated the gonococcus in the areas. The commonest examples are found in diphtheria, typhoid fever and acute endocarditis. The foci may be the starting points of patches of fibrous myocarditis.

III. Fragmentation and Segmentation.—This condition was described by Renaut and Landouzy in 1877. Two forms are met with: (1) Segmentation. The muscle fibres have separated at the cement line. (2) Fragmentation. The fracture has been across the fibre itself, and perhaps at the level of the nucleus. Longitudinal division is unusual. Although the condition doubtless arises in some instances during the death agony, as in sudden death by violence, in others it would seem to have clinical and pathological significance. It is found associated with other lesions, fibrous myocarditis, infarction and fatty degeneration. J. B. MacCallum distinguished a simple from a degenerative fragmentation. The first takes place in the normal fibre, which, however, shows irregular extensions and contractions. The second succeeds degeneration in the fibre. Hearts the seat of marked fragmentation are lax, easily torn, the muscle fibres widely separated, and often pale and cloudy.

IV. Parenchymatous Degeneration.—This is usually met with in fevers, or with endocarditis or pericarditis, and in infections and intoxications generally. It is characterized by a pale, turbid state of the cardiac muscle, which is general, not localized. Turbidity and softness are the special features. It is the softened heart of Laënnec and Louis. Stokes speaks of an instance in which "so great was the softening of the organ that when the heart was grasped by the great vessels and held with the apex pointing upward, it fell down over the hand, covering it like a cap of a large mushroom." There is a degeneration of the muscle fibres; sometimes the change in the fibres is extreme and no trace of the striae can be detected.

V. Fatty Heart.—Under this term are embraced fatty degeneration and fatty overgrowth or infiltration.

(*a*) *Fatty Degeneration.*—The frequency and importance of this condition have probably been greatly overestimated and the designation has been loosely used. Microscopically visible fat does not necessarily mean fatty degeneration, and it is a question whether fatty and fibrous changes can be differentiated. There is no question of its occurrence in phosphorus poisoning and pernicious anemia, but in general a clinical diagnosis of fatty degeneration is most uncertain and there are no symptoms or signs peculiar to it.

(*b*) *Fatty Overgrowth or Infiltration.*—This is usually a simple excess of the normal subpericardial fat, termed *cor adiposum* by the older writers. In pronounced instances the fat infiltrates between the muscular substance and, separating the strands, may reach even to the endocardium. In corpulent persons there is always much pericardial fat. It forms part of the general obesity and occasionally leads to dangerous impairment of the contractile power of the heart. The entire heart may be enveloped in a thick sheeting of fat through which not a trace of muscle substance can be seen. On section the fat infiltrates the muscles, separating the fibres, and in some places there may be complete substitution of fat for the muscle substance. In rare instances the fat may be in the papillary muscles. The heart is usually much relaxed and the chambers are dilated.

VI. Other Degeneration.—(*a*) *Brown Atrophy.*—This is a common change in the heart muscle, particularly in chronic valvular lesions and in the senile heart. When advanced the color of the muscles is a dark reddish brown, and the consistence is usually increased. The fibres present an accumulation of yellow brown pigment chiefly about the nuclei. (*b*) *Amyloid degeneration* occasionally occurs in the intermuscular connective tissue and in the blood vessels, not in the fibres. (*c*) The *hyaline transformation of Zenker* occurs in prolonged fevers. The affected fibres are swollen, homogeneous, translucent, and the striae are faint. (*d*) *Calcareous degeneration* occasionally occurs in the myocardium and the muscle fibres are infiltrated with lime salts.

VII. Functional Basis of Myocardial Insufficiency.—The cause of insufficiency may be in disturbance of one or more of the functions of the heart muscle. In many cases it is probable that more than one is affected. In some cases the disturbance is temporary and complete recovery follows, as seen in auricular fibrillation or heart block occurring with acute infectious diseases. Here inflammatory changes or disturbance from toxins may be responsible. The most striking common disturbance of function is seen in auricular fibrillation. The importance of structural changes which are usually responsible for the disturbances of function must be remembered.

Symptoms.—The clinical features of *chronic myocarditis* as a rule are slight until some degree of myocardial insufficiency is present. There may be no symptoms whatsoever and sudden death occur. The most common early symptom is some shortness of breath on exertion. Some patients complain of precordial discomfort or there may be attacks of severe pain. Fatigue, vertigo, irritability, insomnia, digestive disturbance and the appearance of hemorrhoids may be suggestive although not characteristic. Unusual effort, or an acute infection, such as bronchitis, may bring on evidence of the myocardial disease. In many cases, the presence of chronic myocarditis is brought to our attention in a routine examination or one made for other complaints. Enlargement of the heart, perhaps with some alteration in the character of the sounds, an abnormal response to exercise tests, arteriosclerosis and hypertension, perhaps with evidence of renal disease, are significant. The electrocardiographic study may give positive evidence of myocardial change but a normal tracing does not exclude disease.

The symptoms complained of by patients with *myocardial failure* are as follows: (*a*) Cardiovascular system: Pain in the cardiac area or extending to the shoulders and down the arms, a sense of weight in the precordium; palpitation is a rare complaint. (*b*) Respiratory system: Dyspnea at rest or on exertion, or orthopnea, Cheyne-Stokes respiration, cough, loss of voice from pressure of a dilated left auricle on the left recurrent laryngeal nerve, hemoptysis (from lung infarcts). (*c*) Central nervous system: sleeplessness, mental symptoms, delusions, melancholia, and especially toward the end stupor and drowsiness. (*d*) Cyanosis, pallor, edema and occasionally purpura in the lower limbs. (*e*) Alimentary system: The stasis in the abdominal organs in right heart failure produces loss of appetite, indigestion, flatulence, vomiting, constipation, diarrhea, abdominal pain, hemorrhoids, etc. (*f*) Renal system: The urine is scanty, high colored, and contains albumin.

Examination of the *heart* may reveal an apex beat which is feeble, outside the nipple line, diffuse, and whose maximum intensity is not easily localized. The pulsation may be marked on inspection and cover a very wide area; arterial pulsation in the neck in left heart failure may be great; in right heart failure the jugular veins may be very dilated. On percussion the cardiac area may be much increased to the right or to the left, or both. On auscultation the sounds may be difficult to hear, or feebler than normal. With the muscular insufficiency there is often a *relative insufficiency* of the mitral and tricuspid valves, rarely of the aortic and pulmonic valves. If the patient is seen for the first time in an attack of decompensation, it may be impossible to decide whether a mitral insufficiency is relative (that is from inability of the valves to close the relaxed orifice) or due to organic valvular disease. In many elderly patients with arteriosclerosis and hypertrophy, the murmur of relative insufficiency may be loud and intense. An exact diagnosis of the valvular lesion is of no great practical importance; the muscular insufficiency is the important factor. Gallop rhythm may be present. The pulse may show great variations; marked failure may exist with a full bounding pulse; more usually it is feeble with diminished tension; it may be irregular, intermittent, slow, or rapid. The vital capacity is much reduced from the normal 3,500-4,000 to 1,500-2,000 cc. (J. H. Pratt).

When *dilatation* occurs there are gallop rhythm, shortening of diastole, and a systolic murmur at the apex or the first sound may be short and much like the second. Shortness of breath on exertion is an early feature in many cases, and anginal attacks may occur. There is sometimes a tendency to syncope, and the patient may wake in the early morning with an attack of severe dyspnea. These "spells" may be associated with nausea and alternate with others in which there are anginal symptoms. These are the cases, too, in which for weeks there may be mental symptoms. The patient has delusions and may even become maniacal. Toward the close Cheyne-Stokes breathing may occur. It was described in the following terms by John Cheyne (*Dublin Hospital Reports,* vol. ii, p. 221, 1818): "For several days his breathing was irregular; it would entirely cease for a quarter of a minute, then it would become perceptible, though very low, then by degrees it became heaving and quick, and then it would gradually cease again: this revolution in the state of his breathing lasted about a minute, during which there were about thirty acts of respiration." It is seen more frequently in hypertensive and uremic states than in myocardial degeneration alone.

The *blood pressure* in myocardial insufficiency shows no uniform figures. The systolic pressure may be high even with a failing heart. In serious degrees of myocardial affection it is usually low. In cases in which there has been hypertension the maximum may be lower or higher than the normal for the patient. Probably in early stages of failure the heart is stimulated to increased energy and the maximum pressure overcompensates the circulatory defect.

Myocardial failure may be predominantly of one side and naturally this is of the left ventricle more often than of the right. With failure of the *left ventricle* there are signs of disturbance in the pulmonary circulation, much more marked than in the peripheral vessels. Dyspnea, paroxysmal cardiac dyspnea and edema of the lungs may be marked and the vital capacity is reduced. Gallop rhythm, especially protodiastolic, pulsus alternans and accentuation of the pulmonic second sound are found frequently. With failure of the *right ventricle* the signs of venous congestion are prominent, fullness of the veins of the neck and arms, enlargement of the liver and edema of the legs. Digestive disturbances may be marked and hemorrhoids may appear.

Fatty infiltration exists in very obese persons but produces no symptoms until the muscular fibre is so weakened that dilatation occurs. These patients may for years present a feeble but regular pulse; the heart sounds are weak and muffled, and a murmur may be heard at the apex. Attacks of dyspnea are not uncommon, and the patient may suffer from bronchitis.

Myocardium in Hyperthyroidism.—This is important from the side of the thyroid disease but also because the predominent features may suggest cardiac disease and the other and causal condition be overlooked. There is frequently the complaint of palpitation coming on in attacks, tachycardia with extra systoles often being found, and sometimes paroxysmal auricular fibrillation. There is overaction of the heart with a short forcible apex impulse, sometimes a thrill and a first sound which may suggest mitral stenosis. There may be hypertension. The size of the heart determined by X-ray study is less than the physical examination suggests and pulsation in the pulmonary artery may be marked. The thyroid gland may not seem enlarged. With suspicion of thyroid disease, all the studies required for the diagnosis of this should be made. Rest and digitalis may have little influence on the cardiac condition.

Following an *operation* a variety of disturbing conditions occur which should be carefully studied. Sometimes what is regarded as "acute dilatation" occurs with very rapid heart action. Some are paroxysmal auricular tachycardia, auricular fibrillation or auricular flutter. Pressure on the vagus or on the eyes may correct paroxysmal auricular flutter.

Cardioptosis.—In this the heart is narrow, lies vertically and is low in position. It is found in the subnormal type with arterial hypoplasia, a tendency to undernutrition and vasomotor instability. Dilatation occurs readily with any slight infection or disturbance and is easily overlooked owing to the small size of the heart with which a normal extent of dulness represents enlargement. They respond quickly to rest and digitalis.

Functional Tests.—There are many of these, the principle being to have the patient perform certain exercises, such as hopping on one leg, bending over, etc., and then studying the circulatory response. The exercise chosen should be suitable for the age and habits of the patient. The extent of response (pulse rate, blood pressure) and the length of time it persists are important points. But every patient is constantly doing "functional tests" in his daily life, which careful inquiry should elicit. There is a reduction in the pulmonary vital *capacity* in cardiac insufficiency as a result of engorgement of the pulmonary vessels, pleural effusion, infarct, etc.

We may group the cases of myocardial failure as follows:

(1) Those in which sudden death occurs with or without previous indications of heart trouble. Sclerosis of the coronary arteries exists—in some with recent thrombus and white infarcts; in others with extensive fibroid disease. Some cases of sudden death may be due to deficiency in the coronary blood supply due to sudden lowering of the diastolic pressure. Many patients never complain of cardiac distress, but, as in the case of Chalmers, the celebrated Scottish divine, enjoy unusual vigor of mind and body

(2) Cases in which there are cardiac arrhythmia, shortness of breath on exertion, attacks of dyspnea, sometimes anginal attacks, collapse symptoms with sweats and slow pulse, and occasionally marked mental symptoms.

(3) Cases with general arteriosclerosis and hypertrophy and dilatation of the heart. They are often robust men of middle age who have worked hard and lived carelessly. Dyspnea, cough and swelling of the feet occur early, and the patient comes under observation with gallop rhythm or an irregular heart with an apex systolic murmur. Recovery from the first or second attack is the rule. It is a common form of myocardial disease.

(4) Following *hypertension* there is marked hypertrophy of the left ventricle and often sclerosis of the coronary arteries. Myocardial failure is a common result; some die from cerebral vascular lesions or renal lesions. The term *hypertensive heart disease* does not seem to be of particular advantage. The myocardial features do not differ essentially from those of myocardial failure with normal or low blood pressure. It does suggest the course of events.

Diagnosis.—The diagnosis of *chronic myocarditis* may be suggested by the features mentioned before or made in a routine examination; the electrocardiographic study may be important. In *myocardial insufficiency* the symptoms are the best aid in early diagnosis. The response to exertion is important, always remembering the normal ability of the patient. Shortness of breath, distress and precordial discomfort or pain, with increased cardiac rate are significant. The distress at first is on exertion, later when at rest or for some time after exertion. With the condition well marked there is rarely much difficulty.

The X-ray study may give aid particularly in estimating the changes in the various chambers of the heart. The circulatory changes in the lungs can be estimated as passive congestion gives marked shadows.

Prognosis.—Each case must be judged on its own merits, special notice being taken of the age, probable origin, and anatomical basis of the insufficiency. With disturbance of rhythm the nature of this should be determined as it has an important bearing on the outcome. Permanent inversion of the T wave in leads I and II is of grave outlook. Alteration of the QRS complex in all the derivations is serious. Low voltage changes in all three leads are of serious import. The outlook in affections of the myocardium in advanced life is extremely grave. Patients recover, however, in a surprising way from serious attacks, particularly those of the third group.

Treatment.—Some patients never come under treatment; the first are the final symptoms. Other patients with marked failure, if treated on general lines, recover quickly. Much more difficult is the management of those patients in whom there is marked disturbance of function as heart block, auricular fibrillation or alternation of the heart.

The patient with *chronic myocarditis* without symptoms should lead a sensible life with avoidance of over-exertion and strain as far as possible. Rest of mind and freedom from anxiety are important, if more difficult to secure. The diet should be simple and excess of fluid intake avoided. If he is overweight, this should be reduced gradually. The bowels should be kept regular by simple measures. A period of rest each day is advisable and 10 hours of the 24 should be spent in bed. Sufficient sleep is important for which sedatives may be necessary. Any focal infection and anemia should be treated. Should digitalis be given? This must be decided for each patient but the majority, especially if there is hypertrophy, seem to be helped by it. Small amounts are usually enough, such as one or two grains of the leaves once or twice a day. This may be taken constantly or for two or three weeks in each month as the results indicate.

The following are the measures in the treatment of myocardial failure:

(*a*) Rest.—This is essential whenever there is myocardial failure; the patient should be in bed in the most comfortable position. With severe dyspnea he may be more comfortable in a chair.

(*b*) Diet.—In acute conditions it is usually well to limit this in amount, especially the fluids. With marked passive congestion liquid diet may be advisable; otherwise small amounts of simple food may be given at short intervals. In any case with dilatation it is well to limit the total daily intake of fluids to 1,500 cc. A "dry diet" for a few days is sometimes useful. It is usually wise to avoid large amounts of carbohydrates but these patients often do well with considerable amounts of sugar. The giving of glucose, perhaps with insulin, is sometimes useful but not always, which suggests that the indications for its use are not clear. One method is to give 5 units of insulin before the morning and evening meal and 25 grams of glucose with the meal. It is hoped that the nutrition of the heart muscle may be helped by this procedure.

(*c*) The Relief of the Embarrassed Circulation.

(1) *By Venesection.*—In dilatation, when venous engorgement is marked and there is orthopnea with cyanosis, the abstraction of 10 to 20 ounces of blood is indicated. This is the occasion in which timely venesection may save the patient's life. It is particularly helpful in the dilated heart of arterio-sclerosis.

(2) *By Depletion through the Bowels.*—This is particularly valuable when dropsy is present. The salines are to be preferred; before breakfast from half an ounce to an ounce of Epsom salts may be given in concentrated form. This usually produces liquid evacuations. The compound jalap powder in half dram (2 gm.) doses, or elaterin (gr. 1/10 0.006 gm.) may be employed for the same purpose. Even when the pulse is feeble cathartics are well borne, and they deplete the portal system rapidly and efficiently.

(3) *Remedies Which Aid the Heart.*—Of these the most important is *digitalis,* which was introduced into practice by Withering. The indication for its use is insufficiency of the heart muscle, most especially when auricular fibrillation is present. Broken compensation, no matter what valvular lesion is present, is the signal for its use. It slows and increases the force of the contractions. High blood pressure is not a contra-indication. The beneficial effects are best seen in cases of mitral disease with auricular fibrillation. On theoretical grounds it has been urged that its use is not so advantageous in aortic insufficiency, since it prolongs diastole and leads to greater distention. This need not be considered, and digitalis may be as serviceable in this as in any other condition associated with dilatation. It may be given in the form of the leaves or the tincture; it is a matter of indifference if the drug is good. The dosage varies according to the condition. In severe cases one to two drams (4-8 cc.) of the tincture is given at once followed by 20 minims three times a day. In less severe cases 20-30 minims (1.3-2 cc.) are given three times a day until a definite effect is produced. The weight of the patient should be considered. Free purgation is an advantage before digitalis is begun. The very large dosage should not be given as a routine and toxic effects should be avoided. The leaf (gr. i corresponding to 10 minims of the tincture) may be employed in place of the tincture. If there is vomiting, the tincture can be given by rectum in 100 cc. of warm water. The use of "active principles" is not advised. If there is auricular fibrillation it is well to continue the use of digitalis indefinitely in the best dosage for that patient. The opinion that digitalis is of use in auricular fibrillation only is not correct, and it will be found beneficial in other conditions, sometimes when there are but few symptoms and perhaps fewer signs of myocardial insufficiency.

Digitalis can be used to advantage in conditions in which there is no definite loss of compensation. Patients who have had myocardial failure often do well to take the drug steadily. The dosage must be determined for each patient; one or two grains of the leaves once a day may be enough. The same applies to patients in whom there is reason to expect a loss of compensation some time in the future, *e.g.* with marked hypertrophy. The steady administration of small doses of digitalis is often useful in them.

Ill effects rarely follow digitalis. Toxic effects are seen in the production of nausea and vomiting, apparently due to a reflex action conveyed to the vomiting centre from the heart by the sympathetic fibres and probably by the vagus (Hatcher). There may be marked slowing of the heart, heart block of varying degree or alternation of the heart beat. Disturbances of vision of various kinds may occur, altered color vision, blurred vision and scotomas. These subside on the withdrawal of the digitalis and are rarely serious. There are patients who require and take digitalis uninterruptedly for years. When there is dyspnea on exertion and cardiac distress, from 5 to 10 minims (0.3 to 0.6 cc.) three times a day may be advantageously given for prolonged periods. In severe conditions and if there is vomiting it may be necessary to give digitalis intramuscularly. Some of the special fluid preparations of digitalis suitable for hypodermic use should be employed in doses of ℳ 15-30 (1-2 cc.). There is risk in giving digitalis intravenously and this should be used only in a severe emergency.

Of other remedies strophanthus may be of service, the tincture being given in doses of 15 minims (1 cc.) but its effect is uncertain when given by mouth. In severe conditions strophanthin gr. 1/200 (0.00032 gm.) can be given intravenously and repeated once or twice at intervals of 12 to 24 hours. The intramuscular is safer than the intravenous administration. Convallaria, adonis vernalis and sparteine are recommended as substitutes for digitalis, but their inferiority is so manifest that their use is rarely indicated. Ouabain may be given intravenously, 0.5 mg. (gr. 1/120) for the first dose and 0.25 mg. (gr. 1/240) each day until a total dosage of 2-3 mg. is given. Drugs, such as caffeine, diuretin and theocin, are useful in case of edema for their diuretic effect.

When anemia is marked iron should be given in full doses and arsenic may be given also.

Thyroidectomy.—The work of Blumgart *et al.* has shown that complete removal of the thyroid gland may result in great improvement in patients with marked cardiac disease. The removal of the thyroid gland reduces metabolism and lessens the work of the heart. The *whole gland* has to be removed.

Special Treatment.—(*a*) *Dropsy.*—The improved circulation under the influence of digitalis increases the amount of urine and favors resorption of fluid. Cathartics, by depleting the portal circulation, promote the absorption of fluid from the lymph spaces and lymph sacs. To these measures the use of caffeine, theobromin, diuretin and theocin may be added. Theophyllin preparations may be useful, especially in arteriosclerotic patients as they may aid by dilating the coronary arteries. Metaphyllin is given in doses of gr. i-ii (0.065-0.13 gm.) three times a day. Salyrgan may be used, care being taken to study the renal condition as it is a mercurial and may damage the kidney. It is given intravenously or intramuscularly in doses of 0.5-1 cc. every 3 or 4 days. Ammonium chloride is often given at the same time in doses of 30 to 60 grains (2-4 gm.) daily. Novasurol (merbaphen) is used as salyrgan but is more toxic. In some cases, however, it is not relieved, and the legs may be punctured by aspirating needles, with rubber tubing attached, which are inserted and left for hours; they often drain away large amounts. This is better than scarification. Canton flannel bandages may be applied to the edematous legs. With marked hydrothorax or ascites tapping is advisable before digitalis is given.

(*b*) Dyspnea.—The patients are usually unable to lie down and should have a comfortable bed-rest—if possible, one with lateral projections, so that in sleeping the head can be supported as it falls over. The chest should be carefully examined, as hydrothorax is a common cause. There are cases of mitral regurgitation with recurring hydrothorax, usually on the right side, which require relief by tapping over long periods. For nocturnal dyspnea, particularly with restlessness, morphia is invaluable and may be given without hesitation. The value of the calming influence of opium and its derivatives in cardiac insufficiency is not sufficiently recognized. There are instances of cardiac dyspnea unassociated with dropsy, especially with hypertension, in which nitroglycerine or sodium nitrite is of service, given in increasing doses. Oxygen may give some relief.

(*c*) Palpitation and Cardiac Distress.—With great hypertrophy and distressing throbbing, aconite is of service in doses of from 1 to 3 drops every two or three hours. An ice bag over the heart is also of service. For pain, often marked in aortic lesions, sodium iodide in 10-grain (0.6 gm.) doses, three times a day, or nitroglycerine may be tried. Small blisters are sometimes advantageous. An important cause of palpitation and distress is abdominal distention for which suitable measures must be used.

(*d*) Gastric Symptoms.—The patients who do badly and fail to respond to digitalis are often those in whom nausea and vomiting are prominent. The liver is often greatly enlarged; there is stasis in the hepatic vessels, and little can be expected of drugs until the venous engorgement is relieved. If vomiting persists, it is best to give ice, small quantities of milk and lime water, and alkaline drinks. The bowels should be freely moved and drugs given by rectum or hypodermically.

(*e*) Cough and Hemoptysis.—The former is almost a necessary concomitant of myocardial insufficiency, owing to engorgement of the pulmonary vessels and more or less bronchitis. It is allayed by measures directed rather to the heart than to the lungs. Hemoptysis may be beneficial. An army surgeon, invalided during the American Civil War on account of hemoptysis, supposed to be due to tuberculosis, had for years, with mitral insufficiency and enlarged heart, many attacks of hemoptysis. His condition was invariably better after an attack. It is rarely fatal, except in some cases of acute dilatation, and seldom calls for special treatment.

(*f*) Sleeplessness.—A distressing feature is disturbed sleep. Patients may wake suddenly with throbbing of the heart, often in an attack of nightmare. Subsequently, when compensation has failed, it is also a worrying symptom. The sleep is broken, restless, and frequently disturbed by frightful dreams. Sometimes a dose of spirit of chloroform with spirit of camphor will give a quiet night. The compound spirit of ether, Hoffmann's anodyne, though unpleasant, is frequently useful when compensation has partially failed and the patients suffer from restless nights. Paraldehyde, chloral hydrate and barbital are sometimes serviceable, but it is best, if these fail, to resort to morphia without hesitation.

(*g*) Renal Symptoms.—With broken compensation the urinary secretion is diminished, and the amount may sink to 5 or 6 ounces in the day. Digitalis usually increases the flow. A brisk purge may be followed by increased secretion. The combination of digitalis, squill and calomel is sometimes effective when digitalis alone has failed. Diuretin in doses of 15 grains (1 gm.), theocin (gr. v, 0.3 gm.) or theobromine (gr. v, 0.3 gm.) three times a day is sometimes useful.

The DIET in chronic cardiac diseases may be difficult to regulate. Retention of the chlorides is an important factor in edema. In the intervals between attacks a salt free diet as far as possible should be used. Starchy foods and articles likely to cause flatulency should be forbidden.

Syphilitic Heart Disease.—The treatment of myocardial insufficiency is as in other forms. The treatment for the syphilis requires caution and judgment. At first mercury, usually best by inunction, and sodium iodide (gr. 10, 0.6 gm.) should be given. Later bismuth can be used. Arsenic preparations should be given with great caution and in small doses. Neoarsphenamine may be begun with a dose of 0.1 gm. and, if well taken, the dose can be gradually increased.

Thyrotoxic Heart Disease.—Rest and sufficient sleep should be secured. Digitalis should be given cautiously; some patients are harmed by it. The proper treatment for Graves' disease should be given. Quinidine may be given for auricular fibrillation, especially if present after operation.

Paroxysmal Cardiac Dyspnea ("Cardiac Asthma").—This usually occurs at night but may follow exertion. The patients are usually over 50 years of age, and arteriosclerosis, myocardial disease, nephritis, hypertension, and coronary artery disease, some or all, are present. A sudden rise in blood pressure, an aortic reflex, increased respiration and diminished blood supply to the myocardium during sleep are suggested as causes. Syphilis may be responsible in younger patients. Stasis of blood in the lungs and failure of one or the other ventricle are usually found. The onset is usually sudden with severe dyspnea, so that the patient has to sit up and cough; the sputum is often bloody. There may be pulmonary edema. The pulse rate is usually increased and there may be a marked rise in blood pressure. The attacks may last for some hours and are of grave significance as death may occur. In the *treatment* of an attack morphia (gr. 1/4, 0.016 gm.) and atropine (gr. 1/100, 0.00065 gm.) should be given hypodermically and repeated if necessary. Larger amounts of atropine should be given if there is pulmonary edema. The use of vasodilators may give relief, especially if there is an increase in pressure. With marked distention of the veins, venesection is useful. Digitalis is usually of benefit. These patients should take a very small evening meal and no late supper.

CORONARY ARTERY OCCLUSION

Occlusion occurs rarely from embolism and is usually associated with marked sclerosis of the vessels. In some cases a *thrombus* is found at autopsy but in other cases the exact mechanism of the occlusion is not clear. Changes in the artery, slowing of the blood stream and possibly a greater tendency to agglutination of the platelets are factors in the process. In the early stages there is hyperemia with coagulation necrosis. The muscle affected becomes softer and necrotic. If the infarct is extensive and includes the whole thickness of the wall, rupture may occur, usually in from two to three weeks. This should be kept in mind with regard to exertion at this time. If the infarct involves the inner surface of the ventricle a mural thrombus may form and emboli may be detached to block large arteries if on the left side or to cause pulmonary infarction if on the right side. If the infarct involves the outer surface of the myocardium, a fibrinous exudate forms; a friction rub is heard if its situation permits. With recovery there is fibrosis but regeneration of muscle fibres does not occur. A "scar" results and if the wall is weak an aneurism may form.

As to *sex,* males predominate. With regard to *age,* it occurs especially in patients over 50 but more cases seem to be occurring in younger persons and below the age of 40. In earlier life embolism is more common. Arteriosclerosis is common and many of the patients have hypertension. A considerable number have had attacks of precordial pain. As to exciting causes we know little. Exertion may be a factor but not infrequently the attack begins with the patient at rest.

Symptoms.—There are all grades of severity from attacks so mild that the patient does not have to give up activity to those of maximum severity with sudden death. The attack of average severity has distinctive features. The *onset* is usually sudden, but may be gradual, and often occurs during sleep. There is not the same relation to effort as in angina pectoris. The pain is very severe, felt in the lower sternal region and often for some distance to the right and left. It may be felt in the epigastrium. The pain is usually constant and persists, unless relieved, for hours or days. It may radiate or remain local. It is not relieved by an ordinary dose of morphia. *Dyspnea* is present in some degree and may be marked in patients who have little or no pain. *Vomiting* is common. There are signs of *shock;* there is a curious pallor, perhaps with cyanosis and severe sweating. The patient may be restless and throw himself about. There may be marked apprehension. The *heart* shows an increase in rate which may not come on immediately. It may show an increase in size and the impulse is feeble. The sounds are distant and feeble and there may be gallop rhythm or other disturbance of rhythm. The *blood pressure* usually shows a marked drop which may come on suddenly or be delayed for a couple of days. A localized *pericardial friction* rub is heard in some cases, usually not before the second or third day. *Fever* is common, usually appearing on the second day and rarely being over 102°. It persists for varying periods, subsiding gradually. *Leukocytosis* occurs and may appear promptly; counts of 10,000 to 15,000 are usual with a high percentage of polynuclear cells. The picture is that of a patient who is "hard hit"; exhaustion may be marked.

Electrocardiogram.—Studies should be made as soon as possible and repeated daily, if possible, for a week to ten days. The most striking changes are in the R-T interval and the T deflection. There may be alterations in the QRS group. The changes are evident within several hours after the onset and vary frequently in the first two or three days which is helpful in differentiating acute coronary occlusion from conditions which resemble it. The fourth lead, the direct chest lead, may show changes characteristic of this condition when the usual leads are normal.

Certain other features may be marked. In the *lungs* there may be marked congestion and perhaps edema. Râles are heard at the bases very commonly. The *liver* may be enlarged and tender, with edema of the feet and albuminuria. These are more probable if the right heart is involved. Dyspnea may be very marked.

The *course* depends largely on the extent of infarction and the previous condition of the myocardium. In some patients the most critical period is at the onset and for a short time after; in others the signs of shock are not specially marked at first, but the condition of the heart becomes much worse a few days later.

Diagnosis.—In typical cases there is little difficulty. The distinction from *angina pectoris* may give difficulty in cases lacking clear-cut features of either. The onset in angina is due to definite causes, not in coronary occlusion; the pain in angina is upper sternal, in occlusion, lower sternal; the duration in angina is short and the pain is relieved promptly by vasodilators and morphia, in occlusion the pain persists and is not relieved by vasodilators or by the usual dose of morphia. Fever, leukocytosis, marked change in the heart, and a fall in blood pressure are not found in angina. The difficulty comes in mild cases of coronary occlusion without typical features. The electrocardiogram may be of aid. It is safer to regard a doubtful case as coronary occlusion than to take the opposite view and make light of the symptoms.

Pulmonary infarction may give a picture much like coronary occlusion; they may occur together. The situation of the pain, bloody sputum, definite signs in the lung and the X-ray study should give the diagnosis of pulmonary infarction. An *acute abdominal* condition may be suggested. Formerly coronary occlusion was mistaken for this but with the emphasis laid on it, the more common error now is to diagnose an abdominal condition as occlusion. The pain of occlusion may be in the abdomen with muscular rigidity. Consideration of the difficulty and especially the findings in the heart are important. The previous history may be of value. The occurrence of upper abdominal pain, perhaps not severe, in a middle aged patient, especially after meals, should suggest the possibility of coronary occlusion, perhaps of mild degree.

Prognosis.—This must always be uncertain as regards the ultimate outlook; no one can predict the future as regards recurrences. The degree of injury to the myocardium is important and much depends on the efficiency of the muscle elsewhere than in the infarct. Time has taught us that the outlook is more favorable than we thought some years ago. As to the outcome of an attack it is well to be cautious and not too encouraging or too pessimistic. The evidence of the injury to the myocardium is the most important element and next in importance is the treatment given.

Treatment.—Absolute rest is essential. This should be secured by morphia given hypodermically, the first dose being one-half grain. If there is not prompt relief, one-third of a grain should be given. The repetition must depend on the condition but always give enough to secure comfort. Atropine may be added if there are signs of pulmonary congestion. Vasodilators should not be given. The patient should be kept warm and heat employed if there is shock. *Oxygen* is often helpful, even if there is no cyanosis. It should be given for some time and not stopped suddenly. The diet should be liquid and not over 1200 cc. given in 24 hours, unless large amounts of fluid have been lost by sweating. The bowels can be left alone for two or three days and then an oil enema given followed by a simple enema if necessary. Mineral oil can be given to secure soft stools; straining must be avoided.

The use of *digitalis* requires judgment. As a rule it should not be given unless there is evidence of marked myocardial failure and passive congestion. Caffeine may be given in an emergency and dextrose intravenously. After the acute features are over a sedative, such as phenobarbital, and theobromine (gr. v, 0.3 gm.) or metaphyllin (gr. 1½, 0.1 gm.) may be given for some time.

If the heart rate is very rapid, quinidine (gr. iii, 0.2 gm.) may be given every 8 hours.

The time of complete rest should be six weeks and longer if the attack was very severe or evidence of myocardial damage is marked. The increase in activity should be very gradual. The diet can be increased steadily. Vitamin C is advised in full doses. Small doses of digitalis may be useful during convalescence. After recovery a careful study of the patient's limits of exertion should be made and he should be impressed with the importance of keeping within them.

ENDOCARDITIS

Inflammation of the lining membrane of the heart is usually confined to the valves, so that the term is practically synonymous with valvular endocarditis. It occurs in several forms—*acute*, characterized by the presence of vegetations with loss of continuity or of substance in the valve tissues; *subacute;* and so-called *chronic* (better *sclerotic*) with a slow sclerotic change, resulting in thickening, puckering and deformity. A common form is an acute process occurring on sclerotic valves, already damaged—the so-called recurring endocarditis. The term "chronic endocarditis" is established by custom, but the process is sclerotic rather than inflammatory.

ACUTE ENDOCARDITIS

This may occur in rare instances as a primary, independent affection but in the great majority of cases it is a complication in various infective processes, so that in reality the disease does not constitute an etiological entity. For convenience of description we speak of a simple or benign, and a bacterial, malignant, ulcerative or infective endocarditis.

Etiology.—Simple endocarditis does not constitute a disease of itself, but is invariably found with some other affection. The most frequent cause is *rheumatic fever*. Bouillaud first emphasized the frequency of the association of simple endocarditis with rheumatic fever. Tonsillitis may be complicated with endocarditis. Of the specific diseases of childhood it is perhaps most common in scarlet fever, while it is rare in measles, diphtheria and smallpox. In typhoid fever it occurred in 6 of 1,500 cases.

In *pneumonia* both simple and malignant endocarditis occur. In 100 autopsies at the Montreal General Hospital there were 5 instances of the former. Among 61 cases of endocarditis studied bacteriologically, pneumococci were found in 21 (Marshall). Of 517 fatal cases of acute endocarditis, 115 were with pneumonia—22.3 per cent. (E. F. Wells). Acute endocarditis may occur in pulmonary tuberculosis and was found in 12 of 216 postmortems.

In *chorea* simple warty vegetations are found on the valves in a large majority of all fatal cases, in 62 of 73 collected cases. There is no disease in which, postmortem, acute endocarditis has been so frequently found. The endocarditis of *syphilis* possibly belongs here. Little is known of the early stages but it probably occurs both in acute and recurrent forms. It is usually observed in late stages. And, lastly, simple endocarditis is met with in diseases associated with progressive debility, as cancer, gout, and nephritis.

Subacute Bacterial Endocarditis. This develops in valves which have been damaged by previous endocarditis, usually rheumatic, or is associated with congenital lesions. The organism is the *Streptococcus viridans* in 90 per cent or over of the cases. The influenza bacillus and the gonococcus are found in the remainder. The most frequent age is between 20 and 30 years.

MALIGNANT, SEPTIC OR ULCERATIVE ENDOCARDITIS is met with: (*a*) As a primary disease of the lining membrane of the heart or of its valves.

(*b*) In pneumonia, in various fevers, in septic processes and most frequently as an infection on old sclerotic valves. In a majority of cases it is a local process in an acute infection. Congenital lesions are very prone to the severer forms of endocarditis, particularly affections of the pulmonary valves and the margins of an imperfect ventricular septum.

The existence of a primary endocarditis has been doubted; but there are instances in which persons previously in good health, without any history of affections with which endocarditis is usually associated, have been attacked by a severe infection. In one case death occurred on the sixth day and no lesions were found other than those of malignant endocarditis.

The simple endocarditis of rheumatic fever or of chorea rarely progresses into the malignant form. Of all acute diseases complicated with severe endocarditis pneumonia probably heads the list. Gonorrhea is a much more common cause than has been supposed. The affection may complicate erysipelas, septicemia (from whatever cause) and puerperal fever.

Morbid Anatomy.—SIMPLE ENDOCARDITIS is characterized by the presence on the valves or on the lining membrane of the chambers of minute vegetations, ranging from 1 to 4 mm. in diameter, with an irreguar and fissured surface, giving a warty or verrucose appearance. Often these little cauliflower-like excrescences are attached by very narrow pedicles. They are more common on the left side than the right, and on the mitral more often than on the aortic valves. The vegetations are on the line of closure of the valves—*i. e.*, on the auricular face of the auriculoventricular valves, a little distance from the margin, and on the ventricular side of the sigmoid valves. It is rare to see swelling or macroscopic evidence of infiltration of the endocardium in the neighborhood, or redness, even when they occur upon valves the seat of sclerotic changes, in which capillary vessels extend to the edges. With time the vegetations may increase greatly in size, but in simple endocarditis the size rarely exceeds that mentioned. Hirschfelder showed experimentally that they may form with great rapidity, even in a few hours.

The vegetations are composed of blood plates, leukocytes and fibrin in varying proportions. At a later stage they appear as small outgrowths of connective tissue. The transition of one form into the other can often be followed. The process consists of a proliferation of the endothelial cells and the cells of the subendothelial layer which invade the fresh vegetation, and ultimately entirely replace it. The blood cells and fibrin disintegrate and are gradually removed. Even when the vegetation has been entirely converted into connective tissue it is often found at autopsy to be capped with a thin layer of fibrin and leukocytes.

Micro-organisms may be found associated with the vegetations. They tend to be entangled in the granular and fibrillated fibrin or in the older ones to cap the apices.

Subsequent Changes.—(*a*) The vegetations may become organized and the valve restored to a normal state (?). (*b*) The process may extend, and a simple may become an ulcerative endocarditis. (*c*) The vegetations may be broken off and carried in the circulation to distant parts. (*d*) The vegetations become organized and disappear, but they initiate a nutritive change in the valve tissue which ultimately leads to *sclerosis,* thickening, and deformity. The danger in simple endocarditis is not immediate, but remote, and consists in the process which results in sclerosis of the valves.

Subacute Bacterial Endocarditis.—In this the lesion, which may be large or small, rarely ulcerates and if this occurs it is usually in the aortic valves. It involves the mitral more often than the aortic orifice and very rarely the right heart. The chordae tendineae are often involved and there may be mural endocarditis. Emboli are often detached. Glomerular changes may be found in the kidneys. If healing occurs there is fibroid change, possibly with calcareous deposit.

Malignant Endocarditis.—Practically in every case of this form vegetations are present. In it the loss of substance in the valve is more pronounced, the deposition—thrombus formation—from the blood is more extensive, and the organisms are present in greater number and often show increased virulence. This form is often found in heart valves already the seat of chronic changes or congenital disease.

There is much loss of substance, which may be superficial and limited to the endocardium, or, what is more common, it involves deeper structures, and not very infrequently leads to perforation of a valve, the septum or even of the heart itself. The affected valve shows necrosis, with more or less loss of substance; the tissue is devoid of preserved nuclei and presents a coagulated appearance. Upon it a mixture of blood plates, fibrin and leukocytes enclosing masses of micro-organisms is found. The subjacent tissue often shows sclerotic thickening and always infiltration with exuded cells.

Parts Affected.—The following figures, taken from the Goulstonian lectures (Osler) give an approximate estimate of the frequency with which in 209 cases different parts of the heart were affected in malignant endocarditis: Aortic and mitral valves together in 41; aortic valves alone in 53; mitral valves alone in 77; tricuspid in 19; the pulmonary valves in 15; and the heart walls in 33. In 9 instances the right heart alone was involved, in most cases the auriculoventricular valves.

Mural endocarditis is seen most often at the upper part of the septum of the left ventricle. Next in order is endocarditis of the left auricle on the postero-external wall. The vegetations may extend along the intima of the pulmonary artery into the lung. A common result of the ulceration is the production of valvular aneurism. In three-fourths of the cases the affected valves present old sclerotic changes. The process may extend to the aorta, producing extensive endarteritis with multiple acute aneurisms.

Associated Lesions.—The associated changes are those of the primary disease, those due to embolism, and the changes in the myocardium. In the endocarditis of septic processes there is the primary local lesion—an acute necrosis, a suppurative wound or puerperal disease.

The changes due to *embolism* are striking, but it is remarkable that in some instances, even with endocarditis of a markedly ulcerative character, there may be no trace of embolic processes. The *infarcts* may be few in number—only one or two, perhaps, in the spleen or kidney—or they may exist in hundreds throughout various parts of the body. They may present the ordinary appearance of red or white infarcts of a suppurative character. They are most common in the spleen and kidneys, though they may be numerous in the brain, and in many cases are abundant in the intestines. In right sided endocarditis there may be infarcts in the lungs. In many of the cases there are innumerable miliary abscesses. Acute suppurative *meningitis* was met with in 5 of 23 Montreal cases, and in over 10 per cent of 209 cases from the literature. Acute suppurative parotitis may occur. Lastly, the accompanying *myocarditis* plays an important rôle. The valvular insufficiency in acute endocarditis is probably not due to the row of little vegetations, but to the myocarditis, with resulting relative insufficiency.

Indeterminate Forms.—Under this heading Libman includes: (1) Atypical forms of verrucous endocarditis and (2) cases described as *terminal endocarditis* (diabetes, nephritis, etc.).

Bacteriology.—In malignant endocarditis, cocci—hemolytic streptococci, staphylococci, pneumococci and gonococci—are the most frequent. More rarely, especially in simple vegetative endocarditis, the bacilli of tuberculosis, typhoid fever and anthrax have been encountered. The colon bacillus has been found, and Howard described a case of malignant endocarditis due to an attenuated diphtheria bacillus. Marshall in 61 cases found the pneumococci in 21, streptococci alone or with other bacteria in 26 and staphylococcus aureus in 12. The meningococcus may cause endocarditis. Combined infections are not uncommon. In the subacute bacterial form the *Streptococcus viridans* is the common organism. As a rule no organisms are found in the simple endocarditis in chronic diseases, as tuberculosis, nephritis, etc. They may have been present and died out.

Symptoms.—The clinical course and the signs of SIMPLE ENDOCARDITIS are not characteristic. The majority of cases are latent and there is no indication of cardiac mischief. Endocarditis is frequently found postmortem in persons in whom it was not suspected during life. There are certain features, however, by which its presence is indicated with a degree of probability. The patient, as a rule, does not complain of any pain or cardiac distress. In rheumatic fever, the symptoms to excite suspicion would be increased rapidity of the heart, perhaps slight irregularity, and an increase in the fever, without aggravation of the arthritis. Rows of tiny vegetations on the valve segments seem a trifling matter to excite fever, and it is difficult in the endocarditis of febrile processes to say definitely in every instance that an increase in the fever depends upon this complication; but a study of recurring endocarditis shows that the process may be associated for weeks or months with fever from 100° to 103°. Palpitation may be marked and is a symptom upon which certain authors lay great stress.

The *diagnosis* rests upon physical signs, which are notoriously uncertain. A murmur in a case of fever is often taken as proof of the existence of endocarditis—a common mistake due to the fact that a murmur is common to it and to a number of other conditions. At first there may be only a slight roughening of the first sound, which may gradually increase to a distinct murmur. The apex systolic murmur is often the result of *myocarditis.* It may not be present in the endocarditis of chronic maladies as tuberculosis and carcinoma, since in them muscle involvement is less common (Krehl). Reduplication and accentuation of the pulmonic second sound are frequent. An aortic diastolic murmur is good evidence of endocarditis.

It is difficult to give a satisfactory clinical picture of MALIGNANT ENDOCARDITIS because the modes of onset are so varied and the symptoms so diverse. Arising in the course of some other disease, there may be simply an increase of the fever or a change in its character. In a majority of cases there are certain general features, such as irregular pyrexia, chills, toxemia, leukocytosis, sweating, delirium, and gradual failure of strength. Various clinical forms have been described depending on the most marked features, such as septic, typhoid and cerebral.

Embolic processes may give special features, such as delirium, coma or paralysis from involvement of the brain or its membranes, pain in the side and local peritonitis from infarction of the spleen, hematuria from implication of the kidneys, impaired vision from retinal hemorrhage and suppuration and even gangrene in various parts.

The "*septic form*" usually occurs in connection with an external wound, the puerperal process, acute necrosis or gonorrhea. There are rigors, sweats, irregular fever, and all the signs of septic infection. The heart symptoms may be completely masked by the general condition and attention called to them only by the occurrence of embolism. Optic neuritis is not uncommon, and was present in 15 cases of chronic septic endocarditis (Faulkner) and in four of these recurrent retinal hemorrhages occurred.

The "*typhoid form*" has a less irregular fever, early prostration, delirium, somnolence and coma, diarrhea, sweating, which may be of a drenching character, petechial and other rashes, and occasionally parotitis. The heart lesion may be completely overlooked and in some instances careful examination has failed to discover a murmur.

In the "*cerebral form*" the clinical picture may simulate a meningitis or meningitis may occur. There may be acute delirium or a variety of psychical changes, coma, paralysis or aphasia.

Certain special features may be mentioned. The *fever* is not always of a remittent type, but may be high and continuous. *Petechial rashes* are common and the similarity is strong to certain cases of typhoid and cerebrospinal fever. In one case the disease was thought to be hemorrhagic smallpox. There may be small hemorrhages in the palms and soles. Erythematous rashes are not uncommon. The sweating may be most profuse, exceeding that in pulmonary tuberculosis. *Diarrhea* is not necessarily associated with embolic lesions in the intestines. *Jaundice* has been observed and some cases have been mistaken for acute yellow atrophy. Cases with chronic valve disease usually present no difficulty in diagnosis. *Blood cultures* are usually positive and should be repeated if negative at first.

The *course* is varied, depending largely upon the nature of the primary trouble. Except in the disease grafted upon chronic valvulitis the course is rarely beyond five or six weeks. A rapidly fatal case was described by Eberth, the duration of which was scarcely two days.

Subacute Bacterial Endocarditis.—Due particularly to the work of Libman this has become a well recognized group. The clinical picture is varied; the prominent signs given by Libman are: (1) endocarditis; (2) multiple arterial embolism; (3) bacteria in the blood; and (4) fever. Certain other features are important: (*a*) marked progressive *anemia;* (*b*) *hemorrhagic* features, especially petechial; some cases of chronic purpura may belong here; (*c*) painful *cutaneous nodes,* red raised spots on the skin of the hands and feet lasting a few days (Osler nodes); (*d*) marked *renal* disease, due to embolism (embolic focal nephritis); (*e*) marked *splenic enlargement;* (*f*) *arthritis;* (*g*) symptoms from the *nervous system,* cerebral or meningeal; (*h*) *clubbing* of the fingers; and (*i*) brown *pigmentation* of the face. The renal changes are especially in the glomeruli and are embolic. Renal insufficiency is a common cause of death. The anemia is of the secondary type and usually the leukocytes are normal or diminished. Tenderness over the sternum may be found and be most marked in the bacteria-free stage.

As to the *course,* Libman's studies show that the patients with a positive blood culture nearly all die. If positive are followed by negative cultures, death usually occurs within a few months. In patients in whom the cultures are negative some are otherwise like those with positive cultures, others gradually lose the fever but die later, and in still others, fever may be absent for long periods. In the last group there has usually been previous endocarditis and anemia and renal disease are common. The duration may be from a few months to two years. There are all grades of severity and some cases are very mild. Some are very *acute* with a picture much like malignant endocarditis. Possibly some of these are instances of a double infection with hemolytic and nonhemolytic streptococci. There are occasional recurrent cases.

In many cases the process is engrafted on an old, sometimes an unrecognized, valve lesion. The *onset* may be insidious with indefinite symptoms, fatigue, general malaise and anorexia. At first fever may be the only feature; in a few cases there are chills at the onset or recurring chills may arouse the suspicion of malaria. The patient may keep at work with fever and perhaps an occasional sweat. The murmur of the old valve lesion may show no change, and even with the most extensive disease of the mitral cusps the heart's action may be little disturbed. For months, fever and progressive weakness may be the most marked features. It is in such cases that the embolic phenomena are of special aid in diagnosis. Hematuria or tender skin nodes may be suggestive. The emboli in the conjunctivae, or on the fingers and toes, occur as small painful red areas. With involvement of the aortic segments the signs of a progressive lesion are more common. There is marked secondary anemia and usually leukocytosis of considerable degree. Blood cultures should be taken at intervals and the cultures kept for some time as the organisms may grow slowly. Large amounts of blood should be used in order to secure uniform samples which make discovery more likely.

Diagnosis.—In many cases this is very difficult; in others, with marked embolic symptoms, it is easy. From simple endocarditis the subacute and malignant forms are readily distinguished, though confusion occasionally occurs in the transitional stage, when a simple is developing into a malignant form. The constitutional symptoms are graver, the fever is higher, rigors are common, and septic symptoms occur. Some of the cases not associated with puerperal processes or bone disease are confounded with typhoid fever. A differential diagnosis may be impossible until blood cultures or specific reactions are positive. Points which may guide us are: The more abrupt onset in endocarditis, the absence of any regularity of the pyrexia in the early stage and the cardiac features. Oppression and shortness of breath may be early symptoms. Rigors, too, are not uncommon. There is a marked leukocytosis in infective endocarditis. Between pyemia and malignant endocarditis there are practically no differential features, for the disease really constitutes an *arterial pyemia* (Wilks). In acute cases resembling the fevers the diagnosis of typhus, undulant, typhoid or cerebrospinal fever may be made. The intermittent pyrexia has led to the diagnosis of malaria but this disease can be excluded by the blood examination. Blood cultures aid greatly and are necessary for an etiological diagnosis. In the *subacute* form, a period of study may be necessary, especially if blood cultures are negative, and particular watch should be kept for the special features of this form. The occurrence of obscure fever in a patient with a heart lesion should immediately put the practitioner on his guard.

Prognosis.—In acute simple endocarditis the outlook for recovery is good as regards life, except in severe cases of carditis in rheumatic fever, but there is likely to be permanent damage of the valve. In the subacute bacterial form, death usually results. In 1934, Libman stated that he had seen 17 recoveries. The malignant form is practically always fatal.

Treatment.—We know no measures by which in rheumatic fever, chorea, or the eruptive fevers endocarditis can be prevented. As many cases arise, particularly in children, in mild forms of these diseases, it is well to insist upon rest and quiet, and to bear in mind that an acute endocarditis, though in its immediate effects mild, is ultimately serious. This is enforced by the observations of Sibson that on a system of absolute *rest* the proportion of cases of rheumatic fever attacked by endocarditis was less than of those who were not so treated. It is doubtful in rheumatic fever whether the salicylates reduce the liability to endocarditis. Considering the extremely grave after-results of simple endocarditis in children, the question arises whether it is possible to do anything to avert the onset of progressive sclerosis of the affected valve. Caton recommends: (1) Prolonged rest in bed for three months; (2) a series of small blisters over the heart; and (3) iodide of potassium in moderate doses for many months. If there is much vascular excitement an ice-bag may be placed over the heart. The treatment of the subacute bacterial and malignant endocarditis is practically that of septicopyemia—useless and hopeless in a majority of the cases. Blood transfusion, which entails some risk, should be done only if severe anemia demands it, not with any idea of influencing the infection. We have never seen any benefit from the transfusion of blood from a donor to whom a vaccine made from the organism obtained from the patient had been given. It may result in sudden death. Proof is lacking that antiseptic drugs given intravenously are of value. The same may be said of serum and vaccines. Capps advises sodium cacodylate (gr. i-iv, 0.06-0.24 gm. daily, intravenously) in the subacute bacterial form. It is given until there is a garlic odor to the breath.

CHRONIC SCLEROTIC ENDOCARDITIS

Definition.—A sclerosis of the valves leading to shrinking, thickening and adhesion of the cusps, often with the deposition of lime salts, with shortening and thickening of the chordae tendinae, leading to insufficiency and to narrowing of the orifice. It may be primary, but is more often secondary to acute endocarditis, particularly the rheumatic form.

Etiology.—It is a mistake to regard every case of sclerotic valve as a sequel to an acute endocarditis. Long ago Roy and Adami called attention to the possibility that sclerosis of the valve segments might be a sequel of high pressure. The preliminary endocarditis may be a factor in weakening the valve, the progressive thickening of which may be a direct consequence of the strain. As age advances the valves begin to lose their pliancy, show slight sclerotic changes and foci of atheroma and calcification. The toxins of the specific fevers may initiate the change. A very important factor in the case of the aortic valves is *syphilis*. The strain of prolonged and heavy muscular exertion may play a part. In the aortic segments it may be only the valvular part of a general arteriosclerosis.

The *frequency* of sclerotic endocarditis may be gathered from the following figures: In various autopsy series the percentage has ranged from four to nine. The relative frequency of involvement of the valves is thus given in the collected statistics of Parrot: The mitral orifice in 621, aortic in 380, tricuspid in 46, and pulmonary in 11. This gives 57 instances in the right to 1,001 in the left heart.

Morbid Anatomy.—Vegetations such as occur in acute endocarditis are not present. In the early stage, the edge of the valve is a little thickened and perhaps presents a few small nodular prominences, which in some cases may represent the healed vegetations of the acute process. In the aortic valves the tissue about the corpora Arantii is first affected, producing a slight thickening with an increase in the size of the nodules. The substance of the valve may lose its translucency with a grayish opacity and slight loss of its delicate tenuity. In the auriculoventricular valves these early changes are seen just within the margin and here it is not uncommon to find swellings of a grayish red, somewhat infiltrated appearance, almost identical with the similar structures on the intima of the aorta in arteriosclerosis. Even early there may be yellow or opaque white subintimal fatty degenerated areas. As the sclerotic changes increase, the fibrous tissue contracts and produces thickening and deformity of the segment, the edges of which become round, curled, and incapable of that delicate apposition necessary for perfect closure. An aortic valve may be narrowed one fourth or even one third across its face, the most extreme grade of insufficiency being induced without any special deformity and without narrowing of the orifice. In the auriculoventricular segments a simple process of thickening and curling of the edges of the valves, inducing a failure to close without forming any obstruction to the normal course of the blood-flow, is less common. Still, we meet with instances at the mitral orifice, in which the edges of the valves are curled and thickened, so that there is extreme insufficiency without any material narrowing of the orifice. More frequently, as the disease advances, the chordae tendinae become thickened, first at the valvular ends and then along their course. The edges of the valves at their angles are gradually drawn together and there is a narrowing of the orifice, leading to more or less stenosis. Finally, in the sclerotic and necrotic tissues lime salts are deposited and may even reach the deeper structures of the fibrous rings, so that the entire valve becomes a dense calcareous mass. The chordae tendinae may gradually become shortened, greatly thickened, and in extreme cases the papillary muscles are implanted directly upon the sclerotic valve. The apices of the papillary muscles usually show marked fibroid change. In all stages the vegetations of simple endocarditis may be present, and the severe ulcerative forms often attack these sclerotic valves.

Chronic *mural* endocarditis produces cicatricial-like patches of a grayish white appearance which are sometimes seen on the muscular trabeculae of the ventricle or in the auricles. It often occurs with myocarditis.

The endocarditis of the *fetus* is usually of the sclerotic form and involves the valves of the right more frequently than those of the left side.

CHRONIC VALVULAR DISEASE

Effects of Valve Lesions.—The general influence on the work of the heart may be briefly stated as follows: The changes in the valves induce insufficiency or stenosis, which may exist separately or in combination. The narrowing retards the normal flow and the insufficiency permits the blood current to take an abnormal course. The result in the former case is difficulty in the expulsion of the contents of the chamber through the narrow orifice; in the other, the overfilling of a chamber by blood flowing into it from an improper source as in mitral insufficiency, when the left auricle receives blood both from the pulmonary veins and from the left ventricle. In both instances the effect is dilatation of a chamber, and to expel the normal amount of blood from a dilated chamber a relatively greater amount of energy is required, which by various adjustments the muscle is stimulated to do.

The cardiac mechanism is fully prepared to meet ordinary grades of dilatation which constantly occur during sudden exertion. A man at the end of a hundred yard race has his right chambers greatly dilated and his reserve cardiac power worked to its full capacity. The slow progress of sclerotic changes brings about a gradual, not an abrupt, insufficiency, and the moderate dilatation which follows is at first overcome by the ordinary reserve strength of the heart muscle. Gradually a new factor is introduced. The constant increase in the energy put forth by the heart is a stimulus to the muscle fibres to increase in bulk and probably also in number; the heart hypertrophies, and the effect of the valve lesion becomes *compensated.* The equilibrium of the circulation is in this way maintained.

The nature of the process is illustrated in the accompanying diagram, from Martius. The perpendicular lines in the figures represent the power of work of the heart. While the muscle in the healthy heart (Diagram I) has at its disposal the maximal force, *a c*, it carries on its work under ordinary circumstances (when the body is at rest) with the force *a b* and *b c* is the reserve force by which the heart accommodates itself to greater exertion.

If there be a gross valvular lesion, the force required to do the ordinary work of the heart (at rest) becomes very much increased (Diagram II). But in spite of this enormous call for force, insufficiency of the muscles does not necessarily result, for the working force required is still within the limits of the maximal power of the heart, a_1 b_1 being less than a_1 c_1. The muscle accommodates itself to the new condition by making its reserve force mobile. If nothing further occurred, this could not be permanently maintained, for there would be left over for emergencies only the small reserve force b_1 y. Even at rest the heart would be using continuously almost its entire maximal force. Any slight exertion requiring more extra force than that represented by the small value, b_1 y (say the effort required on going upstairs) would

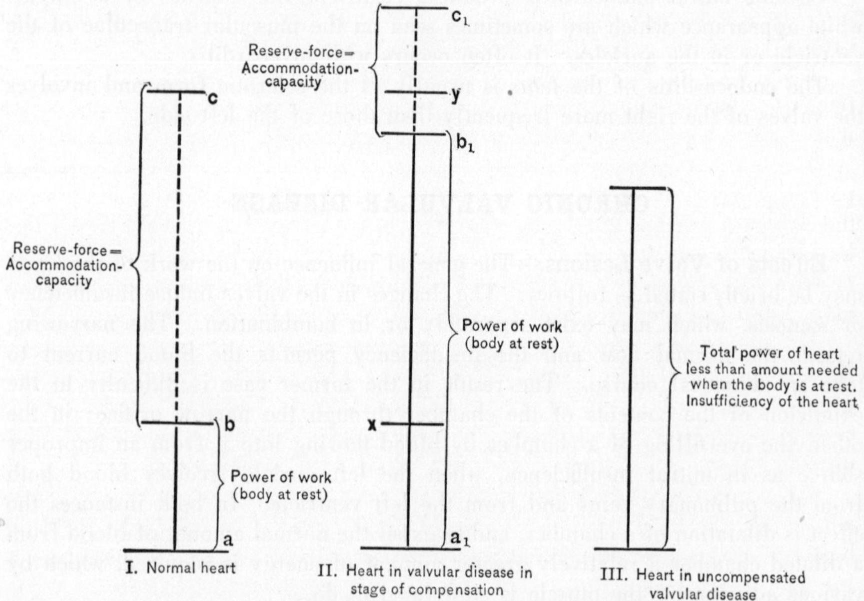

Fig. 12.—Diagrammatic Presentation Showing the Force of the Heart for Work under Normal Conditions and in Valvular Lesions.

bring the heart to the limit of its working power, and dyspnea would appear. Such a condition does not last long. The working power of the heart gradually increases. More and more exertion can be borne without causing dyspnea, for *the heart hypertrophies.* Finally, a new, more or less permanent condition is attained, in that the hypertrophied heart possesses the maximal force, a_1 c_1. Owing to the increase in volume of the heart muscle, the total force of the heart is greater *absolutely* than that of the normal heart by the amount y c_1. It is, however, *relatively* less efficient, for its reserve force is much less than that of the healthy heart. Its capacity to accommodate itself to unusual calls is permanently diminished.

Turning to the disturbances of compensation, it is to be borne in mind that any heart, normal or diseased, can become insufficient whenever a call upon it exceeds its maximal working capacity. The liability to such disturbance will depend, above all, upon the accommodation limits of the heart—the less the width of the latter, the easier will it be to go beyond the heart's efficiency. A comparison of Diagrams I and II will make it clear that the heart in valvular disease will become insufficient much earlier than the heart of a healthy individual. The heart in valvular disease, on account of its small reserve force, has to do maximal or nearly maximal work far more frequently than the normal heart. The power of the heart may become decreased to the amount necessary simply to carry on its work when the body is at rest, or it may cease to be sufficient even for this. The reserve force gained through the compensatory process may be entirely lost (Diagram III).

AORTIC INSUFFICIENCY

This best-defined and most easily recognized of valvular lesions was first carefully studied by Corrigan, whose name it sometimes bears.

Etiology and Morbid Anatomy.—It is more frequent in males than in females, affecting chiefly men at the middle period of life. The ratio which it bears to other valve diseases has been given as from 30 to 50 per cent.

There are six groups of cases: I. Those due to *congenital malformation*, particularly fusion of two of the cusps—most commonly those behind which the coronary arteries are given off. It is possible that such aortic valves may be competent but a great danger is the liability of the malformed segments to sclerotic changes. Of 17 cases all presented sclerotic changes, and the majority had, during life, the clinical features of chronic heart disease.

II. *Endocarditic Group.*—Endocarditis may produce an acute insufficiency by ulceration and destruction of the valves; the aortic valves may be completely eroded away. In the valvulitis of rheumatic fever, the insufficiency is caused by nodular excrescences at the margins or in the valves, which may ultimately become calcified; more often it induces a slow sclerosis.

III. *Syphilis.*—This is the most important cause, certainly in young adults and middle-aged patients. In a series of 200 cases in the Jefferson Hospital, Regester found about 60 per cent due to syphilis. The spirochetes may be found in the valves. The process begins in the aorta and involves the valves secondarily by extension or causes dilatation of the aortic ring with relative insufficiency. Some of the supposed cases of cure of aortic endocarditis may be instances of the latter.

IV. *Arteriosclerotic Group.*—A common cause of insufficiency is a slow, progressive sclerosis of the segments, resulting in a curling of the edges. It may be associated with general arteriosclerosis. The condition of the valves is such as has been described in chronic endocarditis. It may be noted, however, how slight a grade of curling may produce serious insufficiency. Associated with the valve disease is, in a majority of cases, a more or less advanced arteriosclerosis of the arch of the aorta, one serious effect of which may be a narrowing of the orifices of the coronary arteries. The sclerotic changes are often combined with atheroma which may exist at the attached margin of the valves without inducing insufficiency. In other instances insufficiency may result from a calcified spike projecting from the aortic attachment into the body of the valve, and so preventing its proper closure. Anatomically one can usually recognize the arteriosclerotic variety by the smooth surface, the rounded edges and the absence of excrescences.

V. Insufficiency may be induced by *rupture of a segment*—a very rare event in healthy valves, but not uncommon in disease, either from excessive effort or from the ordinary strain on a valve eroded and weakened by ulcerative endocarditis or damaged by syphilis.

VI. *Relative insufficiency*, due to dilatation of the aortic ring and adjacent arch, is very infrequent. It occurs in extensive sclerosis of the ascending portion of the arch with great dilatation just above the valves. The valve segments are usually involved with the aorta but the changes in them may be slight. In aneurism just above the aortic ring relative insufficiency of the valve may be present. Whether aortic insufficiency occurs from dilatation of the left ventricle has been much discussed—a relative incompetency similar to that which occurs at the pulmonary orifice. There are cases in which transient diastolic murmurs occur with dilatation of the heart. J. B. MacCallum, whose untimely death was a great loss to science, described a sphincter-like band of muscle encircling the opening of the left ventricle into the aorta, and relaxation of this ring muscle may cause insufficiency of the valve.

Insufficiency may be combined with various grades of narrowing, particularly in the endocarditic group. In a majority of the cases of the arteriosclerotic form there is no stenosis but with aortic stenosis there is almost without exception some grade, however, slight, of insufficiency.

Effects.—The direct effect of aortic insufficiency is the regurgitation of blood from the aorta into the ventricle, causing an overdistention of the cavity and a reduction of the blood column; that is, a relative anemia in the arterial tree. The amount returning varies with the size of the opening. The double blood flow into the left ventricle causes dilatation of the chamber, and finally hypertrophy, the grade depending upon the lesion. In this way the valve defect is compensated, and, as with each systole a larger amount of blood is propelled into the arterial system, the regurgitation of a certain amount during diastole does not, for a time at least, seriously impair the nutrition of the peripheral parts. For a time there is little or no resistance offered to the blood flow from the auricle—the ventricle accommodates itself readily to the extra amount, and there is no disturbance in the lesser circulation. In acute cases with rapid destruction of the segments or rupture there may be the most intense dyspnea and even profuse hemoptysis. The distress may be extreme in cases of rupture of a valve.

In this lesion dilatation and hypertrophy reach their most extreme limit. The heaviest hearts on record are described in this affection. The so-called bovine heart, *cor bovinum*, may weigh 35 or 40 ounces, or, as in a case of Dulles's, 48 ounces. The dilatation is usually extreme and is in marked contrast to the condition in pure aortic stenosis. The papillary muscles may be greatly flattened. The mitral valves are usually not seriously affected, though the edges may present slight sclerosis, and there is often *relative insufficiency*, owing to distention of the mitral ring. Dilatation and hypertrophy of the left auricle are common, and secondary enlargement of the right heart occurs in all cases of long standing. In the arteriosclerotic and syphilitic groups there is an ever present possibility of narrowing of the orifices of the coronary arteries or an extension of the sclerosis to them, leading to fibroid myocardial degeneration. In the endocarditis cases the intima of the aorta may be perfectly smooth. The so-called *dynamic dilatation* of the arch is best seen in these cases. A young girl, whose case had been reported as one of aneurism, had forcible pulsation and a tumor which could be grasped above the sternum

—postmortem the innominate artery did not admit the little finger and the arch was not dilated!

The effect on the blood supply of the *coronary arteries* is important as they miss the effect of the blood pressure during diastole, which aids in keeping the coronary vessels full. The influence on the myocardium is evident. The arteries of the body usually present more or less sclerosis due to the strain which they undergo during the forcible ventricular systole. The systolic pressure is usually increased but this is not always present.

Symptoms.—The condition is often discovered accidentally in persons who have not presented any features of cardiac disease. Headache, dizziness and a feeling of faintness on rising quickly are among the early symptoms. Palpitation and distress on slight exertion are common. Long before any signs of failing compensation, *pain* may be a marked feature. It is extremely variable and may be of a dull, aching character confined to the precordia but more frequently it is sharp and radiating, and transmitted up the neck and down the arms, particularly the left. Disease of the aorta is often responsible for pain. Angina pectoris is more frequent with this than any other valve lesion. Anemia is common, much more so than in aortic stenosis or mitral affections. Distressing dreams and disturbed sleep occur more in this than in other forms of valvular disease.

Mental symptoms are often seen with this lesion or the patients may be irritable and difficult to manage; toward the close there may be delirium, hallucinations and morbid impulses. It is important to bear this in mind, for patients occasionally display suicidal tendencies.

Physical Signs.—*Inspection* shows a wide area of forcible impulse with the apex beat in the sixth or seventh interspace, and perhaps as far out as the anterior axillary line. In young subjects the precordia may bulge. In very slight insufficiency there may be little or no enlargement. On *palpation* a diastolic thrill is occasionally felt but is not common. The impulse is usually strong and heaving, unless in dilatation, when it is wavy and indefinite. Occasionally two or three interspaces over the heart are depressed with systole from atmospheric pressure. *Percussion* shows a great increase in the heart dulness, chiefly downward and to the left.

Auscultation.—A diastolic murmur is heard at the base of the heart and propagated down the sternum. It may be feeble or inaudible at the aortic cartilage, and is often heard best at midsternum opposite the third costal cartilage or along the left border of the sternum. It is usually blowing and prolonged, or "long drawn," as the phrase is. It is produced by the reflux of blood into the ventricle. In some cases it is loudly transmitted to the axilla at the level of the fourth interspace, not by way of the apex. The second sound may be heard or be replaced by the murmur, or with a dilated arch the second sound may have a ringing metallic or booming quality and the diastolic murmur is well heard, or even loudest, over the manubrium. Occasionally over the carotid artery the second sound is distinctly audible when absent at the aortic cartilage and, according to Broadbent, it is at the carotid that we must listen for the second aortic sound, for when heard it indicates that the regurgitation is small in amount, and is consequently a favorable prognostic element. In the larger arteries a systolic thud or shock may be heard and sometimes a double murmur.

The first sound may be clear at the base; more commonly there is a soft, short, systolic murmur. In the arteriosclerotic group the systolic murmur is, as a rule, short and soft, while in the endocarditic group, in which the valve segments are united and sometimes calcified, the systolic murmur is rough and may be accompanied by a thrill.

At the apex, or toward it, the diastolic murmur may be faintly heard, propagated from the base. With full compensation the first sound is usually clear at the apex; with dilatation there is a loud systolic murmur of relative mitral insufficiency, which may disappear as the dilatation lessens.

Flint Murmur.—A second murmur at the apex, to which attention was called by the late Austin Flint, is not uncommon. It is of a rumbling, echoing character, occurring in the middle or latter part of diastole, and limited to the apex region. It is less intense than the murmur of mitral stenosis, and may be associated with a thrill. It is probably caused by the impinging of the regurgitant current from the aortic orifice on the large, anterior flap of the mitral valve, so as to cause interference with the entrance of blood at the time of auricular contraction. The condition is thus essentially the same as in a moderate mitral stenosis. This murmur is present in about half of the cases of uncomplicated aortic insufficiency (Thayer). It is very variable, disappearing and reappearing without apparent cause. The sharp, first sound and abrupt systolic shock, so common in true mitral stenosis, are rarely present, while the pulse is characteristic of aortic insufficiency.

Arteries.—The examination of the arteries is of great value. *Visible pulsation* is more commonly seen in the peripheral vessels in this than in any other condition. With the ophthalmoscope the retinal arteries are seen to pulsate. Not only is the pulsation evident, but the characteristic *jerking quality* is apparent. The throbbing carotids may lead to the diagnosis of aneurism. In many cases pulsation can be seen in the suprasternal notch and the abdominal aorta may lift the epigastrium with each systole. In severe cases with great hypertrophy, particularly with anemia, the vascular throbbing may be of an extraordinary character, jarring the whole front of the chest, causing the head to nod, and even the tongue may throb rhythmically. To be mentioned with this is the *capillary pulse,* seen very often in aortic insufficiency, best under the thumb nail or by drawing a line upon the forehead, when the margin of hyperemia on either side alternately blushes and pales. In extreme grades the face or the hand may blush visibly at each systole. It is met with also in profound anemia, occasionally in neurasthenia, and in conditions of great relaxation of the peripheral arteries. Pulsation may also be present in the peripheral veins. On palpation the characteristic *collapsing* or *Corrigan* pulse is felt. The pulse wave strikes the finger forcibly with a quick jerking impulse and immediately recedes or collapses. This is sometimes best appreciated by grasping the arm at the wrist and holding it up. The pulse may be delayed—*i. e.,* there is an appreciable interval between the beat of the heart and the pulsation in the radial artery, which varies according to the extent of the regurgitation.

The systolic pressure is variable and is often high; the diastolic is low and sometimes can not be obtained. This disproportion—a *high pulse pressure*—is characteristic. The systolic pressure in the femoral is higher than in the brachial artery. The sphygmographic tracing is very characteristic, showing the high ascent, the sharp top, and the quick drop in which the dicrotic notch and wave are very slightly marked.

The studies of Stewart and of W. G. MacCallum showed that the low position of the dicrotic notch in the descending arm of the pulse wave and the collapsing pulse are not due, as was formerly supposed, to the regurgitation in the left ventricle, but to dilatation of the peripheral arteries, which is a sort of protective adaptation under the vasomotor influences.

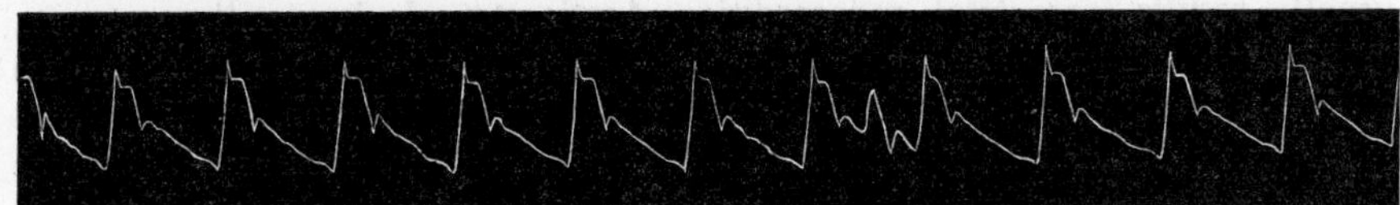

Fig. 13.—Pulse Tracing in Aortic Insufficiency; an Extra Systole is Shown.

Aortic insufficiency may be fully *compensated* for years and the patients may not suffer any inconvenience; it is often found accidentally. So long as the hypertrophy equalizes the valvular defect there may be no symptoms and the individual may take moderate exercise without distress. The cases which last the longest are those in which the insufficiency follows endocarditis and is not part of a general arteriosclerosis. The age at the time of onset is important as in youth the lesion is not often from sclerosis, and the coronary arteries are unaffected. Coexistent lesions of the mitral valve tend to disturb compensation early. Pure aortic insufficiency is consistent with years of average health and with a tolerably active life. Alterations in the electrocardiogram may aid in prognosis. Increase in the P-R interval and the QRS complex, inversion of the T wave in Lead II, and lack of correspondence in the routine findings are of serious import.

With the onset of myocardial changes, with increasing degeneration of the arteries, particularly with a progressive sclerosis of the arch and involvement of the orifices of the coronary arteries, the compensation becomes disturbed. The insufficiency of the circulation is seen first on the arterial side in occasional fainting, giddiness, or mental irritability and enfeeblement; later there may be mitral regurgitation and embarrassment of the right heart.

AORTIC STENOSIS

Definite aortic stenosis is a rare lesion. It may occur with insufficiency and probably in almost every case of stenosis there is some leakage.

Etiology and Morbid Anatomy.—In the milder grades there is adhesion between the segments, which are so stiffened that during systole they cannot be pressed back against the aortic wall. The process of cohesion between the segments may go on without great thickening, and produce a condition in which the orifice is guarded by a comparatively thin membrane, on the aortic face of which may be seen the primitive raphes separating the sinuses of Valsalva. In some instances this membrane is so thin and presents so few traces of sclerotic changes that the condition looks as if it was congenital. More commonly the valve segments are thickened and rigid with a cartilaginous hardness. In advanced cases they may be represented by calcified masses obstructing the orifice, through which a circular or slit-like passage is seen. The older the patient the more likely it is that the valves will be rigid and calcified.

We may speak of a *relative stenosis* when with normal valves and ring the aorta immediately beyond is greatly dilated. A stenosis due to involvement of the aortic ring in sclerotic changes without lesion of the valves is referred to by some authors but we have never met with an instance. A subvalvular stenosis, the result of endocarditis in the mitrosigmoidean sinus, usually results from fetal endocarditis. Aortic stenosis is usually met with at a more advanced period of life than insufficiency, and the most typical cases are associated with extensive arterial changes in old men.

Owing to the obstruction the ventricle works against increased resistance and its walls become hypertrophied, usually at first with little or no dilatation. In this condition are the most typical instances of concentric hypertrophy, in which, without much, if any, enlargement of the cavity, the walls are greatly thickened. The systole is prolonged, even as much as twenty-five per cent. There may be no changes in the other cardiac cavities if compensation is well maintained. The amount of blood propelled through the narrow orifice may be smaller than normal, though when compensation is good the pulse may be of medium volume.

Symptoms.—The condition may be latent for an indefinite period, as long as hypertrophy is maintained. Early symptoms are due to defective blood supply to the brain, dizziness and fainting. Palpitation, pain about the heart, and anginal symptoms are not so marked as in insufficiency. Many cases in old people have symptoms pointing rather to general arterial disease. Cheyne-Stokes breathing is not uncommon with or without anemia.

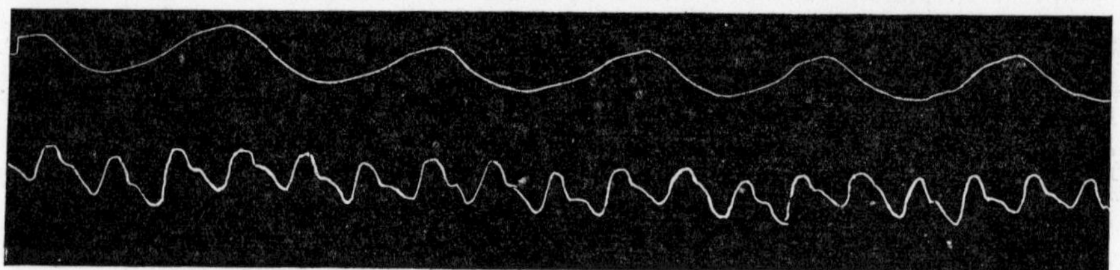

FIG. 14.—PULSE TRACING IN AORTIC STENOSIS.

PHYSICAL SIGNS.—*Inspection* may fail to reveal any cardiac impulse, particularly in old men with rigid chest walls and emphysematous lungs. Under these circumstances there may be a high grade of hypertrophy without any visible impulse. Even when the apex beat is visible, it may be feeble and indefinite. In many cases the apex is displaced downward and outward, and the impulse looks strong and forcible.

Palpation reveals in many cases a *thrill* at the base of the heart of maximum force in the aortic region felt best at full expiration. The apex beat may not be palpable or there may be a slow, heaving, forcible impulse.

Percussion never gives the same wide area of dulness as in aortic insufficiency and its extent depends largely on the state of the lungs.

Auscultation.—A rough systolic murmur is heard with maximum intensity at the aortic area and propagated into the great vessels. One of the last lessons learned by the student is to recognize that a systolic murmur at the aortic area does not necessarily mean stenosis. Roughening of the valves or of the intima of the aorta, and hemic states are much more frequent causes. In aortic stenosis the murmur has a harsher quality, is louder and more frequently musical than in the conditions just mentioned. When compensation fails the murmur may be soft and distant. The second sound is rarely heard at the aortic area, owing to the thickening and stiffness of the valve. A diastolic murmur is not uncommon. The *pulse* in pure aortic stenosis is small, usually of good tension, with a slow rise, well sustained, regular, and perhaps slower than normal.

Diagnosis.—With an extremely rough or musical systolic murmur of maximum intensity at the aortic region and transmitted to the vessels of the neck, hypertrophy of the left ventricle, a systolic thrill, and a hard, slow pulse of moderate volume, which in a tracing gives a curve of slow rise, a broad, well sustained summit and slow decline, a diagnosis of aortic stenosis can be made with some degree of certainty, particularly in an elderly patient. In aortic insufficiency a systolic murmur is usually present, but has neither the intensity nor is it accompanied by a thrill. With dilatation of the aorta, the murmur may be harsh or musical; but the existence of a second sound, accentuated and ringing, usually differentiates this condition.

MITRAL INSUFFICIENCY

Etiology.—Insufficiency of the mitral valve ensues: (*a*) From changes in the segments whereby they are contracted and shortened, usually combined with changes in the chordae tendineae, or with more or less narrowing of the orifice. (*b*) As a result of changes in the walls of the ventricle, either dilatation, so that the valve segments fail to close an enlarged orifice, or changes in the muscular substance, so that the segments are imperfectly coapted during the systole—*muscular insufficiency*. The common lesions producing insufficiency result from endocarditis, which causes a gradual thickening at the edges of the valves, contraction of the chordae tendineae, and union of the edges of the segments, so that in a majority of cases there is not only insufficiency, but some narrowing as well. Except in children, we rarely see the mitral leaflets curled and puckered without narrowing of the orifice. Calcareous plates at the base of the valve may prevent perfect closure of the segments. (*c*) From sclerosis of the valves, not due to endocarditis but with general arteriosclerosis, especially in elderly patients. It is possible that this occurs in some cases of syphilis.

In long-standing cases the entire mitral structures are converted into a firm calcareous ring. From *valvular insufficiency* the condition of *muscular insufficiency* must be carefully distinguished. It is met with in dilatation of the left ventricle and in weakening of the muscle in fevers and anemia.

Morbid Anatomy.—The effects of mitral insufficiency are as follows: (*a*) The imperfect closure allows blood to regurgitate from the ventricle into the auricle, so that at the end of diastole this chamber contains not only the blood from the lungs, but also that regurgitated from the left ventricle. This necessitates dilatation, and, as increased work is thrown upon it in expelling the augmented contents, hypertrophy as well.

(*b*) With each systole of the left auricle a larger volume of blood is forced into the left ventricle, which dilates and subsequently hypertrophies.

(*c*) During diastole, as blood is regurgitated into the auricle from the left ventricle, the pulmonary veins are less readily emptied. In consequence the right ventricle expels its contents less freely, and in turn becomes hypertrophied and dilated.

(*d*) Finally, the right auricle also is involved, its chamber is enlarged, and its walls are increased in thickness.

(*e*) The effect upon the *pulmonary vessels* is to produce dilatation both of the arteries and veins—often in long-standing cases, atheromatous changes; the capillaries are distended, and ultimately brown induration is produced. Perfect compensation may be effected, chiefly through the hypertrophy of both ventricles, and the effect upon the peripheral circulation may not be manifested for years, as a normal volume of blood is discharged from the left heart at each systole. The time comes, however, when, owing either to increase in the grade of incompetency or to failure of compensation, the left ventricle is unable to send out its normal volume. For years this congested condition may be limited to the lesser circulation, but finally the tricuspid valves become incompetent, and the systemic veins are engorged. This leads to passive congestion and, when extreme, to edema.

Muscular insufficiency is rarely followed by such perfect compensation. There may be in acute destruction of the aortic segments an acute dilatation of the left ventricle with relative mitral incompetency, great dilatation of the left auricle, and intense engorgement of the lungs from which profuse hemorrhage may result. In these cases there is little chance for the establishment of compensation. In cases of hypertrophy and dilatation of the heart, without valvular lesions, the insufficiency of the mitral valve may be extreme and lead to great pulmonary congestion, engorgement of the systemic veins, and cardiac dropsy, which can not be distinguished from that of mitral insufficiency due to lesion of the valve itself. In *chronic nephritis* the left ventricle may gradually fail, leading to relative mitral insufficiency and passive congestion, similar to that due to lesion of the valve itself. Adherent pericardium, especially in children, may lead to like results.

Symptoms.—During the development of the lesion, unless the insufficiency comes on acutely, the compensatory changes go hand in hand with the defect, and there are no subjective symptoms. So, also, in the stage of perfect compensation, there may be an extreme grade of mitral insufficiency with enormous hypertrophy, yet the patient may not be aware of the existence of heart trouble, and suffer no inconvenience except perhaps a little dyspnea on exertion. It is only when the compensation has not been perfectly effected, or, having been so, is broken that the patients begin to be troubled. The symptoms may be divided into two groups:

(*a*) The *minor* manifestations while compensation is still good. Patients with marked insufficiency often have a congested appearance of the face, the lips and ears have a bluish tint, and the venules on the cheeks may be enlarged—signs in many cases very suggestive. In long standing cases, particularly in children, the fingers may be clubbed, and there is shortness of breath on exertion. This is one of the most constant features and may exist for years. Owing to the passive congestion of the lungs these patients are liable to bronchitis or hemoptysis. There may also be palpitation. As a rule, however, in well balanced lesions in adults, this period of full compensation is not associated with symptoms which call the attention to an affection of the heart, and with care the patient may reach old age in comparative comfort without having to curtail seriously his pleasures or his work.

(*b*) Sooner or later comes a period of *broken compensation* (myocardial insufficiency) in which the most intense symptoms are those of venous engorgement. There are palpitation, weak, irregular action of the heart and signs of dilatation. The irregularity may be due to extra systoles or auricular fibrillation. Dyspnea is an especial feature and there may be cough. A distressing symptom is the cardiac "sleep-start," in which, just as the patient falls asleep, he wakes gasping and feeling as if the heart were stopping. There is usually slight cyanosis, and even slight jaundice. The most marked symptoms are those of venous stasis. The congestion of the pulmonary vessels accounts in part for the dyspnea. There is cough, often with bloody or watery expectoration. Edema usually sets in, beginning in the feet and extending to the body and the serous sacs. Right sided hydrothorax may recur and require repeated tapping. The urine is usually scanty and albuminous, and contains casts and sometimes blood cells. With judicious treatment compensation may be restored and the serious symptoms pass away. Patients usually have recurring attacks of this kind, and die with a general dropsy; or there is progressive dilatation of the heart. Sudden death in these cases is rare. Some cases of mitral disease reach what may be called the *hepatic stage,* when the predominant features are due to the secondary changes in the liver.

PHYSICAL SIGNS.—*Inspection.*—In children the precordia may bulge and there may be a large area of visible pulsation. The apex beat is to the left of the nipple, in some cases in the sixth interspace, in the anterior axillary line. There may be a wavy impulse in the cervical veins, which are often full, particularly when the patient is recumbent.

Palpation.—The force of the impulse depends largely upon the stage. In full compensation it is forcible and heaving; when myocardial insufficiency is present, usually wavy and feeble.

Percussion.—The dulness is increased and there may be an extensive transverse area of heart dulness. It does not extend so much upward along the left margin of the sternum as beyond the right margin and to the left of the nipple line.

Auscultation.—At the apex there is a systolic murmur which wholly or partly obliterates the first sound. It is loudest here, and has a blowing, sometimes musical character, particularly toward the latter part. It is transmitted to the axilla and may be heard at the back, in some instances over the entire chest. There are cases in which the murmur is heard best along the left border of the sternum. Usually at the apex the transmitted second sound may be heard. Occasionally there is also a soft, sometimes a rough or rumbling presystolic murmur. As a rule, in extreme mitral insufficiency from valvular lesion with great hypertrophy of both ventricles, there is heard only a loud blowing murmur during systole. A murmur of mitral insufficiency may vary a great deal, according to the position of the patient. An important sign is an accentuated pulmonary second sound.

The *pulse*, during the period of full compensation, may be full and regular, often of low tension. With the first onset of symptoms it may become irregular, a feature which persists and is usually due to auricular fibrillation.

The three important physical signs of mitral regurgitation are: (*a*) Systolic murmur of maximum intensity at the apex, propagated to the axilla and heard at the angle of the scapula; (*b*) accentuation of the pulmonary second sound; (*c*) evidence of enlargement of the heart, particularly increase in the transverse diameter, due to hypertrophy of both ventricles.

Diagnosis.—The diagnosis is often made on insufficient grounds and the mere presence of an apex systolic murmur is not sufficient. Cardiorespiratory murmurs should be recognized as of no significance. Soft murmurs heard during fever or in patients with anemia are not evidence of mitral disease. There is a systolic murmur which begins after a definite clear interval following the first sound, about midway between the two sounds, which is probably not a sign of disease of the valve. A patient may have it for many years with no symptoms and without any cardiac change. It usually gives trouble in an insurance examination. We can make theories as to its production but it is not evidence of disease.

We can make a diagnosis of mitral insufficiency when there is enlargement of the left ventricle, without any other explanation, and passive congestion in the lungs. We can watch a patient go through an attack of rheumatic fever with evidence of endocarditis and signs of mitral insufficiency (at first there may be doubt as to organic damage or relative insufficiency) and as years go on note enlargement of the ventricle. Later the signs of mitral stenosis may appear, which is positive proof that the valve has been damaged. But from a murmur alone we should be chary of diagnosing organic mitral insufficiency.

It is not always possible to say whether an insufficiency is due to lesion of the valve segment or to relative incompetency. The character of the murmur, the propagation, the accentuation of the pulmonary second sound, and the hypertrophy may not be sufficient. The history is sometimes of greater value than the examination. The cases most likely to lead to error are those of dilatation and hypertrophy (in which the systolic murmur may be of great intensity) with hypertension. The result of treatment observation for some days usually makes the diagnosis clear.

MITRAL STENOSIS

Etiology.—There are two groups of cases, one following an acute endocarditis, the other the result of a slow sclerosis of the valves without any history of rheumatic fever or other infection. It is more common in females than in males. This is not easy to explain, but rheumatic fever and chorea occur more frequently in girls. In a surprising number of cases of what the French call *pure* mitral stenosis no recognizable etiological factor can be discovered. This has been regarded by some as favoring the view that they may be of congenital origin, but congenital affections of the mitral valve are notoriously rare. Some suggest congenital syphilis but this seems unlikely. The possible influence of tonsillitis is difficult to estimate. While met with at all ages, stenosis is certainly most frequent in young adult women.

Morbid Anatomy.—The valve segments and chordae may be fused together, the result of endocarditis. The condition varies a good deal, according to the amount of atheromatous change. In many cases the curtains are so welded together and the whole valvular region so thickened that the orifice is reduced to a mere chink—*button-hole contraction.* In nonendocarditic cases the curtains are not much thickened, but narrowing has resulted from gradual adhesion at the edges, and thickening of the chordae tendineae, so that from the auricle it looks cone-like—the so-called *funnel-shaped variety.* Cases in which the valve segments are slightly deformed, but the orifice is considerably narrowed, are regarded by some as possibly of congenital origin. The involvement of the chordae tendineae is usually extreme and the papillary muscles may be inserted directly upon the valve. In moderate grades of constriction the orifice admits the tip of the index finger; in more extreme forms the tip of the little finger; and occasionally one finds a specimen in which the orifice seems almost obliterated. The heart is not greatly enlarged, rarely weighing more than 14 or 15 ounces. The left ventricle is sometimes small and may look very small in comparison with the right ventricle, which forms the greater portion of the apex. In cases in which there is stenosis with insufficiency the left ventricle may be moderately dilated and hypertrophied.

White thrombi may be found in the appendix of the left auricle. Occasionally a large part of the auricle is occupied by an antemortem thrombus. Still more rarely the remarkable *ball thrombus* is found, in which a globular concretion, varying in size from a walnut to a small egg, lies free in the auricle.

The left auricle discharges its blood with greater difficulty and in consequence dilates, and its walls increase in thickness. Although the auricle is unfitted to compensate an extreme lesion, the probability is that for some time during the gradual production of stenosis the increasing power of the walls counterbalances the defect. In 36 cases of well-marked stenosis Samways found the auricle hypertrophied in 26, dilatation coexisting in 14. Eventually the tension is increased in the pulmonary circulation and extra work thrown on the right ventricle, which gradually hypertrophies. Relative incompetency of the tricuspid valve and congestion of the systemic veins supervene.

Symptoms.—Mitral stenosis may for years be efficiently compensated by the hypertrophy of the right ventricle. Many persons with this lesion present no symptoms. They may for years be short of breath on going upstairs, but carry on ordinary activity without discomfort. Hemoptysis is not infrequent and may recur for years. The *pulse* is smaller in volume than normal, and often irregular (auricular fibrillation). Vegetations may be whipped off into the circulation and cause hemiplegia or aphasia, or both. This is not uncommon in women. Patients with mitral stenosis may survive this accident for an indefinite period.

Physical Signs.—*Inspection.*—There is often a flush on the cheeks, and clubbing of the fingers is common. The lower sternum and adjoining costal cartilages are often prominent, owing to hypertrophy of the right ventricle. The apex beat may be ill defined but usually it is not far beyond the nipple line, and the chief impulse is over the lower sternum and adjacent cartilages. Often in thin-chested persons there is pulsation in the third and fourth left interspaces close to the sternum. When compensation fails, the impulse is much feebler, and the veins of the neck may show marked pulsation or the right jugular stand out as a prominent tumor. In the later stage there is great enlargement with pulsation of the liver.

Palpation reveals in a majority of the cases a well defined, presystolic *thrill,* which is best felt, as a rule, at the apex or a little inside it. It is of a rough, grating quality, often peculiarly limited in area, most marked during expiration, and terminates in a sharp, sudden *shock,* synchronous with the impulse. This most characteristic sign is pathognomonic of mitral stenosis and is perhaps the only instance in which the diagnosis of a valvular lesion can be made by palpation alone. It is often variable and may be brought out by exercise. The impulse is felt most forcibly over the lower sternum and in the fourth and fifth left interspaces. An impulse is felt in the third and fourth interspaces, or in rare cases even in the second, from the conus arteriosus of the right ventricle; even in the most extreme grades of mitral stenosis there is never such tilting forward of the auricle as would enable it to produce an impression on the chest wall.

Percussion gives an increase in dulness to the right of the sternum but not usually a great increase beyond the left nipple line. There may be dulness in the left interscapular region.

Auscultation.—The findings are varied and puzzling combinations of sounds and murmurs may be heard. At the apex or a little inside it, often in a very limited region, is heard a rough, vibratory or purring presystolic murmur, cumulative or crescendo in character, often of short duration, which teminates abruptly in the loud snapping first sound. This murmur is synchronous with the thrill and the shock with the first sound. The murmur may occupy the entire period of diastole, or the middle or only the latter half. A difference can often be noted between the earlier and later parts of the murmur, when it occupies the entire time. In some cases a soft diastolic murmur is heard after the second sound at the apex. This may increase and merge into the presystolic murmur. Often there is a peculiar rumbling or echoing quality, which in some instances is heard only over a single bell-space of the stethoscope. The administration of amyl nitrite may bring out the murmur more clearly. Some hold that the crescendo murmur is due to regurgitation and that the murmur occurs before the systolic sound but not before the contraction. It may persist with auricular fibrillation. In line with this, what is regarded as the true presystolic murmur is often faint, of low pitch and separated from the following sound or murmur. It is absent in auricular fibrillation; it may coexist with the crescendo murmur. A rumbling, echoing presystolic murmur at the apex is heard in some cases of aortic insufficiency (Flint murmur), occasionally in adherent pericardium with great dilatation of the heart, and in upward dislocation of the organ. The Graham Steell murmur of *relative pulmonary insufficiency* may be heard in the pulmonic area.

A systolic murmur may be heard at the apex or along the left sternal border, often of extreme softness and audible only when the breath is held. Sometimes the systolic murmur is loud and distinct and is transmitted to the axilla. The pulmonic second sound is loudly accentuated and often reduplicated. It may be transmitted far to the left and be heard with great clearness beyond the apex. With good compensation the second sound is heard at the apex; its disappearance suggests the approach of decompensation. The sharp, snapping first sound which follows the presystolic murmur is not easy to explain. It can scarcely be a valvular sound produced chiefly at the mitral orifice, since it may be heard with great intensity when the valves are rigid and calcified. It has been suggested that it is a loud snap of the tricuspid valves caused by the powerful contraction of the hypertrophied right ventricle. Broadbent thinks it may be due to the abrupt contraction of a partially filled left ventricle. The sound may be audible at a distance from the patient (Graves). In one case the first sound was audible six feet from the chest wall.

These signs are characteristic only of the stage in which compensation is maintained. The murmur may be soft, almost inaudible, and only brought out after exertion. Finally there comes a period in which, with the establishment of auricular fibrillation, the signs change. This is due to the absence of contraction of the auricle. Thus a presystolic murmur may disappear as there is not the usual difference in pressure in the auricle and ventricle at the time when the auricle should be contracting. With the auricle paralyzed the murmur is more likely to be heard early in diastole. Difference in rate may cause marked changes in the time and character of the murmur. In patients over 45 or 50, hypertension is fairly common.

Sometimes in the apex region a sharp first sound or gallop rhythm may be heard. The systolic shock may be present after the disappearance of the thrill and the characteristic murmur. If partial heart block occurs a complicated set of signs results as the auricle is contracting more often than the ventricle. With recovery of compensation and with increasing vigor of contraction of the right ventricle and left auricle, the presystolic murmur reappears. At this stage the nature of the valve lesion may be entirely overlooked. *Auricular fibrillation* is the rule in the arrhythmia of mitral stenosis.

Pressure of the enlarged auricle on the left recurrent laryngeal nerve, causing paralysis of the vocal cord on the corresponding side, has been described and the diagnosis of aneurism of the arch of the aorta may be made. Fetterolf and Norris concluded that it is not due to pressure from the left auricle directly, but to squeezing of the nerve between the pulmonary artery and the aortic arch, and that the paralysis is due to the neuritis so excited.

The X-ray examination shows a prominence in the region of the pulmonary artery and the dilated left auricle may be evident when the patient is examined in the oblique position. Inflammatory affections of the lungs or pleura seriously disturb the right heart, and these patients stand pneumonia badly. Many patients with mitral stenosis do not have dropsy. The liver may be greatly enlarged, and in the late stages ascites is not uncommon, particularly in children.

TRICUSPID VALVE DISEASE

Tricuspid Regurgitation.—This results very rarely from endocarditis. Nearly always the condition is a relative insufficiency, and secondary to a mitral lesion or myocardial insufficiency. It happens in a sound heart as a "safety valve" action when the pressure in the right heart is excessive, as in severe exertion. It occurs in conditions of the lungs which obstruct the circulation, such as fibrosis and emphysema, particularly with chronic bronchitis. The symptoms are those of obstruction in the lesser circulation with venous congestion in the systemic veins. The signs are:

(*a*) Systolic regurgitation of the blood into the right auricle and the transmission of the pulse wave into the veins of the neck. If the regurgitation is slight or the contraction of the ventricle is feeble there may be no venous throbbing, but in other cases there is marked systolic pulsation in the cervical veins. Marked pulsation in these veins occurs when the valves become incompetent. Slight oscillations are not uncommon when the valves are intact. The distention is sometimes enormous, particularly during coughing, when the right jugular at the root of the neck may stand out, forming a prominent ovoid mass. Occasionally the regurgitant pulse wave may be widely transmitted and be seen in the subclavian and axillary veins, and even in the subcutaneous veins over the shoulder or in the superficial mammary veins.

The regurgitant pulsation may be transmitted to the hepatic veins, causing pulsation of the liver. This is best appreciated by bimanual palpation. The pulsation may be readily distinguished, as a rule, from the impulse from the ventricle or that transmitted from the aorta.

(*b*) The second important sign is a systolic murmur of maximum intensity over the lower sternum. It is usually a soft, low murmur, often distinguished from a coexisting mitral murmur by differences in quality and pitch, and may be heard to the right as far as the axilla. Sometimes it is very limited in its distribution. Percussion usually shows increase in dulness to the right of the sternum, and the impulse in the lower sternal region is forcible. In the great majority of cases the symptoms are those of the associated lesions. In fibrosis of the lung and chronic emphysema the failure of the right ventricle may lead to cardiac dropsy.

Tricuspid Stenosis.—The condition is rare and not often recognized in life. Of 26,000 medical admissions in the Johns Hopkins Hospital there were only 8 with clinical or postmortem diagnosis of this condition; and in 3,500 autopsies, only 5 cases were found, all in females. Of 195 collected cases, there were 141 females, 38 males, 16 sex unknown. In a majority of the cases —104—the mitral and tricuspid were affected together, in 14 the tricuspid alone, in 64 the tricuspid and aortic. A definite history of rheumatism was present in only 66 cases (Futcher).

The *diagnosis* is not often made; extreme cyanosis and dyspnea are common, and toward the end the ordinary signs of cardiac failure. Among the important physical signs are *presystolic pulsation* in the jugular veins and in the enlarged liver. A presystolic thrill may be felt at the tricuspid area with a marked systolic shock. The cardiac dulness is increased to the right, and a rumbling presystolic murmur may be present over the lower sternum with an extension to the right border.

PULMONARY VALVE DISEASE

Murmurs in the pulmonic region are extremely common; lesions of the valves are exceedingly rare. Balfour well called the pulmonic area the region of "auscultatory romance." A systolic murmur is heard here under many conditions—(1) very often in health, in thin-chested persons, particularly in children, during expiration and in the recumbent posture; (2) when the heart is rapid, as in fever and after exertion; (3) it is a favorite situation of the cardiorespiratory murmur; (4) in anemic states; and (5) the murmur of mitral insufficiency may be well heard along the left sternal margin.

Stenosis is almost invariably a congenital anomaly and is one of the most important congenital cardiac affections. The valve segments are usually united, leaving a small, narrow orifice. In adults cases occasionally occur. The congenital lesion is commonly associated with patency of the ductus Botalli and imperfection of the ventricular septum. There may also be tricuspid stenosis. Acute endocarditis not infrequently attacks the sclerotic valves. The physical *signs* are extremely uncertain. There may be a systolic murmur with a thrill best made out to the left of the sternum in the second intercostal space. This murmur may be like that of aortic stenosis, but is not transmitted into the vessels. It may be transmitted to the left shoulder. The pulmonary second sound is weak or obliterated, or replaced by a diastolic murmur. Usually there is hypertrophy of the right heart.

Pulmonary Insufficiency.—This rare lesion was originally described by Morgagni. Pitt analysed 109 cases from the Guy's Hospital Reports, of which 60 had infectious endocarditis, 18 were due to a dilated pulmonary artery, 14 to pulmonary stenosis, 14 to aortic aneurism, 13 to abnormality in the number of the valves, and 6 unclassified. Pitt makes two groups, one with a rapid course, sometimes with definite symptoms pointing to the heart but the signs to general septicemia. In the second group the cardiac symptoms are marked, dyspnea, cough, etc., and the physical signs are definite.

The *signs* are those of regurgitation into the right ventricle, but, as a rule, it is difficult to differentiate the murmur from that of aortic insufficiency, though the maximum intensity may be in the pulmonic area. The absence of the vascular features of aortic insufficiency is important. Both Gibson and Graham Steell called attention to the possibility of leakage through these valves in cases of great increase of pressure in the pulmonary artery, and to a soft diastolic murmur heard under these circumstances. Relative pulmonary insufficiency is probably of rare occurrence.

Combined Valvular Lesions.—Valvular lesions are more often combined than single. This is particularly the case in congenital disease. In children mitral and aortic lesions, the result of rheumatic fever, are common. Pure mitral insufficiency and pure mitral stenosis may exist for years, but in time the tricuspid becomes involved. Aortic valve lesions are more commonly uncombined than mitral lesions. The added lesion may be hurtful or helpful. A stenosis may lessen the regurgitation in aortic insufficiency; and a narrowing of the mitral orifice may be beneficial in mitral regurgitation.

Prognosis in Valvular Disease.—The question is entirely one of efficient compensation. So long as this is maintained the patient may suffer no inconvenience, and even with a serious valve lesion the function of the heart may be little, if at all, disturbed. Practitioners should remember that the best judgment may be gathered from inspection and palpation rather than from auscultation. *The myocardium is more important than the valve.* A murmur *per se* is of little or no moment in determining the prognosis in any given case. There is a group of patients who present only a systolic murmur over the body of the heart or at the apex, in whom the left ventricle is not hypertrophied, the rhythm is normal, and who have not had rheumatic fever.

Among the conditions influencing prognosis are: (*a*) AGE.—Children under ten are bad subjects. Compensation is well effected, and they are free from many influences which disturb compensation in adults. The coronary arteries are healthy and nutrition of the heart muscle can be readily maintained. Yet, in spite of this, the outlook is usually bad. The valve lesion itself is apt to be progressive and the limit of cardiac reserve is early reached. There seems to be proportionately a greater degree of hypertrophy and dilatation. Among other factors of this period are insufficient food in the poorer classes, the recurrence of rheumatic attacks, and the existence of pericardial adhesions. The outlook in a child who can be carefully supervised and prevented from damaging himself by overexertion is better than in one who is constantly overtaxing his circulation. The valvular lesions at, or subsequent to, puberty are more likely to be permanently and efficiently compensated. Sudden death from heart disease is very rare in children.

(*b*) SEX.—Women bear valve lesions, as a rule, better than men, owing partly to the fact that they live quieter lives, partly to the less common involvement of the coronary arteries, and to the greater frequency of mitral lesions. Pregnancy and parturition are disturbing factors, but are less serious than some writers would have us believe.

(*c*) VALVE AFFECTED.—The relative prognosis of the different valve lesions is difficult to estimate and each case must be judged on its own merits. *Aortic insufficiency* is unquestionably the most serious; yet for years it may be perfectly compensated. Favorable circumstances are a moderate hypertrophy and the absence of symptoms of cardiac distress, extensive arteriosclerosis and angina. The prognosis rests largely with the condition of the coronary arteries. Rheumatic lesions of the valves, inducing insufficiency, are less apt to be associated with endarteritis at the root of the aorta; and in such cases the coronary arteries may escape for years. When aortic insufficiency is a part of disease at the root of the aorta, the coronary arteries are almost invariably involved, and the outlook is much more serious. This is often the case in syphilis. Sudden death is not uncommon, from acute dilatation during exertion, or from blocking of a coronary artery. The liability of this form to be associated with angina pectoris also adds to its severity. *Aortic stenosis* is comparatively rare, most common in elderly men, and is, as a rule, well compensated.

In mitral lesions the outlook on the whole is more favorable than in aortic insufficiency. *Mitral insufficiency*, when well compensated, has a better prognosis than mitral stenosis. Except aortic stenosis, it is the lesion most often met with in patients over sixty years. The patients who last the longest are those in whom the valve orifice is more or less narrowed, as well as incompetent. There is no valve lesion so poorly compensated and so rapidly fatal as that in which the mitral segments are gradually curled and puckered until they form a narrow strip around a wide mitral ring—a condition specially seen in children. In some cases of mitral insufficiency the defect is thoroughly balanced for thirty or forty years, without distress or inconvenience. Even with great hypertrophy the compensation may be most effective. Women may pass safely through repeated pregnancies, though here they are liable to accidents associated with the severe strain.

In *mitral stenosis* the prognosis is usually regarded as less favorable but our experience places this lesion almost on a level, particularly in women, with mitral insufficiency. The observations of Levine suggest that hypertension in patients over 45 years of age is favorable. The figures given by Broadbent indicate that the age at death in mitral stenosis is comparatively advanced. Of 53 fatal cases from St. Mary's Hospital, thirty-three was the age for males, and thirty-eight for females. These women often pass through repeated pregnancies with safety. There is always the risk of cerebral embolism.

The outlook depends principally on the condition of the *myocardium*. With evidence of muscular insufficiency the prognosis is always grave. The *etiological* factor is important, thus rheumatic fever or syphilis may have caused serious myocardial mischief. The prognosis in syphilitic aortic disease is always serious. Every case must be judged separately, and all the circumstances carefully balanced. The development of auricular fibrillation, alternation of the heart, etc., must be taken into account. There is no question which requires greater experience and more mature judgment, and the most experienced are sometimes at fault. The following conditions justify a favorable prognosis: Good general health and good habits; no exceptional liability to rheumatic fever; origin of the valvular lesion independently of degeneration; existence of the valvular lesion without change for over three years; sound ventricles, of moderate frequency and general regularity of action; the absence of serious forms of arrhythmia; sound arteries, with a normal tension; and freedom from passive congestion.

Treatment.—(*a*) Stage of Compensation.—A common error is to administer drugs, such as digitalis, on the discovery of a murmur. If the lesion has been found accidentally, it may be best not to tell the patient, but rather an intimate friend. Often it is necessary to be frank in order that the patient may take preventive measures. He should lead a quiet, regulated, orderly life, free from excitement and worry, and the risk of sudden death makes it imperative that the patient suffering from aortic disease should be warned against overexertion and hurry. An ordinary wholesome diet in moderate quantities should be taken; tobacco may be allowed in moderation, but alcohol should be interdicted or used in small amount. Exercise should be regulated by the feelings of the patient. So long as no cardiac distress or palpitation follows, moderate exercise will prove beneficial. Any focus of infection should be treated and any acute infection treated with great care. The skin should be kept active by a daily bath. Hot baths should be avoided and the Turkish bath forbidden. With full-blooded corpulent individuals, an occasional saline purge should be taken. Patients with valvular lesions should not go to very high altitudes. The act of coition has risks, particularly in aortic disease. Knowing that the causes which most disturb compensation are acute infections, overexertion, mental worry and malnutrition, the physician should give suitable instructions in each case. The decision as to whether the risk of *pregnancy* should be taken is often difficult. It should be forbidden if there has been evidence of myocardial failure. With good compensation it is for the patient to decide after full consideration of the dangers.

(*b*) Stage of Broken Compensation.—The break may be immediate and final, as when sudden death results from acute dilatation or from coronary artery occlusion, or it may be gradual. Irregularity is not necessarily an indication of failing compensation but demands an accurate diagnosis. Serious failure of compensation is indicated by signs of dilatation, cyanosis, gallop rhythm, or certain forms of arrhythmia, with or without edema. These are dependent on the myocardium and the measures indicated are those for myocardial insufficiency. In mitral stenosis, valvulotomy has been done successfully (Cutler and Levine).

SPECIAL PATHOLOGICAL CONDITIONS

ANEURISM OF THE HEART

Aneurism of a valve results from acute endocarditis, which produces softening or erosion and may lead to perforation of the segment or to gradual dilatation of a limited area under the influence of the blood pressure. The aneurisms are usually spheroidal and project from the ventricular face of an aortic valve. They are much less common on the mitral segments. They frequently rupture and produce extensive destruction and insufficiency.

Aneurism of a Coronary Artery.—This is very rare. The aneurism is usually single and on the first inch of the left coronary. There are two groups, mycotic and arteriosclerotic. Rupture occurred in half the reported cases. There are no positive symptoms or signs.

Aneurism of the walls results from the weakening due to fibroid myocarditis, infarction from coronary artery occlusion, or occasionally follows acute mural endocarditis, which more commonly leads to perforation. It has followed a stab wound, a gumma of the ventricle and, according to some authors, pericardial adhesions. The left ventricle near the apex is usually the seat, because here fibrous degeneration is most common. Of 90 cases, 59 were situated here (Legg). In the early stages the anterior wall of the ventricle, near the septum, sometimes the septum itself, is slightly dilated, the endocardium opaque, and the muscular tissue sclerotic. In a more advanced stage the dilatation is pronounced and layers of thrombi occupy the sac. Ultimately a large rounded tumor may project from the ventricle and attain a size equal to that of the heart. There may be a number of aneurismal bulgings. Rupture occurred in 7 of Legg's cases.

The *signs* are indefinite. Occasionally there is marked bulging in the apex region and the tumor may perforate the chest wall. In mitral stenosis the right ventricle may bulge and produce a visible pulsating tumor below the left costal border, which has been mistaken for cardiac aneurism. When the sac is large and presses upon the heart, there may be a marked disproportion between the strong cardiac impulse and the feeble pulsation in the peripheral arteries. The X-ray study may aid in diagnosis.

RUPTURE OF THE HEART

This rare event is usually associated with infarction, fatty infiltration or myocardial degeneration. In some instances acute softening from occlusion of a coronary artery, suppurative myocarditis or a gummatous growth has been the cause. The majority of the patients are over sixty years of age. Schaps reports a case in an infant of four months associated with an embolic infarct of the left ventricle. Harvey, in his second letter to Riolan (1649), described the case of Sir Robert Darcy, who had distressing pain in the chest and syncopal attacks with suffocation, and finally cachexia and dropsy. Death occurred in one of the paroxysms. The wall of the left ventricle of the heart was ruptured, "having a rent in it of size sufficient to admit any of my fingers, although the wall itself appeared sufficiently thick and strong."

The rent may occur in any of the chambers, but is most frequent in the left ventricle on the anterior wall, not far from the septum. Rupture of the interventricular septum may occur, usually after infarction. The accident usually takes place during exertion. There may be no preliminary symptoms and without any warning the patient may fall and die in a few moments. In other instances there may be a sense of anguish and suffocation, and life may be prolonged for several hours. In a Montreal case, the patient walked up a steep hill after the onset of symptoms and lived for thirteen hours. In one case the patient lived for eleven days.

NEW GROWTHS AND PARASITES

Primary neoplasm is extremely rare. Secondary tumors may be single or multiple, and are usually without symptoms, even when the disease is extensive. In one case in the right ventricle a mass was found which involved the anterior segment of the tricuspid valve and partly blocked the orifice. There were numerous cancerous emboli in the pulmonary artery. In another instance the heart was greatly enlarged, owing to masses of colloid cancer the size of cherries. Mediastinal neoplasm may penetrate the heart, though it is remarkable how extensive disease of the mediastinal glands may be without involvement of the heart or vessels. There are no characteristic symptoms or signs.

Cysts are rare. They are found in different parts, and are filled either with a brownish or a clear fluid. Blood cysts occasionally occur. Both the *Cysticercus cellulosae* and echinoccus cysts occur occasionally.

WOUNDS AND FOREIGN BODIES

Wounds of the heart may be caused by external injuries, by foreign bodies passing from the esophagus, or by therapeutic puncture.

(*a*) Bullet wounds are common. Recovery may take place and bullets may be encysted in the organ. Stab wounds are still more common. A medical student, on a spree, passed a pin into his heart. The pericardium was opened and the head of the pin was found outside of the right ventricle. It was grasped and an attempt made to remove it, but it was withdrawn into the heart and, it is said, caused the patient no further trouble (Moxon).

(*b*) Hysterical girls sometimes swallow pins and needles, which, passing through the esophagus and stomach, are found in various parts of the body. A remarkable case was reported by Allen J. Smith of a girl from whom several dozen needles and pins were removed, chiefly from subcutaneous abscesses. Several years later she died of heart disease and needles were found in the tissues of the adherent pericardium.

(*c*) Puncture of the heart has been done as a therapeutic procedure but is not without risk. Hemorrhage may take place from the puncture, though it is not often extensive.

CONGENITAL AFFECTIONS OF THE HEART

These have only a limited clinical interest, as in a large proportion the anomaly is not compatible with life, and in others nothing can be done to remedy the defect or even to relieve the symptoms. Congenital affections result from interruption of the normal course of development or from inflammatory processes—endocarditis; sometimes from both.

General Anomalies.—Of general anomalies of development the following conditions may be mentioned: *Acardia,* absence of the heart; *double heart,* which has occasionally been found in extreme grades of fetal deformity; *dextrocardia,* in which the heart is on the right side, either alone or as part of a general transposition of the viscera; *ectopia cordis,* associated with fission of the chest wall and of the abdomen. The heart may be situated in the cervical, pectoral or abdominal regions. Except in the abdominal variety, the condition is very rarely compatible with extrauterine life. Occasionally the child lives for some months, and the heart may be seen and felt beating beneath the skin in the epigastric region.

Anomalies of the Cardiac Septa.—The septa of both auricles and ventricles may be defective, in which case the heart consists of but two chambers, the *cor biloculare* or reptilian heart. In the septum of the auricles there is a very common defect, *patent foramen ovale,* owing to the fact that the membrane closing the foramen ovale has failed at one point to become attached to the ring, and leaves a valvular slit. Neither this nor the small cribriform perforations of the membrane are of any significance.

The *foramen ovale* may be patent without a trace of membrane closing it. In some instances this exists with other serious defects, such as stenosis of the pulmonary artery or imperfection of the ventricular septum. In others the patent foramen ovale is the only anomaly, and in many instances it does not appear to cause any embarrassment, having been found in persons who have died of various affections. The ventricular septum may be absent, the condition known as *trilocular heart.* Much more frequently there is a small defect in the upper portion of the septum, either in the situation of the membranous portion known as the "undefended space" or in the region just anterior to this. This is frequently associated with narrowing of the pulmonary orifice or of the conus arteriosus of the right ventricle.

Apart from the instances in association with narrowing of the orifice of the pulmonary artery, or of the conus, there are cases in which defect of the *membranous septum* is the only lesion, a condition not incompatible with long and fairly active life. The late Professor Brooks of the Johns Hopkins University knew from early manhood that he had heart trouble, but he accomplished an extraordinary amount of work, and lived to be about 60. Imperfect septum was the only lesion. The physical signs are fairly distinctive with usually some evident enlargement of the heart, and a murmur described by Roger as follows: "It is a loud murmur, audible over a large area, and, commencing with systole, is prolonged so as to cover the normal tic-tac. It has its maximum at the upper third of the precordial region. It is central, like the septum, and from this central point gradually diminishes in intensity in every direction. The murmur does not vary at any time, and it is not conducted into the vessels." In some cases there is a distinct systolic intensification of this loud continuous murmur.

Congenital Heart Block.—Recent reviews accept about 30 cases. It may occur with a patent interventricular septum. A slow pulse in a young child should suggest this diagnosis. The average heart rate is 50; one case had a ventricular rate of 75. Stokes-Adams attacks are rare. The prognosis depends more on other abnormalities than on the heart block, as apparently it does not tend to shorten life.

Anomalies and Lesions of the Valves.—Numerical anomalies of the valves are not uncommon. The semilunar segments at the arterial orifices may be increased or diminished in number. Supernumerary segments are more frequent in the pulmonary artery than in the aorta. Four, or sometimes five, valves have been found. The segments may be of equal size, but, as a rule, the supernumerary valve is small. Instead of three there may be only two semilunar valves, the *bicuspid condition;* this is more frequent in the aortic valve. Of 21 instances only 2 occurred at the pulmonary orifice. Two of the valves have united, and from the ventricular face show no trace of division or else a slight depression where the union has occurred. From the aortic side there is usually some trace of division into two sinuses of Valsalva. There has been discussion as to the origin of this, whether it is an anomaly or due to endocarditis, fetal or postnatal. The combined segment is usually thickened, but the fact that this anomaly is met with in the fetus without a trace of sclerosis or endocarditis shows that it may, in some cases at least, result from a developmental error.

Patent ductus arteriosus.—The ductus should close as respiration is established but may not do so. In this event a systolic murmur can be heard with maximum intensity in the second left interspace close to the sternum, accompanied by a systolic thrill. These are found in the first years of life, say five. Later a diastolic murmur is added which is loud, heard generally over the thorax and loudest in the second and third left interspaces. There is a thrill also. These give a continuous machinery murmur. An area of dulness is found above the third left rib close to the sternum (Gerhardt's triangle of dulness). This can be seen in a skiagram. There are no symptoms from this lesion alone and if they are present there is another cause for them. Before the diastolic murmur appears, pulmonary stenosis may give difficulty but right ventricular enlargement is generally present. The lesion in itself is harmless and restriction of activity is not indicated. In *coarction of the aorta* there is a stenosis between the left subclavian artery and the ductus arteriosus. The condition may be latent and the symptoms are variable. The vascular signs depend on the inequality of the circulation in the upper and lower parts of the body and the dilated collateral vessels in the upper part of the body. The femoral pulse is absent or retarded and diminished, with decreased blood pressure in the legs, in contrast to hypertension in the arms and a full radial pulse, often unequal on the two sides. The X-ray study may show erosion of the ribs. The heart is usually enlarged. The symptoms and signs tend to progress.

Anomalies of the auriculoventricular valves are not often met with.

Fetal endocarditis may occur either at the arterial or auriculoventricular orifices. It is nearly always of the chronic or sclerotic variety and very rarely of the warty or verrucose form. There are little nodular bodies, sometimes six or eight in number, on the mitral and tricuspid segments—the nodules of Albini—which represent the remains of fetal structures, and must not be mistaken for endocardial outgrowths. The little rounded, bead-like hemorrhages of a deep purple color, which are common on the heart valves of children, are also not to be mistaken for the products of endocarditis. In fetal endocarditis the segments are usually thickened at the edges, shrunken and smooth. In the mitral and tricuspid valves the cusps are united and the chordae tendineae thickened and shortened. In the semilunar valves all trace of the segments has disappeared, leaving a stiff membranous diaphragm perforated by an oval or rounded orifice. It is sometimes difficult to say whether this has resulted from fetal endocarditis or is an error in development. In many instances the processes are combined; an anomalous valve becomes the seat of sclerotic changes. According to Rauchfuss, endocarditis is more common on the right side of the heart only because the valves are more often the seat of developmental errors.

Lesions at the Pulmonary Orifice.—*Stenosis* is one of the commonest and most important of congenital heart affections. A slow endocarditis causes gradual union of the segments and narrowing of the orifice so that it admits only a small probe. In some cases the smooth membranous condition of the combined segments suggests faulty development. In some instances vegetations occur. The condition is compatible with life for many years, and in a considerable proportion of the cases of congenital heart disease above the tenth year this lesion is present. With it there may be defect of the ventricular septum. Pulmonary tuberculosis is a common cause of death. Obliteration or *atresia* of the pulmonary orifice is a less frequent but more serious condition than stenosis. It is associated with persistence of the ductus arteriosus and patency of the foramen ovale or defect of the ventricular septum with hypertrophy of the right heart. *Stenosis of the conus arteriosus* of the right ventricle exists in a considerable proportion of the cases of pulmonary stenosis. At the outset a developmental error, it may be combined with sclerotic changes. The ventricular septum is imperfect, the foramen ovale usually open, and the ductus arteriosus patent. The lesions at the pulmonary orifice constitute the most important group and of 631 instances of congenital anomalies analyzed by Maude Abbott, 150 cases came under this category.

Congenital lesions of the aortic orifice are not very infrequent. Abbott analyzed 28 cases of stenosis and atresia; stenosis of the left conus arteriosus may also occur, a condition not incompatible with prolonged life. Ten of the 16 cases tabulated by Dilg were over thirty years of age.

Transposition of the large arterial trunks is a not uncommon anomaly. There may be no hypertrophy, cyanosis or heart murmur.

Symptoms of Congenital Heart Disease.—There are two groups of cases: (1) The cyanotic group (venous-arterial shunt), "morbus caeruleus," and (2) The noncyanotic group (arterial-venous shunt). Under the former comes pulmonary stenosis which with defect of the ventricular septum at the base, dextroposition of the aorta and hypertrophy of the right ventricle makes the *"tetralogy of Fallot."* In the second group, patent ductus arteriosus, patent foramen ovale and defect of the ventricular septum are the most common. Marked physical signs and few symptoms are found in this group. In the cyanotic group *dyspnea* on exertion and *cough* are common symptoms. A great increase in the number of the red corpuscles is common, and they may reach 8 or 9 million. There may be nucleated red cells and great variation in size and shape. The children rarely thrive and often display a lethargy of both mind and body. The fingers and toes are *clubbed* to a degree rarely met with in any other affection. The cause of the *cyanosis* has been much discussed. Morgagni referred it to the general congestion of the venous system due to obstruction. Deficient aeration of the blood owing to diminished lung function may be an important factor. A view, often attributed erroneously to William Hunter, was that the discoloration was due to the admixture in the heart of venous and arterial blood; but lesions may permit of very free mixture without producing cyanosis. Variot suggested a disturbance of the whole circulatory system, and particularly vasomotor paresis and malaeration of the red cells. Probably a variety of causes may be responsible but the essential feature is deficient aeration of the blood by direct passage of venous blood into the arterial tree or by obstruction to the entrance of venous blood into the pulmonary circulation.

Diagnosis.—In children, *cyanosis,* with or without enlargement of the heart, and the existence of a *murmur,* are sufficient, as a rule, to determine the presence of a congenital heart lesion. The cyanosis gives no clue to the precise nature of the trouble, as it is common to many lesions and may be absent in certain conditions. The murmur is usually systolic. It is not always present, and there are instances of complicated congenital lesions with normal heart sounds. In two or three instances fetal endocarditis has been diagnosed *in gravida* by a rough systolic murmur, and corroborated subsequent to the birth of the child. Hypertrophy is present in a majority of the cases of congenital defect. The fatal event may be caused by abscess of the brain. For a full discussion the student is referred to the monograph of Dr. Maude Abbott in our System of Medicine.

The conclusions of Hochsinger are as follows:

"(1) In childhood, loud, rough, musical heart murmurs, with normal or only slight increase in the heart dulness, occur only in congenital heart disease. The acquired endocardial defects with loud heart murmurs in young children are almost always associated with great increase in the heart dulness. In the transposition of the large arterial trunks there may be no cyanosis, no heart murmur, and an absence of hypertrophy.

"(2) In young children heart murmurs with great increase in the cardiac dulness and feeble apex beat suggest congenital changes. The increased dulness is chiefly of the right heart, whereas the left is only slightly altered. In acquired endocarditis in children, the left heart is chiefly affected and the apex beat is visible; the dilatation of the right heart comes late and does not materially change the increased strength of the apex beat.

"(3) The entire absence of murmurs at the apex, with their evident presence in the region of the auricles and over the pulmonary orifice, is always an important element in differential diagnosis, and points rather to septum defect or pulmonary stenosis than to endocarditis.

"(4) An abnormally weak second pulmonic sound associated with a distinct systolic murmur is a symptom which in early childhood is only to be explained by the assumption of a congenital pulmonary stenosis.

"(5) Absence of a palpable thrill, despite loud murmurs which are heard over the whole precordial region, is rare except with congenital defects in the septum, and it speaks, therefore, against an acquired cardiac affection.

"(6) Loud, especially vibratory systolic murmurs, with the point of maximum intensity over the upper third of the sternum, associated with a lack of marked symptoms of hypertrophy of the left ventricle, are very important for the diagnosis of a persistence of the ductus Botalli, and can not be explained by the assumption of an endocarditis of the aortic valve."

Treatment.—The child should be warmly clad and guarded from all circumstances liable to excite bronchitis. There are two dangers from which the patient should be protected, *strain* and *infection*. A careful life such as is suitable for a child with rheumatic heart disease, attention to areas of focal infection and avoidance of general infections are important. In the attacks of urgent dyspnea with lividity venesection is advisable. Saline cathartics are useful. Digitalis must be used with care; it is sometimes beneficial in the later stages. When compensation fails, the indications for treatment are those of myocardial insufficiency in acquired cardiac disease.

ANGINA PECTORIS

Definition.—A symptom-complex characterized by paroxysmal attacks of pain, usually thoracic, associated with vascular changes.

History.—In 1768 Heberden described a "disorder of the breast," to which he gave the name of "Angina Pectoris." Before this date Morgagni had described definite cases. The association with coronary artery disease was early shown by Jenner. John Hunter died in an attack. The connection with aortitis as demonstrated by Corrigan and Allbutt, the recognition of extrapectoral forms, and the introduction of nitrites in treatment by Lauder Brunton are important contributions of the nineteenth century.

Etiology.—It is not common in the public wards of hospitals but is rather a disease of the better classes. The occurrence of the anginal syndrome in pernicious anemia is of interest; the attacks are usually not severe.

Sex and Age.—The syndrome is much more common in males, six to one in our series. The ages from 50 to 70 show the largest number of cases but it is not uncommon from 40 to 50. In earlier life, syphilitic aortitis is a factor.

Race.—The disease seems to be relatively more frequent in the United States. Jews appear to be particularly prone.

Occupation.—It is not an affection of the working classes. A life of stress and strain, particularly of worry, seems to predispose to it, and this is perhaps why it is so common in our profession. From John Hunter onward a long list of distinguished physicians have been its victims.

Cardiovascular Disease.—In persons under forty syphilis is an important feature, causing an aortitis, often limited to the root of the vessel. Whatever the cause, arteriosclerosis predisposes to angina. A majority of the patients have sclerosis, many high blood pressure. Business and professional men leading lives of great strain, and eating, drinking, and smoking to excess, form a large proportion of angina cases.

HEREDITY.—The disease may occur in members of three generations, as in the Arnold family.

Imitative Features.—Outbreaks of angina-like attacks have been described. After the death of one member of a family from the disease, another may have somewhat similar attacks. Two of his physicians had angina after Senator Sumner's fatal attack. One of them died within two weeks; the other, a young man, recovered completely.

Pathology.—There is no definite lesion which can be regarded as responsible. In the great majority there are alterations in the aorta and coronary arteries. The changes in the coronary arteries may be limited to the orifices, with a fairly normal vessel wall otherwise. In the majority the arteries show changes throughout. Aortitis may be prominent in younger subjects, often syphilitic. In some instances no lesions have been found. In one case a man aged 26 had attacks, which were regarded as functional, on and off for two years. Death occurred after a series of paroxysms. The aorta was small, otherwise there were no changes.

Pathogenesis.—No generally accepted explanation of the phenomena of the attack has been offered and probably various factors may be responsible. It has been regarded as a "neuralgia" of the cardiac nerves, a cramp of the heart-muscle, or of parts of it, a manifestation of myocardial ischemia, the result of some chemical or physicochemical agent, or an expression of tension of the ventricular walls. The intermittent claudication theory of Allan Burns may be defined as a state in which an artery admits enough blood to a muscular structure for quiet work, but not enough for increased work, so that the contractile function of the muscle is disturbed and pain results. Sir James Mackenzie regarded the disease as an expression of cardiac exhaustion and also of a susceptible nervous system. The pain is a viscerosensory reflex; the feeling of constriction a visceromotor reflex. Reid suggests that failure of reflex dilatation of the peripheral vascular system may cause a sudden rise of pressure in the aorta and left ventricle. The increased tension irritates the nerve supply. It has been termed "The cry of distress of the cardiac plexus." Probably various factors operate in different patients. Reflex influences, as from the stomach or gallbladder and particularly from the esophagus, seem to be responsible in some cases. The removal of a diseased gallbladder may result in complete disappearance of angina pectoris.

We owe much to Sir Clifford Allbutt for his studies on the disease, which should be consulted by every student. His explanation is that in the large proportion of cases the attacks are due to disease of the thoracic aorta, especially in its outer coat where there are sensory end-organs regulating blood pressure. Tension of the first portion of the aorta is an important factor. The coronary arteries and myocardium have little to do with the pain but much with the mortality. Sudden death may be from vagus inhibition. There is strong evidence that this explanation is correct in certain cases. Very similar attacks of pain occur in acute and in some cases of chronic aortitis. In many cases aortic pain can be clearly distinguished from cardiac pain; some patients have both and recognize the difference. The picture produced by occlusion of the coronary arteries can usually be distinguished from angina pectoris; the symptoms due to coronary artery disease otherwise are practically those of myocardial degeneration. It is well to realize that the cause of severe thoracic pain may be difficult to determine.

A number of conditions may be responsible for an attack. (1) *Physical exertion* in almost any form. Walking on the level *slowly*, the patient may be comfortable but increase beyond a certain pace or going up a slight grade brings on an attack. Some patients are affected by walking against a wind or fast driving in an open motor car. Any sudden exertion or hurry does the same. (2) *Emotion* and *excitement*. These are important causes, anger or annoyance being likely to cause an attack. (3) *Cold*. This may be shown on general chilling or by going out on a cold day, on taking a cold bath or even on washing the face in cold water. (4) *Digestive disturbance*, especially with distention after a heavy meal, is a common cause. Numerous other causes may operate, such as stooping over, straining at stool, coitus, etc. In nearly all there is the influence of strain either physical or mental.

Myocardial insufficiency is not a cause and the features of this are not present in angina pectoris. With myocardial failure or coronary occlusion the features of angina disappear in the majority of cases. The localization of the pain is often that of disease of the aorta and not of the myocardium. Space does not allow full discussion of the theories advanced. No one explanation covers all cases and angina pectoris may be regarded as a symptom-complex in which many factors may participate.

Symptoms.—Various classifications have been made but these are not satisfactory. Attacks of varying severity occur and it is important to recognize this. In the mildest form there is a feeling of substernal tension, uneasiness, or distress, rising at times to positive pain, usually associated with emotion, sometimes with exertion, but soon passing off. There may be slight pallor or a feeling of faintness. When rising to speak in public there may be a feeling of substernal tension—it is a common experience—which passes off. Muscular effort, as in climbing a hill, may bring on the sensation. In the high pressure life a man may experience for weeks or months this sense of substernal tension, not pain, and without accurate localization or radiation, and not increased by exercise or emotion. It is, as one patient expressed it, a "hot-box" indicating too great pressure and too high speed. It is away after the night's rest, and may disappear entirely when the "harness" is taken off.

In patients who show the usual features of angina pectoris, the two special features are the existence in a large proportion of all the cases of organic disease of heart or vessels and the liability to sudden death. An exciting cause of the attack can usually be traced. John Hunter used to say that "his life was in the hands of any rascal who chose to worry him," and his fatal attack occurred in a fit of anger.

Phenomena of the Attack.—The patient is seized with agonizing pain, usually about the upper sternum, and a sense of constriction, sometimes of extreme degree. In some cases the pain begins in the periphery (neck or arm) and travels to the thorax. The pain usually radiates to the left shoulder and down the left arm. It may radiate to the left back, to the neck, angle of the jaw or to the scalp. The extent of referred pain varies greatly. It may radiate down both arms or to the right arm only. There may be numbness of the fingers or in the cardiac region. The face is usually pallid and may assume an ashy gray tint, and not infrequently there is profuse *sweating.* The paroxysm lasts from several seconds to a minute or two, during which, in severe attacks, the patient feels as if death were imminent. As pointed out by Latham, there are two elements in it, the pain—*dolor pectoris*—and the indescribable feeling of anguish and sense of imminent dissolution—*angor animi.* The patient remains immobile. There are great distress and anxiety, and the patient may drop dead in the attack or pass away in syncope. The condition of the heart during the attack is variable; the pulsations may be uniform and regular. The pulse tension may be increased, but it is surprising, even in cases of extreme severity, how slightly the character of the pulse may be altered. After the attack there may be eructations or the passage of a large quantity of clear urine. The patient usually feels exhausted, and for a day or two may be badly shaken; in other instances in an hour or two he feels himself again. Dyspnea is not a usual feature. The electrocardiogram may show changes in the ventricular complexes or no change at all.

Death may occur in the first attack, as in the case of Thomas Arnold. Paroxysms may occur for many years before the fatal attack. The so-called *status anginosus* is probably always due to coronary artery occlusion.

There is a *chronic* form in which attacks occur irregularly. John Hunter's first seizure was in 1773, and he had many in the 20 years before his death. Sometimes life is a terrible burden, as any emotion or effort may bring on an attack. Sometimes, after paroxysms of great severity recurring for months, or even for so long as two years, complete recovery takes place.

Extrapectoral Features.—In the attack the pain usually radiates up the neck and down the left arm. The pain may begin in the left arm, or in the jaw, even in the front teeth, or in one testis. Sometimes the pain remains in these distant parts, and yet the attack presents, as noted by Heberden, all the features of angina. The attack may begin with agonizing pain in the left leg or in the left pectoral muscle. The entire features of the attack may be subdiaphragmatic—the so-called *angina abdominis.* These cases are rare and should be carefully studied to exclude coronary artery occlusion.

Tender areas may be found on pressure on the sternum and the second to fourth ribs on the left side, occasionally on the right side. They may persist for some time. There may be alteration of sensation over different areas. The blood pressure may be high or low. It may be extraordinarily high—340 mm. Hg in one case. *Cerebral features* are not common, but unconsciousness, transient monoplegia, or hemiplegia and aphasia may occur.

Diagnosis.—In typical severe attacks there is rarely any difficulty, especially if an attack is observed or a good description is obtained. In all cases careful inquiry should be made as to the situation and radiation of the pain, as well as its character. The pain of angina is referred to the upper sternum in the majority of cases; pain felt about the apex or over the lower precordium or sternum is probably not anginal. The sense of constriction, the attitude and color of the patient, and sweating are important. In *coronary occlusion,* the onset is without apparent cause, the signs of shock or collapse are more marked, the heart action is very weak, the pulse is rapid and small, the blood pressure usually drops to low figures, there may be leukocytosis and fever; the pain persists for a longer period and is not relieved by nitrites. Pericarditis may be found. The diagnosis of *abdominal angina* may be possible only if an attack is observed and coronary artery occlusion excluded. In cases of less severe thoracic pain, particularly if not localized, the diagnosis may be very difficult. Careful inquiry should be made as to causal factors, as the influence of exertion and emotion is important, with thorough study for other causes of pain. Attacks of thoracic pain in women, especially those with an anxiety neurosis, may give difficulty. There may be marked vasomotor features, the patients are often restless, and the pain persists for some time, longer than in the usual attack of angina pectoris. Attacks of thoracic pain in patients with severe rheumatic heart disease should be studied carefully before they are termed angina. It is a good rule to treat doubtful cases as if they were angina. The occurrence of attacks of moderate or slight severity must be remembered.

Prognosis.—In men under 40 syphilis must be suspected, and with appropriate treatment recovery may be complete (see the Lumleian Lectures (Osler, *Lancet,* 1910, I). In men in the 5th and 6th decades who have lived the high pressure life a change of habits may bring relief; but, as Walshe remarked, "the cardinal fact in real angina is its uncertainty." Even after attacks of the greatest severity recovery is possible. The circumstances that bring on an attack are important. The angina that follows any slight exertion is, as a rule, more serious than that which comes on with severe effort or is excited by emotion; yet one patient who could never dress without having what he called "angor de toilette" lived for 11 years. The electrocardiogram may be normal and is not diagnostic of angina pectoris. It gives information as to the state of the myocardium, and irregularity or spreading of the QRS complex in all leads and inversion of the T wave are regarded as serious indications. The cardiovascular condition is of the first importance in prognosis. Very high blood pressure, advanced arteriosclerosis, marked disease of the aorta, valvular disease and myocardial weakness are of serious import. Some patients have no obvious signs of cardiac disease. In cases associated with gastric or gallbladder disease or prostatitis in males, after correction of these conditions, the attacks may disappear. In women the forms with marked vasomotor disturbance as a rule do well, and when neurotic or hysterical manifestations are prominent the outlook is good.

There are three modes of dying in angina—one, as Walshe says, "is sudden, instantaneous, coeval with a single pang." The functions of life stop abruptly, and with a gasp all is over. Ventricular fibrillation may be the cause. In a second mode, following a series of attacks, the heart grows weaker and the patient dies in a progressive asthenia; while in a third there is a gradually induced cardiac insufficiency with dyspnea.

Treatment.—Prolonged rest is important for four to six weeks and the general treatment should be much the same as for aneurism. Every effort should be made to reduce anxiety and sources of irritation. Factors which induce an attack should be avoided. The diet should be simple and the bowels kept freely open. If there are any signs of myocardial insufficiency, even without loss of compensation, an occasional course of digitalis is advisable. Syphilitic cases require active treatment—neoarsphenamine in small doses followed by mercury and iodide. In the neurotic cases with a recognition of the disturbance in the vasomotor system a rest cure and hydrotherapy are indicated. Ergotin grs. ii (0.13 gm.) three times a day is useful in vasomotor instability. It is always well to give iodide in the dosage found best for the patient. The effect of vasodilators should be tried and the one used which is most useful. Many patients do well by taking sodium nitrite (gr. i, 0.06 gm. three times a day) regularly and carrying nitroglycerine with them so that it can be taken at once (gr. 1/100-gr. 1/50) on any feeling of discomfort or pain. The taking of nitroglycerine and morphine at the first sign of an attack is often successful in preventing severe manifestations. The use of theobromine or theophylline compounds is sometimes of benefit.

In the *attack* inhalation of nitrite of amyl, introduced by Lauder Brunton, may give instant relief. In the recurring terrible paroxysms it may lose its effect, but many patients are relieved promptly, and it gives comfort and confidence to carry the *perles.* Nitroglycerine tablets (gr. 1/100) should be carried by the patient and one or two put under the tongue at the first feeling of pain. Morphia should be used freely when vasodilators fail and attacks recur with great frequency. Chloroform may have to be used, and is always helpful, never harmful. Treatment by radium and X-ray has been used; some favorable results have been reported.

Surgical.—The variety of the procedures, the majority of which involve sympathectomy, is remarkable and this suggests that no one of these operations can be regarded as established. But a large percentage of successful results should not be expected. More is to be hoped for from paravertebral alcohol injections of the thoracic nerve roots on the left side. In some cases there is no doubt that "the danger signal" is removed but these procedures hold out hope for some patients. Total removal of the thyroid gland is useful in some cases. It should be done only after careful consideration.

DISEASES OF THE ARTERIES

ACUTE ARTERITIS

This occurs most often with acute infections, especially rheumatic and typhoid fever. In the aorta it may follow infectious endocarditis or infection may occur through the vasa vasorum in septicemia or pyemia, or spread from bronchial lymph nodes or the pericardium. It may be associated with bacterial (mycotic) aneurisms.

Symptoms.—If the process is in the aorta, any symptoms are part of the general process and cannot be separated. If in the peripheral arteries the vessel may be tender on pressure or there is severe pain, sometimes with redness and swelling. The pulse may be obliterated in the artery below and the limb becomes cold and white. The results depend on the collateral circulation very largely; gangrene does not always follow. In *treatment* little can be done beyond keeping the part thoroughly warm and relieving pain.

ARTERIOSCLEROSIS

The conception of arteriosclerosis as an independent affection—a general disease of the vascular system—is due to Gull and Sutton. Arteriosclerosis in one sense is not a disease but comprises changes which may occur with or follow many diseases. The term designates anatomical changes rather than a clinical condition in itself. The clinical features result mainly from interference with the blood supply of organs or tissues, and the resulting disturbance of function. Any classification of its forms must be morphological and not clinical; the effort to separate too many forms causes confusion.

Definition.—A vascular lesion characterized by pathological thickening of the arterial walls, due probably to various factors, with an inflammatory reaction and degenerative changes as important elements, while hyperplastic and involutionary processes play a part; no one process is entirely responsible. In the large vessels the changes are often designated as atheroma; in the smallest vessels as obliterative endarteritis.

Etiology.—Among the important factors are the following:

(*a*) Hypertension.—The blood pressure depends upon five factors: The heart pump supplies the force; the elastic coats of the large arteries store and convert an intermittent into a continuous stream; the small arteries act as sluices or taps regulating the control to different parts; the capillary bed is the irrigation field over which the nutritive fluid is distributed, and the drainage system is represented by the veins and lymph channels.

Galen first grasped the fact that life depends upon the maintenance of a due pressure in these irrigation fields: "Many canals dispersed throughout all the parts of the body convey to them blood as those of a garden convey moisture, and the intervals separating those canals are wonderfully disposed by nature in such a way that they should neither lack a sufficient quantity of blood for absorption, nor be overloaded at any time with an excessive supply."

The blood pressure varies greatly in different individuals and in the same individuals under varying conditions. The normal pressure is from 120 to 130 mm. of mercury, but in persons over 50 it is often from 130 to 150 mm. A permanent pressure above 160 mm. may be called high, but there are great regional variations.

The relation of hypertension to arteriosclerosis has been much discussed. There are three groups of cases. (1) The simple high tension without signs of arterial or renal disease—what Clifford Allbutt called *hyperpiesia*. In this condition, met with in individuals otherwise healthy, the blood pressure is permanently high—above 180—but, so far as can be ascertained, there are no arterial, cardiac or renal changes. It is difficult to exclude internal, not discernible alterations in the splanchnic and other vessels, since vascular disease may be very localized. Clinically the group is well defined and very important. The tendency is to advance to the second group unless the hypertension disappears. The condition is met with frequently in those who lead high pressure lives.

The exact cause of this high tension we do not know. Some have attributed it to overactivity of the adrenals, and it does occur with certain adrenal tumors, but it is much more likely that the primary difficulty is somewhere in the capillary bed—in that short space in which the real business of life is transacted. Probably *diffuse hyperplastic sclerosis* is often responsible, beginning first in the smaller vessels of the kidney and spleen. However produced, the important point is that this hypertension leads to arteriosclerosis. Major emphasized the possible influence of the guanidine bases.

(2) In the second group the hypertension is associated with arteriosclerosis with consecutive cardiac and renal disease.

(3) In the third group the high tension is secondary to forms of chronic nephritis in association with cardiovascular disease.

(*b*) As an INVOLUTION PROCESS arteriosclerosis is natural with old age, and is the expression of the natural wear and tear to which the tubes are subjected. Longevity is a vascular question, which has been well expressed in the axiom that "a man is only as old as his arteries." To a majority of men death comes primarily or secondarily through this portal. The onset of what may be called physiological arteriosclerosis depends, firstly upon the quality of arterial tissue (vital rubber) which the individual has inherited, and secondly upon the wear and tear to which he has subjected it. That the former plays a most important rôle is shown in the cases in which arteriosclerosis sets in early in life in individuals in whom none of the recognized etiological factors can be found. Thus a man of forty may present vessels as much degenerated as is usual at eighty. Entire families sometimes show this tendency to early arteriosclerosis, which can not be explained in any other way than that in the makeup of the machine bad material was used for the tubing. The influence of heredity plays a considerable part but more commonly the arteriosclerosis results from the bad use of good vessels. The influence of infection, general or focal, is often an additional factor.

(*c*) INTOXICATIONS.—Alcohol, lead and gout play a rôle, although the precise mode of their action is not clear. They may act by increasing the peripheral resistance in the smaller vessels and so raising the blood pressure, or possibly, as Bright taught, they alter the quality of the blood and render more difficult its passage through the capillaries. The toxins of disturbed metabolism or of infections may produce degenerative changes in the media and adventitia. Thayer called attention to the frequency of arterial changes as a sequence of typhoid fever.

(*d*) ENDOCRINE DISTURBANCE.—This is seen especially with the menopause but other factors are probably concerned.

(*e*) OVEREATING.—This plays an important part in inducing arteriosclerosis. It is associated with obesity in many cases. An increase of cholesterol in the blood plasma may have an influence. George Cheyne's advice is always applicable.

(*f*) STRESS AND STRAIN.—There are men in the fifth decade who have not had syphilis or gout, who have eaten and drunk with discretion, and in whom none of the ordinary factors are present—men in whom the arteriosclerosis seems to come on as a direct result of a high pressure life.

(*g*) OVERWORK OF THE MUSCLES may act by increasing the peripheral resistance and by raising the blood pressure.

(*h*) RENAL DISEASE.—The relation between the arterial and kidney lesions has been much discussed. There are two groups of cases, one in which the arteriosclerosis is primary, and the other in which it is secondary to a primary affection of the kidneys.

(*i*) Syphilis causes a special form of arterial degeneration.

Morbid Anatomy.—The affection is met with most frequently in the aorta and its main branches. It is comparatively less frequent in the mesenteric and rare in the pulmonary arteries. Several forms may be recognized:

(*a*) NODULAR.—The aorta presents in the early stages numerous flat projections, yellowish or yellowish white in color, particularly about the orifices of the branches. The initial change is in the intima, probably due to bacterial toxins, and the lesions in many ways resemble those of the next group. In the early stage these patches do not involve the entire intima. In more advanced stages the patches undergo atheromatous changes. The material undergoes softening and breaks up into granular material, consisting of molecular débris—the so-called atheromatous abscess. Klotz has called attention to the frequency of nodular endarteritis about the orifices of the intercostal arteries in young people, usually in association with acute infections.

(*b*) DIFFUSE ARTERIOSCLEROSIS.—In this form, the "arterio-capillary fibrosis" of Gull and Sutton, well termed diffuse hyperplastic sclerosis, met with usually in middle-age, the affection is widespread throughout the arteries. The essential lesion is a thickening of the intima in the smaller arteries, which is uniform in the circumference. In the arterioles the first change is swelling and proliferation of the endothelial cells, which undergo hyaline swelling with the production of fatty granules. Gradually the cell outline is lost and the protoplasm replaced by fat. The nuclei disappear. The fatty degeneration stops where the arteriole joins the parent vessels, in which the intima is thickened with the same hyaline change, and there may be great increase in the elastic tissue. The changes in the endothelium are an essential part of the process; the hyaline change may be inflammatory or degenerative. Hypertrophy of the media occurs more in the larger vessels. There is difference of opinion as to the relative part played by inflammatory and degenerative processes. There is much to be said for the view that bacterial toxins play a large part in the etiology. In this group the heart hypertrophies and fibrous myocarditis is often present. The kidneys are sclerotic, may be increased in size and are usually firm. In places the surface may be rough, or present atrophied depressed areas of a deep red color.

(*c*) SENILE ARTERIOSCLEROSIS.—In this the larger arteries are dilated and tortuous, the walls thin and stiff, and the smaller vessels, as the radials, converted into rigid tubes like pipe-stems. The intima of the aorta may be occupied by rough, calcareous plaques, with fissures and loss of substance. There may be subendothelial softening with the formation of atheromatous ulcers on which thrombi may deposit. In the smaller vessels, there are degeneration and calcification of the media—the so-called Monckeberg type.

(*d*) SYPHILITIC ARTERIOSCLEROSIS.—In the aorta this is usually a mesaortitis with definite characteristics. Macroscopically it may be limited in extent, localized at the root of the aorta, or about the orifice of an aneurism, or there is a band of an inch in width on some portion of the tube, while other parts are normal. In other instances the intima is involved, not with the usual plaque-like areas of atheroma, but there are shallow depressions and short transverse or longitudinal puckerings sometimes with a stellate arrangement; or the intima is pitted and scarred with depressions and linear sulci. Microscopically the most important changes are in the media and adventitia: (1) perivascular infiltration of the vasa vasorum; (2) small-celled infiltration in areas of the media, with (3) splitting, separation, and destruction of elastic fibres and the muscle cells. The intima over these areas may be perfectly normal, but often shows signs of thickening with fatty degeneration and the production of hyaline. Similar changes have been described by Klotz in the larger blood vessels in congenital syphilis. The specific nature of this mesaortitis has been determined by the detection of the spirochetes. Other forms affecting the smaller vessels are referred to under syphilis.

(*e*) SCLEROSIS OF THE PULMONARY ARTERY is met with in various conditions: (1) With high tension in the pulmonary circulation, particularly in emphysema and mitral disease. (2) Gummatous arteritis has been met with (Warthin). (3) Primary sclerosis is not uncommon in India (Leonard Rogers). (4) With chronic tuberculosis and thickened pleura. (5) Congenital cardiac lesions with a communication between the two sides. Aneurismal dilatation may be present. Syphilis is a factor in some cases in which dyspnea, cyanosis, polycythemia, repeated hemoptysis, angina with enlargement of the heart and chronic passive congestion are features (*"Ayerza's disease"*).

In many cases of arteriosclerosis the condition is not confined to the arteries, but extends not only to the capillaries but also to the veins, and may properly be termed an *angiosclerosis.*

(*f*) SCLEROSIS OF THE VEINS—*phlebosclerosis*—is not an uncommon accompaniment of arteriosclerosis. It is seen in heightened blood pressure, as in the portal system in cirrhosis of the liver and in the pulmonary veins in mitral stenosis. The affected vessels are usually dilated, and the intima shows a compensatory thickening, which is particularly marked in those regions in which the media is thinned. The new formed tissue in the endophlebitis may undergo hyaline degeneration and is sometimes extensively calcified. Without arteriosclerosis the peripheral veins may be sclerotic, usually in conditions of debility, but not infrequently in young persons.

SYMPTOMS.—The early symptoms are interesting. Stengel has called attention to the pallor, and there may be dyspeptic symptoms. It is remarkable with what rapidity the disease may progress. The peripheral arteries may stiffen and grow old in a couple of years.

The combination of hypertension, palpable thickening of the arteries, hypertrophy of the left ventricle, and accentuation of the aortic second sound is common in one form of arteriosclerosis. From the period of establishment the course may be very varied. For years the patient may have good health, and be in a condition analogous to that of a person with a well compensated valvular lesion. There may be no renal symptoms, or there may be a larger amount of urine, with transient albuminuria, and now and then hyaline casts. The subsequent history is extraordinarily diverse, depending upon the territory in which the sclerosis is most advanced, or upon the accidents which are so liable to happen, and the symptoms may be cardiac, cerebral, renal, etc. In some cases there is a rapid loss of weight.

(*a*) *Cardiac.*—Involvement of the coronary arteries may lead to various results—occlusion with sudden death, fibroid degeneration, aneurism of the heart and rupture. An important group of symptoms results from the dilatation which finally gets the better of the hypertrophy. The patient presents the features of cardiac insufficiency and when he comes under observation for the first time the signs may suggest chronic valvular disease, with a loud blowing murmur at the apex. Many terminate in this way.

(*b*) *Blood Pressure.*—This depends upon the degree of peripheral resistance and the force of the ventricular contraction. Hypertension may exist for a time with little arteriosclerosis; but, as a rule, when the hypertension has been persistent, sclerosis and high tension are found together. On the other hand, a *low* or *normal* pressure may be present when arteriosclerosis is the primary condition.

(*c*) The *cerebral* symptoms are varied and embrace those of many degenerative diseases, acute and chronic (which follow sclerosis of the smaller branches) and cerebral hemorrhage. Syphilis should always be considered. Transient hemiplegia, monoplegia or aphasia may occur in advanced arteriosclerosis. The attacks are often brief, lasting twenty-four hours or less and recovery may be perfect. Recurrence is the rule, and a patient may have a score or more attacks of aphasia, or in a couple of years there may be half a dozen transient hemiplegic attacks or one or two monoplegias, or paraplegia for a day or two. These cases seem best explained on the view of transient spasm. Vertigo occurs frequently, and may be simple, or associated with slow pulse and syncopal or epileptiform attacks—the Stokes-Adams syndrome. The X-ray study may show changes in the abdominal aorta.

(*d*) *Renal* symptoms supervene in a large number of cases. A sclerosis, patchy or diffuse, is present in a majority of the cases at autopsy, and the condition is practically that of contracted kidney. It is seen typically in the senile form, and not infrequently develops early in life as a direct sequence of the diffuse variety. It is often difficult to decide clinically (and the question is one upon which good observers might not agree in a given case) whether the arterial or the renal disease has been primary.

(*e*) *Abdominal Arteriosclerosis.*—This may be associated particularly with overeating and chronic overtaxing of the stomach and intestines. The condition is not uncommon, and the sclerosis of the splanchnic vessels may be out of all proportion to that elsewhere. The *symptoms* are indefinite, sometimes resembling those of the ordinary neurosis with marked constipation, features by no means certainly associated with sclerosis; on the other hand, there is much more reason to connect the attacks of severe abdominal pain as in lead colic, with spasm of the vessels in this condition. Cases of angina pectoris with abdominal pain may be due to angiospasm of the sclerotic vessels.

(*f*) *Gangrene* of the extremities may be due directly to vascular disease or to the dislodgment of thrombi. Sudden transient paralysis of the legs may occur.

(*g*) *Sclerosis of the Vessels of the Legs.*—(1) *Intermittent Claudication.*—The main symptom is pain in the legs, after walking for a few minutes or on walking fast, which may pull the patient "up short" or gradually reach a point at which motion is impossible. The patient rarely falls and after resting for a few minutes he can again walk. The attacks are similar to those of angina pectoris; as one patient expressed it—"there is no difference in the sensation, it is only in the place." (2) *Cramp* of the muscles may occur, and aggravate the pain, sometimes in paroxysms of severe intensity, or nocturnal cramp may be troublesome. (3) Numbness, tingling and sensations of cold are common, and when dependent the feet may become deeply congested; they become white when elevated. (4) *Ulcers* of the toes which may be painful. (5) Sudden *gangrene* which may be due to thrombosis. (6) Superficial *phlebitis.* (7) Absence of the pulse at the ankle and perhaps in the popliteal artery. The femoral pulse may be diminished. Routine examination of the arteries of the leg and foot should be made. The arteries of the feet may be felt as hard cords without pulsation.

Diagnosis.—The recognition of thickening of the arterial walls is usually easy but care should always be taken to feel the radial artery when empty of blood. The temporal artery is often prominent in thin persons without being much thickened. Palpation should always include several arteries in addition to the radial—the brachial, temporal, femoral and the arteries of the foot. Search should be made for alteration in the aorta (dilatation) and the retinal arteries should be inspected. The diagnosis should include the blood pressure, the state of the kidneys and the heart. Diagnosis of the form of arteriosclerosis is possible to some extent. Calcareous deposits may be felt or show in X-ray plates. In the cases with hypertension and renal changes, the sclerosis is usually of the diffuse hyperplastic form.

In vascular disease of the arms and legs it is important to decide the parts played by mechanical obstruction and vascular spasm. In the foot the posterior tibial nerve is anesthetized with procaine (just below the anterior malleolus) and the effect on the surface temperature, in the area of distribution of the nerve, is observed. If there is no increase then vasoconstriction plays no part. If a rise to 30.5° C. occurs, spasm is the main factor. Other methods of study are (1) the oscillometer, (2) the skin temperature, (3) the response to the histamine test (1-1000 solution) as shown by the flare and wheal, (4) the rate of absorption of saline solution injected intradermally and (5) the X-ray study of the arteries.

Prognosis.—This depends greatly on the renal and myocardial condition. With advanced disease in either or both the ultimate outlook is grave. The distribution of the vascular changes is not uniform and signs of special involvement in one organ are more serious than thickening of the peripheral vessels. In rapidly advancing cases the outlook is grave. If the process is stationary and due to some past disease, such as typhoid fever, there is little change in the life expectation if the myocardium and kidneys are not damaged. The association of obesity or diabetes adds to the gravity of the outlook.

Treatment.—In the late stages the conditions must be treated as they arise in the various viscera. In the early stages, before any local symptoms are manifest, the patient should be enjoined to live a quiet well regulated life, avoiding excesses in food and drink. The adjustment of the patient's life as regards business or his profession, stress and worry, and disturbing factors must be accomplished in the best possible way. Ordinary exercise is beneficial and the patient should not limit his physical activity unless there are other reasons for it. If the patient is overweight this should be reduced gradually. The diet should be of simple food, quantity being more important than quality. A moderate amount of protein should be taken as it is usually harmful to reduce this too much. The intake of salt should be kept down; a sufficient amount is added in cooking without using it at table. It is usually best to explain frankly the condition of affairs, and so gain his intelligent cooperation. Special attention should be paid to the bowels and urine, and the skin kept active by daily baths. Alcohol in all forms should be prohibited. A visit every year to one of the mineral springs is usually serviceable. It is an advantage if the winter can be spent in a warm climate. If there has been a syphilitic history the persistent use of iodide is indicated; indeed, even in hilitic cases it seems to do good. It is best given in small doses, (0.3 to 0.6 gm.). Whenever the blood pressure is high nitroglycer- m nitrite may be given to relieve symptoms rather than with any hope lly influencing the disease. With involvement of the vessels of the should be taken to keep the leg and foot as warm as possible, trauma e avoided, especially in cutting the nails, and the feet should be kept very clean. Dry heat may be used and diathermy has been employed. The use of postural exercises, as in Buerger's disease, and placing the foot and leg in cold and hot water alternately may be helpful. With ulcer or gangrene the usual measures are employed. If spasm is predominant, on theoretical grounds, lumbar sympathectomy should be useful but the results are doubtful. The same may be said of peri-arterial sympathectomy.

THROMBO-ANGIITIS OBLITERANS—*Buerger's Disease*

Definition.—A vascular disease, involving arteries and veins with thrombosis, pain, intermittent claudication, edema, ulceration and gangrene. Vasomotor spasm is common, probably most in the early stages. We owe to Buerger the first complete study of the disease.

Etiology.—The disease occurs predominantly in males and usually in middle age. The essential cause is unknown but an infectious factor is strongly suggested. Against this is the sex occurrence. Tobacco may be a contributing factor; certainly the majority of the patients have used it to excess, especially cigarettes. The disease occurs in some who have never used tobacco. As to *race,* it occurs in those of the Hebrew race in a large percentage, especially Russian and Polish, but also in other races. Negroes may be an exception.

Pathology.—There is an inflammatory lesion of the arteries and veins with thrombus formation. The artery, vein and nerve may be involved in an inflammatory, indurated mass. The thrombus becomes organized with canalization. Arteriosclerotic changes are present. The acute process involves local areas from time to time. There may be phlebitis, sometimes migratory, of the superficial veins. The nerves in the involved areas may show a neuritis. Some studies suggest that there is a tendency to concentration of the blood.

Symptoms.—The onset is usually gradual with pain in the leg and foot. One side is involved first and the other usually follows after a variable interval. There is coldness of the leg and intermittent claudication. With the inflammatory process there may be local pain and swelling. Later there are changes due to the interference with the blood supply. The foot is cyanotic when allowed to hang down and pale when elevated. The pulsation in the arteries is reduced or absent. Trophic lesions follow with fissures or ulcers, often about the nails, onychia and gangrene. The pain usually is greatly aggravated with these developments. *Phlebitis* of the superficial veins is common and may occur before the arteries are involved. It may be migratory or repeated attacks occur.

While the legs are most frequently involved, the disease involves the arms not infrequently but rarely alone, usually with the legs. A similar lesion occurs elsewhere than in the arms and legs, especially in the coronary and mesenteric vessels. Coronary occlusion occurs in some of these patients. Some patients have disturbance of vision and marked changes have been found in the retinal vessels.

Diagnosis.—Raynaud's disease should not cause difficulty, especially with a period of observation. In the cases of disturbance of the circulation due to arteriosclerotic changes, there is not the degree of pain in Buerger's disease. The special tests to determine the state of the circulation are important. They are particularly useful in the early stages.

Early diagnosis and prompt treatment with improvement suggest a favorable outlook. When ulceration or gangrene has appeared the prognosis is serious, especially for saving the limb.

Treatment.—The patient should be in bed with dry heat used constantly. The use of tobacco is forbidden. Postural exercises and hydrotherapy with alternating heat and cold are useful. Sodium citrate solution (250 cc. of a 2 per cent solution) or physiological salt solution (250 cc.) is given intravenously every second day for a month. After a month the injections are given every third day, or fourth day, and the patient is allowed to be in a wheel chair. Foreign protein therapy is also used; typhoid vaccine is given every two or three days (25 million is the first dose and this is increased by 25 million in each dose until 12 are given).

If there is a definite element of vasoconstriction, and this is usually marked in the early stages, *sympathetic ganglionectomy* (second to fourth lumbar ganglia) has proved useful. *Adrenalectomy* has given favorable results in some cases but only if there is not marked blocking of the large arteries and the collateral circulation is capable of vasodilatation. The tests after anesthesia determine this. With gangrene, unless slight and responding to treatment, amputation is indicated. It may be necessary also if there is very severe pain which can not be controlled. In all stages measures have to be employed for the relief of pain; morphia is often required, for a time at any rate.

ALTERATION IN BLOOD PRESSURE

Variations in blood pressure do not constitute diseases but result from disturbances in many diseased conditions. The arterial pressure depends on (1) the power of contraction of the left ventricle, (2) the volume of blood forced into the aorta, (3) the condition of the arteries, especially their elasticity, (4) the vasomotor tone, particularly in the capillaries, (5) the peripheral resistance and (6) the viscosity of the blood. The blood pressure is not fixed in health but varies especially with exercise and nervous disturbance.

Hypertension.—To warrant this term, the increase in pressure must be permanent, and a systolic pressure of 160 may be taken as an arbitrary figure for the minimum of hypertension.

Etiology.—Clinically it occurs in a variety of conditions, always remembering that there may be a combination of factors. The most important are: (1) *Hypertrophy* of the left ventricle. (2) *Essential hypertension, hyperpiesia.* The cause of this is obscure but it often leads to changes in the vessels and to renal changes, which may terminate in chronic nephritis with hypertension. This sequence of events is proved; the mechanism of the process is doubtful in many cases. (3) *With renal disease.* The maximum figures are found in this group, especially in chronic interstitial nephritis. (4) With some cases of *arteriosclerosis,* especially in those termed diffuse hyperplastic sclerosis. (5) With *endocrine* gland disturbance. This includes many puzzling cases. Hypertension in women about the menopause is comparatively common. In some cases it may last for some months or a year and then disappear. Certain tumors of the adrenal glands (paraganglioma) cause paroxysmal hypertension. (6) With *intracranial* conditions causing increased intracranial pressure, such as hemorrhage. (7) With *increased volume of blood.* (8) With increased *viscosity* of the blood. (9) With *obesity.*

Pathogenesis.—This is obscure in many cases and there are probably several factors. (1) *Mechanical.* These operate in hypertrophy of the ventricle and in the nephritic-sclerotic group. (2) *Nervous.* The effect is apparently through the vasomotor system and possibly by influences on the endocrine glands. (3) *Chemical* and *toxic.* Of these we know very little and it is here perhaps that much of the etiology lies. The view that excessive secretion of epinephrine is often responsible has little to support it. What part bacterial toxins play is a question but low-grade long continued infections may be important. Major finds increased amounts of guanidine bases in the blood.

Symptoms.—These are variable and difficult to separate from those due to other conditions. In many cases there are none; the individual is in good health and the hypertension is discovered accidentally. Headache, vertigo, feelings of fullness in the head and flushing are common complaints. *Acute paroxysmal hypertension* is seen as a rule in patients with hypertension and myocardial disease. Some are cases of syphilitic disease of the aorta and aortic valves. The onset of symptoms is usually acute with great distress and dyspnea. Some have pain with the features of angina pectoris. Sweating is common. The blood pressure may rise from 200 to 280 or 300 systolic and the diastolic increase also. Vasodilator drugs may give relief but morphia hypodermically is much more effective. The distress and increase in pressure may occur together or the latter may occur first. The heart rate may increase or remain unchanged. What may be termed "hypertension hypochondriasis" is frequent. The patients suffer more from knowing that hypertension is present than from the hypertension itself. They study their blood pressure figures as some do those of the stock market. The physical findings may show only high pressure and in temporary cases there may be nothing more. Usually changes in the arteries are evident, or appear later, with cardiac hypertrophy and renal changes. In many cases the hypertension is only part of the picture. The *diagnosis* of hypertension offers no difficulty but should not be made on one reading unless there are definite cardiac, renal or cerebral changes. The diagnosis of the cause demands careful study.

In *malignant hypertension* there are severe headache, often great loss of weight, marked retinal changes, marked hypertension with the diastolic pressure much increased, and a progressive course. The duration is about two years but may be less. A study of the arterioles in a portion of excised muscle shows the characteristic changes.

Prognosis.—This depends principally on the cause and the extent of disease in the circulatory and renal systems. Marked increase in the diastolic pressure is generally of serious significance. The long duration of life in some patients with hypertension should always be kept in mind.

Treatment.—The etiology should be studied, any causal factors removed if possible and other lesions properly treated. Any focus of infection should be removed. How much should the patient be told as to the hypertension and the figures? Good judgment is needed to decide this, but it is rarely wise to frighten him with talk of hemorrhage, etc. A frank explanation of the condition and the reasons for the treatment advised is usually wise, with the advice not to have the pressure taken frequently. Often the question arises as to how much reduction in work is advisable. Each patient is a special problem but in general it is wise to advise cutting down the amount of business or work, especially if it involves worry and strain. Mental rest and quiet, so far as they can be secured, are important. Long hours of physical rest are useful. Exercise, short of fatigue, is helpful, best in the form of walking, golf, etc. A good vacation, often well spent at one of the springs, is an advantage. One day a week in bed on a low diet is useful. The *diet* should not be too much restricted, as the mistake of too much reduction in protein is often made. The *quantity* of food should be reduced in the majority. Meat, poultry or fish may be taken once a day in moderate amounts; eggs need not be forbidden. Tea and coffee are to be used in moderation; alcohol should not be taken. Water should be taken fairly freely, especially before meals. It is well to reduce the amount of salt; none should be added to the food. If the patient is overweight, by proper diet and exercise, this should be reduced. In such patients it is well to reduce the carbohydrate intake.

Bathing in tepid or warm water is usually best. The bowels should be kept well open, for which a saline before breakfast is often useful. A weekly dose of blue mass (gr. 5-10, 0.3-0.6 gm.) or mercury and chalk powder (gr. 5, 0.3 gm.) at bedtime for two successive nights is often beneficial. Some patients do well with irrigations of the colon once or twice a week in addition. A *sedative,* such as phenobarbital is generally helpful. The use of *vasodilators* is sometimes of value in relieving symptoms, especially headache and dizziness. Nitroglycerine, sodium nitrite and erythrol tetranitrate are the most useful. The dose must be decided for each patient. Sodium sulphocyanate in doses of gr. v (0.3 gm.) has been used but its value is slight. Hyperventilation by deep breathing exercises has been employed. In patients at the menopause, ovarian extract may be effectual. Iodide is rarely beneficial.

Hypotension.—A persistent systolic figure below 110 may be regarded as hypotension. There are two groups of cases: (1) Essential or Primary Hypotension, which is natural for the individual and (2) Secondary Hypotension, due to a number of causes.

Etiology of Secondary Hypotension.—(1) Weakness of the *left ventricle.* (2) *Vasomotor disturbance,* especially in some infections, as typhoid fever, and in general nervous debility. (3) In some cases of *arteriosclerosis.* (4) In *anemia.* (5) In conditions in which the amount of blood is decreased as after hemorrhage or severe diarrhea. (6) In some *endocrine gland disturbances.* Special interest belongs to the question of *adrenal insufficiency* which may be a factor in some cases. (7) With *cachexia* and *malnutrition.* (8) In *shock.*

Symptoms.—Headache and dizziness are common, especially on getting up suddenly from a recumbent position or on stooping. Weakness is common and fatigue is easily produced. *Syncope* may occur frequently and especially on changing from the recumbent to the upright position. There may be a marked drop in blood pressure. Special interest attaches to the *white line* produced by gently drawing the nail over the skin of the body. It appears slowly and may persist for some minutes. Some regard it as diagnostic of adrenal insufficiency but this is doubtful. Vasomotor instability is often marked. Evidence of disturbance in the sympathetic nervous system is usually present. As a rule there is a less proportionate fall in the diastolic than in the systolic and pulse pressures. The symptoms in the secondary group are difficult to separate from those of the associated condition. In "*postural hypotension*" there is a marked fall of pressure, often with vertigo, when the patient stands. The application of a tourniquet to the legs or making movements of the legs may raise the pressure. Influence of the carotid sinus and aortic nerves is suggested.

Essential Hypotension is comparatively common and in the majority of patients does not cause any symptoms. However, if anything occurs to cause a drop in pressure their margin of safety is low and symptoms may be marked. Some are of the thin, visceroptotic build and subject to vasomotor disturbances but by no means all and hypotension may be normal in a strong energetic individual. In the "feeble" type of individual there is usually nervous instability with fatigue both physical and nervous. The basal metabolism may be low.

Prognosis.—In the essential form the hypotension is usually permanent and probably conduces to longevity as there is a minimum of wear and tear on the circulation. In the secondary forms the outlook depends on the associated condition.

Treatment.—This may be etiological as in myocarditis or anemia. Every effort should be made to improve the general health. Exercise has to be carefully ordered as these patients are easily fatigued; simple exercises which can be done with the patient lying down are useful. An abdominal support may give much comfort. Rest should be ample and an hour or two of rest in the day is an advantage. Cool baths or sponging with brisk rubbing is helpful. Drugs sometimes help but often have no effect. Ergot, as the fluid extract (ʒ ss, 2 cc.) or ergotin (gr. ii, 0.13 gm.), is often useful. Pituitary extract (gr. ii, 0.13 gm.) is worth a trial. Adrenal gland therapy can be tried as the whole gland extract (gr. 5, 0.3 gm.). The preparations of the adrenal cortex may prove to be useful. Ephedrine may be given in doses of 50 milligrams. Some of these patients have a low blood sugar and the taking of dextrose tablets at times when fatigue is felt may be of benefit. Digitalis is not indicated except for myocardial insufficiency.

AORTITIS

Acute Aortitis.—This is much more common than is usually recognized. It occurs in acute infections but especially in septicemia and rheumatic fever, particularly in children who have aortic endocarditis. Of greatest importance is its occurrence in syphilis.

Pathology.—The process may be diffuse or most evident in slightly raised areas which at first are soft and later harder and with a yellow tinge. The first portion of the arch is most often affected and this may involve the orifices of the coronary arteries. If the aorta was previously diseased, all stages of atheroma may be found.

Symptoms.—*Pain* is common, usually referred to the upper part of the sternum and sometimes radiating into the arms. There may be dyspnea and a sense of thoracic oppression. In the syphilitic form, pain is the outstanding symptom, sometimes with the characters of angina pectoris. In other forms the pain is merged in the symptoms of the primary condition, especially in the acute infections.

Signs.—There may be marked pulsation in the neck, especially in the suprasternal notch, where the aorta may be seen and felt, and in the first and second interspaces. There is dulness over the manubrium and in the first two interspaces, both to right and left. The second sound may have a musical bell-like quality, sometimes very characteristic. The *syphilitic* form as a rule shows in addition the signs of aortic insufficiency.

Diagnosis.—The main requisite is that the condition be kept in mind. It is unrecognized because not considered. The X-ray study shows enlargement of the aorta. Difficulty arises in the diagnosis between *organic* and *dynamic* dilatation. The latter occurs especially in rheumatic fever and thyrotoxicosis. Time may be required to decide as later examinations show if there is permanent enlargement. A positive Wassermann reaction or other evidence of syphilis gives the diagnosis of this form.

Prognosis.—The condition in itself probably does not shorten life but may lead to permanent damage of the aortic orifice and to chronic aortitis. In the syphilitic forms the amount of change depends somewhat on early diagnosis and proper treatment.

The treatment is that of the etiological condition.

Chronic Aortitis.—(Dilatation of the Aorta).—This is a common condition, frequently overlooked. The diffuse dilatation is sometimes described under aneurism but deserves separate mention. It was first described by Hodgson in 1815 as "preternatural permanent enlargement of the cavity of an artery." It is often associated with aortic insufficiency, a combination which the French term *maladie de Hodgson*.

Etiology.—It is much more common in males and the colored race shows a high incidence. There are several groups: (1) As a result of infection and acute aortitis a permanent dilatation remains especially in rheumatic fever and syphilis. (2) As part of a general arteriosclerosis in which the aorta is specially involved. (3) In the aged it is common as part of advanced arterial degeneration.

Pathology.—The extent of dilatation varies greatly and may involve only a portion of the arch, extend throughout the whole extent of the aorta or only to where the aorta passes through the diaphragm. The orifices and part of the vessels given off from the aorta may be involved in the dilatation. The aorta shows all grades of gross atheromatous change.

Symptoms.—There are several groups: (1) Latent cases, especially in the aged. (2) The symptoms due to cardiac disease predominate, especially myocardial insufficiency or aortic insufficiency. (3) A group with features suggestive of angina pectoris, not surprising in view of the disease of the first part of the aorta. The pain may radiate down either arm or sometimes down both. The common complaints are of pain, dyspnea and cough.

Signs.—The neck may be full with distended veins and a collar of pulsation above the clavicles and sternum. Pulsation in the suprasternal notch is common. The manubrium may be lifted and pulsation in the upper two interspaces is often seen. The order of frequency is second right, second left, first right and first left interspace. This pulsation is usually diffuse and can rarely be felt distinctly. The aorta may be felt above the sternum or with the finger behind it. *Dulness* is very important, over the manubrium and adjoining interspaces. It is continuous with the heart dulness in most cases but not always. The width of the dulness in the first interspaces may be 8 to 14 cm. and the extent may vary from time to time. On *auscultation* the second sound often has an amphoric bell-like quality, which is diagnostic if present. The murmur of an associated aortic insufficiency may have the same quality. The blood pressure is low in the majority. Arteriosclerosis is usually and aortic insufficiency (relative or permanent) often present. The *pressure signs* are as in aneurism, inequality of the pupils, laryngeal paralysis, tracheal tug, inequality of the radial pulses and dysphagia.

Diagnosis.—The main point is to know of the condition and look for it. The diagnosis from aneurism or displacement of the aorta is difficult in a few cases; the X-ray study will decide. In some cases a carotid artery, usually the right, is curved, owing to its point of origin being higher, and forms a prominence above the clavicle, which may be mistaken for an aneurism. The pain may suggest angina pectoris but is rarely so severe, often lasts for a considerable time, and is not so often caused by exertion; mild exertion sometimes relieves the pain. Sweating is rare.

Treatment.—A quiet even life with avoidance of strain, physical or mental, a limited diet, open bowels, and the treatment of symptoms are the main points. If syphilis is responsible, treatment should be given but usually the damage is beyond repair. Vasodilators are useful for pain.

ANEURISM

Definition.—A tumor containing blood or blood clot in direct communication with the cavity of the heart, the surface of a valve, or the lumen of an artery.

History.—Galen knew external aneurism well, and in the second century A. D., Antyllos devised his operation of incising and emptying the sac inclosed between ligatures. Internal aneurism was recognized by Fernelius in the 16th century and Vesalius was very familiar with it. Ambroise Paré suggested the relation of aneurism to syphilis, which was insisted upon in the great monograph of Lancisi in 1728. Morgagni in 1761 described very fully the symptoms and morbid anatomy. The modern views date from the studies of Helmstedter and Köster. The researches of Eppinger, Thoma, and Welch emphasized the importance of the changes in the media.

Classification.—The following classification may be adopted:

I. True aneurism, in which one or more of the coats of the vessel form the wall of the tumor: (*a*) *Dilatation aneurism*—(1) Limited to a certain portion of the vessel, fusiform, cylindroid; (2) extending over a whole artery and its branches—cirsoid aneurism. (*b*) *Circumscribed saccular aneurism*, the common form of aneurism of the aorta. (*c*) *Dissecting aneurism,* with splitting of the media, and occasionally with the formation of a new tube.

II. False aneurism, following a wound or the rupture of an artery or of a true aneurism, causing a diffuse, or circumscribed, hematoma.

III. Arteriovenous aneurism, either with direct communication between an artery and vein, or with the intervention of a sac, *varicose aneurism.*

IV. Special forms, as the parasitic, erosion, traction and mycotic.

Etiology.—Predisposing Causes.—*Age.*—In the young and in the very old the disease is rare, but it may occur at any age. Richy collected 41 cases (1923) of aneurism of the thoracic aorta below the age of 19 years. Only two cases were syphilitic and nearly half were mycotic, usually with rheumatic fever. Congenital aneurism usually occurs in the cerebral arteries.

Sex.—Males are attacked much more frequently than females—5 to 1.

Race and Locality.—Lucke and Rea in the collected statistics of 160,145 autopsies found 1,452 cases of aneurism (1 in 110). The proportion was higher in the United States than in Great Britain, Scandinavia, Germany or Austria. The disease is more common in Great Britain than on the Continent. Among about 19,000 postmortems at Vienna there were 230 cases of aneurism, while among 18,678 at Guy's Hospital there were 325 cases. It is much more common among the negroes of North America than among the whites. In India aneurism is rare, though syphilis and arterial disease are common. Possibly, as Roger suggests, the low blood pressure in the natives may have some influence.

Occupation.—Soldiers, sailors, draymen, iron and steel workers, and dock workers are particularly prone. This is due to the effect of strain on a vessel damaged by syphilis.

Determining Causes.—I. *Acute Infections.*—In the specific fevers areas of degeneration are common in the aorta. Fortunately in most instances they are confined to the intima, but occasionally, as in typhoid fever, the changes may be in the media. *The* infection with which aneurism is especially connected is *syphilis*—a fact recognized in the eighteenth century by Lancisi and by Morgagni, and dwelt upon specially in 1876 by F. H. Welch, of the British Army. All recent figures show a very high percentage of syphilis and it is rare not to find a positive Wassermann reaction in an aneurismal patient. Other infections play a very minor rôle. With rheumatic fever, pneumonia, and septicemia, the mycotic aneurism may occur.

II. The second factor is *strain,* particularly that associated with sudden and violent muscular effort. The media is the protecting coat of the artery, and during a violent effort, laceration or splitting of the intima may occur over a weak spot. If small this leads to a local bulging of the media and the gradual production of a sac, or the tear of the intima may heal completely, or a dissecting aneurism may form. In other instances a widespread mesaortitis leads to gradual, diffuse distention of the artery. This type of aneurism, frequent in the aged, may follow ordinary chronic atheroma.

III. *Occasional Causes.*—(*a*) *Embolism:* The emboli may consist of vegetations or calcified fragments from the valves. This form, often multiple, is met with in infective endocarditis, in which the emboli probably pass to the vasa vasorum, causing mesaortitis with weakening of the wall; but in the smaller vessels the aneurisms are caused by the direct lodgment of the emboli which infect and weaken the wall. (*b*) *External Injury:* A blow on the chest, a sudden fall, or the jar of an accident may cause a rupture of the intima over a weak spot in the aorta, with the production of a dissecting or sacculated aneurism. (*c*) *External Erosion:* A tuberculous focus may involve the wall of the aorta; or a bullet lodged near the wall of an artery may weaken it and aneurism follows. (*d*) In the horse there is a *parasitic aneurism* common in the mesenteric vessels, due to growth in them of *Strongylus armatus*. (*e*) Thoma described a "traction" aneurism in the concavity of the arch at the point of insertion of the ductus Botalli.

Morbid Anatomy.—NUMBER.—Usually there is one aneurism, but three or four or even a dozen may be present. Multiple cup-shaped tumors in the aorta are always syphilitic. The mycotic are usually multiple and in the peripheral vessels there may be a dozen or more.

FORM.—There are two great types—one in which the lumen of the vessel is dilated, and the other in which a limited section of the wall gives way with the formation of a sac. Typical cylindrical and spindle shaped aneurisms are seen in the aorta and in the vessels of the second and third dimensions. The sacculated form is the more common. They are either flat, saucer-shaped, or cup-shaped, or sometimes beyond a very narrow orifice is a cylindrical tumor of variable size, from a pin's head in the smaller vessels, as in the brain, to a huge sac which may fill one-half of the chest.

VESSELS AFFECTED.—Of a series of 551 cases studied by Crisp, the thoracic aorta was involved in 175, abdominal aorta in 59, femoral-iliac in 66, popliteal in 137, innominate in 20, carotids in 25, subclavians in 23, axillary in 18. The other smaller vessels are rarely attacked. Of late years aneurism of the external vessels appears to be much less frequent.

ANEURISM OF THE AORTA

A. Aneurism of the Thoracic Aorta.—For purposes of discussion this part of the vessel may be divided into the sinuses of Valsalva, ascending, transverse, and descending portions.

(*a*) ANEURISM OF THE SINUSES OF VALSALVA is most frequent in young syphilitic subjects. There may be pouching of one or all three sinuses; the aortic ring is apt to be involved with aortic insufficiency. The special features are: (1) It is often *latent*, causing sudden death by perforation into the pericardium. (2) It is a medicolegal aneurism met with in coroner's cases. (3) Angina pectoris is not uncommon with it. (4) Aortic insufficiency is often associated. (5) In a majority of cases syphilitic mesaortitis is present.

(*b*) ANEURISM OF THE ASCENDING ARCH.—Along the convex border aneurism frequently arises and may grow to a large size, either passing out into the right pleura or forward, pointing at the second or third interspace, eroding the ribs and sternum, and producing an external tumor. Here the sac may compress the superior vena cava, causing engorgement of the vessels of the head and arm; sometimes it compresses the subclavian vein and causes enlargement and edema of the right arm. Perforation may take place into the superior vena cava. In rare instances, when the aneurism springs from the concave side of the vessel, the tumor may appear to the left of the sternum. Large aneurisms in this situation may displace the heart down and to the left, and sometimes compress the inferior vena cava, causing swelling of the feet and ascites. The right recurrent laryngeal nerve is often compressed. The innominate artery is rarely involved. Death commonly follows from rupture into the pericardium, pleura or superior cava; less commonly from rupture externally, sometimes from syncope.

(*c*) Aneurism of the Transverse Arch.—The direction of growth is most commonly backward, but the sac may grow forward, erode the sternum, and form a large tumor. The sac presents in the middle line and to the right of the sternum much more often than to the left, which occurred in only 4 of 35 aneurisms in this situation (O. A. Browne). Even when small and producing no external tumor it may cause marked *pressure signs,* involving the trachea and esophagus, and giving rise to cough, often paroxysmal, and dysphagia. The left recurrent laryngeal nerve is often involved. A small aneurism from the lower or posterior wall of the arch may compress a bronchus, inducing bronchorrhea, bronchiectasis and suppuration in the lung—a process sometimes termed "aneurismal phthisis." Occasionally enormous aneurisms arise in this situation, and grow into both pleurae, extending between the manubrium and the vertebrae; they may persist for years. The sac may be evident at the sternal notch. The innominate artery, less commonly the left carotid and subclavian, may be involved, and the radial or carotid pulse absent or retarded. The thoracic duct may be compressed.

The ascending and transverse portions of the arch are not infrequently involved together, usually without the branches; the tumor grows upward, or upward and to the right.

(*d*) Aneurism of the Descending Portion of the Arch.—This may be the traction aneurism of Thoma. The sac projects to the left and backward, and often erodes the vertebrae from the third to the sixth dorsal, causing great pain and sometimes compression of the spinal cord. Dysphagia is common. Pressure on a bronchus may induce bronchiectasis, with retention of secretions, and fever. A tumor may appear externally in the region of the scapula, and attain an enormous size. Death may occur from rupture into the pleura, or the sac may grow into the lung and cause hemoptysis.

(*e*) Aneurism of the Descending Thoracic Aorta.—This is the least common situation of aortic aneurism. The larger number occur close to the diaphragm, the sac lying upon or to the left of the bodies of the lower dorsal vertebrae, which are often eroded. It may be latent, in 3 of 14 cases (Osler), and is often overlooked; pulmonary and pleural symptoms are common. Pain in the back is severe; dysphagia is not infrequent. Slow leaking may cause symptoms suggestive of an acute abdominal condition. The sac may reach an enormous size and form a subcutaneous tumor in the left back.

Symptoms.—Broadbent made the useful division of aneurisms of *symptoms* and aneurisms of *physical signs;* the former is more commonly seen when the transverse arch is involved, the latter when the ascending portion. There may be no symptoms. A man may present a tumor which has eroded the chest wall without pain or any discomfort but this is rare.

An important feature in thoracic aneurism is *pain,* particularly marked in deep seated tumors. It is usually paroxysmal, sharp, and lancinating, often very severe when the tumor is eroding the vertebrae, or perforating the chest wall. In the latter case after perforation the pain may cease. Anginal attacks are not uncommon, particularly in aneurisms at the root of the aorta. Frequently the pain radiates down the left arm or up the neck, sometimes along the upper intercostal nerves. Superficial tenderness may be present. *Cough* results from direct pressure on the trachea or is associated with bronchitis. The sputum in these cases is abundant, thin, and watery; subsequently it becomes thick and turbid. *Paroxysmal cough* of a peculiar brazen, ringing character is a characteristic feature in some cases, particularly when there is pressure on the recurrent laryngeal nerves; the cough may have a peculiar wheezy quality—the "goose cough."

Dyspnea, which is common in aneurism of the transverse portion, is not necessarily associated with pressure on the recurrent laryngeal nerves, but may be due to compression of the trachea or a bronchus. It may occur with marked stridor. Loss of voice and hoarseness occur from pressure on the recurrent laryngeal, usually the left, inducing paralysis or spasm of a vocal cord. Paralysis of an abductor on one side may be present without any symptoms. It is more particularly when paralytic contractures supervene that attention is called to laryngeal symptoms.

Dysphagia may be due to spasm or direct compression. A tube or sound should never be passed in these cases, as the esophagus may be almost eroded and perforation of the sac has taken place.

Heart Symptoms.—The heart is hypertrophied in less than one-half of the cases and this is due to conditions other than the aneurism. The aortic valves are sometimes incompetent, either from disease of the segments, generally syphilitic, or stretching of the aortic ring.

Physical Signs.—INSPECTION.—A good light is essential; cases are often overlooked owing to a hasty inspection. The face is often suffused, the conjunctivae injected, and the veins of the chest and one arm engorged. The pupils may be unequal. In many instances inspection is negative. On either side of the sternum there may be abnormal pulsation which should be looked for carefully. Three sorts of pulsation may be seen: (1) A general shock, such as is seen in violent throbbing of the heart or of an aneurism. In anemia, in neurasthenia and in great hypertrophy this widespread shock may suggest aneurism. (2) A diffuse localized impulse which may be caused by a deep-seated aneurism but which is met with also in tumors, in pulsating pleurisy and in a few cases without evident cause. (3) The punctate, heaving true aneurismal impulse which when of any extent is visibly expansile. It is most frequent above the third rib to the right of the sternum, in the second left interspace, over the manubrium, and behind in the left interscapular region. When the innominate is involved the throbbing may be seen at the right sterno-clavicular joint and above it. An external *tumor* is present in many cases, projecting through the upper part of the sternum or to the right, sometimes involving the sternum and costal cartilages on both sides, forming a swelling the size of a cocoanut or larger. The skin is thin, often blood stained, or it may have ruptured, exposing the laminae of the sac. The apex beat may be displaced, particularly when the sac is large. It is more commonly due to dislocation than to enlargement of the heart.

PALPATION.—The area and degree of pulsation may be best determined by palpation. When the aneurism is deep seated and not apparent externally, the bimanual method should be used, one hand upon the spine and the other on the sternum. There may be only a diffuse impulse. When the sac has perforated the chest wall the impulse is, as a rule, forcible, slow, heaving and expansile. It may be more forcible than the apex beat. The resistance may be great if there are thick laminae beneath the skin; more rarely the sac is soft and fluctuating. There may be a diastolic *shock,* often of great intensity, which is a valuable sign of aneurism. A systolic thrill is sometimes present. The pulsation is sometimes felt in the suprasternal notch.

PERCUSSION.—The small and deep seated aneurisms are in this respect negative. In the larger tumors, there is an area of dulness, the position of which depends upon the part of the aorta affected. Aneurisms of the ascending arch grow forward and to the right, producing dulness on one side of the manubrium; those from the transverse arch produce dulness in the middle line, extending toward the left of the sternum, while aneurisms of the descending portion most commonly produce dulness in the left interscapular region. The note is flat and there is a feeling of increased resistance.

AUSCULTATION.—Adventitious sounds are not always heard. Even in a large sac there may be no murmur. Much depends upon the thickness of the laminae of fibrin. An important sign, particularly if heard over a dull region, is a ringing, accentuated second sound. A systolic murmur may be present; sometimes a double murmur, in which case the diastolic is usually due to aortic insufficiency. A systolic murmur alone is of little moment. A continuous humming top murmur with systolic intensification is heard when the aneurism communicates with the vena cava or the pulmonary artery.

Among OTHER PHYSICAL SIGNS of importance are retardation of the pulse in the arteries beyond the aneurism, or in those involved in the sac. There may be a marked difference between the right and left radial, both in volume and time. The blood pressure on the two sides may be unequal. A sign of large thoracic aneurism is obliteration of the pulse in the abdominal aorta and its branches. Attention was called to this in a patient who had aortic insufficiency. There was a well-marked diastolic murmur, but in the femorals and abdominal aorta no pulsation could be found. Examination of the back showed a large area of pulsation in the left scapular region. The sac probably was large enough to act as a reservoir annihilating the pulse wave and converting the intermittent into a continuous stream.

A condition suggestive of pneumothorax may be caused by compression of one bronchus by the sac (Newton Pitt). Air passes beyond the obstruction, but has difficulty in getting out, so that the lung is gradually distended, causing enlargement of the side with a hyperresonant note and absence of breath sounds. The X-ray picture may alone decide the diagnosis.

The *tracheal tugging* was described by Oliver. The patient should be in the erect position with the mouth closed and the chin low. The cricoid cartilage is grasped between the finger and thumb or the ends of two fingers are hooked under it and steady pressure made upward. A pull or tug on the trachea is felt. Sometimes it is visible. This is a sign of great value in the diagnosis of deep-seated aneurisms, though it may occasionally be felt in tumors, in the extreme pulsation of aortic insufficiency and in dilatation of the aorta. The trachea may be pushed to one side.

Occasionally a systolic murmur may be heard in the trachea, or even at the patient's mouth, when opened. This is either the sound conveyed from the sac, or is produced by the air as it is driven out of the trachea during systole. Altered signs in one lung are common effects of pressure.

Hemorrhage may come from (*a*) soft granulations in the trachea at the point of compression, in which case the sputum is blood tinged, but large quantities of blood are not lost; (*b*) from rupture of the sac into the trachea or a bronchus; (*c*) from perforation into the lung or erosion of the lung tissue. The bleeding may be profuse, rapidly proving fatal, and is a common cause of death. It may persist for weeks or months, in which case it is hemorrhagic weeping through the sac, which is exposed in the trachea. In some instances, even after a profuse hemorrhage, the patient recovers and may live for years. A man with thoracic aneurism, who had several brisk hemorrhages, died four years after, having in the meantime enjoyed average health. Death from hemorrhage is relatively more common in aneurism of the third portion of the arch and of the descending aorta.

Venous compression may involve one subclavian or the superior vena cava. A curious phenomenon is clubbing of the fingers of one hand, sometimes without any special distention or venous engorgement. Tumors of the arch may involve the pulmonary artery, producing compression, or in some instances adhesion of the pulmonary segments and insufficiency of the valve; or the sac may rupture into the artery, producing instantaneous death.

Pupil Signs.—These may be due to pressure on the *sympathetic,* which may cause dilatation of one pupil from irritation and contraction when the nerve is paralyzed. Flushing of the side of the face and ear, increased temperature and sweating may be present. As Ainley Walker and Wall have shown, the anisocoria is frequently due to vascular conditions—with low blood pressure in one carotid the pupil on that side is dilated, with high pressure contracted, and in 26 cases of aneurism they found a relation between the state of the pupil and the arteries on the same side. In some cases the anisocoria is a syphilitic manifestation.

An X-ray study should be made in all doubtful cases. The fluoroscope gives an accurate picture of the situation, the size and the relation to the heart. Even a small sac may be seen. Tortuosity of the aorta, due to arteriosclerosis, may suggest aneurism, particularly with the fluoroscope.

Diagnosis.—Aneurism of the aorta may be confounded with: (*a*) The violent throbbing impulse of the arch in aortic insufficiency.

(*b*) *Simple Dynamic Pulsation.*—This leads to error in the abdominal more often than in the thoracic aorta.

(*c*) *Dilatation* of the arch has many of the features of aneurism. The X-ray examination may be required to decide the diagnosis.

(*d*) In *curvature* of the *spine* there may be great displacement of the aorta, so that it pulsates forcibly on one side of the sternum.

(*e*) *Solid Tumors.*—When the tumor projects externally and pulsates the difficulty may be considerable. In tumor the heaving, *expansile* pulsation is absent, and there is not that sense of force and power which is so striking in a perforating aneurism. A diastolic shock is not felt. Auscultatory signs are less definite, as large aneurisms may occur without murmurs and murmurs may be heard over tumors. The greatest difficulty is in deep seated thoracic tumors. The physical signs may be indefinite. The ringing aortic second sound is rarely, if ever, heard over tumor. Tracheal tugging is a valuable sign.

Pressure phenomena are less common in tumor. The general appearance of the patient in aneurism is better than in tumor, in which there may be cachexia and enlargement of the glands in the axilla or in the neck. The X-ray study is most important. The result of the Wassermann reaction is of aid. Occasionally cancer of the esophagus simulates aneurism, producing pressure on the left bronchus.

(*f*) *Pulsating Pleurisy.*—In *empyema necessitatis,* if the projecting tumor is in the neighborhood of the heart and pulsates, the condition may be mistaken for aneurism. The absence of a heaving, firm impulse and of a diastolic shock would, with the history and the existence of a pleural effusion, determine the diagnosis. If necessary, puncture may be made with a fine needle. In a majority of the cases of pulsating pleurisy the throbbing is diffuse and widespread, moving the whole side. The X-ray study is of value.

Prognosis.—The outlook is always grave. Life may be prolonged for some years, but the patients are in constant jeopardy. Spontaneous cure is not very infrequent in the small sacculated tumors. The cavity becomes filled with laminae of firm fibrin, which become dense and hard, the sac shrinks considerably, and finally lime salts are deposited in the old fibrin. The laminae of fibrin may be on a level with the lumen of the vessel, causing complete obliteration of the sac. The cases which rupture externally, as a rule, run a rapid course, although there are exceptions; the sac may contract, become firm and hard, and the patient may live for years. The cases which last longest are those in which a saccular aneurism projects from the ascending arch. The aneurism may be enormous and yet life be prolonged for years. A remarkable instance is the case of dissecting aneurism reported by Graham. The patient was invalided after the Crimean War with aneurism of the aorta, and for years was under the observation of J. H. Richardson, of Toronto, under whose care he died in 1885. The autopsy showed a healed aneurism of the arch, with a dissecting aneurism extending the whole length of the aorta, which formed a double tube.

Treatment.—In a large proportion of cases this can only be *palliative* but in every instance measures should be taken which promote clotting and consolidation in the sac. In any series of cured aneurisms a majority of the patients have not been known to be subjects of the disease but the obliterated sac has been found postmortem.

The most satisfactory plan in early cases, when it can be carried out thoroughly, is the modified Valsalva method advised by Tufnell, of Dublin, the essentials of which are rest and a restricted diet. The *rest* should, as far as possible, be absolute. The reduction of the daily number of heart beats, when a patient is recumbent and without exertion, amounts to many thousands, and is one of the principal advantages of this plan. Mental quiet should also be secured. The *diet* advised by Tufnell is extremely rigid—a total of 10 ounces of solid food and 8 ounces of fluid a day. It is not possible to keep to such amounts for any long period but the intake should be as small as possible. The bowels should be kept freely open and straining at stool avoided. This treatment should be pursued for several months, but usually it is impossible to carry it out for more than a few weeks at a time. It is adapted only to the saccular form, and in large sacs communicating with the aorta by a comparatively small orifice the chances of consolidation are fairly good. Calcium lactate (60 grains, 4 grams, a day) may be given. The patient with symptoms should be at rest on a low diet. At all times he should live a quiet life, avoiding overexertion, fatigue and strain. The bowels should be kept regular, and constipation and straining carefully avoided. Of drugs, iodide of sodium is of great value. It may be given in doses of from 5 to 20 grains (0.3 to 1.3 gm.) three times a day. The most striking effect of iodide is the relief of pain. Although the damage is done, yet it is well to give specific treatment. A thorough course of mercury or bismuth should be given and repeated as often as indicated. Neoarsphenamine should be given very cautiously and the effect carefully watched. There is risk with its use and the initial dose should be not more than 0.1 gram.

When the tumor is large, or there seems little prospect of consolidation, it is better to advise a man to go on quietly with his occupation. Our profession has offered many examples of good work by men with aortic aneurism who wisely preferred to die in harness.

Other Conditions.—Pressure on veins causing engorgement, particularly of the head and arms, is sometimes promptly relieved by free *venesection,* and, at any time, in attacks of dyspnea with lividity, bleeding may be done with great benefit. The nitrites may be given if the blood pressure is high, but rest and low diet, restriction of fluids and free purgation are usually more effectual than drugs in reducing blood pressure. In the final stages morphia is, as a rule, necessary. Chloroform inhalations may be necessary. The question of tracheotomy sometimes comes up in cases of urgent dyspnea. If it is due to bilateral abductor paralysis the trachea may be opened, but this is extremely rare, and urgent dyspnea is usually caused by pressure about the bifurcation. When the sac appears externally and grows large, an ice-bag or a belladonna plaster may be applied but wiring and electrolysis are most useful. In some instances an elastic support may be used with advantage.

Surgical Measures.—Consolidation may be promoted in the sac by the combination of wiring and electrolysis. Moore, in 1864, first wired a sac, putting in 78 feet of fine wire. Corradi proposed the combined method of wiring with electrolysis, which was first used by Burresi in 1879. H. A. Hare did the operation 35 times without any accident. He emphasized the importance of employing a gold platinum wire without too much spring (silver is not suitable), of using the positive pole in the aneurism and not giving too strong a current (5 milliamperes at the beginning, gradually increased to 50, and then decreased to 5 again, the current being passed for about 50 minutes). Wire should be used which snarls and does not coil. A wire which coils tends to press against the aneurismal wall. In nearly all of Hare's patients there was marked benefit, the duration of which was variable. One patient lived for nine years. The decrease in the size of the aneurism is often marked but the relief of pain is a striking feature. The most favorable cases are those in which the aneurism is sacculated, which can usually be determined by the X-ray study. A carotid artery-internal jugular vein anastomosis (end-to-end, not lateral) has been helpful in some cases.

B. Aneurism of the Abdominal Aorta.—Of 233 cases collected by Nixon, 207 were in males, 26 in females; 121 were between the ages of twenty-five and forty-five. Nixon reported a case in a syphilitic girl of twenty. There were 16 cases among 16,000 admissions at the Johns Hopkins Hospital.

Pathology.—The sac is most common just below the diaphragm in the neighborhood of the celiac axis. The tumor may be fusiform or sacculated, and is sometimes multiple. Projecting backward, it erodes the vertebrae and may cause numbness and tingling in the legs and finally paraplegia, or it may pass into the thorax and burst into the pleura. More commonly the sac is on the anterior wall and projects forward as a definite tumor in the middle line or a little to the left. The tumor may project in the epigastric region (most common), in the left hypochondrium, in the left flank or in the lumbar region. When high up beneath the diaphragm it may attain considerable size without being apparent on palpation. If it ruptures into the retroperitoneal tissues a tumor in the flank may be formed gradually, which enlarges with very little pulsation. It may be mistaken for sarcoma or abscess, and an operation may be performed.

The chief *symptom* is pain, very often of a neuralgic nature, passing round to the sides or localized in the back, and more persistent and intense than in any other variety of aneurism. Gastric symptoms, particularly vomiting, may be early and deceptive features.

Diagnosis and Physical Signs.—Inspection may show marked *pulsation* in the epigastric region, sometimes a definite tumor. A thrill is not uncommon. The pulsation is forcible, expansile, and sometimes double when the sac is large. On palpation a *definite tumor can be felt.* Though usually fixed, the aneurism may be freely movable. If large, there is some dulness on percussion, which usually merges with that of the left lobe of the liver. On auscultation, a systolic murmur is, as a rule, audible, and is sometimes best heard at the back. A diastolic murmur is occasionally present, usually very soft in quality. No pulsation, however forcible, no thrill, however intense, no murmur, however loud, justifies the diagnosis of abdominal aneurism unless there is a *definite tumor which can be grasped and which has an expansile pulsation.* Attention to this rule will save many errors. Retardation of the pulse in the femoral artery is common. The *throbbing abdominal aorta* was well described by Morgagni and Laënnec, and called by Allan Burns the "preternatural pulsation in the epigastrium." It is met with (*a*) in nervous women often associated with enteroptosis and pain, and sometimes, as Morgagni pointed out, with vomiting of blood. (*b*) In anemia particularly after severe hemorrhage, in which the throbbing may shake the patient and the bed. (*c*) In aortic insufficiency. (*d*) In sclerosis of the abdominal aorta. A common mistake is to regard this throbbing aorta as aneurism. The vessel may appear dilated and may be grasped in the hand. A tumor of the pylorus, of the pancreas, or of the left lobe of the liver may be lifted with each impulse of the aorta and be confounded with aneurism. The absence of the forcible expansile impulse and the examination in the knee elbow position, in which the tumor, as a rule, falls forward, and the pulsation is not then communicated, suffice for differentiation.

Prognosis.—The outlook is bad but a few cases heal spontaneously. Death may result from (*a*) complete obliteration of the lumen by clots; (*b*) compression paraplegia; (*c*) rupture (which occurred in 152 of the 233 cases in Nixon's series) either into the pleura, retroperitoneal tissues, peritoneum, or the intestines, most commonly into the duodenum; (*d*) embolism of the superior mesenteric artery, producing intestinal infarction.

Treatment.—This is the same as in thoracic aneurism. With an aneurism low down pressure was successfully applied by Murray, of Newcastle. It must be kept up for many hours under anesthesia. The plan is not without risk, as patients have died from bruising and injury of the sac. Nine cases in our series were treated surgically. In two the wiring and electrolysis were followed by great improvement; one man lived for three years.

C. Dissecting Aneurism.—The majority of aneurisms of the aorta begin with a split or crack of the intima over a spot of syphilitic mesaortitis. Once this split has started the aorta may rupture in all its coats, or an aneurism may form at the site, or the fracture of the intima, though large and often circumferential, may heal; or the blood may extend between the coats, separating them for many inches, or in the entire extent, forming a dissecting aneurism; and, lastly, such a dissecting aneurism may heal perfectly.

Spontaneous rupture of the aorta is not very infrequent. Klotz (1932) collected 40 cases from the literature below the age of 40; 9 were 20 years of age or under. The majority, perhaps all, are associated with some degree of dissecting aneurism. There is a peculiar noninflammatory mucoid degeneration of the media, the reason for which is obscure. Syphilis plays no part in it. Usually there is agonizing pain with features of shock, and death may take place instantly; but in fully half of the cases there are two characteristic stages, the first corresponding to the rupture of the inner coats, the second eight to ten hours, or as long as fifteen days later, to fatal rupture of the external layer.

Dissecting aneurism is uncommon. There were only two cases in 16 years at the Hopkins Hospital, where aneurism is exceptionally frequent. The primary split is most frequently in the arch, not far above the valves, and is in the form of a transverse, or vertical, clean cut incision. The extent of the separation of the coats is variable. If the adventitia is reached, rupture is certain to take place, as only the structures of the middle coat can resist for any time the pressure of the blood. The blood may pass for several inches, separating the media, and then burst internally or externally. In other cases the dissection reaches from the ascending arch to the bifurcation, even passing down into the vessels of the leg. The splitting of the coats may reach to all the subdivisions of the aorta. The symptoms are those spoken of under rupture; but a remarkable condition may follow, leading to:

Healed Dissecting Aneurism.—The earlier observers of this regarded it as an anatomical anomaly of a double aorta. The outer tube formed by the dissecting aneurism may extend the entire length of the aorta, occupying the full circumference. The most extraordinary feature is that the outer tube may present a perfectly smooth and natural appearance, and be lined with a new intima. The condition may last for many years.

ANEURISM OF THE BRANCHES OF THE ABDOMINAL AORTA

The **celiac axis** is not infrequently involved in aneurism of the first portion of the abdominal aorta. The *splenic artery* is occasionally the seat of aneurism. This rarely causes a tumor large enough to be felt; sometimes, however, the tumor is of large size. In a man, aged thirty, who had an illness of several months' duration, there was a tumor in the left hypochondriac region, the dulness of which merged with that of the spleen. There was no pulsation, but it was thought that a murmur was heard. The chief symptoms were vomiting, severe epigastric pain, occasional hematemesis, and finally severe hemorrhage from the bowels. An aneurism of the splenic artery the size of a cocoanut was situated between the stomach and the transverse colon. The sac contained densely laminated fibrin. It had perforated the colon. Of 39 cases of aneurism on the branches of the abdominal aorta collected by Lebert, 10 were of the splenic artery.

Of aneurism of the *hepatic artery* Friedenwald and Tannenbaum collected 65 cases (1922) of which 45 were extrahepatic. Rupture took place in 45 cases, in 33 into the abdominal cavity and in 21 into the bile passages. Infections other than syphilis play the main part in etiology. Pain, gastro-intestinal hemorrhages, jaundice and fever are common features, so that it is usually mistaken for gallbladder disease or ulcer. Ligation of the artery may be done but is rarely successful.

Aneurism of the *superior mesenteric artery* is not very uncommon. The diagnosis is scarcely possible from aneurism of the aorta. Plugging of the branches or of the main stem may cause infarction of the bowel. The diagnosis may be possible only after the abdomen is opened.

Renal Artery.—Many are false aneurisms and trauma is a frequent cause. Pulsation and a *bruit* are not always present. Operation is often successful.

Pulmonary Artery.—Primary aneurism of the trunk is very rare. The forms are: (*a*) Of the trunk and main branches. Most of the patients are in the third and fourth decades and syphilis is the important factor. Warthin demonstrated spirochetes in atherosclerosis with aneurism. (*b*) Acute embolic aneurism, which may be multiple with septic thrombi in the veins or endocarditis of the right side of the heart. (*c*) The small aneurisms in the walls of pulmonary cavities, already considered.

MYCOTIC OR BACTERIAL ANEURISMS

Etiology.—These are due to bacterial infection and have two modes of origin. (1) *Intravascular.* In the majority the infection comes from bacterial endocarditis, in 187 of 217 cases collected by Stengel and Wolferth (1923). Other sources are infections in the lungs and bones. The most frequent organisms are nonhemolytic streptococci. Emboli play an important part, being carried in the vasa vasorum, or lodging, especially at a bifurcation, and infecting the wall. Direct infection by bacteria in the blood stream is rare. (2) *Extravascular.* In this the infection may come from an abscess or an infected lymph node. The adventitia is first affected. The ages in the series varied from 4 to 74 years; the majority were in the second, third and fourth decades.

Pathology.—In the series of 217 cases, in 49 cases more than one aneurism was found. The aorta was involved in 66 cases, especially in the arch; the intracranial arteries in 34; the pulmonary artery in 6 and its branches in 8 cases. The size is usually small, not larger than a walnut, and rupture occurs frequently. The intima may be quite normal to the edge of the aneurism.

Symptoms.—Sometimes the occurrence of embolism is noted first, followed very soon by an aneurism, or the aneurism may be discovered first. There is usually severe pain with local redness and swelling. Expansile pulsation may be present. The condition may be mistaken for phlebitis at first.

Treatment.—If the aneurism occurs with endocarditis the outlook is hopeless and symptomatic treatment is indicated. With an infection which is mild or subsiding, operation may be done on a superficial artery. Stengel and Wolferth report a case of healing of a mycotic aneurism.

ARTERIOVENOUS ANEURISM

In this form, known to Galen, but first accurately described by the great William Hunter, there is abnormal communication between an artery and a vein. When a tumor lies between the two it is known as *varicose aneurism;* when there is a direct communication without tumor the vein is chiefly distended and the condition is known as *aneurismal varix.*

While it occurs in the aorta, it is much more common in the peripheral arteries as a result of stab or gunshot wounds.

An aneurism of the ascending portion of the aorta may open directly into the vena cava. Cyanosis, edema, and great distention of the veins of the upper part of the body are the most frequent signs, and develop, as a rule, with suddenness. A thrill is present in some cases. A continuous murmur with systolic intensification is of great diagnostic value. Thurman (Medico-Chirurgical Transactions, 1840) gave the first accurate account of this murmur and the characteristic type of cyanosis. There is only one condition with which it could be confounded, viz., the remarkable cyanosis of the upper part of the body which follows crushing accidents to the thorax. Perforation between the aorta and pulmonary artery causes much the same features. In a few cases an aneurism of the abdominal aorta perforates the inferior vena cava —edema and cyanosis of the legs and lower half of the body, and the distinctive thrill and murmur are present.

In the *arteriovenous* aneurisms which follow wounds of the peripheral arteries the features are characteristic. First, the veins enlarge as the arterial blood flows under high pressure into them. The affected limb may be greatly swollen and in a young person may lengthen, and the growth of hair is increased. Secondly, a strong *thrill* is felt, of maximum intensity at the site of the aneurism, but sometimes felt at the most distant parts of a limb. Thirdly, a characteristic continuous *murmur* with systolic intensification is heard. In the external arteries the condition may persist for years before disability is caused by enlargement of the veins and swelling of the limb. Marked change in the heart may occur with enlargement and myocardial failure, so that treatment should not be delayed. Surgical treatment by a skilled operator is indicated.

Periarteritis Nodosa

An inflammatory lesion of the smaller arteries, beginning in the outer coats, with hyaline degeneration of the media, and formation of secondary aneurisms with thrombosis and rupture. The nodular syphilitic arteritis should not be included in this group. It was described first by Kussmaul and Maier in 1866. Singer found 130 cases in 1927.

The *etiology* is probably infectious. Tonsillitis may precede the attack. The disease appears to be a subacute infection with forms of staphylococci and streptococci (Klotz). Syphilis is not a factor. The smaller arteries are involved, the lesions being exudative or degenerative. The adventitia, media and intima are affected; the media may show necrosis. Aneurism, hemorrhage and thrombosis occur. The nodular tumors vary in numbers from a dozen to many hundreds and may be visible. They differ in structure from the other forms of nodular arteritis, the syphilitic and mycotic.

The disease runs the course of a septic process with fever, weakness, anemia, muscular and joint pains, epigastric pain, vomiting, diarrhea, purpura, asthenia and emaciation. There is usually leukocytosis and occasionally eosinophilia. The *local* features depend on the vessels affected; the coronary and renal arteries are often involved. Abdominal signs are common, with pain, vomiting, and diarrhea with melena. Pancreatitis or rupture of an ulcer has been simulated. The lesions in the peripheral arteries may cause severe pain and suggest neuritis. Small nodules in the skin or subcutaneous tissues occur in about 20 per cent of the cases. Removal and examination of the nodule establishes the diagnosis. Otherwise the *diagnosis* is difficult. The picture may be so varied that many conditions are suggested, especially some acute abdominal condition. The *course* has an average duration of two months. Recovery has occurred. Treatment is symptomatic.

DISEASES OF THE VEINS

Superior Vena Cava.—Obstruction may result from many causes. (1) Aortic aneurism which may compress the vessel or perforate it. (2) Pressure of mediastinal tumors. (3) Chronic mediastinitis. (4) Tuberculosis of mediastinal lymph nodes or by extension from the lung. (5) Thrombosis. (6) Syphilis and extension of pericarditis are suggested. There is venous obstruction in the head, neck, arms and thoracic wall down to about the fifth rib and distention of the collateral circulation. The cerebral congestion may cause headache and vertigo. There may be marked dyspnea. The condition is usually chronic and the course and treatment depend on the associated condition. When due to rupture of an aneurism the symptoms are very acute and death usually results promptly.

Inferior Vena Cava.—Thrombosis usually results from compression of the vein or from the extension of thrombi from other vessels. Occasional instances have occurred with acute infectious diseases. As to the clinical features there may be little change in the terminal stages of other diseases. Usually there is well-marked edema of the legs and of the back without ascites. This edema may be unilateral. Occasionally there is a decrease in the amount of urine due to involvement of the renal veins. If the patients survive, an extensive collateral circulation is established which is generally marked in the superficial veins. If the circulation is carried on by the deeper veins alone, diagnosis may not be possible. It may be that compression where the vena cava passes through the diaphragm is a not infrequent cause.

PHLEBITIS AND THROMBOPHLEBITIS

It is difficult to distinguish between phlebitis alone and phlebitis with thrombus formation. Probably some thrombosis is present in nearly all cases. Two divisions of phlebitis are made: (1) plastic or simple phlebitis and (2) suppurative phlebitis. The terms endo- and periphlebitis suggest the origin of the process.

Plastic Phlebitis.—The clinical picture shows great variation depending on the size of the vein affected and the extent of thrombosis.

Etiology.—(1) With infectious disease as typhoid fever. (2) With or following local infection, as tonsillitis. (3) Postoperative, especially with operations in the lower abdomen and pelvis. (4) Puerperal. (5) Traumatic. (6) Toxic. It is difficult to speak with certainty as to this group as a mild infection is difficult to exclude. The phlebitis of gout may belong here. (7) Secondary to thrombosis. It is possible that with changes in the blood, thrombosis may occur and phlebitis result secondarily, as in polycythemia and chlorosis. (8) In thrombo-angiitis obliterans. (9) Stasis. The influence of this is seen especially in the left iliac or femoral vein. (10) Syphilis.

Symptoms.— *Pain* is present with tenderness over the affected vein. Over superficial veins there may be redness, swelling and local heat. The vein may be felt as a hard cord. If a large vein is involved with thrombosis, edema of the limb is usually marked. The general features vary; fever and leukocytosis are common. With involvement of small veins, as in the feet, there may be little more than pain. In *thrombophlebitis migrans* there are recurrent attacks which involve a local area of superficial veins in the arms and legs, later veins of the viscera may be involved. There is marked local redness and tenderness with swelling, also fever. There may be long intervals between attacks. The cause is obscure; gout and syphilis are suggested while some cases are apparently with thrombo-angiitis obliterans. The *course* of plastic phlebitis is usually slow and weeks are required for recovery. The complication most dreaded is pulmonary embolism, more frequent in some forms, as the postoperative. The ultimate result, as in femoral thrombophlebitis, depends on the extent of canalization in the thrombus and the collateral circulation. The leg may be permanently enlarged and give some disability.

Treatment.—Rest is essential and should be complete. Massage and unnecessary handling and movement should be strictly forbidden. The limb should be elevated and in as comfortable a position as possible. In the diet it is advised to limit the calcium intake and so milk should not be given. With phlebitis in a leg, the bowels should be kept freely open to avoid pressure from the colon. Locally an ice-bag, lead and opium lotion or belladonna ointment may be applied. The period of rest depends on the severity of the attack. Passive motion may be begun after all signs of inflammation have subsided and active motion later. Support by an elastic bandage is advisable in the leg and this should be kept up for some months.

Suppurative Phlebitis.—This may be part of a septicemia or the infection may have reached the vein from an infected area adjoining. There are features of the original infection and if the phlebitis involves a surface vein the local signs are marked. Fever, chills, a rapid pulse and toxic features occur. Septic emboli carry the infection elsewhere. In certain cases, surgical treatment may be successful.

Thrombosis.—It is difficult to separate this from phlebitis as they usually occur together. Either may be primary. In altered conditions of the blood, as in chlorosis, or with marked slowing of the current thrombosis may occur primarily. However, in the great majority of cases it is secondary to phlebitis. The thrombus may act by causing obstruction or portions of it may be detached and act as emboli. If the thrombus is infected with pyogenic organisms, septic emboli are set free and septicopyemia results. In the surface veins the features are as mentioned under phlebitis.

VENOUS BLOOD PRESSURE

The normal venous pressure varies within a wide range, 40 to 150 mm. (usually from 60 to 80) of water. A venous pressure varying from 140 to 280 mm. of water is common in cardiac decompensation. There is apparently no relation between the range of venous and arterial pressure. Increased venous pressure is in cardiac failure. In congestive heart failure involving the right heart it can be measured by venous pressure determinations. When left heart failure is present, the pressure is increased in the lesser circulation and no method is available for measuring this type of failure alone. The estimation of venous pressure is valuable in differentiating dyspnea which is cardiac in origin from other forms. It is helpful in pneumonia in determining what part circulatory weakness takes in causing symptoms. It may be of aid in deciding as to the value of venesection. The venous pressure is normal in bronchial asthma and chronic conditions of the lungs, such as emphysema, etc., unless there is failure of the right side of the heart.

ANGIOMATOSIS: TELANGIECTASIA

Definition.—A disease with multiple telangiectases from which bleeding occurs. There are multiple localized dilatations of the capillaries and venules from which spontaneous hemorrhages occur—not due to disease of the blood.

Classification.—The following groups are made by Madden (1934). (1) Primary, which includes the hereditary forms and certain cases of familial bleeding. (2) Secondary, which may include bleeding in a variety of diseases which may cause endarteritis or injure the vasomotor system. In this group heredity plays no part. The area of bleeding has no special situation but the mucous membranes are affected less often than in the primary form. (3) Nevoid, which may be congenital or appear later. The so-called spider angiomata belong here. They occur especially with chronic jaundice and disappear if it clears; in leukemia they are usually permanent. The most important of all these is the primary form.

Angiomatosis (*Telangiectasia*) *Hereditary—familial form.*—The condition occurs in both sexes, may be transmitted by either sex and behaves as a Mendelian dominant. Goldstein (1931) found mention in the literature of over 90 families with 550 members affected. The lesions may be present at birth and usually increase in number with age. As a rule they are most numerous on the face and on the mucous membrane of the mouth and nose. The defect is described as a lack of the muscular and elastic tissue in the dilated vessels. Slight trauma or congestion may cause bleeding and the absence of retraction of the vessels favors its prolongation. In some cases bleeding does not occur until youth or even adult life.

Symptoms.—Hemorrhage is the striking feature, epistaxis being most frequent. It may occur spontaneously or be due to trauma or congestion. The coagulation and bleeding time, fragility of the red cells and calcium content of the blood are normal. The blood platelets are usually stated to be normal but some low counts are reported. Anemia may result from the hemorrhage. In addition to epistaxis, bleeding may occur from the skin, respiratory, digestive, or urinary tracts, and intracranially. Some cases of "essential hematuria" may be due to this.

The *telangiectases* may not be noted until adult life. They may appear as spider networks of capillaries, dilated vessels, red areas or blebs, or as nevi. They are most common about the face and in the nose and mouth; they are rare elsewhere except on the finger tips. Rare findings are splenomegaly and intolerance to blood transfusion. Death may result from hemorrhage, intracranial or elsewhere.

The *Lindau syndrome* shows pial angiomas which may show calcification, seen in roentgenograms, in the walls of affected vessels or in thrombosed areas. Glaucoma occurs also. The relationship of this syndrome is doubtful.

Diagnosis.—The *diagnosis* depends on heredity, hemorrhage and the presence of telangiectasia. As bleeding may occur and few or no telangiectases be visible the diagnosis may be missed. A thorough study should prevent error.

In *prevention*, those having this disease should not have children. *Treatment* of the hemorrhage is difficult unless the bleeding area can be seen when the cautery may be useful. Radium and X-rays have been used for nevi and applied also over the spleen.

SECTION XI

DISEASES OF THE GLANDS OF INTERNAL SECRETION

Introduction.—Disturbances in the endocrine glands may be due to hyper-, hypo- or dysfunction. The results may be shown in various ways: (1) the features caused by disturbance in the gland specially involved, (2) secondary disturbances in other endocrine glands, as they are all bound together, causing a multiglandular syndrome, (3) involvement of the sympathetic nervous system and, through this, widespread influence on many organs and (4) symptoms and signs due to increase in size. There seem to be special relations between certain glands, which may take the form of inhibition or of stimulation. The possibility of *antihormones* has to be considered. It may be that they are produced by the injection of gland stimulating substances. Possibly injected protein may stimulate the formation of antihormones. At present we can say little regarding them.

The endocrine glands influence growth, metabolism, reproduction and many bodily processes, especially with the sympathetic nervous system. The thyroid is stimulated by the sympathetic system proper, and it lowers the threshold of sympathetic stimulation. In early life it may be that the thymus acts as a check; if it persists, certain changes result. The thyroid and pituitary particularly influence growth until the sex glands become active. In later life the acceleration glands, such as the thyroid, tend to have less influence. Throughout there may be disturbing factors of which psychical, metabolic, and toxic, especially bacterial, are the most important. The factors originating in the psychical life act through the sympathetic system, the metabolic in various ways, often through nutrition, and the toxic by influencing the glands and their secretions. Tumors, often adenomata, usually cause hyperfunction. In all a vicious circle may be established. The pituitary gland is the most important one with its influence on the gonads, thyroid, adrenals and pancreas. In development and sex activity, the pituitary, gonads and adrenal cortex play an essential part. In carbohydrate metabolism the adrenal medulla and islands of Langerhans have an important relationship. But in general it is well to be cautious in diagnosing multiglandular disturbance; one gland is usually particularly at fault.

DISEASES OF THE SUPRARENAL BODIES AND CHROMAFFIN SYSTEM

Introduction.—Of the two parts of the suprarenal bodies, (1) the *medulla* belongs to the chromaffin system, which includes a similar tissue scattered in the sympathetic ganglia and the carotid glands, and (2) the *cortex* of mesodermal origin. The chromaffin bodies produce an internal secretion, *epinephrine*, with important effects on the circulation and on the sympathetic system. Epinephrine is regarded as a stimulant to the sympathetic system, as having a vasoconstrictor effect on some arteries and a dilator effect on the bronchi; it also causes an increase in the amount of sugar in the blood by conversion of liver glycogen to glucose. In some way it influences the pigment metabolism of the skin and possibly the muscular vigor. Disturbance in function of the *medulla* is known particularly through the disease described by Addison. The *cortex* bears some relation to the sexual organs as shown by the sex anomalies that develop with tumors and by the enlargement during pregnancy. With some new growths of the cortex there is precocity with special effects on the genitalia and secondary sex characters. The female shows masculine characteristics. The cortex is necessary to life; animals may live, apparently without difficulty, after removal of the medulla.

Glycosuria is caused by the injection of epinephrine, and in animals a form of arteriosclerosis, probably due to the high blood pressure. Many theoretical conceptions have been entertained of the relation between a defect of the adrenal secretion and asthenic affections, and it is suggested that adrenal insufficiency plays an important rôle in acute infections, in tuberculosis, and many wasting diseases, with which it is interesting to note that increased pigmentation may be associated. It is difficult to obtain positive evidence as to such relationships and they are difficult to prove.

ADDISON'S DISEASE

Definition.—A disease characterized by muscular and vascular asthenia, gastro-intestinal disturbance, and pigmentation of the skin; due to tuberculosis or atrophy of the adrenals, or to degenerative changes in the chromaffin system generally. Probably changes in the cortex are chiefly responsible for the changes; both adrenals must be involved to cause the disease.

The recognition of the disease is due to Addison of Guy's Hospital, whose monograph on "The Constitutional and Local Effects of Disease of the Suprarenal Capsules" was published in 1855.

Etiology.—The disease is rare. Only 17 cases were seen in 21 years in the United States (Osler). In large clinics a year or more may pass without a case. Males are more frequently attacked than females. The majority of cases occur between the twentieth and fortieth years. In a congenital case the child lived for eight weeks, and the adrenals were found large and cystic. In a few cases a blow on the abdomen or back has preceded the onset. A certain number of cases have been associated with Pott's disease. An increase in the disease in France was reported during the Great War.

Morbid Anatomy.—There is rarely emaciation or anemia. Rolleston thus summarizes the condition of the suprarenal bodies in Addison's disease:

"1. The fibrocaseous lesion due to tuberculosis—far the commonest condition found. 2. Simple atrophy. 3. Chronic interstitial inflammation leading to atrophy. 4. Malignant disease invading the capsules, including Addison's case of malignant nodule compressing the suprarenal vein. 5. Blood extravasated into the suprarenal bodies. 6. No lesion of the suprarenal bodies themselves, but pressure or inflammation involving the semilunar ganglia.

"The first is the only common cause of Addison's disease. The others, with the exception of simple atrophy, may be considered as very rare."

The nerve cells of the semilunar ganglia have been found degenerated and deeply pigmented, and the nerves sclerotic. The ganglia are not uncommonly entangled in the cicatricial tissue about the adrenals. The chromaffin cells in the sympathetic ganglia and in the abdominal plexuses generally disappear.

Amyloid changes may occur in the adrenals and these may possibly be responsible for extensive degeneration. The cases of extensive destruction of the glands without Addison's disease are explained by a persistence of the chromaffin structures elsewhere, while extensive involvement of the extracapsular chromaffin system may be sufficient to cause the symptoms, the adrenals themselves being intact.

Few changes of importance are found in other organs. The spleen is occasionally enlarged; the thymus may be persistent and the lymph nodes and tonsils enlarged. The thyroid gland may show changes. The other organs show only the alterations associated with a protracted illness.

Symptoms.—In the words of Addison, the characteristic symptoms are "anemia, general languor or debility, remarkable feebleness of the heart's action, irritability of the stomach, and a peculiar change of color in the skin." The onset is, as a rule, insidious. The feelings of weakness usually precede the pigmentation. In other instances the gastro-intestinal symptoms, the weakness and the pigmentation come on together. Loss of weight is common. There are a few cases in which the course is acute, following a shock or some special depression. There are several important features:

(*a*) Pigmentation.—This, as a rule, first attracts the attention of the patient's friends. The coloration ranges from a light yellow to a deep brown or even black. In typical cases it is diffuse, but always deeper on exposed parts and in regions where the normal pigmentation is more intense, as the areolae of the nipples and about the genitals and anus; also wherever the skin is compressed or irritated. At first it may be confined to the face and hands. Occasionally it is absent. Patches showing atrophy of pigment, leucoderma, may occur. The pigmentation occurs on the mucous membranes of the mouth, conjunctivae and vagina but it is not distinctive and is common in the negro. A patchy pigmentation of the serous membranes has often been found. Over the diffusely pigmented skin there may be little mole-like spots of deeper pigmentation, and on the trunk, particularly on the lower abdomen, it may be "ribbed" like the sand of the seashore.

(*b*) Gastro-intestinal Symptoms.—The disease may set in with attacks of nausea and vomiting, spontaneous in character. There may be marked aversion to fatty foods. Towards the close there may be pain with retraction of the abdomen, and even features suggestive of peritonitis. Anorexia may be extreme. The gastric symptoms are variable; occasionally they are absent. Attacks of diarrhea are frequent and come on without obvious cause.

(*c*) Asthenia, the most characteristic feature, may be manifested early as a feeling of inability to carry on the ordinary occupation, or the patient may complain constantly of feeling tired. There may be an extreme degree of muscular prostration in an individual apparently well nourished, whose muscles feel firm and hard. The cardiovascular asthenia is manifest in a feeble action of the heart, which may come on in paroxysms, in attacks of vertigo, or syncope, in one of which the disease may prove fatal. The blood pressure is low and may fall to 70 or 80 mm. of Hg.

Headache is frequent; convulsions occasionally occur. Pain in the back may be an early symptom and there may be pain on pressure in the costolumbar angle. Anemia, specially referred to by Addison, is not common. In a majority the blood count is normal. The sugar content of the blood is low in some cases. Renal insufficiency may occur with an increase in the nitrogen of the blood.

The termination is by syncope, which may occur early in the course, by gradual progressive asthenia, or by the development of tuberculous lesions. A noisy delirium with urgent dyspnea may precede the fatal event. These acute disturbances are always serious.

Diagnosis.—Pigmentation is not confined to Addison's disease. The following conditions may show pigmentation; some of which, *e.g.*, *a* and *b*, are due to disturbance in the chromaffin system.

(*a*) *Abdominal growths*—tubercle, cancer, or lymphoma. In tuberculosis of the peritoneum pigmentation is not uncommon.

(*b*) *Pregnancy*, in which the discoloration is usually limited to the face. Uterine disease is a common cause of a patchy melasma.

(*c*) *Hemochromatosis*, associated with cirrhosis of the liver, pigmentation of the skin, and diabetes.

(*d*) In overworked persons of constipated habit there may be a patchy staining of the face and forehead.

(*e*) The vagabond's discoloration, caused by the irritation of lice and dirt, may reach a high grade and has been mistaken for Addison's disease.

(*f*) In rare instances there is deep pigmentation in melanotic cancer.

(*g*) In certain cases of *exophthalmic goitre* abnormal pigmentation occurs.

(*h*) In rare cases the pigmentation in *scleroderma* is general.

(*i*) In the face there may be an extraordinary degree of pigmentation due to innumerable small black comedones. If not seen in a very good light, the face may suggest argyria. Pigmentation of an advanced grade may occur in chronic ulcer of the stomach and in dilatation of the organ.

(*j*) *Argyria* has sometimes been mistaken for Addison's disease.

(*k*) *Arsenic* may cause a most intense pigmentation of the skin.

(*l*) With arteriosclerosis and chronic heart disease there may be marked melanoderma.

(*m*) In *pernicious anemia* the pigmentation may be marked.

(*n*) There is a form of deep pigmentation, usually in women, which persists for years without any special impairment of health. The pigmentation is a little more leaden than is usual in Addison's disease.

(*o*) In *ochronosis* there may be a deep melanotic pigmentation of the face and hands.

(*p*) In von Recklinghausen's disease the pigmentation may be uniform and suggestive of adrenal disease.

In any case of unusual pigmentation these conditions must be excluded; the diagnosis of Addison's disease is scarcely justifiable without the asthenia. In many instances it is difficult early in the disease to arrive at a definite conclusion. The low blood pressure, nausea and gastric irritability are important. A salt-free diet may decrease the symptoms but also may be dangerous. As the lesion of the capsules is often tuberculous, in doubtful cases the tuberculin test may be used. With tuberculosis there may be calcification of the adrenals which can be recognized by an X-ray study.

Prognosis.—The disease is usually fatal. The cases in which pigmentation is slight or does not occur run a more rapid course. There are acute cases which, with great weakness, vomiting and diarrhea, prove fatal in a few weeks. In a few cases the disease is much prolonged, even to six or ten years. In rare instances recovery has taken place in the past and periods of improvement, lasting many months, may occur. The use of the active cortical extracts should improve the outlook.

Treatment.—When asthenia appears the patient should be confined to bed and sudden efforts and muscular exercise should not be allowed. Fatal syncope may occur at any time. For the diarrhea large doses of bismuth may be given and for the irritability of the stomach simple diet and alkalies. The diet should be light and nutritious; sugar should be given freely. Sodium chloride should be given freely, up to 20 grams a day. As the disease is often tuberculosis an open-air treatment may be carried out. If there is any evidence of syphilis, specific treatment should be given cautiously.

Adrenal Therapy.—The so-called Muirhead treatment, which originated at the Mayo Clinic, consists in giving the dried gland by mouth in large doses and epinephrine hypodermically in as large doses as possible. This treatment has been of benefit. More recently there is the use of the cortical extracts (Swingler and Pfiffner, and Hartman) which may be regarded as substitution therapy. The employment of these extracts intravenously is particularly important in collapse. The dose of the cortical extract must be guided largely by the condition of the patient in acute conditions and by the results in the maintenance dose.

In case of dehydration, normal saline solution with 5 per cent glucose, intravenously in amounts of 500 to 1000 cc. is useful.

OTHER AFFECTIONS OF THE SUPRARENAL GLANDS

Lesions of the Adrenal Cortex.—Remarkable changes in the secondary sexual characters have been associated with tumors and other lesions of this part—the so-called suprarenal genital syndrome. Pseudohermaphroditism has been found in connection with hyperplasia of the cortex. The reverse may occur. Premature puberty, with the development of the secondary sexual characters, obesity and overgrowth of hair, may appear as early as the fifth or sixth year. *Progeria* (premature senility of children), described by Hastings Gilford, is associated with *defect* of the cortex. A tumor may lead to the condition known in women as virilismus or hirsutismus, in which a growth of hair occurs on the face, the voice becomes masculine, and the muscular strength may increase. Later, there may be emaciation, pigmentation, and mental changes. The majority of cases come on after puberty. There is usually amenorrhea, the uterus is small and the ovaries may show degeneration. There are instances of mild virilism, some coming on after the menopause, in which obesity may be marked. Some of these cases may be primarily basophil adenoma of the pituitary (Cushing). In all cases of virilism the possibility of an adrenal tumor and its removal should be considered.

Hyper- and Hypofunction of the Adrenals.—The state of our knowledge is too uncertain to make it worth while to discuss the conditions grouped under the term hyper- and hypo-epinephrinemia. In *acute adrenal insufficiency* there may be abdominal pain with diffuse tenderness, marked prostration, malaise, vomiting, a small soft pulse, low blood pressure, hypoglycemia and sometimes diarrhea, convulsions, coma and death. The suggestion of Sergent that the "white line," is an evidence of adrenal insufficiency has not been supported, but in some cases of asthenia and low blood pressure the response to the administration of adrenal gland substance is prompt. That certain disturbances come under these headings can not be doubted but much work is necessary before they can be accurately stated.

Hemorrhage.—*Acute hemorrhagic adrenalitis* presents a picture somewhat like acute pancreatitis—a sudden onset with pain, vomiting, profound prostration and death within a few days. The cause is obscure; it may be infectious. It occurs most often in young children. In other cases convulsions occur or a typhoid state with profound asthenia results. The disease may be associated with fever and purpura, both cutaneous and visceral.

Chronic Cortical Insufficiency.—Anorexia, which may be marked, asthenia, loss of weight, often extreme, hypotension and mental apathy are the main features. Pigmentation is not always present. There may be pain, weakness and paresthesias of the arms and legs, and sometimes polyneuritis. Trophic ulcers may appear. The adrenal glands show degenerative lesions in the cortex. The *diagnosis* from Addison's disease may be difficult. Pituitary disease has to be considered. The *treatment* should be as in Addison's disease.

Tumors.—Stevens (1923) collected 75 cases of adenocarcinoma of the gland of which one-third were in infants or young children. Metastases occurred early and were usually widespread. Weakness, gastro-intestinal disturbance and pain were the commonest symptoms. The pain usually extended up to the corresponding shoulder and across the abdomen. Pigmentation, hematuria (possibly due to pressure on the renal vein) and overgrowth of hair were found occasionally. Successful removal has been done. In children excessive genital development with overgrowth of hair and obesity has been found due to hyperfunction of the adrenal cortex. The tumors of the adrenal medulla are: (1) Neuroblastoma. (*a*) The "Pepper type" has metastases to the liver, abdominal lymph nodes and lungs. (*b*) The "Hutchison type" has metastases to the skull, orbit (with exophthalmos) and long bones. (*c*) The "Goldzeiher type" has a severe form of anemia, much like pernicious anemia. (2) Ganglioneuroma. These are rare and rarely have metastases. (3) Paraganglioma. These may cause paroxysmal hypertension with headache, nausea, vomiting and weakness. They may be associated with diabetes. The younger the patient the less is the differentiation of the tumor elements. Tumors of the bones of the skull and orbits in a young child suggest chloroma or metastases from a tumor of the adrenal medulla. There are rare cases of tumor of the medulla in which paroxysmal attacks of hypertension occur, with dyspnea, oppression and pulmonary edema occasionally. Overaction of the medulla is suggested. Removal of the tumor has relieved the symptoms.

Carotid Glands.—Situated at the bifurcation of the carotid arteries, these bodies, each about the size of a grain of wheat, belong to the chromaffin group. They are of interest as the seat of tumors, benign at first but which may become malignant. The situation at the bifurcation of the carotid artery, movable laterally but not vertically, single, smooth, not tender or painful, a transmitted pulsation with a thrill and a murmur, bulging of the wall of the pharynx, slow growth and long duration, are the important features. Removal has been done but with considerable risk.

DISEASES OF THE THYMUS GLAND

The thymus has little resemblance to the other ductless glands and must be classed as an epithelial rather than as a lymphoid organ. At birth the thymus gland weighs about 12 grams; from the first to the fifth year about 23 grams; from the sixth to the tenth year about 26 grams; from the eleventh to the fifteenth year about 37½ grams, and from the sixteenth to the twentieth year about 25½ grams, after which it undergoes a gradual atrophy (Hammar). Involution not taking place, a "persistent thymus" remains.

There may be a relationship between the thymus and the sex glands. The work of Rowntree *et al.* shows that thymus extract accelerates the rate of growth and development in rats, hastens the onset of adolescence in the offspring of the treated rats, and increases fertility. The use in succeeding generations seems to increase the effect.

HYPERTROPHY OF THE THYMUS

The size of the gland varies so greatly that it is not easy to define the limits between persistency and enlargement. Between the manubrium sterni and the vertebral column in an infant of eight months the distance is only 2.2 cm. (Jacobi), so that it is easy to understand how an enlarged gland may induce what Warthin called "thymic tracheostenosis." There appear to be, as this author suggests, three groups of cases:

(*a*) *Thymic stridor*, either congenital or developing soon after birth, varying in intensity and aggravated by crying and coughing.

(*b*) *Thymic asthma*, sometimes known as Kopp's or Miller's asthma, is an exaggerated and more persistent form of the stridor. While much dispute exists as to this form, there seems no doubt as to its occurrence, as there are cases in which complete relief has followed removal of the gland or X-ray therapy.

(*c*) Lastly, in some cases sudden death has occurred, usually in connection with the condition of lymphatism about to be described.

Persistence of the gland has been met with in many affections, such as Graves' disease, Addison's disease, acromegaly, myasthenia gravis, rickets, etc. Many observers regard the association of an enlargement with Graves' disease as more than accidental and as a sort of compensatory process.

ATROPHY OF THE THYMUS

This is met with accidentally in children, especially as Ruhräh has shown, in marasmus and chronic wasting disorders. Of other morbid conditions, *hemorrhages* are not uncommon. Inflammation of the gland (*thymitis*) may occur by infection from neighboring tissues. Mediastinal tumors may originate in the remnants of the thymus; dermoid tumors and cysts have been met with; tuberculosis and syphilis of the gland are occasionally seen. The condition in congenital syphilis, in which there are fissure-like cavities in the gland filled with purulent fluid, is probably postmortem softening.

STATUS THYMICOLYMPHATICUS: LYMPHATISM

Definition.—A combination of constitutional anomalies among which are hyperplasia of the lymphoid tissues and of the thymus, hypoplasia of the cardiovascular system, and peculiarities of configuration.

Formerly the condition was regarded as specially important in young children, but it is found both in children and adults. In Bellevue Hospital, 457 cases were found among 5,652 autopsies (8 per cent). Of these only 92 were below the age of twenty years (Symmers). In young adults lymphatism is common. Borst and Grace found lymphatic hyperplasia in 56 per cent of 2,000 men killed in action and in 86 per cent of those aged 19 and 20.

Among the results of the condition are: (1) A liability to sudden death. This may be from several causes. (*a*) *Anaphylaxis.* Necrosis occurs in the lymphoid tissues with resulting sensitization. With further necrosis a fatal attack may result. (*b*) *Cerebral hemorrhage.* The hypoplastic arteries rupture easily, as from slight trauma, a point of medicolegal importance. (*c*) In young children sudden death may result from pressure of the enlarged gland ("thymic death"), but this is very rare. (2) Increased susceptibility to acute infections and decreased resistance to them, particularly endocarditis, pneumonia, cerebrospinal fever and sepsis. (3) In women there is increased danger in childbirth. (4) Psychical instability. The subjects form a considerable proportion of cases of drug addiction and suicide.

Pathology.—Symmers describes two forms—status lymphaticus and recessive status lymphaticus. The former shows well-developed changes in the lymphoid tissues and occurs at an age when these structures are active. The recessive form shows atrophic changes in the lymphoid structures which vary with the time of involution. Of 249 cases, 118 were instances of status lymphaticus, 89 of the recessive form and 42 were borderline cases, tending toward recession. In the status lymphaticus form the thymus was hyperplastic, the average weight being about 25 gm. No instance was found of death being due to pressure from the thymus. Histologically the thymus showed hyperplasia, which may be extreme. Necrotic changes were marked in the lymph nodes, especially in the cases of sudden death from slight causes. This is regarded by Symmers as being in close relation to anaphylaxis.

Symptoms.—Children with lymphatism are often fat, may be anemic and flabby but are usually regarded as in good health. The tonsils are often enlarged and adenoids are present. They have little resistance to infections and are easily upset by trifling ailments. They are often subject to nasal catarrh, mouth breathing is common, and vasomotor changes are frequent. The spleen may be enlarged. The blood may show a marked lymphocytosis. The *enlarged thymus* may be shown by dulness over the upper sternum and to each side of it which shifts upward with extreme retraction of the head (Boggs). There may be bulging or the gland may be felt in the episternal notch. The X-ray shadow may be distinct. In these cases there may be attacks, often after a fit of temper or a crying spell, in which the child shows noisy breathing, stridor and cyanosis. Respiration may stop for some seconds or death may occur.

After puberty in males the main points are: (1) A slender thorax, rounded arms and thighs, and a suggestion of the feminine type. (2) A soft delicate skin. (3) A scanty growth of hair on the face, especially on the upper lip and chin, and in the axillae, with a feminine distribution of pubic hair. (4) The external genitals may be poorly developed; some are cryptorchids. (5) The cervical and axillary glands may be palpable. In *females* the main features are: (1) A slender thorax and extremities. (2) A soft delicate skin. (3) Scanty axillary and pubic hair. (4) Hypoplasia of the genital organs.

Diagnosis.—Suspected cases should be carefully examined before any operation. The enlargement of the superficial glands, of the tonsillar tissues and of the spleen is easily determined. The adult forms are readily recognized from the general characteristics.

Treatment.—In children it is well to reduce the sugar and starch in the duct to a minimum, giving skim milk, eggs, meat, green vegetables and fruits. A general tonic treatment with iron and arsenic should be given. A large thymus causing compression may require removal but treatment by X-rays is often successful. In the adult forms there is no special treatment.

TUMORS OF THE THYMUS GLAND

These are rare, the majority being sarcomata. Symmers and Vance divide tumors of the thymic parenchyma into those originating from the predominant cell of the adult thymus, the lymphocyte, and those from the early predominant epithelial cell. The latter are very rare and occur in patients over 50. The lymphocytic tumors occur earlier in life; many are in children. The symptoms are usually those of pressure and are variable. Early diagnosis, especially aided by X-rays gives a chance of removal. Otherwise X-ray or radium therapy is indicated.

DISEASES OF THE THYROID GLAND

CONGESTION

At puberty, in girls, often at the onset of menstruation, the gland enlarges; in certain women the neck becomes fuller at each menstruation, and it was an old idea that the gland enlarged at or after defloration. From mechanical causes, as tight collars or repeated crying, the gland may swell for a short time. Slight enlargement is common in acute infections.

THYROIDITIS

Acute Thyroiditis is nearly always secondary to some infection and may be simple or purulent. It occurs with typhoid fever, smallpox, measles, pneumonia, mumps, influenza, and after tonsillectomy. Epidemics have been reported. It is rare in ordinary hospital practice.

Symptoms.—The whole gland may be involved or only one lobe. There are swelling, pain on pressure, redness, and, when suppuration occurs, softening or fluctuation. The pressure signs may be acute and severe. In suppurative cases the tenderness is marked and the diagnosis from cellulitis may be difficult. Often the acute inflammation subsides spontaneously. Myxedema has followed destruction of the entire gland by acute suppuration.

Treatment.—Sedatives may be required for discomfort. Iodine should not be used in any way. An ice-bag should be applied locally. With signs of suppuration free drainage should be secured.

Chronic Thyroiditis.—This may follow the acute form. A chronic fibrosis may progress to myxedema. There is a *primary chronic thyroiditis* (also termed sclerotic or woody), known also as Riedel's struma, which occurs in either sex, between the ages of 20 and 40, without previous thyroid disease. There is inflammation, with the formation of dense connective tissue which involves the deep tissues of the neck and may compress the trachea and recurrent laryngeal nerves. Sections usually show very little thyroid tissue. The onset is with swelling of the neck, which increases rapidly; the mass is hard, smooth, and firmly fixed to the deeper structures. There is rarely pain or tenderness. Owing to the hardness of the mass, it may be regarded as malignant. Spontaneous disappearance has occurred. If treatment is necessary on account of signs of pressure, the least possible interference is wise as myxedema has followed removal of the slight remaining thyroid tissue and treatment by X-rays. The condition termed *struma lymphomatosa* (Hashimoto) is probably a modification of the same process.

TUMORS OF THE THYROID

Of these the most important are: (*a*) *Infective granulomata*—tuberculosis, actinomycosis and syphilis, which are rare. Tuberculosis may be mistaken for exophthalmic goitre. Swelling of the gland may occur in recent syphilitic infection, and gummata in the congenital form. (*b*) *Malignant tumors* are more common than statistics usually indicate. Wilson, from the Mayo Clinic, states that among 16,558 thyroid operations, 207 cases of malignant disease were found; in addition there were 83 inoperable cases. Carcinoma is much more common than sarcoma. It is more frequent in women and occurs especially in the fifth decade. It seems to be more common in areas of endemic goitre. Adenomas play an important part in the etiology and so the history of recent growth in a previous nodular tumor is frequent. In a certain number the growth is slow. There is usually a progressive increase in the size of the thyroid, which is often irregular. With this, signs of pressure on the larynx, trachea and esophagus are common. *Pain* is not uncommon and there may be a good deal of cardiovascular disturbance. In later stages the tumor is large and the surface veins are distended. The skin may become adherent and pressure signs are marked. Erosion of the trachea or esophagus may occur. Metastases are common, especially in the lungs and bones. The *diagnosis* has to be made from adenoma and operation should be done if there is any doubt. Rapidity of growth, hardness and fixation of the mass are important. *Treatment* is surgical and should not be delayed. The use of radium or X-rays is advisable after operation and as a palliative measure.

ABERRANT AND ACCESSORY THYROIDS

In various places, from the root of the tongue to the arch of the aorta, fragments of thyroidal tissue have been found. These aberrant portions of the gland may enlarge and undergo cystic degeneration. In the mediastinum they may form large tumors, and in the pleura an accessory cystic thyroid may occupy the upper portion, and in one case the cystic gland filled nearly the entire side. The so-called *lingual thyroid* is not uncommon, varying in size from a hemp seed to a pea, usually free in the deep muscles of the tongue, or attached to the hyoid bone. When enlarged the *lingual goitre* may form a tumor of considerable size. The true thyroid gland has been absent, and removal of the lingual goitre has been followed by myxedema.

SIMPLE GOITRE

Definition.—A chronic enlargement of the thyroid gland, due to lack of iodine, occurring sporadically or endemically.

Distribution.—Goitre is widely distributed throughout North America. In England it is common in certain regions; the Thames valley, the Dales, Derbyshire, Sussex, and Hampshire. In Switzerland, in the mountains of Germany and Austria, the mountainous districts of France, and in the Pyrenees the disease is very prevalent. The areas of endemic goitre seem to be extending.

Etiology.—The disease is rarely congenital except in very goitrous districts. Cases are most common at or about puberty, and the tendency diminishes after the twentieth year. Women are much more frequently attacked than men, in a proportion of 6 or 8 to 1. The disease occurs at every latitude and in every altitude, in valleys and in plains, and in various climates. It seems to be less prevalent by the seashore.

In the diffuse colloid goitre of adolescence there is probably exhaustion of the thyroxin with a resulting stimulation of the thyroid. The formation of thyroxin is disturbed from *shortage of iodine.* Infection may influence the exhaustion of thyroxin in the tissues. It is suggested that bacteria in the digestive tract may influence the absorption of iodine. There is a goitrogenous substance in cabbage. The essential cause is lack of or imperfect utilization of a sufficient amount of iodine.

Morbid Anatomy.—Usually the whole gland is involved, but one lobe only may be attacked. There are various changes which may be combined: (1) Parenchymatous, in which there is a general increase in the thyroid tissue; (2) an increase in the amount of colloid; (3) cystic, in which the cysts contain colloid material; hemorrhage may occur into the cysts; and (4) a great increase in fibrous tissue. There is an increase in the colloid material of the follicles. Degenerations of various kinds are common, particularly cystic, in which there are many large and small cavities with colloid contents. In some of these cystic forms there are papillary ingrowths into the alveoli. Sometimes extensive hemorrhages occur in the gland.

Symptoms.—The increase in size is usually insidious and in many cases there are no symptoms and the only complaint is of the disfigurement from the enlargement. Symptoms are due to *pressure;* the trachea may be flattened, usually from an enlarged isthmus, or narrowed by circular compression. The symptoms are more or less marked stridor and cough, which may persist for years without special aggravation. They may occur with very large glands, with the small encircling goitre, or with a goitre beneath the sternum. Pressure on the recurrent nerves may cause attacks of dyspnea, particularly at night, and the voice may be altered. Pressure on the vagus is not common. Sometimes there is difficulty in swallowing, and the veins of the neck may be compressed. The heart may be involved, possibly from pressure on the vagi. Other cardiac disturbances probably mean hyperthyroidism. The basal metabolism may be below normal (10 to 15 per cent). This is altered very rapidly by giving thyroid gland or thyroxin. The *diagnosis* of enlargement of the gland rarely gives difficulty unless it is intrathoracic. Care should be taken to recognize hyperthyroidism if present. With *intrathoracic goitre* there are dyspnea and choking sensations, especially with movement, and the patient sleeps with the head high. Dulness, decreased movement of the larynx on swallowing, laryngeal paralysis, venous obstruction, and signs of bronchial compression may be found. The X-ray study is important. Sometimes the tumor may appear and disappear.

Acute colloid goitre occurs, usually in boys about puberty. It may cause serious pressure and require operation. The use of thyroxin intravenously is advised.

Prognosis.—Many cases in the young get well; too often the tumor persists, but it may disappear on a change of locality.

Prevention.—The brilliant work of Marine and his associates has shown that in a great majority of cases simple goitre can be prevented by the administration of iodine. Amounts of 5 grains (0.3 gm.) of the iodide given twice weekly for a month, in the spring and autumn, are usually sufficient.

Treatment.—Iodine in some form is used extensively, and often is curative. Its effect is to stimulate the gland to a healthy action. In young people 2 to 5 grains (0.13 to 0.3 gm.) of iodide may be given daily. Iodine injections into the gland are not advisable. Iodine may be applied externally as an ointment (5 per cent). The use of X-rays is not advisable as a rule. When the gland is large or there are signs of pressure, surgical measures are indicated.

HYPOTHYROIDISM (*Cretinism and Myxedema*)

Definition.—A constitutional affection due to insufficiency of the thyroid gland, characterized by a myxedematous condition of the subcutaneous tissues and mental disturbance, and anatomically by atrophy of the thyroid gland.

While under hypothyroidism we have cretinism and myxedema as entities, there are grades of hypothyroidism of such mild character that they hardly deserve the designation of myxedema. The features are very varied and may not suggest thyroid disease. Fatigue, often like that of neurasthenia, headache (which may be like migraine) and diffuse pains, often about the joints, and sometimes abdominal, are common. Vasomotor disturbances of various kinds, sometimes in the nasal mucous membrane, and urinary disturbances may be found. The weight is not always increased. The basal metabolism may be about –10 to –15, sometimes lower. The typical features of myxedema are generally lacking. In some of these patients the disturbance may not be primarily in the thyroid gland, rather in the pituitary gland. The blood cholesterol may be high. In some cases in women about the menopause there may be arthritic disturbance.

History.—As early as 1859 Schiff had noted that in the dog removal of the gland was followed by certain symptoms. Gull described "a cretinoid change in women," and in the eighties the observations of Ord and other English physicians separated a well defined entity called "myxedema."

Kocher (in 1883) reported that 30 of his first 100 thyroidectomies had been followed by a characteristic picture, to which he gave the name "cachexia strumipriva," an observation made in the previous year by the Reverdins, who had recognized the relation of this change to the disease known as "myxedema." The researches of Horsley, and the investigation of the Clinical Society of London, made it clear that the changes following complete removal of the gland (cachexia strumipriva), myxedema, and sporadic cretinism, were one and the same disease, due to insufficiency of the thyroid gland. Schiff and Horsley demonstrated that animals could be saved by the transplantation of the glands. Then came the discovery of George Murray and Howitz that feeding with thyroid extract replaced the gland function, and cured the disease. The first patient given thyroid by Murray in 1891 died in 1919, aged 74, from heart disease. The activity of the gland is connected with the metabolism of iodine, of which the maximum amount in the gland does not exceed 25 milligrams.

Kendall isolated the active principle, *thyroxin,* which contains 65 per cent of iodine. It is an amino-acid which enters into reaction and is regenerated so that it can repeat the process. It acts as does thyroid extract in myxedema. There is a quantitative relation between thyroxin and the rate of basal metabolism.

The outcome of a host of researches has been the recognition of the enormous importance of the internal secretion of the gland, which is essential for normal growth in childhood, and has a marked influence on metabolism. It stimulates both vegetative nervous systems.

Etiology.—This is clear in the cases of complete removal of the gland or when atrophy of the remaining portion of the gland occurs. Probably atrophy is responsible in the cases occurring after exophthalmic goitre and infections. In cretinism usually one or both parents have thyroid disease. In some cases the gland is absent. In myxedema a number of factors may be operative: (1) at the *menopause* it is not uncommon; (2) with frequent childbearing and sometimes with pregnancy; (3) following acute infections; (4) with other endocrine disturbances, and (5) in old age. Females are much more often affected than males and especially between 40 and 50.

Clinical Forms.—There are three groups of cases—cretinism, myxedema proper, and operative myxedema. To Felix Semon is due the credit of recognizing that these are one and the same condition.

CRETINISM.—Two forms are recognized—the sporadic and the endemic. In the *sporadic* form the gland may be congenitally absent, or is atrophied after one of the specific fevers, or the condition develops with goitre. The disease is not very uncommon; the histories of 58 cases were collected in a few years in the United States and Canada (Osler). It is more common in females than in males—35 in the series.

Morbid Anatomy.—Absence of the gland or complete fibrous atrophy is the common condition. Goitre with any trace of gland tissue is rare. There is delay in the appearance of the centres of ossification. Arrest of development, a brachycephalic skull in the endemic, and a dolichocephalic in the sporadic form, are the chief skeletal changes.

Symptoms.—Hypothyroidism should be suspected in all children overweight at birth, nine pounds or over. In such children signs of delayed bone development should be looked for by an X-ray study. Otherwise the condition is rarely recognized before the child is six months old and often not until later. These children usually lose weight from malnutrition; by the age of two years they are under size and under weight. The development of bone is retarded. The child does not grow normally and is not bright mentally. The tongue looks large and hangs out of the mouth. The hair may be thin and the skin very dry. Usually by the end of the first year and during the second year the signs become very marked. The face is large and bloated, the eyelids are puffy and swollen; the alae nasi are thick, the nose is depressed and flat. Dentition is delayed, and the teeth which appear decay early. The abdomen is swollen, the legs are thick and short, and the hands and feet undeveloped and pudgy. The face is pale and sometimes has a waxy, sallow tint. The fontanelles remain open; there is muscular weakness, and the child can not support itself. In the supraclavicular regions are large pads of fat. The child may lapse into imbecility.

In cases in which the atrophy of the gland follows a fever the condition may not come on until the fourth or fifth year, or later. This is really, as Parker determined, a *juvenile myxedema.* In a few of the sporadic forms cretinism develops with an existing goitre. It may retard development, bodily and mental, without ever progressing to complete imbecility.

Endemic Cretinism.—This occurs wherever goitre is very prevalent, as in parts of Switzerland, Savoy, Tyrol, and the Pyrenees. It formerly prevailed in parts of England. The clinical features are the same as in the sporadic form, stunted growth and feeble mind, plus goitre.

The *diagnosis* in a typical instance is very easy after one has seen a case or good illustrations. Infants sometimes become flabby, lose their vivacity, or show a protuberant abdomen and lax skin with slight cretinoid appearance. These milder forms may be due to transient functional disturbance. Other causes of defective development, especially syphilis, should be excluded. It may be difficult to determine the basal metabolism but the effect of giving thyroid extract is of great aid in diagnosis. The *prognosis* depends on the time when treatment is begun; if early the child may become normal. In older children there may be improvement but a normal condition does not follow often. Cretins usually die young from intercurrent disease.

Myxedema of Adults (*Gull's Disease*).—Women are much more frequently affected than men—in a ratio of 6 to 1. The disease may affect several members of a family, and it may be transmitted through the mother. In some instances there has been first the appearance of exophthalmic goitre. The symptoms of myxedema may disappear during pregnancy or may develop postpartum. Myxedema and exophthalmic goitre may occur in sisters. Extreme forms are not as common in America as in England. C. P. Howard collected 100 American cases, of which 86 were in women.

The *onset* is usually insidious with mental dulness and loss of memory. *Obscure pains,* especially in the legs, are common; they are aggravated by rubbing or pressure. The pain is situated in the skin and subcutaneous tissues and is marked on pinching the skin. In other cases, due to involvement of the ligaments, there may be relaxation of the joints, causing pain and conditions such as flatfoot or lordosis. The clinical features are marked increase in the general bulk of the body, a firm, inelastic swelling of the skin, which does not pit on pressure; dryness and roughness, which tend with the swelling to obliterate the lines of expression in the face; imperfect nutrition of the hair; local tumefaction of the skin and subcutaneous tissues, particularly in the supraclavicular region. Perspiration is usually much decreased. The physiognomy is altered: the features are coarse and broad, the lips thick, the nostrils broad and thick and the mouth enlarged. The hair of the eyebrows is often scanty, especially on the outer part. Over the cheeks, sometimes the nose, there is a reddish patch. There is a striking slowness of thought and movement. The memory becomes defective, the patients grow irritable and suspicious, and there may be headache. In some instances there are delusions and hallucinations, leading to dementia. The gait is heavy and slow. The temperature may be below normal and the patients often suffer in cold weather. The pulse is usually slow and the blood pressure low. Constipation is generally marked. Hemorrhage sometimes occurs, probably due to decreased coagulability of the blood. There is often a moderate secondary anemia with a normal leukocyte count. The blood cholesterol is high. Albuminuria is sometimes present, more rarely glycosuria. The tendon reflexes give a slow movement and greater stimulation than normal is needed to elicit a response. Death is usually due to some intercurrent disease, most frequently tuberculosis (Greenfield). The thyroid gland is diminished in size and may be completely atrophied and converted into a fibrous mass. The subcutaneous fat is abundant, and in some instances a great increase in the mucin has been found. The larynx is also involved. Myocardial insufficiency of various grades is not uncommon. The *heart* may be considerably enlarged but the rate is often slow. There is interstitial edema. Small P and QRS complexes with low amplitude of the T waves is common. Under treatment the enlargement may disappear. Arteriosclerosis is not uncommon.

The basal metabolism is reduced 20 to 40 per cent below the normal.

The course is slow but progressive, and extends over ten or fifteen years. A condition of acute and temporary myxedema may develop with enlargement of the thyroid and may follow exophthalmic goitre. The symptoms of the two diseases have been combined. In one case a young man increased in weight enormously during three months, then had tachycardia with tremor and active delirium and died within six months of the onset.

Operative Myxedema; Cachexia strumipriva.—This sometimes follows extirpation of the thyroid. If a small fragment of the thyroid remains, or if there are accessory glands, the symptoms do not develop. Operative myxedema is very rare in America.

The *diagnosis* of marked myxedema is easy, as a rule. The general aspect —the subcutaneous swelling and the pallor—suggests nephritis, which may be strengthened by casts and albumin in the urine; but the solid character of the swelling, the exceeding dryness of the skin, the yellowish white color, the low temperature, the loss of hair, the dull, listless mental state and the low basal metabolism should differentiate the conditions. In dubious cases not too much stress should be laid upon the supraclavicular swellings. There may be marked fibrofatty enlargements in this situation in healthy persons. In mild cases the diagnosis is often overlooked because myxedema is not considered. The basal metabolism and the results of thyroid therapy are important. *The frequency of mild forms should be remembered.*

Jelliffe points out that in some cases tabes dorsalis may be diagnosed owing to the pains, unequal and sluggish pupils, myotonia, and decreased patellar and tendon Achilles reflexes.

Hypothyroidism should be considered in children who are dull and backward, in women who have symptoms suggesting a premature menopause, in obesity, and in those with constipation the cause for which is obscure.

Treatment.—The patients suffer in cold and improve in warm weather. They should be kept at an even temperature, and, if possible, move to a warm climate during the winter months. Repeated warm baths with massage are useful. Our art has made no more brilliant advance than in the cure of the disorders due to hypothyroidism. That we can to-day rescue children otherwise doomed to helpless idiocy—that we can restore to health the victims of myxedema—is a triumph of experimental medicine for which we are indebted largely to Horsley and his pupil Murray. Transplantation of the gland was first tried; then Murray used an extract subcutaneously. Hector Mackenzie in London and Howitz in Copenhagen introduced the method of feeding. The gland is efficacious in a majority of the cases of myxedema in infants or adults. It makes little difference how it is administered. The dried gland is the most convenient and it is well to begin with 1 grain (0.065 gm.) three times a day. The dose is increased or decreased until the proper dose is found. Care should be taken to be sure of the strength of the preparation which is given. In many cases there are no unpleasant symptoms; in others there are irritation of the skin, restlessness, rapid pulse, delirium and in rare instances tonic spasms, the condition to which the term *thyroidism* is applied. The results, as a rule, are unparalleled by anything in the whole range of curative measures. A poor, feeble-minded, toad-like caricature of humanity may be restored to mental and bodily health. Loss of weight is one of the first and most striking effects; one patient lost over 30 pounds within six weeks. The skin becomes moist, the urine is increased, the perspiration returns, the temperature rises, the pulse rate quickens, the mental torpor lessens and the basal metabolism increases. Ill effects are rare. In all grades of hypothyroidism the dosage of thyroid extract must be studied and decided by results. Di-iodothyronine has been employed with good results in doses of 50 to 75 mg. daily.

The treatment must be carried out in two stages—one, early, in which full doses are given until the cure is effected; the other, the permanent use of small doses sufficient to preserve the normal metabolism. In cretinism it seems necessary to keep up the treatment indefinitely as relapse may follow the cessation of the use of the extract.

ADENOMATOUS GOITRE

In the human thyroid there are usually groups of undeveloped thyroid cells; with the need for increased activity these "rests" grow and form the adenomata often present in simple goitre. They are very variable in size and number. The frequent association of colloid and adenomatous goitre is to be noted. The simple adenomatous goitre may be diffuse or nodular. It usually develops about or soon after puberty and may persist indefinitely without causing symptoms. In other cases toxic symptoms may appear years later (toxic adenomatous goitre). Probably a variety of causes may be responsible, such as nervous disturbance and infections.

In *simple adenomatous goitre* the picture is very much the same as in simple goitre but the gland may be more irregular and nodular in places.

In *toxic adenomatous goitre* additional features are added. As a rule this happens only after many years of enlargement of the gland and so the patients are usually forty years of age or over. The onset is usually gradual and for a time the symptoms may not be marked. *Fatigue* is of special importance. The features are much like those of Graves' disease with certain differences. There may be exophthalmos but the other eye signs are slight. Tremor may be absent or coarse. The tachycardia is not so marked and is more often influenced by sleep or digitalis. Hypertension (especially increase in the diastolic pressure) and myocardial degeneration (auricular fibrillation) are more common. Vasomotor disturbances are less marked. The thyroid gland is large and often irregular; it does not often show pulsation, thrill or murmur. The psychical features are less marked and loss in weight is gradual. The basal metabolism is increased.

In **diagnosis,** the history of goitre for many years and the clinical features are usually sufficient, particular importance belonging to increased basal metabolism, which is often the deciding factor. The distinction from "neurasthenic" conditions may be difficult and often depends more on a careful study than on any special test, except basal metabolism. As patients with toxic goitre are resistant to the usual effects of quinine, 10 grain (0.6 gm.) doses may be given four times a day for several days. The absence of any of the usual results suggests hyperthyroidism.

The **prognosis** is variable and depends on the severity of the symptoms and the myocardial damage. It is essentially a chronic condition.

The **prevention** is that of simple goitre and it is to be hoped that by the administration of iodine or iodide many cases can be prevented.

The **treatment** is essentially surgical. Attention should be given to foci of infection. Treatment by X-rays or radium is usually not effectual. Iodine has little influence or may increase the nervous symptoms.

It may be mentioned that there is not a universal agreement that toxic adenomatous goitre should be separated from Graves' disease.

EXOPHTHALMIC GOITRE (*Graves', Basedow's, or Parry's Disease*)

Definition.—A disease characterized by goitre, exophthalmos, tachycardia, and tremor, associated with a perverted or hyperactive state of the thyroid gland and increased activity of the vegetative nervous system.

The essential nature of Graves' disease is in doubt. The thyroid changes, which represent extreme stimulation of the gland, may be entirely *secondary* and result from various causes. It may be a question of too much thyroxin production or the formation of an abnormal substance; Plummer suggests an incomplete thyroxin molecule. The disturbed function of the thyroid may be associated with a lack of iodine. Excessive administration of thyroid extract does not cause exophthalmic goitre. A distinction should be made between hyperthyroidism and Graves' disease. Not all cases of overactivity of the gland go on to exophthalmic goitre, but it is probable that the possibility of this exists. It may be difficult to classify the borderline cases.

Historical Note.—In the posthumous writings of Caleb Hillier Parry (1825) is a description of 8 cases of Enlargement of the Thyroid Gland in Connection with Enlargement or Palpitation of the Heart. In the first case, seen in 1786, he also described the exophthalmos: "The eyes were protruded from their sockets, and the countenance exhibited an appearance of agitation and distress, especially in any muscular movement." The Italians claim that Flajani described the disease in 1800. Moebius states that his original account is meagre and inaccurate, and bears no comparison with that of Parry. If the name of any physician is to be associated with the disease, undoubtedly it should be that of the distinguished old Bath physician. Graves described the disease in 1835 and Basedow in 1840.

Etiology.—*Age.*—In Sattler's collection of 3,477 cases only 184 were under the age of sixteen. *Sex.*—The proportion of females is greatly in excess; in Sattler's collected cases the ratio was 5.4 to 1.

The exciting causes are probably varied and in many cases two or more are concerned. The acute infections, focal infections, previous thyroid disease and particularly nervous disturbances are factors. The influence of worry, anxiety, mental shock and severe fright is evident in some cases. A psychical factor seems to be a sufficient cause in certain patients. Other glands may be concerned. Deficiency of the adrenal glands and gonads is suggested which in turn may be caused by disturbance in the pituitary gland.

A *family predisposition* may exist and several members may be affected. Warthin suggested that there is a distinct pathological constitution, "a Graves' constitution," a congenital tendency which may remain quiescent. A constitutional defect of the thymicolymphatic (Graves') constitution is present in all cases of Graves' disease and toxic adenoma. There is a "juvenile morphology and rapid functional reactions." Neurogenic or toxic factors may determine the occurrence of the disease. Certainly there does not seem proof that the features of Graves' disease are due to hypersecretion.

Pathology.—The essential change consists in increased activity of the gland, which enlarges as a result of hyperplasia and shows increased vascularity. The normal colloid is greatly reduced or absent. The epithelial cells of the follicles show proliferation and the lymphadenoid tissue is increased. These changes may occur only in limited areas of the gland. The enlargement occasionally results in mechanical disturbance. The increased secretion causes definite results: (1) There is a great increase in metabolism; (2) other endocrine glands are affected, and (3) the sympathetic nervous system is stimulated. The active principle—thyroxin—was isolated by Kendall. In many cases there is enlargement of the thymus, which may play a part in the lymphocytosis usually found (30-60 per cent) with decrease in the neutrophiles. Myxedema may develop in the late stages, and there are transient edema and in a few cases scleroderma, which indicate that the nutrition of the skin is involved. The degree of hyperthyroidism and dysthyroidism may be difficult to determine. The relative amounts of each may vary. The response to iodine therapy depends on the influence on dysthyroidism. Some cases may be termed "thyroid instability."

Symptoms.—Acute and chronic forms may be recognized. In the acute form the disease may progress with great rapidity. In a patient of J. H. Lloyd's, of Philadelphia, a woman, aged thirty-nine, who had been healthy, but whose friends had noticed that her eyes looked rather large, was suddenly seized with intense vomiting and diarrhea, rapid action of the heart, and great throbbing of the arteries. The eyes were prominent and the thyroid gland enlarged and soft. The gastro-intestinal symptoms continued, the pulse became more rapid, and the patient died on the third day of the illness. The acute cases show marked toxemia but not always delirium.

More frequently, the onset is gradual and the disease is chronic. Toxic symptoms usually appear within a year. There are five principal features—tachycardia, exophthalmos, enlargement of the thyroid, tremor and increased basal metabolism. Persistent fatigue is a frequent early symptom.

Tachycardia.—Rapid heart action is the most constant phenomenon. The pulse rate at first may be not more than 95 or 100, but when the disease is established it may be from 140 to 160, or even higher. The increase is most marked in the sympathicotonic cases. Irregularity is usually due to auricular fibrillation. Auricular flutter may occur. In a well developed case the visible area of cardiac pulsation is much increased and the action is heaving and forcible. There is probably nothing specific in the cardiac condition. There is increased work due to increased metabolism and perhaps decreased glycogen content. There is marked visible pulsation in the arteries. The capillary pulse is readily seen, and there are few diseases in which one may see at times with greater distinctness the venous pulse in the veins of the hands. The throbbing pulsation may be felt even in the finger tips. Vascular erythema is common—the face and neck are flushed and there may be a widespread erythema. The blood pressure varies; there may be an early stage of hypertension followed by hypotension. In some patients hypertension may return after a time. Murmurs are usually heard, a loud systolic at the apex and base. The heart sounds may be very intense. In rare instances they may be heard at some distance from the patient; according to Graves, as far as four feet. Attacks of acute dilatation may occur with dyspnea, cough and a frothy bloody expectoration.

Exophthalmos.—A characteristic facial aspect is given by the staring expression, caused in part by protrusion of the eyeballs, but more particularly by retraction of the lids exposing the sclerae. The exophthalmos, which may be unilateral, usually follows the vascular disturbance. The protrusion may become very great and the eye may even be dislocated from the socket, or both eyes may be destroyed by panophthalmitis. The vision is normal. Graefe noted that when the eyeball is moved downward the upper lid does not follow it as in health (Graefe's sign). The palpebral aperture is wider than in health, owing to spasm or retraction of the upper lid. The patient winks less frequently than in health (Stellwag's sign). There is marked tremor of the lids and they contract spasmodically in advance of the elevating eyeball. Moebius called attention to disturbance of convergence of the two eyes. The majority of the eye signs are autonomic in origin. Changes in the pupils and in the optic nerves are rare.

ENLARGEMENT OF THE THYROID is the rule but may be absent. It may be general or in only one lobe, and is rarely so large as in ordinary goitre. The swelling is firm but elastic. There are rarely pressure signs. The vessels are usually much dilated, and the gland may pulsate. A thrill may be felt and a double murmur is common and pathognomonic (Guttmann).

TREMOR was really first described by Basedow. It is involuntary, fine and about eight to the second. It is important in the diagnosis of early cases.

The *basal metabolism* shows a marked increase and this is an important aid in diagnosis. In very severe cases the increase may be 75 per cent or over, in severe cases 50 to 75 per cent and in milder forms from 20 to 50 per cent. Boothby in a study of 2,332 cases of exophthalmic goitre found in 94 per cent a basal metabolism of +20 or over, in 5 per cent between +11 and +20 and in 1 per cent normal. In 1,425 patients with adenoma and toxic features, 68 per cent were +20 or over and 32 per cent +11 to +20; in adenoma without hyperthyroidism the findings were within normal limits in all.

Other features are anemia, emaciation and slight fever. The blood shows lymphocytosis. The blood *cholesterol* is decreased and the degree of this is a good guide to the progress of the disease. Attacks of vomiting and diarrhea may occur; the latter may be severe and distressing, recurring at intervals and without evident cause. Great complaint is made of the forcible throbbing in the arteries, often accompanied with flushes of heat and profuse perspiration. An erythematous flushing is common. Pruritus may be a severe and persistent symptom. Multiple telangiectases have been described. Solid, infiltrated edema is not uncommon and may be transitory. A remarkable myxedematous state may supervene. Pigmentary changes are common and may be patchy or generalized. The coexistence of scleroderma and Graves' disease has been noted. Irritability of temper, change in disposition, and mental depression may occur. There is often marked emotional disturbance. An important complication is acute toxicosis, in which the patient may die in a few days. Weakness of the muscles is not uncommon, particularly a feeling of "giving way" of the legs. If the patient holds the head down and is asked to look up without raising the head, the forehead remains smooth and is not wrinkled, as in a normal individual (Joffroy). A feature noted by Charcot is a great diminution in the electrical resistance, which may be due to the saturation of the skin with moisture owing to the vasomotor dilatation (Hirt). There may be decreased hydrochloric acid in the stomach. The spleen may be enlarged in chronic cases. The emaciation may be extreme. Glycosuria and albuminuria are not infrequent and true diabetes may occur. In women the menstrual function may be disturbed. The influence of pregnancy on the disease is variable.

The course is usually chronic, lasting several years, and often with remissions. After persisting for six months or a year the symptoms may disappear. There are instances in which the symptoms came on with great intensity, following fright, and disappeared again in a few days.

Prognosis.—Statistics are misleading, as only the severe cases come under hospital treatment. Probably 65 per cent of the patients make a good recovery and 10 to 12 per cent die. Certain others go on to some degree of chronic invalidism. There are often periods of remission. In the hands of competent surgeons the mortality from operation is low and the results are excellent. The same may be said of X-ray therapy in properly selected cases. Treatment early in the course improves the outlook.

Diagnosis.—The typical cases are easily recognized but the difficulty comes with the partially developed forms and hyperthyroidism. The patient should be kept at rest and carefully studied. If the giving of thyroid extract (gr. i-ii, 0.06-0.12 gm.) for a few days increases the symptoms and pulse rate, it is significant. In acute cases syphilis should be excluded. The test of Goetsch which consists in the response to the injection of epinephrine (0.5 cc.) is sometimes of value. An increase in the pulse rate and blood-pressure and aggravation of the general symptoms are the important points. It may aid in the diagnosis from early tuberculosis which may show features suggestive of hyperthyroidism. The response to quinine hydrobromide may be of value: 10 grains (0.6 gm.) are given three times a day and usually within a few days the normal individual has symptoms of cinchonism. They do not appear in exophthalmic goitre. Certain signs should suggest the possibility of hyperthyroidism: (1) tachycardia, (2) rapid emaciation without evident cause, (3) diarrhea without evident cause, (4) lymphocytosis, and (5) nervous disturbance otherwise difficult to explain. Diagnosis in the borderline cases depends more on careful study and observation than on any single test. The most important point is the increase in basal metabolism, but this should be done by a competent worker and the necessity of repeated tests realized. An increase of at least 15 per cent is necessary to have significance.

There is a group in which many of the features of Graves' disease are present but the basal metabolism is normal. Such cases represent "*autonomic imbalance*" (List, Hyman and Kessel). The most frequent feature is tachycardia, next coming thyroid enlargement. Tremor and eye signs are less common. A normal basal metabolism is the important diagnostic point.

Treatment.—It is usually well to try medical treatment before surgery is considered. Halfway measures should not be considered; the patient should be in bed, at absolute rest and excitement and irritation avoided. Any causes of worry should be corrected if possible. Long hours of sleep should be secured by sedatives if necessary. Any focus of infection should be treated. Tobacco, alcohol, tea and coffee should be forbidden. The patients should be liberally fed and sufficient food given to equalize the increased metabolism. In the diet, milk, buttermilk and foods prepared with milk should figure largely. Cereals, eggs, butter, bread or toast, vegetables and fruits may be given. Meat broths and meat are not to be given; small amounts of chicken may be taken occasionally. Water should be taken freely, best as distilled water, but, if not available, boiled water. An ice-bag should be applied over the heart. Of internal remedies, belladonna and ergot seem helpful in some cases. Quinine hydrobromide (gr. 10, 0.6 gm. three times a day) is often useful. Iodine in the form of Lugol's solution (♏ x, 0.6 cc.) is useful but should be given in severe cases only if operation is to be done. It may be given in mild cases. There may be marked improvement with its use and a trial of it is advisable before operation. The application of the X-rays or radium has been successful in many cases.

Surgical Treatment.—Operation is indicated, (1) when there are compression signs, (2) when there is no gain under a proper trial of medical treatment and (3) when medical treatment causes improvement but there is not complete recovery. Severe toxicosis is usually a contra-indication to surgery. Removal of part of the thyroid gland offers the best hope of permanent cure. It is remarkable with what rapidity all the symptoms may disappear after partial thyroidectomy. A second operation may be necessary in severe cases. Ligature of the arteries may be enough. Excision of the superior cervical ganglia of the sympathetic has one beneficial result, *viz.*, the production of slight ptosis, which obviates the staring character of the exophthalmos.

DISEASES OF THE PARATHYROID GLANDS

The parathyroid bodies occur, as a rule, in two pairs on either side of the lateral lobes of the thyroid gland; small ovoid structures from 6 to 8 mm. in length. The parathyroid gland hormone has an influence on calcium and phosphorus metabolism. With increased production of the hormone there is an increase of serum calcium, a decrease of serum phosphorus and an increase in the excretion of both in the urine. Removal of the parathyroid glands results in a fall in serum calcium, a rise in the serum phosphorus and a fall in the excretion of both in the urine. As nearly all the calcium of the body is in the bones, hyperfunction of the parathyroids leads to withdrawal of calcium from the bones and they become porous. The increased excretion of calcium and phosphorus in the urine may cause renal damage and lead to the formation of calculi. *Hypoparathyroidism* is an important cause of tetany. It may be that the parathyroids are concerned in some of the other conditions in which tetany occurs. This is sufficient warrant for considering this disease here, though it may result from other causes.

TETANY

Definition.—Hyperexcitability of the neuromuscular system with bilateral chronic or intermittent spasms of the muscles of the extremities. There are definite changes in the calcium metabolism, in many cases due to disturbance in the function of the parathyroid glands.

Etiology.—It occurs in epidemic form, particularly in the spring, sometimes with slight fever and behaves like an acute infection. It may occur in, or follow, the infections, typhoid fever, measles, etc. Of 8 cases reported by C. P. Howard, 4 were with dilatation of the stomach, 2 with hyperacidity, 1 with chronic diarrhea, and 1 with lactation. In adults the gastro-intestinal group is the most common, usually with vomiting, loss of hydrochloric acid, dehydration and alkalosis. It may follow successive pregnancies—the "nurse's contracture" of Trousseau.

In children it is common with rickets and in gastro-intestinal affections of artificially fed infants associated with wasting. Laryngospasm and child crowing are usually manifestations of tetany. In infantile tetany hemorrhages into the parathyroid glands have been found. Forced breathing, as in acute diseases, hysteria, early anesthesia and with excessive exercise, may cause alkalosis and tetany follows. The same may result from overdosage of sodium bicarbonate. There is disturbance of the acid-base equilibrium. In cases of thyroidectomy in which the parathyroids have been removed, hypoparathyroidism follows. This is permanent if all parathyroid tissue is removed. In some cases the condition is temporary suggesting that enough parathyroid tissue is left; it may undergo hyperplasia. Idiopathic hypoparathyroidism occurs but is probably very rare.

Morbid Anatomy.—Atrophy, hemorrhages, adenomas, cysts and inflammations have been found in the parathyroids but the glands have been found normal in fatal cases.

Symptoms.—The tonic spasms occur chiefly in the upper extremities; the arms are flexed across the chest with the hands in the so-called "obstetric" position, the proximal phalanges flexed, the middle and distal extended with the thumb contracted in the palm. The legs are extended with plantar flexion of the feet and toes. The muscles of the face are not so often involved, but there may be trismus and spasm of the muscles of expression. The spasms may last only for a few hours or persist for days or weeks, recurring in paroxysms. Contracture of the back muscles is rare; occasionally there are general convulsions. Laryngospasm may occur with noisy inspiration. Pain is variable, sometimes being severe. The pulse may be quickened and the temperature raised. Disturbance of sensation is rare. In chronic cases, the skin looks tense or drawn, there may be edema, the hair falls out, and the teeth may subsequently show defects in the enamel. Perinuclear cataract may follow a prolonged attack, Certain additional features are present:

Trousseau's sign is thus described—"So long as the attack is not over, the paroxysm may be reproduced at will. This is effected by compressing the affected parts, either in the direction of their principal nerve trunks, or over their blood-vessels so as to impede the arterial or venous circulation." The spasm is caused by pressure on the nerves. It may be elicited months, or even years, after an attack. It is not always present.

Chvostek's phenomenon depends on an increased excitability of the motor nerves. A slight tap on the facial will throw the muscles into spasm, sometimes only limited groups. It is sometimes seen in debilitated children who have not had tetany and may occur in healthy children.

Erb's phenomenon is due to increased electrical excitability of the motor nerves. In normal infants a cathodal opening contraction is not caused by a current of less than 5 milliamperes; contraction is obtained in tetany with much less. Anodal hyperexcitability is also present, especially in latent tetany, but it may occur in normal infants and in other conditions.

Diagnosis.—The disease is readily recognized. Between the attacks, or even long after, the signs may be obtained. The common carpopedal spasm of debilitated infants is regarded by some as mild tetany. The predisposing factors, gastro-intestinal disease, thyroidectomy, pregnancy, etc., should be borne in mind. There is rarely any difficulty in differentiating tetanus, epilepsy or functional cramps. Hysterical spasm may give difficulty.

Prognosis.—Postoperative cases may prove fatal. Death in the gastro-intestinal forms is usually from the primary conditions. Recovery is the rule in children. The cause is an important element in prognosis. The use of parathyroid hormone has improved the outlook in cases due to hypoparathyroidism.

Treatment.—In children the condition with which the tetany is associated should be treated. Baths and cold sponging often relieve the spasm as promptly as in child-crowing. Calcium should be given freely. In acute conditions calcium chloride can be given intravenously (10 cc. of a 10 per cent solution), and repeated as necessary. Calcium lactate (gr. x-xv, 0.6 to 1 gm.) is given three times a day. Milk and vitamin D should be given freely; the latter aids the absorption of calcium. Parathormone is given intramuscularly in doses of 10 to 50 units. It should always be used in acute cases. It may lose its effect after prolonged use. The blood calcium should be followed to avoid hypercalcemia. Excessive alkaline therapy should be avoided. Ammonium chloride (gr. 30-90, 2-6 gm. a day) has proved useful, probably by correcting alkalosis.

In gastric tetany, especially when due to dilatation of the stomach, the mortality is high, and recovery without operative interference is rare. Regular, systematic lavage with large quantities of saline or mildly antiseptic solutions is sometimes beneficial.

HYPERPARATHYROIDISM

This may result from overfunction of the parathyroids with hyperplasia but more frequently is associated with the presence of parathyroid adenomata. The removal of these has resulted in cessation of the hyperfunction. Hyperparathyroidism causes the disease described by von Recklinghausen, in 1891, as generalised osteitis fibrosa cystica.

Osteitis Fibrosa Cystica.—This shows softening of the bones with areas of cystic degeneration, possibly gross deformity of bones and fractures, with hypercalcemia and decreased blood phosphorus.

Etiology.—Hyperparathyroidism is the cause, due to hyperplasia or adenomata of the parathyroid glands. Females are affected about twice as often as males. The most common age is from 35 to 55.

Symptoms.—The onset may be with thirst and polyuria. There is complaint of pain in the bones, particularly in the back, pelvis and legs. There may be marked tenderness in the hands. Deformity slowly increases. The head may enlarge and be held in flexion; the spine is shortened. There may be tender areas in the bones and fractures occur easily, sometimes spontaneously. Marked muscular weakness and hypotonia occur. Nausea, vomiting and abdominal cramps may be present. There is decreased electrical excitability of the muscles. Emaciation and cachexia follow in severe cases. The blood shows a high serum calcium (12 to 23 mg. per 100 cc.) and a low phosphorus content (1 to 2.7 mg.). The calcium excretion in the urine is increased from slight amounts to eight times the normal. The radiograms show marked decalcification with a granular mottling and sometimes the presence of cysts. The picture is distinctive. In some cases the disease is described as local. Renal changes are common and *calculi* are present in a number of the patients. Tumors in the neck are felt in a small proportion of the cases.

Diagnosis.—This has to be made from osteomalacia, Paget's disease, multiple myeloma, fragilitas ossium and carcinoma of the bone. The study of the blood, especially the calcium content which is above 12, and the X-ray findings are distinctive.

Prognosis.—This depends on the possibility of correcting the cause, as other treatment is not effectual.

Treatment.—This consists in removal of the hyperfunctioning parathyroid tumors. There may be great difficulty in finding the parathyroid glands. With hyperplasia alone, portions of the glands should be removed. If temporary hypoparathyroidism results, parathormone and calcium should be given. Every effort should be made to nourish the patient and calcium and phosphorus should be given freely to supply the loss, with vitamin D. Pain may require sedatives. Care should be taken to avoid fractures so far as is possible.

DISEASES OF THE PITUITARY GLAND

The pituitary gland consists of two lobes, (*a*) an anterior lobe, originating from the roof of the pharynx which has a glandular structure with three types of cells, acidophilic, basophilic and neutrophilic; it is necessary for life; and (*b*) a smaller posterior lobe which arises from the floor of the third ventricle and is composed (1) of a central neuroglial portion (pars nervosa) and (2) an investment of epithelial cells (pars intermedia). Removal of the posterior lobe may cause little disturbance.

Modern knowledge of the functions of the gland began with the studies of Marie on its relation to acromegaly and gigantism. Then Schäfer and Oliver discovered that injection of an extract of the gland caused a rise in blood pressure. Since these observations an enormous amount of work has been done, and we now appreciate the remarkable influence of this complicated structure which may be regarded as the most influential of all the endocrine glands. It is the dominating partner. It is important in the influences which it exerts on other glands and on development, reproduction and metabolism.

The *hormones* produced in the *anterior* lobe are (1) a growth hormone, (2) a sex hormone or hormones (Prolan A and B), (3) thyrotropic hormone, (4) pancreaticotropic hormone, (5) adrenotropic hormone and (6) parathyrotropic hormone. The sex hormone is not specific; that is from male or female it stimulates the gonads of both sexes. The thyrotropic hormone stimulates the secretion of thyroxin and increases metabolism. There may be a lactogenic hormone. The *posterior* lobe produces two hormones at least; one raises blood pressure and has an influence on renal secretion (vasopressin) and the other stimulates contraction of the uterus and smooth muscle of the bowel (oxytocin). The extract of the posterior lobe is termed Liquor Pituitarii, U.S.P. It is used in diabetes insipidus. The result of the injection into animals of pituitary gland extracts in causing severe gastritis and possibly necrosis of the gastric mucous membrane is of interest especially with Cushing's observations on acute gastric lesions in some of his patients who had been operated on.

The close relationship of the pituitary to the diencephalon is important. This area, with such important nuclei, may be responsible for much disturbance at a distance, possibly often through the autonomic system. It is suggested that by a system of veins passing up from both lobes of the pituitary, much of the hormone material may act directly on the nervous system. By its influence on other glands many diseases may occur or be influenced.

Disturbances in the function of the pituitary gland are not clearly grouped into the effects of deficiency and excess, though one can differentiate states of hyper- and hypopituitarism. Owing to the situation of the gland it is very liable to feel the effect of pressure from neighboring or even distant lesions, so that disturbance of function may be due not only to a primary involvement, but to secondary compression. There are *neighborhood symptoms* due to enlargement of the gland, especially headache, alteration in the visual fields, optic atrophy and sometimes convulsive seizures. The results of disturbance of the secretion of hormones are very varied; some cases are clear cut while others are very complicated. A number of groups may be recognized.

(*a*) Cases of tumor growth showing signs of distortion of neighboring structures, and the constitutional effects of altered glandular activity. The X-rays show changes in the configuration of the pituitary fossa; there are pressure signs on the adjacent cranial nerves, bitemporal hemianopia, optic atrophy and oculomotor palsies. Uncinate fits are not unusual. The *convulsive seizures* usually begin during adolescence and the patients show features of under-activity of the gland with X-ray evidence of pituitary change. There is a form of *headache* associated with pituitary disturbance.

(*b*) Cases in which the neighborhood manifestations are pronounced but the constitutional features are slight. The regional signs of tumor are marked, but there may be slight or transient evidence of disturbed glandular activity, perhaps only disturbed carbohydrate metabolism with adiposity.

(*c*) Cases in which the neighborhood manifestations are absent or slight, though the glandular symptoms are unmistakable. The gland is not so large as to cause regional symptoms. There are skeletal changes either of over- or undergrowth. Disturbance of carbohydrate metabolism is often associated with the early stages of acromegaly, or there is a great increase in tolerance. In some cases there is a tendency to the deposition of fat, subnormal temperature, drowsiness, slow pulse, dry skin, loss of hair, and a high tolerance for sugars. Most cases of acromegaly fall in this group and show at first evidences of hyperpituitarism, and later of insufficiency. In the adult, adiposity, high sugar tolerance, subnormal temperature, psychic manifestations, and sexual infantilism of the reversive type indicate hypopituitarism and may exist without regional symptoms of tumor.

(*d*) Hypophysial symptoms may be shown by patients with internal hydrocephalus from any cause, and this dyspituitarism may result from a lesion, inflammatory or neoplastic, in the neighborhood of the third ventricle.

These are the most important of the groups but there are also cases with manifestations indicating involvement of other internal secretions with that of the hypophysis, and a large group in which transient hypophysial symptoms occur as in pregnancy, cranial injuries and infectious diseases.

Disturbances in the function of the pituitary gland may lead to remarkable changes in growth; *hyperpituitarism* may lead to gigantism, when the process antedates ossification of the epiphyses—the *Launois type;* to acromegaly when it is of later date; *hypopituitarism* to adiposity, with skeletal and sexual infantilism when the process originates in childhood—the *Fröhlich type;* to adiposity and sexual infantilism of the reversive type when originating in the adult. Much remains to be done in clearing the relations of the types of infantilism—the Lorain, the Brissaud, the pancreatic, the intestinal—to the internal secretions.

ACROMEGALY

Definition.—A syndrome characterized by increase in size of the face and extremities associated with hyperfunction (excess of the growth hormone) of the anterior lobe of the pituitary gland. If it antedates ossification of the epiphyses this leads to gigantism, and in the adult leads to overgrowth of the skeleton and other changes which we know as acromegaly.

Etiology.—It is a rare disease and rather more frequent in women. It affects particularly persons of large size. Twenty per cent of acromegalics are above six feet in height when the symptoms begin, and fully 40 per cent of giants are acromegalics (Sternberg). Trauma, the infections, and emotional shock have preceded the onset of the disease. There is overactivity of the acidophilic cells of the anterior lobe.

Pathology.—Practically all of the cases show changes in the pituitary gland, hyperplasia, adenoma, fibroma, or sarcoma, causing distention of the sella turcica and, in the late stages, pressure on surrounding structures; the symptoms are in part due to disturbance of the function of the gland (the other cells may be destroyed), and in part to pressure on adjacent parts.

The bones show the most striking changes; there is a general enlargement of the extremities, but the skeleton is more or less affected. The enlargement, due to a periosteal growth, is most evident in the hands and feet. The bones of the face are always involved. The orbital arches, frontal prominences, zygoma, malar, and nasal bones are increased in size; the lower jaw is elongated, thickened, and the teeth separated. The X-ray picture shows characteristic changes in the sella turcica. The skin and subcutaneous tissues are thickened and hypertrophy is seen in the soft parts of the face. The brain has been found large, but the most important changes are those due to pressure at the base. The internal organs have been found enlarged.

Symptoms.—When the pituitary gland is involved in tumor growth, which is common in acromegaly, the symptoms may be grouped into those due to mechanical effects and those associated with perversion of the secretion.

(*a*) Regional Symptoms.—*Headache* is common, usually frontal, and often very severe. Somnolence has been noted and may be the first symptom. Ocular features occur in a large proportion of the cases, diminution of the fields of vision, bitemporal hemianopia, optic atrophy, and, in late stages, pressure on the third nerve and abducens. One eye only may be affected. Exophthalmos may occur. Deafness is not infrequent. Irritability, marked change in the disposition, great depression and progressive dementia have been noted. Epistaxis and rhinorrhea may be present.

(*b*) Symptoms due to the perversion of the internal secretion itself form the striking features of the disease. The patient's friends first notice a gradual increase in the features, which become heavy and thick; or the patient himself may notice that he takes a larger size of hat, or with the progressive enlargement of the hands a larger size of gloves. The enlargement of the extremities does not interfere with their free use.

The hypertrophy is general, involving all the tissues, and gives a curious spadelike character to the hands. The lines on the palms are much deepened. The wrists may be enlarged, but the arms are rarely affected. The feet are involved like the hands and are uniformly enlarged. The big toe, however, may be much larger in proportion. The nails are usually broad and large, but there is no curving, and the terminal phalanges are not bulbous. The joints may be painful and neuralgia is common. The head increases in volume, but not as much in proportion as the face, which becomes much elongated and enlarged in consequence of the increase in the size of the superior and inferior maxillary bones. The latter increases greatly in size, and often projects below the upper jaw. The alveolar processes are widened and the teeth are often separated. The soft parts increase in size, and the nostrils are large and broad. The eyelids are sometimes greatly thickened, and the ears enormously hypertrophied. The tongue may be greatly enlarged. Late in the disease the spine may be affected and the back bowed—kyphosis. The bones of the thorax may progressively enlarge. With this increase in size the skin of the hands and face may appear normal. Sometimes it is slightly altered in color, coarse, or flabby, but it has not the dry, harsh appearance of the skin in myxedema. The muscles are sometimes wasted. Asthenia is common. In cases without tumor, the progress may cease and the condition remain stationary. It does not necessarily shorten life.

Also associated with disturbance of the function of the gland is glycosuria, noticed in many cases and common in the early stages; in the advanced stages there is a high tolerance for sugar. Symptoms on the part of other ductless glands are common. Thyroid disturbance is not rare, usually hypothyroidism, but thyrotoxicosis may occur. Myxedema or a flabby obesity may occur late. Amenorrhea is an early symptom in women. Impotence is common in advanced cases in men. The blood pressure, basal metabolism and temperature are usually low.

Diagnosis.—This rarely offers difficulty; hypertrophic pulmonary osteoarthropathy and osteitis deformans are the conditions most likely to be confused. The general features and an X-ray study should prevent confusion.

Treatment.—In cases due to tumor, surgical measures are indicated. Otherwise X-ray therapy should be used and in cases of hyperplasia this may be effectual if used early. Glandular therapy is not very successful. With evidence of posterior lobe disturbance, as shown by polyuria, the posterior lobe extracts should be used. Glycosuria may require treatment as in diabetes mellitus. With marked thyroid gland disturbance the usual treatment should be given. Sedatives have to be given for pain.

Gigantism.—This is due to overfunction of the anterior lobe of the pituitary with an excess of the growth hormone beginning in childhood. It may be associated with a pituitary tumor, in which case surgery may be useful. Otherwise X-ray therapy should be employed.

Simmonds' Disease.—This syndrome, described by Simmonds in 1914, hypophysial cachexia, is due to atrophy of the anterior lobe of the pituitary and characterised by cachexia, premature senility, generalised atrophy and asthenia. The onset is usually between the ages of 30 and 40 and it occurs more frequently in women. Infection by an embolus, especially in puerperal sepsis, syphilis and granuloma may be causal. The *clinical features* are asthenia, emaciation and general decreased bulk, loss of hair and teeth, sometimes thirst and polyuria. There is susceptibility to cold with lowered basal metabolism. Amenorrhea and sterility occur in the female and loss of sexual desire and power in the male. The skin is pale and wrinkled. The bones atrophy. Lethargy and coma may occur towards the end. The disease is usually progressive but some patients live for many years. In *treatment*, anterior pituitary extracts should be used energetically.

Pituitary Basophilism (*Cushing's disease*).—This like acromegaly, is a hyperpituitary disorder with secondary polyglandular manifestations. It is characterized by a plethoric adiposity limited to the face, neck and trunk, purplish lineae atrophicae, hypertrichosis, sexual dystrophy, hypertension, skeletal decalcification and hyperglycaemia.

Etiology.—The disease is more common in young females but may occur at any age. Some of its features (*e.g.*, hypertension, adiposity and glycosuria) may be due to secretory excitation of the tuberal nuclei. The secondary effects on other ductless glands (thyroid, parathyroid, pancreatic islets and adrenal cortex) are shown by a low basal metabolic rate, high calcium elimination, glycosuria and symptoms suggesting hyperadrenalism.

Clinical features.—Early features in females are amenorrhea, plethoric adiposity sparing the extremities, and hypertrichosis of face and body. Osteomalacia leading to kyphosis and loss of height may be marked, and suggest parathyroid disease. A moderate polycythemia may occur. The glycosuria may be difficult to control by insulin. Pains in the back and abdomen are common and asthenia may be marked. Cardiac hypertrophy and arteriosclerosis are late features, and renal sclerosis has been described. The disease may have spontaneous remissions but death usually occurs from intercurrent infections, pulmonary edema or apoplexy.

Diagnosis.—The clinical syndrome is striking and there should be little difficulty in its recognition. Differential diagnosis from hyperparathyroidism or hyperadrenalism may in some cases be difficult.

Treatment.—Irradiation of the pituitary body has been found to be of benefit in some cases. Since the gland is rarely enlarged by the adenoma, surgery is not likely to be indicated.

Laurence-Biedl Syndrome.—This is characterized by *adiposity, retinitis pigmentosa, mental deficiency* and *polydactylism.* It may be familial but apparently is not hereditary. The cause is obscure. In some patients changes in the sella turcica have been found, suggesting that the pituitary gland may be involved; others regard it as perhaps due to a lack of development, possibly of centres in the midbrain and involving the pituitary gland. The *diagnosis* should not offer difficulty. The results of *treatment* are variable. Some patients undoubtedly have been helped by thyroid gland extract and pituitary gland extract, either of the whole gland or the anterior lobe. It is generally an advantage to reduce the overweight. The mental condition of one of our patients improved considerably under thyroid treatment; the basal metabolism was normal.

DISEASES OF THE PINEAL GLAND

"That there is a small gland in the brain in which the soul exercises its functions more particularly than in the other parts" was the opinion of Descartes. The condition termed *macrogenitosomia praecox* shows premature physical and psychical development, especially in the sex characteristics. What we know now is derived chiefly from clinical cases. But the nature of the internal secretion, if any, is unknown. Some hold that disturbance of this gland may be associated with muscular dystrophy. Rowntree *et al* by injection of pineal gland extract in rats have produced precocious development, especially gonadal, with increased growth of hair in the offspring; the animals are dwarfed. This suggests a relationship to the thymus gland by which marked changes in growth may be produced.

Disease of the gland, usually tumor, may cause (1) pressure symptoms, which may be due partly to disturbance of the pituitary gland; (2) focal symptoms, due to involvement of the cranial nerves, particularly those of the eyes, (3) features believed to be due to internal secretion disturbance, as sexual precocity, carbohydrate tolerance, obesity and increase in the growth of hair. In some cases there have been signs of meningitis.

DISEASES OF THE SEX GLANDS

The endocrine part of the testicle is represented by the *interstitial cells* of Leydig and of the ovary by the interstitial cells and the cells of the corpus luteum. The secretions influence the development of the secondary sexual characters. *Hyperfunction* causes premature sexual development in both sexes. *Hypofunction* is shown (1) in eunuchs, in whom there is complete loss of the glands, and (2) in eunochoids, in whom there is insufficiency of the glands. In eunuchs there is lack of genital development, the body is large and fat, there is scanty growth of hair, and the psychical state is altered. In females whose ovaries are removed after puberty the features of the artificial menopause appear. *Eunochoids* differ according as the insufficiency occurred before or after puberty. There is usually involvement of other glands, especially the pituitary, with a multiglandular syndrome. The individuals are usually tall and fat with absence of secondary sexual characters. The genitals show hypoplasia, and sterility, with disturbance of the sexual function, is the rule. In treatment, glandular extracts may be used, pituitary in the male and ovarian in the female.

Female sex hormones.—The injection of fatty substances extracted from the ovaries brings on estrus in animals after removal of the ovaries. The substance, named estrin, was found in the ovary and placenta. Later it was found in the urine of pregnant women and lower animals. The substance has been crystallised and belongs to the sterols. Partial hydrogenation increases its activity. The corpus luteum hormone is a diketone and has also been found in the urine of pregnant females. By injections of both hormones menstruation can be produced in women who have had both ovaries removed. If a woman has a uterine mucosa, menstruation can be induced. It seems probable that by the use of these hormones menstrual and menopausal disturbances can be helped, especially metrorrhagia. They may also be useful in some cases of lack of development and infantilism.

INFANTILISM

Definition.—A disturbance in growth with persistence of infantile or puerile characters and a retardation of development, bodily and mental.

Etiology.—It is difficult to make a satisfactory classification of the causes or of the cases of infantilism—in some no cause is evident, in others the failure in development has followed obvious disease, and there are cases directly dependent upon loss of some internal secretion.

I. Cachetic infantilism is not uncommon, as any serious chronic malady may delay development. Children with *hookworm* disease may reach the age of 20 or older before puberty occurs. *Syphilis* is a common cause. *Renal Dwarfism* occurs in children with nephritis in whom the renal disease may appear to have been congenital or to have begun soon after birth. There may be polyuria with deficient growth and bony deformities of which knock-knee is often the first noted. It has occurred with congenital cystic kidneys. Rickets may be present. Despite the renal sclerosis and nitrogen retention, hypertension does not occur. Where malaria is very prevalent delayed sexual development is not uncommon and it is not infrequent in congenital heart disease. There is a toxic infantilism due to the action of alcohol and lead. The influence of lack of vitamins may be important.

II. The Hormonic Type.—There are several varieties directly dependent upon disturbance of the internal secretions. The most important are:

(*a*) Thyroidal or Cretinoid Infantilism.—This has been described.

(*b*) The Fröhlich type, dystrophia adiposogenitalis, due to hypofunction of the pituitary gland, probably of both lobes, is characterized by great obesity and genital hypoplasia. The symptoms are due to a secretory deficit, for they are capable of experimental reproduction by partial glandular extirpation in animals (Cushing). This syndrome usually appears in childhood but may begin in adult life. The obesity is of the pituitary type, most marked about the pelvis. There is amenorrhea in females and impotence in males. There may be a tumor or cyst of the pituitary, pressure on the gland or atrophy. In *diagnosis* the characteristic obesity and lack of development, both genital and of the secondary sex characters, are suggestive. There may be increased sugar tolerance and low basal metabolism. It is a mistake to regard every fat child with slow genital development as having this disease. In *treatment* if a tumor or cyst is present surgery is indicated. Otherwise glandular therapy should be used, best by injection, although benefit seems to have resulted from the extract of the whole pituitary gland given by mouth. The *Brissaud type* is probably due to dyspituitarism. A round, chubby face, underdeveloped skeleton, prominent abdomen, large layer of fat over the whole body, rudimentary sexual organs, no growth of hair except on the head, and absence of the second dentition, are the prominent features of this form.

(*c*) Pancreatico-intestinal Type.—Cases of infantilism associated with intestinal changes are described. Bramwell thought the pancreas was at fault, and his patients improved under treatment with pancreatic extract. Some may be instances of the coeliac disease.

(*d*) Pituitary Infantilism (*So-called Lorain Type*).—"In this variety the figure is so small that, at first sight, it looks like that of a child. When the patient is stripped, however, his outlines are seen to be those of an adult, and not those of childhood. The head is proportionately small, and the trunk well formed; for the shoulders are broad compared to the hips, and the bony prominences and the muscles stand out distinctly. We have before us a miniature man (or woman, as the case may be), and not one who has retained the characteristics of childhood beyond the proper time. There is, indeed, no growth of facial, pubic or axillary hair, yet the genital organs, though small, are well shaped and quite large enough for the size of the body. The intelligence in both sexes is generally normal" (John Thomson). The cause is probably associated with disturbance of the anterior lobe of the pituitary with lack of the growth and sex hormones. In treatment, anterior pituitary preparations should be tried.

III. Progeria.—Under this term Hastings Gilford described a condition in children of incomplete development (infantilism) with premature decay. The facial appearance, the attitude, the loss of hair, wasting of the skin, are those of old age, and postmortem extensive fibroid changes are found, particularly in the arteries and kidneys. The condition is apparently due to disease of the anterior pituitary lobe and may be an exaggerated form of pituitary infantilism.

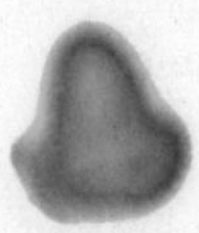

SECTION XII

DISEASES OF THE NERVOUS SYSTEM

SYSTEM DISEASES

INTRODUCTION

There are certain diseases of the nervous system which are confined, if not absolutely, still in great part, to definite tracts (combinations of neurones) which subserve like functions. These tracts are called *systems,* and a disease confined to one of them is a *system disease.* If more than one system is involved, the process is called a combined system disease. Just what diseases should be classed under these names has caused much discussion. We can not speak positively; our knowledge is not sufficiently accurate, either as to the exact limits of the systems, or the nature and extent of the process in the several diseases. It may be said that the nervous system is composed of two great systems of neurones, the afferent or sensory system and the efferent or motor system, and the connections between them.

Tabes dorsalis is a disease confined at its onset to the afferent system, and progressive muscular atrophy is one of the efferent system. Several theories have been advanced to explain why a disease should be limited to a definite system of neurones. One view is based upon the idea that in certain individuals one or the other of these systems has an innate tendency to undergo degeneration; another assumes that neurones with a similar function have a similar chemical construction (which differs from that of neurones with a different function) and this is taken to explain why a toxin should show a selective action for a single functional system of neurones.

DISEASES OF THE AFFERENT OR SENSORY SYSTEM

TABES DORSALIS

(*Locomotor Ataxia; Posterior Spinal Sclerosis*)

Definition.—An affection characterized clinically by sensory disturbances, incoordination, trophic changes, and involvement of the special senses, particularly the eyes. Anatomically there is degeneration of the root fibres of the posterior columns of the cord, of the posterior roots, and at times of the spinal ganglia and peripheral nerves. Degenerations have been described in the brain, particularly the cortex cerebri, in the ganglion cells of the cord, and in the endogenous fibres of the posterior columns.

Etiology.—It is a widespread disease, more frequent in cities than in the country. Among 16,562 cases in the neurological dispensary of the Johns Hopkins Hospital there were 201 cases of tabes. Males are attacked more frequently than females, the proportion being nearly 10 to 1. The disease is not very uncommon in the negro in the United States. It is a disease of adult life, the great majority of cases occurring between the thirtieth and fiftieth years. There are a good many cases of the existence of the disease in both husband and wife, and a few in which the children are also affected. Occasionally cases are seen in young men, and it may occur in children with congenital syphilis. *Syphilis* is *the* important cause. The interval between the syphilitic infection and the first symptoms of tabes is variable. Five to fifteen years is the period in one-half the cases. Intervals from two to twenty-five years occur.

Pathology.—Posterior spinal sclerosis, although the most obvious gross change, is not an adequate description. The posterior fibres are of two kinds, those with their cell bodies outside the cord in the spinal ganglia, the so-called exogenous, or root fibres, and those which arise from cells within the cord, the endogenous fibres. These two sets occupy fairly well-determined regions, and a study of early cases of tabes has shown that the exogenous or root fibres are first affected. The fibres of the dorsal roots enter the cord in two divisions, an external and an internal; the former is composed of fibres of small calibre, which, in the cord, make up Lissauer's tract, and occupy the space between the apex of the dorsal cornua and the periphery of the cord, and really do not form part of the dorsal columns. They are short, soon entering the gray matter, and do not seem to be affected, or only slightly so, in early cases.

The larger fibres enter the cord by the internal division, just medial to the cornua, in what is known as the root entry zone. Some enter the gray matter of the spinal cord almost directly and others after a longer course, while still others run in the cord to the medulla, to end in the nuclei of the dorsal columns. That it is the coarse posterior root fibres which are first affected in tabes is generally admitted, but there is much divergence of opinion as to the character and location of the initial process.

Nageotte calls attention to the frequency of a transverse, interstitial neuritis of the posterior roots just after they have left the ganglia and are still surrounded by the dura, and he believes that this is the primary lesion. Obersteiner and Redlich laid stress on inflammation of the pia mater over the dorsal aspect of the cord, which involves the root fibres as they pass through. They point out that it is just here that the dorsal roots are most vulnerable, for at this point—that is, while surrounded by the pia—they are almost completely devoid of their myelin sheaths. Changes in the blood vessels of the cord, of the pia, and of the nerve roots have been described in early tabes, and Marie and Guillain advanced the belief that the changes in the cord are due to syphilis of the posterior lymphatic system which is confined to the dorsal columns of the cord, the pia mater over them and the dorsal roots.

With the Marchi stain, degeneration of the root fibres in the root-entry zone is a constant finding in early cases. This change is radicular in the sense that it varies in intensity with the different roots and is most marked in the sacral and lumbar regions. The degeneration is not found in the dorsal roots, but begins within the cord just beyond where the root fibres lose their neurilemma and their myelin sheaths. Degenerated fibres may be traced into the dorsal gray matter and among the ganglion cells of the columns of Clarke. The long columns which ascend the cord also degenerate.

In more advanced cases, there are degeneration of the dorsal roots and some alteration of the cells in the spinal ganglia. The fibres distal to the ganglia are practically normal, although at times the sensory fibres, at the periphery of a limb, show degeneration. Within the cord, the exogenous fibres are diseased; there is also degeneration in the endogenous system of fibres. Optic atrophy is frequent and other cranial nerves may be affected by an interstitial inflammation of the proximal parts of the nerves.

The disease occasionally spreads beyond the sensory system in the cord, and in advanced cases the cells in the ventral horns may be degenerated in association with muscular atrophy. Mott very generally found more or less marked changes in the pyramidal fibres; these he believed to be evidence of changes in the cerebral cortex. Degeneration of the cortex may exist, but even when mental symptoms are absent, or very mild, similar slight changes have been described, just as in general paresis, without marked tabetic symptoms, there may be degeneration of the dorsal columns. The close association of tabes and general paresis will be considered later.

Symptoms.—For convenience, these are considered under three stages—the incipient or pre-ataxic, the ataxic and the paralytic.

Incipient Stage.—The onset differs very widely in the different cases, and mistakes in diagnosis are often made early in the disease. The following are the most characteristic initial symptoms:

Pains, usually of a sharp stabbing character; hence, the term lightning pains. They last for only a second or two and are most common in the legs or about the trunk, and tend to follow dorsal root areas. They dart from place to place. The pains may not be severe. They usually come in attacks in which the pains are repeated frequently, always with a sudden onset. At times they are associated with a hot burning feeling and often leave the affected area painful to pressure, and occasionally herpes may follow. The intensity of the pain varies from a sore, burning feeling of the skin to a pain so intense that, were it not for momentary duration, it would exceed human endurance. They occur at irregular intervals, and are prone to follow excesses or to come on when health is impaired. When typical, these pains are practically pathognomonic. Gastric and other crises may occur. Paresthesia may be among the first symptoms—numbness of the feet, tingling, etc.—and at times a sense of constriction about the body. Hyperesthesia is common on the trunk, especially in the lower part, and with it the abdominal reflexes may be very active. There may be areas over which there is marked tenderness on any stimulus, especially cold. There may be subjective loss of sensation in various areas. Muscular hypotonia may be an early feature.

Objective sensory changes appear *early* and are always present if subjective pain has been present for any time. The areas may be very sensitive to stimuli and with this there may be decreased pain sensibility. The disturbances are variable but pain and temperature sensations are often affected. The areas specially involved are (1) on the nose, (2) on the feet, (3) about the anus, (4) a band around the thorax and (5) on the inner surfaces of the arms. In suspicious cases these areas should be carefully studied.

Ocular Signs.—(*a*) *Optic atrophy.* This occurs in about 10 per cent of the cases, and is often an early and even the first sign. There is a gradual loss of vision, which in a majority of cases leads to total blindness. This appears to be secondary to a syphilitic meningitis. (*b*) *Ptosis,* which may be double or single. (*c*) *Paralysis* of the external muscles of the eye. This may be of one muscle or of all the muscles of the eye. The paralysis is often transient, the patient complaining of double vision for a certain period. (*d*) *Argyll-Robertson* pupil, in which there is loss of the iris reflex to light but contraction during accommodation. The pupils are often small—spinal myosis—and may be unequal or irregular.

Bladder Symptoms.—The first warning may be difficulty in emptying the bladder or incontinence, especially at night. Decrease in sexual desire and power may be an early symptom.

Trophic Disturbances.—These usually occur later, but at times they are early, and one's attention may be called to the trouble by a perforating ulcer or a characteristic Charcot joint.

Loss of the Deep Reflexes.—This important sign may occur years before the development of ataxia. Even alone it is of great moment, since it is very rare to find individuals in whom the knee and ankle jerks are normally absent. The combination of loss of either of these with one or more of the features mentioned above, especially the lightning pains and ptosis or Argyll-Robertson pupil, is practically diagnostic. These reflexes gradually decrease, and one may be lost before the other, or disappear first in one leg.

These initial features may persist for years without incoordination. The patient may look well and feel well, and be troubled only by the lightning pains or one of the other subjective symptoms. Progressive nerve deafness and paralysis of the vocal cords, with the laryngeal muscles paralyzed or paretic, may occur. The disease may never progress beyond this stage, and when optic atrophy develops early and leads to blindness, ataxia rarely, if ever, supervenes, an antagonism noted by many authors.

Ataxic Stages.—*Motor Symptoms.*—The ataxia, which comes on gradually, is believed to be due to a disturbance or loss of the afferent impulses from the muscles, joints and deep tissues. A disturbance of the muscle sense can usually be demonstrated. One of the first indications is inability to get about readily in the dark or to maintain equilibrium when washing the face with the eyes shut. When the patient stands with the feet together and the eyes closed, he sways and has difficulty in maintaining his position (Romberg's sign), and he may be quite unable to stand on one leg. He does not start off promptly at the word of command. On turning quickly he is apt to fall. He has more difficulty in descending than ascending stairs. Gradually the characteristic *ataxic gait* develops. The normal man walks by faith, the tabetic by sight. The patient, as a rule, walks with a stick, the eyes are directed to the ground, the body is thrown forward, and the legs are wide apart. In walking, the leg is thrown out violently, the foot is raised too high and is brought down in a stamping manner with the heel first, or the whole sole comes in contact with the ground. Ultimately the patient may be unable to walk without the assistance of two canes. This gait is very characteristic. The incoordination is not only in walking, but in the performance of other movements. If the patient is asked, when in the recumbent posture, to touch one knee with the other foot, the irregularity of the movement is very violent. Incoordination of the arms is less common, but usually develops in some grade. It may in rare instances exist before the incoordination of the legs. It may be tested by asking the patient to close his eyes and to touch the tip of the nose or the tip of the ear with the finger, or with the arms thrust out to bring the tips of the fingers together. The incoordination may be noticed early by difficulty in buttoning the collar or performing one of the acts of dressing.

With marked incoordination there is but little loss of muscular power. The grip of the hands may be strong and firm, the power of the legs may be unimpaired, and their nutrition, except toward the close, may be unaffected.

There is a remarkable muscular relaxation (*hypotonia*) which enables the joints to be placed in positions of hyperextension and hyperflexion. It gives sometimes a marked backward curve to the legs.

Sensory Symptoms.—The lightning pains may persist. They vary greatly in different cases. Some patients are rendered miserable by them; others escape altogether. Common symptoms are tingling, "pins and needles," particularly in the feet, and areas of hyperesthesia or anesthesia. The patient may complain of a change in sensation in the soles of the feet, as if cotton was interposed between the floor and the skin. Sensory disturbances occur less frequently in the hands. Objective sensory disturbances can usually be found and almost every variety of disturbance of tactile, pain and temperature sense has been described. Bands of a moderate grade of anesthesia about the trunk are not uncommon; they are apt to follow the distribution of spinal segments. The most marked disturbances are usually on the legs. Retardation of the sense of pain is common, and a pin prick on the foot is first felt as a simple tactile impression, and the sense of pain is not perceived for a second or two or may be delayed for several seconds. The pain felt may persist. A curious phenomenon is the loss of the power of localizing pain. If the patient is pricked on one limb he may feel it on the other (allocheiria), or a pin prick on one foot may be felt on both feet. Pruritius may occur over the areas affected by the pains. The muscular sense, usually affected early, becomes much impaired. This may be present in the pre-ataxic stage. The vibration sense is often decreased in the legs and over the sacrum.

Reflexes.—The loss of the knee and ankle jerks, the latter usually first, is an important sign but occasionally they are retained, and in these cases the lumbar segments are little if at all involved. The skin reflexes are often increased early but may be diminished later when the tactile sense is lost. The plantar reflex is usually normal unless there is sclerosis of the pyramidal tracts. The oculocardiac reflex is often absent.

Special Senses.—Ataxia is rare with optic atrophy. Deafness may occur, due to lesion of the auditory nerve and there may be attacks of vertigo. Olfactory symptoms are rare. W. B. Swift has drawn attention to ataxic speech with "a slovenly indistinct enunciation that shows partially in the vowels but predominantly in the consonants." Suggested tests are "e" (as in ell), "t," "journals" and "Time and tide wait for no man."

Visceral Symptoms.—Among the remarkable sensory disturbances are the *tabetic crises*, severe paroxysms of pain referred to various areas; thus, ocular, laryngeal, gastric, nephritic, rectal, urethral, and clitoral crises have been described. The most common are the gastric and laryngeal. *Gastric crises* may occur early and persist as the most prominent feature. The onset is usually sudden, with severe pain in the epigastrium, radiating to the back and behind the sternum. Vomiting follows and may be independent of food. Hematemesis and intestinal hemorrhages may occur. Pallor, sweating, cold extremities and a small pulse are associated, and in rare instances death occurs in collapse. The blood pressure may be very high (Barker) and the condition may be associated with angiospasm in the gastric and mesenteric vessels. The X-ray examination shows spasmodic contractions of the stomach. No special change may be found at autopsy. In the laryngeal crises there may be true spasm with dyspnea and noisy inspiration. A patient may die in the attack. There are also nasal crises, associated with sneezing fits. The contrary condition may occur, that is, absence of pain from visceral lesions, as rupture of a gastric ulcer, and render diagnosis very difficult.

The *sphincters* are frequently involved. Early in the disease there may be a retardation in voiding or incontinence. Later there is retention, and cystitis may occur. Unless great care is taken the inflammation may extend to the kidneys. Constipation is common. Later the sphincter ani is weakened. The sexual power is usually lost in the ataxic stage.

Trophic Changes.—Herpes, edema, ecchymosis or sweating may occur in the course of the pains. Alteration in the nails may occur. A perforating ulcer may develop on the foot, usually beneath the great toe. A perforating buccal ulcer has been described. Onychia may prove troublesome.

Arthropathies (Charcot Joints).—Anatomically there are: (1) enlargement of the capsule with thickening of the synovial membranes and effusion; (2) slight enlargement of the ends of the bones, with small exostoses; (3) a dull velvety appearance of the cartilages, with atrophy in places. The knees are most frequently involved. The spine is affected in rare instances, usually in the lumbar region. Trauma, with loss of pain sense, is an important element in the causation. A striking feature is the usual absence of pain. Occasionally there is pain from the distended soft parts and skin but not from the bones. Suppuration may occur, also spontaneous fractures. *Atrophy* of the muscles, usually a late manifestation, may be localized and associated with neuritis or due to involvement of the ventral horns.

Aneurism and aortic insufficiency are not uncommonly present. Both are associated syphilitic manifestations.

Cerebral Symptoms.—Hemiplegia may develop at any stage of the disease, more commonly when it is well advanced. It may be due to hemorrhagic softening from disease of the vessels, to progressive cortical changes or rarely to coarse syphilitic disease. The lost knee jerk may return on the affected side. Hemianesthesia is sometimes present.

Cerebrospinal Fluid.—The examination is of great value; the findings are: (1) *Cell content.* Lymphocytosis is found in about 90 per cent, the number of cells usually being between 40 and 60, and rarely over 100. The higher counts are found when irritative symptoms are marked. With an arrest of the process the counts are lower. (2) *Globulin.* This is positive in 90-95 per cent. In old quiescent cases there may be no increase. (3) *Wassermann reaction.* This is nearly always positive but may be negative in quiescent cases. The blood Wassermann test is positive in about 70 per cent. (4) *Colloidal gold reaction.* This is present in 85-90 per cent (a midzone reaction) and aids in diagnosing tabes from paresis. A paretic curve in a patient with signs of tabes points to the possible development of paresis subsequently.

PARALYTIC STAGE.—After persisting for an indefinite number of years the patient may become bedridden and paralyzed when he is likely to be carried off by an intercurrent affection, such as pyelonephritis or pneumonia.

Juvenile tabes is more frequent in girls and usually due to congenital syphilis. Optic atrophy is comparatively common, while pains, ataxia and visceral lesions are less frequent than in adults.

COURSE.—A patient may remain in the pre-ataxic stage for an indefinite period; and the loss of knee jerks and atrophy of the optic nerves may be the sole indications of the disease. In such cases incoordination rarely develops. In a majority of cases the progress is slow, and after six or eight years, sometimes less, the ataxia is well marked. The symptoms vary a good deal; thus, the pains, which may have been excessive at first, often lessen. The disease may remain stationary for years; then exacerbations occur and it makes rapid progress. Occasionally the process seems to be arrested. There are instances of what may be called acute ataxia, in which, within a year or even less, the incoordination is marked, and the paralytic stage may develop within a few months. The disease itself rarely causes death, and after becoming bedridden the patient may live for fifteen or twenty years.

Diagnosis.—In well marked cases there is no difficulty but one should not wait for the loss of reflexes or pupil signs to make the diagnosis. The *pains* are suggestive, especially with a history or evidence of syphilis. The greatest importance in early diagnosis attaches to disturbances of *sensation,* for which a careful search should be made. The most useful test is the response to the prick of a pin, shown by delay in perception, decreased sensation, or unusual sensations. Certain areas are especially important; the earliest loss is usually on the legs, most marked distally, decreasing toward the trunk and usually not corresponding to root distribution. There is often a zone of analgesia around the trunk, most often on the upper thorax. The ulnar border of the arms may be affected or the centre of the face, including the nose and adjoining parts of the cheeks. This may involve the greater part of the face—the tabetic mask. Absence of pain when the calf muscles are compressed and hypotonia are aids. Decrease of vibration sense is of value. The early ocular palsies are of great importance. A squint, ptosis or the Argyll-Robertson pupil may be the first sign, and exist with the loss only of the ankle or knee jerk. Loss of the knee jerk does occasionally occur in healthy individuals. The study of the spinal fluid is of great aid, especially the result of the Wassermann test and the colloidal gold reaction.

The diseases most likely to be confounded with tabes dorsalis are: (*a*) PERIPHERAL NEURITIS.—The steppage gait of arsenical, alcoholic or diabetic neuritis is unlike that of tabes. There is a paralysis of the feet, and the leg is lifted high so that the toes may clear the floor. The use of the word *ataxia* in this connection should not be continued. In the rare cases in which the muscle sense is particularly affected and in which there is true ataxia, the absence of the lightning pains and eye signs, with the history make the diagnosis clear. In diphtheritic paralysis the early loss of the knee jerk and the eye signs may suggest tabes, but the history, the existence of paralysis of the throat, and the absence of pains render a diagnosis easy.

(*b*) Combined Sclerosis.—Marked incoordination with spastic paralysis occurs in this condition. In a majority of the cases this is distinguished by the absence of pains and eye signs, but it may be a manifestation of the cord lesions in taboparalysis.

(*c*) Cerebral Disease.—In diseases involving the afferent tracts ataxia is prominent at times. It is usually unilateral or limited to one limb; this, with the history and the associated symptoms, excludes tabes.

(*d*) Cerebellar Disease.—The cerebellar incoordination has only a superficial resemblance to that of tabes, and is more a disturbance of equilibrium than a true ataxia; the knee jerk is usually present, there are no lightning pains or sensory disturbances; while, on the other hand, there are signs suggestive of an intracranial lesion.

(*e*) Syphilitic affections involving the dorsal columns of the cord may be associated with incoordination and resemble tabes very closely.

(*f*) General Paresis.—Though of identical origin and often associated, it is of great practical importance to determine, if possible, whether the type is to be spinal or cerebral, for when this is established, it does not often change. The difficulty arises in the early stage, when any alteration in the mental characteristics is of the utmost significance. Loss of the deep reflexes and lightning pains speak for tabes; active reflexes, with ocular changes, especially optic atrophy, are suggestive of paresis.

(*g*) Visceral crises and neuralgic symptoms may lead to error, and in middle-aged men with severe, recurring attacks of abdominal pain, it is always well to bear in mind the possibility of tabes.

Prognosis.—Complete recovery can not be expected, but arrest of the process is not uncommon and a marked amelioration is frequent. Optic nerve atrophy has this hopeful aspect—that incoordination rarely follows and the progress of the spinal symptoms may be arrested. On the other hand, mental symptoms are more likely to follow. The optic atrophy itself is occasionally checked. On the whole, the prognosis is bad. There is more hope that in early cases the course may be arrested. Death may be from some cardiovascular complication, from tuberculosis, pneumonia or pyelonephritis.

Treatment.—To arrest the progress and to relieve, if possible, the symptoms are the objects which the practitioner should have in view. A quiet, well-regulated method of life is essential. It is not well, as a rule, for a patient to give up his occupation so long as he is able to keep about and perform ordinary work, provided there is no evident mental change. Tabetics have for years conducted large businesses, and there have been several notable instances in our profession of men who have risen to distinction in spite of the existence of this disease. Care should be taken in the diet, particularly if gastric crises have occurred. Attention should be given to the bladder and bowels. Excesses of all sorts, more particularly *in baccho et venere*, should be carefully avoided. A man in the pre-ataxic stage should not marry.

As soon as tabes is diagnosed or strongly suspected active treatment should be given; mercury is probably of more value than arsphenamine. A thorough course of mercurial inunctions should be given (20 to 30) and neoarsphenamine given intravenously (0.3-0.6 gm.) once a week for six weeks. This sequence should be repeated once or twice and its further repetition decided by the condition. Iodides should be given steadily in full dosage. The treatment should be carried out persistently and the spinal fluid studied frequently as improvement in this is a good indication. The various forms of intraspinal treatment seem of no value and may be harmful. In some cases the giving of mercury by inunction followed by spinal puncture weekly, in which as much fluid is withdrawn as possible, has proved of benefit. The use of tryparsamide is not advised.

For the pains, complete rest in bed and counterirritation to the spine may be employed. The severe spells which come on particularly after excesses of any kind are often relieved by a hot bath or by a Turkish bath. For the severe recurring attacks of lightning pains spinal root cocainization may be tried. Cannabis indica, acetylsalicylic acid, phenacetine, etc., are sometimes useful. Suppositories of codeine (gr. 1, 0.06 gm.) and extract of belladonna (gr. ½, 0.03 gm.) may give relief. In the severe paroxysms of pain and the crises morphia may be necessary but its use should be as infrequent as possible. Electricity is of very little benefit. For gastric crises, chloretone (gr. v-x, 0.3-0.6 gm.) or tincture of iodine (♏ x, 0.6 cc.) may be given. The dorsal spinal nerve roots of the seventh, eighth, ninth, and tenth have been divided with good results. The laryngeal crises are rarely dangerous. An application of cocaine may be made or a few whiffs of chloroform or nitrite of amyl may be given. In all cases of tabes with hypertension the prolonged use of nitroglycerine, given until the physiological effect is produced, is of service in allaying pain and diminishing the frequency of the crises. Its use must be guarded when there is aortic insufficiency. The bladder demands constant care. When it can not be perfectly emptied the catheter should be used. Tincture of belladonna (♏ v-x, 0.3-0.6 cc.) is useful when there is incontinence. The *Charcot joint* should be given rest and immobilised. Aspiration is advisable if there is much effusion. Care should be given to the feet if there is trophic disturbance.

Frenkel's method of *reeducation* often helps the patient to regain to a considerable extent the control of the voluntary movements. The patient is first taught, by repeated systematic efforts, to perform simple movements; from this he goes to more and more complex movements. This should be directed and supervised by a trained teacher, as the result depends upon the skill of the teacher as much as upon the perseverance of the patient.

GENERAL PARESIS AND TABOPARALYSIS

The majority of cases of tabes run their course with practically no mental symptoms, and patients with general paresis may never present symptoms that suggest tabes. For practical purposes we should keep the distinction clearly in mind, and it seems best to consider them separately. There is, however, a group of cases in which the symptoms of the two diseases are associated in every combination for which the name "taboparalysis" is used.

General Paresis

Definition.—A chronic meningo-encephalitis caused by the spirochete of syphilis, often associated with other local changes leading to mental disturbances and finally to dementia and paralysis.

Etiology.—The average interval from the syphilitic infection is 10 to 20 years. Males are affected much more frequently than females. It occurs chiefly between the ages of thirty and fifty-five, although it may begin in childhood as the result of congenital syphilis. Not infrequently both husband and wife are affected, or one has paresis and the other tabes. Statistics show that it is more common in the lower classes of society, but in America in general medical practice the disease is certainly more common in the well-to-do classes.

Morbid Anatomy.—The dura is often thickened, and its inner surface may show the various forms of hypertrophic pachymeningitis. The pia is cloudy, thickened and adherent to the cortex. The cerebrospinal fluid is increased in the meningeal spaces, especially in the meshes of the pia, and at times to such an extent as to resemble cysts. The brain is small, and weighs less than normal. The convolutions are atrophied, especially in the anterior and middle lobes. In acute cases the brain may be swollen, hyperemic, and edematous. The brain cortex is usually red, and, except in advanced cases, it may not be atrophied, the atrophy of the hemispheres being at the expense of the white matter. The lateral ventricles are dilated to compensate for the atrophy of the brain, and the ependyma may be granular.

In many cases changes are present in the spinal cord and peripheral nerves. There are the typical tabetic changes. There may be degeneration of the pyramidal systems of fibres secondary to the cortical changes. Most commonly there is a combination of these two processes. Foci of hemorrhage and softening, dependent upon coarse vascular changes, are not infrequently found, but are not typical of the disease. There are various views as to the nature of the changes. The vascular theory is that from an inflammatory process starting in the sheaths of the arterioles there is a diffuse parenchymatous degeneration with atrophic changes in the nerve cells and neuroglia. The syphilitic toxin causes degeneration in the nervous tissues with secondary changes in the neuroglia and vascular systems. The spirochetes are found in the brain tissue and rarely in the cord.

Symptoms.—Prodromal Stage.—Irritability, inattention to business amounting sometimes to indifference or apathy, and sometimes a *change in character*, marked by acts which may astonish the friends and relatives, are usually the first indications. There may be unaccountable fatigue after moderate physical or mental exertion. Instead of apathy or indifference there may be an extraordinary degree of physical and mental restlessness. The patient is continually planning and scheming, or may launch into extravagances of the wildest character. A common feature at this period is the display of an unbounded egoism. He boasts of his personal attainments, his property or his position in life. There may be indications of moral perversion, manifested in offences against decency or the law, many of which acts show a suspicious effrontery. Forgetfulness is common, and may be shown in inattention to business details and in the minor courtesies of life. At this period there may be no motor phenomena. The onset is usually insidious, although in some cases epileptiform or apoplectiform seizures are the first signs. Attacks of hemicrania, like ophthalmic migraine, may occur. Among the early motor features are tremor of the tongue and lips in speaking, slowness of speech, and hesitancy with mixing of syllables or letters. Inequality of the pupils, temporary paresis of the eye muscles with diplopia, the Argyll-Robertson pupil, optic atrophy, and changes in the deep reflexes, may precede the mental symptoms for years.

Second Stage.—This is characterized in brief by mental exaltation or excitement and a progress in the motor symptoms. "The intensity of the excitement is often extreme, acute maniacal states are frequent; incessant restlessness, obstinate sleeplessness, noisy, boisterous excitement, and blind, uncalculating violence especially characterize such states" (Lewis). It is at this stage that the delusion of grandeur becomes marked and the patient believes himself to be possessed of countless millions or to have reached the most exalted sphere possible in profession or occupation. This expansive delirium is, however, not characteristic of general paresis. Besides, it does not always occur, but in its stead there may be marked melancholia or hypochondriasis, or, in other instances, alternate attacks of delirium and depression.

The *facies* has a peculiar stolidity, and in speaking there is marked tremulousness of the lips and facial muscles. The tongue is also tremulous, and may be protruded with difficulty. The speech is slow, interrupted, and blurred. Writing becomes difficult on account of unsteadiness of the hand. Letters, syllables, and words may be omitted. The subject matter of the patient's letters gives valuable indications of the mental condition. In many instances the pupils are unequal, irregular, sluggish, sometimes large. Important features in this stage are apoplectiform seizures and paralysis. There may be slight syncopal attacks in which the patient turns pale and may fall. Some of these are *petit mal.* In the apoplectiform seizure the patient falls suddenly, becomes unconscious, the limbs are relaxed, the face is flushed, the breathing stertorous, the temperature increased and death may occur. Epileptiform seizures are more common than apoplectiform. There may be a definite aura. The attack usually begins on one side and may not spread. There may be twitchings in the facial or brachial muscles. Typical Jacksonian epilepsy may occur. Recurring attacks of *aphasia* are not uncommon, and paralysis, either monoplegic or hemiplegic, may follow the seizures, or may come on with great suddenness and be transient. In this stage the gait becomes impaired, the patient trips readily, has difficulty in going up or down stairs, and the walk may be spastic or occasionally tabetic. This may be progressive. The deep reflexes are usually increased but may be lost. Bladder or rectal symptoms gradually develop. The patient becomes helpless, bedridden, and completely demented, and unless care is taken may suffer from bedsores. Death occurs from exhaustion or some intercurrent affection. Spinal cord features may come on with or precede the mental troubles. There are cases in which one is in doubt for a time whether the symptoms indicate tabes or general paresis, and it is well to bear in mind that every feature of pre-ataxic tabes may exist in the early stage of general paresis.

Cerebrospinal Fluid.—The findings are as follows: (1) *Cell content.* A lymphocytosis is present in 98-100 per cent and the average content is 30-60 cells. (2) *Globulin.* This is practically always positive. (3) *Wassermann reaction.* This is positive in nearly every case and usually there is a strong reaction with small amounts. The blood reaction is positive in 98-100 per cent. (4) *Colloidal Gold reaction.* This is nearly always positive, in 98-100 per cent, with a typical paretic curve (a first-zone reaction).

Taboparalysis.—Emphasis has been laid on the identity of the processes underlying tabes and general paresis, the spinal cord in the first case receiving the full force of the attack, and the brain in the second. It is suggested that stress determines the location of the process; men whose occupations require much bodily exercise are apt to have tabes, while those whose activities are largely mental suffer from paresis. Usually when the cord features are pronounced the brain symptoms remain in abeyance, and the reverse is also true. There are exceptions, and cases of well-marked tabes may later show the typical symptoms of paresis, but even then the ataxia, if it is not of too high a grade, may improve.

Optic atrophy, when it occurs in the pre-ataxic stage of tabes, usually indicates that the ataxia will not be pronounced, but it is frequently followed by mental symptoms. Mott states that about 50 per cent of his asylum cases of taboparalysis had preceding optic atrophy so that it is of grave significance. The mental symptoms may be delayed for years.

Made up of a combination of features of the two conditions, the *symptom complex* of taboparalysis varies greatly. It may begin as tabes with lightning pains, Argyll-Robertson pupil, loss of the deep reflexes, etc., to have the mental symptoms added later; or, on the other hand, cord symptoms may come on after the patient has shown marked mental changes. The symptoms from the first may be so combined that the name taboparalysis is applicable. Absent knee jerks, ocular palsies or pupillary signs may precede the breakdown for years, but none has so grave a significance in regard to the mental state as optic atrophy. Other types of alienation may occur with tabes, and the mistake must not be made of regarding them all as general paresis.

Diagnosis.—The recognition of general paresis in the earliest stage is extremely difficult, as it is often impossible to decide that the slight alteration in conduct is anything more than one of the moods or phases to which most men are at times subject. Syphilis should always be excluded in adults showing signs of psychoneurosis. The description by Folsom is an admirable presentation of the characters of the early stage: "It should arouse suspicion if, for instance, a strong, healthy man, in or near the prime of life, distinctly not of the 'nervous,' neurotic, or neurasthenic type, shows some loss of interest in his affairs or impaired faculty of attending to them; if he becomes varyingly absent-minded, heedless, indifferent, negligent, apathetic, inconsiderate, and, although able to follow his routine duties, his ability to take up new work is, no matter how little, diminished; if he can less well command mental attention and concentration, conception, perception, reflection, judgment; if there is an unwonted lack of initiative, and if exertion causes unwonted mental and physical fatigue; if the emotions are intensified and easily change, or are excited from trifling causes; if the sexual instinct is not reasonably controlled; if the finer feelings are even slightly blunted; if the person regards with a placid apathy his own acts of indifference and irritability and their consequences, and especially if at times he sees himself in his true light and suddenly fails again to do so; if any symptoms of cerebral vasomotor disturbances are noticed, however vague or variable."

There are cases of *cerebral syphilis* which closely simulate general paresis. The mode of onset is important, particularly since paralytic symptoms are usually early in syphilis. The affection of the speech and tongue is not present. Epileptic seizures are more common and more liable to be cortical or Jacksonian in character. The expansive delirium is rare. While symptoms of general paresis are not common with gummata or gummatous meningitis, paresis may follow closely upon the syphilitic infection. Postmortem in such cases there may be nothing more than a general arteriosclerosis and diffuse meningo-encephalitis, which may present nothing distinctive. Cases occur in which typical syphilitic lesions are combined with the ordinary lesions of general paresis. There are certain forms of lead encephalopathy which resemble general paresis. *Tumor* may sometimes simulate progressive paresis, but in the former the signs of increase of intracranial pressure are usually present. The findings in the spinal fluid are important.

Cytodiagnosis.—Changes in the cerebrospinal fluid are important. Lymphocytosis is the rule and is usually associated with a marked globulin reaction. It is the expression of a subacute or chronic inflammatory process. The syphilitic triad—tabes, paresis, and cerebrospinal lues—is suggested by lymphocytosis in the spinal fluid. Positive reactions, cytological and chemical, are among the earliest somatic signs, and may clear up obscure cases of tabes and paresis, at the time when diagnosis is most difficult.

Prognosis.—As a rule the progress is slowly downward and the course terminates in a few years, although it is occasionally prolonged ten or fifteen years. There may be remissions in which the patient is able to resume his occupation. The outlook is more favorable with present treatment.

Treatment.—The patient should be in a hospital and every effort made to improve the general health. The most useful measures are fever therapy and the use of tryparsamid. Fever therapy may be given by the inoculation of malarial fever, typhoid vaccine or diathermy. The general condition should be carefully studied before any one is used. Serious vascular or renal disease, etc., suggests caution. In the malarial therapy the patient is infected by tertian malaria and an average of 10 or 12 paroxysms may be allowed. Then the patient is given quinine. Typhoid vaccine is given intravenously with an initial dose of 25 million organisms; this is gradually increased. Tryparsamid should not be used in patients with retinal changes. The method is to give 3 gm. of tryparsamid in 15 cc. of sterile freshly distilled water intravenously once a week for eight doses. After five to eight weeks a second similar course is given and if necessary a third course. The serological findings are carefully followed. Retinal changes should be watched for and the drug stopped if there is disturbance of vision. Mercury or bismuth and iodides may be given in addition. Intraspinal treatment and the use of arsphenamine are not indicated. Careful nursing and the orderly life of an asylum are necessary in a great majority of the cases. For sleeplessness and the epileptic seizures bromides may be used. Prolonged remissions, which are not uncommon, may be erroneously attributed to the action of remedies.

DISEASES OF THE EFFERENT OR MOTOR TRACT

PROGRESSIVE (CENTRAL) MUSCULAR ATROPHY

(*Poliomyelitis anterior chronica; Amyotrophic Lateral Sclerosis; Progressive Bulbar Paralysis*)

Definition.—A disease characterized by a chronic degeneration of the motor tract, usually of the whole, but at times limited to the lower segment.

Associated with it is a progressive atrophy of the muscles, with more or less spastic rigidity.

Three affections belong in this category: (*a*) Progressive muscular atrophy of spinal origin; (*b*) amyotrophic lateral sclerosis; and (*c*) progressive bulbar paralysis. A slow atrophic change in the motor neurones is the anatomical basis, and the disease involves, in many cases, the cortical, bulbar and spinal centres. There may be simple muscular atrophy with little or no spasm, or progressive wasting with marked spasm and great increase in the reflexes. There may be signs of involvement of the motor nuclei in the medulla—a glossolabio-laryngeal paralysis; in others, with atrophy (especially of the arms) a spastic condition of the legs and bulbar phenomena, tremors develop and signs of a cortical lesion. These stages may be traced in the same case. For convenience, bulbar paralysis is considered separately, and *progressive muscular atrophy* and *amyotrophic lateral sclerosis* are taken together.

History.—The disease is known as the Aran-Duchenne type of progressive muscular atrophy and as Cruveilhier's palsy, after the French physicians who described it. Luys and Lockhart Clarke first demonstrated that the cells of the ventral horns of the spinal cord were diseased. Charcot separated two types—one with simple wasting of the muscles, due, he believed, to degeneration confined to the ventral horns (and to this he restricted the name progressive muscular atrophy—type, Aran-Duchenne); the other, with spastic paralysis of the muscles followed by atrophy. As the anatomical basis for this he assumed a primary degeneration of the pyramidal tracts and a secondary atrophy of the ventral horns. To this he gave the name of amyotrophic lateral sclerosis. There is little evidence to show that any such sharp distinction can be made between these two diseases.

Etiology.—The cause is doubtful. Syphilis is associated with some of the cases and this form of atrophy has occurred in tabes dorsalis. It is more frequent in males than in females and affects adults, usually after the thirtieth year, though occasionally younger persons are attacked. Cases of progressive muscular atrophy in early life belong as a rule to the dystrophies. The Werdnig-Hoffman type is a familial affection and does not belong here. The spastic form may develop late in life—after seventy—as a senile change.

Morbid Anatomy.—The essential change is a slow degeneration of the motor path, involving particularly the lower motor neurones. The upper neurones are also involved, either first, simultaneously, or at a later period. Associated with the degeneration in the cells of the ventral horns there is a degenerative atrophy of the muscles. The following are the important anatomical changes: (*a*) The gray matter of the cord shows the most marked alteration. The large ganglion cells of the ventral horns are atrophied, or, in places, have entirely disappeared, the neuroglia is increased, and the medullated fibres are much decreased. The fibres of the ventral nerve roots passing through the white matter are wasted. (*b*) The ventral roots outside of the cord are also atrophied. (*c*) The muscles affected show degenerative atrophy, and the intermuscular branches of the motor nerves are degenerated. (*d*) The degeneration of the gray matter is rarely confined to the cord, but extends to the medulla, where the nuclei of the motor cerebral nerves are involved. (*e*) In a majority of cases there is sclerosis in the ventrolateral tracts, the lateral pyramidal tracts particularly are diseased, but the degeneration is not confined to them, but extends into the ventrolateral ground bundles. The direct cerebellar and the ventrolateral ascending tracts are spared. The degeneration in the pyramidal tracts extends to the brain to the motor cortex, the cells of which are degenerated. (*f*) In those cases in which no sclerosis has been found in the pyramidal tracts there has been a sclerosis of the ventrolateral ground bundle (short tracts).

Symptoms.—Irregular pains, sensory disturbances or feelings of stiffness may precede the onset of the wasting which is usually gradual. The hands are usually first affected, and there is difficulty in performing delicate manipulations. The muscles of the ball of the thumb waste early, then the interossei and lumbricales, leaving marked depressions between the metacarpal bones. Ultimately the contraction of the flexor and extensor muscles and the extreme atrophy of the thumb muscles, the interossei, and lumbricales produce the clawhand—*main en griffe* of Duchenne. The flexors of the forearm are usually involved before the extensors. In the shoulder girdle the deltoid is first affected; it may waste before the other muscles of the arm. The trunk muscles are gradually attacked; the upper part of the trapezius long remains unaffected. Owing to the weakness of the muscles which support it, the head tends to fall forward. The platysma myoides is unaffected and often hypertrophies. The arms and the trunk muscles may be much atrophied before the legs are attacked. The face muscles are usually attacked late.

Ultimately the intercostal and abdominal muscles may be involved, the wasting proceeds to an extreme grade, and the patient may be actually "skin and bone," and, as "living skeletons," the patients are seen in "museums" and "side-shows." Deformities and contractures result, and lordosis is almost always present. Fibrillary twitching is common and may occur in muscles which are not attacked. It is an important sign but not a characteristic feature. The irritability of the muscles is increased. Sensation is unimpaired, but the patient may complain of numbness and coldness of the affected limbs. The electrical reactions progressively diminish and may disappear. In cases of rapid wasting and paralysis the reaction of degeneration may be obtained. The excitability of the nerve trunks may persist after the muscles cease to respond. The loss of power is usually proportionate to the wasting.

Amyotrophic Spastic Form.—The foregoing description applies to the cases in which the atrophy and paralysis are flaccid—*atonic,* as Gowers called it. In other cases, those which Charcot described as amyotrophic lateral sclerosis, spastic paralysis precedes the wasting. The reflexes are greatly increased. It is one of the conditions in which a jaw clonus may be obtained. The most typical condition of spastic paraplegia may result. On starting to walk, the patient seems glued to the ground and makes ineffectual attempts to lift the toes; then four or five short, quick steps are taken on the toes with the body thrown forward; and finally he starts off, sometimes with great rapidity. Some of the patients can walk up and down stairs better than on the level. The wasting is never so extreme as in the atonic form, and the loss of power may be out of proportion to it. The sphincters are unaffected. Sexual power may be lost early. A flaccid atrophic paralysis with increased reflexes is the common finding. The differences depend upon the relative extent of involvement of the upper and lower motor segments and the time of the involvement of each. The condition may be unilateral.

As the degeneration extends upward an important change takes place from the occurrence of bulbar symptoms, which may, however, precede the spinal manifestations. The lips, tongue, face, pharynx and larynx may be involved. The lips may be affected and articulation impaired for years before serious symptoms occur. In the final stage there may be tremor, the memory fails, and a condition of dementia supervenes.

Diagnosis.—Progressive (central) muscular atrophy begins, as a rule, in adult life, without hereditary or family influences (the early infantile form being an exception), and usually affects first the muscles of the thumb, and gradually involves the interossei and lumbricales. Fibrillary contractions are common, electrical changes occur, and the deep reflexes are usually increased. These usually distinguish it from the other forms of muscular wasting. It is well to remember that the earliest and most marked indication of *cervical rib* may be atrophy of the small muscles of the hand. In *syringomyelia* the sensory disturbances, as a rule, make the diagnosis clear, but when these are absent or but little developed it may be very difficult to distinguish the disease. Neoplasm of the cord or spine or pachymeningitis may give difficulty but a careful study, especially of the spinal fluid, observation for a short time and the absence of fibrillation should prevent error.

Bulbar Paralysis (Glossolabiolaryngeal Paralysis)

When the disease affects the motor nuclei of the medulla first or early, it is called bulbar paralysis, but it has practically no independent existence, as the spinal cord is sooner or later involved.

Symptoms.—The disease begins with slight defect in the speech, and difficulty in pronouncing the dentals and linguals. The paralysis starts in the tongue, and the superior lingual muscle gradually becomes atrophied, and finally the mucous membrane is thrown into transverse folds. In the process of wasting the fibrillary tremors are seen. Owing to the loss of power in the tongue, the food is with difficulty pushed back into the pharynx. The saliva may be increased and is apt to accumulate in the mouth. When the lips become involved the patient can neither whistle nor pronounce the labial consonants. The mouth looks large, the lips are prominent and there is constant drooling. The food is masticated with difficulty. Swallowing becomes difficult, owing partly to regurgitation into the nostrils, partly to the involvement of the pharyngeal muscles. The muscles of the vocal cords waste and the voice becomes feeble, but the laryngeal paralysis is rarely so extreme as that of the lips and tongue.

The **course** is slow but progressive. Death may result from an aspiration pneumonia, sometimes from choking, more rarely from involvement of the respiratory centres. The mind usually remains clear. The patient may become emotional. In a majority of the cases the disease is only part of a progressive atrophy, either simple or associated with a spastic condition. In the later stage of amyotrophic lateral sclerosis the bulbar lesions may paralyze the lips long before the pharynx or larynx becomes affected.

The **diagnosis** is readily made, either in the acute or chronic form. The involvement of the lips and tongue is usually well marked, while that of the palate may be long deferred. In *pseudobulbar paralysis* bilateral disease of the motor cortex in the lower part of the ascending frontal convolution, or about the knee of the internal capsule may interfere with the supranuclear paths, causing paralysis of the lips and tongue and pharynx, which closely simulates a lesion of the medulla. Sometimes the symptoms appear on one side, but they may develop suddenly on both sides. Bilateral lesions have usually been found, but the disease may be unilateral. There is arteriosclerosis and the bulbar features are usually sequels of hemiplegic attacks.

Acute bulbar paralysis may be due to (*a*) hemorrhagic or embolic softening in the pons and medulla; (*b*) acute inflammatory softening, analogous to poliomyelitis, occurring occasionally as a postfebrile affection as after diphtheria, and after severe electric shocks. It usually comes on very suddenly and the symptoms may correspond closely to those of an advanced case of chronic bulbar paralysis. The sudden onset and the associated symptoms make the diagnosis easy. In these acute cases there may be loss of power in one arm, or hemiplegia, sometimes alternate hemiplegia, with paralysis on one side of the face and on the other side of the body. (*c*) In poliomyelitis and encephalitis there are cases with acute bulbar symptoms.

Treatment.—The disease is incurable. The downward progress is slow but certain, though in a few cases a temporary arrest may take place. Trauma, fatigue and cold should be avoided. If syphilis is present, specific treatment does not result in much benefit. Systematic massage is useful in the spastic cases.

SPASTIC PARALYSIS OF ADULTS

(*Primary Lateral Sclerosis*)

Definition.—A gradual loss of power with spasm of the muscles of the body, the lower extremities being first and most affected, unaccompanied by muscular atrophy, sensory disturbance, or other symptoms. A systemic degeneration of the pyramidal tracts is assumed.

Symptoms.—The general symptoms of spastic paraplegia in adults are very distinctive. The patient complains of feeling tired, of stiffness in the legs, and perhaps of pains of a dull aching character in the back or in the calves. There may be no definite loss of power, even when the spastic condition is well established. In other instances there is definite weakness. The stiffness is felt most in the morning. In a well developed case the gait is most characteristic. The legs are moved stiffly and with hesitation, the toes drag and catch against the ground, and, in extreme cases, when the ball of the foot rests upon the ground a distinct clonus develops. The legs are kept close together, the knees touch, and in certain cases the adductor spasm may cause cross-legged progression. On examination, the legs may at first appear tolerably supple, perhaps flexed and extended readily. In other cases the rigidity is marked, particularly when the limbs are extended. The spasm of the adductors of the thigh may be so extreme that the legs are separated with great difficulty. With this extreme rigidity the patient usually loses the power of walking. The nutrition is well maintained; the muscles may be hypertrophied. The reflexes are greatly increased. The slightest touch upon the patellar tendon produces an active knee jerk. The rectus clonus and the ankle clonus are easily obtained. In some instances the slightest touch may throw the legs into violent clonic spasm, to which Brown-Séquard gave the name of spinal epilepsy. The superficial reflexes are also increased. The arms may be unaffected for years, but occasionally they become weak and stiff at the same time as the legs.

The *course* is progressively downward. Years may elapse before the patient is bedridden. Involvement of the sphincters, as a rule, is late; occasionally it is early. The sensory symptoms rarely progress, and the patients may retain good nutrition. Ocular symptoms are rare.

Diagnosis.—This, so far as the clinical picture is concerned, is readily made, but it is often very difficult to determine accurately the nature of the underlying pathological condition. A history of syphilis is present in many cases. After a fairly typical clinical course some cases at autopsy have shown very different conditions—transverse myelitis, multiple sclerosis, cerebral tumor, etc. General paresis may begin with symptoms of spastic paraplegia, and Westphal believed that it was only in relation to this disease that a primary sclerosis of the pyramidal tracts occurred. In any case the diagnosis of primary systemic degeneration of the pyramidal tract is doubtful.

Treatment.—Not much can be done to check the progress. Division of the posterior nerve roots is permissible when the motor weakness is due chiefly to spasticity. A number of patients have been operated upon successfully. The same has been done in the spasticity with bilateral athetosis.

SECONDARY SPASTIC PARALYSIS

Following any lesion of the pyramidal tract there may be a spastic paralysis; thus, in a transverse lesion of the cord, whether from slow compression (as in caries), chronic myelitis, the pressure of tumor, chronic meningomyelitis or multiple sclerosis, degeneration takes place in the pyramidal tracts below the point of disease. The legs become stiff and rigid, and the reflexes increase. In compression paraplegia if the transverse lesion is complete, the limbs may be flaccid, without increase in the reflexes—*paraplégie flasque* of the French. The condition of the patient in these secondary forms varies very much. In chronic myelitis or multiple sclerosis he may be able to walk but with a characteristic spastic gait. In compression myelitis, in fracture or in caries, there may be complete loss of power with rigidity.

It may be difficult or even impossible to distinguish these cases from those of primary spastic paralysis. Reliance is to be placed upon the associated symptoms; when these are absent no definite diagnosis as to the cause of the spastic paralysis can be given.

Syphilitic Spinal Paralysis.—Erb described a symptom group under the term syphilitic spinal paralysis. The points upon which he laid stress are a very gradual onset with a development finally of the features of a spastic paresis; the tendon reflexes are increased, but the muscular rigidity is slight in comparison with the exaggerated deep reflexes. There is rarely much pain, and the sensory disturbances are trivial, but there may be paresthesia and the girdle sensation. The bladder and rectum are usually involved, and there is sexual failure or impotence. And, lastly, improvement is not infrequent. A majority of instances of spastic paralysis of adults not the result of slow compression of the cord are associated with syphilis and belong to this group.

HEREDITARY AND FAMILIAL DISEASES

MUSCULAR DYSTROPHIES: MYOPATHIES

Definition.—Muscular wasting, with or without an initial hypertrophy, beginning in various groups of muscles, usually progressive and dependent on primary changes in the muscles or the neuromuscular endings.

Etiology.—There is a familial tendency—the disease occurring in two or more generations—or several members of the same generation may be affected. Members of the same family may be attacked through several generations: as many as 20 or 30 cases have been described in five generations. Males are more frequently affected than females. In families, persons of the same sex are usually attacked, but unaffected females may transmit the disease. In Erb's cases 44 per cent showed no heredity. The disease usually sets in before puberty, but the onset may be as late as the twenty-fifth year, or even later. The creatine metabolism is abnormal; creatine is not retained in the muscles.

Pathology.—There is a progressive atrophy of the muscle fibres with an increase of fibrous tissue and fat. In the pseudohypertrophic form the increase in connective tissue is marked so that the size is increased. In other cases atrophy may predominate.

Symptoms.—Clumsiness in the movements of the child is the first symptom noticed and on examination certain muscles or groups of muscles seem to be enlarged, particularly those of the calves. The extensors of the leg, the glutei, the lumbar muscles, the deltoid, triceps and infraspinatus, are the next most frequently involved, and may stand out with great prominence. The muscles of the neck, face, and forearm rarely suffer. Sometimes only a portion of a muscle is involved. With this hypertrophy of some muscles there is wasting of others, particularly the lower portion of the pectorals and the latissimus dorsi. The attitude when standing is very characteristic. The legs are far apart, the shoulders thrown back, the spine is greatly curved, and the abdomen protrudes. The gait is waddling and awkward. In getting up from the floor the position assumed, so well known by Gowers' figures, is pathognomonic. The patient first turns over in the all-fours position and raises the trunk with his arms; the hands are then moved along the ground until the knees are reached; then with one hand upon a knee he lifts himself up, grasps the other knee, and gradually pushes himself in the erect posture, as it has been expressed, by climbing up his legs. The striking contrast between the weakness and the powerful looking pseudohypertrophic muscles is very characteristic. The enlarged muscles may, however, be relatively strong.

The course is slow, but progressive and usually not over ten years. Wasting proceeds and finally all traces of the enlarged condition of the muscles disappear. At this late period distortions and contractions are common. The muscles of the shoulder girdle are nearly always affected early, so that with the hands under the arms, when one endeavors to lift the patient, the shoulders are raised to the level of the ears, and one gets the impression that the child is slipping through. These "loose shoulders" are very characteristic. The abnormal mobility of the shoulder blades gives them a winged appearance, and the arms seem much longer than usual when they are stretched out.

There are no sensory symptoms. The atrophic muscles do not show the reaction of degeneration except in extremely rare instances.

Clinical Forms.—A number of forms have been described, depending upon the age at onset, the muscles first affected, the occurrence of hypertrophy, heredity, etc., but there is no sharp division between the forms. The following are the more important:

I. *The pseudohypertrophic type* of Duchenne, most common in childhood and in family groups. The hypertrophy of the muscles is the striking feature, whether a true hypertrophy or a lipomatosis. There is also a juvenile type with atrophy, affecting chiefly the shoulder girdles and upper arms. Isolated cases occur in adults.

II. *The facioscapulohumeral type* of Landouzy-Dejerine. The face is first involved, causing the myopathic facies, the lips prominent, the upper one projecting, the eyes cannot be closed, nor the forehead wrinkled, the smile is transverse, from inaction of the levators of the lip. Later the shoulder-girdle muscles are involved, the scapulae are winged, the upper arms wasted, and lastly, the thigh muscles. With all this there may be no hypertrophy, though often, if carefully sought, there will be found areas of enlargement—the so-called muscle balls. This form may begin in adults.

III. *The thigh muscle type* of Leyden, Moebius and Zimmerlin, in which the disease starts in the extensors of the thighs which are deeply involved before other groups of upper arms and trunk are attacked.

In all forms, when the muscles of the trunk become involved, there is flattening of the chest and the peculiar "*wasp-waist*" described by Marie.

Diagnosis.—The muscular dystrophies can usually be distinguished readily from the other forms of muscular atrophy.

(*a*) In the cerebral atrophy loss of power usually precedes the atrophy.

(*b*) Progressive (central) muscular atrophy begins in the small muscles of the hand, the reaction of degeneration is present and fibrillary twitchings occur in both the atrophied and nonatrophied muscles. The central atrophies come late in life, the dystrophies, as a rule, early. In the progressive muscular dystrophies heredity plays an important rôle. In the rare cases of early infantile spinal muscular atrophy occurring in families the symptoms are so characteristic of a central disease that the diagnosis presents no difficulty.

(*c*) In the neuritic muscular atrophies, due to lead or trauma, seen for the first time when the wasting is marked there is often difficulty, but the absence of family history and the distribution are important, while the paralysis is out of proportion to the atrophy. Sensory symptoms may be present.

(*d*) Progressive neural muscular atrophy. Here heredity is also a factor, and the disease usually begins in early life, but the distribution of atrophy and paralysis, which is at first confined to the periphery of the extremities, helps to distinguish it from the dystrophies.

Prognosis.—The outlook in the primary muscular dystrophies is bad. The wasting progresses uniformly, uninfluenced by treatment.

Treatment.—By massage the progress may be occasionally retarded. Glycocoll may be given (10 to 20 gm. daily) with ephedrine. The amino-acid apparently aids the formation and retention of creatine in the muscles. Epinephrine and pilocarpine have been given with symptomatic benefit. The general health should be carefully looked after, moderate exercise allowed with friction of the muscles with oil, and when the patient becomes bedfast, as is inevitable sooner or later, care should be taken to prevent contractures in awkward positions. Sugar should be given freely in all the muscular dystrophies.

FAMILIAL SPINAL MUSCULAR ATROPHY
(*Werdnig-Hoffman*)

A rare disease which may be hereditary as well as occurring in a family without disease in the ascendants. Anatomically there is marked degeneration of the anterior horns in the spinal cord, of the anterior roots, and less marked changes in the peripheral nerves, with widespread atrophy of the muscular fibres. While in many cases the disease resembles muscular dystrophy, anatomically it appears to be a progressive central muscular atrophy. The onset is in the first year, sometimes prenatal, often within two months of birth. There is weakness of the trunk muscles and later in the limbs. The paralysis is followed by atrophy of the muscles which may show fibrillary tremors. The trunk muscles finally become completely paralyzed and death may result from paralysis of the intercostal muscles and diaphragm or from bulbar paralysis. The course is progressive and the later the onset the longer the course. In the prenatal cases or those beginning soon after birth the course is rapid. Death usually occurs within a year. The *diagnosis* from amyotonia congenita may be difficult but in this the paralysis is not complete and tends to improve. There is no treatment of any value.

PROGRESSIVE NEURAL MUSCULAR ATROPHY
(*Peroneal Muscular Atrophy—Charcot-Marie-Tooth*)

The peroneal type, described first by Charcot, Marie, and Tooth, is a hereditary and familial disease beginning in childhood, affecting first the muscles of the peroneal group, leading to clubfoot. The disease seems to occupy a position between central muscular atrophy and the muscular dystrophies, resembling the latter in the early onset and familial character, and the former in the occurrence of fibrillary twitchings, the presence of electrical changes and the implication of the small muscles of the hand. Anatomically sclerosis of the posterior and posterolateral columns, atrophy of the cells of the anterior horns and alterations of the peripheral nerves are found.

The essential feature is implication of the distal with normal proximal portions of the limbs, which gives a very characteristic picture. There is great decrease of the electrical excitability. Ocular symptoms are rare; occasionally there is atrophy of the optic nerves. The disease should be suspected in cases of acquired clubfoot. In *treatment*, general care, avoidance of fatigue, massage and electricity, and light splints at night to reduce deformity are useful. Tenotomy should not be done.

PROGRESSIVE INTERSTITIAL HYPERTROPHIC NEURITIS

This is a familial disease beginning, as a rule, in infancy with a combination of the symptoms of tabes and muscular atrophy. Anatomically there is sclerosis of the posterior columns of the cord with interstitial hypertrophic neuritis. It was first described by Dejerine and Sottas, and, though rare, a good many families have been reported, one by Marie in which seven children were affected. The spinal cord lesions resemble those of tabes, and result from degeneration of the posterior nerve roots. The hypertrophy of the nerves is of a unique type. The affected muscles waste completely and there is replacement by fibrous tissue.

The *symptoms* begin in early life and are: (*a*) Incoordination very like that of tabes dorsalis, only as the disease progresses the gait is steppage; (*b*) sensory disturbances, sometimes pains which are fulgurant in character; (*c*) muscular atrophy, limbs and face, in the former chiefly distal and in the legs extending up to the lower third of the thigh. The feet are usually in the varus position; kyphoscoliosis is also present. (*d*) Ocular symptoms are marked—myosis, Argyll-Robertson sign. (*e*) The peripheral nerves are hypertrophied, sometimes double the normal size, smooth and not painful, those of the lower limbs being chiefly involved. The optic and olfactory nerves escape. The peculiar distribution usually gives the diagnosis. The disease should be suspected in acquired double clubfoot. In *treatment* exercises should be used suitable for the strength; fatigue should be avoided. Massage and electricity are useful. Heavy apparatus should be avoided and tenotomy not done. Light splints should be worn at night to lessen the deformity.

HEREDITARY ATAXIA (*Friedreich's Ataxia*)

Definition.—A familial disease occurring in childhood characterized by locomotor and static ataxia, speech disturbances and nystagmus, and anatomically by degeneration of the posterolateral and spinocerebellar tracts. In 1863 Friedreich first reported six cases.

Etiology.—It is a family disease; the 143 cases analyzed by Griffiths occurred in 71 unrelated families. Males are most frequently attacked, 86 to 57 in Griffiths' series. Direct inheritance occurs and was noted in 33 cases. The onset is usually before puberty, but may be as late as the 25th year. The cause is unknown. The disease belongs to Gowers' abiotrophies, an inherited weakness, lack of vitality in certain sections of the nervous system, leading to early degeneration.

Morbid Anatomy.—Both cord and cerebellum have been reported smaller than usual. The posterior meninges may be thickened. The important change is a complete sclerotic degeneration of the posterolateral tracts forming the most typical example of combined degeneration. Gowers' tract and the direct cerebellar are always involved.

Symptoms.—The incoordination begins in the legs, and the gait is swaying, irregular, and more like that of a drunken man without the characteristic stamping gait of the true tabes. Romberg's sign may or may not be present. The ataxia of the arms occurs early and is very marked; the movements are almost choreiform, irregular and somewhat swaying. In a voluntary movement the action is overdone, the prehension is clawlike, and the fingers may be spread or overextended just before grasping an object. The hand frequently moves about an object for a moment, and then suddenly pounces upon it. There are irregular, swaying movements of the head and shoulders. There is in many cases what is known as *static ataxia*, that is, ataxia of quiet action. It occurs when the body is held erect or when a limb is extended—irregular, oscillating movements of the head and body or of the extended limb.

The muscle tone depends on the relative degeneration in the posterior roots and pyramidal tracts; the former tends to abolish and the latter to increase it. The same governs the tendon reflexes; they are usually absent, sometimes early, but if the pyramidal tracts are specially affected the reflexes persist. The plantar reflex shows an extensor response. The skin and eye reflexes are normal. Sensory symptoms are not usually present. The cerebrospinal fluid is normal.

Nystagmus is a characteristic feature. Atrophy of the optic nerve rarely occurs. Disturbance of *speech* is common; usually slow and scanning; it may be explosive. The expression is often dull; the mental power is, as a rule, maintained, but late in the disease becomes impaired. A striking feature is early deformity of the feet, pes cavus. The big toe is flexed dorsally on the first phalanx. Scoliosis is common.

The course is progressive but slow. As the disease advances, paralysis comes on and may ultimately be complete. Some of the patients never walk.

Diagnosis.—This is not difficult when several members of a family are affected. The onset in childhood, the curious form of incoordination, the loss of knee jerks, the early deformity of the feet, the position of the great toe, scoliosis, nystagmus, and speech disturbance make up an unmistakable picture. With hereditary chorea it has certain similarities, but usually this disease does not set in until after the 30th year.

Treatment.—The disease is incurable but every effort should be made to keep up the general health. The patients should not be put to bed unless this is absolutely necessary as inactivity often does harm. Comfortable boots for the deformed feet should be worn. Educational training of the muscular movements as in tabes is useful.

HEREDITARY CEREBELLAR ATAXIA (*Marie*)

This closely resembles Friedreich's ataxia in so far as the ataxia, nystagmus and speech disturbances are concerned. It differs in (1) a later onset (after twenty) in many cases; (2) the ataxia is more purely cerebellar; (3) there is spasticity of the legs with increased knee jerks; (4) there is no talipes or scoliosis; and (5) optic atrophy and ocular palsies are common with the occasional presence of the Argyll-Robertson pupil. Marie regarded the lesion as atrophy of the cerebellum but the lesions may be more widely spread and resemble the Friedreich form. In the form termed *spinocerebellar* or Sanger Brown's ataxia there is degeneration of the spinocerebellar tracts and less marked change in the dorsal columns. The pyramidal tracts are usually not affected. The ataxia, speech disturbance and movements are like those in the Friedreich form but the onset is later in life, nystagmus is rare, ocular paralyses occur, optic atrophy is common and scoliosis does not occur.

There are other forms of cerebellar ataxia resembling those discussed. (1) Primary progressive cerebellar ataxia shows degeneration of the cortex cells of the cerebellum and of the connecting fibres with the central nuclei. The cerebellum is reduced in size. The onset is in middle life. Ataxia, nystagmus, speech disturbance and irregular movements occur. The reflexes are normal.

(2) In the form described by Dejerine and Thomas the lesions are more widespread, involving the olivary bodies, the pons and cerebellar peduncles. Atrophy of the cerebellum occurs. The onset is usually in middle age. The features are much like the preceding form.

FAMILIAL SPASTIC PARALYSIS

Definition.—A familial, abiotrophic, disease, involving chiefly the pyramidal tracts. It is sometimes hereditary.

Etiology.—It begins in children, usually after the seventh year; the onset may be delayed until the twentieth: three or four members of a family may be attacked; boys more often than girls in the proportion of 88 to 51 (Deléarde and Minet). In some families in which the disease has been hereditary, the females have escaped. Mild cases in a family may exist with increase of the reflexes as the only symptom.

Pathology.—The spinal degeneration is chiefly in the pyramidal tracts of the lumbar and lower thoracic regions. In the late stages the lesions may be those of a combined sclerosis with involvement of the direct cerebellar tracts. Imperfect development of the cord (agenesia) may be a factor.

Symptoms.—Early exaggeration of the knee jerks may precede any paralysis or weakness; gradually there are spasticity and Babinski's sign, with contractures and paralysis. The abdominal reflexes disappear. It is important to rule out the cases with mental features and Little's disease. The paralysis may extend to the upper limbs, and eyes and speech are involved. In others again there is atrophy of the muscles, and the picture is not unlike amyotrophic lateral sclerosis, or a disseminated sclerosis. Very different pictures may be presented by affected children in the same family.

CHRONIC HEREDITARY CHOREA

(*Huntington's Chorea*)

Definition.—A hereditary disease characterized by irregular movements, disturbance of speech and progressive mental deterioration.

History.—In 1863 Lyon described it as chronic hereditary chorea. In 1872 George Huntington, whose father, grandfather, and great-grandfather had treated cases, gave in three brief paragraphs its salient features—heredity, late onset, and mental changes. The disease is more common in the United States than in Europe. Davenport studied the four great family complexes of Long Island, Connecticut, and Massachusetts "which show nearly 1000 cases of Huntington's chorea, and yielding the remarkable results that practically all can be traced back to some half-dozen individuals, including three (probable) brothers who migrated to America in the XVIIth century."

Inheritance.—It never skips a generation. The age of onset does not appear to vary, averaging from thirty-five to thirty-eight. The mental type is usually hyperkinetic. Among 3000 persons related to the 962 cases studied by Davenport, there were many other nervous disorders—epilepsy in 39, infantile convulsions in 19, and feeble-mindedness in 73.

Pathology.—There is marked destruction of the smaller ganglion cells of the globus pallidus system which have a coordinating and inhibitory control over the larger motor cells. When this is lost chorea results (Hunt). The large cell system of the globus pallidus stands in relation to the paralysis agitans syndrome and the small cell system to the chorea syndrome. The other findings are varied. Meningeal thickening and atrophy of the cortex, with a loss of cells, have been present in some cases. Arteriosclerotic changes are common in older subjects.

Symptoms.—Difficulty in performing delicate actions with the hands, as in writing or buttoning a collar, may be the earliest indication, or there are slight involuntary movements of the head and face. When well established, the movements are slower than in Sydenham's chorea, irregular and incoordinate. The face muscles are early involved, causing involuntary grimaces. The gait is irregular and swaying, not unlike that of a drunken man. The speech is slow and the syllables blurred. The reflexes, not altered at first, are later increased. Certain biotypes have been observed by Davenport. Thus the tremors may be absent and the mental condition present, or the muscular movements may be present without mental defects. The chorea may not progress and the onset may be early in life. He found family differences in all these points.

The mental changes may come early, outbreaks of temper and excitement are common, alternating with periods of depression. Usually a progressive failure of the mental powers leads to complete dementia. Dreading a terrible fate, suicide in certain members of the families is not surprising.

Prevention.—Davenport's study shows how much more serious the disease is than we had hitherto thought. It is transmitted through males and females, and Davenport states that there is no evidence of any abstention from or selection against marrying in the members of the large group of hereditary choreas studied by him. There is no efficient treatment.

PROGRESSIVE LENTICULAR DEGENERATION

(*Wilson's Disease: Hepatolenticular Degeneration*)

Definition.—A familial, not hereditary, extrapyramidal disease usually coming on early in life, characterized by tremor and spasticity with bilateral changes in the lenticular nuclei and cirrhosis of the liver.

Described by Wilson in 1912, it is apparently the same condition which Gowers designated *tetanoid chorea* and resembles the *pseudosclerosis* of Westphal and Strümpell. The onset is between the ages of 10 and 25 years. As to pathogenesis Wilson suggests the selective action of some toxin possibly due to the hepatic cirrhosis. The lenticular nuclei show degeneration with cavitation and atrophy. The process may extend more widely to the internal capsule, motor cortex, basal ganglia and pyramidal tracts. The cirrhosis of the liver is marked and of a mixed type.

The main features are disturbance of motor functions, rigidity, difficulty in deglutition and speech, emotional disturbances and a terminal dementia. There are no true paralyses, sensory symptoms or changes in the reflexes. The involuntary movements may be of the nature of tremor, choreiform or athetoid; they involve the extremities and are often increased on effort. There are muscular rigidity, weakness, spasticity and painful muscular contractions. When the patient grasps an object he may have difficulty in relaxing his hold.

As the disease progresses contractures and progressive emaciation are marked. The patient becomes helpless and is unable to use the arms and legs or turn in bed. The hepatic cirrhosis does not seem to cause any symptoms but there may be repeated attacks of acute hepatitis. A curious annular brownish-green pigmentation of the cornea has been noted in some cases. The disease is progressive with a course in acute cases of a few months and in chronic forms of two to seven years. There is no specific treatment.

PERIODIC PARALYSIS

Definition.—A recurring paralysis, lasting from a few hours to a few days, affecting members of the same family, with abolition of the faradic excitability of both muscles and nerves. Death may occur in an attack.

History.—After a few scattered references, the disease was accurately described in 1885 by Westphal and Oppenheim. Family groups then began to be recognized, and now a large number of cases have been studied.

Etiology.—The majority have occurred in groups but sporadic cases occur. Holtzapple reported seventeen cases in four generations. Many members of this family suffered from migraine. Transmission is either through the male or female; the disease may skip a generation.

Pathology.—Nothing definite is known. Winternitz could find no organic lesions in two fatal cases in the family reported by Holtzapple. Naturally auto-intoxication has been suggested, and extensive researches into metabolism have been made. Diminution of creatinin excretion has been determined. In some respects the disease is similar to Myasthenia gravis, in which there are attacks of transient paralysis. Westphal regarded the disease as a vasomotor neurosis associated with migraine, which was such a striking feature in Holtzapple's cases. Temporary collapse of the vessels is met with in this condition, and Holtzapple suggests that this may occur in the anterior horns. Disturbance of the myoneural junction may be suggested.

Symptoms.—The clinical picture is similar in all recorded cases. The paralysis involves, as a rule, the arms and legs, but may be general below the neck. It comes on in healthy persons without apparent cause, and often during sleep. At first there may be weakness of the limbs, a feeling of weariness and sleepiness, but rarely with sensory symptoms. The paralysis, beginning in the legs, to which it may be confined, is usually complete within the first twenty-four hours. The neck muscles are sometimes involved, and occasionally those of the tongue and pharynx. The cerebral nerves and the special senses are, as a rule, unaffected. The temperature is normal or subnormal, and the pulse slow. The deep reflexes are diminished, sometimes abolished, and the skin reflexes may be enfeebled. The faradic excitability of both muscles and nerves is reduced or abolished. Improvement begins within a few hours or a day or two, the paralysis disappearing completely and the patient becoming perfectly well. The attacks usually recur at intervals of one to two weeks, but they may return daily. They generally cease after the fiftieth year. There may be dilatation of the heart during the attack.

Treatment.—A low protein diet is advisable and free elimination should be ensured. Potassium bromide (gr. 30, 2 gm.) with caffeine citrate (gr. ii, 0.13 gm.) has been of value early in the attack and potassium citrate in full doses may shorten or abort an attack. The use of glycocoll and ephedrine is worth a trial.

AMAUROTIC FAMILY IDIOCY

(*Tay-Sachs' Disease*)

Definition.—A family disease of infancy characterized by mental impairment progressing to idiocy, progressive muscular weakness, macular changes in the retina and a fatal termination.

History.—In 1881 Warren Tay reported a group of cases characterized by muscular weakness, macular lesions, and death before the age of two years. B. Sachs extended our knowledge of this rare disease.

Etiology.—It occurs usually, but not exclusively, in Hebrew children. The etiology is unknown. Syphilis plays no part. Consanguinity of the parents may be a factor. The most typical cases occur in infancy. There is a *late infantile* form beginning about the age of three years without the cherry red spot but usually with optic atrophy. The so-called *juvenile* form begins from the eighth to the twelfth year and is probably closely related to the infantile form. This shows no predilection for the Hebrew race. It may be that the children are born with a nervous system so inadequate that the cells, after performing their function for a few years or months, undergo complete degeneration. The disease comes into the category of Gowers' abiotrophies. Probably the condition termed *familial retinocerebral degeneration* with mental deterioration, nystagmus and optic atrophy is closely related.

Pathology.—There is marked agenesia of the brain, with degenerative changes in the large pyramidal cells, and swelling of the dendrites. The degenerative changes are widely spread throughout the gray matter of the brain, the cord, and the spinal ganglia (Schaffer). The retinal changes are due to a similar degeneration in the ganglion cells.

Symptoms.—Healthy at birth, and to the third or fourth month, the child then begins to be listless, moving the limbs very little, and, as time goes on, is not able to hold up the head or sit up. The muscles are flaccid, rarely spastic. There is progressive failure of vision and examination of the fundus shows a disappearance of the nerve cells of the retina and a *cherry red spot* in the region of the macula. Within a year a hitherto well-developed baby becomes marantic, completely blind, and death occurs as a rule before the end of the second year. The disease must be distinguished from the ordinary diplegias and paraplegias. It is not always easy as spasticity may be present, but the retinal changes are distinctive. There is no treatment.

Related to the Tay-Sachs' disease is the remarkable familial macular degeneration without dementia in which the disease starts about puberty.

MYOCLONIC EPILEPSY

This is a familial disorder, beginning in childhood with epilepsy, chiefly nocturnal, and followed by myoclonic attacks and progressive dementia. A majority of the cases have occurred in family groups and often in degenerate stock. Single cases may occur in normal families. Nothing is known of the causation; Lundborg suggests a thyroid origin. The changes found in the brain cortex have been those of chronic epilepsy and dementia.

Symptoms.—The onset, in childhood, is with nocturnal epilepsy, which in a year or two is followed by myoclonia, sometimes preceded by tremor. All the voluntary muscles are involved in short, quick, clonic spasms, which progressively increase in intensity. The child may at first have good and bad days, the latter following, as a rule, nights with severe epileptic seizures. The myoclonia grows worse and the patient falls into a state of dementia. The severe myoclonia attacks lead up to genuine epileptic seizures. There is a strong psychic feature which is intensified if the patient knows he is watched; bright lights, sounds, and handling the muscles have the same effect (Lundborg). The familial character and the nocturnal epilepsy separate it from the essential myoclonia of Friedreich. The treatment is that of epilepsy.

DISEASES OF THE MENINGES

The spinal membranes may be affected separately but inflammatory processes often involve both. The process may be inflammatory (suppurative), hemorrhagic or hypertrophic. Inflammation of the dura mater is termed pachymeningitis and of the pia mater leptomeningitis, but usually the comprehensive term meningitis is used. The symptoms and signs produced are due to involvement of the nerves and spinal cord rather than to changes in the meninges.

DISEASES OF THE DURA MATER (*Pachymeningitis*)

(1) **External Pachymeningitis.**—Cerebral.—Hemorrhage often occurs as a result of fracture. Inflammation of the external layer of the dura is rare. Caries of the bone, either extension from middle-ear disease or due to syphilis, is the principal cause. In the syphilitic cases there may be a great thickening of the inner table and a large collection of pus between the dura and the bone. Occasionally the pus is infiltrated between the two layers of the dura mater or may extend through and cause a dura-arachnitis.

The *symptoms* are indefinite. In acute cases signs of irritation are present. In the syphilitic cases there may be a small sinus communicating with the exterior. Compression symptoms may occur with or without paralysis.

Spinal.—An acute form may occur in syphilitic affections of the bones, with retropharyngeal abscess, in tumors, and in aneurism. There are irritation of the nerve roots involved and compression of the cord. The chronic form is more common, and is a constant accompaniment of tuberculous caries of the spine. The internal surface of the dura may be smooth, while the external is rough and covered with caseous masses. The entire dura may be surrounded, or the process may be confined to the ventral surface.

(2) **Internal Pachymeningitis.**—This occurs in four forms: (1) Pseudomembranous, (2) purulent, (3) hypertrophic and (4) hemorrhagic. Pseudomembranous inflammation of the lining membrane of the dura is not usually recognizable, but an example of it came under observation as a secondary process in pneumonia. Purulent pachymeningitis may follow an injury, but is more commonly the result of extension from inflammation of the pia. It is remarkable how rarely pus is found between the dura and arachnoid membranes.

The hypertrophic form is usually syphilitic; the dura mater may be greatly thickened and involve the nerve roots and cord.

Hemorrhagic Internal Pachymeningitis.—CEREBRAL FORM.—This remarkable condition, first described by Virchow, is very rare in general medical practice. During ten years no case came to autopsy at the Montreal General Hospital but in the postmortem room of the Philadelphia Hospital, which received material from a large almshouse and asylum, the cases were not uncommon. As to the frequency in asylum work, in 1,185 postmortems at the Government Hospital for the Insane, Washington, there were 197 cases with "a true neomembrane of internal pachymeningitis" (Blackburn). Of these cases, 45 were chronic dementia, 37 general paresis, 30 senile dementia, 28 chronic mania, 28 chronic melancholia, 22 chronic epileptic insanity, 6 acute mania, and 1 case imbecility.

It has been found in profound anemia and diseases of the blood vessels, and has followed the acute fevers—typhoid fever in a child (Barker). It may occur in badly nourished cachectic children (Herter).

Pathology.—There is venous hemorrhage into the subdural space and trauma is probably often responsible. Practically we see one of three conditions: (*a*) subdural vascular membranes, often of extreme delicacy; (*b*) simple subdural hemorrhage; (*c*) a combination of the two, vascular membrane and blood clot. The vascular membrane may exist without a trace of hemorrhage—simply a fibrous sheet of varying thickness, permeated with large vessels, which may form beautiful arborescent tufts. There are instances in which the subdural hemorrhage is found alone, but in some of these the hemorrhage may have destroyed all trace of the vascular membrane. In some cases a series of laminated clots are found, forming a layer from 3 to 5 mm. in thickness. Cysts may occur within this membrane. The source of the hemorrhage is probably the dural vessels. Some hold that the bleeding comes from the vessels of the pia mater, but in the early stage there is no evidence of this; on the other hand, the highly vascular subdural membrane may be covered with the thinnest possible clot, which has evidently come from the dura. The subdural hemorrhage is often associated with atrophy of the convolutions, and it is held that this is one reason why it is so common in the insane, especially in general paresis and dementia senilis. It occurs also in various cachectic conditions in which cerebral wasting is common. König found in 135 cases of hemorrhagic pachymeningitis that 23 per cent accompanied tuberculosis.

The **symptoms** are indefinite, or there may be none at all, especially when the hemorrhages are small or have occurred very gradually, and the diagnosis can not be made with certainty. Headache has been prominent in some cases, and when the condition exists on one side there may be hemiplegia. The most helpful signs for diagnosis, indicating that the hemorrhage in an apoplectic attack is *meningeal,* are (1) those referable to increased intracranial pressure, (slowing and irregularity of the pulse, vomiting, coma, contracted pupils, reacting to light slowly or not at all) and (2) paresis and paralysis, gradually increasing, with symptoms which point to a *cortical* origin. Extensive bilateral disease may exist without any symptoms whatever.

The *spinal fluid* may be bloody but this is not always the case. It is not a little curious that coma may come on and be the chief feature when anatomically the condition is a laminated hematoma evidently of long standing.

Spinal Form.—The spinal *internal pachymeningitis*, described by Charcot and Joffroy, involves chiefly the cervical region (*P. cervicalis hypertrophica*). The space between the cord and the dura is occupied by a firm, concentrically arranged, fibrinous structure, which arises within, not outside, the dura mater. It is anatomically identical with the cerebral internal hemorrhagic pachymeningitis. The *etiology* is unknown; syphilis has existed in a few cases. The cord is usually compressed; the central canal may be dilated—hydromyelus—and there are secondary degenerations. The *nerve roots* are involved and are damaged and compressed. The extent is variable. It may be limited to one segment, but more commonly involves a considerable portion of the cervical enlargement. Some cases present characteristic *symptoms*. There are intense neuralgic *pains* in the course of the nerves whose roots are involved. They are chiefly in the arms and in the cervical region, and vary greatly in intensity. There may be hyperesthesia with numbness and tingling; atrophic changes may develop, and there may be areas of anesthesia. Gradually motor disturbances appear; the arms become weak and the muscles atrophied, particularly in certain groups, as the flexors of the hand. The extensors remain intact, so that the clawhand is gradually produced. The grade of atrophy depends much upon the extent of involvement of the cervical nerve roots, and in many cases the atrophy of the muscles of the shoulders and arms becomes extreme. The condition is one of cervical paraplegia, with contractures, flexion of the wrist, and typical *main en griffe*. Usually before the arms are greatly atrophied there are the symptoms of the second stage—involvement of the legs and the gradual production of a spastic paraplegia, due to secondary changes in the cord.

The disease runs a chronic course, lasting, perhaps, two or more years. In a few instances recovery has taken place. The disease is to be distinguished from amyotrophic lateral sclerosis, syringomyelia and tumors. From the first it is separated by the marked severity of the initial pains in the neck and arms; from the second by the absence of the sensory changes characteristic of syringomyelia. From certain tumors it is very difficult to distinguish; in fact, the fibrinous layers form a tumor around the cord.

The condition known as *hematoma* of the dura mater may occur at any part of the cord, or, in its slow, progressive form—pachymeningitis hemorrhagica interna—may be limited to the cervical region. It is sometimes extensive, and may coexist with a similar condition of the cerebral dura. Cysts may occur filled with hemorrhagic contents. The *treatment* of these conditions depends upon the cause. With injury or caries operation may be indicated. If syphilis is responsible active treatment should be given.

DISEASES OF THE PIA MATER

(*Acute Cerebrospinal Leptomeningitis*)

Etiology.—Under cerebrospinal fever and tuberculosis the two most important forms have been described. Other conditions with which meningitis is associated are: (1) *The acute fevers*, more particularly pneumonia, influenza, erysipelas and septicemia; less frequently smallpox, typhoid fever, scarlet fever, etc. (2) *Injury or disease of the bones of the skull.* In this group the most frequent cause is necrosis of the petrous portion of the temporal bone in chronic otitis. (3) *Extension from disease of the nose.* Meningitis has followed perforation of the skull in sounding the sinuses, suppurative sinusitis and necroses of the cribriform plate. (4) As a *terminal infection* in chronic nephritis, arteriosclerosis, heart disease and the wasting diseases of children.

The following table of the chief acute forms may be useful:

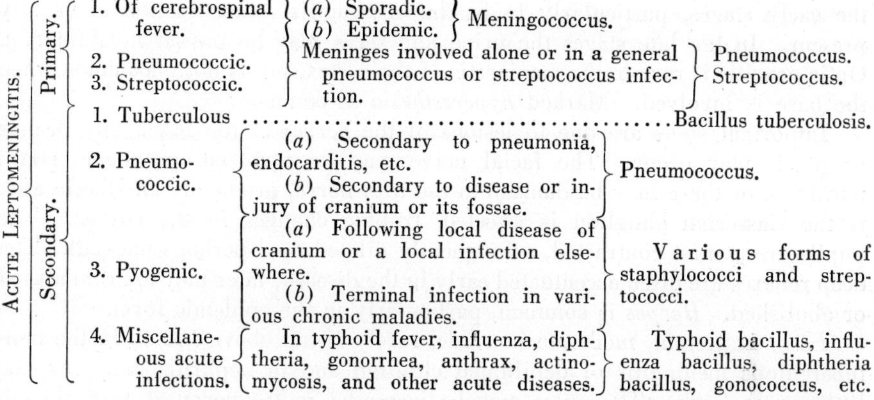

Acute Leptomeningitis.			
Primary.	1. Of cerebrospinal fever.	(a) Sporadic. (b) Epidemic.	Meningococcus.
Primary.	2. Pneumococcic. 3. Streptococcic.	Meninges involved alone or in a general pneumococcus or streptococcus infection.	Pneumococcus. Streptococcus.
Secondary.	1. Tuberculous	....	Bacillus tuberculosis.
Secondary.	2. Pneumococcic.	(a) Secondary to pneumonia, endocarditis, etc. (b) Secondary to disease or injury of cranium or its fossae.	Pneumococcus.
Secondary.	3. Pyogenic.	(a) Following local disease of cranium or a local infection elsewhere. (b) Terminal infection in various chronic maladies.	Various forms of staphylococci and streptococci.
Secondary.	4. Miscellaneous acute infections.	In typhoid fever, influenza, diphtheria, gonorrhea, anthrax, actinomycosis, and other acute diseases.	Typhoid bacillus, influenza bacillus, diphtheria bacillus, gonococcus, etc.

Morbid Anatomy.—The basal or cortical meninges may be chiefly attacked. The degree of involvement of the spinal meninges varies. In the form with pneumonia and ulcerative endocarditis the disease is bilateral and usually limited to the cortex. In extension from disease of the ear it is often unilateral and may be accompanied with abscess or thrombosis of the sinuses. In the nontuberculous forms in children, in the meningitis of chronic nephritis, and in cachectic conditions the base is usually involved. In the cases secondary to pneumonia the effusion beneath the arachnoid may be very thick and purulent. The ventricles may be involved, though in these forms they rarely present the distention and softening found in tuberculous meningitis. In large series the tuberculous and meningococcus forms are by far the most frequent.

Symptoms.—Cortical meningitis is not to be recognized by any symptoms from a condition which may be produced by the toxins of many of the specific fevers. In so-called cerebral pneumonia, unless the base is involved and the nerves affected, the disease is unrecognizable since identical symptoms may be produced by engorgement of the meninges. In typhoid fever, in which meningitis is very rare, the twitchings and retraction of the neck are usually associated with toxemia or meningism, not with true meningitis.

A knowledge of the *etiology* is important. Thus, in middle-ear disease the development of high fever, delirium, vomiting, convulsions, and retraction of the head is extremely suggestive of meningitis or abscess. *Headache,* which may be severe and continuous, is the most common symptom. While the patient remains conscious this is usually the chief complaint, and even when semicomatose he may groan and place his hand on his head. In the fevers, particularly in pneumonia, there may be no complaint of headache. *Delirium* is frequently early and most marked when the fever is high. Photophobia is often present. *Convulsions* are less common in simple than in tuberculous meningitis. In the simple meningitis of children they may occur. Epileptiform attacks which come and go are highly characteristic of direct irritation of the cortex. Rigidity and spasm or twitchings of the muscles are more common. Stiffness and retraction of the muscles of the neck are important signs; but they are not constant, and occur most often when the inflammation is extensive on the meninges of the cervical cord. There may be trismus, gritting of the teeth or spastic contraction of the abdominal muscles. *Vomiting* is common in the early stages, particularly in basilar meningitis. Constipation is usually present. In the late stages the urine and feces may be passed involuntarily. Optic neuritis is rare in the meningitis of the cortex, but is not uncommon when the base is involved. Marked *hyperesthesia* is common.

Important signs are due to lesions of the *nerves* at the base. Strabismus or ptosis may occur. The facial nerve may be involved, producing slight paralysis, or there may be damage to the fifth nerve, producing anesthesia and, if the Gasserian ganglion is affected, trophic changes in the cornea. The pupils are at first contracted, subsequently dilated, and perhaps unequal. The deep reflexes are often accentuated early in the disease; later they are diminished or abolished. *Herpes* is common, particularly in the epidemic form.

Fever is present, moderate in grade, rarely rising above 103°. In the non-tuberculous meningitis of debilitated children and in nephritis there may be little or no fever. The pulse may be increased in frequency at first, though this is unusual. One striking feature is the slowness of the pulse in relation to the fever, even in the early stages. Subsequently it may be irregular and still slower. Very rapid emaciation often occurs. *Kernig's sign* is described under cerebrospinal fever. There may be a concomitant reflex of one leg when passive flexion is made of the other or when the neck is bent forward there is flexion of the legs both at the knees and hips or of all four extremities (Brudzinski's sign). *Lumbar puncture* is exceedingly valuable for diagnosis. The sugar in the spinal fluid is reduced or absent. A turbid fluid usually indicates an acute nontuberculous meningitis. At first the fluid may be only opalescent. As a rule a preponderance of polymorphonuclear leukocytes is present with the meningococcus or pyogenic organisms; a mononuclear exudate occurs in tuberculosis or poliomyelitis. In tuberculous meningitis the fluid is usually clear; in only one of 69 cases was it opalescent (Connal). The causal organism may be found in the spinal fluid.

Diagnosis.—The discussion under cerebrospinal fever applies. One should decide first if meningitis is present, and next the etiology. In both a study of the cerebrospinal fluid is the most important aid. Concussion, which is often a traumatic encephalitis, may suggest meningitis.

Treatment.—The patient should be kept as quiet as possible and causes of irritation removed. An ice-bag should be applied to the head. Sedatives should be given if the patient is conscious and suffering. The bowels should be freely moved. Warm baths or packs may be given every three hours. Hexamine in doses of 60 grains (4 gm.) daily may be tried, as Crowe has shown that it is excreted in the cerebrospinal fluid and inhibits the growth of organisms in the meninges. When the causal organism is determined serum treatment may be used if available. The meningococcus form has been discussed. With a meningitis due to Types I and II pneumococcus the serum should be used freely both intraspinally and intravenously. In meningitis due to the influenza bacillus the use of serum is indicated. In the streptococcus and staphylococcus forms the serum should be tried.

Lumbar and cisternal puncture, as a therapeutic measure, is of great value, relieving the headache and sometimes reducing the fever.

MENINGISM.—This is a condition in which there are symptoms of meningitis, but postmortem the characteristic pathological changes are not present. It is practically the condition described as meningeal irritation, and is most frequent in the acute fevers of children, particularly in pneumonia and typhoid fever, sometimes in alcoholism and in middle-ear disease. Lumbar puncture usually gives a large amount of clear, sterile fluid, under increased pressure and sometimes showing a slight increase in the number of cells. While many disturbances are due to the fluid being under increased pressure, *subnormal pressure* may be responsible for symptoms. Headache, dizziness, and possibly dullness (semicomatose) may be due to deficiency of cerebrospinal fluid. Similar features may be seen after lumbar puncture. The condition is corrected, usually rapidly, by subcutaneous saline injections.

ACUTE ASEPTIC MENINGITIS.—This has an acute onset with the usual signs of meningitis. The cranial nerves are rarely involved. The spinal fluid shows increased pressure; it may be clear or cloudy. The cells average 100-250; polymorphonuclears may predominate early but usually there is lymphocytosis. The protein is increased; the sugar content is about normal. Fever persists for 7 to 10 days. The prognosis is good. Repeated lumbar puncture should be done.

CHRONIC LEPTOMENINGITIS.—This is rarely seen apart from syphilis or tuberculosis, in which the meningitis is associated with the growth of the granulomata in the meninges and about the vessels. The symptoms are extremely variable, depending upon the situation of the growth. The meningococcus meningitis may run a very chronic course, but of all forms the posterior basic may be the most protracted, as cases may have a duration of a year or more.

MENINGOMYELO-ENCEPHALITIS

ACUTE POLIOMYELITIS (*Heine-Medin Disease*)

Definition.—An acute infection characterized anatomically by widespread lesions of the nervous system, with special localization in many cases in the anterior horns of the gray matter in the spinal cord—hence the common name, poliomyelitis anterior. There are two views as to the essential nature of the disease. One is that it is exclusively an infection of the nervous system; the other that there is a general infection, which is supported by the lymphatic hyperplasia (not found in experimental animals).

History.—In 1840 von Heine separated this type from other forms of paralysis and in 1887 Medin called attention to its occurrence in widespread epidemics. Serious outbreaks have occurred in many parts of the United States and Canada. The incidence of the disease has increased in Great Britain and Europe; in Sweden and Norway and parts of Austria it has assumed epidemic proportions. In 1916 in the U. S. registration area there were 7,130 deaths and 1,370 in 1930.

Etiology.—In its epidemic behavior the disease closely resembles cerebrospinal fever. Sporadic cases occur in all communities and under at present unknown conditions increase at times to epidemic proportions. It prevails especially in the late summer and autumn.

Age is an important element; a majority of cases occur in young children. The more prevalent the epidemic the greater the proportion of young adults attacked. Males and females are about equally attacked.

The degree of infectiousness from person to person is slight, and in this it resembles cerebrospinal fever and pneumonia. So far as we know, the disease is transmitted almost entirely by healthy carriers.

The cause is probably a filterable virus. In Flexner's studies, monkeys inoculated with the twentieth generation of the culture developed typical experimental poliomyelitis. The infective agent is present in the brain and spinal cord, in the nasopharyngeal secretions and in the blood. The disease is inoculable into monkeys and may be transmitted from one animal to another. It has been transmitted by intracerebral injection of an emulsion made from flies which had fed on the spinal cord of a monkey dead of the disease. An important point is that the virus passes from the central nervous system in the monkey to the nasal mucosa and vice versa, and the application of the virus to this part is a ready means of inoculation. The path of invasion is apparently by the axones from the peripheral nerve terminals in the nasal mucous membrane. Some hold that infection occurs by the gastro-intestinal tract, at any rate in some cases. Digestive disturbance may be an early feature.

Morbid Anatomy.—The lesions are widespread in the nervous system. It is not an affection limited to the anterior horns of the gray matter of the spinal cord, but a widespread poliomyelo-encephalomeningitis.

Swelling of the spleen and a marked general hyperplasia of the lymphoid apparatus are found. The cerebrospinal fluid is usually increased but clear. The pia mater is hyperemic but without exudate. Cases with pronounced cerebral symptoms show swelling and flattening of the convolutions, with hyperemia of the gray matter and here and there small hemorrhages. The changes in the spinal cord are very characteristic. The meninges are moist, the pia is hyperemic, sometimes with small capillary hemorrhages. On section the cut surface bulges, the gray matter is hyperemic, appearing as a reddened H, or the redness is limited to the anterior horns, which may show spots of hemorrhage. These changes may be localized to the swellings of the cord or extend throughout its entire extent. Microscopically there is small-celled infiltration about the vessels of the meninges, most marked in the lumbar and cervical swellings. The infiltration extends into the fissures of the cord and follows the blood-vessels. The meningeal implication is much more intense than indicated macroscopically. In the cord the smaller blood vessels are distended, hemorrhages occur in the gray matter; there is marked perivascular infiltration, chiefly of lymphocytes, which collect about the vessels, forming definite foci. Sometimes the majority of the cells are polymorphonuclear leukocytes. The ganglion cells, usually those of the anterior horns, degenerate and gradually disappear, probably secondary to the acute vascular alterations and toxemia. Hyperemia, edema and infiltration are marked. After the inflammation subsides, the nerve cells may be destroyed, or only damaged so that some recovery is possible. Sclerotic changes follow in the affected areas. The muscles innervated from the damaged areas atrophy depending on the amount of destruction of the nerve cells. In fatal cases there are changes in the medulla and pons of much the same nature, but the ganglion cells rarely show such widespread destruction.

Symptoms.—The incubation period is probably 3 to 10 days. There are three stages: (1) An initial period of general infection which lasts from a few hours to 3 or 4 days and varies in severity. There may be fever, malaise, drowsiness, evidence of meningeal irritation, hyperesthesia, twitching, irritability and gastro-intestinal symptoms. Nasopharyngeal symptoms may occur. (2) Invasion of the subarachnoid space—*meningitic stage*. This is of short duration with signs of meningeal irritation, stiffness of the neck and back, hyperesthesia and changes in the spinal fluid. There is pain on flexing the spine. (3) *Paralytic stage* when the anterior horn cells are affected. This may be the first manifestation which is observed. Prodromal symptoms are more common in the epidemic form. The *paralysis* is of the flaccid form, with loss of the deep reflexes in affected areas and subsequent atrophy. The paralysis is usually most widespread at the onset and gradually lessens. The temporary paralysis is due to inflammatory and toxic changes while the permanent paralysis depends on destruction of nerve cells. In the early stages there is usually a well-marked polymorphonuclear leukocytosis. Among the forms are:

(*a*) Abortive Form.—There are rare cases with slight symptoms and indications of cerebrospinal irritation, but without any motor disturbances. The symptoms pass away and the diagnosis remains doubtful, nor would suspicion be aroused were it not for other cases. The presence of specific immune bodies in the blood of these patients has been shown.

(*b*) Common Poliomyelitic or Spinal Form.—There is paresis before the paralysis or the paralysis is abrupt in its onset and reaches its maximum in a very short time, showing the characteristic irregularity and lack of symmetry. The legs are involved more often than the arms. Paralysis of the trunk muscles occurs often. One or both arms may be affected, or one arm and one leg, or both legs. In the arm the paralysis is rarely complete, the upper-arm muscles may be most affected or the lower-arm group muscles acting functionally together, with centres near each other in the spinal cord, are paralyzed together. Careful examination usually shows some degree of weakness to be more widespread than appears at first sight. Disturbances of sensation occur, especially tenderness of the muscles. The bladder and rectum are rarely involved but there may be retention of urine.

(*c*) Progressive Ascending Form.—A certain number of cases, particularly in epidemics, run a course similar to Landry's paralysis, with which, no doubt, some of them have been confounded. The disease begins in the legs with the usual symptoms, the paralysis extends upward, involving the arms and the trunk, and death may occur with bulbar symptoms from the third to the fifth day. In the Swedish epidemic of 1905 of the 159 cases which died within the first two weeks, 45 presented this form.

(*d*) Bulbar Form.—In this the cranial nerves are involved and a wide variety of lesions may result. There may be difficulty in breathing and swallowing with paralysis of the ocular, facial, lingual or pharyngeal muscles. The onset may be sudden. The picture depends upon the extent and distribution of the lesions in the medulla and pons. A fatal result is common. The course in this form may be very short.

(*e*) Meningitic Form.—This is important, as the cases simulate and may be mistaken for cerebrospinal fever. The picture is of an acute meningitis—headache, pain and stiffness in the neck, vomiting, pain and rigidity in the back, drowsiness and unconsciousness. The disease may begin with the paralytic features and show the meningeal complications later. Convulsions and Kernig's sign may be present. The two diseases may prevail at the same time and only the careful examination of the cerebrospinal fluid may give the diagnosis.

(*f*) Cerebral Form.—Here the picture is that which we recognize as the acute encephalitis or polio-encephalitis of children, a description of which we owe to von Strümpell. The disease sets in suddenly, with fever, vomiting and convulsions, followed by paralysis of one side of the body or one limb. Many patients die, others recover and present the usual after-picture of the cerebral hemiplegia of children. A large proportion of these cases probably results from this form. Athetosis and epilepsy may be sequels.

(*g*) Cerebellar Form.—In this there is marked ataxia with retraction of the head and rigidity of the neck, but not necessarily nystagmus. Acute vestibulitis may give a similar picture for a few days, but complete bilateral deafness follows.

(*h*) Polyneuritic Form.—In this the patients complain much more of pain, particularly in the form which simulates polyneuritis. There is loss of the tendon reflexes and disturbance of sensation. There is pain in the affected limbs, particularly on movement, with tenderness on pressure on the nerves and on the muscles; the paralysis may extend, involving chiefly the peripheral extensor muscle groups, and be followed by rapid wasting.

(*i*) Transverse Myelitic Form.—Following slight fever and indisposition, the features may be those of a transverse myelitis, a complete flaccid paraplegia. Of two cases of this type in young adults, in one recovery was complete, and in the other with a very small amount of residual paralysis.

Anomalous forms are common during an epidemic. The muscles of respiration may be involved early, the diaphragm alone may be paralyzed, or the intercostals or the muscles of the palate and pharynx. Involvement of the facial muscles, usually a slight weakness, may be present, and in 5 of 90 cases studied by F. R. Fraser the facial muscles alone were involved. In one instance ptosis was the only paralytic symptom on admission. Remarkable forms occur quite unlike the classical picture. In one case there was paralysis of one side of the soft palate with slight fever; the serum of this patient protected a monkey from intracerebral injection of the poliomyelitic virus. There may be slight fever with general spasticity of the muscles and tremor or rigidity of the muscles with coma. Herpes zoster may occur.

Spinal Fluid.—This usually shows increase both in amount and pressure; it may be clear or slightly hazy. There is an increase in the number of cells, which may be from 15 or 20 up to 1200 per c.mm. The largest number are usually mononuclears; occasionally a larger number of polymorphonuclears is found early. The albumin and globulin are usually increased. The amount of glucose and chloride is normal. The Wassermann reaction may be the only means of diagnosing the condition from syphilis.

Course.—Usually within a few days the extent of paralysis lessens and the improvement is rapid for a short time; after this it is slow but may continue for months or years. The residual paralysis is usually less than seemed probable at first. Return of the reflexes is a hopeful sign. The atrophy becomes evident in a few weeks from the onset. The affected limbs show less development as the patient grows older, and the deformity is usually most marked in the leg. The reaction of degeneration is present in the atrophied muscles. Early in the course the muscles lose the faradic response.

Diagnosis.—In the stages before paralysis appears, this is difficult; a variety of signs suggesting irritation of the nervous system is suggestive. There may be marked gastro-intestinal disturbance. The occurrence of an epidemic and the findings in the cerebrospinal fluid are suggestive. When paralysis occurs in the ordinary spinal cases there is rarely any difficulty. An important point to remember is that during epidemics the disease presents an extraordinary number of forms. Some cases run a course like an acute infection, others have the picture of Landry's paralysis, in others again meningeal symptoms predominate, or there may be hyperesthesia and pain, with the picture of a polyneuritis.

It is not improbable that some obscure cases of meningitis are instances of poliomyelitis. The same may be said of the acute encephalitis in children causing hemiplegia. The complexity of the symptoms makes the diagnosis difficult, so that the study of the spinal fluid is important. The diagnosis from peripheral neuritis may be very difficult. Loss of the vibration sensation is more common in peripheral neuritis, and later the electrical changes and the reaction of degeneration may be distinctive.

Prognosis.—The mortality varies greatly in different epidemics. It was 27 per cent in New York City in 1916. The fatal cases are usually of the ascending, bulbar and meningeal types. As regards the muscles, complete loss of response to faradism means severe atrophy. If it is never completely lost the outlook is good and even extreme paralyses may disappear. The prognosis for the paralysis is not easy to determine. Formerly, we thought that residual paralysis would remain if any large number of muscle groups were involved, but cases of severe and widespread involvement may recover gradually and completely. Second attacks and relapses are very rare.

Prophylaxis.—The patient should be isolated, the discharges and articles used carefully disinfected, and special care taken of the nasal and pharyngeal discharges. It does not seem necessary to enforce a quarantine against those who come into relation with the patients. Active immunization appears to be possible and if effectual will be a great boon. The intramuscular injection of 10 to 20 cc. of convalescent serum may be useful.

Treatment.—The patient should be at rest and given the usual treatment during the febrile stage. Salicylates can be given for pain and discomfort with codeine or morphine if necessary. Hexamine should be given in doses of gr. 20-30 (1.3-2 gm.). Lumbar puncture should be done at once and repeated in twelve hours if much fluid is obtained. The puncture should be repeated daily for three or four days. The spinal fluid should be drained freely. If there is respiratory difficulty atropine should be given freely, and with respiratory failure the Drinker respirator should be used or artificial respiration carried on. In the meningeal form hot packs are useful. Blood serum from one who has recovered from the disease, if available, is useful in the early stages intraspinally and intravenously. Intraspinally less should be given than the amount of fluid removed. Intravenously 40 cc. can be given to children up to two years and up to 80 cc. to children ten years of age. It should be given in the preparalytic stage if this is recognized. Serum tinged with hemoglobin should be given intramuscularly.

The muscles involved should be given as complete rest as possible and kept in a relaxed position. The affected limbs should be wrapped in cotton wool and placed in the position which gives the greatest physiological rest, so that they are not stretched by opposing muscles. Voluntary movements should not be allowed for some weeks. If the spinal muscles are involved, the patient should not sit up without proper support. Educational movements and the use of apparatus demand the greatest care not to fatigue the muscles. Careful massage and passive movements may be practised. There is no evidence that electricity is of any value and it may do harm by exciting contractions in normal muscles. Fatigue is harmful and should be guarded against for many months. Careful study should be made of the best forms of reeducation movements for each patient.

The muscle itself as a factor has been emphasized by William MacKenzie of Melbourne as biologically it is all important in treatment. The disease really destroys muscle adjustments, and one of the first things to do is to place the muscle at physiological rest in the zero position, in which it is itself relaxed, and both its own action, and that of its opponent prevented. Massage, he urges, should not be given too early, until, for example, the patient can elevate the upper limb when sitting up, and the heel when lying on the back. Persistent gradual reeducation of the muscles yields remarkable results. Passive movements may be used and with toys a child may be encouraged to use the muscles of any group which still act. The treatment of residual deformities is a question of orthopedic surgery.

EPIDEMIC ENCEPHALITIS

(*Encephalitis lethargica; Epidemic Polio-encephalitis*)

Definition.—An infectious disease, with protean manifestations, chiefly in the central nervous system, characterized by lethargy, paralysis of the cranial nerves (usually the third), and in some cases, spinal and neuritic features.

There are various forms such as the typical epidemic form, Australian X disease, Japanese form and that seen in the St. Louis epidemic of 1933. Encephalitis in acute infectious diseases seems to be more common in recent years.

History.—There are records of outbreaks suggesting this disease in 1712 in Germany and in 1890 in parts of southern Europe (to which the name Nona was given). Cases occurred in Austria and France in 1916 and in England in the spring of 1918. The disease was widely spread, only a few cases occurring in each locality, sometimes two or three in the same house. The disease was recognized in the United States about the end of 1918.

Etiology.—Males and females are attacked in about equal numbers. In striking contrast to poliomyelitis it is rare in young children and most common in young adults; cases in patients over the age of fifty are not uncommon. While the disease has resemblances to poliomyelitis, they are distinct entities. There have been very few epidemics in institutions. The agent was proved to be a virus in the St. Louis epidemic of 1933. Infection is probably from *carriers* and by the nasal mucosa.

Pathology.—The brain may have a pink or rose color and is hyperemic. Hemorrhages in the meninges and in the region of the basal ganglia may be found. The situation of the lesions varies markedly and the midbrain, pons, and basal ganglia are particularly involved, especially the substantia nigra. Lesions occur in the cortex, cerebellum and spinal cord. There is vascular congestion with marked lymphocytic infiltration about the vessels and cellular infiltration of the nerve tissues with edema. The areas of extravascular infiltration may form visible foci. The lesions occur in nodular and diffuse forms. The nerve cells show degeneration which may be very local and irregularly distributed. Thrombosis and necrosis are rare. The cranial nerve paralyses are due to involvement of the nuclei and congestion and infiltration have been described in the roots of the cranial and spinal nerves. The gray matter at the base of the brain is particularly involved. The meninges may show inflammation. The lesions are like those found in rabies and sleeping sickness. The spinal cord lesions are usually slight. The lethargy may be toxic but is possibly mechanical due to interruption of stimuli in the thalamus, which is frequently involved. The later changes involve (1) the vessels with hyaline and calcareous degeneration of the media and adventitia especially and particularly in certain areas, especially the substantia nigra, (2) hydrocephalus, chronic or intermittent, from imperfect drainage of the ventricles, and (3) meningeal thickening.

Clinical Features.—These comprise the features of an infectious disease with the special manifestations due to the lesions in the nervous system. When the marked possibilities of variation in the situation of these lesions are considered, the diverse results and the polymorphous character of the symptoms and signs can be understood. It is natural that different forms are described in consequence. Lethargy is not characteristic of all; there is a very definite myoclonic form. In all the involvement of the cranial nerves is important. There may be very few symptoms in the early stages.

The incubation period is variable and uncertain. Prodromal symptoms range from a few hours to a week, and are chiefly headache, lethargy, stiffness in the back, diffuse pains, and catarrhal features. The general features are of an acute infection. There is usually fever at the onset which, as a rule, is not high and does not last long but in some cases persists for weeks. It may disappear and recur. Headache, general malaise, and gastro-intestinal disturbance are common. There may be vomiting and constipation is generally marked. Local pains may be marked, probably due to involvement of the nerve roots. A number of local manifestations may occur, such as sweating, salivation, dysphagia, hiccough and retention of urine. Convulsions are rare. The signs due to involvement of the nervous system are of the greatest variety and all kinds of variations and combinations are seen.

Lethargy, present in many cases, comes on as a rule gradually, occasionally very suddenly, and is generally not more than a stupor and heaviness, from which the patient can be roused, the so-called "anergic apathy," but in others it is much deeper, passing into coma. As the disease progresses, the patient presents a dull apathetic look. The wrinkles are smoothed, the muscles of the face may be moved with great difficulty, or there may be definite bilateral facial paralysis. The arms are flexed and catalepsy is not uncommon. When roused the patient may answer simple questions intelligently. In some cases the picture is very different. Active delirium or violent mania may be present. Persistent insomnia may occur, about which the patient may not specially complain. There may be excitement or a condition of euphoria. Some patients talk incessantly; others are irritable and restless. In some cases the drowsiness combined with ataxia suggests alcoholic intoxication. The speech may be blurred and difficult; this depends on the degree of involvement of the facial muscles. Tremors, twitchings, and choreiform movements may occur, and persist long into convalescence.

Cranial Nerves.—These are nearly always involved at some time and to some degree even if transient and slight. A history of double vision is common. The pupils may show inequality, irregularity, and a sluggish reaction to light, or the Argyll-Robertson sign. Ptosis is common, often bilateral and sometimes overlooked on account of the lethargy. Paralysis of the eye muscles is frequent; it may be so slight as to be made out with difficulty or diplopia and strabismus may be marked. The third nerve is most frequently involved, the sixth frequently. Nystagmus is common. The seventh nerve is frequently affected; the process is usually unilateral. Involvement of the other cranial nerves is not as common.

Disturbance of Movement.—There may be the greatest variety of disturbance of muscular movement. Fibrillary tremors and twitching are common. Involuntary movements may involve a small area; thus there may be rhythmical movements of small extent about the forehead or face. They are often seen in the lower thorax or abdomen; one rectus muscle may show it. Of special interest is the *myoclonic form* in which there are widespread rhythmical contractions. The onset may be with severe pain. The contractions may be so marked that the patient is thrown out of bed. The muscles of the abdomen and legs are specially involved. Some cases of prolonged hiccough may be due to this. In other cases the movements are athetoid or choreiform, or resemble those of paralysis agitans. Slowness of movement with rigidity is common, giving a mask-like appearance of the face and immobility of the body. Paralysis of all kinds may occur; spasticity with increased deep reflexes and an extensor plantar response may be found.

Sensory disturbances are rare. There may be pain, particularly on pressure of the muscles, and there is sometimes hyperesthesia. The reflexes may vary greatly from day to day; the knee jerks may be abolished for a time. Sphincter features are sometimes present. Dysphagia has been recorded.

Forms.—For convenience various forms are described, much as in poliomyelitis, and it is evident that the possible combinations are many. (1) So-called "abortive" cases with mild or transient manifestations. These are probably common. (2) Cases with general features but no localizing signs. The latter may be very slight and of short duration but are rarely absent entirely. (3) The *lethargic* form, usually with localizing signs. (4) *Psychical* forms in which delirium and mental features predominate; paralysis or myoclonus may appear later. (5) *Labyrinthian* form with vertigo or loss of equilibrium. (6) *Cerebellar* form, with a picture of acute cerebellar ataxia. (7) *Bulbar* form. (8) *Meningeal* form. Meningitis may be closely simulated and in case of hemorrhage, the spinal fluid may contain blood. (9) *Neuritic* form. (10) *Spinal* form. This may show paralyses like poliomyelitis or a picture like myelitis. (11) *Myoclonic* form. (12) There is a form much like *myasthenia* *gravis.* (13) Some cases show features of multiple sclerosis. (14) A *hemorrhagic* form is described. Hemorrhages may occur in the nervous system, from the mucous surfaces or in the skin.

Respiratory disturbances are common, spasmodic cough, transient attacks of dyspnea, rapid or slow respiration, especially the former, periods of apnea, respiratory tics, and sniffling.

Signs suggestive of *meningeal* involvement occur. The cerebrospinal fluid is, as a rule, clear with 10 to 20 cells per c.mm. (rarely 100 cells), mostly mononuclears, the globulin little, if at all, increased. The sugar is increased. The colloidal gold test may give a luetic curve.

The **course** is extremely variable and the disease may persist for months. There are acute fatal cases. In some cases recovery takes from months to two years. Relapses or exacerbations may occur. Of special importance are the *sequels* which occur in great variety and in many combinations. Among them are psychical changes, which may progress to dementia, alterations in disposition and conduct, headache, marked neurasthenic states and insomnia. Disturbances of the sympathetic system may be marked. Respiratory disturbances have been observed. Nocturnal excitement has been noted, especially in children. Organic changes may be shown by ptosis, pupillary changes, nystagmus, strabismus, facial asymmetry, difficulty in speech or swallowing, paralysis of an extremity, and pyramidal tract involvement. Tremors are common, of the tongue, facial muscles or extremities. A large group shows *postencephalitic parkinsonism,* which may appear after an interval, with an expressionless face and alteration in the attitude with tremors and disturbance of gait. The tremors are variable; some are choreiform or athetoid. The outlook in these cases is very grave as regards recovery. Tics and torsion spasm are seen. Diabetes insipidus and obesity have followed an attack.

Diagnosis.—Typical cases offer no difficulty. Special watch should be kept for the cranial nerve paralysis which may be of short duration. The following conditions deserve mention: (1) Poliomyelitis. The similarity may be marked but the spinal fluid usually shows more marked changes. (2) Psychoses characterized by stupor, lethargy or catalepsy. (3) Tuberculous meningitis in which the spinal fluid findings are not characteristic. (4) Acute syphilitic meningo-encephalitis and endarteritis. (5) Botulism. (6) Cerebral hemorrhage or thrombosis may be simulated by some cases of encephalitis. (7) Status epilepticus. (8) Uremia. (9) Other forms of encephalitis. The diagnosis may be made by the sequels after an unrecognized attack.

Prognosis.—An acute onset with rapid development of severe toxemia, marked delirium, high fever, coma and marked myoclonic features is of grave omen. The mortality is probably about 20 to 25 per cent in the acute stages. Sudden death occurs especially in the bulbar form. The ultimate prognosis is uncertain and the frequency of sequels renders the outlook for complete recovery always doubtful.

Treatment.—The patient should be isolated and carefully nursed, care being taken to avoid bed sores; nasal and rectal feeding may be required and special care should be taken to keep the mouth and throat clean. Special care is to be given to the bowels, which should be kept freely open. Retention of urine should be avoided. Lumbar puncture should be done at once and repeated daily for some days, the number of times being governed by the results. There is no specific treatment. Sodium salicylate intravenously has been reported as helpful. Sedatives may be required for headache or pain. The insomnia is resistant and full doses of hypnotics may be necessary. In convalescence, hot baths, massage and passive motion may be used for rigidity. As much encouragement as possible should be given. For the Parkinsonian syndrome hyoscine hydrobromide in doses up to gr. 1/50 (0.0013 gm.) three times a day, tincture of belladonna and stramonium in full doses may be useful. Atropine has been effective in some of the cases with respiratory disturbances. Phenobarbital seems to be beneficial in some patients.

MYELITIS

ACUTE MYELITIS

Etiology.—Acute myelitis affecting the cord in a limited or extended portion—the gray matter chiefly, or the gray and white matter together, is met with: (*a*) As an independent affection probably due to infection, and leading to rapid loss of power with the symptoms of an acute ascending paralysis. Some of these cases are unusually widespread acute forms of poliomyelitis. There is an acute hemorrhagic form with high fever, the relation of which to other forms is uncertain. (*b*) As a sequel of the infectious diseases, such as smallpox, typhus, measles, and gonorrhea. (*c*) There is a form described as *acute benign infectious myelitis,* usually after infection of the upper respiratory tract, in which recovery is generally rapid and complete. (*d*) As a result of *trauma,* either fracture of the spine or very severe muscular effort. Concussion without fracture may produce it, but this is rare. Acute myelitis scarcely ever follows railway accidents. (*e*) In diseases of the *bones* of the spine, either caries or cancer. This is a more common cause of localized acute transverse myelitis than of the diffuse affection. (*f*) In disease of the cord, such as *tumors* and *syphilis;* in the latter with gummata, in which case it is usually a late manifestation, or it may follow within a year of the primary affection. In the syphilitic form the process may be secondary to vascular disease or to meningeal involvement. In cases of long standing marked sclerosis results, and in a transverse lesion there is ascending and descending secondary degeneration.

Morbid Anatomy.—In localized acute myelitis affecting white and gray matter, as met with after accident or an acute compression, the cord is swollen, the pia injected, the consistence greatly reduced, and on incising the membrane an almost diffluent material may escape. In less intense grades, on section at the affected area, the distinction between the gray and white matter is lost, or is extremely indistinct. There are cases with the appearances of an acute hemorrhagic myelitis.

Symptoms.—(*a*) Acute Diffuse Myelitis.—This form is in the epidemic poliomyelitis, or occurs with syphilis or one of the infectious diseases, or is seen in a typical manner in the extension from injuries or from tumor. The onset, though scarcely so abrupt as in hemorrhage, may be sudden; a person may be attacked on the street and have difficulty in getting home. In some instances, the onset is preceded by pains in the legs or back, or a girdle sensation is present. It may be marked by chills, occasionally by convulsions; fever is usually present from the beginning—at first slight, but subsequently it may become high.

The *motor* functions are rapidly lost, sometimes as quickly as in Landry's paralysis. The paraplegia may be complete, and, if the myelitis extends to the cervical region, there may be impairment of motion, and ultimately complete loss of power in the arms as well. The sensation is lost but there may at first be hyperesthesia. The *reflexes* in the initial stage are increased, but in acute central myelitis, unless limited to the thoracic and cervical regions, the reflexes are usually abolished. The rectum and bladder are paralyzed. Trophic disturbances are marked; the muscles waste rapidly; the skin is often congested, and there may be localized sweating. The temperature of the affected limbs may be lowered. Acute bed sores may occur and sometimes a multiple arthritis is present. In these acute cases the general symptoms become greatly aggravated, the pulse is rapid, there is delirium, the fever increases, and may reach 107° or 108° F.

The *course* of the disease is variable. In very acute cases death follows in from five to ten days. The cases following the infectious diseases, particularly the fevers and sometimes syphilis, may run a milder course.

(*b*) Acute Transverse Myelitis.—The symptoms naturally differ with the situation of the lesion.

(1) Acute transverse myelitis in the *thoracic region*, the most common situation, produces a very characteristic picture. The symptoms of onset are variable. There may be initial pains or numbness and tingling in the legs. The paralysis may set in quickly and become complete within a few days; but more commonly it is preceded for a day or two by sensations of pain, heaviness and dragging in the legs. The paralysis of the legs is usually complete, and if at the level, say, of the sixth thoracic vertebra, the abdominal muscles are involved. Sensation may be partially or completely lost. At the onset there may be numbness, tingling, or even hyperesthesia in the legs. At the level of the lesion there is often a zone of hyperesthesia. A girdle sensation may occur early, and when the lesion is in this situation it is usually felt between the ensiform and umbilical regions. The reflexes are variable. There may at first be abolition; subsequently, those which pass through the segments lower than the one affected may be exaggerated and the legs may show spastic rigidity. It does not always happen, however, that the reflexes are increased here, for in a total transverse lesion of the cord they are usually entirely lost. That this is not due to the preliminary shock is shown by the fact that the abolition may be permanent. The muscles become extremely flabby, waste, and lose their faradic excitability, and the sphincters lose their tone. The temperature of the paralyzed limbs is variable. It may at first rise, then fall and become subnormal. Lesions of the skin and bed sores are not uncommon. There is at first retention of urine, and subsequently spastic incontinence. If the lumbar centres are involved, there are vesical symptoms from the outset. The urine is alkaline and may become ammoniacal. The bowels are constipated and there is usually incontinence of feces.

(2) *Transverse Myelitis of the Cervical Region.*—If the lesion is at the level of the sixth or seventh cervical nerves, there is paralysis of the arms, more or less complete, sometimes sparing the muscles of the shoulder. Gradually

there is loss of sensation. The paralysis is usually complete below the point of lesion, but there are rare instances in which the arms only are affected, the so-called cervical paraplegia. In addition there are features which are more characteristic of transverse myelitis in the cervical region, such as vomiting, hiccough, and slow pulse, which may sink to 20 or 30, pupillary changes—myosis—sometimes attacks of dysphagia, dyspnea, or syncope.

The *course* of complete transverse myelitis depends upon its cause. Death may result from extension. Segments of the cord may be completely and permanently destroyed, in which case there is persistent paraplegia. The pyramidal fibres below the lesion undergo secondary degeneration, and there is an ascending degeneration of the dorsal median columns. If the lower segments of the cord are involved the legs may remain flaccid. In some instances a transverse myelitis of the thoracic region involves the ventral horns above and below the lesion, producing flaccidity of the muscles, with wasting, fibrillary contractions and the reaction of degeneration. More commonly in the cases which last many months there is more or less rigidity with spasm or persistent contraction of the flexors of the knee. The *prognosis* is always serious as regards complete recovery. The syphilitic cases usually make the best recovery if recognized early and properly treated.

The *diagnosis* of myelitis is rarely difficult. As in the acute ascending paralysis of Landry, and certain cases of multiple neuritis, it presents a rapid and progressive motor paralysis. From the former it is distinguished by more marked involvement of sensation, trophic disturbances, paralysis of bladder and rectum, rapid wasting, electrical changes and fever. From acute cases of *multiple neuritis* it may be more difficult to distinguish, as the sensory features may be marked, though there is rarely, if ever, in multiple neuritis complete anesthesia; the wasting, moreover, is more rapid in myelitis. The bladder and rectum are rarely involved—though in exceptional cases they may be—and, most important of all, trophic changes, bullae, bed sores, etc., are not seen in multiple neuritis. An *etiological* diagnosis is important, especially for treatment. Syphilis should always be considered; the spinal fluid study is usually definite. The possibility of pressure from disease of the vertebrae or by tumor has to be excluded.

Treatment.—In the rapidly advancing form due either to a diffuse inflammation in the gray matter or to transverse myelitis, the important measures are scrupulous cleanliness, care and watchfulness in guarding against bed sores, and the avoidance of cystitis. In an acute onset in a healthy subject the spine may be cupped. Counterirritation is of doubtful advantage. No drugs have any influence upon acute myelitis, except in subjects with syphilis, in which case bismuth or mercury and iodide should be given energetically. Mercury seems to be much more useful than arsphenamine, which may be given in the intervals between courses of mercury. Arsenic and strychnine may be used in the later stages. When the muscles have wasted, massage is beneficial in maintaining their nutrition. The patient should make every effort to perform muscular movements himself and thus aid improvement. Electricity should not be used in the early stages. It is of no value in the transverse myelitis in the thoracic region with retention of the nutrition in the muscles of the leg.

ACUTE ASCENDING (LANDRY'S) PARALYSIS

Definition.—An acute ascending flaccid paralysis beginning in the legs and spreading upwards, with loss of reflexes and no marked disturbance of sensation. The termination is in complete recovery or death, in which case no gross nervous system lesions are found.

Etiology and Pathology.—The disease occurs most commonly in males between the twentieth and thirtieth years. It has followed the specific fevers and various organisms have been isolated. One form of poliomyelitis has an acute course and a picture similar to Landry's paralysis. Spiller in a rapidly fatal case found destructive changes in the peripheral nerves and alterations in the cell bodies of the ventral horns. He suggests that the toxic agent acts on the lower motor neurones as a whole, and that possibly no lesions were found in some cases because the more delicate histological methods were not used. It has much similarity to acute polyneuritis.

Symptoms.—Weakness of the legs, gradually progressing, often with tolerable rapidity, is the first symptom. In some cases within a few hours the paralysis of the legs becomes complete. The muscles of the trunk are next affected, and within a few days, or even less in more acute cases, the arms are also involved. The neck muscles are next attacked, and finally the muscles of respiration, deglutition and articulation. The reflexes are lost, but the muscles neither waste nor show electrical changes. The sensory symptoms are variable; in some cases tingling, numbness, and hyperesthesia have been present. In the more characteristic cases sensation is intact and the sphincters are uninvolved. The spinal fluid shows no specific features. Enlargement of the spleen has been noted. *Bulbar* symptoms may be early and there are cases in which the picture has been acute *descending* paralysis. The course is variable. It may prove fatal in less than two days or persist for a week or two weeks. In a large proportion of the cases the disease is fatal, usually by respiratory failure. One patient was kept alive for 41 days by artificial respiration (C. L. Greene).

Diagnosis.—This is difficult, particularly from certain forms of multiple neuritis, and if we include in Landry's paralysis the cases in which sensation is involved distinction between the two affections is impossible. We apparently have to recognize the existence of a rapidly advancing motor paralysis without involvement of the sphincters, without wasting or electrical changes in the muscles, without trophic lesions, and without fever—features sufficient to distinguish it from an acute myelitis or spreading poliomyelitis. It is doubtful whether these characters always enable us to differentiate the cases of multiple neuritis. The cases of poliomyelitis with an acute ascending paralysis should not be difficult to recognize during an epidemic.

Treatment.—The comfort of the patient should be studied; frequent change of position is useful. An effort should be made to give sufficient food. The bowels should be kept open and retention of urine avoided. Lumbar puncture should be done and repeated daily for some days. Sedatives may be required for discomfort or pain. Atropine is advised, especially in view of excessive bronchial secretion; gr. 1/100 (0.0006 gm.) can be given four times a day. Artificial respiration or the respirator should be used if necessary, in the hope that the paralysis has reached the height and will soon subside. Convalescence requires no special treatment; massage is useful.

DEGENERATIVE MYELITIS

POSTEROLATERAL SCLEROSIS: SUBACUTE COMBINED DEGENERATION

Definition.—A disorder with symptoms referable to degeneration of the posterior and lateral columns of the cord, occasionally occurring without obvious cause, but most commonly an associated lesion of Addisonian anemia; it occurs also with chronic toxemias and prolonged subinfections.

Etiology.—The disease is most frequent between fifty and sixty, rarely occurs before thirty, may occur in the aged and affects the sexes equally. The exact etiology is in doubt but some toxic agent is supposed to be responsible. It occurs most often with pernicious anemia but sometimes with secondary anemia and with toxic states as in poisoning from ergot and in cachectic conditions.

Pathology.—The essential change involves the white matter of the cord and brain stem. No increase in neuroglia occurs. The posterior and lateral columns are specially involved and the clinical picture varies with the relative changes in them. There may be areas of degeneration elsewhere, which may take the form of an annular sclerosis, especially in the middorsal region. The nerve cells are affected secondarily. Perhaps the same cause is responsible for the anemia (when present) and the cord changes. In some cases the cord changes antedate the anemia.

Symptoms.—The onset is insidious and usually with *sensory* disturbances in the fingers and toes; numbness and tingling are common with a variety of other sensations. Loss of pain sense may antedate loss of touch. The sensory disturbance advances from the legs to the trunk and in late stages may be absolute. Loss of muscle sense, vibration sense and of sense of position may be early. Some patients have pains, much like those of tabes, and a girdle sensation is common. *Motor* disturbance may appear early but usually follows the sensory symptoms. The legs are easily tired, the feet drag, and gradually rigidity of the legs comes on. The conditions found will depend on the relative involvement of the posterior and lateral columns. There may be ataxia with the rigidity. The *reflexes* are exaggerated with an extensor plantar response. As the posterior columns become involved, the spasticity lessens and flaccid paralysis replaces it. The paraplegia may become complete with absence of the knee jerk, an extensor plantar response and muscular atrophy. The arms as a rule are not markedly involved and may show sensory changes only. The sphincters are affected in the later stages.

The deep *reflexes* are usually increased in the early and absent in the late stages. The extensor response to plantar stimulation may appear early and is persistent. The skin reflexes are usually increased. Trophic changes in the skin and nails are common. In the late stages mental disturbances may appear. If *anemia* is present there are the usual blood features. The anemia may follow the cord disease. There is absence of free hydrochloric acid in the stomach. The *course* is variable with an average length of about two years. There are acute cases of short duration and mild forms which persist for years. Remissions occur but the ultimate outcome is fatal.

In the *secondary* variety there may be few or no symptoms in patients long bedridden. When fully developed there are (1) muscular hypotony, (2) loss of the knee jerk, and (3) ataxia, due to involvement of the posterior columns; or (1) muscular hypertony, (2) exaggerated deep reflexes and positive Babinski sign, and (3) motor weakness due to degeneration of the pyramidal tract (L. F. Barker).

Diagnosis.—In the early stages the sensory disturbances should excite suspicion. Syphilis and multiple sclerosis should be excluded. Spinal tumor and tabes may be suggested but care should prevent difficulty. The flaccid form may resemble polyneuritis but the Babinski sign and absence of tenderness should distinguish them. Friedreich's ataxia should not cause confusion.

Treatment.—Any focus of infection should be treated. Anemia should be treated very vigorously. Liver extract should be given intramuscularly or ventriculin in full dosage. The use of iron is advised by some, Blaud's mass, 150 grains daily for 2 or 3 months, or ferrous sulphate 10 grains a day. Vitamins, especially B, should be given freely (yeast). Thyroid gland extract is said to be of benefit in some cases. It is well to give dilute hydrochloric acid. Special attention should be given to prevent infection or bed sores, and infection of the bladder avoided as long as possible. Sedatives may be required for pain. Sleep is sometimes disturbed by spasms for which barbital or phenobarbital may be given.

"Central Neuritis."—This name has been given by Scott to a disease in adults occurring in Jamaica, which perhaps belongs here. The early features are inflammation of the eyes and later changes in the mouth followed by diarrhea and marked changes in the nervous system. In the latter the first symptoms are sensory disturbances in the feet and legs, followed by incoordination and loss of control over the legs. The knee jerks are absent. Death usually occurs from inanition with diarrhea and true paralysis does not occur. In those who recover there is disturbance of vision, deafness and a peculiar steppage gait. Histologically the nervous system showed general changes, perivascular infiltration, degeneration and fibrosis. The disease suggests some form of toxemia. The term "central neuritis" was given by Adolf Meyer to a "parenchymatous systemic degeneration, mainly in the nervous system," found in alcoholic, senile and cachectic states, and in depressive psychoses at the time of involution. The features are fever, diarrhea, emaciation, twitching and rigidity of the extremities, and changed reflexes. Mentally there is an anxious agitation with delirium or stupor.

SENILE SPASTIC PARALYSIS

Unlike the Deacon's "Wonderful One-Hoss Shay," the wear and tear incident to daily use tells more on one part of the machine than another. Like Dean Swift "Some go at the top first, others in their legs, others again in both simultaneously." While the whole nervous system may show decay—"the golden bowl broken and the silver cord loosened"—an early sign of old age is the lessening of the control over the muscles, evidenced by tremor and inability to perform the finer movements with the same precision. The gait becomes tottering, the steps uncertain, and at last the use of the legs is lost for walking, though every muscle group may be put in action. Or one may watch the gradual onset of a spastic paraplegia—a progressive weakness with spasticity and greatly increased reflexes. The steps are short, the feet not lifted from the ground, and the gait uncertain; yet in many cases the strength of the muscles is maintained. The sphincters are not, as a rule, affected. Arteriosclerosis is usually present and in premature senility the vessels of the legs may be very sclerotic and the arteries of the feet obliterated. Typical intermittent claudication may precede the paraplegia.

COMPRESSION OF THE SPINAL CORD

(*Compression Myelitis*)

Definition.—Interruption of the functions of the cord by compression.

Etiology.—Caries of the spine, new growths, aneurism, and parasites are the important causes of slow compression. Caries of the spine is in a majority of instances tuberculous and associated with angular curvature. The involvement of the cord is due to pachymeningitis externa, to abscess or in rare cases to direct spicules of bone. There may be a tuberculous pachymeningitis without caries. The injury to the cord may be from interference with the blood supply and edema, the effects of which are temporary if the condition is relieved. If there is thrombosis of the vessels with resulting necrosis, the damage is permanent. In a few cases it is due to syphilis and occasionally to extension of disease from the pharynx. It is most common in early life, but may occur after middle age. It may follow trauma. Compression may result from aneurism of the thoracic aorta or the abdominal aorta, in the neighborhood of the celiac axis. Malignant growths of the spine frequently cause a compression paraplegia. A retroperitoneal sarcoma or the growths of Hodgkin's disease may invade the vertebrae. More commonly the involvement is secondary to cancer of the breast. Of parasites, the echinococcus and the cysticercus may occur in the spinal canal.

Symptoms.—These may be due to changes in the bones, nerves, and cord. Many symptoms are due to compression of the blood vessels.

Vertebral.—In malignant disease and aneurism erosion of the bodies may take place without producing deformity of the spine. Fatal hemorrhage may follow erosion of the vertebral artery. In caries it is the rule to find more or less deformity, amounting often to angular curvature. The compression of the cord is rarely if ever the direct result of this bony kyphosis but is due to thickening of the dura, the presence of inflammatory products between this membrane and the bodies of the vertebrae. The spinous processes of the affected vertebrae are tender on pressure, and pain follows jarring movements or twisting of the spine. There may be extensive tuberculous disease without much deformity, particularly in the cervical region. With aneurism or tumor pain is a constant and agonizing feature.

Nerve Root Symptoms.—These result from compression of the nerve roots as they pass out between the vertebrae. In caries, even when the disease is extensive and the deformity great, radiating pains from compression involvement of the roots are rare. Pains are more common in cancer of the spine and may be agonizing. There may be acutely painful areas—the *anesthesia dolorosa*—in regions of the skin which are anesthetic to tactile and painful impressions. The nerve trunks are not tender. Trophic disturbances may occur, particularly herpes. Pressure on the ventral roots may give rise to wasting of the muscles supplied by the affected nerves. This is most noticeable in disease of the cervical or lumbar regions.

CORD SYMPTOMS.—(*a*) *Cervical Region.*—The caries may be between the axis and the atlas or between the latter and the occipital bone. In such instances a retropharyngeal abscess may be present, giving rise to difficulty in swallowing. There may be spasm of the cervical muscles, the head may be fixed, and movements may be impossible or cause great pain. In a patient in the Montreal General Hospital movement was liable to be followed by transient, instantaneous paralysis of all four extremities, owing to compression of the cord. In one of these attacks the patient died.

In the lower cervical region there may be signs of interference with the ciliospinal centre and dilatation of the pupils. Occasionally there is flushing of the face and ear of one side or unilateral sweating. Deformity is not so common, but healing may take place with the production of a callus of enormous breadth, with complete rigidity of the neck.

(*b*) *Thoracic Region.*—The deformity is here more marked and pressure symptoms are more common. The time of onset of the paralysis varies very much. It may be early, even before the curvature is manifest, and it is noteworthy that Pott first described the disease that bears his name as "a palsy of the lower limbs which is frequently found to accompany a curvature of the spine." More commonly the paralysis is late, occurring many months after the curvature. The paraplegia is slow in its development; the patient at first feels weak in the legs or has sensory disturbance, numbness, tingling, pins and needles. The girdle sensation may be marked, or severe pains in the course of the intercostal nerves. The legs are frequently drawn up, sometimes in spasm, the reflex spinal automatism. Motion is, as a rule, more quickly lost than sensation. The paraplegia is usually spastic, with exaggerated reflexes. There is an extensor plantar response. Abolition of the reflexes is rarely met with in compression from caries as the transverse lesion is rarely complete. The paraplegia may persist for months, or even more than a year, and recovery be possible.

(*c*) *Lumbar Region.*—In the lower dorsal and lumbar regions the symptoms are practically the same, but the sphincter centres are involved and the reflexes are not exaggerated.

(*d*) *Old Lesions of Cord.*—Following trauma in Pott's disease the dura may be much thickened, the cord narrowed and embedded in cicatricial tissue.

Rapid compression of the cord usually results from fracture or dislocation. The extent of injury to the cord is variable, depending on the amount of bone injury. Marked compression causes a flaccid paralysis, loss of sensation and reflexes below the lesion and retention of urine followed by incontinence. Bladder infection and bed sores are common. The outlook is always serious. If there is complete division of the cord, operation should not be done; if there is some function remaining, laminectomy should be done. Operation is indicated if the signs show injury of the cauda equina.

Diagnosis.—The X-ray picture is of first importance. The injection of lipiodol by cisternal or lumbar puncture and finding by the X-rays the distance to which it spreads is useful in determining the site. Caries is by far the most frequent cause of slow compression of the cord and when there are external signs the recognition is easy. There are cases in which the exudation in the spinal canal between the dura and the bone leads to compression before there are any signs of caries, and if the root symptoms are absent it may be extremely difficult to arrive at a diagnosis. In compression the spinal fluid may show a marked increase in albumin without any increase in the cells; xanthochromia may be present but occurs in other conditions. Persistent lumbago is a symptom of importance in masked Pott's disease, particularly after injury. Brown-Séquard's paralysis is more common in tumor and in injuries than in caries. Pressure on the nerve roots, too, is less frequent in caries than in malignant disease. The cervical form of pachymeningitis produces a pressure paralysis. Following removal of the breast for carcinoma, even after long intervals, recurrence in the vertrebrae may cause pressure on the spinal nerves or on the cord. There may be no local recurrence. Neuralgic pains in the neck or back, or in the course of the sciatic, often associated with obscure nervous symptoms, suggesting hysteria, may be present for months before any signs of paralysis or of recurrence elsewhere. The persistence of the pains and their intensity should arouse suspicion. Paraplegia may come on, not often with deformity, and the pains may be of terrible intensity, well deserving the name *paraplegia dolorosa.*

Treatment.—In compression by aneurism or metastatic tumors the condition is hopeless. In the former the pains may not be very severe but in the latter morphia is always necessary. Compression by caries is often successfully relieved even after the paralysis has persisted for a long period. When caries is recognized early, rest and support to the spine by various methods may do much to prevent paraplegia. When paralysis has occurred, rest with extension gives the best hope of recovery. It is to be remembered that restoration may occur after compression of the cord has lasted for months or even more than a year. Patients have been cured by recumbency alone, enforced for weeks or months; the extradural and inflammatory products are absorbed and the caries heals. In earlier days brilliant results were obtained by suspension, a method introduced by J. K. Mitchell in 1826, and pursued with success by his son, Weir Mitchell. The suspension methods have been superseded by those of hyperextension during recumbency with the use of plaster jackets to secure immobility. Forcible correction of the deformity under anesthesia is not recommended. In protracted cases, after these methods have had a fair trial, operation is usually advisable and has in many instances been successful. The occurrence of abscess or a sudden increase in deformity with signs of greater pressure indicate the need of operation. In meningeal tumors a laminectomy should be done. In old traumatic lesions operation may be indicated for severe nerve root pains. The general treatment of caries is that of tuberculosis.

DIFFUSE SCLEROSES

General Remarks.—The supporting tissue of the central nervous system is the neuroglia, derived from the ectoderm. The meninges are composed of true connective tissue derived from the mesoderm, a little of which enters the brain and cord with the blood vessels. The neuroglia plays a large part in pathological process within the central nervous system, but changes in the connective tissue elements may also be important. A convenient division of the cerebrospinal scleroses is into degenerative, inflammatory and developmental forms.

The *degenerative scleroses* comprise the largest and most important subdivision, in which the following groups may be made: (*a*) The common secondary Wallerian degeneration which follows when nerve fibres are cut off from their trophic centres; (*b*) toxic forms, among which may be placed the scleroses from lead and ergot, and the scleroses of the dorsal columns, due in a large proportion of cases to syphilis; (*c*) the sclerosis associated with change in the smaller arteries and capillaries.

The *inflammatory scleroses* embrace a less important and less extensive group, comprising secondary forms which follow irritative inflammation about tumors, foreign bodies, hemorrhages and abscess. Possibly a similar change may follow the primary, acute encephalitis, which Strümpell held is the initial lesion in the cortical sclerosis in infantile hemiplegia.

The *developmental scleroses* are believed to be of a purely neurogliar character, and embrace the growth about the central canal in syringomyelia and some hold the sclerosis of the dorsal columns in Friedreich's ataxia.

MULTIPLE (INSULAR: DISSEMINATED) SCLEROSIS

Definition.—A chronic affection of the brain and cord, characterized by localized areas in which the nerve elements are more or less replaced by neuroglia. This may occur in the brain or cord alone, more commonly in both. Probably the initial lesion is an inflammatory one.

Etiology.—It is most common in young persons and in females. The onset is most often between 15 and 30 years of age. Several members in a family may be attacked. It is much less common in the United States than in Great Britain; only 91 cases among 12,000 patients (Collins) against 159 among 2568 cases in three years at the National Hospital, London. The etiology is obscure; trauma, fatigue, cold, exposure, intoxications and infections have all been mentioned. Syphilis plays no part.

Morbid Anatomy.—The sclerotic areas are widely and irregularly distributed. The patches are most abundant in the neighborhood of the ventricles, and in the pons, cerebellum, basal ganglia and medulla. The cord may be only slightly involved or there may be many areas throughout its length. The cervical region is apt to be most affected. The nerve roots and the branches of the cauda equina are often attacked. In recently invaded areas there are inflammatory areas showing infiltration with mononuclear cells around the blood vessels with edema. Degeneration of the medullary sheaths occurs, with the persistence for some time of the axis-cylinders. There is marked proliferation of the neuroglia, the fibres of which are denser and firmer. Secondary degeneration, although relatively slight, does occur.

Symptoms.—When the irregular distribution and number of the lesions are considered, it is easy to realize that the clinical manifestations may show a great variety in character and combination. The early inflammatory and vascular lesions may cause *temporary disturbance* only, so that the symptoms are of short duration. The tendency is for the sclerosis to increase so that the injury becomes permanent and, therefore, the clinical features become more constant. Two main forms are described; the first (the more frequent) shows acute exacerbations at intervals with alternating quiescent periods, and the second a progressive course. The onset varies; it may be slow and gradual or with some sudden condition which may be temporary. Among the early manifestations are some disturbance of sensation, dragging of one foot, nystagmus, some disturbance of vision, such as diplopia, or of the bladder function (frequency, precipitate micturition, retention, or incontinence). There may be weakness of one or both legs, especially when fatigued, with irregular pains and stiffness. There may be transient dimness of vision or decrease of acuteness of vision, a central scotoma, or *retrobulbar neuritis.*

As the disease progresses certain features are usually present: (*a*) *Motor signs.* Weakness in the legs and stiffness, usually increased to a spastic paraplegia with the signs of a pyramidal lesion, increase of the deep reflexes, loss of the abdominal and cremasteric reflexes and an extensor plantar response. The gait may be spastic or also ataxic. The arms are usually affected less than the legs.

(*b*) *Volitional or intention tremor.* There is no weakness of the arms, but on attempting to pick up an object there is tremor or rapid oscillation. A patient may be unable to lift a glass of water to the mouth. The tremor may be marked in the legs, and in the head, which shakes as he walks. When the patient is recumbent the muscles may be perfectly quiet. On attempting to raise the head from the pillow, trembling comes on at once.

(*c*) *Scanning speech.* The words are pronounced slowly and separately, or the individual syllables may be accentuated. (*d*) *Nystagmus,* rapid and horizontal, is more common in multiple sclerosis than in any other affection of the nervous system. (*e*) *Ocular signs.* Some have been mentioned. The occurrence of double vision is important. Optic atrophy is common. Pallor of the temporal half of the disk is often seen. (*f*) *Mental changes.* These are common in the later stages, shown by defective memory, emotional disturbance and lack of control. Some of these, with vague complaints for which no basis is found, are often responsible for the common error of regarding this disease as hysteria.

Sensation is not affected markedly in the majority of cases. The vibration sense may be lost. The sphincters, as a rule, are unaffected until the later stages. Vertigo is common, and there may be sudden apoplectiform attacks, as in general paresis. The presence of the extensor plantar reflex and absence of the abdominal reflexes are common.

The *course* is variable and the remarkable remissions must be emphasized. Some are steadily progressive. In the later stages the patient usually becomes helpless from the paralysis of the legs, which are often in spastic flexion. Sphincter control is lost and bed sores are frequent.

Diagnosis.—For the early diagnosis three important signs are loss of abdominal reflexes, weakness of the abdominal muscles and pallor of the temporal sides of the optic disks (L. F. Barker). The history of transient disturbances is important, especially diplopia, numbness and weakness. Volitional tremor, scanning speech, and nystagmus form a characteristic symptom-group, but this classical triad is less common than the irregular forms which easily escape recognition. Paralysis agitans, combined sclerosis, neurosyphilis, compression of the cord, certain cases of general paresis and hysteria may simulate the disease very closely. Of all organic diseases of the nervous system disseminated sclerosis in its early stages is most commonly taken for hysteria. The points in the differentiation are spastic weakness of the legs, pallor of the optic disk, absence of the abdominal reflexes, the Babinski sign, nystagmus, bladder disturbances, and the volitional tremor. The tremor in hysteria is not volitional but the diseases may coexist. If in doubt, suspend judgment. Unilateral cases are recorded. The spinal fluid may show a mid-zone colloidal gold curve with a negative Wassermann reaction. There may be an increase in the cells and globulin.

Pseudosclerosis—the Westphall-Strümpell disease—is a rare condition simulating multiple sclerosis and not often distinguished from it during life. Mental changes are more pronounced, the tremor is more exaggerated, the nystagmus not always present, and the gait more ataxic. It sets in earlier, sometimes in the first decade, and in a majority of the cases no lesions have been found postmortem.

The PROGNOSIS is unfavorable. Ultimately, the patient, if not carried off by some intercurrent affection, becomes bedridden. In 200 cases the average duration was twelve years; 3 recovered (Bramwell).

TREATMENT.—No known treatment has any certain influence on this disease. Arsenic may be given. Avoidance of fatigue, physical and mental, is important. In acute stages there should be absolute rest but otherwise activity, short of fatigue, is advisable. Massage, hot baths and muscular reeducation help some patients. Benefit has resulted from opening the spinal canal (Elsberg). *Fever therapy* by malarial fever or using foreign protein may be tried but diathermy seems more useful. It should be employed as early as possible but not with patients over 50 years of age. Incontinence of urine may be helped by belladonna.

Miliary sclerosis is a term which has been applied to several different conditions. Gowers mentions a case in which there were grayish red spots at the junction of the white and gray matters, in which the neuroglia was increased. There is also a condition in which, on the surface of the convolutions, there are small nodular projections, varying from a half to five or more millimetres in diameter.

Diffuse sclerosis may involve an entire hemisphere, or a single lobe, in which case the term *sclérose lobaire* has been applied by the French. It is not important in general practice, but is most frequent in idiots and imbeciles. In extensive sclerosis of one hemisphere the ventricle is usually dilated. The symptoms depend upon the region affected. There may be considerable sclerosis without symptoms or much mental impairment. In a majority of cases there is hemiplegia or diplegia with imbecility or idiocy.

Tuberose Sclerosis.—Described by Bourneville in feeble-minded children, and regarded as a pathological curiosity, it has been shown to be a definite type of disease, which is sometimes recognized clinically. Imbecility and epilepsy are present, without, as a rule, paralysis. Anatomically there are remarkable tuberous tumors, embedded in the cortex cerebri, ranging in size from a pea to a walnut, white in color, and very hard. There is an overgrowth of the neuroglia and of large ganglionic cells. A peculiarity, which may enable the disease to be recognized, is the occurrence of congenital tumors in other organs, heart, kidneys and skin. Adenoma sebaceum of the face, small, closely-set growths about the nose and cheeks, often with a vascular matrix, is the most common. Renal tumors were found in 19 of 29 cases.

DIFFUSE AND FOCAL DISEASES OF THE SPINAL CORD

TOPICAL DIAGNOSIS

From the symptoms presented by a spinal cord lesion it is possible to determine more or less accurately not only the level but also the transverse extent of the segmental involvement. The effects of injury or disease may be circumscribed and involve the gray matter of the segment or the tracts running through it; it may be more extensive and involve the cord in a given level in its entire transverse extent; finally, there are cases in which only one lateral half of the cord is implicated. It is well to have a definite routine in the examination, for each factor may be helpful in determining the site and character of the lesions. Some of the more important points are: (1) *subjective sensations,* particularly the characters and seat of pain, if any be present, such as the radiating pains of dorsal root compression; (2) the patient's *attitude,* as the position of the arms in cervical lesions, the character of the respiration, whether diaphragmatic, etc.; (3) *motor symptoms,* the groups of paralyzed muscles and their electrical reaction; (4) *sensory symptoms,* including tests for tactual, thermic, and painful impressions, for muscle sense, bone sensation, vibration sense, etc.; (5) the condition of the *reflexes,* both the tendon and skin reflexes as well as those of the pupil, etc.; (6) the surface temperature and condition of the skin, which gives an indication of *vasomotor* disturbance. The table on pages 971-973 and the figures on pages 974 and 975 will be useful while making an examination.

Focal Lesions.—A lesion involving a definite part of the gray matter destroying the cell bodies of the lower motor neurones and leading to degeneration of their axis-cylinder processes, is accompanied by a loss of power to perform certain definite movements. Thus in anterior poliomyelitis the only symptom may be a flaccid paralysis, and the seat of the lesion is revealed by the muscles involved. If from injury or disease a lesion involves more than the gray matter and, for example, if the neighboring fibres of the pyramidal tract be affected there may be in addition a spastic paralysis of the muscles whose centres lie in the lower levels of the cord. The degree of such a paralysis depends upon the intensity of the lesion of the pyramidal tract and may vary from a slight weakness in dorsal flexion of the ankle to an absolute paralysis of all the muscles below the lesion. Again, if the afferent tracts are affected sensory symptoms may be added to the motor palsy. There may be disturbances of pain and temperature sense alone or touch also may be affected. This, however, is rare except in serious lesions. The upper border of disturbed sensation often indicates most clearly the level of the disease, especially when this is in the thoracic region where the corresponding level

Localization of the Functions in the Segments of the Spinal Cord

Segment.	Striped Muscles.	Reflex.	Skin Fields (cf. Figs. 15 and 16).
I, II and III C.	Splenius capitis. Hyoid muscles. Sternomastoid. Trapezius. Diaphragm (C III–V). Levator scapulae (C III–V).	Hypochondrium (?). Sudden inspiration produced by sudden pressure beneath the lower border of ribs (diaphragmatic).	Back of head to vertex. Neck (upper part).
IV C.	Trapezius. Diaphragm. Levator scapulae. Scaleni (C IV–T I). Teres minor. Supraspinatus. Rhomboid.	Dilatation of the pupil produced by irritation of neck. Reflex through the sympathetic (C IV–T I).	Neck (lower part to second rib). Upper shoulder.
V C.	Diaphragm. Teres minor. Supra- and infraspinatus (C V–VI). Rhomboid. Subscapularis. Deltoid. Biceps. Brachialis anticus. Supinator longus (C V–VII). Supinator brevis (C V–VII). Pectoralis (clavicular part). Serratus magnus.	Scapular (C V–T I). Irritation of skin over the scapula produces contraction of the scapular muscles. Supinator longus and biceps. Tapping their tendons produces flexion of forearm.	Outer side of shoulder and upper arm over deltoid region.
VI C.	Teres minor and major. Infraspinatus. Deltoid. Biceps. Brachialis anticus. Supinator longus. Supinator brevis. Pectoralis (clavicular part). Serratus magnus (C V–VIII). Coracobrachialis. Pronator teres. Triceps (outer and long heads). Extensors of wrist (C VI–VIII).	Triceps. Tapping elbow tendon produces extension of forearm. Posterior wrist. Tapping tendons causes extension of hand (C VI–VII).	Outer side of forearm, front and back. Outer half of hand (?).
VII C.	Teres major. Subscapularis. Deltoid (posterior part). Pectoralis major (costal part). Pectoralis minor. Serratus magnus. Pronators of wrist. Triceps. Extensors of wrist and fingers. Flexors of wrist. Latissimus dorsi (C VI–VIII).	Scapulohumeral. Tapping the inner lower edge of scapula causes adduction of the arm. Anterior wrist. Tapping anterior tendons causes flexion of wrist (C VII–VIII).	Inner side and back of arm and forearm. Radial half of the hand.

LOCALIZATION OF THE FUNCTIONS IN THE SEGMENTS OF THE SPINAL CORD (*Continued*)

SEGMENT.	STRIPED MUSCLES.	REFLEX.	SKIN FIELDS (CF. FIGS. 15 AND 16).
VIII C.	Pectoralis major (costal part). Pronator quadratus. Flexors of wrist and fingers. Latissimus. Radial lumbricales and interossei.	Palmar. Stroking palm causes closure of fingers.	Forearm and hand, inner half.
I T.	Lumbricales and interossei. Thenar and hypothenar eminences (C VII–T I).		Upper arm, inner half.
II to XII T.	Muscles of back and abdomen. Erectores spinae (T I–LV). Intercostals (T I–T XII). Rectus abdominis (T V–T XII). External oblique (T V–XII). Internal oblique (T VII–L I). Transversalis (T VII–L I).	Epigastric. Tickling mammary region causes retraction of epigastrium (T IV–VII). Abdominal. Stroking side of abdomen causes retraction of belly (T IX–XII).	Skin of chest and abdomen in oblique dorsoventral zones. The nipple lies between the zone of T IV and T V. The umbilicus lies in the field of T X.
I L.	Lower part of external and internal oblique and transversalis. Quadratus lumborum (L I–II). Cremaster. Psoas major and minor (?).	Cremasteric. Stroking inner thigh causes retraction of scrotum (L I–II).	Skin over lowest abdominal zone and groin.
II L.	Psoas major and minor. Iliacus. Pectineus. Sartorius (lower part). Flexors of knee (Remak). Adductor longus and brevis.		Front of thigh.
III L.	Sartorius (lower part). Adductors of thigh. Quadriceps femoris (L II–L IV). Inner rotators of thigh. Abductors of thigh.	Patellar tendon. Tapping tendon causes extension of leg. "Knee jerk."	Front and inner side of thigh.
IV L.	Flexors of knee (Ferrier). Quadriceps femoris. Adductors of thigh. Abductors of thigh. Extensors of ankle (tibialis anticus). Glutei (medius and minor).	Gluteal. Stroking buttock causes dimpling in fold of buttock (L IV–V).	Mainly inner side of thigh and leg to ankle.
V L.	Flexors of knee (ham string muscles) (L IV–S II). Outward rotators of thigh. Glutei. Flexors of ankle (gastrocnemius and soleus) (L IV–S II). Extensors of toes (L IV–S I). Peronaei.		Back of leg, and part of foot.

Localization of the Functions in the Segments of the Spinal Cord (*Continued*)

Segment.	Striped Muscles.	Reflex.	Skin Fields (cf. Figs. 15 and 16).
I to II S.	Flexors of ankle (L V–S II). Long flexor of toes (L V–S II). Peronaei. Intrinsic muscles of foot.	Foot reflex. Extension of Achilles tendon causes flexion of ankle (S I–II). Ankle clonus. Plantar. Tickling sole of foot causes flexion of toes or extension of great toe and flexion of others.	Back of thigh, leg and foot; outer side.
III to V S.	Perineal muscles. Levator and sphincter ani (S I–III).	Vesical and anal reflexes.	Skin over sacrum and buttock. Anus. Perineum. Genitals.

of motor paralysis is not easily demonstrated. It is unusual for cutaneous anesthesia in organic lesions of the cord to extend above the level of the second rib and the tip of the shoulder, for this represents the lower border of the skin-field of the fourth cervical (see sensory charts), and a lesion of this level sufficient to cause sensory disturbances would probably occasion motor paralyses as well and affect respiration. The demonstrable upper border of the anesthetic field may not quite reach that which represents the level of the lesion. This is due to the functional overlapping of the segmental skin fields (Sherrington) and applies more to touch than to pain and temperature. There is often a narrow zone of hyperesthesia above the anesthetic region.

Complete Transverse Lesions.—When the transverse lesion is total and the lower part of the cord is cut off entirely from above, there is complete sensory and motor paralysis to the segmental level of the injury. Certain features are as follows: (1) Total flaccid paralysis of muscles below the level of the lesion. (Spastic paralysis indicates that the lesion is incomplete.) (2) Rapid wasting of the paralyzed muscles with loss of faradic excitability. (3) The sphincters lose their tone and there is dribbling of urine. (4) There is total anesthesia to the level of the lesion (the zone of hyperesthesia is rarer). Riddoch, by the study of cases of complete division of the spinal cord from war injuries, has shown that under favorable conditions the portion of the cord caudal to the lesion not only recovers its reflex functions but becomes highly excitable. Three stages may be recognized: (1) A stage of muscular flaccidity, (2) a stage of reflex activity, and (3) a stage of gradual failure of the reflex functions of the isolated portion of the cord.

Unilateral Lesions (*Brown-Séquard Paralysis*).—The *motor* symptoms, which follow lesions limited to one lateral half of the cross section of the spinal cord, are confined to one side of the body; they are on the same side as the lesion. At the level of the lesion, owing to destruction of cell bodies of the lower system of neurones, there will be flaccid paralysis and atrophy of those muscles whose centres of innervation lie at this level. Owing to degeneration of the pyramidal tract, the muscles whose centres are at lower levels,

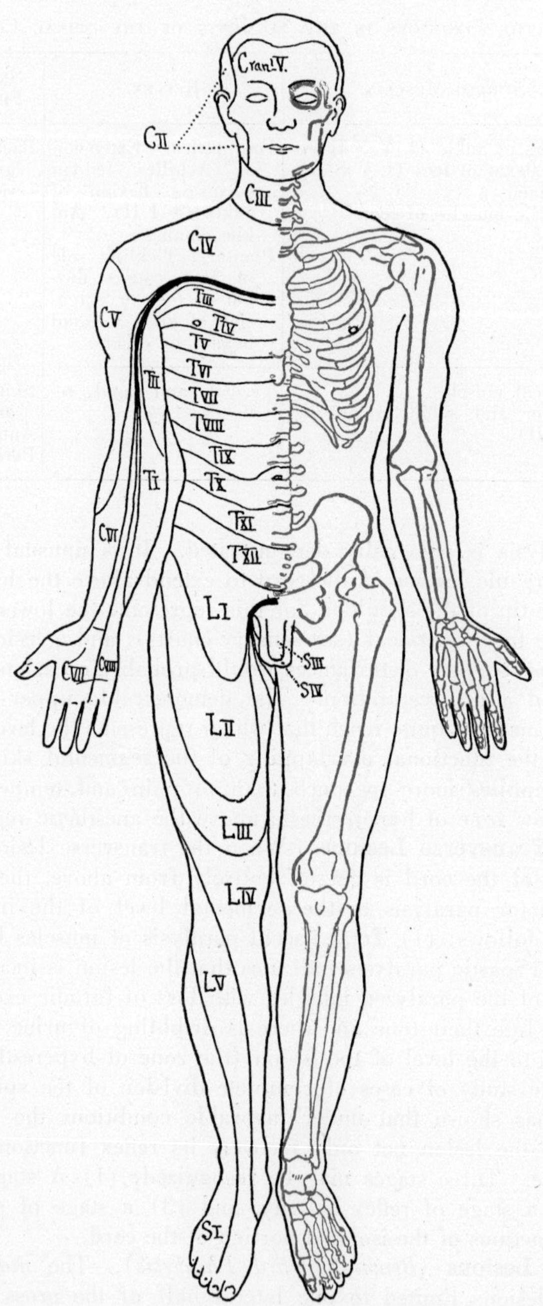

Fig. 15.—Anterior Aspect of the Segmental Skin Fields of the Body, Combined from the Studies of Head, Kocher, Starr, Thorburn, Edinger, Sherrington, Wichmann, Seiffer, Bolk, Cushing, and Others.

Heavy lines represent levels of fusion of dermatomes and the pre-axial and postaxial lines of the limbs.

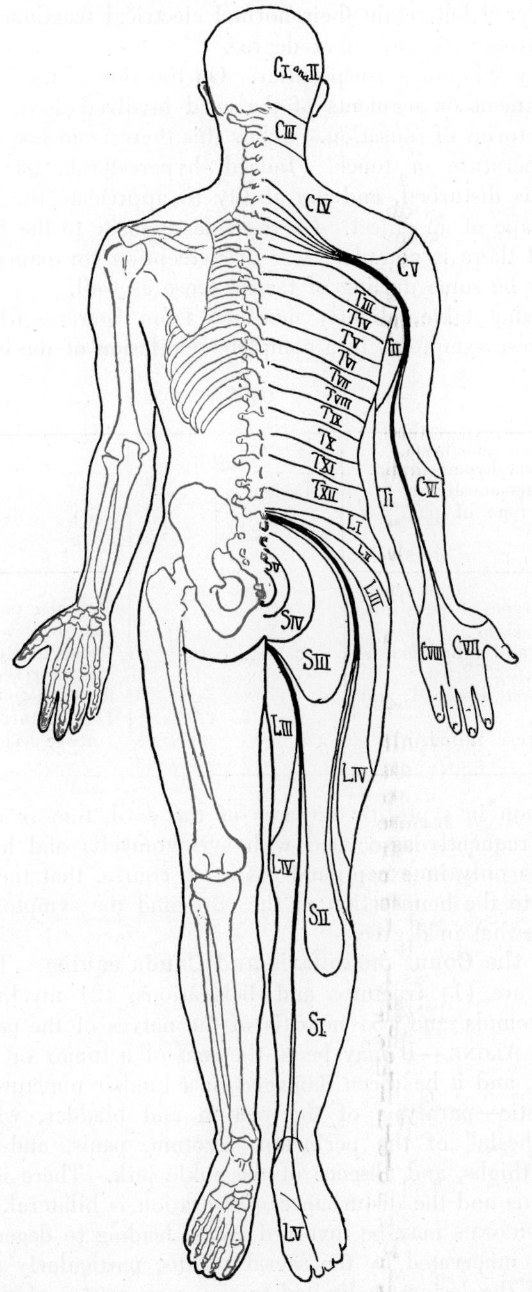

Fig. 16.—Posterior Aspect of the Segmental Skin Fields of the Body.

are also paralyzed but retain their normal electrical reactions, become spastic, and do not atrophy to any great degree.

The *sensory* symptoms are peculiar. On the side of the lesion corresponding to the segment or segments of the cord involved there is a zone of anesthesia to all forms of sensation. Below this there is no loss in the perception of pain, temperature or touch. Indeed, hyperesthesia has been described. Muscle sense is disturbed, and the ability to appreciate the size, consistency, weight and shape of an object. On the side opposite to the lesion and nearly up to its level there is complete loss of perception for pain and temperature and there may be some dulling of tactile sense as well.

The following table, slightly modified from Gowers, illustrates the distribution of these symptoms in a complete semilesion of the cord:

Cord

Zone of cutaneous hyperesthesia. Zone of cutaneous anesthesia. Lower segment type of paralysis with atrophy.	Lesion.	
Upper segment type of paralysis. Hyperesthesia of skin. Muscular sense and allied sensations impaired. Reflex action first lessened and then increased. Surface temperature raised.		Muscular power normal. Loss of sensibility of skin to pain and temperature. Muscular sense normal. Reflex action normal. Temperature same as that of above lesion.

It is common in syphilitic diseases of the cord, tumors and stabwounds, and is not infrequently associated with syringomyelia and hemorrhages into the cord. It is only in exceptional cases, of course, that the lesion is absolutely limited to the hemisection of the cord and the symptoms consequently may vary somewhat in degree.

Lesions of the Conus medullaris and Cauda equina.—The chief lesions of this region are (1) fractures and dislocations, (2) myelitis, (3) tumors, (4) gunshot wounds, and (5) neuritis of the nerves of the cauda.

(1) CONUS ALONE.—It may be in the seat of a tumor or a focal myelitis or hemorrhage, and it has been damaged in a lumbar puncture. The features are characteristic—paralysis of the rectum and bladder, with the "riding-breeches anesthesia" of the perineum, scrotum, penis, and postero-internal aspects of the thighs, and absence of the ankle jerk. There is less pain than in caudal lesions and the disturbance of sensation is bilateral.

(2) The EPICONUS may be involved alone, leading to degenerative atrophy of the muscles innervated by the sacral plexus, particularly the peronei and the glutei. "If the lesion be limited to the gray matter of the epiconus, the Achilles reflex is abolished, but the knee jerk can be elicited and the sphincters remain unaffected" (Barker).

(3) CAUDA EQUINA.—An unusual number of cases followed bullet and shell wounds in the late war. The picture varies with the level of the lesion, from complete paralysis of all the muscles of the legs with anesthesia, includ-

ing the genitals, but if below the second sacral roots, there is no paralysis of the lower limbs, but there is the typical saddle-shaped anesthesia. The caudal lesions are more often unilateral and the neuralgic pains are more severe.

Of tumors of the cauda mention must be made of the diffuse giant tumors described by Collins and Elsberg, with well marked caudal and conus symp-

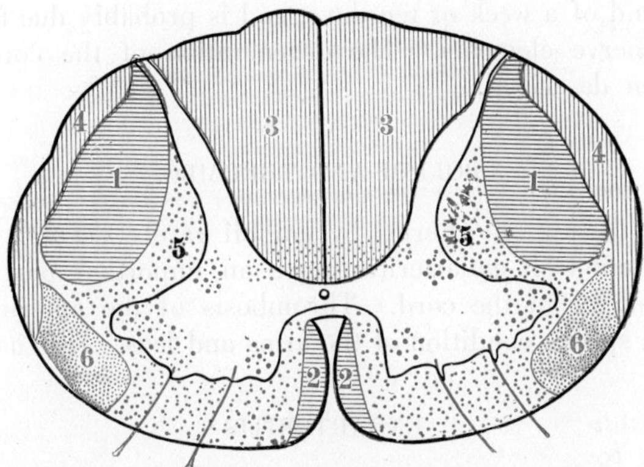

Fig. 17.—Diagram of Cross-section of the Spinal Cord, Showing Motor, Red, and Sensory, Blue, Paths.

1, Lateral pyramidal tract. 2, Ventral pyramidal tract. 3, Dorsal columns. 4, Direct cerebellar tract. 5, Ventrolateral ground bundles. 6, Ventrolateral ascending tract of Gowers. (Van Gehuchten, colored.)

toms. There is also a remarkable *neuritis* in which the caudal roots are swollen and the nerves degenerated, in association with a high grade of local arteriosclerosis. The symptoms in the cases reported by Kennedy and Elsberg were pain, sphincter involvement and sensory changes in the sacral roots.

AFFECTIONS OF THE BLOOD VESSELS

CONGESTION

Apart from actual myelitis, we rarely see congestion of the spinal cord, and, when we do, it is usually limited to the gray matter or to a definite portion of the organ. The white matter is rarely found congested, even when inflamed. The gray matter often has a reddish pink tint, but rarely a deep reddish hue, except with myelitis. If we know little anatomically of congestion of the cord, we know less clinically, for there are no characteristic features.

ANEMIA

So, too, with this state. There may be extreme grades of anemia without symptoms. There is no reason to suppose that such sensations as heaviness in the limbs and tingling are especially associated with anemia.

Profound anemia follows ligature of the aorta. Within a few moments after the application of a ligature paraplegia came on (Herter). Paralysis of the sphincters occurred, but less rapidly. Observations by Halsted on occlusion of the abdominal aorta in dogs showed that paraplegia occurs in a large percentage of cases, many of which recover as the collateral circulation is established. In fatal cases Gilman found extensive alterations in the cell bodies of the lower part of the cord with degenerations. This is of interest in connection with the occasional rapid development of a paraplegia after profuse hemorrhage, usually from the stomach or uterus. It may come on at once or at the end of a week or ten days, and is probably due to an anatomical change in the nerve elements. The degeneration of the cord in pernicious anemia has been described.

EMBOLISM AND THROMBOSIS

Blocking of the spinal arteries by emboli rarely occurs. Thrombosis of the smaller vessels with endarteritis plays an important part in many acute and chronic changes in the cord. Thrombosis of the anterior spinal artery gives a bilateral spastic condition of the arms and legs. It is usually syphilitic.

ENDARTERITIS

It is remarkable how frequently in persons over fifty the arteries of the spinal cord are found sclerotic. The following forms may be met with: (1) A nodular peri-arteritis or endarteritis associated with syphilis and sometimes with gummata of the meninges; (2) an arteritis obliterans, with great thickening of the intima and narrowing of the lumen, involving chiefly the medium and larger-sized arteries. Miliary aneurisms or aneurisms of the larger vessels are rarely found in the spinal cord. Attacks of transient paraplegia may be due to spasm or other changes in the vessels of the cord. In the remarkable neuritis of the cauda equina described by Kennedy and Elsberg there is marked sclerosis of the arteries.

HEMORRHAGE INTO THE SPINAL MEMBRANE; HEMATORACHIS

In meningeal "apoplexy," as it is called, the blood may lie between the dura mater and the spinal canal—extrameningeal hemorrhage—or within the dura mater—intrameningeal hemorrhage.

Extrameningeal hemorrhage occurs usually as a result of traumatism. The exudation may be extensive without compression of the cord. The blood comes from the large plexuses of veins which may surround the dura. The rupture of an aneurism into the spinal canal may produce extensive and rapidly fatal hemorrhage.

Intrameningeal hemorrhage is a less frequent result of trauma but in general is perhaps rather more common. It is rarely extensive from causes acting directly on the spinal meninges themselves. Scattered hemorrhages may occur in acute fevers, and there may be much extravasation in malignant smallpox. It may be into the theca alone and along the spinal nerve roots. Bleeding may occur in convulsive disorders, such as epilepsy, tetanus and strychnia poisoning, and has been recorded with difficult parturition and in purpura. The most extensive hemorrhages occur from rupture of an aneurism at the base of the brain, either of the basilar or vertebral artery. In ventricular hemorrhage the blood may pass from the fourth ventricle into the spinal meninges. In cranial fractures, particularly of the base of the skull, the resultant hemorrhage almost always finds its way into the subarachnoid space about the cord and may be demonstrated by the withdrawal of bloody fluid by a lumbar puncture. On the other hand, hemorrhage into the spinal meninges may possibly ascend into the brain.

Symptoms.—The symptoms in moderate grades may be slight and indefinite. The spinal features suggest lumber puncture and the nature of the fluid, flowing under pressure, determines the presence of hemorrhage. In the nontraumatic cases the hemorrhage may come on suddenly or after a day or two of uneasy sensations along the spine. As a rule, the onset is abrupt, with sharp pain in the back and symptoms of irritation in the course of the nerves. There may be muscular spasms, or paralysis may come on suddenly, either in the legs alone or both in the legs and arms. In some instances the paralysis develops more slowly and is not complete. There are no signs of cerebral disturbance. The clinical picture varies. If the hemorrhage is in the *lumbar* region, the legs alone are involved, the reflexes may be abolished, and the action of the bladder and rectum is impaired. If in the *thoracic* region, there is more or less complete paraplegia, the reflexes are usually retained, and there are signs of disturbance in the thoracic nerves, such as girdle sensations, pains and sometimes herpes. In the *cervical* region the arms as well as the legs may be involved; there may be difficulty in breathing, stiffness of the muscles of the neck, and occasionally pupillary signs. In a case of influenza-pneumonia there was bilateral spastic rigidity associated with extensive hemorrhage into the theca spinalis and along the nerve roots. There was no free blood in the canal. Branson reports two cases, probably influenza, with bloody fluid (40-50 cc.) withdrawn under considerable pressure. The spinal symptoms were slight and both patients recovered.

The *diagnosis* from hemorrhage into the cord is made by the signs of irritation preceding the paralysis, which is usually less marked. The study of the spinal fluid distinguishes it from meningitis. The *prognosis* depends much upon the cause. Recovery may take place in the traumatic cases and in those associated with the infectious diseases. The *treatment* depends largely on the cause. Lumbar puncture should be repeated as indicated.

HEMORRHAGE INTO THE SPINAL CORD; HEMATOMYELIA

Most frequently a result of traumatism, intraspinal hemorrhage is naturally more common in males and during the active period of life. In some cases no cause can be found. Cases have followed cold or exposure; it occurs also in tetanus and other convulsive diseases, and hemorrhage may be associated with tumors, syringomyelia or myelitis. A direct injury to the spine is by far the most common cause. Acute flexure of the neck, often without fracture or dislocation of the vertebrae, is the most common form of accident. There were many such cases during the war. The level of the lesion, for this reason, is most frequently in the lower cervical region.

Anatomical Condition.—The extent of the hemorrhage may vary from a small focal extravasation to one which finds its way in columnar fashion a considerable distance up and down the cord. The bleeding primarily takes place into the gray matter, and this as a rule suffers most, but the surrounding medullated tracts may be thinned out and lacerated.

Symptoms.—As one side of the cord is usually involved more than the other, the Brown-Séquard syndrome is common. The symptoms are sudden in onset, and leave the patient with hyperesthesia and a paralysis which becomes spastic and is most marked on one side, while anesthesia, chiefly to pain and temperature, is most marked on the opposite side of the body. Often a distressing hyperesthesia, usually a "pins and needles" sensation, may be present for many days, but there is rarely acute pain of the radiating or root type. As hematomyelia is most frequent in the lower cervical region, in addition a brachial type of palsy is common, with flaccid and atrophic paralysis of the muscles innervated from the lowest cervical and first thoracic segments. The hemorrhage may occur in segments farther down the cord, the lumbar enlargement being affected next in frequency to the lower cervical. The segmental level of the paralysis necessarily varies accordingly.

The condition may prove rapidly fatal, particularly if the extravasation is bilateral and extends high enough in the cord to involve the centres for the diaphragm. More frequently there is a more or less complete recovery with a residual palsy of the arm and a partial anesthesia, corresponding to the level of the lesion, and some spasticity of the leg.

Diagnosis.—In the traumatic cases this is comparatively easy, and it is important to recognize them, as they are often needlessly subjected to operation under the belief that they are instances of acute compression. Myelitis and poliomyelitis have to be excluded. The residual symptoms in old cases may closely simulate those in syringomyelia.

Treatment.—Absolute rest is important and the patient should be disturbed as little as possible. Special care must be given the skin to prevent bed sores and to the bladder to prevent cystitis. If lumbar puncture is done for diagnosis, the least amount necessary should be removed. Treatment of the paralyzed parts should not be begun for six weeks after the hemorrhage, when electricity, gentle massage and passive movements are indicated.

TUMORS OF THE SPINAL CORD AND ITS MEMBRANES

SYRINGOMYELIA (GLIOMA, GLIOMATOSIS)

Definition.—A gliosis about the central canal, either forming a local tumor, or more often a diffuse growth associated with cavity formations, extending lengthwise, and sometimes communicating with the central canal.

Dilatation of the central canal—hydromyelus—must be distinguished from syringomyelia; it is a congenital anomaly; only rarely do the cavity formations of syringomyelia represent the distended canal itself.

Morbid Anatomy.—The lower cervical and upper dorsal regions are the usual seat. They are: (1) either a diffuse gliosis or at one level a definite tumor from which the growth extends for some inches, causing enlargement of the cord. (2) Tube-like cavities, extending for a variable distance, usually in the dorsal aspect and sometimes involving only one cornu. The processes leading to the formation of the cavities are various, such as hemorrhage and thrombotic degenerations, evidences of which may be present. The wall of the tubes may be smooth and lined with ependymal cells. (3) Degenerative changes in other parts of the cord due to pressure.

Symptoms.—Men are more often affected, 133 of 190 cases collected by Schlesinger. The disease begins, as a rule, before the thirtieth year. The symptoms vary with the seat and extent of the disease. A typical case beginning in the lower cervical region presents the following features: (1) Lower motor neurone involvement, with a progressive atrophy of the muscles of the hands and arms, and sometimes fibrillary tremors, so that the Aran-Duchenne disease is suspected. The typical clawhand may exist. As the disease progresses, there is degeneration of the pyramidal tracts with a spastic paraplegia, so that the picture suggests amyotrophic lateral sclerosis.

(2) *Sensory changes;* (*a*) pains of the nerve root type, chiefly in the arms; (*b*) the syringomyelic *dissociation of sensation,* in which the sense of touch is retained, while those of heat and pain are lost. The muscle sense is not disturbed. The loss of temperature sense may be early, and a patient's fingers may be burnt by a cigarette.

(3) *Trophic* changes, as destructive whitlows, with atrophy of the terminal phalanges (Morvan's disease), vasomotor swelling of the hands, thickening of the skin, sweating and arthropathies, which latter occur in about 10 per cent of the cases. While this is the common form, there may be no disturbance of sensation for years, only the amyotrophic type of paralysis; there may be general anesthesia to pain and temperature, with very little motor disturbance; and there is a form with bilateral spastic diplegia.

Marked scoliosis may be present, a feature not easily explained. The analgesia and loss of thermic sense are due to involvement of the peri-ependymal gray matter and the posterior horns. The tactile sensations travel in the posterolateral regions of the cord which are rarely involved. Disturbance of the cervical sympathetic is common. With higher involvement there may be nystagmus, diplopia or atrophy of the tongue.

The *diagnosis* is easy in well pronounced cases, but when the motor features predominate, it may not be possible to distinguish the disease from amyotrophic muscular paralysis. With the widespread anesthesia hysteria is simulated; while the combination of anesthesia and loss of the finger tips may suggest leprosy. A *cervical rib* may give very similar features; the two conditions may coexist. In a few instances the gliosis extends to the medulla with the production of bulbar symptoms. The *course* is variable and there may be no change for long periods. The tendency is to slow progression.

Treatment.—Care should be taken to avoid injury and local infection. Active treatment by mercury, given by inunction, and iodide is advised. X-ray exposures over the spine have been followed by improvement. Laminectomy with drainage of the cavity fluid has been of benefit, but there is danger from an anesthetic. Cervical puncture has been done.

TUMORS OF THE CORD AND MENINGES

Tumors may be situated within the membranes (intradural) and in the spinal cord (intramedullary) or outside it (extramedullary). Extradural tumors usually involve the vertebrae and are commonly metastatic carcinomas.

The intramedullary tumors are usually gliomas. A majority are extramedullary, and originate on the dura or pia in the blood vessels or on the nerve roots. Schlesinger's tabulation of 400 cases shows that the growths in order of frequency are tubercle, fibroma and syphiloma. Rarer forms are lipoma, psammoma, neuroma, myxoma and angioma. A few cases of aneurism and echinococcus cyst have been reported. There is an occasional diffuse sarcomatous tumor which tends to spread up and down.

Symptoms.—Localized persistent *pain,* perhaps with occasional remission in severity is an important and usually the first symptom. Subjective sensory disturbances follow with many varieties of paresthesia. The pain, due to root involvement, is on the same side as the lesion, but paresthesia, due to compression, may be on either or both sides. In some cases with a small tumor from the pia or arachnoid on the anterior aspect or posterior between the nerve roots, pain may be of late occurrence. (1) *Irritation*—sensory and motor. Pressure on the posterior roots causes pain, unilateral or bilateral, at the level of the distribution of the nerves. Hyperesthesia with a sense of burning is common. In the cervical region the sympathetic fibres may be involved. Only in a few cases are sensory features absent. *Motor* irritation due to pressure on the anterior roots and anterolateral columns causes spontaneous spasms of the muscles, rarely of the arms, very often of the legs, and they constitute an important sign. Suddenly, without the patient's knowledge, the legs are drawn up, sometimes in pain, the thighs flexed on the abdomen, the legs on the thighs and foot, and especially the big toe on the ankle. It is a reflex of spinal automatism similar to that described by Sherrington in the decerebrated animal. It is the "defensive" reflex of Babinski, but Sherrington's term is preferable. It may be excited by stimulating the skin of the leg or foot, but the important point is the automatic type of the reflex and its significance as a sign of pressure irritation on the cord, at any stage early or late of the process.

(2) *Compression.*—Anesthesia may occur in the region of distribution of the nerve root or roots involved; atrophy of the muscles may follow pressure on the anterior roots. Pressure on the cord may produce the features of a hemilesion with a Brown-Séquard syndrome. Gradually, after months or even years, the compression is complete with a spastic paraplegia and all the features of a spinal automatism. All stages from nerve root irritation to a total transverse lesion may be followed through a period of months or years.

The situation of the growth is determined by the root levels involved, and it is to be remembered that the tendency is usually to locate it below the actual situation. The X-rays are often of great value in determining the nature of the pressure, particularly in excluding disease of the vertebrae.

Spinal Fluid.—From an extensive study Sprunt and Walker describe two forms of xanthochromia, in one of which the color is due to dissolved hemoglobin, the fluid does not coagulate, and the amount of globulin is small. This is more common with brain tumor. In a larger group the fluid is clear yellow, coagulates, and has a large amount of globulin and no hemoglobin—the *Froin syndrome;* it is a compression sign, associated with the isolation of a culdesac, in which the fluid stagnates. It suggests spinal tumor or intradural inflammation. Lumbar puncture may give a clear normal fluid. The leukocytes may be increased; the chief point is the xanthochromia.

Diagnosis.—The order of progress is usually pain, paresthesia, paralysis. Most tumors are lateral. Ventral or ventrolateral tumors are most likely to give indefinite features. Posterior tumors have root pains and posterior column disturbances particularly. In the segment diagnosis the level of the sensory change is the most important point. When constant and severe root pains are associated with a progressive paralysis, the diagnosis may be easily made. Caries may cause identical symptoms, but the radiating pains are rarely so severe. Cervical meningitis simulates tumor very closely and in reality produces identical effects, but the slow progress and the bilateral character from the outset may distinguish it. Syphilitic meningomyelitis may resemble tumor and present radiating pains, a sense of constriction, and progressive paralysis. Syringomyelia may give a similar picture. A radiogram may be of aid if the vertebrae are infiltrated by the growth. The nature of the tumor can rarely be indicated with precision. With a syphilitic history gumma may be suspected, or, with coexisting tuberculous disease, a solitary tubercle. Tumors of the cord itself cause loss of power and sensation below the lesion. There may be paresthesia before the anesthesia or pains in the legs. Occasionally there is dissociation of sensation which aids in the diagnosis of extramedullary tumors. The picture varies greatly depending on the parts of the cord first and most involved.

Treatment.—It is difficult to say which rouses greater admiration—the brilliant diagnosis of the clinician or the technique of the surgeon, the combination of which enabled Gowers and Horsley to remove, for the first time and with permanent success, a tumor of the spinal cord. The report of this case should be read to his class by every teacher of neurology (Medico-Chir. Soc. Trans., London, LXXI, 1888). In syphiloma recovery is possible, even after complete paraplegia. The hopeful cases are the isolated growths springing from the membranes, and operation has been followed by an ever increased percentage of recovery.

DIFFUSE AND FOCAL DISEASES OF THE BRAIN

TOPICAL DIAGNOSIS

In many regions disease may exist without causing symptoms—the so-called *silent areas*. Other areas at once give symptoms. These are the cortical motor centres and the associated sensory centres, the speech centres, the centres for the special senses, and the tracts which connect these cortical areas with each other and with other parts of the nervous system. The following is a brief summary of the effects of lesions from the cortex to the spinal cord:

The Cerebral Cortex.—(*a*) *Destructive lesions* of the motor cortex cause *paralysis* in the muscles of the opposite side. The paralysis is at first flaccid, later spastic, the extent depending upon that of the lesion It is apt to be limited to the muscles of the head or of an extremity, giving rise to the cerebral monoplegias. One group of muscles may be more affected than others, especially in lesions of the highly differentiated area for the arm. It is uncommon to find all the muscle groups of an extremity equally involved in cortical monoplegia. In small bilateral symmetrical lesions monoplegia of the tongue may result without paralysis of the face. A lesion may involve centres lying close together or overlapping one another, thus producing associated monoplegias—*e. g.*, paralysis of the face and arm, or of the arm and leg, but not of the face and leg without the arm. Very rarely the whole motor cortex is involved with paralysis of the opposite side—cortical hemiplegia.

Adjoining and posterior to the motor area is the region of the cortex in which the impulses concerned in general bodily sensation (cutaneous sensibility, muscle sense, visceral sensations) first arrive (the somesthetic area). Combined with the muscular weakness there is usually some disturbance of sensations, particularly of those of the muscular sense. In lesions of the

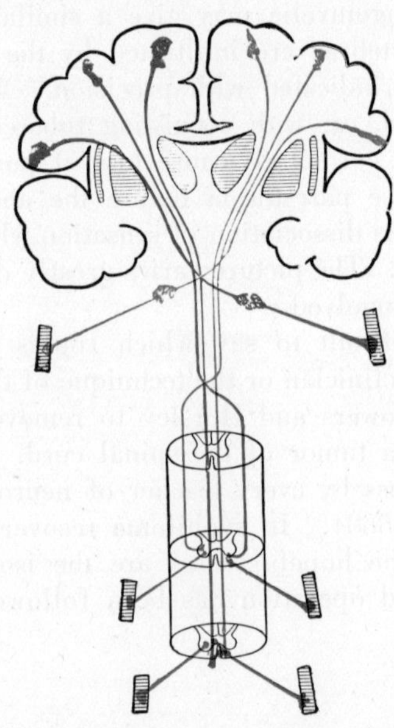

Fig. 18.—Diagram of Motor Path from Each Hemisphere, Showing the Crossing of the Path, Which Takes Place in the Upper Segment Both for the Cranial and Spinal Nerves. (Van Gehuchten, colored.)

superior parietal lobe the stereognostic sense is very often affected. The sense of touch, pain and temperature may be lowered, but not markedly unless the superior and inferior parietal lobules are involved in subcortical lesions. Paresthesias and vasomotor disturbances are common accompaniments of paralyses of cortical origin.

(*b*) *Irritative lesions* cause localized spasms. The most varied muscle groups corresponding to particular movement forms may be picked out. If the irritation be sudden and severe, attacks of Jacksonian epilepsy may occur. These may be preceded and accompanied by subjective sensory impressions. Tingling or pain, or a sense of motion in the part, is often the *signal symptom* (Seguin), and aids in determining the seat of the lesion.

When lesions are both destructive and irritative, there are combinations of the symptoms produced by each. For instance, certain muscles may be paralyzed, and those represented near them in the cortex may be the seat of localized convulsions, or the paralyzed limb itself may be at times subject to convulsive spasms, or muscles which have been convulsed may become paralyzed. The close observation of the sequence of the symptoms in such cases often makes it possible to trace the progress of a lesion involving the motor cortex. The most frequent cause is a developing tumor, though sometimes local thickenings of the membranes of the brain, small abscesses, minute hemorrhages, or fragments of a fractured skull are responsible.

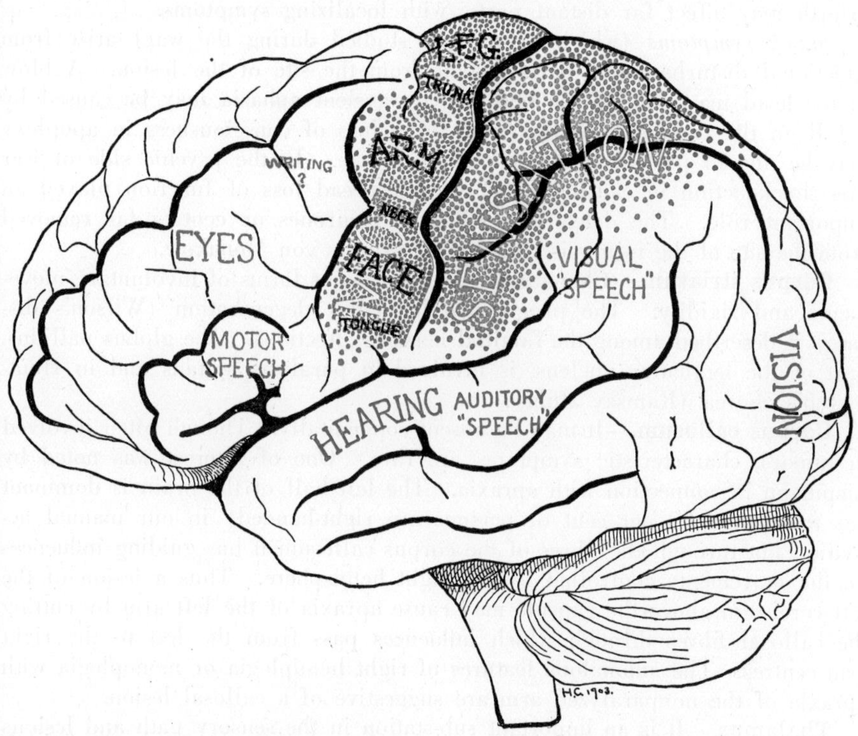

Fig. 19.—Diagrammatic Representation of Cortical Localization in the Left Hemisphere, Showing the Speech Centres.

The motor areas determined by unipolar faradic excitation of the anthropoid cortex (Sherrington and Grünbaum) are here shown stippled in red and lie anterior to the Rolandic fissure. The sensory areas presumably lie posterior to this fissure and are roughly indicated in blue without accurate delineation. Lying as it does on the upper surface of the hemisphere, the leg area should not be visible on a lateral view such as is given here.

Centrum semiovale.—Lesions may involve either projection fibres (motor or sensory) or association fibres. If the involvement of the motor path causes paralysis, this has the distribution of a cortical palsy when the lesion is near the cortex, and of a paralysis due to a lesion of the internal capsule when it is near that region. Other systems of fibres running in the centrum semiovale may be involved, causing sensory disturbances—hemianesthesia and hemianopia—and if the lesion is in the left hemisphere, one of the different forms of aphasia may accompany the paralysis.

Two other features may be associated with a cortical or indeed with any lesion. *Neighborhood symptoms* are produced by pressure. A tumor may cause disturbance of function in adjacent centres, or interrupt motor or sensory paths. A hemorrhage often causes transient symptoms which clear up after the clot shrinks. Transient disturbances of the speech centres and temporary involvement of the paths in the internal capsule are common effects. *Distal symptoms* are produced in two ways. The pressure of a tumor in the frontal lobe may influence the function of the motor centres or a pituitary growth may affect far distant parts, with localizing symptoms.

Shock symptoms (which were much studied during the war) arise from functional disturbance of parts distant from the site of the lesion. A blow in the head may abolish the knee jerk; transient aphasia may be caused by a fall on the right side of the head. The loss of consciousness in apoplexy may be due in part to the shock of the stroke. In the psychic side of war this shock action in causing local or widespread loss of function played an important rôle. The deleterious effect on neurones or centres far removed from the site of the injury is called *diaschisis* by von Monakow.

Corpus striatum.—Changes here cause various forms of involuntary movements and rigidity. The progressive lenticular degeneration (Wilson's disease) is described among the familial nervous affections. The globus pallidus, part of the lenticular nucleus, is involved in paralysis agitans and in Huntington's chorea (Ramsay Hunt).

Corpus callosum.—It may be absent congenitally. Though often involved in tumors, characteristic symptoms are rare. One of interest was noted by Liepmann in connection with apraxia. The left half of the brain is dominant (as more than 90 per cent of persons are right-handed) in our manual activities, but through the fibres of the corpus callosum it has guiding influences on the movements controlled by the right hemisphere. Thus a lesion of the left cerebrum above the capsule may cause apraxia of the left arm by cutting the callosal fibres through which influences pass from the left to the right arm centres. The anomalous features of right hemiplegia or monoplegia with apraxia of the nonparalyzed arm are suggestive of a callosal lesion.

Thalamus.—It is an important sub-station in the sensory path and lesions of this part are associated with athetoid and choreic movements.

The *thalamic syndrome* consists of: (1) Contralateral hemianesthesia, sometimes with severe pains; (2) irregular movements—ataxic, choreic, or athetoid; and, (3) as the lesion progresses, hemiparesis, but the plantar reflex may remain flexor. Lesions of the posterior third may involve the optic radiations causing bilateral homonymous hemianopia. Control of the voluntary movements with loss of the mimic associated movements of the lower half of the face in laughing and crying suggests a thalamic lesion.

In *hemiballismus* there are incoördinated twisting and rolling movements of half the body. The condition is attributed to disease of the corpus luysi.

Internal Capsule (Fig. 20).—Through this pass within a rather narrow area all, or nearly all, of the projection fibres (motor and sensory) which are connected with the cerebral cortex. Since here all the fibres of the upper motor segment are gathered together in a compact bundle, a lesion in this region is apt to cause complete hemiplegia of the opposite side, followed later by contractures; and if the lesion involves the hinder portion of the posterior limb there is also hemianesthesia, including even the special senses. As a rule, however, lesions of the internal capsule do not involve the whole structure. The disease usually affects the anterior or posterior portions, and even in instances in which at first the symptoms point to total involvement there is often a disappearance of a large part of the phenomena after a short time. Thus, when the pyramidal tract is destroyed the arm may be affected more than the leg, or *vice versa.* The facial paralysis is usually slight, though if the lesion be well forward in the capsule the paralysis of the face and tongue may be marked.

The bilaterally innervated muscles of the upper face, of mastication, of deglutition, phonation, and of the trunk muscles are very slightly involved. The patient can wrinkle the forehead, and close the eye on the affected side, but the muscles may be weak, as shown by lessened respiratory movement on the paralyzed side.

Hemianesthesia alone without involvement of the motor fibres is rare. There is usually also at least partial paralysis of the leg. When the retrolenticular portion of the capsule is destroyed the hemianesthesia is accompanied by hemianopia, disturbance of hearing, and sometimes of smell and taste. Hemianesthesia with pain, hemichorea, marked tremor or hemiathetosis—thalamic syndrome—after a capsular hemiplegia point to involvement of the thalamus or the hypothalamic region.

Capsular lesions when pure are not usually accompanied by aphasic symptoms, alexia or agraphia. A "subcortical" motor aphasia may result if the lesion is bilateral, as in pseudobulbar paralysis, or if on the left side it is so extensive as to destroy the fibres connecting Broca's convolution with the opposite hemisphere, as well as the pyramidal fibres on the same side.

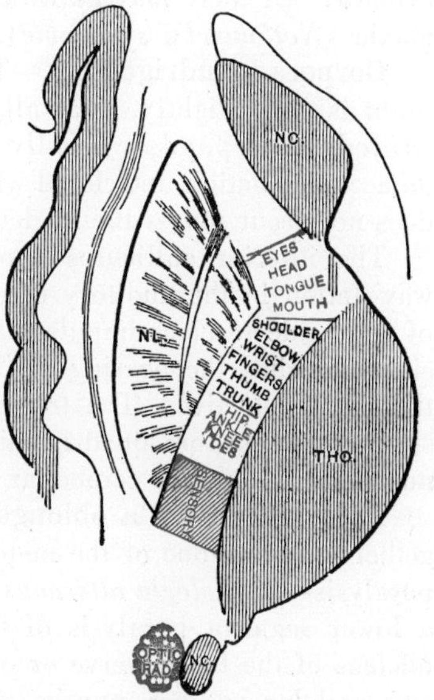

Fig. 20.—Diagram of Motor and Sensory Representation in the Internal Capsule.

NL., Lenticular nucleus. NC., Caudate nucleus. THO., Optic thalamus. The motor paths are red and black, the sensory are blue.

Crura (Cerebral Peduncles).—From this level through the pons, medulla, and cord the upper and lower motor segments are represented, the first by the fibres of the pyramidal tracts and by the fibres which go from the cortex to the nuclei of the cerebral nerves, the latter by the motor nuclei and the nerve fibres arising from them. Lesions often affect both motor segments, and produce paralysis having the characteristics of each. Thus a single lesion may involve the pyramidal tract and cause a spastic paralysis on the opposite side of the body, and also involve the nucleus or the fibres of one of the cerebral nerves, and so produce a lower segment paralysis on the same side as the lesion—crossed paralysis. In the crus the third and fourth cerebral nerves run near the pyramidal tract, and a lesion of this region is apt to involve them or their nuclei, causing partial paralysis of the muscles of the eye on the same side as the lesions, combined with a hemiplegia of the opposite side (*Weber-Gubler syndrome*) (Fig. 21, 3).

The optic tract also crosses the crus and may be involved, giving hemianopsia in the opposite halves of the visual fields.

If the tegmentum be the seat of a lesion which does not involve the base of the peduncle (or pes) there may be disturbances of cutaneous and muscular sensibility, ataxia, disturbances of hearing, or oculomotor paralysis. An oculomotor paralysis of one side, accompanied by a hemiataxia of the opposite side, appears to be especially characteristic of a tegmental lesion (*Benedikt's syndrome*). Or there may be with the crossed paralysis the features of cerebellar ataxia (*Nothnagel's syndrome*).

Corpora quadrigemina.—The chief functions are visual and auditory. Sight is only slightly, if at all, disturbed when the superior colliculus is destroyed. The pupil is usually widened, and the reactions, both to light and on accommodation, interfered with. Apparently actual paralysis of eye muscles does not occur unless the nucleus of the third nerve is also injured.

The inferior colliculus (posterior quadrigeminal body) is an important way-station in the auditory conduction path. Since the central auditory path of each side receives impulses from both ears, lesion of the colliculus on one side may dull the hearing on both sides, though the opposite ear is usually the more defective. The tremor and ataxia which sometimes accompany lesions of the corpora quadrigemina are probably due to involvement of the red nucleus and superior cerebellar peduncles.

Pons and Medulla oblongata.—Lesions involving the pyramidal tract, together with any one of the motor cerebral nerves of this region, cause crossed paralysis—*hemiplegia alternans.* A lesion in the lower part of the pons causes a lower segment paralysis of the face on the same side (destruction of the nucleus of the facial nerve or of its root fibres) and a spastic paralysis of the arm and leg on the opposite side (injury to pyramidal tract) (Fig. 21, 4). This is referred to as alternate hemiplegia or the Millard-Gubler type. The abducens, the motor part of the trigeminus, and the hypoglossus nerves may also be paralyzed in the same manner. When the central fibres to the nucleus of the hypoglossus are involved a peculiar form of anarthria results. If the nucleus itself be diseased, swallowing is interfered with.

When the sensory fibres of the fifth nerve are interrupted, together with the sensory tract for the rest of the body, which has already crossed the middle line, there is a crossed sensory paralysis—*i.e.,* disturbed sensation in the distribution of the fifth on the side of the lesion, and of all the rest of the body on the opposite side—*hemianesthesia cruciata.*

A paralysis of the external rectus muscle of one eye and of the internal rectus of the other eye (conjugate paralysis of the muscles which turn the eyes to one side), in the absence of a "forced position" of the eyeballs, is highly characteristic of certain lesions of the pons. In such cases the internal rectus may still be capable of functioning on convergence, or when the eye to which it belongs is tested independently of that in which the external rectus is paralyzed. This form, known as the Foville type of hemiplegia alternans, is found, as a rule, only when the lesion lies just in front of the abducens or involves the nucleus itself, or includes, besides the root fibres of the abducens, that portion of the formatio reticularis that lies between them and the fasciculus longitudinalis medialis (von Monakow). The facial nerve is often involved in these paralyses.

In lesions of the pons the patient often has a tendency to fall toward the side on which the lesion is, probably on account of implication of the middle peduncle of the cerebellum. Still more frequent is the simple motor hemiataxia which is often accompanied by a dissociated sensory disturbance, pain and temperature being affected, while touch remains normal. The muscular sense may also be involved. Only when the lesion is very extensive are there disturbances of hearing.

So small is the space in which important paths and nuclei are crowded that a lesion of the medulla may involve the motor tract on both sides, causing total bilateral paralysis—tetraplegia, usually due to thrombosis or to a small hemorrhage. Or the arm on one side and the leg on the other may be involved—hemiplegia cruciata.

Cerebellum.—As "the head ganglion of the proprioceptive system" (Sherrington) to this lesser brain converge the impulses of deep sensibility, and from it pass the impulses which control the tone of the muscles and their coordination when in action. In addition to its influence in maintaining equilibrium, the cerebellum has an important rôle in regulating and controlling voluntary movements. This is concerned with the muscular tone, the direction and measurement of movements, the maintenance of attitudes, and the control of coordinated movements. Hence disturbance of coordination, nystagmus, hypotonia, asthenia, ataxia (cerebellar) and volitional tremor result from diseased conditions. The disturbance may affect special functions. Ramsay Hunt described a condition, *Dyssynergia cerebellaris progressiva* or chronic progressive cerebellar tremor, in which there is a generalized volitional tremor which begins locally and gradually progresses. There is a progressive degeneration of the structures which control and regulate the muscular movements. When at rest and with the muscles relaxed the tremor ceases. Other symptoms of cerebellar disease, such as vertigo, ataxia, nystagmus and seizures are absent.

Unilateral Lesions.—As the functions of each lobe are homolateral, the symptoms are on the same side, and are negative not irritative in character. They may be grouped as follows (Gordon Holmes):

(1) *Disturbance of Muscle Tone.*—The limbs flop about in an unnatural way, and the muscles are soft and flabby. The hypotonia is so marked that the thigh can be flexed on the abdomen and the heel placed on the buttock very easily. In walking the arm swings inertly, and if the forearms are held vertically, the wrist on the affected side falls passive in extreme flexion.

(2) *Asthenia* was a feature almost constant in the war cases. It is noted when the patient holds the arms outstretched or raises a weight, and is well shown by the dynamometer. The movements are slow, a delay in initiation and in relaxation. The affected limbs tire easily.

(3) *Ataxia.*—In direction, force and range, the purposive movement errs, and with the eyes open. With the arm outstretched, asked to touch the nose with the index finger, he will bring it to the chin, and with undue force. Natural movements may be decomposed (Babinski), *e.g.*, when asked to touch the knee with the heel, instead of flexing thigh and leg together, the hip is first flexed and then the knee. This *asynergia* is due to a lack of the proper

association of agonists, antagonists and fixating muscles. The movements are ill measured (*dysmetria*), particularly quick movements, in both force and aim, and not along the shortest possible line. Tremor may occur in the moving limb, sometimes "intention" in character, or static, as in slight oscillations of the head when at rest; more characteristic is the tremor occurring in maintaining an attitude and involuntary movement (*Astasia*).

(4) *The Rebound Phenomenon.*—With elbows supported the patient pulls each hand towards his mouth against the resistance of the observer who holds the wrist. If let go suddenly, the hand on the affected side flies to the mouth often with great force, while the other is arrested almost immediately by the antagonists. This is a striking and valuable test.

(5) *Adiadokocinesis.*—In executing alternate movements as in rapid pronation and supination of the elbow, the homolateral limb moves more slowly, less regularly, and tires earlier, and there may be adventitious movements of the fingers.

(6) With *vertigo* the tendency is to fall towards the affected side, but the sensation of displacement may be of self or of external objects. It seems a more constant symptom in tumor than in injury.

(7) *The Pointing Test* (Bárány).—With closed eyes the patient is asked with his extended forefinger to touch the observer's finger held at some distance above the bed, and then as he brings the finger down to the bed and slowly up again the finger deviates outwardly.

(8) *Attitude and Gait.*—The head tends to be flexed towards the side of the lesion and rotated to the opposite side; and the body may be concave to the side of the lesion. On standing he is shaky and unsteady, and tends to fall towards the affected side, often with a feeling as if he were pulled over. The attitude may be very striking, the head and trunk inclined to the affected side, the spine concave to it, with the pelvis tilted, the shoulder lifted, the trunk rotated and held stiff. There is no Romberg sign. In walking he mistrusts the affected leg, which is usually rotated outwards, the foot may be dragged or raised unnaturally and brought to the floor with a flop. Stumbling towards the affected side, he makes efforts to control the tendency to fall. When asked to stop, he can not pull up suddenly. The arm on the affected side hangs inertly, without the normal swing.

(9) *Ocular Disturbances.*—In wounds there is early deviation of the eyes to the opposite side—or "skew deviation," the homolateral eye down and in, the other up and out. Fixation nystagmus is the rule in injury, and the oscillations are slower and larger when the patient looks to the affected side. How far it is due to coexisting labyrinthine lesion is not determined.

Among minor features to be mentioned are a slow, "sing-song" speech, the words are blurred, the articulation nasal and the end syllables explosive. The homolateral reflexes may for a time be absent. As a rule the knee jerk is less brisk, and has a pendulum character. The superficial reflexes are not changed. Sensation in any form is unchanged.

Bilateral lesions show disturbances similar to those described above, but speech is more disturbed, the muscles of the trunk and neck are very hypotonic, and naturally when standing the maintenance of equilibrium is much more difficult. The features so characteristic of unilateral lesion are not essentially changed when the *vermis* is involved, unless perhaps the tremor is more marked. The effects of cortical and nuclear lesions do not appear to differ. The war experience does not support the view of special cortical localization, or of the existence of local centres for movement in different directions (Bárány). The clinical observations confirm Luciani's conclusion that *atonia, asthenia,* and *astasia* form a characteristic cerebellar triad.

APHASIA

Under the general term aphasia—with agnosia and apraxia—is included the loss of the memories of the vocal, written, manual and other signs and symbols by which we communicate with our fellows and indicate our knowledge of the nature and use of things. As in all voluntary movements speech requires not only a motor but a sensory apparatus, and we have, as composing the speech mechanism, a sensory or receptive part as well as a motor or emissive part. These two parts are associated with the higher centres underlying the intellectual process, and are controlled by them. The problems of aphasia are probably the most complicated that exist in disease.

The muscles which are used in the production of articulate speech are many and widely distributed. These muscles are active in other less complicated movements; for instance, respiration, crying, sucking, etc., and these comparatively simple movements are represented in the gray matter of the lower motor segment in the pons, medulla and spinal cord. The association of neurones upon which these movements depend is made during fetal life, and is in good working order at the time of birth.

As the child's brain grows and takes control of the spinal centres through the medium of the pyramidal tracts, other more complex movements are developed and special neurones are set apart for this purpose. There is, then, a rerepresentation (Hughlings Jackson) of the finer movements of these muscles in the upper motor segment. They are localized in the central convolution about the lower part of the Rolandic fissure.

This group of movements, which are in part congenital and in part acquired during the early months of life, is that from which the delicate movements of articulate speech are developed. The structures upon which these movements depend make the *primary* or *elementary speech mechanism.*

The cortical centres are in the lower third of the central convolution on both sides of the brain. They are bilaterally acting centres, and a lesion limited to either one should not produce marked or permanent defects in speech. This is true for the right side, but on the left Broca's convolution is so closely situated that it or its connecting fibres are usually injured at the same time, and aphasia results. The path from the cortical centres is made up of the motor fibres which go to the nuclei of the pons and medulla, and in the internal capsule is situated near the knee. As in the cortex, a unilateral lesion here causes only slight disturbances of speech due to difficult articulation, following weakness of the opposite side of the face and tongue. On the left side, if the lesion is so near the cortex as to involve the fibres which connect Broca's convolution with the primary speech mechanism, *subcortical motor aphasia* is produced. Bilateral lesions (usually in the internal capsule, but at times in the cortex) cause speechlessness, with paralysis of the muscles of articulation—pseudobulbar paralysis. To these speech defects Bastian gave the name *aphemia* and Marie, *anarthria*.

The lower segment of the primary speech mechanism is made up of the motor nuclei in the medulla, etc., and the peripheral nerves arising from them. Lesions here, if extensive enough—as, for instance, in progressive bulbar paralysis—may cause speechlessness—anarthria (Bastian); but usually they are more limited, giving various disturbances of articulation.

The Auditory Speech Centre.—As the child learns to speak there is developed in the cortex of the brain an association of centres which takes control of the primary speech mechanism. The child is constantly hearing objects called by names, and he learns to associate certain sounds with the look, feel, taste, etc., of certain things. When he hears such a sound he gets a more or less clear mental picture, or, in other words, he has developed certain auditory memories. These memories of the sounds of words are stored in what is called the *auditory speech centre*. This centre, which in the majority of people is the controlling speech centre, is situated on the left side in right-handed people and on the right side in those who are left-handed. The afferent impressions arising in the ears reach the transverse gyri of the temporal lobes, those from each ear going to both sides of the brain. From each of these primary auditory centres impulses are sent to the auditory speech centre in the temporal lobe of the left hemisphere. The exact location of this so-called centre is not accurately determined, but it is thought to occupy the first and perhaps part of the second temporal convolutions. Marie denies all speech centres, but places the cortical region, which has to do with the intellectual processes underlying language, rather vaguely in the left temporoparietal lobe. This he designates "Wernicke's zone," a lesion of which alone can produce aphasia. The child endeavors, and by repeated efforts learns, to make the sounds that he hears, and he first becomes able to repeat words, then to speak voluntarily. To do this, he has to learn certain very delicate movements, and so there is developed a special motor centre for speech in which these movements are localized.

The Motor Speech Centre.—This was placed by Broca, and those who immediately followed him, in the posterior part of the left third frontal convolution. It is around this—Broca's centre—that the discussion started by Marie has been most heated. Marie and his followers deny that this portion of the brain has anything to do with speech, and insist that the so-called motor aphasia is merely a "combination of aphasia (of which they admit but one type, that due to lesions of Wernicke's zone) with anarthria." Anarthria they think of as a speech disturbance without any intellectual defect, due to a lesion of their lenticular zone, an ill-defined area in the centre of the brain.

Marie's position has been much discussed, and many excellent observers have come to the rescue of the old view which accepts Broca's convolution as the motor speech centre. The studies of cases of apraxia, which seem to have determined a centre in the left frontal lobe for certain purposive movements, as in the use of objects, gestures, etc., have lent support to the importance of Broca's convolution.

The motor speech centres and the corresponding area in the right brain are connected either directly by special motor fibres with the bulbar nuclei, or, as is more probable, indirectly, through the medium of the cortical centres of the primary speech mechanism in the lower part of the Rolandic region on both sides.

The speech centres are in close connection with the rest of the brain cortex, and in this way they take part in the general mental activities, of which, indeed, the speech processes form a large part. Some authors have assumed that the several sensory elements which go to make a concept are brought together in a special region of the brain, and here, as it were, united by a name. This is called "the centre for concepts," or "naming centre" (Broadbent), but most writers have followed Bastian in considering that the supposition of such a centre is unnecessary.

The mechanism which has been described is that which is developed in uneducated people and in children before they have learned to read and write, and is of primary importance in all speech processes. As the child learns to read he associates certain visual impressions with the speech memories he has acquired, and then adds to his concepts the visual memories of written or printed symbols. These memories are stored in the visual speech centre.

The Visual Speech Centre.—This is placed by nearly all authors in the angular and supramarginal convolutions on the left side, where it is believed visual impressions from both occipital lobes are combined in speech memories. Von Monakow denies such a special centre, but holds that visual speech memories are dependent upon the direct connection of the general visual centres in both occipital lobes with the speech sphere. That speech defects result from injury to the angular and supramarginal convolutions, he admits; but he thinks these are due to an interruption of fibre tracts which lie beneath and not to a destruction of a cortical centre. The distinction is, therefore, of more theoretical than practical importance. Marie includes this region in his Wernicke's zone.

In learning to write, the child develops certain delicate movements of the arm and hand, and thus acquires another method of externalizing his speech activities. Whether or not this requires the development of a separate writing centre, apart from the general Rolandic arm centre, or is brought about by an evolution of the latter through the medium of Broca's convolution, is a vexed question. Gordinier recorded a case of total agraphia, with no sensory or motor speech aphasia, in which a tumor occupying the foot of the second left frontal convolution was found at autopsy. *Agraphia* is a special form of apraxia. The movements of writing are learned under the influence of visual impressions in association with other speech memories, although there is a more direct path, which is used in copying unknown characters. Just as the movements of articulate speech are constantly under the control of auditory memories, so are the movements of writing regulated by visual memories; but in this case the other speech memories are of great importance.

With the development of the associations which underlie reading and writing, the speech mechanism may be said to be complete, although its activities are capable of practically endless extension, as when music or foreign languages are learned.

It will be seen that the cortical speech centres—the speech sphere of the French—occupy the part of the brain near the Sylvian fissure, and that they all receive their blood from the Sylvian artery. Speaking broadly, the posterior part of this region is sensory and the anterior is motor. The sensory areas are near the optic radiation and the motor are near the general motor tracts, and so, with lesions of the posterior part, hemianopia is apt to be associated with the speech disturbance while hemiplegia occurs with disease of the anterior area. These associations often help to distinguish a sensory from a motor aphasia, but each type has special characteristics.

Auditory Aphasia.—Most people in mentally recalling words do so by means of their auditory speech memories—*i. e.*, they think of the sound of the words, and, in voluntary speech, it is probable that the will acts on the motor centre indirectly through the auditory centre. This centre is also necessary for reading in such persons. There are persons, however, in whom the mental processes are carried on by visual memories, and in these "visuals" the visual speech centres take the predominant place in speech usually occupied by the auditory centres.

Complete abolition of all the auditory speech memories by destruction of the first temporal convolution causes the most extensive disturbances of speech. Such a person is unable to comprehend speech, either spoken or printed. Voluntary speech is much disturbed, and although at first he may talk, his speech is nothing but a jargon of misplaced words, and he soon becomes speechless. Writing is also lost, and he can neither repeat words nor write at dictation. He may be able to copy.

Lesions are often only partial, and the resultant disturbance may be simply a difficulty in speech due to the loss of nouns or to the transposition of words (*paraphasia*), the writing showing the same defect. The patient usually understands what he hears and reads, and can repeat words and write at dictation. Bastian called this condition "amnesia verbalis." It may be so pronounced that voluntary speech and writing are nearly lost, even when the auditory memories can still be aroused by new afferent impressions and he is able to understand what is said to him and what he reads. He can usually repeat and read aloud.

The afferent paths, which reach the auditory speech centre from the two primary auditory centres, may be destroyed. A lesion to do this must be in the white matter beneath the first temporal convolution on the left side. Such a lesion blocks all auditory impressions coming to the centre, and the patient is not able to understand anything said to him, cannot repeat words or write from dictation. As the cortical centres are not disturbed, and the auditory speech memories are still present, there is no disturbance of voluntary speech or writing, and the patient can read perfectly. This is pure word deafness or subcortical sensory aphasia.

Visual Aphasia.—Destruction of the visual centre in the angular and supramarginal convolutions causes a loss of the visual speech memories, and the patient is unable to read printed or written characters. He is unable to write—agraphia—and he can not copy. His understanding of spoken words is good, and voluntary speech is normal or only slightly paraphasic.

A subcortical lesion involving the afferent fibres going to the visual speech centre causes pure word-blindness (subcortical alexia)—*i.e.*, there is inability to understand written or printed words. Voluntary speech and writing are good. The patient can not read his own writing except by aid of muscle-sense impression, in retracing the letters, either voluntarily or passively. Associated with this is always hemianopia.

Word-deafness and word-blindness are often combined, and at times it is not only the tracts that connect the primary auditory and visual centres with the speech spheres, but also those which associate them with the other sensory centres in the formation of concepts, that are diseased. In this case the patient has lost not only his auditory and visual speech memories, but also all of his memories which have to do with hearing and sight. He has mind-deafness and mind-blindness—*i.e.*, he is unable to recognize objects when he hears or when he sees them. Further, there may be a dissociation of all the sensory centres from each other or from the higher psychical centre, which is practically the same thing, in which case the patient is entirely unable to recognize objects or use them properly—*i.e.*, he has sensory apraxia or agnosia.

Motor Aphasia.—Lesions of the motor speech zone, possibly in rare cases of Broca's convolution alone, more commonly of a wider area, cause loss of the power of speech. The patient may be absolutely dumb, or he may have retained one or two words or phrases, which is believed to be due to the activity of the corresponding region of the right brain. He will make no effort to repeat words. His mind is comparatively clear, and he understands what is said to him, but reads poorly. He has not a clear mental picture of words. This is tested by asking him to squeeze the observer's hand or to make expiratory efforts as many times as there are syllables in a well-known name. It is not often easy to obtain coöperation in this test.

Voluntary writing is usually lost in cortical motor aphasia, and many authors believe that writing movements are controlled from this centre. Others, who believe that there is a special writing centre, contend that a lesion strictly limited to the motor speech centre would not cause agraphia, and cite cases which seem to support their view. If there is much disturbance of internal speech, writing must be impaired.

Subcortical motor aphasia is described as due to the destruction of the fibres which join Broca's convolution to the primary speech mechanism. Lesions which have produced this type of aphasia have been in the white matter of the left hemisphere near Broca's convolution. These would be within Marie's lenticular zone. There is complete loss of the power of speech without any disturbance of internal speech. The patient's mental processes are not disturbed, and he can write perfectly if the hand is not paralyzed.

Cases of aphasia are rarely simple and it is often impossible to classify them accurately. The problems involved are exceedingly complicated, and the student must not suppose that cases are as straightforward as the various diagrams appear to indicate. A majority are very complex, but with patience the diagnosis of the variety can often be worked out. The following tests should be used, after the presence or absence of paralysis is determined and whether the patient is right- or left-handed: (1) The power of recognizing the nature, uses, and relations of objects—*i.e.*, whether agnosia and apraxia are present or not; (2) the power to recall the name of familiar objects seen, smelled or tasted, or of a sound when heard, or of an object touched; (3) the power to understand spoken words; (4) the capability of understanding printed or written language; (5) the power of appreciating and understanding music; (6) the power of voluntary speech—in this it is to be noted particularly whether he misplaces words or not; (7) the power of reading aloud and of understanding what he reads; (8) the power to write voluntarily and of reading what he has written; (9) the power to copy; (10) the power to write at dictation; and (11) the power of repeating words.

The *medicolegal aspects* of aphasia are of great importance. No general principle can be laid down, but each case must be considered on its merits. Langdon, in reviewing the whole question, concludes: "Sanity established, any legal document should be recognized when it can be proved that the person making it can understand fully its nature by any receptive channel (*viz.*, hearing, vision or muscular sense), and can, in addition, express assent or dissent with certainty to proper witnesses, whether this expression be by spoken speech, written speech or pantomime."

Prognosis.—In young persons the outlook is good, and the speech is gradually restored apparently by the development of other portions of the brain. The opposite hemisphere often takes part in this. In adults the condition is less hopeful, particularly in complete motor aphasia with right hemiplegia. The patient may remain speechless, though capable of understanding everything, and attempts at reeducation may be futile. Partial recovery may occur, and the patient may be able to talk, but misplaces words. In sensory aphasia the condition may be only transient, and the different forms rarely persist alone without impairment of the powers of expression.

The *education* of an aphasic person requires the greatest care and patience, particularly if, as often happens, he is emotional and irritable. It is best to begin by the use of detached letters, and advance slowly to words of only one syllable. Children often make rapid progress, but in adults failure is only too frequent, even after the most painstaking efforts. In right-sided hemiplegia with aphasia the patient may be taught to write with the left hand.

AFFECTIONS OF THE BLOOD VESSELS

ARTERIOSCLEROSIS—CEREBRAL FEATURES

(1) Transient Paralysis.—With hypertension and sclerotic vessels attacks of aphasia, monoplegia and hemiplegia occur, with the following characters: they are transient, leave no permanent damage and recur. Pure cases of motor aphasia are met with—a twelve to twenty-four hour inability to speak, without any mental disturbance. Monoplegia of the arm alone, or with the face, is more common than hemiplegia. A patient may have scores of attacks over many years. Numbness and tingling or twitching of the angle of the mouth or the hand may precede an attack. One patient had transient hemianopia. Sudden paraplegia may come on and last part of a day. Coming down the gangway of a steamer, a friend who had had many attacks of monoplegia suddenly lost power in the legs, and had to be carried. He could walk next day. Another dropped in the street, and when seen twelve hours later, the paralysis was just disappearing and the reflexes obtainable. These are not attacks of intermittent claudification. Hypertensive attacks may be responsible. The possible influence of increased concentration or viscosity of the blood, as from vomiting or diarrhea, should be considered. It may also have an influence in apoplexy. It is important to prevent dehydration in old persons. Inman emphasized the importance of *slowing* of the cerebral circulation in explaining the temporary disturbances in arteriosclerosis and as also favoring thrombosis. He warns against fatigue and suggests exercises, with the patient lying down, especially of the abdominal muscles, to aid the splanchnic circulation.

(2) Convulsions may occur with the above attacks or independently. The attack rarely has the graded features of true epilepsy, but there are widespread clonic movements, with unconsciousness for a few minutes to an hour. There may be daily attacks and transient paralysis may follow on aphasia. The general condition may remain good and the mental state undamaged.

(3) Psychical Changes.—Following a convulsion, the patient may be dazed and "not himself" for some hours. A remarkable feature in many cases is the retention of exceptional mental vigor. A transient mental outburst may replace, as it were, the motor attack. One subject of innumerable monoplegias would waken at night, stamp about the room, tear up books and papers, all the time talking to himself. He would know nothing about it in the morning. Similar outbursts occurred in the day. A transient cloud may pass over the mind before the onset of hemiplegia. Returning from a game of golf, a man did not know his house or recognize his wife and surroundings. After a good night's rest he woke with weakness of the right side and confusion of speech which had gone by the evening.

As the disease progresses, the mental state may fail, but in contradistinction to the presenile and senile types of dementia, many of these patients keep a clear mind and there are none of the features of Binswanger's *dementia presenilis* or of Alzheimer's disease. An explanation of these attacks is not easy. Their frequency and the rapid restoration of function rule out destructive lesions. Possibly they are due to spasm of the arteries and a temporary ischemia, a view strongly supported by similar attacks in Raynaud's disease, or to a temporary edema.

Clinically there are three groups of cases: (1) The arteriosclerosis of middle-aged men; (2) the senile form; and (3) special presenile forms.

(1) ARTERIOSCLEROSIS (see p. 860 under diseases of the arteries).

(2) SENILE ARTERIOSCLEROSIS.—Old age is largely a question of the blood vessels, but the wear and tear of life affects different parts in different persons. With the progressive weakening of the mental powers as age advances, widespread changes in the arteries, both basal and cortical, are found. Often it is not a question of the petrol tank—the blood supply—but the whole machine is worn out. A real mental vigor may exist with advanced arteriosclerosis. A man of sixty in full practice at the bar died suddenly of angina pectoris. The basal arteries were pipestems, and the smaller cortical vessels creaked under the knife!

In a normal old age the convolutions waste, the pigment granules and the lime salts increase, the meninges become cloudy, the cortical arteries thicken, the glia in the gray matter increases particularly about the smaller vessels, and there are the areas of atrophy, as described by Marie, Peck and others. With these organic changes the mental grip fails, the memory weakens, the emotions are less under control, and year by year in a slow process of devolution the last stage of all is reached, second childhood—babyhood rather—as the man ends as he began, with only a vegetative system.

This happy, normal process with "mild gradations of decay," recognized by all except the senile himself, bears out Plato's dictum that "old age is an easy death." But it may be far otherwise, and "the evening of life may be a stormy and unhappy period." The peculiarities of the individual become more marked and to an unpleasant degree; he becomes egotistical, emotional and suspicious, or careless in the minor proprieties of life and intensely selfish. The most pathetic of martyrdoms are the miseries endured by children in the unrequited, unappreciated devotion to an irritable, egotistical, self-centered senile parent. But the pity of it is that the worst troubles may not be intensification of any personal peculiarities, but terrible perversions of character of a distressing nature. The man of active useful life may be depressed to distraction by the thought of the failure he has been; the godly man is worried over his lost soul; the moral teacher and saintly soul may become a lecher; or the loving affectionate husband a brutal tyrant.

3. Special Types.—While in normal old age there is nothing local, on the other hand, the senility may be chiefly local and affect the brain at a comparatively early age. The changes are usually those of normal old age, and associated with loss of judgment, emotional perversions and progressive mental impairment. The cardiovascular and renal conditions play an important rôle in these cases (Southard). Various forms have been described,—the *presbyophrenia* of Wernicke—characterized by "marked disturbances of the recording faculty, with retention for a long time of orderly thought and judgment . . . and tendency to confabulation" (Barker). Binswanger's *dementia presenilis* begins between the ages of 40 and 50, with loss of memory, apathy, etc., without syphilis or the somatic feature of *general paresis*. *Alzheimer's* disease is a slow dementia with focal symptoms, aphasia and apraxia, and in addition to the regressive changes in the vessels and glia, a peculiar condition of the neurofibrils. Southard and Alford called attention to a group of senile dementias (14 of 42 cases specially studied) of obscure etiology, which do not come in these types as the vessels are not sclerotic and the convolutions are not atrophied.

HYPEREMIA AND ANEMIA

Less and less stress is now laid on these conditions. The symptoms usually referred to active hyperemia in the infectious diseases are due to the action of toxic agents rather than to changes in the circulation.

Anemia.—The anatomical condition of the brain is very striking. The membranes are pale, only the large veins are full, the small vessels over the gyri are empty, and an unusual amount of cerebrospinal fluid is present. On section both the gray and white matter look extremely pale and the cut surface is moist. Very few *puncta vasculosa* are seen.

Symptoms.—The effects of sudden anemia of the brain are well illustrated by the ordinary fainting fit. When the symptoms are the result of hemorrhage, there are drowsiness and giddiness; flashes of light, dark spots before the eyes, and noises in the ears; the respiration becomes hurried; the skin is cool and covered with sweat; the pupils are dilated, there may be vomiting, headache, or delirium, and gradually, if the bleeding continues, consciousness is lost and death may occur with convulsions. In the more chronic forms, such as result from anemia, a condition of irritable weakness results. Mental effort is difficult, the slightest irritation is followed by undue excitement, the patient complains of giddiness and noises in the ears, or there may be hallucinations or delirium. These symptoms occur in an extreme grade as a result of prolonged starvation, and a similar condition is seen in certain cases of arteriosclerosis, when the brain is poorly nourished.

An interesting set of symptoms, to which the term *hydrencephaloid* was applied by Marshall Hall, occurs in the anemia and debility produced by prolonged diarrhea in children. The child is in a semicomatose condition with the eyes open, the pupils contracted, and the fontanelle depressed. In the earlier period there may be convulsions. The coma may gradually deepen, the pupils become dilated, and there may be strabismus and even reaction of the head, symptoms which closely simulate those of basilar meningitis.

EDEMA OF THE BRAIN

Whether it occurs as a clinical entity is doubtful. As a secondary process it occurs under the following conditions: In general atrophy of the convolutions, in which case the edema is represented by an increase in the cerebrospinal fluid and in that of the meshes of the pia. In extreme venous dilatation from obstruction, as in mitral stenosis or tumors, there may be congestive edema, in which, with great filling of the blood vessels, the substance of the brain is unusually moist. The most acute edema is a local process around tumors and abscesses. The symptoms of compression following concussion or contusion, as shown by Cannon, are frequently attributable to cerebral edema due to change in osmotic pressure. An intense infiltration, local or general; may occur in nephritis, and to it certain uremic symptoms may be due. There is a form, "wet brain," found in alcoholics.

Anatomical Changes.—These are not unlike those of anemia. When the edema follows progressive atrophy, the fluid is chiefly within and beneath the membranes. The brain substance is anemic and moist and has a wet, glistening appearance, which is very characteristic. In some instances the edema is more intense and local, and the brain substance may look infiltrated with fluid. The amount of fluid in the ventricles is usually increased.

Symptoms.—These are in great part those of lessened blood flow and are not well defined. Some of the cerebral features of uremia may depend upon it. Cases have been reported in which unilateral convulsions or paralysis occurred in chronic nephritis, and in which the condition appeared to be associated with edema of the brain. The older writers laid great stress upon an apoplexia serosa, which may have been a general edema of the brain. Some cases of transient paralysis or aphasia may be caused by edema.

Treatment.—Associated conditions require the proper treatment. Lumbar puncture is indicated and should be repeated when necessary. The bowels should be freely moved by salines. In the "wet brain" of alcoholism ergot in full doses is useful.

CEREBRAL HEMORRHAGE

The bleeding may come from branches of either of the two great groups of cerebral vessels—the *basal,* comprising the circle of Willis and the central arteries passing from it and from the first portion of the cerebral arteries, or the *cortical group,* the anterior, middle and posterior cerebral vessels. In a majority of cases the hemorrhage is from the central branches, more particularly from those given off by the middle cerebral arteries in the anterior perforated spaces, and which supply the corpora striata and internal capsules. One of the largest of these branches which passes to the third division of the lenticular nucleus and to the anterior part of the internal capsule, the lenticulostriate artery, is so frequently involved in hemorrhage that it was called by Charcot *the artery of cerebral hemorrhage.* Hemorrhages from this and from the lenticulothalamic artery include more than 60 per cent of all cerebral hemorrhages. The bleeding may be into the substance of the brain, to which alone the term cerebral apoplexy is applied, or into the membranes (meningeal hemorrhage); both are usually included under the terms intracranial or cerebral hemorrhage.

Etiology.—High blood pressure and arterial disease in persons over forty years of age are the main factors.

Age.—After thirty the liability increases with each decade. It may be congenital as in the child of a woman dead of typhoid fever. It occasionally occurs in children from rupture of a small aneurism, but before the age of thirty it is very uncommon. Of 154 cases at St. Bartholomew's Hospital traceable to arterial changes there was no case under thirty; the maximum for both sexes was at the fifty-sixth year. After sixty the numbers appear to decline, but if "due correction is made for the age-distribution of a population, the liability of the individual to this form of death increases steadily up to old age" (F. W. Andrewes). Before the fifth decade hemorrhage is rare; then in the fifth and sixth decades cases progressively increase in number.

Sex.—There is a marked preponderance of males.

Heredity.—Formerly thought to be a very important factor, heredity influences the incidence in rendering members of families in which the blood vessels degenerate early more liable to cerebral hemorrhage. What was known as the apoplectic habitus, or build, is still spoken of, by which we mean a stout, plethoric person of medium size with a short neck.

Special Factors.—Individuals with progressive renal disease and consecutive arteriosclerosis and hypertrophy of the heart are particularly liable to cerebral hemorrhage. Alcohol, immoderate eating, prolonged muscular exertion, syphilis, and gout are antecedents in many cases. Endocarditis may lead indirectly to apoplexy by causing embolism and aneurism of the vessels of the brain. Hemorrhage may occur with new growths. Cerebral hemorrhage occurs occasionally in the specific fevers and in leukemia.

The actual exciting cause is not always evident. The attacks may be sudden without any preliminary symptoms. In other instances straining efforts or overaction of the heart may cause a rupture. Some cases occur during sleep or follow slight trauma. The records of University College Hospital analyzed by Ernest Jones indicate that in none of 123 cases did the attack come on through excessive bodily effort.

Morbid Anatomy.—Direct Changes.—The lesions are almost invariably in the cerebral arteries, in which the following changes may lead to it:

(*a*) The rupture of miliary aneurisms is a common cause. They occur most frequently on the central arteries, but also on the smaller branches of the cortical vessels. On section they may be seen as localized, small dark bodies, about the size of a pin's head. Sometimes they are seen in numbers upon the arteries when withdrawn from the anterior perforated spaces.

(*b*) Aneurism of the branches of the circle of Willis. These are by no means uncommon, and will be considered subsequently.

(*c*) Endarteritis and periarteritis in the cerebral vessels most commonly lead to hemorrhage by the production of aneurisms, either miliary or coarse. There are instances in which the most careful search fails to reveal anything but diffuse degeneration of the cerebral vessels.

(*d*) Whether hemorrhage ever occurs by *diapedesis* without actual rupture is doubtful. It is tempting to assume this explanation in certain mild cases with slight signs. Possibly it does in purpura.

(*e*) In persons over sixty the hemiplegia may depend upon small areas of softening in the gray matter—the *lacunae* of Marie—varying in size from a pin's head to a pea or a small bean, grayish red in tint. The lenticular nucleus is particularly apt to be involved. The blood vessels are always diseased.

The hemorrhage may be meningeal, cerebral or intraventricular.

Meningeal hemorrhage may be outside the dura, between dura and arachnoid, or between the arachnoid and the pia mater. The following are the chief causes: Fracture of the skull, in which case the blood usually comes from the lacerated meningeal vessels, sometimes from the torn sinuses. In these cases the blood is usually outside the dura or between it and the arachnoid. The next most frequent cause is rupture of aneurisms on the larger cerebral vessels. The blood is usually subarachnoid. An intracerebral hemorrhage may burst into the meninges. A special form of meningeal hemorrhage is found in the newborn, associated with injury during birth. And lastly, meningeal hemorrhage may occur in the constitutional diseases and fevers. The blood may be in a large quantity at the base and extend into the cord or upon the cortex. Owing to the frequency of aneurisms in the middle cerebral vessels, the Sylvian fissures are often distended with blood.

Intracerebral hemorrhage is most frequent in the neighborhood of the corpus striatum, particularly toward the outer section of the lenticular nucleus. The hemorrhage may be small and limited to the lenticular body, the thalamus, and the internal capsule, or it may extend to the insula. Hemorrhages confined to the white matter—the centrum semiovale—are rare. Localized bleeding may occur in the crura or in the pons. Hemorrhage into the cerebellum usually comes from the superior cerebellar artery. The extravasation may be limited to the substance or may rupture into the fourth ventricle. It is suggested that primary necrosis of nervous tissue may be responsible for hemorrhage.

Ventricular Hemorrhage.—This is rarely primary, coming from the vessels of the plexuses or of the walls. More often it is secondary, following hemorrhage into the cerebral substance. It is not infrequent in early life and may occur during birth. Of 94 cases collected by Edward Sanders, 7 occurred during the first year, and 14 under the twentieth year. In adults it is almost always caused by rupture of a vessel in the neighborhood of the caudate nucleus. The blood may be found in one ventricle only, but more commonly it is in both lateral ventricles, and may pass into the third ventricle and through the aqueduct of Sylvius into the fourth ventricle, forming a complete mould in blood of the ventricular system. In these cases the clinical picture may be that of "*apoplexie foudroyante.*"

Multiple Hemorrhages.—Of 128 nontramuatic cases at the Cook County Hospital there were 28 with discrete multiple hemorrhages. The most common form is hemorrhage into the basal ganglia and into the pons; the next, bilateral basal hemorrhage. In the brain compression following hemorrhage, the blood pressure rises; this increased intracranial tension is doubtless the cause of rupture in other vessels weakened by disease. The pontine arteries seem specially susceptible, as the small terminal vessels come off at right angles to a very large trunk (Phyllis Greenacre).

Subsequent Changes.—If the hemorrhage is of any extent there is compression of the brain, which, with a secondary edema, may play a part in causing coma. The blood gradually changes in color, and ultimately the hemoglobin is converted into hematoidin. Inflammation occurs about the area, limiting it, and ultimately a definite wall may be produced, inclosing a cyst with fluid contents. In other instances a cyst is not formed, but the connective tissue proliferates and leaves a pigmented scar. In meningeal hemorrhage the effused blood may be gradually absorbed and leave only a staining of the membranes. In other cases, particularly in infants, when the effusion is cortical and abundant, there may be localized wasting of the convolutions and the production of a cyst in the meninges. Possibly porencephaly may arise in this way. Secondary degeneration follows, involving various tracts according to the location of the hemorrhage and the damage done by it to nerve cells or their medullated axones.

Symptoms.—Primary.—Premonitory indications are rare. As a rule, the patient is seized while in full health or in the performance of some every day action, occasionally an action requiring strain or extra exertion. There may be headache, sensations of numbness or tingling or pains in the limbs, or even choreiform movements in the muscles of the opposite side, the so-called prehemiplegic chorea. In other cases temporary disturbances of vision and of associated movements of the eye muscles have been noted, but none of the prodromata of apoplexy (the so-called "warnings") are characteristic. Transient aphasia or monoplegia may precede the attack. The onset may be with sudden loss of consciousness and complete relaxation of the extremities. This is common with hemorrhage into the ventricles. In such instances the name *apoplectic stroke* is particularly appropriate. In other cases it is more gradual and the loss of consciousness may not occur for a few minutes after the patient has fallen, or after the paralysis of the limbs is manifest. In the typical apoplectic attack the condition is as follows: There is deep unconsciousness; the patient can not be roused. The face is injected, sometimes cyanotic, or of an ashen gray hue. The pupils vary; usually they are dilated, sometimes unequal, and always, in deep coma, inactive. If the hemorrhage be so located that it can irritate the nucleus of the third nerve the pupils are contracted (hemorrhages into the pons or ventricles). The respirations are slow, noisy, and accompanied with stertor. Sometimes Cheyne-Stokes rhythm may be present. The chest movements on the paralyzed side may be restricted, in rare instances on the opposite side. The cheeks are often blown out during expiration, with spluttering of the lips. The pulse is usually full, slow, and of increased tension. The temperature may be normal, but is often subnormal. In basal hemorrhage the temperature may be high. The urine and feces are usually passed involuntarily. Convulsions are not common. It may be difficult to decide whether the condition is apoplexy with hemiplegia or sudden coma from other causes. An indication of hemiplegia may be discovered in the difference in the tonus of the muscles on the two sides. If the arm or the leg is lifted, it drops "dead" on the affected side, while on the other it falls more slowly. The lack of muscular tone of the paralyzed limb may be determined by inspection; the muscle mass of the thigh acts like a semifluid sac and takes the shape determined by gravity. In a patient lying or sitting on a firm support, the thigh of the paralyzed limb is broadened or flattened, while that on the normal side has a more rounded contour. Rigidity may be present, especially in some cases of middle meningeal hemorrhage. In watching the movements of the facial muscles in the stertorous respiration it will be seen that on the paralyzed side the cheek is blown out in a more marked manner. The head and eyes may be turned to one side—conjugate deviation. Sudden death is exceptionally rare and death hardly ever occurs under some hours.

In other cases, in which the onset is not so abrupt, the patient may not lose consciousness, but in a few hours there is loss of power, unconsciousness comes on gradually, and deepens into profound coma—ingravescent apoplexy. The attack may occur during sleep; the patient may be found unconscious or wakes to find that the power is lost on one side. Small hemorrhages in the territory of the central arteries may cause hemiplegia without loss of consciousness. In old persons the hemiplegia may be slight and follow a transient loss of consciousness, and is usually most marked in the leg. It is associated with other senile changes. This form is often due to the presence of lacunar softening.

Usually within forty-eight hours after the onset, sometimes within from two to six hours, there is fever with some constitutional disturbance associated with inflammatory changes about the hemorrhage and absorption of the blood. The period of inflammatory reaction may continue for from one week to two months. The patient may die in this reaction, or, if consciousness has been regained, there may be delirium or recurrence of the coma. At this period early rigidity may develop in the paralyzed limbs and trophic changes occur, such as sloughing or the formation of vesicles. The most serious of these is the sloughing eschar of the lower part of the back, or on the paralyzed side, which may appear within forty-eight hours of the onset and is usually of grave significance. The common congestion at the bases of the lungs is regarded by some as a trophic change.

Conjugate Deviation.—In a flaccid paralysis the eyes and sometimes the head may be turned away from the paralyzed side, that is, the eyes look toward the cerebral lesion. This is almost the rule in hemiplegia, When, however, convulsions or spasm occur or the state of so-called early rigidity, the conjugate deviation of the head and eyes may be in the opposite direction; that is to say, the eyes look away from the lesion and the head is rotated toward the convulsed side.

Hemiplegia.—When consciousness is restored and the patient improves, a unilateral paralysis may persist due to the destruction of the motor area or the pyramidal tract in any part of its course. Hemiplegia is complete when it involves face, arm, and leg, or partial when it involves only one or other of these parts. This may be the result of a lesion (*a*) of the motor cortex; (*b*) of the pyramidal fibres in the corona radiata and in the internal capsule; (*c*) of a lesion in the cerebral peduncle; or (*d*) in the pons Varolii. The situation of the lesions and their effects are given in Fig. 21. Vascular lesions are perhaps the most common cause, but tumors and areas of softening may also induce it. The special details of the hemiplegia may be considered. The face (except in lesions in the lower part of the pons) is involved on the same side as the arm and leg. This results from the fact that the facial muscles stand in precisely the same relation to the cortical centres as those of the arm and leg. The signs of facial paralysis are usually well marked. There may be a slight difficulty in elevating the eyebrows or in closing the eye on the paralyzed side, or in rare cases, the facial paralysis is complete, but the movements may be present with emotion, as laughing or crying. The facial paralysis is partial, involving only the lower portion of the nerve, so that the orbicularis oculi and the frontalis muscles are much less involved than the lower branch. The hypoglossal nerve also is involved. In consequence, the patient can not put out the tongue straight, but it deviates toward the paralyzed side, inasmuch as the geniohyoglossus of the sound side is unopposed. In a few cases the protrusion is toward the side of the lesion, a fact not easily explained. With right hemiplegia there may be aphasia. Even without marked aphasia difficulty and slowness in speaking are common.

The arm is, as a rule, more completely paralyzed than the leg. The loss of power may be absolute or partial. In severe cases it is at first complete. In others, when the paralysis in the face and arm is complete, that of the leg is only partial. The face and arm may alone be paralyzed, while the leg escapes. Less commonly the leg is more affected than the arm, and the face may be only slightly involved.

Certain muscles escape in hemiplegia, particularly those associated in symmetrical movements, as those of the thorax and abdomen, which Broadbent explains by supposing that as the spinal nuclei controlling these movements on both sides constantly act together they may, by means of this intimate connection, be stimulated by impulses coming from only one side of the brain. Hughlings Jackson pointed out that in quiet respiration the muscles on the paralyzed side act more strongly than the corresponding muscles, but that in forced respiration the reverse condition is true.

The degree of *permanent paralysis* after a hemiplegic attack varies greatly. When the restitution is partial, it is always certain groups of muscles which recover rather than others. Thus in the leg the residual paralysis concerns the flexors of the leg and the dorsal flexors of the foot—*i.e.*, the muscles which are active in the second period of walking, shortening the leg, and bringing it forward while it swings. The muscles which lift the body when the foot rests upon the ground, those used in the first period of walking, include the extensors of the leg and the plantar flexors of the foot. These "lengtheners" of the leg often recover almost completely when the paralysis is due to lesions of the pyramidal tract. In the arms the residual paralysis usually affects the muscle groups which oppose the thumb, those which rotate the arm outward, and the openers of the hand. As a rule, there is at first no wasting of the paralyzed limbs.

Crossed Hemiplegia.—A paralysis in which there is loss of function in a cerebral nerve on one side with loss of power (or of sensation) on the opposite side of the body is called a crossed or alternate hemiplegia. It is met with in lesions, commonly hemorrhage, in the crus, the pons, and the medulla.

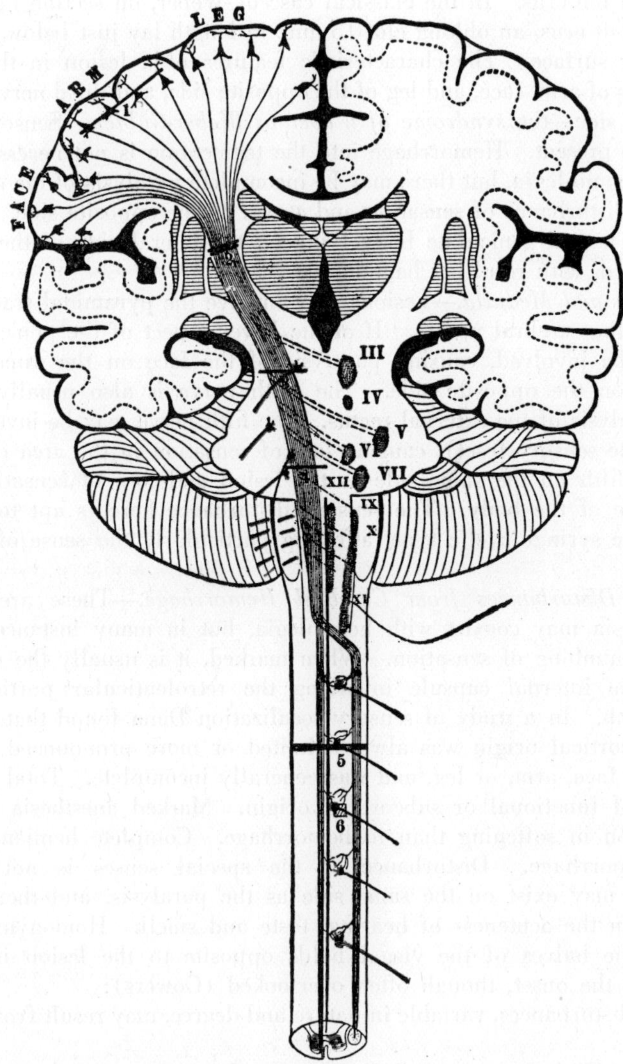

FIG. 21.—DIAGRAM OF MOTOR PATH FROM LEFT BRAIN.

The upper segment is black, the lower red. The nuclei of the motor cerebral nerves are shown on the right side; on the left side the cerebral nerves of that side are indicated. A lesion at 1 would cause upper segment paralysis in the arm of the opposite side—cerebral monoplegia; at 2, upper segment paralysis of the whole opposite side of the body—hemiplegia; at 3 (in the crus), upper segment paralysis of the opposite face, arm, and leg, and lower segment paralysis of the eye-muscles on the same side—crossed paralysis; at 4 (in the lower part of the pons), upper segment paralysis of the opposite arm and leg, and lower segment paralysis of the face and external rectus on the same side—crossed paralysis; at 5, upper segment paralysis of all muscles represented below lesion, and lower segment paralysis of muscles represented at level of lesion—spinal paraplegia; at 6, lower segment paralysis of muscles localized at seat of lesion—anterior poliomyelitis. (Van Gehuchten, modified.)

(*a*) *Crus.*—The bleeding may extend from vessels supplying the corpus striatum, internal capsule, and optic thalamus, or the hemorrhage may be primarily in the crus. In the classical case of Weber, on section of the lower part of the left crus, an oblong clot 15 mm. in length lay just below the medial and inferior surface. The characteristic features of a lesion in this locality are paralysis of arm, face, and leg of the opposite side, and third nerve paralysis of the same side—the *syndrome of Weber* or *Weber-Gubler.* Sensory changes may also be present. Hemorrhage into the tegmentum is not necessarily associated with hemiplegia, but there may be incomplete paralysis of the oculomotor nerve, with disturbance of sensation and ataxia on the opposite side. The optic tract or the lateral geniculate body lying on the lateral side of the crus may be compressed, with resulting hemianopia.

(*b*) *Pons and Medulla.*—Lesions may involve the pyramidal tract and one or more of the cerebral nerves. If at the lower aspect of the pons, the facial nerve may be involved, causing paralysis of the face on the same side and hemiplegia on the opposite side. The sixth nerve is also usually involved, causing paralysis of the external rectus. The fifth nerve may be involved, with the fillet (the sensory tract), causing loss of sensation in the area of distribution of the fifth on the same side as the lesion and loss of sensation on the opposite side of the body. The sensory disturbance here is apt to be dissociated, of the syringomyelic type, affecting particularly the sense of pain and temperature.

Sensory Disturbances from Cerebral Hemorrhage.—These are variable. Hemianesthesia may coexist with hemiplegia, but in many instances there is only slight numbing of sensation. When marked, it is usually the result of a lesion in the internal capsule involving the retrolenticular portion of the posterior limb. In a study of sensory localization Dana found that anesthesia of organic cortical origin was always limited or more pronounced in certain parts, as the face, arm, or leg, and was generally incomplete. Total anesthesia was either of functional or subcortical origin. Marked anesthesia was much more common in softening than in hemorrhage. Complete hemianesthesia is rare in hemorrhage. Disturbance of the special senses is not common. Hemianopia may exist on the same side as the paralysis, and there may be diminution in the acuteness of hearing, taste and smell. Homonymous hemianopia of the halves of the visual fields opposite to the lesion is frequent shortly after the onset, though often overlooked (Gowers).

Psychic disturbances, variable in nature and degree, may result from cerebral hemorrhage.

Reflexes.—With deep coma due to increased intracranial pressure the knee jerks and abdominal reflexes may be absent on both sides with a bilateral extensor plantar reflex. Later they may return on the nonhemiplegic side. On the hemiplegic side the lost reflexes may return only after weeks. As to the time of return, especially of the patellar reflexes, marked differences are observable. The deep reflexes later are increased on the paralyzed side, and ankle clonus may be present. Plantar stimulation gives an extensor response in the great toe (Babinski's sign) or dorsal flexion of the foot on irritating the skin over the tibia (Oppenheim's sign). The other superficial reflexes are usually diminished. The sphincters are not affected.

The *course* depends upon the situation and extent of the lesion. If slight, the hemiplegia may disappear completely within a few days or a few weeks. In severe cases the rule is that the leg gradually recovers before the arm, and the muscles of the shoulder girdle and upper arm before those of the forearm and hand. The face may recover quickly.

Except in the very slight lesions, in which the hemiplegia is transient, changes take place which may be grouped as

SECONDARY.—These correspond to the chronic stage. In a patient in whom little or no improvement takes place within eight or ten weeks it will be found that the paralyzed limbs undergo certain changes. The leg, as a rule, recovers enough power to enable the patient to get about, although the foot is dragged. Occasionally a recurrence of severe symptoms is seen, even without a new hemorrhage. In both arm and leg the condition of *secondary contraction* or *late rigidity* comes on, always most marked in the arm which becomes permanently flexed at the elbow and resists all attempts at extension. The wrist is flexed upon the forearm and the fingers upon the hand. The position of the arm and hand is very characteristic. There is frequently, as the contractures develop, a great deal of pain. In the leg the contracture is rarely so extreme. The loss of power is most marked in the muscles of the foot and, to prevent the toes from dragging, the knee in walking is much flexed, or more commonly the foot is swung round in a half circle.

The *reflexes* are greatly increased at this stage. These contractures are permanent and incurable, and are associated with a secondary descending sclerosis of the motor path. There are cases in which rigidity and contracture do not occur, but the arm remains flaccid, the leg having regained its power. This *hémiplégie flasque* of Bouchard is found most commonly in children. Among other secondary changes are: Tremor of the affected limbs, postparalytic chorea, athetosis, arthropathies on the affected side, muscular atrophy and thin glossy skin of the hemiplegic limb.

Atrophy of the muscles may occur, thought to be due in some cases to secondary alterations in the gray matter of the ventral horns; but atrophy may follow as a direct result of the cerebral lesion, the ventral horns remaining intact. These atrophies are most common in cortical lesions involving the domain of the third main branch of the Sylvian artery, and in central lesions involving the lenticulothalamic region. Their explanation is not clear. The wasting of cerebral origin, which occurs most frequently in children and leads to hemiatrophy of the muscles with stunted growth, is to be sharply separated from the hemiatrophy of the muscles of the adult following within a relatively short time upon the hemiplegia.

Basal hemorrhage.—This shows disturbances of consciousness, severe occipital headache, rigidity of the neck, Kernig's sign, cranial nerve paralysis and blood-stained cerebrospinal fluid, varying from bright red to yellow.

Diagnosis.—There are three groups of cases which offer difficulty:

(1) Cases in which the onset is gradual, a day or two elapsing before the paralysis is fully developed, are readily recognized, though it may be difficult to determine whether the lesion is due to thrombosis or hemorrhage.

(2) In the sudden apoplectic stroke in which the patient rapidly loses consciousness the difficulty in diagnosis may be still greater, particularly if the patient is in deep coma when first seen.

The first point to be decided is the existence of hemiplegia. This may be difficult, although, as a rule, even in deep coma the limbs on the paralyzed side are more flaccid and drop instantly when lifted; whereas on the nonparalyzed side the muscles retain some degree of tonus. One cheek may puff or one side of the mouth splutter in expiration. The reflexes may be decreased or lost on the affected side and there may be conjugate deviation of the head and eyes. Rigidity in the limbs on one side is in favor of a hemiplegic lesion. It is difficult in a majority of these cases to say whether the lesion is due to hemorrhage, embolism, or thrombosis.

(3) Large hemorrhage into the ventricles or into the pons may produce sudden loss of consciousness with complete relaxation, simulating coma from uræmia, diabetes, alcoholism, opium poisoning or epilepsy.

The previous history and the mode of onset may give valuable information. In *epilepsy* convulsions have preceded the coma; in *alcoholism* there is a history of constant drinking, while in *opium poisoning* the coma develops more gradually, the pupils are small and the respirations slow. With *diabetic coma* the breath often smells of acetone. *Sunstroke,* pernicious forms of *malaria* and *carbon monoxide poisoning* may give difficulty. In *ventricular hemorrhage* the coma is sudden and comes on rapidly. The hemiplegic symptoms may be transient, quickly giving place to complete relaxation. Convulsions occur in some cases, and may lead one astray—as in a case of ventricular hemorrhage in a puerperal patient, in whom, naturally enough, the condition was thought to be uremic. Rigidity is often present. In hemorrhage into the *pons* convulsions are frequent. The pupils may be strongly contracted, conjugate deviation may occur, and the temperature is apt to rise rapidly. The contraction of the pupils in pontine hemorrhage naturally suggest opium poisoning. The difference in temperature in the two conditions is a valuable diagnostic point. The apoplectiform seizures of general paresis have usually been preceded by abnormal mental symptoms, and the associated hemiplegia is seldom permanent.

The cerebral attacks in *Stokes-Adams disease* may resemble apoplexy very closely. One stout patient, the subject of many attacks, had been bled so often that he had a label inside his coat—"Do not bleed me in an attack."

It may be impossible at first to give a definite diagnosis. In emergency cases the physician should be particularly careful about the following points: The examination of the head for injury or fracture; the urine should be tested for albumin and sugar, and studied microscopically; a careful examination should be made of the limbs with reference to the degree of relaxation or the presence of rigidity, and the condition of the reflexes; the state of the pupils should be noted and the temperature taken. The odor of the breath (alcohol, acetone, etc.) should be noted. The most serious mistakes are made with patients who are drunk at the time of the attack, a combination by no means uncommon. Under these circumstances the diagnosis of alcoholic coma may be made. It is best to regard each case as serious and to bear in mind that this is a condition in which, above all others, mistakes are common.

In *meningeal hemorrhage,* as from ruptured aneurism, the attack is sudden, with pain in the head, rapid loss of consciousness, bilateral flaccidity or difficulty in determining the existence of hemiplegia, rapid rise in temperature, and the presence of blood under high pressure in the spinal fluid.

Apoplexy with a sudden onset, deep coma, increasing symptoms, fever and respiratory disturbance is usually from hemorrhage. A definite sign is the finding of blood in the cerebrospinal fluid (care should be taken not to mistake blood due to the puncture as indicating hemorrhage).

Prognosis.—From cortical hemorrhage, unless extensive, the recovery may be complete without contracture. This is more common when the hemorrhage follows injury than when it results from disease of the arteries. Infantile meningeal hemorrhage may produce idiocy or spastic diplegia. Large hemorrhages into the corona radiata, and especially those which rupture into the ventricles, rapidly prove fatal. The hemiplegia with lesions of the internal capsule, from rupture of the lenticulostriate artery, is usually persistent and followed by contracture. When the retrolenticular fibres of the internal capsule are involved there may be hemianesthesia, and later, especially if the thalamus be implicated, hemichorea or athetosis.

In any case the following symptoms are of grave omen: deep coma at the onset; persistence or deepening of the coma during the second and third day; rapid rise in temperature within the first forty-eight hours after the initial fall. In the reaction which takes place on the second or third day the temperature usually rises, and its gradual fall on the third or fourth day with return of consciousness is a favorable indication. The rapid formation of bed sores is a serious sign. The occurrence of albumin and sugar, if abundant, in the urine is unfavorable.

When consciousness returns and the patient is improving, the question is anxiously asked as to the paralysis. The extent of this can not be determined for some weeks. With slight lesions it may pass off entirely. If persistent at the end of a month some grade of permanent palsy is certain to remain, and gradually the late rigidity supervenes.

The *treatment* is discussed on page 1014.

SUBARACHNOID HEMORRHAGE

Aneurisms are especially important in the arteries at the base of the brain. The varieties are (1) *arteriosclerotic*, (2) *syphilitic*, which are rare, (3) *mycotic*, and (4) those usually described as *congenital*, in which there is a defect in the media. The last generally occur where a vessel divides, are usually about the size of a currant and have been termed "berry" aneurisms. Rupture gives the syndrome of:

Spontaneous subarachnoid hemorrhage.—This is more common than we formerly recognized. It may occur at any age but usually in youth or young adult life. There may have been severe exertion previously. Exposure to sunlight has been suggested but, as Adie showed, some cases of supposed heat stroke are instances of subarachnoid hemorrhage. The *onset* is sudden with headache and vertigo, perhaps with nausea and vomiting, followed by stupor or loss of consciousness. The headache is very severe and occipital. The patient may be irritable and restless, show photophobia and be difficult to examine. In severe cases, complete coma and convulsions are followed by death. Otherwise signs of meningeal irritation appear, with rigidity of the neck, severe pain on deep pressure in the occipital region and Kernig's sign. The pupils are variable in size and may be unequal. The deep reflexes are variable. There may be involvement of the cranial nerves. Retinal hemorrhages, sometimes very large, may be found and edema of the disk. There may be some fever and leukocytosis. There may be a large amount of albumin in the urine and glycosuria in some cases. The signs suggest a serious cerebral lesion with meningeal irritation. The *spinal fluid* is uniformly and usually heavily blood stained.

The *course* is variable; if favorable the symptoms clear but there is always the danger of further bleeding. In unfavorable cases the coma increases, fever becomes higher and death follows. In general the outlook is fairly good. Some patients show curious psychical disturbances for some time after recovery.

There has been much interest in the possibility of recognizing the presence of these aneurisms before rupture. Some patients give a history suggesting migraine. Focal pressure symptoms would be difficult to interpret. If the aneurism was unusually large it might cause pressure and suggest an intracranial tumor.

Diagnosis.—With coma there are many possibilities of error. *Uremia,* if there is much albumin in the urine, *diabetic coma,* if there is glycosuria, and *heat stroke. Encephalitis* has been the diagnosis in some cases. The value of lumbar puncture is evident. With the finding of bloody fluid, trauma being excluded, hemorrhage into the ventricle and cerebral hemorrhage which has ruptured into the ventricle or subarachnoid space have to be considered. With hemorrhage into the ventricle the onset is sudden with deep coma, repeated general tonic spasms or complete flaccidity. Fever occurs rapidly and the blood pressure increases. Death usually follows in a short time. There is much the same picture with cerebral hemorrhage which ruptures into a ventricle.

Treatment.—This requires good judgment in the use of *lumbar puncture;* on the one hand is the need of relieving intracranial pressure, on the other the danger of causing further bleeding. There are differences of opinion; one suggests daily lumbar puncture for a few days and then every second day until the fluid is clear; the other advises repetition of lumbar puncture only when signs of intracranial pressure demand it. The latter seems the better plan. In any event the spinal fluid should be allowed to run very slowly and not more than 20 cc. removed at one time. It is suggested that an hour be taken to secure this amount. *Sedatives* are usually required; morphia should be given cautiously and bromide or one of the barbiturates is safer. The diet should be liquid and not more than 1000 cc. given daily. Dextrose (100 cc. of a 25 per cent solution) can be given intravenously and magnesium sulphate by mouth to reduce the intracranial pressure. Convalescence should be prolonged and the patient allowed to resume activity very gradually.

EMBOLISM AND THROMBOSIS

(*Cerebral Softening*)

Embolism.—Embolism occurs more frequently in women, owing, no doubt, to the greater frequency of mitral stenosis. The embolus usually enters the carotid, rarely the vertebral artery. In the great majority of cases it comes from the left heart and is a vegetation of a fresh endocarditis or, more commonly, of a recurring endocarditis, or from the segments involved in an ulcerative process. Less often the embolus is a portion of a clot which has formed in the auricular appendix. Portions of clot from an aneurism, thrombi from atheroma of the aorta, or from the pulmonary veins, may also cause blocking of the branches of the circle of Willis. In the puerperal condition cerebral embolism is not infrequent. It may occur in women with heart disease, but in some instances the heart is uninvolved, and the condition is associated with the formation of clots in the heart or pulmonary veins. A majority of cases of embolism occur in heart disease, 89 per cent (Saveliew). Cases are rare in the acute endocarditis of rheumatic fever, chorea and febrile conditions. It is much more common in the endocarditis which attacks old sclerotic valves. The embolus most frequently passes to the left middle cerebral artery and less often to the posterior cerebral and vertebral. A large plug may lodge at the bifurcation of the basilar. Embolism of the cerebellar vessels is rare.

Thrombosis.—This occurs (1) about an embolus, (2) as the result of a lesion of the arterial wall (either endarteritis with or without atheroma or, particularly, the *syphilitic* arteritis), (3) in aneurisms, both large and miliary, (4) as a direct result of abnormal conditions of the blood as in the anemia of hemorrhage, chlorosis, septicemia and the cachexia of cancer and (5) with new growths. The influence of focal infection may be important. The arterial changes which lead to thrombosis and hemorrhage are practically the same. Thrombosis occasionally follows ligation of the carotid artery. The thrombosis is most common in the middle cerebral and basilar arteries. It is suggested that softening of limited areas, sufficient to induce hemiplegia, may be caused by sudden collapse of cerebral arteries from cardiac weakness or marked hypotension.

Anatomical Changes.—The embolus may retract, so that the blood flow is restored, or be carried on and lodge in a smaller vessel; in either case improvement occurs. In many instances a secondary thrombosis follows which may be extensive. In both embolism and thrombosis *edema* occurs which, as in hemorrhage, causes pressure and so is a cause of coma. Degeneration and softening of the territory supplied by the vessels are the ultimate result in both embolism and thrombosis. Blocking in a terminal artery may be followed by infarction, in which the territory may be deeply infiltrated with blood (hemorrhagic infarction) or be pale, swollen, and necrotic (anemic infarction). Gradually the process of *softening* proceeds, the tissue is infiltrated with serum and the nerve fibres degenerate and become fatty. The neuroglia is swollen and edematous. The color of the softened area depends upon the amount of blood. Formerly much stress was laid upon the difference between *red*, *yellow*, and *white* softening. The red and yellow are seen chiefly on the cortex. Sometimes red softening is particularly marked in embolism and about tumors. The gray matter shows many punctiform hemorrhages. There is a variety of yellow softening, common in elderly persons, in the gray matter, in spots from 1 to 2 cm. in diameter, sometimes angular in shape, the edges cleanly cut, and the softened area represented by a turbid, yellow material. White softening occurs most frequently in the white matter, and is seen best about tumors and abscesses. Inflammatory changes are common in and about the softened areas. When the embolus comes from an infected focus, as in ulcerative endocarditis, suppuration may follow. The final changes vary greatly. The degenerated tissue elements are gradually removed, and if the region is small may be replaced by connective tissue and the formation of a scar. If large, the resorption results in the formation of a cyst.

The position and extent of the softening depend upon the obstructed artery. An embolus which blocks the middle cerebral at its origin involves not only the arteries to the anterior perforated space, but also the cortical branches, and in such a case there is softening in the neighborhood of the corpus striatum, as well as in part of the region supplied by the cortical vessels. The freedom of anastomosis between these branches varies. Thus, in embolism of the middle cerebral artery in which the softening has involved only the territory of the central branches, blood may reach the cortex through the anterior and posterior cerebrals. When the middle cerebral is blocked (as is perhaps oftenest the case) beyond the point of origin of the central arteries, one or other of its branches is usually most involved. The embolus may lodge in the vessel passing to the third frontal convolution, or in the artery of the ascending frontal or ascending parietal; or lodge in the branch passing to the supramarginal and angular gyri, or enter the lowest branch distributed to the upper convolutions of the temporal lobe. Instances occur of softening limited to a part, at any rate, of the territory supplied by these arteries. Some of the most accurate focalizing lesions are produced in this way.

There is greater freedom of communication in the cortical branches of the different arteries than is usually admitted, but the absence of softening in some instances in which smaller branches are blocked shows how complete may be the compensation, probably by the capillaries. The dilatation of the collateral branches may take place very rapidly; thus a patient with chronic nephritis died twenty-four hours after the hemiplegic attack. There were recent vegetations on the mitral valve and an embolus in the right middle cerebral artery just beyond the first two branches. The central portion of the hemisphere was swollen and edematous. The right anterior cerebral was greatly dilated, and its diameter was nearly three times that of the left.

Symptoms.—Extensive thrombotic softening may exist without any symptoms and it is not uncommon in postmortems on elderly persons to find areas of softening scattered over the convolutions. It may take place in the "silent" regions without exciting any symptoms. When the central or cortical branches of the middle cerebral arteries are involved the symptoms are similar to those of hemorrhage from the same arteries. Permanent or transient hemiplegia results. When the central arteries are involved the softening in the internal capsule is commonly followed by hemiplegia. Certain peculiarities are associated with embolism and thrombosis respectively. The results of thrombosis are probably more variable than those of embolism.

In *embolism* the patient is usually the subject of heart trouble, or there exist some of the conditions already mentioned. The onset is sudden, without premonitory symptoms but sometimes with intense headache. When the embolus blocks the left middle cerebral artery the hemiplegia is associated with aphasia. In *thrombosis*, on the other hand, the onset is more gradual; the patient has previously complained of headache, vertigo, tingling in the fingers; the speech may have been embarrassed for some days; the patient has had loss of memory or is incoherent, or paralysis begins at one part, as the hand, and extends slowly, and the hemiplegia may be incomplete or variable. Abrupt loss of consciousness is much less common, and when the lesion is small consciousness is retained. In thrombosis due to syphilitic disease, the hemiplegia may come on gradually without any disturbance of consciousness.

The hemiplegia following thrombosis or embolism has practically the characteristics, both primary and secondary, described under hemorrhage.

The following may be the effects of blocking the different vessels: (*a*) *Vertebral.* The left branch is more frequently plugged. The effects are involvement of the nuclei in the medulla and symptoms of acute bulbar paralysis. It rarely occurs alone; more commonly with:

(*b*) *Blocking of the Basilar Artery.*—When this is entirely occluded, there may be bilateral paralysis from involvement of both motor paths. Bulbar symptoms may be present; rigidity or spasm may occur. The temperature may rise rapidly. The symptoms, in fact, are those of apoplexy of the pons.

(*c*) The *posterior cerebral* supplies the occipital lobe on its medial surface and the greater part of the temporosphenoidal lobe. If the main stem be thrombosed there is hemianopia with sensory aphasia. Localized areas of softening may exist without symptoms. Blocking of the main occipital branch or of the artery passing to the cuneus, may be followed by hemianopia. Hemianesthesia may result from involvement of the posterior part of the internal capsule. With thrombosis of a branch of the posterior cerebral of one hemisphere and a branch of the middle cerebral of the other the most pronounced instances of apraxia occur.

(*d*) *Internal Carotid.*—The symptoms are variable. The vessel is ligated without risk in a majority of cases; in other instances transient hemiplegia follows; in others again the hemiplegia is permanent. These variations depend on the anastomoses in the circle of Willis. If these are large and free, no paralysis follows, but if the posterior and anterior communicating vessels are small or absent the paralysis may persist. Blocking of the internal carotid within the skull by thrombosis or embolism is followed by hemiplegia, coma, and usually death. The clot is rarely confined to the carotid itself, but spreads into its branches and may involve the ophthalmic artery.

(*e*) *Middle Cerebral.*—This is the vessel most commonly involved, and if plugged before the central arteries are given off, permanent hemiplegia usually follows from softening of the internal capsule. Blocking of the branches beyond this point may be followed by hemiplegia, which is more likely to be transient, involves chiefly the arm and face, and if the lesion be on the left side is associated with aphasia. There may be plugging of the individual branches passing to the inferior frontal (producing motor aphasia if the disease be on the left side), to the anterior and posterior central gyri (usually causing total hemiplegia), to the supramarginal and angular gyri (giving rise, if on the left side, probably without exception to the so-called visual aphasia (alexia), usually also to right-sided hemianopsia), or to the temporal gyri (in which event with left sided thrombosis word-deafness results).

(*f*) *Anterior Cerebral.*—No symptoms may follow, and even when the branches which supply the paracentral lobule and the top of the ascending convolutions are plugged the branches from the middle cerebral are usually able to effect a collateral circulation. Monoplegia of the leg may result. Hebetude and dullness of intellect may follow obstruction of the vessel.

(*g*) *Cerebellar.*—Usually the posterior inferior cerebellar artery is affected. There is severe vertigo, with vomiting and rotating movements. The patient can not stand or sit; he must lie. After the acute features are over there are the signs of a unilateral cerebellar lesion. There are disturbances of sensation due to a lesion of the spinothalamic tract. There may be signs of disturbance of the medulla.

Prognosis.—In embolism this depends on the extent of tissue which is deprived of blood supply; hence the collateral circulation is important. It is often impossible to decide this. In thrombosis the outlook is probably best in the syphilitic cases if early diagnosis and active treatment are possible. In cases due to other forms of arterial disease the ultimate outlook is grave as the lesions are likely to lead to further vascular damage. The outlook for the paralysis is much as in hemorrhage.

Treatment of Hemorrhage, Thrombosis and Embolism.—The patient should be placed in bed, with his head moderately elevated and the neck free. He should be kept absolutely quiet. If there are dyspnea, stertor, and signs of mechanical obstruction to respiration, he should be turned on his side. This lessens the liability to congestion of the lungs. Venesection seems to be indicated theoretically in cases of hemorrhage with high pressure, but practically is of no value and is not advisable except that with marked cyanosis in plethoric subjects it is sometimes useful. A rapid rise of arterial tension usually indicates an endeavor to counteract increasing intracranial pressure. The indication under these circumstances is the relief of the intracranial pressure by craniotomy and removal of the clot, if this is possible. This is particularly applicable in subdural hemorrhage. An ice-bag may be placed on the head and hot bottles to the feet. The bowels should be freely opened, by calomel or elaterin followed by magnesium sulphate, which by mouth or rectum often gives marked relief to the symptoms of increased intracranial pressure from any cause. Counterirritation to the neck or to the feet is not necessary. Catheterization may be required, especially if the patient remains long unconscious.

Special care should be taken to avoid bed sores; and if bottles or hot water bags are used, they should not be too hot, since blisters may be readily caused. Stimulants are not necessary, unless the pulse becomes feeble and signs of collapse supervene. During recovery the patient should be still kept entirely at rest, even in the mildest attacks remaining in bed for at least fourteen days. An ice-bag should still be kept to the head. The diet should be light and the bowels kept open. Attention should be paid to the position of the paralyzed limb or limbs, which if swollen may be wrapped in cotton batting or flannel. Small doses of iodide (gr. v, 0.3 gm.) may be given.

In *thrombosis* or *embolism* venesection is not indicated, as it rather promotes clotting. If, as is often the case, the heart's action is feeble and irregular, small doses of digitalis may be given. The bowels should be kept open, but it is not well to purge actively, as in hemorrhage.

In thrombosis with syphilitic disease of the arteries, most frequent in men between twenty and forty (in whom the hemiplegia often sets in without loss of consciousness), active antisyphilitic treatment is indicated; mercury and iodide should be given in full dosage. Practically these are the only cases of thrombosis in which we see satisfactory results from treatment.

Very little can be done for the *hemiplegia* which remains. The damage is too often irreparable and permanent, and it seems improbable that iodide or any remedy hastens in the slightest degree Nature's dealing with the blood clot. Passive movements or massage, and later reeducation should be used systematically, in order to maintain the nutrition of the muscles and prevent contractures if possible. Massage should not be begun until at least ten days after the attack. It is doubtful if electricity is of much value; some regard it as more likely to do harm by increasing spasticity. The patient should be encouraged to perform simple movements and exercise himself, and attempt to walk when the acute features are over. When contractures occur, passive movements and massage are useful, and it has been suggested that tendon transplantation, or cross suture of nerves, may cause improvement. There is always the possibility of another attack and the patient should lead a quiet life with a simple diet, keeping the bowels open and avoiding undue exertion and emotional disturbance as much as possible.

In a case of complete hemiplegia the friends should at the outset be told frankly that the chances of full recovery are slight. Power is usually restored in the leg sufficient to enable the patient to get about, but in the majority of instances the finer movements of the hand are permanently lost. In permanent hemiplegia in older persons some mental weakness may follow the attack, and the patient become irritable and emotional.

ANEURISM OF THE CEREBRAL ARTERIES

Miliary aneurisms are not included, but reference is made only to aneurism of the larger branches. The condition is not uncommon. There were 12 instances in 800 autopsies in the Montreal General Hospital. This is a considerably larger proportion than in Newton Pitt's collection from Guy's Hospital, 19 times in 9,000 inspections.

Etiology.—Males are more frequently affected than females. The disease is most common at the middle period of life. One of the Montreal cases was a lad of six and Pitt describes one at the same age. The chief causes are (*a*) congenital defects, (*b*) endarteritis, simple or syphilitic, which leads to weakness of the wall and dilatation, and (*c*) embolism. These aneurisms are often found with endocarditis. Pitt concluded that it is exceptional to find cerebral aneurism unassociated with fungating endocarditis. The embolus disappears and dilatation follows the secondary inflammatory changes in the vessel.

Morbid Anatomy.—The middle cerebral branches are most frequently involved. In 166 cases (statistics of Osler, Lebert, Durand, and Bartholow) the middle cerebral was involved in 49, basilar in 44, internal carotid in 24, anterior cerebral in 14, posterior communicating in 8, anterior communicating in 11, vertebral in 7, posterior cerebral in 6, inferior cerebellar in 3. The size of the aneurism varies from that of a pea to that of a walnut. The hemorrhage may be meningeal with very slight laceration of the brain substance, or, as Coats has shown, entirely within the substance.

Symptoms.—The aneurism may attain considerable size and cause no symptoms. In a majority the first sign is rupture and fatal apoplexy. Distinct symptoms are most frequently caused by aneurism of the internal carotid, which may compress the optic nerve or the commissure, causing neuritis or paralysis of the third nerve. A murmur may be audible. Aneurism in this situation may cause irritative and pressure symptoms at the base of the brain or bilateral temporal hemianopia. Aneurism of the vertebral or the basilar may involve the nerves from the fifth to the twelfth. A large sac at the termination of the basilar may compress the third nerves or the crura. In some cases the aneurism ruptures through a very small opening and the blood escapes slowly. The process tends to go on to death, but recovery has occurred.

The *diagnosis* may be made if its possibility is considered. The larger sacs produce the symptoms of tumor and their rupture is usually fatal. The treatment is that of cerebral hemorrhage.

THROMBOSIS OF THE CEREBRAL SINUSES AND VEINS

The condition may be primary or secondary. Lebert (1854) and Tonnele were among the first to recognize the condition clinically.

Primary thrombosis of the sinuses and veins is rare. It occurs (*a*) in children, particularly during the first six months of life, usually in connection with diarrhea. Gowers believed that it is frequent, and that thrombosis of the veins is not an uncommon cause of infantile hemiplegia.

(*b*) With chlorosis and anemia, the so-called *autochthonous sinus thrombosis.* Of 82 cases of thrombosis in chlorosis, 78 were in the veins and 32 in the cerebral sinuses. The longitudinal sinus is most frequently involved. The thrombosis is usually associated with venous thromboses elsewhere and the patients die in one to three weeks, but recovery may occur.

(*c*) In the terminal stages of cancer, tuberculosis, and other chronic diseases thrombosis may occur in the sinuses and cortical veins. To the coagulum in these conditions the term marantic thrombus is applied.

Secondary thrombosis is much more frequent and follows extension of inflammation from contiguous parts to the sinus wall. The common causes are disease of the internal ear, fracture, compression of the sinuses by tumor, abscess or suppurative diseases outside the skull, particularly erysipelas, carbuncle and parotitis. In secondary cases the lateral sinus is most frequently involved. Of 57 fatal cases in which ear disease caused death with cerebral lesions, in 22 thrombosis existed in the lateral sinuses (Pitt). Tuberculous caries of the temporal bone may be responsible. The thrombus may be small or fill the entire sinus and extend into the internal jugular vein. In more than half of these instances the thrombus was suppurating. The disease spreads from the necrosis on the posterior wall of the tympanum by the petrosomastoid canal. It is not so common in mastoid disease.

Symptoms.—*Primary thrombosis* of the *longitudinal* sinus may occur without exciting symptoms and is found accidentally postmortem. There may be mental dulness with headache. Convulsions and vomiting may occur. In other instances there is nothing distinctive. In the chlorosis cases the head symptoms are usually marked. The patient may be dull and stupid, with vomiting, dilatation of the pupils and double choked disks. In other cases the patients have headache, vomiting and delirium. Paralysis or paresis may be present. Bristowe reported a case in an anemic girl of nineteen, who had convulsions, drowsiness and vomiting. Tenderness and swelling developed in the position of the right internal jugular vein, and a few days later on the opposite side. Phlebitis occurred later in the right leg. The patient recovered. Such symptoms in anemia should lead to the suspicion of cerebral thrombosis. In infants the diagnosis can rarely be made.

In thrombosis of the *cavernous* sinus there is prominence of the eyes with edema of the orbit, conjunctiva and face. There is disturbance of vision with swelling of the disk and hemorrhages. Paralysis of the ocular muscles may occur. With involvement of the *lateral* sinus the thrombus may extend to the jugular vein and be palpable.

In the *secondary thrombi* the symptoms are commonly those of septicemia and in over 70 per cent of Pitt's cases death was due to pulmonary pyemia. This author draws the following conclusions: (1) The disease spreads oftener from the posterior wall of the middle ear than from the mastoid cells. (2) The otorrhea is generally of some standing, but not always. (3) The onset is sudden, the chief symptoms being pyrexia, rigors, pains in the occipital region and in the neck, associated with a septicemic condition. (4) Well-marked optic neuritis may be present. (5) The appearance of acute local pulmonary mischief or of distant suppuration is almost conclusive of thrombosis. (6) The average duration is about three weeks, and death is generally from pulmonary pyemia. The chief points in the diagnosis may be gathered from these statements.

Associated with thrombosis of the *lateral sinus* there may be venous stasis and painful edema behind the ear and in the neck. The external jugular vein on the diseased side may be less distended than on the opposite side, since owing to the thrombus in the lateral sinus the internal jugular vein is less full than on the normal side, and the blood from the external jugular can flow more easily into it.

Treatment.—This from the medical side is symptomatic. Care should be taken not to allow clothing to press on the neck and to avoid bending the neck. If signs of meningitis appear, in lumbar puncture as little fluid as is necessary should be removed. Surgical measures should be carried out early. The secondary forms, especially those following disease of the middle ear, often do well and many lives have been saved by operation after extensive sinus thrombosis.

CEREBRAL PALSIES OF CHILDREN

Introduction.—There are three great groups: I. Those due to *prenatal* factors, *agenesia cerebri, microcephalus, porencephaly, congenital cysts, etc.* II. *Natal* or *intrapartum* which includes the large group of birth palsies due to meningeal hemorrhage, etc.; and III. The *postnatal* group of which the larger proportion is due to acute encephalitis between the second and sixth year, leading to hemiplegia. In all these cerebral palsies there are three important factors: (1) Disturbance to some extent of the normal mental development, (2) paralysis, and (3) spasticity in greater or less degree.

A number of important conditions may be grouped together for convenience of description—aplasia cerebri, meningeal hemorrhage, spastic diplegia, Little's disease, bilateral athetosis, etc.

I. Aplasia (Agenesia) cerebri.—This is due to failure of development of the cerebral cortex due to intra-uterine conditions. Nothing abnormal may be noted at birth, which has not been delayed or assisted by instruments. The head may be small and the sutures may close early. Then it is noticed that the child does not develop normally in the use of the muscles; the movements are irregular but not athetoid. The head wobbles, the child does not sit up, the dentition is delayed, and by the second year, the failure of development is evident. The arms and legs may become stiff and bilateral spastic rigidity supervene. More often the limbs remain relaxed, the child may learn to walk in an awkward way but full power over the movements is never acquired, and the child settles into a state of idiocy. Anatomically the brain is small, the convolutions ill-developed, and there may be areas of lobular sclerosis, sometimes the remarkable tuberose form.

II. Meningeal Hemorrhage (*With conservative paraplegia spastica cerebralis (Heine); Little's disease; Tetraplegia spastica*).—Heine, one of the founders of modern orthopedics, recognized the cerebral origin of many of the palsies of children; and Little subsequently called attention to the "influence of abnormal parturition, difficult labors, premature birth and asphyxia on the mental and physical condition of the child, especially in relation to deformities." In 1885 Sarah McNutt's careful studies correlated the meningeal hemorrhage with the subsequent palsies as recognized by Heine and Little.

The causes are: (1) Tearing of the veins from pressure on the head in a contracted pelvis and in forceps delivery. (2) Asphyxia. Extreme stasis causes rupture of veins at the point of entrance to the longitudinal sinus (Cushing). (3) Hemorrhage may be with a hemorrhagic condition of the newborn.

The hemorrhage is from the pia, usually over the cortex and widely spread. It may be more on one side than the other, and may extend over the cerebellum. The brain substance may be softened or compressed, and present foci of hemorrhage. The hemorrhage may be extradural, and even extend into the spinal cord. First birth, premature birth, foot presentation, but above all, the indiscriminate and careless use of the forceps are the causal factors. There is much wisdom in the dread expressed by Shandy Senior, of the dangers of compression of the delicate and fine web of the brain.

Symptoms.—*Early.*—The asphyxia may be protracted. Unusual torpor, absence of the natural crying, inability to take the breast, flaccidity of the limbs, sometimes with rigidity on one side or convulsions, unequal and dilated pupils, and slow breathing with signs of atelectasis are suggestive features. There may be hemorrhages elsewhere if the condition is associated with the hemorrhagic disease of the newborn. Lumbar puncture may show blood.

Late.—If the child recovers, nothing may be noticed for a few months. Perhaps there are convulsions. The first thing to attract attention is that when the child should begin to walk the limbs are not used readily, and a stiffness of the legs and arms is found. Even at the age of two the child may not be able to sit up, and often the head is not well supported by the neck muscles. The *rigidity,* as a rule, is more marked in the legs, and there is adductor spasm. When supported on the feet, the child either rests on its toes and the inner surface of the feet, with the knees close together, or the legs may be crossed. The stiffness of the arms varies. It may be slight or the rigidity may be as marked as in the legs. When the spastic condition affects the arms as well as the legs, we speak of it as diplegia or tetraplegia; when the legs alone are involved, as paraplegia. There seems no sufficient reason for considering them separately. The spasticity is probably due to changes in the pyramidal system. Constant irregular movements of the arms are not uncommon. The child has great difficulty in grasping an object. The spasm and weakness may be more evident on one side than the other. Strabismus, nystagmus, unequal pupils and optic atrophy may occur. The mental condition is, as a rule, defective and convulsive seizures are common.

III. ACUTE SPORADIC ENCEPHALITIS OF CHILDREN WITH CONSECUTIVE HEMIPLEGIA.—This is an acute infection characterized by fever, convulsions, coma and a consecutive hemiplegia.

Etiology.—Cases of hemiplegia in children's homes and institutions for the feeble-minded fall into two groups—(1) a large one, 95 out of 135 in Osler's series, in which the disease began about the second year, suddenly, in healthy children; and (2) a small one, with a more advanced age of onset, comprising cases of trauma, heart disease, etc. Probably in the majority of cases vascular lesions occurring in an attack of one of the acute infections are responsible. The condition may follow a slight febrile illness during the first year. The incidence in relation to acute poliomyelitis is not known. There did not appear to be an increase of cases during the recent outbreaks.

Pathology.—The motor area of one hemisphere is involved in an acute hemorrhagic lesion, the convolutions swollen and deeply injected, the veins thrombosed, and on section the substance is moist, deep red, and the limitation of the gray matter ill-defined or obliterated. The picture corresponds with Strümpell's polioencephalitis. When the patients come to autopsy years later, sclerosis with atrophy of the motor area is the most common lesion or there is a submeningeal cyst.

Symptoms.—Clinically the disease is sharply defined. A healthy child between the first and fifth years has a convulsion, or a series of them, with fever, possibly vomiting, and then becomes comatose. Preliminary indisposition is rare; headache may be complained of, but without warning the fit, as a rule, is the first symptom. The fever may reach 103°-104°. There may be marked conjugate deviation of the head and eyes: the pupils are usually dilated, and may be unequal. The head may be retracted and naturally meningitis is suspected. In the deep coma the hemiplegia may be—often is—overlooked, but on careful examination the face is seen to be drawn and the arm and leg of one side limp and paralyzed. One of two things happens—the coma persists, the convulsions recur, and the child dies from the second to the fifth day, or the fever drops, the coma lessens, and within a few days the child seems well, but one side is paralyzed.

Complete recovery is rare. The face and arm improve rapidly, the leg lags and drags, as in an ordinary hemiplegia. Speech if disturbed returns. The chief tragedy is a failure to develop mentally, which takes so many of these patients into the feeble-minded homes. The arm of the affected side may not develop but remains shorter and the hand smaller. In other cases recovery is not so complete; both leg and arm are spastic and the latter may present posthemiplegic movements. Sensation is not disturbed. A distressing feature is *epilepsy*, which may occur as pure Jacksonian fits, *petit mal*, or general seizures. Of 135 cases in the series, 41 had epilepsy.

Posthemiplegic Movements.—It was in cases of this sort that Weir Mitchell first described the posthemiplegic movements. They are extremely common and were present in 34 of the series. There may be either slight tremor in the affected muscles, or incoordinate choreiform movements—the so-called posthemiplegic chorea—or, lastly,

Athetosis.—This is a remarkable condition in which there is a combination of spasm with the most extraordinary bizarre movements of the muscles. The patient may not be able to walk. The head is turned from side to side; there are continual irregular movements of the face muscles, and the mouth is drawn and greatly distorted. The extremities are more or less rigid, particularly in extension. On the slightest attempt to move, often spontaneously, there are extraordinary movements of the arms and legs. The patients are often unable to help themselves on account of these movements. The reflexes are increased. The mental condition is variable.

IV. Paralysis Due to Embolism.—This requires no special description as it is practically the same as in adults.

Treatment.—Infants with asphyxia and convulsions have been operated upon soon after birth and cortical clots have been removed. In some cases there has been a complete restoration to health and the usual spastic sequels have not occurred. If there is a hemorrhagic tendency, the use of blood serum is advisable. As the child grows, conditions have to be met—the mental, requiring the care and training necessary for the grade of feeble-mindedness, and the orthopedic treatment of the spasticity, for which much can be done. Passive movements, massage and reeducational exercises are helpful. The educational care in institutions has shown how much patient training is able to help the development of these defective children. In all these patients the degree of development depends very much upon the thorough, painstaking and systematic training of their minds and muscles.

Surgically much may be done by tenotomy and proper apparatus. For the relief of the spasticity operations on the brain are rarely of help. Better results are obtained by nerve resection, and with a high grade of bilateral spasticity, resection of the posterior nerve roots appears to have been helpful. The operation of "sympathetic ramisectomy" (Hunter and Royle) results in decrease of spasticity in muscles. The cases have to be carefully chosen and the best results should follow the operation in spasticity from cortical lesions.

TUMORS, INFECTIONS, GRANULOMATA, AND CYSTS OF THE BRAIN

The most common varieties of new growths within the cranium are:

Infectious Granulomata.—(*a*) *Tubercle* may form large or small growths, usually multiple. Tuberculosis of the glands or bones may coexist, but the tuberculous disease of the brain may occur in the absence of other clinically recognizable tuberculous lesions. The disease is most frequent early in life. The majority of the cases occur under twenty, and many are in children. Of 1,398 cases of verified tumor studied by Cushing, there were 26 tuberculomas. The relative frequency varies greatly in different localities. The nodules are most numerous in the cerebellum and about the base.

(*b*) *Syphiloma* is most common on the cortex cerebri or about the pons. The tumors are superficial, attached to the arteries or the meninges, and rarely grow to a large size. They may be multiple. A gummatous meningitis of the base is common and in this process the oculomotor nerves are often affected. The motor nerves of the eye are particularly prone to syphilitic infiltration, and ptosis and squint are common. The pituitary gland may be involved with symptoms suggestive of diabetes insipidus.

Tumors.—(*c*) *Gliomas.*—These are the most common tumors and occur in all parts of the brain. They are often diffuse but may be encapsulated. The consistence may be much like that of the brain or they may be firm. They are usually very vascular and the vessels are liable to degeneration with resulting hemorrhage, thrombosis and edema. This often accounts for acute features appearing suddenly. The histological appearance varies considerably. They do not give rise to metastases. If necrosis occurs in the tumor, cyst formation may result. Benign and malignant forms occur.

(*d*) *Pituitary adenomas* come next in frequency (about 20 per cent). They may be chiefly neutrophilic, acidophilic or basophilic in character. The tumor effects from pressure are the same.

(*e*) *Meningiomas* (dural endotheliomas) originate in the leptomeninges and compress the brain from without.

(*f*) *Acoustic tumors* originate from the vestibular portion of the eighth nerve and involve the cerebellopontine angle.

(*g*) Other varieties are carcinoma, sarcoma, bony tumors, which grow sometimes from the falx, cholesteatoma, chordoma, and angioma. Fatty tumors are occasionally found on the corpus callosum. There is a remarkable condition, originally described by Rokitansky, in which there is a brownish-black pigmentation of the brain, which may be partly diffuse.

(*h*) *Angiomata* arise from the blood vessels of the meninges and may be associated with nevi of the skin. The nevi in the brain are in no sense metastases from the skin, but benign tumors arising primarily (MacLachlan).

Cysts.—These occur between the membranes and the brain, as a result of hemorrhage or softening. *Porencephalus* is a sequel of congenital atrophy or hemorrhage, or may be due to a development defect. Hydatid cysts have been referred to in the section on parasites. An interesting variety of cyst is that which follows severe injury to the skull in early life. Gliomata often undergo cystic degeneration. Dermoid cyst has been described.

Site.—A majority of all tumors occur in the cerebrum and especially in the centrum ovale. The cerebellum, pons, and membranes are next most often involved. Glioma is more common in the hemispheres and grows slowly. It is usually single. Secondary sarcoma and carcinoma are often multiple.

Symptoms and Signs.—These vary greatly, depending on the position of the tumor, its size, rate of growth, and the occurrence of vascular changes, such as hemorrhage, thrombosis and edema. All tumors are without symptoms for a variable time; it is our business to recognize them at the earliest possible period. The symptoms are of two kinds. (1) *General,* due to increase in intracranial pressure, or (2) *local,* due to effects produced on parts of the nervous system. The following are the most important: *Headache,* either dull, aching, and continuous, or sharp, stabbing, and paroxysmal. It may be diffuse or limited to the back or front and is often remittent. When in the back of the head it may extend down the neck (especially in tumors in the posterior fossa), and when in the front it may be accompanied with neuralgic pains in the face. Occasionally the pain may be very localized and associated with tenderness on pressure. Pressure is the important factor in its production, and small or slowly growing tumors may not cause it.

Choked disk (optic neuritis, papilloedema) should be looked for in every patient presenting cerebral symptoms, for it is the first sign of increased intracranial pressure. Loss of visual acuity usually indicates that optic atrophy has set in. It is usually double, but occasionally is found in only one eye. Growths may attain considerable size without causing choked disk. On the other hand, it may occur with a very small tumor, when this is so situated as to cause internal hydrocephalus. J. A. Martin, from an analysis of the literature with reference to the localizing value, concludes: When there is a difference in the amount of change in each eye it is more than twice as probable that the tumor is on the side of the most marked neuritis. It is constant in tumors of the corpora quadrigemina, present in 89 per cent of cerebellar tumors, and absent in nearly two thirds of the cases of tumor of the pons, medulla and corpus callosum. It is least frequent in cases of tuberculous tumor; most common with glioma and cystic tumors.

Paton and Holmes report upon the eyes of 700 cases of cerebral tumor, concluding that the essential feature of the associated optic neuritis is edema, and in 60 eyes examined histologically the one unfailing change was acute edema, the origin of which they attribute to the venous engorgement.

Vomiting is less constant but with headache and choked disk is of significance. Important points are the absence of definite relation to meals and of digestive disturbances. It may be very obstinate, particularly in growths of the cerebellum and the pons.

Giddiness is often an early symptom, experienced on rising suddenly or turning quickly. It occurs especially with neoplasm in the posterior fossa.

Mental Symptoms.—There is often some change, usually in the direction of dulness. Mania, depressive conditions, delusions, hallucinations and confusional states have been described but are usually late. The patient may act in an unnatural manner, or show stupor and heaviness. The patient may be emotional or silly, or there are symptoms resembling hysteria.

Convulsions, either general and resembling true epilepsy or localized (Jacksonian) in character. Seizures beginning with a gustatory or olfactory aura are common with tumors originating in the infundibular region.

Circulation.—Secondary to increased intracranial pressure there is increased blood pressure. The pulse rate is often slow. Respiration may be slow and sometimes is irregular.

Local Features.—The smaller the tumor and the less marked the general symptoms of cerebral compression the more likely is it that any focal symptoms occurring are of *direct* origin. Localizing features are often misleading. A frontal tumor may have cerebellar features due to increased intercranial pressure which has compressed the cerebellum. The characteristic Bárány cerebellar tests have been present with temporal lobe tumors.

(*a*) *Central Motor Area.*—The symptoms are irritative or destructive in character. *Irritation* in the lower third may produce spasm in the muscles of the face, in the angle of the mouth, or in the tongue. The spasm with tingling may be limited to one muscle group before extending to others, and this Seguin termed the *signal symptom.* The middle third of the motor area contains the centres controlling the arm, and here the spasm may begin in the fingers, the thumb, the muscles of the wrist, or the shoulder. In the upper third of the motor areas the irritation may produce spasm beginning in the toes, in the ankles, or in the muscles of the leg. In many instances the patient can determine accurately the point of origin of the spasm, and there are important sensory disturbances, as numbness and tingling, which may be felt first at the region affected. It is important to determine, first, the point of origin; second, the order or march of the spasm; and third, the subsequent condition of the parts first affected, whether paresis or anesthesia.

Destructive lesions in the motor zone cause paralysis, often preceded by local convulsive seizures; there may be a monoplegia, as of the leg, and convulsive seizures in the arm, often due to irritation. Tumors in the neighborhood of the motor area may cause localized spasms and subsequently, as the centres are invaded by the growth, paralysis occurs. With tumors in the left hemisphere the speech mechanism is apt to be involved if the transverse temporal gyrus or the third frontal convolution and their connecting path are implicated.

(*b*) *Prefrontal Region.*—Neither motor nor sensory disturbance may be present. The general symptoms are often well marked. The most striking feature of growths in this region is a change in character and habits which may progress to stupor or dementia, particularly when the left side is involved. In its extension downward the tumor may involve on the left side the lower frontal convolution and produce aphasia, or in its progress backward cause irritative or destructive lesions of the motor area. Exophthalmos on the side of the tumor may occur and be helpful in diagnosis.

(*c*) Tumors in the *parietal lobe*, particularly on the right side, may grow to a large size without causing any symptoms. There may be word-blindness and mind-blindness when the left angular gyrus and its underlying white matter are involved, and paraphasia. Astereognosis may accompany growths in the parietal lobe.

(*d*) Tumors of the *occipital lobe* produce hemianopia, and a bilateral lesion may produce blindness. Tumors in this region on the left hemisphere may be associated with word-blindness and mind-blindness. In all cases of tumor a careful study should be made of the fields of vision. In addition to the lateral hemianopia there may be remarkable visual hallucinations, and in tumors of the left occipital lobe dissociation of the color sense and inability to find the proper colors of various objects presented.

(*e*) Tumors in the *temporal lobe* may attain a large size without producing symptoms. In their growth they involve the lower motor centres. On the left side involvement of the transverse temporal gyri (auditory sense area) may be associated with word-deafness. In *uncinate seizures* unpleasant hallucinations of taste and smell may occur. Visual disturbances are common.

(*f*) Tumors in the neighborhood of the *basal ganglia* produce hemiplegia from involvement of the internal capsule. Tumors in the optic thalamus may, when small, cause no symptoms, but, increasing, may involve the fibres of the sensory portion of the internal capsule, producing hemianopia and sometimes hemianesthesia. Growths in this situation are apt to cause choked disk early and, growing into the third ventricle, may cause a distention of the lateral ventricles. What has been termed the *thalamic syndrome* may be present—hemianesthesia to pain, touch and temperature, with loss of deep sensibility. With this there may be a very remarkable type of pain, involving the hand and arm and the foot and leg, on the affected side, a sense of burning discomfort rather than sharp pain. Ataxic features are usually present and astereognosis. Motor hemiplegia may be present, and it is unaccompanied by contractures (Dana).

Growths in the *corpora quadrigemina* are rarely limited, but most commonly involve the crura cerebri as well. Ocular symptoms are marked. The pupil reflex is lost and there is nystagmus. In the gradual growth the third nerve is involved as it passes through the crus, in which case there will be oculomotor paralysis on one side and hemiplegia on the other, a combination almost characteristic of unilateral disease of the crus. Ataxia is common.

(*g*) Tumors of the *pons* and *medulla.* The symptoms are chiefly those of pressure upon the nerves emerging in this region. In disease of the pons the nerves may be involved alone or with the pyramidal tract. There may be alternate paralysis—*i.e.,* involvement of the nerves on one side and of the limbs on the opposite side. In tuberculosis (or syphilis) a growth at the inferior and inner aspects of the crus may cause paralysis of the third nerve on one side, and of the face, tongue, and limbs on the opposite side (*syndrome of Weber*). A tumor in the lower part of the pons usually involves the sixth nerve, producing internal strabismus, the seventh nerve, producing facial paralysis, and the auditory nerve, causing deafness. Conjugate deviation of the eyes to the side opposite that on which there is facial paralysis also occurs. When the motor cerebral nerves are involved the paralyses are of the peripheral type (lower segment paralyses).

Tumors of the *medulla* may involve the cerebral nerves alone or cause a combination of hemiplegia with paralysis of the nerves. Paralyses of the nerves are helpful in diagnosis, but one or more of the cerebral nerves may be paralyzed as a result of much increased general intracranial pressure. Signs of irritation in the ninth, tenth and eleventh nerves are usually present, and produce difficulty in swallowing, irregular action of the heart, irregular respiration, vomiting, and sometimes retraction of the head. The hypoglossal nerve is least often affected. The gait may be unsteady or, if there is pressure on the cerebellum, ataxic. Occasionally there are sensory symptoms, numbness and tingling. Toward the end convulsions may occur.

(*h*) Tumors of the *cerebellum* usually give rise to very characteristic features, headache in the occipital region, giddiness, incoordination, nystagmus, ataxia on movement with difficulty in balancing and hence a staggering gait, weakness and hypotonia on the affected side, and early optic neuritis. The head may be tilted to the side of the tumor, and there may be a tendency to fall the same way. When the patient stands on one leg alternately the difference in steadiness is usually evident. *Cystic hemangiomas* of the cerebellum are frequently associated with angiomas and cysts elsewhere (Lindau's Syndrome). Of special importance is the occurrence of an angioma of the retina, which has a familial tendency. The finding of angioma of the retina in a patient with signs of intracranial tumor suggests a hemangioma of the cerebellum.

(*i*) Tumors of the cerebellopontine angle show signs due to pressure on the cranial nerves with signs from the cerebellum when the tumor compresses it. The *acoustic* tumors show disturbance of the eighth with later involvement of the fifth and seventh nerves. Nystagmus occurs with signs of cerebellar involvement later.

Tumors or enlargements of the *pituitary gland* itself, or growths from a congenital *anlage* in its neighborhood which implicate the pituitary gland secondarily, are common. The congenital tumors arise presumably from developmental faults, and show either a teratomatous character or are solid or cystic tumors. There are characteristic signs of pressure upon the neighborhood structures, bitemporal hemianopia being a frequent though not invariable feature. These lesions may occur in patients who have suffered from acromegaly, or who show signs of glandular deficiency or dyspituitarism. The X-ray study is most useful in diagnosis.

Diagnosis.—The frequency of brain tumors should be remembered and a diagnosis made as early as possible. The occurrence of severe, perhaps intermittent, headache with choked disk is always suggestive. With definite general features and local signs the diagnosis should be fairly clear. But an early diagnosis is often very difficult. The patient should be carefully studied and a competent neurologist consulted if there is doubt. As pointed out by R. T. Williamson, progressive hemiplegia, without other symptoms, a paralysis, which gradually becomes more marked day by day and week by week, is almost pathognomonic, even in the absence of choked disk, headache and vomiting. Exceptions to this rule appear to be cerebral abscess and rare instances of polio-encephalitis. It must not be forgotten that severe headache and choked disk may be caused by nephritis. The localization must be gathered from the consideration of the symptoms and signs. Mistakes are most likely to occur with uremia, hysteria, vascular lesions, abscess, serous meningitis, hydrocephalus and general paresis; but careful consideration of all the circumstances usually enables the practitioner to avoid error. The physicians of the National Hospital, London, have drawn attention to the importance of nasal irritation, as shown by the patients rubbing their noses frequently, as suggesting tumor. Care must be taken not to regard improvement under syphilitic treatment as positive evidence of syphilis, as this may occur with other tumors. Lumbar puncture should always be done with due consideration of the dangers and if necessary, as to exclude or prove syphilis, only a small amount of fluid should be removed. As to localization this may be very difficult if the growth is above the tentorium. In this the early signs are of more value than those of late stages. The X-ray study may be of value and should always be done. The introduction of air after the withdrawal of cerebro-spinal fluid may aid in the recognition of certain tumors by the X-ray study (pneumoventriculography).

Prognosis.—Syphilitic tumors alone are amenable to medical treatment. Tuberculous growths occasionally cease to grow and become calcified. The gliomata and fibromata, particularly when the latter grow from the membranes, may last for years. The general tendency is to progress; blindness results from optic neuritis and mental deterioration appears if the duration is sufficient. Death may be sudden, particularly in growths near the medulla; more commonly it is due to coma with increased intracranial pressure.

Treatment.—(*a*) Medical.—Except in syphilis this is palliative only and in syphilis operation should be considered if the signs do not clear rapidly. A Wassermann test of the blood and cerebrospinal fluid should always be made before antiluetic measures are instituted. Treatment with iodide may cause a temporary amelioration of symptoms due to a glioma, so that the therapeutic test is not a dependable one. If syphilis is proved iodide and mercury should be given. Arsphenamine is sometimes given in repeated small doses. The iodide should be given in increasing doses. In tuberculous tumors the outlook is less favorable, though instances of cure are reported, and there is post-mortem evidence that solitary tuberculous tumors may undergo changes and become obsolete. A general tonic treatment is indicated in these cases. The headache usually demands treatment and various analgesic drugs may be given. An ice-cap for the head or, in occipital headache, the application of the Paquelin cautery may be tried. The bromides are not of much use in this headache and, as the last resort, morphia must be given. For the convulsions bromide of potassium is of little service.

(*b*) Surgical.—There is no doubt of the wisdom of referring these patients at once to men who make a special study of neurological surgery. Many tumors of the brain have been successfully removed. If removal is not possible marked amelioration of the pressure symptoms is possible by surgical measures. It is important that they should be instituted early. The most favorable cases are the localized tumors growing from the dura and only compressing the brain substance. Decompression may be done to relieve the headache, which it sometimes does permanently, and to save sight.

INFLAMMATION OF THE BRAIN

ACUTE ENCEPHALITIS

A focal or diffuse inflammation of the brain substance is met with (*a*) as a result of trauma; (*b*) in certain intoxications, alcohol, food and gas poisoning; (*c*) with acute infections, especially measles, mumps, typhus fever and smallpox; (*d*) as one of the rare varieties of poliomyelitis; (*e*) epidemic encephalitis; and (*f*) with infections such as otitis media, pneumonia and endocarditis. The anatomical features are those of an acute hemorrhagic polio-encephalitis. Focal forms are seen in ulcerative endocarditis, in which the gray matter may present deep hemorrhagic areas, firmer than the surrounding tissue. In the fevers there may be more extensive areas, involving two or three convolutions. Localizing symptoms are usually present, though they may be obscured in the severity of the general infection. A typical encephalitis may accompany the meningitis in cerebrospinal fever.

The *symptoms* are not very definite. In severe forms they are those of an acute infection; some cases have been mistaken for typhoid fever. The onset may be abrupt in an individual apparently healthy. Other cases have occurred in convalescence from fevers. The general symptoms are those which accompany all severe acute affections of the brain—headache, somnolence, coma, delirium, vomiting, etc. The *local* symptoms are very varied, depending on the extent of the lesions, and may be irritative or paralytic. Usually fatal within a few weeks, cases may drag on for weeks or months and recover, generally with paralysis. The *treatment* depends greatly on the primary condition.

Postvaccinal Encephalitis.—This has been most prevalent in Holland and Great Britain but cases have occurred the world over. It is most common in childhood and with the first vaccination. It is rare when infants are vaccinated during the first two years of life. The *onset* is about ten days after vaccination. The lesions consist of areas of demyelination especially around the vessels. The onset of symptoms is acute, usually with drowsiness followed by coma. Muscular twitching and convulsions are common. Temporary hemiplegia may occur but ocular paralysis is rare. The Babinski sign is common. The mortality is high, up to 70 per cent. *Treatment* must be symptomatic; lumbar puncture should be done repeatedly.

Traumatic encephalitis, usually the result of a fall or blow on the head, shows hemorrhages which may be on the surface or in the substance of the brain, edema and inflammatory reaction. The danger of increased intracranial pressure is always present. The general features may be marked and increase. Lumbar puncture often gives a blood-stained fluid. Decompression is indicated if the signs of increased intracranial pressure are definite.

In *Encephalitis periaxialis diffusa* (Schilder's Disease) there is usually bilateral involvement of the brain and extensive degeneration of the white matter with demyelination. It occurs in children and young persons. There is cerebral blindness, progressive spastic paralysis and progressive mental deterioration. Unilateral cases may give difficulty in diagnosis. The course may be subacute or chronic but is progressive to death. In "*centrolobar cerebral sclerosis*" there is an acute stage with convulsions, extensive paralysis and speech disturbances, followed by a period of improvement with decrease in the symptoms which passes into a chronic state with various sequels. There is marked overgrowth of neuroglia below the cortex. Some regard this as the same as Schilder's Disease.

SUPPURATIVE ENCEPHALITIS: ABSCESS OF THE BRAIN

Etiology.—Suppuration of the brain substance is rarely primary, but results, as a rule, from extension of inflammation from neighboring parts or infection from a distance through the blood. Instances occur in which it is difficult to assign a cause. The largest number of cases occur between the twentieth and fortieth years, and the condition is more frequent in men than in women. In children under five years of age, the chief causes are otitis media and trauma. There are three important etiological factors.

(*a*) *Trauma.*—Falls upon the head or blows, but more commonly with fracture or punctured wounds. Meningitis is frequently associated.

(*b*) By far the most important infective foci are those which arise in *direct extension from disease of the middle ear*, of the *mastoid cells*, or of the *accessory nasal sinuses.* From the roof of the mastoid antrum the infection readily passes to the sigmoid sinus and induces an infective thrombosis. In other instances the dura becomes involved, and a subdural abscess is formed, which may involve the arachnoid or the pia mater. In another group the inflammation extends along the lymph spaces, or the thrombosed veins, into the substance of the brain. Infection from the tympanic cavity is most likely to cause abscess in the temporal lobe, while infection from the mastoid cells most frequently causes sinus thrombosis and cerebellar abscess.

(*c*) *In Septic Processes.*—Abscess of the brain is not often found in pyemia. In ulcerative endocarditis multiple foci of suppuration are common. Localized bone disease and suppuration in the liver are occasional causes. The specific fevers, bronchiectasis and empyema, may be followed by abscess.

Morbid Anatomy.—The abscess may be solitary or multiple, diffuse or circumscribed. It may be extradural, subdural or in the brain substance. Practically any one of the varieties of pyogenic bacteria may be concerned. Occasionally cultures are sterile. The pus varies in appearance, depending upon the age of the abscess. In early cases it may be mixed with reddish *débris* but in the solitary encapsulated abscess the pus is distinctive, with a greenish tint, an acid reaction, and a peculiar odor, sometimes like that of sulphuretted hydrogen. The brain substance surrounding the abscess is usually edematous and infiltrated. The size varies from that of a walnut to a large orange. In some cases the cavity occupies the greater portion of a hemisphere. Multiple abscesses are usually small. In four-fifths of all cases the abscess is solitary. Suppuration occurs most frequently in the cerebrum, and the temporal lobe is more often involved than other parts, and always on the side of the ear disease. The cerebellum is the next most common seat, particularly in connection with ear disease.

Symptoms.—These may be very obscure. Following injury or operation the disease may run an *acute* course, with fever, headache, delirium, vomiting and rigors. The symptoms are those of suppurative meningo-encephalitis, and it may be very difficult to determine, unless there are localizing signs, whether there is really suppuration in the brain substance. In the cases following *ear disease* the symptoms may at first be those of meningeal irritation. There may be irritability, restlessness, severe headache and aggravated earache. Other striking symptoms, particularly in the more prolonged cases, are drowsiness, slow cerebration, vomiting and optic neuritis. In the chronic form which may follow injury, otorrhea or local lung trouble, there may be a latent period of weeks to several months, or even a year or more. In the "silent" regions, when the abscess becomes encapsulated there may be no symptoms whatever during the latent period. The patient may be under careful observation and no suspicion of suppuration be aroused. Then severe headache, vomiting and fever set in, perhaps with a chill. So, too, after a blow upon the head or a fracture the symptoms may be transient, and months afterward cerebral symptoms of a severe character may develop. In the extradural and subdural cases the features are usually acute and the course is rapid.

The *localization* is often difficult. If situated in or near the motor region there may be convulsions or paralysis, and an abscess in the temporal lobe may compress the lower part of the precentral convolution and produce paralysis of the arm and face, and on the left side cause aphasia. A large abscess may exist in the frontal lobe without causing paralysis, but there is almost always some mental dulness. In the temporal lobe, the common seat, there may be no focalizing symptoms. So also in the parieto-occipital region; though early examination may lead to the detection of hemianopia. In abscess of the cerebellum vomiting is common. If the middle lobe is affected there may be staggering—cerebellar incoordination. Localizing symptoms in the pons and other parts are still more uncertain.

Diagnosis.—In the *acute* cases there is rarely any doubt. A consideration of possible etiological factors is of the highest importance. The history of injury followed by fever, marked cerebral symptoms, the onset of rigors, delirium, and perhaps paralysis, make the diagnosis certain. In chronic ear disease, such cerebral symptoms as drowsiness and torpor, with irregular fever, supervening upon the cessation of a discharge, should excite the suspicion of abscess. Cases in which suppurative processes exist in the orbit, nose or nasopharynx, or in which there has been subcutaneous phlegmon of the head or neck, parotitis, erysipelas, or tuberculous or syphilitic disease of the bones of the skull, should be carefully watched and investigated if cerebral symptoms appear. It is particularly in the *chronic* cases that difficulties arise. The symptoms resemble those of tumor of the brain; indeed, they are those of tumor plus fever. Choked disk, however, so commonly associated with tumor, may be absent. In a patient with a history of trauma or with lung or pleural trouble, who has had slight headache or dizziness, the onset of fever, especially if intermittent and associated with rigors, intense headache and vomiting, points strongly to abscess. The pulse rate in cerebral abscess is usually accelerated, but cases are not rare in which it is slowed. In all forms a leukocytosis may occur. Macewen laid stress upon percussion of the skull as an aid in diagnosis. The note, which is uniformly dull, becomes more resonant when the lateral ventricles are distended in cerebellar abscess and in conditions in which the venae Galeni are compressed. Tenderness of the skull has been noted over the region of the abscess.

It is not always easy to determine whether the meninges are involved and often in ear diseases the condition is a meningo-encephalitis. Sometimes with acute ear disease the symptoms simulate closely cerebral meningitis or abscess. Indeed, Gowers stated that not only may these general symptoms be produced by ear disease, but even distinct optic neuritis.

Prognosis.—This is always serious and the only hope is in successful drainage. Even then complications may appear and cause death.

Treatment.—In ear disease free discharge of the pus should be promoted and careful disinfection practised. The treatment of injuries and fractures comes within the scope of the surgeon. The acute symptoms, such as fever, headache and delirium, must be treated by rest, an ice-cap and sedatives. In all cases, when a reasonable suspicion exists of the occurrence of abscess, the brain should be explored. The cases following ear disease, in which the suppuration is in the temporal lobe or the cerebellum, offer the most favorable chances. The localization can rarely be made accurately and the operator must be guided more by general anatomical and pathological knowledge. In cases of injury the exploration should be over the seat of the blow or the fracture. Hexamine should be given in full dosage.

HYDROCEPHALUS

Definition.—A condition, congenital or acquired, in which there is a great accumulation of fluid within the ventricles of the brain. The cases may be divided into three groups—idiopathic internal hydrocephalus, congenital or infantile, and secondary or acquired.

Idiopathic Internal Hydrocephalus.—A knowledge of this condition explains many anomalous and puzzling cases. An ependymitis causing a serous effusion into the ventricles, with distention and pressure effects, it may be compared to the serous exudates in the pleura or synovial membranes. It is not certain that the process is inflammatory, and Quincke likens it to angioneurotic edema. In very acute cases the ependyma may be smooth and natural looking; in more chronic cases thickened and sodden.

Both children and adults are affected, the latter more frequently. In the acute form the condition is mistaken for tuberculous or purulent meningitis. There are headache, retraction of the neck, and signs of increased intracranial pressure, choked disk, slow pulse, etc. Fever is usually absent, but there are cases with recurring paroxysms. In the chronic form the features are those of tumor—general, such as headache, slight fever, somnolence and delirium; and local, as exophthalmos, optic neuritis, spasms and rigidity of muscles, and paralysis of the cerebral nerves. Exacerbations occur and the symptoms vary in intensity. Recovery may follow and some reported cases of disappearance of symptoms of brain tumor belong in this category.

A variety of this is the *circumscribed serous meningitis* confined to the cerebellopontile angle, due to adhesions of the arachnoid to the cerebellum. Fluid accumulates in the cisterna lateralis. The increased pressure leads to disturbance in function of the nerves in this region, causing the syndrome described by Bárány—tinnitus with deafness, vertigo, occipital headache, facial paralysis and the "pointing error." Other lesions of this region, syphilitic meningitis and tumors, may cause this syndrome.

Chronic Internal Hydrocephalus.—This may be due to obstruction of outflow from the ventricles in the aqueduct of Sylvius (a congenital anomaly) or in the foramina of Magendie and Luschka (usually from inflammation) or to decreased absorption from the subarachnoid space (Dandy and Blackfan).

The lateral ventricles are enormously distended, but the ependyma is usually clear, sometimes a little thickened and granular, and the veins large. The choroid plexuses are vascular, sometimes sclerotic, but often natural looking. The third ventricle is enlarged, the aqueduct of Sylvius dilated, and the fourth ventricle may be distended. The quantity of fluid may reach several litres. It is limpid and contains a trace of albumin and salts. The changes in consequence of the ventricular distention are remarkable. The cerebral cortex is greatly stretched, and over the middle region the thickness may be only a few millimetres without a trace of the sulci or convolutions. The basal ganglia are flattened. The skull enlarges, and the circumference of the head of a child of three or four years may reach 25 or even 30 inches. The sutures widen, Wormian bones develop in them, and the bones of the cranium become exceedingly thin. The veins are marked beneath the skin. A fluctuation wave may sometimes be obtained and Fisher's brain murmur may be heard. The orbital plates of the frontal bone are depressed, causing exophthalmos. The small size of the face, widening somewhat above, is striking in comparison with the enormously expanded skull.

The enlarged head may obstruct labor; more frequently the condition is noticed some time after birth. It has occurred in several members of the same family. Headache is common and convulsions may occur. The reflexes are increased, the child learns to walk late, and ultimately in severe cases the legs become feeble and sometimes spastic. Sensation is much less affected than motility. Choked disk is not uncommon. The mental condition is variable; the child may be bright, but, as a rule, there is some grade of imbecility. The congenital cases usually die within the first four or five years. The process may be arrested and the patient reach adult life. Even when extreme, the mental faculties may be retained, as in Bright's celebrated patient, Cardinal, who lived to the age of twenty-nine, and whose head was translucent when the sun was shining behind him. Care must be taken not to mistake the rachitic head for hydrocephalus. The condition may be associated with other defects, harelip, spina bifida and club-foot.

Dandy has introduced a method of fluoroscopy after the injection of air into the ventricles, the outlines of which are then well seen and the extent but not always the type of hydrocephalus determined.

Acquired Chronic Hydrocephalus.—This is stated to be occasionally primary (idiopathic)—that is to say, it comes on spontaneously in the adult without observable lesion. Dean Swift is said to have died of hydrocephalus, but this seems unlikely. It is based upon the statement that "he (Mr. Whiteway) opened the skull and found much water in the brain," a condition no doubt of *hydrocephalus ex vacuo*, due to the wasting associated with his prolonged illness and paralysis. In nearly all cases there is either a tumor at the base of the brain or in the third ventricle, which compresses the venae Galeni. The passage from the third to the fourth ventricle may be closed, either by a tumor or by parasites. The foramen of Magendie may become closed by meningitis. Chronic inflammation of the ependyma may block the exit of the ventricular fluid. There may be unilateral hydrocephalus from closure of one of the foramina of Monro. In cerebrospinal fever the foramina of exit of the fluid may be occluded, with great distention of the ventricles. These conditions in adults may produce extreme hydrocephalus without any enlargement of the head. Even when the tumor begins early in life there may be no expansion of the skull. In a girl aged sixteen, blind from her third year, the head was not unusually large, the ventricles were enormously distended, and in the Rolandic region the brain substance was only 5 mm. in thickness. A tumor occupied the third ventricle. In other instances the sutures separate and the head gradually enlarges.

The *symptoms* are curiously variable. In the case mentioned there were headaches and gradual blindness; then a prolonged period in which she was able to attend to her studies. Headaches again supervened, the gait became irregular and somewhat ataxic. Death occurred suddenly. In another case there were prolonged attacks of coma with a slow pulse, and on one occasion the patient remained unconscious for more than three months. Gradually progressing optic neuritis without focalizing symptoms, headache, and attacks of somnolence or coma are suggestive symptoms. These cases of acquired chronic hydrocephalus simulate tumor very closely and in some cases can not be diagnosed certainly during life, though the condition may be suspected.

Diagnosis.—There is no difficulty if enlargement of the head is present. The forms secondary to meningitis are usually easily recognized. If due to growths in the brain stem the signs are generally marked. In adults it is difficult to distinguish from intracranial growth.

Prognosis.—This depends largely on the cause. If the course is acute and progressive the outlook is hopeless. In mild cases recovery may follow but there is a danger of mental defect or epilepsy. Remissions of the symptoms may occur, especially in cases of obscure origin.

Treatment.—The use of mercury and iodides is advised by some writers. Various operations have been devised for conveying the fluid to the subtemporal or subcutaneous regions, or connecting the cisterna magna directly with the longitudinal sinus. Decompression may be advisable in some cases.

DISEASES OF THE PERIPHERAL NERVES

NEURITIS

Neuritis may be *localized* in a single nerve, or *general,* involving a large number of nerves—*multiple neuritis* or *polyneuritis.*

Etiology.—*Local neuritis* arises from (*a*) *cold* as, for example, in the facial nerve. (*b*) *Trauma*—wounds, blows, direct pressure on the nerves, the tearing and stretching which follow a dislocation or a fracture, and the hypodermic injection of ether. Under this come the professional palsies, due to pressure in certain occupations. (*c*) *Extension of inflammation* from neighboring parts, as in a neuritis of the facial nerve due to caries in the temporal bone or in arthritis, and occasionally in tumors. (*d*) Some infections, *e.g.*, diphtheria.

Multiple neuritis has a very varied etiology: (*a*) The toxins of *infectious* diseases, as leprosy, diphtheria, typhoid fever, smallpox, etc.; (*b*) the *organic poisons,* such as alcohol and ether, bisulphide of carbon and naphtha, and metallic bodies, as lead and arsenic; (*c*) *cachectic* conditions, as in anemia, cancer, tuberculosis, or marasmus from any cause; (*d*) due to vitamin deficiency; (*e*) metabolic diseases, as in diabetes mellitus; and (*f*) there are cases in which none of these factors prevails, but the disease sets in suddenly after overexertion or exposure to cold.

Morbid Anatomy.—In neuritis due to the extension of inflammation the nerve is usually swollen, infiltrated and red in color. The inflammation may be chiefly *perineural* or it may pass into the deeper portion—*interstitial* neuritis—in which there is an accumulation of lymphoid elements between the nerve bundles. The nerve fibres themselves may not appear involved, but there is an increase in the nuclei of the sheath of Schwann. The myelin is fragmented, the nuclei of the internodal cells are swollen, and the axis cylinders present varicosities or undergo granular degeneration. Ultimately the nerve fibres may be completely destroyed and replaced by a fibrous connective tissue in which much fat is sometimes deposited—*lipomatous neuritis.*

The other form is *parenchymatous* neuritis, in which the changes are like those in the secondary or Wallerian degeneration, which follows when the nerve fibre is cut off from the cell body of the neurone to which it belongs. The medullary substance and the axis cylinders are chiefly involved, the interstitial tissues being but little altered or only affected secondarily. The muscles connected with the degenerated nerves usually show marked atrophic changes, and in some instances the change in the nerve sheath appears to extend directly to the interstitial tissue of the muscles.

Symptoms.—LOCALIZED NEURITIS.—As a rule, the constitutional disturbances are slight. The most important symptom is *pain* of a boring or stabbing character, usually felt in the course of the nerve and in the parts to which it is distributed. The nerve itself is sensitive to pressure, probably, as Weir Mitchell suggested, owing to the irritation of its nervi nervorum. The skin may be slightly reddened or even edematous over the seat of the inflammation. Mitchell described increase in the temperature and sweating in the affected region, and effusion into the joints and herpes. The function of the muscle to which the nerve fibres are distributed is impaired, motion is painful, and there may be twitchings or contractions. The *sensation* of the part may be somewhat deadened, even when the pain is greatly increased. In the more chronic cases of local neuritis, such, for instance, as follow dislocation of the humerus, the pain, which at first may be severe, gradually disappears, though some sensitiveness of the brachial plexus may persist for a long time, and the nerve cords may be firm and swollen. The *pain* is variable—sometimes intense; in others not causing much inconvenience. Numbness and formication may be present and tactile sensation greatly impaired. The motor disturbances are marked. Ultimately there is extreme atrophy of the muscles. Contractures may occur in the fingers. The skin may be reddened or glossy, the subcutaneous tissue edematous, and the nutrition of the nails defective. In some cases subcutaneous nodules develop.

A neuritis limited at first to a peripheral nerve may extend upward—the so-called ascending or migratory neuritis—and involve the larger nerve trunks, or even reach the spinal cord—causing subacute myelitis (Gowers). The condition is rarely seen in the neuritis from cold or in that which follows fevers; it occurs most frequently in traumatic neuritis.

J. K. Mitchell, in his monograph on injuries of nerves, concluded that the larger nerve trunks are most susceptible, and that the neuritis may spread up or down, the former being the most common. The paralysis secondary to visceral disease, as of the bladder, may be due to an ascending neuritis. The inflammation may extend to the nerves of the other side, through the spinal cord or its membranes, or without any involvement of the nerve-centres, the so-called sympathetic neuritis. The *electrical* changes in localized neuritis vary a great deal, depending upon the extent to which the nerve is injured. The lesion may be so slight that the nerve and the muscles to which it is distributed react normally to both currents; or it may be so severe that the *reaction of degeneration* develops within a few days—*i.e.*, the nerve does not respond to stimulation by either current, while the muscle reacts only to the galvanic current and in a peculiar manner. The contraction caused is slow and lazy, instead of sharp and quick as in the normal muscle, and the AC contraction is usually stronger than the KC contraction. Between these extremes there are many grades, and a careful electrical examination is an important aid to diagnosis and prognosis.

The duration varies from a few days to weeks or months. A slight traumatic neuritis may pass off in a day or two, while the severer cases may persist for months or never be completely relieved.

Multiple Neuritis.—The following are the most important groups:

(*a*) *Acute Febrile Polyneuritis.*—The attack follows exposure to cold or overexertion, or, in some instances, comes on spontaneously. The onset resembles that of an acute infectious disease. There may be a definite chill, pains in the back and limbs or joints, so that the case may be thought to be rheumatic fever. The temperature rises rapidly and may reach 103° or 104° F. There are headache, loss of appetite, and the general symptoms of acute infection,

The limbs and back ache. Intense pain in the nerves is by no means constant. Tingling and formication are felt in the fingers and toes, and there is increased sensitiveness of the nerve trunks or of the entire limb. Loss of muscular power, first marked, perhaps, in the legs, gradually comes on and extends with the features of an ascending paralysis. In other cases the paralysis begins in the arms. The extensors of the wrists and the flexors of the ankles are early affected, so that there is foot and wrist drop. In severe cases there is general loss of muscular power, producing a flabby paralysis, which may extend to the muscles of the face and to the intercostals, and respiration may be carried on by the diaphragm alone. The muscles soften and waste rapidly. There may be only hyperesthesia with soreness and stiffness of the limbs; in some cases, increased sensitiveness with anesthesia; in other instances the sensory disturbances are slight. The Argyll-Robertson pupil may be present and the pupils may be unequal. Involvement of the cranial nerves is rare, but the third, fifth and seventh have been involved. The vagus may be attacked and the rapid heart rate is usually attributed to this cause. Involvement of the bladder and rectum is rare, but it does occur and does not necessarily mean involvement of the cord. The clinical picture is not to be distinguished, in many cases, from Landry's paralysis; in others, from the subacute myelitis of Duchenne. There may be considerable difficulty in making a diagnosis.

The *course* is variable. In the most intense forms the patient may die in a week or ten days, with involvement of the respiratory muscles or from cardiac failure. As a rule, in cases of moderate severity, after five or six weeks, the condition remains stationary and then slow improvement begins. The paralysis in some muscles may persist for months and contractures may occur from shortening of the muscles, but even with this the outlook is, as a rule, good, although the paralysis has lasted for a year or more.

(*b*) *Recurring Multiple Neuritis.*—Under the term *polyneuritis recurrens* Mary Sherwood described 2 cases in adults—in one involving the nerves of an arm, in the other both legs. In one patient there were three attacks, in the other two, the distribution in the attacks being identical.

(*c*) *Alcoholic Neuritis.*—This, a most important form of multiple neuritis, was graphically described in 1822 by James Jackson, Sr., of Boston. Wilks recognized it as alcoholic paraplegia, but the starting point of recent researches dates from the observations of Dumesnil, of Rouen. It occurs particularly in steady, quiet tipplers and its appearance may be the first revelation of secret drinking. Vitamin B deficiency may have an important part in the etiology. The onset is usually gradual, and may be preceded for weeks or months by neuralgic pains and tingling in the feet and hands. Convulsions are not uncommon. Fever is rare. The *paralysis* gradually sets in, at first in the feet and legs, and then in the hands and forearms. The extensors are affected more than the flexors, so that there is wrist drop and foot drop. The paralysis may be thus limited and not extend higher in the limbs. In other instances there is paraplegia alone, while in some extreme cases all the extremities are involved. In rare instances the facial muscles and the sphincters are affected. The *sensory* symptoms are very variable. There are cases with numbness and tingling only, without great pain. In other cases there are severe burning or boring pains, the nerve trunks are sensitive, and the muscles are sore when grasped. The hands and feet may be swollen and congested, particularly when held down for a few moments. The cutaneous reflexes, as a rule, are preserved. The deep reflexes are usually lost.

The *course* of these alcoholic cases is, as a rule, favorable, and after persisting for weeks or months improvement gradually begins, the muscles regain their power, and even in the most desperate cases recovery may follow. The extensors of the feet may remain paralyzed for some time, and give to the patient a distinctive walk, the so-called *steppage* gait, characteristic of peripheral neuritis. It is sometimes known as the pseudotabetic gait, although it could not well be mistaken for the gait of tabes. The foot is thrown forcibly forward, the toe lifted high in the air so as not to trip upon it. The entire foot is slapped upon the ground as a flail. It is an awkward, clumsy gait, and gives the patient the appearance of constantly stepping over obstacles. Among the most striking features are the *mental* symptoms. Delirium is common, and there may be hallucinations with extravagant ideas, somewhat like those of general paresis. In some cases the picture is that of delirium tremens, but the most peculiar and almost characteristic mental disorder is that so well described by Wilks, in which the patient loses all appreciation of time and place, and describes with circumstantial details long journeys which, he says, he has recently taken, or tells of persons whom he has just seen. This is the so-called *Korsakoff's syndrome* or psychosis.

(*d*) *Multiple Neuritis in the Infectious Diseases.*—This has been already referred to, particularly in diphtheria, in which it is most common. The outlook is usually favorable and, except in diphtheria, fatal cases are uncommon. Multiple neuritis in tuberculosis, diabetes and syphilis is of the same nature, being probably due to toxemia of some kind. It may follow suppuration anywhere, as septic sore throat, and may occur after superficial septic sores.

(*e*) *The Metallic Poisons.*—Neuritis from *arsenic* may follow: (1) The medicinal use particularly of Fowler's solution. In one case of Hodgkin's disease general neuritis was caused by 10 drams of the solution. In chorea a good many cases have been reported. Changes in the nails are not uncommon, chiefly the transverse ridging. In a young woman who had taken "rough-on-rats" there were remarkable white lines—the leukonychia—running across the nails, without any special ridging. C. J. Aldrich finds that this is not uncommon in chronic arsenical poisoning. (2) The accidental contamination of food or drink. Chrome yellow may be used to color cakes, as in the cases recorded by D. D. Stewart. A remarkable epidemic of neuritis occurred in the Midland Counties of England, which was traced to the use of beer containing small quantities of arsenic, a contamination from the sulphuric acid used in making glucose. (3) A single dose taken by accident or purposely. Pigmentation of the skin is an important distinguishing sign. *Lead* is a much more frequent cause. Neuritis has followed the use of mercurial inunctions. Zinc is a rare cause. In a patient seen with Urban Smith neuritis followed the use of two grains of the sulphocarbolate taken daily for three years. Tea, coffee and tobacco are mentioned as rare causes.

(*f*) *Endemic neuritis,* beri-beri, is considered elsewhere.

Anesthesia Paralysis.—Here may most appropriately be considered the forms of paralysis following the use of anesthetics, or of too long-continued compression during operations. There are two groups of cases:

(*a*) During an operation the nerves may be compressed, either the brachial plexus by the humerus or the musculospiral by the table. The pressure most frequently occurs when the arm is elevated alongside the head or held out from the body. Paralysis of the crural nerves by leg-holders is reported. The too firm application of a tourniquet may be followed by paralysis.

(*b*) Paralysis from cerebral lesions during etherization. Apoplexy or embolism may occur during anesthesia. In Montreal a cataract operation was performed on an old man. He did not recover from the anesthetic and postmortem a cerebral hemorrhage was found. Epileptic convulsions may occur during anesthesia and prove fatal. The possibility of paralysis from loss of blood in operations has to be considered. Paralysis might result from the toxic effects of ether in a very protracted administration.

Angiopathic Paralysis.—Digital compression, the protracted application of the tourniquet and ligation of the main vessel taught us that normal action of the nerves and muscles of a limb is dependent on a good blood supply. In sudden blocking of the femoral artery with an embolus, the pain is not simply at the site of the blockage, but more or less diffuse throughout the limb, which the patient moves with the greatest difficulty. In the numerous war injuries to the arteries, these angiopathic paralyses were not uncommon. In a study of cases of severe wounds of the main vessel of a limb Burrows found the chief symptoms to be: (*a*) subjective changes, numbness, tingling, etc.; (*b*) anesthesia, usually of the glove type; (*c*) paralysis, often complete; (*d*) hardness of the muscles, and (*e*) edema of the limb. With reestablishment of the collateral circulation these may disappear in a few days.

Diagnosis.—The diagnosis of neuritis is often made carelessly and from nothing more than the complaint of pain. Pain in neuritis occurs only when a sensory or mixed nerve is involved. There is pain in the course of the nerve with tenderness or pain on pressure on it, changes in sensation in the area supplied, alteration in the deep reflexes, and muscular weakness and atrophy with altered electrical reactions. A loss of faradic irritability and a marked decrease in galvanic irritability are important signs of multiple neuritis. The relation of the motor and sensory changes is variable. Among the conditions which may lead to error are diseases of the cord, meninges or posterior nerve roots, spondylitis, arthritis, fibrositis, anatomical anomalies, wrong posture, perhaps with muscular strain, and flatfoot.

There is rarely any difficulty in distinguishing the alcohol cases. The wrist and foot drop with congestion of the hands and feet, and the peculiar delirium are characteristic. The rapidly advancing cases with paralysis of all extremities, often reaching to the face and involving the sphincters, probably represent a diffuse involvement of the nervous system, affecting the spinal cord, spinal ganglia and peripheral nerves. The less acute cases, in which the paralysis gradually involves the legs and arms with rapid wasting, simulate closely and may be confounded with the subacute atrophic spinal paralysis of Duchenne. The diagnosis from tabes is rarely difficult. The *steppage* gait is entirely different. There is rarely positive incoordination and the station is good. Foot drop is rare in tabes. The lightning pains are absent and there are usually no pupillary symptoms. The study of the spinal fluid is definite. The etiology is of moment.

Treatment.—Rest in bed is essential and the further ingestion of a causal agent should be prevented. In the acute cases with fever the salicylates and antipyrin are recommended. To allay the intense pain morphia or hot applications of lead water and laudanum are often required. Great care must be exercised in treating the alcoholic form, and the physician must not allow himself to be deceived by the statements of the relatives. It is sometimes exceedingly difficult to get a history of drinking. If there is any tendency to bed sores an air bed should be used or the patient placed in a continuous bath. Gentle friction may be used, and in the later stages, when the atrophy is marked and the pains have lessened, massage is probably the most reliable means at our command. Contractures should be prevented or if present gradually overcome by passive movements and extension. Often with the most extreme deformity from contracture, recovery is, in time, still possible. The interrupted current is useful when the acute stage is passed. Of internal remedies, strychnia is of value and may be given in increasing doses. For syphilis the usual treatment should be given.

NEUROMATA

Tumors situated on nerve fibres may consist of nerve substance proper, the true neuromata, or of fibrous tissue, the false neuromata. The true neuroma usually contains nerve fibres only, or in rare instances ganglion cells. Cases of ganglionic or medullary neuroma are rare; some of them are undoubtedly instances of malformation of the brain substance. In other instances the tumor is, probably, a glioma with cells closely resembling those of the central nervous system. The growths are often intermediate in anatomical structure between the true and the false.

Plexiform Neuroma.—In this remarkable condition the various nerve cords may be occupied by many hundreds of tumors. The disease is often hereditary and usually congenital. The tumors may occur in all the nerves of the body, and, as numbers of them may be made out on palpation, the diagnosis is usually easy. A remarkable case was described by Prudden in which there were 1,182 distinct tumors on the nerves. These tumors are rarely painful, but may cause symptoms through pressure on neighboring structures.

Generalized Neurofibromatosis: von Recklinghausen's Disease: Fibroma Molluscum.—Special attention was directed to this particular form of multiple neuroma by von Recklinghausen in 1882. The disease presents several groups of lesions:

1. Cutaneous.—(*a*) Soft, fibrous nodules, some sessile, others pedunculated, varying in size and greatly in number, are scattered over the skin. They may increase in number as age advances. (*b*) Bluish spots, indicating atrophy of the corium where the fibromata are perforating. (*c*) Pigmentation, in the form of freckles, blotches or diffuse areas. (*d*) Subcutaneous growths, at times of enormous size, causing the condition known as "elephantiasis neuromatosa." Congenital nevi are frequent.

2. Nervous.—Tumors resembling plexiform neuromata may be present on any nerve trunk from the centre to the periphery. The variable situation leads to a variety of sensory or motor phenomena, especially as they may arise from the nerve roots within the spinal canal or cranium. Cases resembling tabes, syringomyelia and spastic paralysis are reported. The patients often show mental changes and disturbance of speech.

3. Bone Lesions.—Changes similar to those of osteomalacia occur in about 7 per cent of the cases.

Other features may be mentioned: Three generations have been affected, or two or three members of a family, or a mother and several children. The lesions may develop during pregnancy and disappear after delivery. Brickner, after whom this syndrome has been named, collected 16 cases. The tumors do not always disappear. Adrian reported a case with multiple myomata of the stomach. A sarcomatous change may occur in the central tumors, but not in the optic and olfactory nerves which have not the sheath of Schwann. There may be associated glioma or other brain tumor.

The nature of the disease is unknown. The occurrence of the pigmentation and the osteomalacia suggest an endocrine disturbance; but the familial and hereditary features point rather to an embryonic origin.

The prognosis depends on the possibility of successful removal of such tumors as are causing greatest inconvenience.

"Tubercula dolorosa."—Multiple neuromata may especially affect the terminal cutaneous branches of the sensory nerves and lead to small subcutaneous painful nodules, often found on the face, breast, or about the joints. They may be associated with tumors of the nerve trunks.

"Amputation Neuromata."—These bulbous swellings may form on the central ends of nerves which have been divided in injuries or operations. They are especially common after amputations. They are due to the tangled coil of axis cylinder processes growing down from the central stump in an effort to reach their former end structures. They are very painful and usually require surgical removal but may recur.

DISEASES OF THE CEREBRAL NERVES

OLFACTORY NERVES AND TRACTS

The functions of the olfactory nerves may be disturbed at their origin, in the nasal mucous membrane, at the bulb, in the course of the tract, or at the centres. The disturbances may be manifested in subjective sensations of smell, complete loss of the sense, and occasionally in hyperesthesia. In the majority of persons the sense of smell is not very keen.

Subjective Sensations; Parosmia.—Hallucinations of this kind are found in the insane and in epilepsy. The aura may be represented by an unpleasant odor, described as resembling chloride of lime, burning rags, or feathers. In a few cases with these subjective sensations tumors have been found in the hippocampi. In rare instances, after injury of the head, the sense is perverted—odors of the most different character may be alike, or the odor may be changed, as in a patient noted by Morell Mackenzie, who for some time could not touch cooked meat, as it smelt to her exactly like stinking fish.

Increased sensitiveness (hyperosmia) occurs chiefly in nervous, hysterical women, in whom it may sometimes be developed so greatly that, like a dog, they can recognize the difference between individuals by the odor alone.

Anosmia; Loss of the Sense of Smell.—This may be produced by: (*a*) Affections of the origin of the nerves in the mucous membrane, which is perhaps the most frequent cause. It is not uncommon with chronic nasal catarrh and polypi. In paralysis of the fifth nerve, the sense of smell may be lost on the affected side, owing to interference with secretion.

(*b*) Lesions of the bulbs or of the tracts. In falls or blows, in caries of the bones, and in meningitis or tumor, the bulbs or the olfactory tracts may be involved. After an injury to the head the loss of smell may be the only symptom. In tabes the sense of smell may be lost, possibly owing to atrophy of the nerves.

(*c*) Lesions of olfactory centres. There are congenital cases in which the structures have not developed. Cases have been reported in which anosmia has been associated with disease in the hemisphere.

To test the sense of smell the pungent bodies, such as ammonia, which act upon the fifth nerve, should not be used, but volatile oils. In all instances a nasal examination should be made, as the condition may be due to local causes. The *treatment* is unsatisfactory even in the cases due to local nasal lesions.

OPTIC NERVE AND TRACT

Lesions of the Retina

These are of importance to the physician, and information of the greatest value may be obtained by a systematic examination of the eye grounds. Only a brief reference can be made to the more important appearances.

Retinitis.—This occurs in certain general affections, more particularly in nephritis, syphilis, leukemia and anemia. The common feature is the occurrence of hemorrhage and the development of opacities. There may also be a diffuse cloudiness due to effusion of serum. The hemorrhages are in the layer of nerve fibres. They vary greatly in size and form, but often follow the course of vessels. When recent the color is bright red, but they gradually change and old hemorrhages are almost black. The white spots are due to fibrinous exudate or to fatty degeneration of the retinal elements, and occasionally to accumulation of leukocytes or to a localized sclerosis.

Albuminuric retinitis occurs in chronic nephritis, particularly in the sclerotic form. The percentage of cases affected is from 15 to 25. There are instances in which these retinal changes occur at a stage when albuminuria may be slight or transient; but in such instances there is a marked arteriosclerosis. Gowers recognized a *degenerative* form (most common), in which, with the retinal changes, there may be scarcely any alteration in the disk; a *hemorrhagic* form, and an *inflammatory* form, in which there is much swelling of the retina and obscuration of the disk. It is noteworthy that in some instances the optic nerve changes predominate over the retinal changes, and one may be in doubt for a time whether the condition is associated with renal or intracranial disease.

Syphilitic Retinitis.—In the acquired form this is less common than choroiditis. In congenital syphilis *retinitis pigmentosa* is sometimes found.

Retinitis in Anemia.—A patient may become blind after a large hemorrhage, either suddenly or within two or three days, and in one or both eyes. Occasionally the loss may be permanent and complete. In some of these instances a neuroretinitis has been found, probably sufficient to account for the symptoms. In the more chronic anemias, particularly the pernicious form, retinitis is common, as determined first by Quincke.

LEUKEMIC RETINITIS.—In this affection the retinal veins are large and distended; there is also a peculiar retinitis, described by Liebreich. It is not very common. There are numerous hemorrhages and white or yellow areas, which may be large and prominent. In one case the retina postmortem was dotted with many small, opaque, white spots, looking like little tumors, the larger of which had a diameter of nearly 2 mm.

Retinitis is also found occasionally in diabetes, in purpura, in chronic lead poisoning, and sometimes as an idiopathic affection.

Functional Disturbances of Vision.—(*a*) TOXIC AMAUROSIS.—This occurs in uremia and may follow convulsions or come on independently. The condition, as a rule, persists only for a day or two. This form of amaurosis occurs in poisoning by lead, alcohol, and occasionally by quinine. It seems more probable that the poisons act on the centres and not on the retina.

(*b*) TOBACCO AMBLYOPIA.—The loss of sight is usually gradual, equal in both eyes, and affects particularly the centre of the field of vision. The eyegrounds may be normal, but occasionally there is congestion of the disks. On testing the color fields a central scotoma for red and green is found in all cases. Ultimately, if the use of tobacco is continued, organic changes may develop with atrophy of the disk.

(*c*) HYSTERICAL AMAUROSIS.—More frequently this is loss of acuteness of vision—amblyopia—but the loss of sight in one or both eyes may apparently be complete. The condition will be mentioned under hysteria.

(*d*) NIGHT-BLINDNESS—NYCTALOPIA—the condition in which objects are clearly seen during the day or by strong artificial light, but become invisible in the shade or in twilight, and *hemeralopia,* in which objects can not be clearly seen without distress in daylight or in a strong artificial light, but are readily seen in a deep shade or in twilight, are rare functional anomalies which may occur in epidemic form.

(*e*) RETINAL HYPERESTHESIA is sometimes seen in nervous patients but is not frequent in actual retinitis. It may occur with albuminuric retinitis and with aortic insufficiency.

Lesions of the Optic Nerve

Optic Neuritis (*Papilloedema; Choked Disk*).—In the first stage there is congestion of the disk and the edges are blurred and striated. In the second stage the congestion is more marked; the swelling increases, the striation also is more visible. The physiological cupping disappears and hemorrhages are not uncommon. The arteries present little change, the veins are dilated, and the disk may swell greatly. In slight grades the swelling gradually subsides and occasionally the nerve recovers completely. In instances in which the swelling and exudate are very great the subsidence is slow, and when it finally disappears there is complete atrophy of the nerve. The retina may participate in the inflammation, which is then a neuroretinitis.

This is of the greatest importance in diagnosis. It may exist in its early stages without any disturbance of vision, and even with extensive changes the sight for a time may be good.

Optic neuritis is seen occasionally in anemia and lead poisoning, more commonly in nephritis as neuroretinitis. It occurs occasionally as a primary idiopathic affection. The frequent connection with intracranial disease, particularly tumor, makes its presence of great value; in over 90 per cent the choked disk is bilateral. It is also found in meningitis, either the tuberculous or the simple form. In meningitis the inflammation may extend down the nerve sheath. In tumor, however, it is probable that mechanical conditions, especially venous stasis, are responsible for the edematous swelling. It often subsides very rapidly after decompression.

Retrobulbar Neuritis.—This occurs most often in multiple sclerosis. It is doubtful how often sinus infection (especially ethmoid and sphenoid) is responsible but it is a factor. Pernicious anemia, diabetes, syphilis, lead, alcohol and tobacco are occasional causes. Infection elsewhere than in the sinuses may be causal. If the lesion is situated so far forward as to involve the papilla there will be papilloedema. Optic atrophy of varying degree may follow.

Optic Atrophy.—This may be: (*a*) A *primary* affection. There is an hereditary form, in which the disease has developed in all the males of a family shortly after puberty. A large number of the cases of primary atrophy are associated with spinal disease, particularly tabes. Other causes which are assigned are diabetes, the specific fevers, methyl alcohol and lead.

(*b*) *Secondary* atrophy results from cerebral diseases, pressure on the chiasma or on the nerves, or, most common, as a sequence of optic neuritis.

The ophthalmoscopic appearances are different in the cases of primary and secondary atrophy. In the former the disk has a gray tint, the edges are well defined, and the arteries look almost normal; whereas in the consecutive atrophy the disk has a staring opaque white aspect, with irregular outlines, and the arteries are very small.

Affections of the Chiasma and Tract

At the chiasma the optic nerves undergo partial decussation. Each optic tract, as it leaves the chiasma, contains nerve fibres which originate in the retinae of both eyes. Thus, of the fibres of the right tract, part have come through the chiasma without decussating from the temporal half of the right retina, the other and larger portion of the fibres of the tract have decussated in the chiasma, coming as they do from the left optic nerve and the nasal half of the retina on the left side. The fibres which cross are in the middle portion of the chiasma, while the direct fibres are on each side. The following are the most important changes from lesions of the tract and chiasma:

Unilateral Affection of Tract.—If on the right side, this produces loss of function in the temporal half of the retina on the right side, and in the nasal half of the retina on the left side, so that there is only half vision, and the patient is blind to objects on the left side. This is termed homonymous hemianopia or lateral hemianopia. The fibres passing to the right half of each retina being involved, the patient is blind to objects in the left half of each visual field. The hemianopia may be partial and only a portion of the half field may be lost. The unaffected visual fields may have the normal extent, but in some instances there is considerable reduction. When the left half of one field and the right half of the other, or *vice versa,* are blind, the condition is known as heteronymous hemianopia.

Disease of the Chiasma.—(*a*) A lesion involves, as a rule, chiefly the central portion, in which the decussating fibres pass which supply the inner

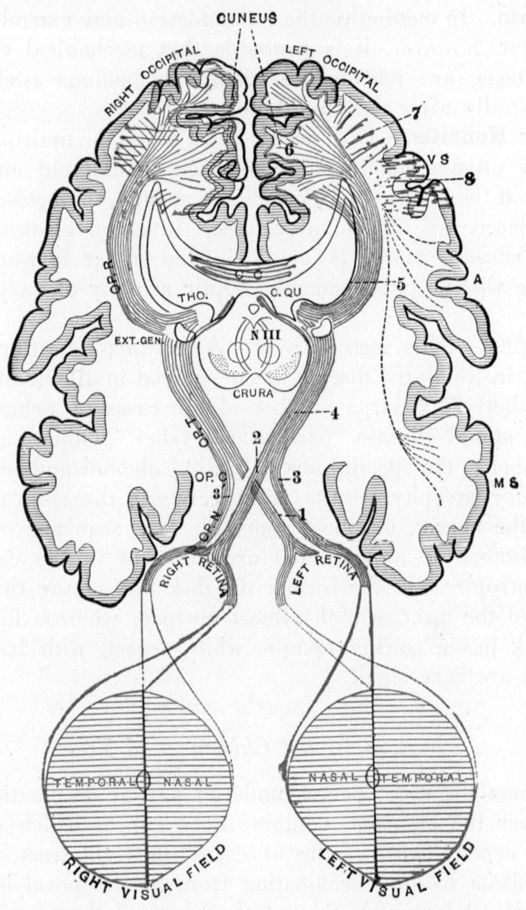

FIG. 22.—DIAGRAM OF VISUAL PATHS. (From Vialet, modified.)

OP. N., Optic nerve. OP. C., Optic chiasm. OP. T., Optic tract. OP. R., Optic radiations. EXT. GEN., External geniculate body. THO., Optic thalamus. C. QU., Corpora quadrigemina. C. C., Corpus callosum. V. S., Visual speech centre. A. S., Auditory speech centre. H. S., Motor speech centre. A lesion at 1 causes blindness of that eye; at 2, bi-temporal hemianopia; at 3, nasal hemianopia. Symmetrical lesions at 3 and 3′ would cause bi-nasal hemianopia; at 4, hemianopia of both eyes, with hemianopic pupillary inaction; at 5 and 6, hemianopia of both eyes, pupillary reflexes normal; at 7, amblyopia, especially of opposite eye; at 8, on left side, word-blindness.

or nasal halves of the retinae, producing in consequence loss of vision in the outer half of each field, or what is known as temporal heminanopia.

(*b*) If the lesion is more extensive it may involve not only the central portion, but also the direct fibres on one side of the commissure, in which case there is total blindness in one eye and temporal hemianopia in the other.

(*c*) Still more extensive disease is not infrequent from pressure of tumors in this region, the whole chiasma is involved, and total blindness results. The different stages in the process may often be traced in a single case from temporal hemianopia, then complete blindness in one eye with temporal hemianopia in the other, and finally complete blindness.

(*d*) A limited lesion of the outer part of the chiasma involves only the direct fibres passing to the temporal halves of the retinae and inducing blindness in the nasal field, or, as it is called, nasal hemianopia. This, of course, is extremely rare. Double nasal hemianopia may occur as a manifestation of tabes and in tumors involving the outer fibres of each tract.

Affections of the Tract and Centres

A lesion of the fibres of the optic path anywhere between the cortical centre and the chiasma will produce hemianopia. The lesion may be situated: (*a*) In the optic tract itself. (*b*) In the region of the thalamus, lateral geniculate body, and the corpora quadrigemina, into which the larger part of each tract enters. (*c*) A lesion of the fibre passing from the centre just mentioned to the occipital lobe. This may be either in the hinder part of the internal capsule or the white fibres of the optic radiation. (*d*) Lesion of the cuneus. Bilateral disease of the cuneus may result in total blindness. (*e*) There is clinical evidence to show that lesion of the angular gyrus may be associated with visual defect, not so often hemianopia as crossed amblyopia, dimness of vision in the opposite eye, and great contraction in the field of vision. Lesions in this region are associated with mind-blindness, a condition in which there is failure to recognize the nature of objects.

The effects of lesions in the optic nerve in different situations from the retinal expansion to the brain cortex are as follows: (1) Of the optic nerve, total blindness of the corresponding eye; (2) of the optic chiasma, either temporal hemianopia, if the central part alone is involved, or nasal hemianopia, if the lateral region of each chiasma is involved; (3) lesion of the optic tract between the chiasma and the lateral geniculate body produces lateral hemianopia; (4) lesion of the central fibres of the nerve between the geniculate bodies and the cerebral cortex produces lateral hemianopia; (5) lesion of the cuneus causes lateral hemianopia; and (6) lesion of the angular gyrus may be associated with hemianopia, sometimes crossed amblyopia, and the condition known as mind-blindness. (See Fig. 22.)

Diagnosis of Lesions of the Optic Nerve and Tract.—This depends much on the associated symptoms. The *significance* of hemianopia varies. There is a functional hemianopia associated with migraine and hysteria. In a considerable proportion of all cases there are signs of organic brain disease. In a certain number of instances of slight lesions of the occipital lobe hemichromatopsia has been observed. The homonymous halves of the retina as far as the fixation point are dulled, or blind for colors. Hemiplegia is common, in which event the loss of power and blindness are on the same side. Thus, a lesion in the left hemisphere involving the motor tract produces right hemiplegia, and when the fibres of the optic radiation are involved in the internal capsule there is also lateral hemianopia, so that objects in the field of vision to the right are not perceived. Hemianesthesia is not uncommon in such cases, owing to the close association of the sensory and visual tracts at the posterior part of the internal capsule. Certain forms of aphasia also occur in many of the cases.

MOTOR NERVES OF THE EYEBALL

Third Nerve (*Nervus oculomotorius*).—The nucleus of origin of this nerve is situated in the floor of the aqueduct of Sylvius; the nerve passes through the crus at the side of which it emerges. Passing along the wall of the cavernous sinus, it enters the orbit through the sphenoidal fissure and supplies all the muscles of the eyeball but the external rectus and superior oblique. Branches pass to the ciliary muscle and the constrictor of the iris. Lesions may affect the nucleus or the nerve in its course and cause paralysis or spasm.

Paralysis.—A nuclear lesion is usually associated with disease of the centres for the other eye muscles, producing general ophthalmoplegia. More commonly the nerve itself is involved in its course, either by meningitis, gumma or aneurism, or is attacked by neuritis, as in diphtheria. Complete paralysis is accompanied by the following features:

Paralysis of all the muscles, except the superior oblique and external rectus, by which the eye can be moved outward and a little downward and inward. There is divergent strabismus. There is *ptosis* or drooping of the upper eyelid, owing to paralysis of the levator palpebrae. The *pupil* is usually dilated. It does not contract to light, and the power of accommodation is lost. The most striking features of this paralysis are the external strabismus, with diplopia or double vision, and the ptosis. In very many cases the affection of the third nerve is partial. Thus the levator palpebrae and the superior rectus may be involved together, or the ciliary muscles and the iris may be affected and the external muscles escape.

There is a remarkable form of *recurring* oculomotor paralysis affecting chiefly women, and involving all the branches of the nerve. In some cases the attacks have come on at intervals of a month; in others a much longer period has elapsed. The attacks may persist throughout life. They are sometimes associated with pain in the head and sometimes with migraine.

Ptosis is a common and important sign. We may here refer briefly to the conditions under which it may occur: (*a*) A congenital, incurable form; (*b*) the form associated with definite lesion of the third nerve, either in its course or at its nucleus. This may come on with paralysis of the superior rectus alone or with paralysis of the internal and inferior recti as well. (*c*) There are instances of complete or partial ptosis associated with cerebral lesions without any other branch of the third nerve being paralyzed. (*d*) Hysterical ptosis, which is double and occurs with other hysterical symptoms. (*e*) Pseudo-ptosis, due to affection of the sympathetic nerve, is associated with symptoms of vasomotor palsy, such as elevation of the temperature on the affected side with redness and edema of the skin. Contraction of the pupil exists on the same side and the eyeball appears to have shrunk into the orbit. (*f*) In idiopathic muscular atrophy, when the face muscles are involved, there may be marked bilateral ptosis. In weak, delicate women there may be a transient ptosis, particularly in the morning, the cause of which is obscure. (*g*) It is common in myasthenia gravis.

Among the most important signs of third-nerve paralysis are those which relate to the ciliary muscle and iris.

Cycloplegia, paralysis of the ciliary muscle, causes loss of the power of accommodation. Distant vision is clear but near objects cannot be properly seen. In consequence the vision is indistinct, but can be restored by the use of convex glasses. This may occur in one or in both eyes; in the latter case it is usually associated with disease in the nuclei. Cycloplegia is an early and frequent sign in diphtheritic paralysis and occurs also in tabes.

Iridoplegia, or paralysis of the iris, occurs in three forms (Gowers):

(*a*) *Accommodation iridoplegia,* in which the pupil does not alter in size during the act of accommodation.

(*b*) *Reflex Iridoplegia.*—The path for the iris reflex is along the optic nerve and tract to its termination, then to the nucleus of the third nerve, and along the trunk of this nerve to the ciliary ganglion, and so through the ciliary nerves to the eyes. Each eye should be tested separately, the other one being covered. The patient should look at a distant object in a dark part of the room; then a light is brought suddenly in front of the eye at a distance of three or four feet, so as to avoid the effect of accommodation. Loss of this iris reflex with retention of the accommodation contraction is known as the *Argyll-Robertson pupil.*

(*c*) *Loss of the Skin Reflex.*—If the skin of the neck is pinched or pricked the pupil dilates reflexly, the afferent impulses being conveyed along the cervical sympathetic. Erb pointed out that this skin reflex is lost usually in association with the reflex contraction, but the two are not necessarily conjoined. In iridoplegia the pupils are often small, particularly in spinal disease, as in the characteristic small pupils of tabes—spinal myosis. Iridoplegia may coexist with a pupil of medium size.

Inequality of the pupils—anisocoria—is not infrequent in syphilis, paresis and tabes. It may occur in perfectly healthy individuals.

Spasm.—Occasionally in meningitis and in hysteria there is spasm of the muscles supplied by the third nerve, particularly the internal rectus and the levator palpebrae. *Nystagmus* is a rhythmical contraction of the eye muscles met with in many congenital and acquired lesions of the brain, particularly in multiple sclerosis. It may be hereditary and has been traced through four generations in association with head nodding (Yawger). Lid nystagmus may also be present. It is met with in albinos. The nystagmus of miners is apparently due to poor light.

Fourth Nerve (*Nervus trochlearis*).—This supplies the superior oblique muscle. In its course around the outer surface of the crus and in its passage into the orbit it may be compressed by tumors, aneurism, or the exudation of basilar meningitis. Its nucleus in the upper part of the fourth ventricle may be involved by tumors or undergo degeneration with the other ocular nuclei. The superior oblique muscle acts to direct the eyeball downward and rotate it slightly. The paralysis causes defective downward and inward movement, often too slight to be noticed. The head is inclined somewhat forward and toward the sound side, and there is double vision when the patient looks down.

Sixth Nerve.—Emerging at the junction of the pons and medulla, it passes forward in a long and exposed course to the orbit, and supplies the external rectus muscle. It is often involved in meningeal exudate, compressed by tumors and possibly involved in an independent neuritis. When paralyzed, there is internal squint with diplopia on attempting to look outwards. The true and the false images are parallel, and grow further apart on looking to the paralyzed side. When the nucleus is involved, the internal rectus of the opposite eye may be paralyzed as the nucleus sends fibres up in the pons to that part of the nucleus of the opposite third nerve which supplies the internal rectus. In one symptom-complex there is a combination of otitis media with paralysis of the sixth nerve. The inflammation travels to the apex of the petrous bone, then to the sixth nerve. The outlook is usually good.

General Features of Paralysis of the Motor Nerves of the Eye.—Gowers divided them into five groups:

(*a*) *Limitation of Movement.*—Thus, in paralysis of the external rectus, the eyeball can not be moved outward. When the paralysis is incomplete the movement is deficient in proportion to the degree of the palsy.

(*b*) *Strabismus.*—The axes of the eyes do not correspond. Thus, paralysis of the internal rectus causes a divergent squint; of the external rectus, a convergent squint. At first this is evident only when the eyes are moved in the direction of the action of the weak muscle. The deviation of the axis of the affected eye from parallelism with the other is called the primary deviation.

(*c*) *Secondary Deviation.*—If, while the patient is looking at an object. the sound eye is covered, so that he fixes the object looked at with the affected eye only, the sound eye is moved still further in the same direction—*e.g.*, outward, when there is paralysis of the opposite internal rectus. This is known as secondary deviation. It depends upon the fact that, if two muscles are acting together, when one is weak and an effort is made to contract it, the increased effort—innervation—acts powerfully upon the other muscle, causing an increased contraction.

(*d*) *Erroneous Projection.*—"We judge of the relation of external objects to each other by the relation of their images on the retina; but we judge of their relations to our own body by the position of the eyeball as indicated to us by the innervation we give to the ocular muscles" (Gowers). With the eyes at rest in the midposition, an object at which we are looking is directly opposite our face. Turning the eyes to one side, we recognize that object in the middle of the field or to the side of this former position. We estimate the degree by the amount of movement of the eyes, and when the object moves and we follow it we judge of its position by the amount of movement of the eyeballs. When one ocular muscle is weak the increased innervation gives the impression of a greater movement of the eye than has really taken place. The mind, at the same time, receives the idea that the object is further on one side than it really is, and in an attempt to touch it the finger may go beyond it. As the equilibrium of the body is in a large part maintained by a knowledge of the relation of external objects to it obtained by the action of the eye muscles, this erroneous projection disturbs the harmony of these visual impressions and may lead to giddiness—*ocular vertigo.*

(*e*) *Double Vision.*—The visual axes do not correspond, so that there is a double image—*diplopia.* That seen by the sound eye is termed the true image; that by the paralyzed eye, the false. In simple or homonymous diplopia the false image is "on the same side of the other as the eye by which it is seen." In crossed diplopia it is on the other side. In convergent squint the diplopia is simple; in divergent it is crossed.

Sympathetic Fibres.—These supply the muscle of Müller, which pushes the eye forward, fibres in the muscle elevating the upper lid and the dilator muscle of the pupil. Stimulation causes widening of the palpebral fissure, exophthalmos and a dilated pupil, as in Graves' disease. Paralysis causes a slight degree of ptosis, enophthalmos and a contracted pupil.

Ophthalmoplegia.—Two forms are recognized—ophthalmoplegia *externa* and *interna* which may occur separately or together.

OPHTHALMOPLEGIA EXTERNA.—The condition is one of more or less complete palsy of the external muscles of the eyeball, due usually to a slow degeneration in the nuclei, but sometimes to pressure of tumors, orbital periostitis or basilar meningitis. It is often, but not necessarily, associated with ophthalmoplegia interna. Of 62 cases in only 11 could syphilis be positively determined (Siemerling). The levator muscles of the eyelids and the superior recti are first involved, and gradually the other muscles, so that the eyeballs are fixed and the eyelids droop. There is sometimes slight protrusion of the eyeballs. The disease is essentially chronic and may last for years. It is found particularly with general paresis, tabes and progressive muscular atrophy. With it may be associated optic atrophy and affections of other cerebral nerves. Occasionally, as noted by Bristowe, it may be functional.

OPHTHALMOPLEGIA INTERNA.—Jonathan Hutchinson applied this term to a progressive paralysis of the internal ocular muscles, causing loss of pupillary action and the power of accommodation. When the internal and external muscles are involved the affection is known as *total ophthalmoplegia,* and in a majority of cases the two conditions are associated. In some the internal form may depend upon disease of the ciliary ganglion.

While, as a rule, ophthalmoplegia is a chronic process, an acute form may be associated with encephalitis or hemorrhagic softening of the nuclei of the ocular nerves. There is usually marked cerebral disturbance in the latter.

Treatment of Ocular Palsies.—It is important to ascertain the cause. The forms associated with tabes are obstinate and resist treatment. Occasionally a palsy, complete or partial, may pass away spontaneously. The cases associated with chronic degenerative changes, as in paresis and bulbar paralysis, are little affected by treatment. On the other hand, in syphilitic cases, specific treatment is often beneficial. Arsenic and strychnia, the latter hypodermically, may be employed. In any case in which the onset is acute with pain, hot fomentations and counterirritation or leeches applied to the temple give relief. Treatment by electricity has been employed without any special effect. The diplopia may be relieved by the use of prisms, or it may be necessary to cover the affected eye with an opaque glass.

FIFTH OR TRIGEMINAL NERVE

Etiology.—Paralysis may result from: (*a*) Disease of the pons, particularly hemorrhage, tumor or sclerosis. (*b*) Injury or disease at the base of the brain. Fracture rarely involves the nerve but meningitis, acute or chronic, and caries of the bone are not uncommon causes. (*c*) The branches may be affected as they pass out—the first division by tumors pressing on the cavernous sinus or by aneurism; the second and third divisions by growths in the sphenomaxillary fossa. (*d*) Primary neuritis, which is rare.

Symptoms.—(*a*) Sensory Portion.—Disease of the fifth nerve may cause loss of sensation in the parts supplied, including the half of the face, the corresponding side of the head, the conjunctiva, the mucosa of the lips, tongue, hard and soft palate, and of the nose of the same side. The anesthesia may be preceded by tingling or pain. The muscles of the face are also insensible and the movements may be slower. The sense of smell is interfered with, owing to dryness of the mucous membrane. The salivary, lachrymal, and buccal secretions may be lessened, and the teeth may become loose. Unless properly guarded an ulcerative inflammation of the eye may follow. *Herpes zoster*, due to virus infection of the Gasserian ganglion, may occur in the region supplied by the nerve, usually the upper branch, and is associated with much pain, which may last for months or years. Corneal ulceration may occur. In herpes zoster there may be slight enlargement of the cervical glands.

(*b*) Motor Portion.—Inability to use the muscles of mastication on the affected side is the distinguishing feature of paralysis of this portion of the nerve. It is recognized by placing the finger on the masseter and temporal muscles, and, when the patient closes the jaw, the feebleness of their contraction is noted. If paralyzed, the external pterygoid can not move the jaw toward the unaffected side; and when depressed, the jaw deviates to the paralyzed side. Motor paralysis of the fifth nerve results from lesions of the nucleus or in the peripheral part of the motor division.

Spasm of the Muscles of Mastication.—*Trismus* may be tonic or clonic, and is an association phenomenon in general convulsions or, more rarely, an independent affection. In the tonic form the jaws are kept close together—lockjaw—or can be separated only for a short space. The muscles of mastication can be seen in contraction and felt to be hard; the spasm is often painful. This tonic contraction is an early sign in tetanus, and is sometimes seen in tetany. A form of this tonic spasm occurs in hysteria. Occasionally trismus follows exposure to cold, and is said to be due to reflex irritation from the teeth, the mouth or caries of the jaw. It may also be a symptom of organic disease due to irritation near the motor nucleus of the fifth nerve.

Clonic spasm of the muscles supplied by the fifth occurs in the form of rapidly repeated contractions, as in "chattering teeth." This is rare apart from general conditions, though cases are on record, usually in women late in life, in whom this isolated clonic spasm of the muscles of the jaw has been found. In another form of clonic spasm sometimes seen in chorea there are forcible single contractions.

The *diagnosis* of disease of the trifacial nerve is rarely difficult but the wide distribution must be remembered. Pain due to disease of the fifth nerve may be regarded as due to lesions of other nerves. The preliminary pain and hyperesthesia of trigeminal neuralgia are sometimes mistaken for ordinary neuralgia. The loss of sensation and the palsy of the muscles of mastication are readily determined. Involvement of one branch means a lesion peripheral to the Gasserian ganglion. In *treatment*, for severe pain sedatives are required and local applications are useful. If there is a suspicion of syphilis, appropriate treatment should be given. Faradization is sometimes beneficial. For herpes zoster the usual treatment should be given.

CLINICAL VARIETIES, DEPENDING ON THE NERVE ROOTS AFFECTED

Trigeminal Neuralgia; Tic Douloureux.—A distinction must be drawn between the minor and major neuralgias of the fifth cranial nerve. The former may be symptomatic of the involvement of the ganglion or one of its branches in some disease process—the pressure of a tumor on the ganglion, carious teeth, sinus infection or injury. There may be referred pains in this area from processes within the cranium. A painful neuralgia may follow an attack of zoster in any division of the fifth nerve.

The *major* trigeminal neuralgia is a primary affection of the Gasserian ganglion. The designation *tic* is not descriptive; there is usually immobility. The sex incidence is about equal; the majority of cases begin between the ages of forty and sixty. No definite etiological factor is evident. The right side is involved in about two-thirds of the cases. Patrick's figures show that the second and third branches are involved more often than the first. It begins most often in the second branch and later two or all three branches may be involved. The *pain* is of sudden onset, usually excruciating and in paroxysms, which may recur, usually not lasting longer than two minutes. The attacks are excited by any external irritation which may be very slight, such as a draught of air, touching the skin, and the movements in speaking, eating or swallowing. The areas over which irritation excites the pain are termed dolorogenetic or "trigger" zones. These do not always correspond to the pain zone. The pain may radiate into the cervical nerves or down the arms. The attacks tend to be of increasing severity and in advanced cases the paroxysms may recur at short intervals in steady succession.

The *diagnosis* is rarely in doubt but minor forms should not be mistaken for the major. The pain in this is paroxysmal, so that a steady pain about the face is probably not trifacial neuralgia. If the area has been rubbed or massaged, or the patient touches it to show where the pain is, the disease is probably not the major form. The disease may be remittent but tends to progress and increase in severity so that life is almost unbearable. There are other forms of facial neuralgia in addition to the trigeminal: (1) Attributed to the *sphenopalatine* (Meckel's) ganglion (Sluder), in which an inflammatory process in the sinuses spreads to the ganglion. There is pain about the eye, root of the nose, and upper jaw back to the mastoid which may spread more widely. The pain is constant or paroxysmal. (2) *Geniculate ganglion.* Hunt has emphasized the involvement of the sensory part of the facial nerve. The auricular herpetic eruption is due to disease of this ganglion. (3) A painful convulsive tic occurs. (4) There is an intractable form in run-down nervous patients, for which no definite cause can be found. (5) *Tumor of the Gasserian ganglion* gives a combination of acute pain with marked impairment of sensation. Many cases show atypical features. Cooper (1933) found 76 cases reported.

Treatment.—The use of heat, including diathermy, may give some relief. Of drugs, chemically pure trichlorethylene may be tried (20 drops are placed on gauze and inhaled three times a day; the liquid should not come in contact with the nose). Alcohol injections into the ganglion or branches are often satisfactory, giving relief for a variable period. Division of the sensory root gives excellent results.

FACIAL NERVE

Paralysis (*Bell's Palsy*).—Etiology.—The facial or seventh may be paralyzed by (*a*) lesions of the cortex—supranuclear palsy; (*b*) lesions of the nucleus itself; or (*c*) involvement of the nerve trunk in its tortuous course within the pons and through the wall of the skull.

(*a*) *Supranuclear paralysis,* due to lesion of the cortex or of the facial fibres in the corona radiata or internal capsule, is, as a rule, associated with hemiplegia. Paralysis is on the same side as that of the arm and leg. It may be due to tumors, abscess, inflammation, or softening in the cortex or in the region of the internal capsule. It is distinguished from the peripheral form by the persistence of the normal electrical excitability of both nerves and muscles and the frequent absence of involvement of the upper branches of the nerve, so that the orbicularis palpebrarum, frontalis and corrugator muscles are spared. In rare instances these muscles are paralyzed. In this form the voluntary movements are more impaired than the emotional. Isolated paralysis—monoplegia facialis—due to involvement of the cortex or of the fibres in their path to the nucleus, is uncommon. The nuclei of origin on either side of the middle line in the medulla are united by decussating fibres with the cortical centre on the opposite side. (See Fig. 21.) A few fibres reach the nucleus from the cerebral cortex of the same side, and this uncrossed path may innervate the upper facial muscles.

(*b*) The *nuclear paralysis* caused by lesions of the nerve centres in the medulla is seen in tumors, encephalitis, chronic softening and hemorrhage. It may be involved in poliomyelitis. In diphtheria this centre may also be attacked. The symptoms are practically similar to those of an affection of the nerve fibre itself—infranuclear paralysis.

(*c*) *Involvement of the Nerve Trunk.*—Paralysis may result from:

(1) Involvement of the nerve as it passes through the pons—that is, between its nucleus in the floor of the fourth ventricle and the point of emergence in the posterolateral aspect of the pons. The specially interesting feature in connection with involvement of this part is the production of what is called alternating or *crossed paralysis,* the face being involved on the same side as the lesion, and the arm and leg on the opposite side, since the motor path is involved above the point of decussation in the medulla (Fig. 21). This occurs only when the lesion is in the lower section of the pons. A lesion in the upper half of the pons involves the fibres not of the outgoing nerve on the same side, but of the fibres from the hemispheres before they have crossed to the nucleus of the opposite side. In this case there would be paralysis of the face and limbs on the side opposite to the lesion. The palsy would resemble the cerebral form, involving only the lower fibres of the facial nerve.

(2) The nerve may be involved at its point of emergence by tumors, particularly by cerebellopontine growths, by gumma, meningitis, or occasionally it may be injured in fracture of the base.

(3) In passing through the Fallopian canal the nerve may be involved in disease of the ear, particularly by caries of the bone in otitis media. This is a common cause. Fibrositis about the nerve may be responsible.

(4) As the nerve emerges from the styloid foramen it is exposed to injuries and blows which may cause paralysis. The fibres may be cut in the

removal of tumors in this region, or the paralysis may be caused by pressure of the forceps in an instrumental delivery.

(5) Exposure to cold acts by inducing a neuritis of the nerve within the Fallopian canal. Reik believes that in most of these cases there is an acute otitis media from which the nerve is involved.

(6) Syphilis is not an infrequent cause, and the paralysis may appear early with the secondary symptoms.

(7) Some cases may result from a virus which causes infection of the geniculate ganglion. In the syndrome described by Ramsay Hunt there is peripheral facial paralysis, vertigo, tinnitus with herpes of the ear and internal auditory meatus. In some cases of facial paralysis the blood contains herpes zoster antibodies.

Facial diplegia is a rare condition occasionally found in affections at the base of the brain, lesions in the pons, simultaneous involvement of the nerves in ear-disease, and in diphtheritic paralysis. Disease of the nuclei or symmetrical involvement of the cortex might also produce it. It may occur as a congenital affection. H. M. Thomas described two cases in one family.

SYMPTOMS.—In the peripheral facial paralysis all the branches of the nerve are involved. The face on the affected side is immobile and can neither be moved at will nor participate in any emotional movements. The skin is smooth and the wrinkles are effaced, a point particularly noticeable on the forehead of elderly persons. The eye can not be closed or the forehead wrinkled, the lower lid droops, and the eye waters. On the affected side the angle of the mouth is lowered, and in drinking the lips are not kept in close apposition to the glass, so that the liquid is apt to run out. In smiling or laughing the contrast is most striking, as the affected side does not move, giving a curious unequal appearance to the two sides of the face. In long-standing cases, when the reaction of degeneration is present, if the patient tries to close the eyes while looking fixedly at an object the lids on the sound side close firmly, but on the paralyzed side there is only a slight inhibitory droop of the upper lid, and the eye is turned upward and outward by the inferior oblique. On asking the patient to show his upper teeth, the angle of the mouth is not raised. In all these movements the face is drawn to the sound side. Speaking may be slightly interfered with, owing to imperfection in the formation of the labial sounds. Whistling can not be performed. In chewing the food, owing to the paralysis of the buccinator, particles collect on the affected side. The paralysis of the nasal muscles is seen on asking the patient to sniff. As the lips are drawn to the sound side, the tongue, when protruded, looks as if it were pushed to the paralyzed side; but on taking its position from the incisor teeth, it will be found in the middle line. The reflex movements are lost in this peripheral form.

When the nerve is involved after the chorda tympani has joined it, the sense of taste is lost in the anterior part of the tongue on the affected side. When the nerve is damaged outside the skull the sense of taste is unaffected. Hearing is often impaired in facial paralysis, most commonly by preceding ear disease. The paralysis of the stapedius muscle may lead to increased sensitiveness to musical notes. Severe *pain* may precede or accompany the paralysis. It is usually in the ear and mastoid region but may radiate to the occipital and trigeminal distribution. The face on the affected side may be swollen.

The *electrical reactions,* which are those of a peripheral palsy, have considerable importance from a prognostic standpoint. Erb's rules are as follows: If there is no change, either faradic or galvanic, the prognosis is good and recovery takes place in from fourteen to twenty days. If the faradic and galvanic excitability of the nerve is only lessened and that of the muscle increased to the galvanic current and the contraction formula altered (the contraction sluggish $AC < KC$), the outlook is relatively good and recovery will probably take place in from four to six weeks; occasionally in from eight to ten. When the reaction of degeneration is present and the mechanical excitability is altered, the prognosis is relatively unfavorable and recovery may not occur for many months.

Course.—This is usually favorable in the common form but not in those due to intracranial lesions or caries of bone. The onset in the form following cold is very rapid, developing perhaps within twenty-four hours, but rarely is the paralysis permanent. Hunt has drawn special attention to *recurrent* facial paralysis which may be on one or alternate sides—"relapsing alternating." In some instances contracture develops as the voluntary power returns, and the natural folds and the wrinkles on the affected side may be deepened, so that on looking at the face one at first may have the impression that the affected side is the sound one. This is corrected at once on asking the patient to smile, when it is seen which side of the face has the more active movement. Aretaeus noted the difficulty sometimes experienced in determining which side was affected until the patient spoke or laughed.

Permanent Facial Paralysis.—One of the distressing sequels is permanent loss of power with immobility and the disfigurement resulting from the overaction of the muscles on the sound side. There are three groups of cases: (1) Those due to *trauma,* especially the birth palsies from injury by forceps. (2) Due to suppurative middle-ear disease, following scarlet fever, diphtheria or sepsis of any kind, such as puerperal fever. (3) In a few cases following the ordinary Bell's paralysis. Even when paralysis exists from childhood, there may be slight voluntary control, and the muscles may respond to faradic stimulus. The facial nerve in reality may have recovered or regenerated, and the disfigurement and loss of function result from over-stretching of the degenerated muscles by the action of their opponents (Turrell).

Diagnosis.—This is usually easy. The distinction between the peripheral and central form is based on facts already mentioned. The diagnosis of the cause may be difficult.

Treatment.—In the cases which result from cold and are probably due to neuritis within the bony canal, hot applications should be made; subsequently counterirritation by iodine or small blisters should be used. If the ear is diseased, free discharge should be obtained. The galvanic current may be employed to keep up the nutrition of the muscles. The positive pole should be placed behind the ear, the negative one along the zygomatic and other muscles. The application can be made daily for a quarter of an hour and the patient can make it himself. Massage in the course of the nerve and of the muscles of the face is also useful. A course of iodide of potassium may be given even when there is no indication of syphilis.

In those cases in which the nerve has been destroyed by an injury, during an operation or from disease, and when there has been no evidence of returning function after a few months, a nerve anastomosis should be performed. For this purpose either the spinal accessory or the hypoglossal nerve may be used. Though the normal conditions may never be completely regained, the motor power will be largely restored and the deformity lessened. Nerve grafting has been done successfully.

Spasm.—This may be limited to a few or involve all the muscles innervated by the facial nerve, and may be unilateral or bilateral. It is known also as *mimic spasm* or *convulsive tic.* Several different affections are usually considered under the name of facial spasm, but we speak here only of the simple spasm of the facial muscles, either primary or following paralysis, and do not include habit spasm in children or the *tic convulsif* of the French.

Gowers recognized two classes—one in which there is an organic lesion, and an idiopathic form. It is thought to be due also to reflex causes, such as the irritation from carious teeth. The disease usually occurs in adults, whereas habit spasm and *tic convulsif,* often confounded with it, are most common in children. True mimic spasm may come on in childhood and persist. When the result of organic disease, there has usually been a lesion of the centre or pressure on the nerve at the base of the brain by aneurism or tumor.

Symptoms.—The spasm may involve only the muscles around the eyes—blepharospasm—in which case there is constant, rapid, quick action of the orbicularis palpebrarum, which, in association with photophobia, may be tonic in character. More commonly the spasm affects the lateral facial muscles with those of the eye, and there is twitching of the side of the face with partial closure of the eye. The frontalis is rarely involved. In aggravated cases the depressors of the angle of the mouth and the platysma myoides are affected. This spasm is confined to one side of the face in a majority of cases, though it may become bilateral. It is increased by emotional causes and by voluntary movements of the face. As a rule, it is painless, but there may be tender points over the course of the fifth nerve, particularly the supraorbital branch. Tonic spasm of the facial muscle may follow paralysis, and is said to result occasionally from cold. The outlook is always dubious. A majority of the cases persist for years and are incurable.

Treatment.—Sources of irritation should be looked for and removed. When a painful spot is present, blistering or the application of the cautery may relieve it. The salicylates, mercury and iodide have seemed to help some patients and should be tried. Injection of alcohol (50 per cent) into the facial nerve has been successful (Patrick). The needle should be introduced with great care and the alcohol injected very slowly until the first signs of weakness of the facial muscles appear. Severe cases may require surgical interference. The nerve may be divided near the stylomastoid foramen and an anastomosis made between it and the spinal accessory.

AUDITORY NERVE

The eighth nerve consists of two separate nerves—the cochlear and vestibular roots. These have different functions, and are best considered separately. The cochlear nerve is connected with the organ of Corti and concerned in hearing. The vestibular nerve is connected with the vestibule and semicircular canals, and has to do with the maintenance of equilibrium.

The Cochlear Nerve

The cortical centre for hearing is in the temporosphenoidal lobe. Primary disease of the auditory nerve in its centre or intracranial course is uncommon. More frequently the terminal branches are affected within the labyrinth. The ears are represented bilaterally in the brain and so a lesion on one side does not cause any marked disturbance, but if the left side is involved this may result in *word-deafness.* A tumor involving the region of the posterior quadrigeminal bodies causes deafness on the same side.

Lesions of the nerve at the base of the brain may result from the pressure of tumors, including the acoustic tumor, syphilis, meningitis, hemorrhage or traumatism. A primary degeneration of the nerve may occur in tabes. Primary disease of the terminal nuclei of the cochlear nerve is rare. A form results from epidemic cerebrospinal meningitis, in which the nerve is frequently involved, causing permanent deafness. In young children the condition results in deafmutism.

Internal Ear.—In a majority of cases with auditory nerve symptoms the lesion is in the internal ear, either primary or the result of extension of disease of the middle ear. Two groups of symptoms may be produced—hyperesthesia and irritation, and diminished function or nervous deafness.

(*a*) Hyperesthesia and Irritation.—This may be due to altered function of the centre as well as of the nerve ending. True hyperesthesia—hyperacusis—is a condition in which sounds, sometimes even those inaudible to other persons, are heard with great intensity. It occurs in hysteria and occasionally in cerebral disease. In paralysis of the stapedius low notes may be heard with intensity. In dyesthesia, or dysacusis, ordinary sounds cause an unpleasant sensation, as commonly happens in connection with headache, when ordinary noises are badly borne.

Tinnitus aurium is a term employed to designate certain subjective sensations of ringing, roaring, ticking and whirring noises in the ear. It is a very common and often a distressing symptom. Certain drugs, such as quinine, may cause it. It is associated with many forms of ear disease and may result from pressure of wax on the drum. It is rare in organic disease of the central connections of the nerve. Sudden intense stimulation of the nerve may cause it. A not uncommon form is that in which the patient hears a continual *bruit* in the ear, and the noise has a systolic intensification, usually on one side. It may suggest an internal aueurism. A systolic murmur may be heard occasionally on auscultation in anemia and neurasthenia. Subjective noises in the ear may precede an epileptic seizure and are sometimes present in migraine. They are common in hypertension and hypotension. Tinnitus in any form, though slight and often regarded as trivial, occasions great annoyance and mental distress, and has driven patients to suicide. The occurrence of tinnitus may vary greatly without evident cause.

The *diagnosis* is readily made; but it is often extremely difficult to determine the cause. The relief of conditions such as anemia or neurasthenia may result in cure. A careful examination of the ear should always be made. One of the most worrying forms is the constant clicking, sometimes audible many feet away from the patient, and due probably to clonic spasm of the muscles connected with the Eustachian tube or of the levator palati. It may persist for years and then disappear suddenly. The pulsating forms of tinnitus, in which the sound is like a systolic murmur, are almost invariably subjective. They often occur in anemia and hypotension. It is to be remembered that in children there is a systolic brain murmur, best heard over the ear, and in some instances appreciable in the adult.

(*b*) Diminished Function or Nervous Deafness.—In testing for nervous deafness, if the tuning fork can not be heard when placed near the meatus, but the vibrations are audible by placing the foot of the tuning fork against the temporal bone, the conclusion may be drawn that the deafness is not due to involvement of the nerve. The vibrations are conveyed through the temporal bone to the cochlea and vestibule. Disturbance of the function of the auditory nerve is not a very frequent symptom in brain disease, but in all cases the function of the nerve should be carefully tested.

The Vestibular Nerve

Our sense of position in space and the control of the balance of the body depend partly on proper function of the vestibular nerve and its central associations in the cerebellum and cerebrum. Disturbance of the relation of the body to space, or of its balance, produces the unpleasant sensation which we call dizziness or vertigo. It results from a discord between the impressions arising in the labyrinth, the cerebellum, the eye muscles and elsewhere, and a failure to coordinate these in the cerebrum. The controlling factor is the vestibular mechanism. The cochlear nerves are often involved simultaneously, producing tinnitus, and nystagmus may be associated.

An apprehension, not a true vertigo, is common in looking from a height, especially in those with disease of the internal ear. True vertigo is always accompanied by a sensation of falling or turning, even when the person is in bed, and if standing, there is incoordination of the muscles, with staggering or falling. The patient may feel that he is moving or the objects about him appear to rotate. The direction in which he falls is variable and of special importance. Nystagmus is often associated and the direction and intensity should be studied.

(1) Auditory (Labyrinthine) Vertigo—Ménière's Syndrome.—In 1861 Ménière described an affection characterized by noises in the ear, attacks of vertigo which may be associated with vomiting and loss of consciousness; in many cases there is progressive loss of hearing. Bárány groups the conditions in which the labyrinth may be affected and vertigo occur under the following heads: (*a*) Acute infectious diseases, influenza, cerebrospinal meningitis, etc. (*b*) Chronic infectious diseases, syphilis particularly. (*c*) Constitutional conditions and intoxications. Hemorrhage into the labyrinth (in leukemia, purpura hemorrhagica, pernicious anemia); chlorosis, thyroid intoxications, arteriosclerosis, etc. (*d*) Tumors and diseases of the central nervous system; tumors of the acoustic nerve, cerebellum, pons, and fourth ventricle, meningitis, cerebellar abscess, multiple sclerosis, tabes, etc. (*e*) Trauma, fracture of the base, etc. (*f*) Hereditary degenerative diseases and malformations of the internal ear. (*g*) Intoxications, alcohol, nicotine, quinine, salicylic acid group, arsenic. To these may be added gas emboli in caisson disease and ordinary emboli. Increase of pressure in the semicircular canals due to disturbance of water metabolism has been suggested.

Symptoms.—The attack usually sets in suddenly with a buzzing noise in the ears and the patient feels as if he were reeling or staggering. He may feel himself to be reeling, or the objects about him may seem to be turning, or the phenomena may be combined. The attack is often so abrupt that the patient falls, though, as a rule, he has time to steady himself by grasping some neighboring object. Consciousness is generally maintained but may be momentarily lost. Ocular symptoms are usually present. Jerking of the eyeballs or nystagmus occurs. The patient becomes pale and nauseated, a clammy sweat breaks out and vomiting may follow. The duration of the attack varies; it may be very short, but usually the patient has to lie quietly for some time, as any movement of the head brings on another attack. Labyrinthine vertigo is usually paroxysmal, coming on at irregular intervals, sometimes of weeks or months; or several attacks may occur in a day.

The *outlook* is uncertain. While some patients recover completely, in others deafness results and the attacks recur at shorter intervals. In aggravated cases the patient constantly suffers from vertigo, and may even be confined to his bed.

Treatment.—A salt free diet with restriction of fluid to a minimum may be helpful. Salicylates should be given freely, perhaps best as acetylsalicylic acid. Bromide is also useful both for the attacks and in prevention, doses of 20 to 30 grains (1.5 to 2 gm.) being given daily. Phenobarbital may be of value. Intracranial division of the eighth nerve has been done and Dandy (1933) reported good results.

Acute Vestibulitis.—In this there is severe vertigo with vomiting and ataxia of a cerebellar form, suggesting bilateral disease of the cerebellum. Permanent deafness on both sides comes on rapidly; the cerebellar features gradually disappear.

Affections of the External and Middle Ears.—Irrigation of the meatus may be followed by giddiness or by a severe Ménière syndrome. Removal of *wax* pressing against the drum may cure a persistent vertigo. All forms of *middle ear disease* may cause vertigo, the suppurative as well as the chronic sclerotic. Noises in the ear are usually present as well. The attacks may be of great severity, but apart from gross brain lesions, death is rare. A patient with chronic deafness and tinnitus had severe vertigo in turning on the left side. There was no suggestion of a central lesion. Death occurred in one of the attacks.

(2) Vertigo in Intracranial Tumors.—The symptom is variable: the largest growth may exist in any region without it—a very small one in a special locality may cause severe attacks. The vestibular fibres may be involved in any part of their course or indirectly compressed. Direct involvement is seen in tumors of the cerebellopontine angle, affecting the eighth and usually the seventh nerves, in cerebellar tumors, and in aneurism.

Vertigo is rarely a focal symptom as it may follow indirect pressure from tumors of the cerebrum.

(3) Ocular Vertigo.—The association of giddiness with ocular defects has long been recognized, and the ocular reflexes of vestibular nerve origin are important in diagnosis. Nystagmus, double vision and paralysis of accommodation may be ocular associations of vertigo. The central connections of the nuclei of the "space nerve" with those of the ocular muscles are very close.

Errors of refraction may cause an irritation and instability of the space nerve centres leading to severe vertigo.

(4) Cardiovascular Vertigo.—Vertigo is common in neurocirculatory asthenia. In cardiac insufficiency giddiness is a frequent complaint particularly with aortic disease. The loss of consciousness in Stokes-Adams' disease may be preceded by vertigo. One of the commonest forms is seen in *hypertension* with arteriosclerosis, very often with tinnitus. It may be slight and noticed only in the morning or on getting up suddenly. In other instances it is one of the most distressing features of sclerosis of the cerebral arteries. Vertigo may precede or accompany the attacks of transient paralysis with asphasia; and with a persistent headache and hypertension it may precede apoplexy. *Hypotension* is also a frequent cause.

(5) Toxic vertigo is described as due to alcohol, tobacco and quinine, to the toxins of the specific fevers and to focal infection. The essential process is a neuritis of the eighth nerve, or a chronic degenerative change, involving cochlea and labyrinth. A high-pitched tinnitus, with progressive deafness, and transient attacks of vertigo, sometimes of the Ménière type, are the usual symptoms. True toxic neuritis of the vestibular nerve is very rare. Gastric, renal and various types of "functional vertigo" have diminished progressively in importance since the studies of Bárány.

DIAGNOSIS.—The nervous, anemic and cardiovascular groups rarely offer any difficulty but the diagnosis from minor epilepsy is not so easy, particularly in the types without spasm. Tinnitus may be present, but it is rare to have loss of consciousness in aural vertigo, in which, also, the actual giddiness is more persistent. The Bárány tests may be applied. A full discussion will be found in Barker's *Clinical Diagnosis,* vol. iii. The vestibular reflexes are as important in some cases as those of the iris.

TREATMENT.—Bromide of potassium, in 20 grains (1.3 gm.) doses three times a day, is sometimes beneficial. If there is a history of syphilis the iodides should be administered. With hypertension nitroglycerin may be given, at first in small doses, but increasing gradually. It is not specially valuable in Ménière's disease, but in the vertigo associated with arteriosclerosis it sometimes acts very satisfactorily. Correction of errors of refraction is sometimes followed by prompt relief.

Endemic Paralytic Vertigo.—In parts of Switzerland and France there is a remarkable form of vertigo described by Gerlier, which is characterized by attacks of paretic weakness of the extremities, bilateral ptosis, remarkable depression, but with retention of consciousness. A somewhat similar syndrome occurs in Japan, where it develops paroxysmally among farm laborers of all ages. It is known as *kubisagari.*

GLOSSOPHARYNGEAL NERVE

The ninth nerve contains both motor and sensory fibres and is also a nerve of the special sense of taste to the tongue. It supplies, by its motor branches, the stylopharyngeus and the middle constrictor of the pharynx. The sensory fibres are distributed to the upper part of the pharynx.

Symptoms.—Of nuclear disturbance we know very little. The pharyngeal symptoms of bulbar paralysis are probably associated with involvement of the nuclei of this nerve. Lesion of the nerve trunk itself is rare, but it may be compressed by tumors or involved in meningitis. Disturbance of the sense of taste may result from loss of function of this nerve, in which case it is chiefly in the posterior third of the tongue. *Glossopharyngeal neuralgia* is rare and characterized by paroxysms of severe pain originating about the tonsil and base of the tongue and referred to the ear and occasionally down the neck. Alcohol injection of the pharyngeal plexus, division of the pharyngeal nerve and intracranial division of the nerve have given relief.

The general disturbances of the sense of *taste* may be briefly mentioned. Loss of the sense of taste—*ageusia*—may be caused by disturbance of the peripheral end organs, as in affections of the mucosa of the tongue. This is common in fever or dyspepsia, in which conditions, as the saying is, everything tastes alike. Strong irritants, such as pepper, tobacco or vinegar, may dull or diminish the sense of taste. Complete loss may be due to involvement of the nerves in their course or in the centres. Perversion of the sense of taste—*parageusia*—is rare except in hysteria and in the insane. Increased sensitiveness is still more rare. There are subjective sensations of taste, as an aura in epilepsy or a hallucination of the insane.

PNEUMOGASTRIC (VAGUS) NERVE

The tenth nerve has an important and extensive distribution, supplying the pharynx, larynx, lungs, heart and alimentary tract. The nerve may be involved at its nucleus along with the spinal accessory and the hypoglossal, forming what is known as bulbar paralysis. It may be compressed by tumors or aneurism, or in the exudation of meningitis, simple or syphilitic. In its course in the neck the trunk may be involved by tumors or in wounds. It has been tied in ligature of the carotid, and has been cut in the removal of deep-seated tumors. The trunk may be attacked by neuritis.

The affections of the vagus are best considered in connection with the distribution of the separate nerves.

Pharyngeal Branches.—With the glossopharyngeal the branches from the vagus form the pharyngeal plexus, from which the muscles and mucosa of the pharynx are supplied. In *paralysis* due to involvement of this either in the nuclei, as in bulbar paralysis, or in the course of the nerve, as in diphtheritic neuritis, there is difficulty in swallowing and the food is not passed on into the esophagus. If one nerve only is involved deglutition is not much impaired. In these cases the food may pass into the larynx, and, when the soft palate is involved, into the posterior nares.

Spasm of the pharynx is usually functional, occurring in hysterical and nervous people. Gowers mentioned a case of a man who could not eat unless alone, on account of the inability to swallow in the presence of others from spasm of the pharynx. This spasm is a well marked feature in rabies, and occurs also in lyssophobia.

Laryngeal Branches.—The superior laryngeal nerve supplies the mucous membrane of the larynx above the cords and the cricothyroid muscle. The inferior or recurrent laryngeal curves around the arch of the aorta on the left side and the subclavian artery on the right, passes along the trachea and supplies the mucosa below the cords and all the muscles of the larynx except the cricothyroid and the epiglottidean. The course of the recurrent laryngeal nerves renders them liable to pressure, particularly by aneurism. The following are the most important forms of paralysis:

(*a*) Bilateral Paralysis of the Abductors.—In this the posterior crico-arytenoids are involved and the glottis is not opened during inspiration. The cords may be close together in the position of phonation, and during inspiration may be brought even nearer together by the pressure of air, so that there is only a narrow chink through which the air whistles with a noisy stridor. This dangerous form of laryngeal paralysis occurs occasionally as a result of cold or may follow a laryngeal catarrh. The posterior muscles have been found degenerated when the others were healthy. The condition may be produced by pressure upon both vagi, or upon both recurrent nerves. As a central affection it occurs in tabes and bulbar paralysis, and also in hysteria. The characteristic symptoms are inspiratory stridor with unimpaired phonation. Possibly some cases of so-called hysterical spasm of the glottis are in reality abductor paralysis.

(*b*) Unilateral Abductor Paralysis.—This frequently results from the pressure of tumors or involvement of one recurrent nerve. Aneurism is the most common cause, though on the right side the nerve may be involved in thickening of the pleura. The left nerve may be affected in mitral stenosis. The symptoms are hoarseness or roughness of the voice with a characteristic cough. Dyspnea is not often present. The cord on the affected side does not move in inspiration. Subsequently the adductors may become involved, in which case phonation is still more impaired.

(*c*) Adductor Paralysis.—This results from involvement of the lateral crico-arytenoid and the arytenoid muscle itself. It is common in hysteria and causes the hysterical aphonia, which may come on suddenly. It may result from catarrh of the larynx or from overuse of the voice. In laryngoscopic examination it is seen, on attempting phonation, that there is no power to bring the cords together.

(*d*) Spasm of the Muscles of the Larynx.—In this the adductor muscles are involved. It is not uncommon in children, and has been referred to as *laryngismus stridulus*. Paroxysmal attacks of laryngeal spasm are rare in the adult, but cases are described in which the patient wakes at night in an attack of intense dyspnea, which may persist long enough to produce cyanosis. Liveing states that they may replace attacks of migraine. They occur in tabes, the laryngeal crises. There is a spastic aphonia, in which, when the patient attempts to speak, phonation is prevented by spasm.

Disturbance of the sensory nerves of the larynx is rare.

(*e*) Anesthesia may occur in bulbar paralysis and in diphtheritic neuritis—a serious condition, as portions of food may enter the trachea. It is usually associated with dysphagia and is sometimes present in hysteria. Hyperesthesia of the larynx is rare.

Cardiac Branches.—The cardiac plexus is formed by the union of branches of the vagi and of the sympathetic nerves. The vagus fibres subserve motor, sensory and probably trophic functions.

Motor.—The fibres which inhibit, control, and regulate the cardiac action pass in the vagi. Irritation may produce slowing of the action. Czermak could slow or even arrest the heart's action for a few beats by pressing a small tumor in his neck against one pneumogastric nerve. There are instances in which persons appear to have had voluntary control over the action of the heart. Cheyne mentions the case of Colonel Townshend, "who could die or expire when he pleased, and yet by an effort or somehow come to life again, which it seems he had sometimes tried before he had sent for us." Slowing of the heart rate has followed accidental ligature of one vagus. Irritation of the nuclei may be accompanied by disturbance of this nerve. On the other hand, when there is complete paralysis of the vagi, the inhibitory action may be abolished and the acceleratory influences have full sway. This is seen in some cases of diphtheritic neuritis and in involvement of the nerve by tumors, or its accidental removal or ligature. Complete loss of function of one vagus may not be followed by any symptoms.

Sensory symptoms on the part of the cardiac branches are very varied. Normally, the heart's action proceeds regularly without the participation of consciousness, but the unpleasant feelings and sensations of palpitation and pain are conveyed to the brain through this nerve. How far the fibres of the pneumogastric are involved in angina it is impossible to say.

Pulmonary Branches.—We know little of the pulmonary branches of the vagi. The motor fibres are stated to control the action of the bronchial muscles. Alterations in the respiratory rhythm are probably due more to changes in the centre than in the nerves themselves.

Gastric and Esophageal Branches.—The muscular movements of these parts are influenced by the vagi and vomiting is induced through them, usually reflexly, but also by direct irritation, as in meningitis. Spasm of the esophagus generally occurs with other nervous phenomena. Pain may be due to cramp of the stomach or to sensory disturbance of this nerve from irritation of the peripheral ends. Some forms of nervous dyspepsia probably depend upon disturbed function of this nerve. The severe gastric crises in tabes are due to central irritation of the nuclei. Vagotonia is an important element in many disorders of the digestive tract.

SPINAL ACCESSORY NERVE

The smaller or internal part of this nerve joins the vagus and is distributed through it to the laryngeal muscles. The larger external part is distributed to the sternomastoid and trapezius muscles.

Paralysis.—The nuclei of the nerve, particularly of the accessory part, may be involved in bulbar paralysis. The nuclei of the external portion, in the cervical cord, may be attacked in degeneration of the motor nuclei of the cord. The nerve may be involved in the exudation of meningitis, or be compressed by tumors or in caries. The *symptoms* of paralysis of the accessory portion which joins the vagus have been given in the account of the palsy of the laryngeal branches of the vagus. Disease or compression of the external portion is followed by paralysis of the sternomastoid and trapezius on the same side. In paralysis of one sternomastoid the patient rotates the head with difficulty to the opposite side, but there is no torticollis, though in some cases the head is held obliquely. As the trapezius is supplied in part from the cervical nerves, it is not completely paralyzed, but the portion which passes from the occipital bone to the acromion is functionless. This is well seen when the patient draws a deep breath or shrugs the shoulders. The middle portion of the trapezius is also weakened, the shoulder droops a little, and the angle of the scapula is rotated inward by the action of the rhomboids and the levator anguli scapulae. Elevation of the arm is impaired, for the trapezius does not fix the scapula as a point from which the deltoid can work.

In progressive muscular atrophy we sometimes see bilateral paralysis of these muscles. Thus, if the sternomastoids are affected, the head tends to fall back; when the trapezii are involved, it falls forward, a characteristic attitude of the head in many cases of progressive muscular atrophy. Gowers suggested that lesions of the accessory in difficult labor may account for those cases in which during the first year of life the child has great difficulty in holding up the head. In children this drooping of the head is an important symptom in cervical meningitis, the result of caries.

The TREATMENT of the condition depends much upon the cause. In the central nuclear atrophy but little can be done. In paralysis from pressure the symptoms may gradually be relieved. The paralyzed muscles should be stimulated by electricity and massage.

Accessory Spasm (*Torticollis; Wryneck*).—The forms of spasm affecting the cervical muscles are best considered here, as the muscles supplied by the spinal accessory are chiefly, though not solely, responsible for the condition.

(*a*) CONGENITAL TORTICOLLIS.—This condition, also known as *fixed* torticollis, depends upon the shortening and atrophy of the sternomastoid on one side. It occurs in children and may not be noticed for several years on account of the shortness of the neck, the parents often alleging that it has only recently come on. It affects the right side almost exclusively. A remarkable circumstance in connection with it is the existence of facial asymmetry, noted by Wilks, which appears to be an essential part of this congenital form. In congenital wryneck the sternomastoid is shortened, hard and firm, and in a condition of more or less advanced atrophy. This must be distinguished from the local thickening in the sternomastoid due to rupture, which may occur at birth and produce an induration. Although the sternomastoid is almost always affected, there are rare cases in which the fibrous atrophy affects the trapezius. This form of wryneck is readily relieved by tenotomy, but the facial asymmetry persists, or may become more evident. Golding-Bird concluded that the facial asymmetry and torticollis are integral parts of one affection which has a central origin, and is the counterpart in the head and neck of infantile paralysis with talipes in the foot.

(*b*) SPASMODIC WRYNECK.—Two varieties occur, the tonic and the clonic, which may alternate in the same case; or, as is most common, they are separate and remain so from the outset. It is most frequent in adults and, according to Gowers, more common in females. In America it seems more frequent in males. There may be a marked neurotic family history, but it is usually impossible to fix upon any definite etiological factor. Some cases have followed cold; others a blow. Brissaud described "mental torticollis," usually seen in neurasthenic patients and elderly persons. It consists of a clonic spasm of the rotators of the head.

The *symptoms* are well defined. In the *tonic* form the contracted sternomastoid draws the occiput toward the shoulder of the affected side; the chin is raised, and the face rotated to the other shoulder. The sternomastoid may be affected alone or with the trapezius. When the latter is implicated the head is depressed still more toward the same side. In long-standing cases these muscles are prominent and very rigid. There may be some curvature of the spine, with the convexity toward the sound side. The cases in which the spasm is *clonic* are much more distressing and serious. The spasm is rarely limited to a single muscle. The sternomastoid is almost always involved and rotates the head so as to approximate the mastoid process to the inner end of the clavicle, turning the face to the opposite side and raising the chin. When with this the trapezius is affected, the depression of the head toward the same side is more marked. The head is drawn somewhat backward; the shoulder is raised by its action. The splenius may be associated with the sternomastoid. Its action is to incline the head and rotate it slightly toward the same side. Other muscles may be involved, as the scalenus and platysma myoides; in rare cases the head may be rotated by the deep cervical muscles. There are cases in which the spasm is bilateral, causing a backward movement. This may be tonic or clonic; in extreme cases the face is horizontal and looks upward.

These clonic contractions may come on without warning, or be preceded by irregular pains or stiffness of the neck. The jerking movements recur every few moments, and it is impossible to keep the head still for more than a minute or two. In time the muscles undergo hypertrophy and may be distinctly larger on one side than the other. In some cases the pain is considerable; in others there is simply a feeling of fatigue. The spasms cease during sleep. Emotion, excitement and fatigue increase them. The spasm may extend from the neck muscles and involve those of the face or arms.

The disease varies much; patients occasionally get well, but the majority persist, and, even if temporarily relieved, the disease frequently recurs. The affection is usually regarded as a functional neurosis, but it is possibly due to disturbance of the cortical centres presiding over the muscles.

Treatment.—Temporary relief is sometimes obtained; a permanent cure is exceptional. Psychotherapeutic treatment has been successful in some cases. In mild cases education in the voluntary relaxation of the affected muscles is useful. Various drugs have been used but rarely with benefit. Occasionally, large doses of bromide lessen the intensity of the spasm. Morphia has been successful in some cases, but there is great danger of establishing a habit. Galvanism may be tried. Counterirritation is probably useless. Fixation of the head mechanically can rarely be borne by the patient. These obstinate cases come ultimately to the surgeon, and the operations of stretching, division and excision of the accessory nerve and division of the muscles have been tried. Temporary relief may follow and is in proportion to the extent of the operation, but, as a rule, the condition returns. Risien Russell thinks that resection of the posterior branches of the upper cervical nerves is most likely to give relief. It may be said that treatment is rarely satisfactory.

(*c*) The NODDING SPASM of children may here be mentioned as involving chiefly the muscles innervated by the accessory nerve. It may be a simple trick, a form of habit spasm, or a phenomenon of epilepsy (*E. nutans*), in which case it is associated with transient loss of consciousness. A similar nodding spasm may occur in older children. In women it may occur with hysteria commonly as part of the so-called salaam convulsion.

HYPOGLOSSAL NERVE

This is the motor nerve of the tongue and for most of the muscles attached to the hyoid bone. Its centre is in the lower part of the medulla.

Paralysis.—(*a*) Cortical Lesion.—The tongue is often involved in hemiplegia, and is protruded towards the paralyzed side.

(*b*) Nuclear and infranuclear lesions result from slow progressive degeneration, as in bulbar paralysis or tabes; occasionally there is acute softening from obstruction of the vessels. The nuclei of both nerves are usually affected together, but may be attacked separately. Trauma, syphilis and lead poisoning are causes. The fibres may be damaged by a tumor, and at the base by meningitis; or the nerve may be involved in the condylar foramen by disease of the skull. It may be involved in a scar or compressed by a tumor in the parotid region. As a result, there is loss of function in the nerve fibres and the tongue undergoes atrophy on the affected side. It is protruded toward the paralyzed side and may show fibrillary twitching.

The *symptoms* of involvement of one hypoglossal are those of unilateral paralysis and atrophy of the tongue. When protruded, it is pushed toward the affected side, and there are fibrillary twitchings. The atrophy is usually marked and the mucous membrane on the affected side is thrown into folds. Articulation is not much impaired in the unilateral affection. When the disease is bilateral, the tongue lies almost motionless in the floor of the mouth; it is atrophied, and can not be protruded. Speech and mastication are extremely difficult and deglutition may be impaired. This is seen in bulbar paralysis and occasionally in progressive muscular atrophy.

The *diagnosis* is readily made and the situation of the lesion can usually be determined, since when supranuclear there is hemiplegia and no wasting of the muscles of the tongue. Nuclear disease is only occasionally unilateral; most commonly bilateral and with bulbar paralysis. The fibres of the hypoglossal may be involved within the medulla after leaving their nuclei. In such a case there may be paralysis of the tongue on one side and paralysis of the limbs on the opposite side, and the tongue, when protruded, is pushed toward the sound side. The *treatment* is that of the causal condition.

Spasm.—This rare affection may be unilateral or bilateral. It is most frequently a part of some other convulsive disorder, such as epilepsy, chorea or spasm of the facial muscles. In some cases of stuttering, spasm of the tongue precedes the explosive utterance of the words. It may occur in hysteria, and is said to follow reflex irritation in the fifth nerve. The most remarkable cases are those of *paroxysmal clonic spasm,* in which the tongue is rapidly thrust in and out, as many as forty or fifty times a minute. The prognosis is usually good.

COMBINED PARALYSIS OF THE LAST THREE AND FOUR CRANIAL NERVES

The war experience widened our knowledge of these cases. There may be: (*a*) *Avelli's syndrome,* palatolaryngeal paralysis from involvement of the ninth and eleventh. With this there may be involvement of the tenth with paralysis of the superior constrictor of the pharynx. When the outer fibres of the spinal accessory are involved, the sternocleidomastoid may be paralyzed on the same side (*Schmidt's syndrome*). (*b*) *Hughlings-Jackson's syndrome.* Involvement of the ix, x, xi, and xii—disturbance of taste and paralysis of the superior constrictor of the pharynx (ix and x); hemianesthesia of the palate and pharynx, sometimes with cough and dyspnea and salivation which may be profuse (x and xi); hemiparalysis of the larynx (xi) with hemiparalysis of the tongue (xii). In wounds of the retroparotidean space or after a parotid bubo, in addition to the hypoglossal, the sympathetic nerves with fibres of the ix, x, and xi may be involved, causing exophthalmos, myosis and sweating, with the combined paralyses known as *Villaret's syndrome.* These combined paralyses may be nuclear caused by syphilis or tuberculous meningitis, by tumor or by injury. In the war cases the lesions were often more extensive, and involvement of the vagus was more common than in the ordinary instances from tumor or meningitis.

DISEASES OF THE SPINAL NERVES

CERVICAL PLEXUS

Occipitocervical Neuralgia.—This involves the nerve territory supplied by the occipitalis major and minor, and the auricularis magnus nerves. The pains are chiefly in the back of the head and neck and in the ear. The condition may follow cold (probably fibrositis) and may be associated with stiffness of the neck or torticollis. It may be due to direct pressure in carrying heavy weights. Unless disease of the bones exists with it or it is due to pressure of tumors, the outlook is usually good. There are tender points midway between the mastoid process and the spine and just above the parietal eminence, and between the sternomastoid and the trapezius.

Affections of the Phrenic Nerve.—Paralysis may follow a lesion in the anterior horns at the level of the third to fifth cervical nerves, or may be due to compression of the nerve by tumors or aneurism. More rarely paralysis results from neuritis, alcoholic, diphtheritic or saturnine.

When the *diaphragm* is paralyzed respiration is carried on by the intercostal and accessory muscles. When the patient is quiet and at rest little may be noticed, but the abdomen retracts in inspiration and is forced out in expiration. On exertion or even on attempting to move there may be dyspnea. If the paralysis sets in suddenly there may be dyspnea and lividity, which is usually temporary (W. Pasteur). Pneumonia or bronchitis seriously aggravates the condition. Difficulty in coughing, owing to the impossibility of drawing a full breath, adds greatly to the danger.

When the phrenic nerve is paralyzed on one side the paralysis may be scarcely noticeable, but inspection and the fluoroscope show that the descent of the diaphragm is much less on the affected side. The *diagnosis* of paralysis is not always easy, particularly in women, who use this muscle less than men, and in whom diaphragmatic breathing is less conspicuous. Immobility of the diaphragm occurs in diaphragmatic pleurisy, large effusions and extensive emphysema. The muscle itself may be degenerated.

Owing to the lessened action of the diaphragm, there is a tendency to stasis at the bases of the lungs, and there may be impaired resonance and signs of congestion. As a rule, however, the paralysis is not confined to this muscle, but is part of a general neuritis or a poliomyelitis, and there are other symptoms of value in determining its presence. The outlook is usually serious. The treatment is that of the neuritis or poliomyelitis. Artificial respiration should be carried on, or the respirator used, if necessary.

Hiccough.—Here may be considered this remarkable symptom, caused by intermittent, sudden contraction of the diaphragm. The mechanism, however, is complex, and while the afferent impressions to the respiratory centre may be peripheral or central the efferent are distributed through the phrenic nerve to the diaphragm, causing the intermittent spasm, and through the laryngeal branches of the vagus to the glottis, causing sudden closure as the air is rapidly inspired. There are various groups:

(*a*) INFLAMMATORY, seen particularly in affections of the abdominal viscera, gastritis, peritonitis, hernia, internal strangulation, appendicitis, suppurative pancreatitis, and in severe forms of typhoid fever.

(*b*) IRRITATIVE, as in direct stimulation of the diaphragm when very hot substances are swallowed, in disease of the esophagus near the diaphragm, and in gastric and intestinal conditions, particularly those with flatus.

(*c*) TOXIC.—In these cases there is usually some general disease, as gout, diabetes or chronic nephritis. Hiccough may be very obstinate in the later stages of chronic nephritis. It may be due to tobacco.

(*d*) Cases in which the cause is in the *nervous system;* hysteria, epilepsy or cerebral tumors. It may be persistent in epidemic encephalitis.

(*e*) From *thoracic* disease, as mediastinitis, mediastinal tumor, pleurisy or pericarditis.

The TREATMENT is often unsatisfactory. Sometimes in the milder forms a sudden reflex irritation will check it at once. A pinch of snuff may be effective. Readers of Plato's Symposium will remember that the physician Eryximachus recommended to Aristophanes, who had hiccough from eating too much, either to hold his breath (which for trivial forms of hiccough is very satisfactory) or to gargle with a little water; but if it still continued, "tickle your nose with something and sneeze; and if you sneeze once or twice even the most violent hiccough is sure to go." The attack must have been of some severity, as it is stated subsequently that the hiccough did not disappear until Aristophanes had resorted to the sneezing.

Ice, a teaspoonful of salt and lemon juice, or salt and vinegar, or a teaspoonful of whisky may be tried. When due to gastric irritation, lavage is sometimes promptly curative. Alkali should be given freely. A hypodermic injection of gr. 1/8 (0.008 gm.) of apomorphia may give prompt relief. The inhalation of carbon dioxide (5 per cent) with oxygen may be successful. A substitute is to hold a paper bag over the mouth and nose, into which the patient breathes for several minutes. Pilocarpine has been recommended. The ether spray on the epigastrium may be effective. Hypodermics of morphia, inhalation of chloroform, the use of amyl nitrite or nitroglycerin have been beneficial. Benzyl benzoate in doses of 30 drops of a 20 per cent solution sometimes is effectual. Galvanism over the phrenic nerve, or pressure on the nerves, applied between the heads of the sternocleidomastoid muscles may be used. Strong traction upon the tongue may give immediate relief. Phrenicotomy has been done in severe prolonged cases. Of ali measures morphia used freely is the best.

BRACHIAL PLEXUS

Cervical Rib.—Frequency.—The anomaly is much more common than indicated in the literature. Sometimes bilateral, it may be complete with bony attachment to the second rib; incomplete, forming a short stump of variable length, or—and this is important—there may be a fibrous band-like attachment from a short rib to the first. It is more common on the left side. Symptoms usually appear between the fifteenth and thirtieth years, and their onset is often due to dropping of the shoulder girdle. Some form of exercise or in women the carrying of a child on the arm may be responsible.

The ribs may be visible, one more plainly than the other, and the subclavian artery, lifted up, may pulsate high in the supraclavicular fossa. This abnormal pulsation and the fullness in the fossa may suggest the presence of the extra rib. The throbbing may be marked enough to suggest aneurism. The rib may be felt, often more marked on one side, even the bifid extremity may be palpable, and the artery felt above the rib sometimes appears longer and larger than normal. Cervical rib may be present on both sides.

Symptoms.—Many patients are unaware of the anomaly; the symptoms, which may come on suddenly, may be grouped as follows:

(1) *Local.* (*a*) Supraclavicular swelling. (*b*) Pulsation. (*c*) Palpable tumor and aneurism.

(2) *Neuritic.* (*a*) Neuralgic pains (supraclavicular, cervical, brachial). (*b*) Paresthesia. (*c*) Local anesthesia. (*d*) Sympathetic nerve features.

(3) *Muscular.* (*a*) Atrophy, in ulnar distribution. (*b*) *Spasm.* (*c*) Intermittent claudication.

(4) *Vascular.* (*a*) Vasomotor changes (ischemia, hyperemia, swelling). (*b*) Local gangrene. (*c*) Aneurism, (i) spurious, (ii) true. (*d*) Thrombosis.

Neuralgic pains occur in the cervical region, sometimes passing up the back of the head; more commonly the pain is in the distribution of the eighth cervical and first dorsal nerve, sometimes only a dull pain and aching with numbness and tingling or even anesthesia. Dissociation of cutaneous sensation, loss of tactile and thermic with retention of pain sense, may be present. The cervical sympathetic may be involved with the usual features. *Muscular atrophy* is usually in the region of distribution of the ulnar nerve. The difference between the two arms may be marked and the interossei wasted, as in progressive muscular atrophy, for which, when bilateral, cases may be mistaken. With pressure on and narrowing of the subclavian, intermittent claudication occurs with numbness, tingling and swelling, sometimes redness of the arm and muscular disability on exertion. At rest the arm is normal and comfortable, but on exertion these features occur; spasm, tonic or clonic, in the muscles of the hand is occasionally seen. The *radial pulses* may be unequal and this may disappear if the arms are raised.

Vasomotor Changes.—Redness with swelling, sometimes cyanosis and mottling, may be present, with changes resembling Raynaud's disease; in a few cases gangrene of the finger tips has followed.

Aneurism.—The subclavian artery may be tilted by the ribs and give a wide area of supraclavicular pulsation. There may be: (1) slight narrowing from pressure, with feeble pulse on the affected side; (2) manifest enlargement of the vessel, fusiform or uniform; or (3) a definite cylindrical aneurism. In 27 of 525 cases collected by Halsted these local changes were present. The dilatation is distal to the point of constriction made by the rib and the scalenus anticus, which Halsted explains by the abnormal play of the blood in the relatively dead pocket beyond the constriction, and the absence of the normal pulse pressure necessary to maintain the integrity of the arterial wall. The nervi arteriorum may be involved.

THROMBOSIS.—This may occur in the vessels beyond the point of constriction, in one case involving suddenly the brachial and later the axillary and subclavian, with the development of an effective collateral circulation.

The relative distribution of the symptoms as given by Halsted from an exhaustive review of the literature was in 63.3 per cent nerve symptoms alone, in 29.4 per cent nervous and vascular symptoms, while 5.3 per cent had only vascular symptoms.

DIAGNOSIS.—This may be made without the X-ray study but this is advisable. A serious difficulty arises when disease of the cord occurs in the subjects of cervical rib, *e.g.*, syringomyelia and progressive muscular atrophy. In cases of prolonged discomfort or pain with vascular or trophic disturbance in the arm, cervical rib should be considered.

TREATMENT.—When accidentally discovered, it is best not to tell the patient. Elevation of the shoulders may give relief. Massage, electricity and other forms of local treatment may be tried. The rib may be removed, but only as a last resort, as the results are not always satisfactory. Division of the scalenus anticus muscle from its insertion may be effectual.

Combined Paralysis.—The plexus may be involved in the supraclavicular region by compression of the nerve trunks as they leave the spine, or by tumors and other morbid processes in the neck. Below the clavicle lesions are more common and result from injuries following dislocation or fracture, sometimes from neuritis. A cervical rib may lead to a pressure paralysis of the lower cord of the plexus. A not infrequent injury in this region follows falls or blows on the neck, which by lateral flexion of the head and depression of the shoulder seriously stretch the plexus. The entire plexus may be ruptured and the arm totally paralyzed. The rupture may occur anywhere between the vertebrae and the clavicle, and involve all the cords of the plexus, or only the upper ones. The so-called "obstetrical palsy" usually results from the forcible separation of the head and neck from the shoulder during delivery, with tearing of the deep cervical fascia and the nerves, involving the roots from above and downwards, so that the injury may vary from a slight lesion of the upper root to complete rupture of the plexus or the tearing of the roots from the cord. In the complete lesion the arm is flaccid and immobile, does not grow, and there is displacement of the head of the humerus; sensory disturbances are rare. The prognosis is bad; only mild cases recover completely. Suturing the broken cords and planting them in the neighboring roots have been followed by good results, but complete recovery rarely if ever follows. Another common cause of lesion of the brachial plexus is luxation of the head of the humerus, particularly the subcoracoid form.

A primary neuritis of the brachial plexus is rare. More commonly the process is an ascending neuritis from a lesion of a peripheral branch, involving first the radial or ulnar nerves, and spreading upward to the plexus, producing gradually complete loss of power in the arm.

Lesions of Individual Nerves of the Plexus.—(*a*) LONG THORACIC NERVE.—*Serratus paralysis* follows injury to this nerve in the neck, usually by direct pressure in carrying loads, and is common in soldiers. It may be due to a neuritis following an acute infection or exposure. Isolated serratus paralysis is rare. It usually occurs with paralysis of other muscles of the shoulder girdle, as in the myopathies and progressive muscular atrophy. Concomitant trapezius paralysis is the most frequent. In the isolated paralysis there is little or no deformity with the hands hanging by the sides. There are slight abnormal obliquity of the posterior border of the scapula and prominence of the inferior angle, but when, as is common, the middle part of the trapezius is also paralyzed the deformity is marked. The shoulder is lower, the inferior angle of the scapula is displaced inward and upward, and the superior angle projects upward. When the arms are held out in front at right angles to the body the scapula becomes winged and stands out prominently. The arm can not, as a rule, be raised above the horizontal. The outlook of the cases due to injury or neuritis is good.

(*b*) CIRCUMFLEX NERVE.—This supplies the deltoid and teres minor and may be involved in injuries, in dislocations, bruising by a crutch, or sometimes by extension from arthritis. Occasionally the paralysis arises from a pressure neuritis during an illness. As a consequence of loss of power in the deltoid, the arm can not be raised. The wasting is usually marked and changes the shape of the shoulder. Sensation may be impaired in the skin over the muscle. The joint may be relaxed and there may be a distinct space between the head of the humerus and the acromion.

(*c*) MUSCULOSPIRAL PARALYSIS; RADIAL PARALYSIS.—This is common, due to the exposed position of the musculospiral nerve. It is often bruised by a crutch, by injuries of the arm, blows or fractures. It may be injured when a person falls asleep with the arm over the back of a chair, or by pressure of the body upon the arm when sleeping on a bench or on the ground. It may be paralyzed by sudden violent contraction of the triceps. It is sometimes involved in a neuritis from cold but this is uncommon. The paralysis of lead poisoning is the result of involvement of certain branches of this nerve.

A lesion when high up involves the triceps, the brachialis anticus, and the supinator longus, as well as the extensors of the wrist and fingers. In lesions just above the elbow the arm muscles and the supinator longus are spared. The most characteristic feature is the wrist drop and the inability to extend the first phalanges of the fingers and thumb. In the pressure palsies the supinators are usually involved and supination can not be accomplished. Sensation may be impaired, or there may be marked tingling, but the loss of sensation is rarely so pronounced as that of motion.

The affection is readily recognized but it is sometimes difficult to say upon what it depends. The sleep and pressure palsies are, as a rule, unilateral and involve the supinator longus. The paralysis from lead is bilateral and the supinators are unaffected. Bilateral wrist drop is a common symptom in many forms of multiple neuritis, particularly the alcoholic; but the mode of onset and the involvement of the legs and arms make the diagnosis easy. The duration and course of musculospiral paralyses are very variable. The pressure palsies may disappear in a few days. Recovery is the rule, even when the affection lasts for many weeks. The electrical examination is of importance in prognosis, and the rules laid down under paralysis of the facial nerve hold good here. The *treatment* is that of neuritis.

(*d*) Ulnar Nerve.—The motor branches supply the ulnar half of the deep flexor of the fingers, the muscles of the little finger, the interossei, the adductor and the inner head of the short flexor of the thumb, and the ulnar flexor of the wrist. The sensory branches supply the ulnar side of the hand—two (or one) and a half fingers on the back, and one and a half fingers on the front. Paralysis may result from pressure, usually at the elbow joint, although the nerve is here protected. Possibly the neuritis in the ulnar nerve in some cases of acute illness may be due to this cause. Owing to paralysis of the ulnar flexor of the wrist, the hand moves toward the radial side; adduction of the thumb is impossible; the first phalanges can not be flexed, and the others can not be extended. In long-standing cases the first phalanges are overextended and the others strongly flexed, producing the clawhand; but this is not so marked as in progressive muscular atrophy. The loss of sensation corresponds to the sensory distribution just mentioned.

(*e*) Median Nerve.—This supplies the flexors of the fingers except the ulnar half of the deep flexors, the abductor and the flexors of the thumb, the two radial lumbricales, the pronators, and the radial flexor of the wrist. The sensory fibres supply the radial side of the palm and the front of the thumb, the first two fingers and half the third finger, and the dorsal surfaces of the same three fingers. This nerve is seldom involved alone. Paralysis results from injury and occasionally from neuritis. There is inability to pronate the forearm beyond the midposition. The wrist can be flexed only toward the ulnar side; the thumb can not be opposed to the tips of fingers. The second phalanges can not be flexed on the first; the distal phalanges of the first and second fingers can not be flexed; but in the third and fourth fingers this action can be performed by the ulnar half of the flexor profundus. The loss of sensation is in the region corresponding to the sensory distribution mentioned. The wasting of the thumb muscles, usually marked in this paralysis, gives a characteristic appearance.

Volkmann's Paralysis.—*Ischemic* paralysis, as it is called, usually follows the pressure of splints and bandages for fracture in the region of the elbow joint. The changes are thought to be due to arrest of the circulation in the muscles, which are hardened and stiff and the flexors of the forearm are contracted. The hand is claw-like with the metacarpophalangeal joints strongly extended and the middle and terminal phalanges strongly flexed. The condition may come on with great rapidity and appears to be a muscular lesion though it is not always possible to exclude pressure on the nerves. The prognosis is good with judicious treatment.

LUMBAR AND SACRAL PLEXUSES

Lumbar Plexus.—The lumbar plexus is sometimes involved in growths of the lymph glands, in psoas abscess, by tumors, and in disease of the vertebrae. The *obturator nerve* is occasionally injured during parturition. When paralyzed the power is lost over the adductors of the thigh and one leg can not be crossed over the other. Outward rotation is also disturbed. The *anterior crural nerve* is sometimes involved in wounds or in dislocation of the hip joint, less commonly during parturition, and sometimes by disease of the bones and in psoas abscess. The special symptoms of affection of this nerve are paralysis of the extensors of the knee with wasting of the muscles, anesthesia of the anterolateral parts of the thigh and of the inner side of the leg to the big toe. This nerve is sometimes involved early in growths about the spine, and there may be pain in its area of distribution. Loss of the power of abducting the thigh results from paralysis of the *gluteal nerve,* which is distributed to the gluteus medius and minimus muscles.

External Cutaneous Nerve.—A peculiar form of sensory disturbance, confined to the territory of this nerve, was first described by Bernhardt in 1895, and a few months later by Roth, who gave it the name of *meralgia paraesthetica.* It may be bilateral. It may be due to a neuritis originating where the nerve passes under Poupart's ligament, just internal to the anterior superior iliac spine. The nerve is usually tender on pressure at this point. In some cases it is due to osteo-arthritis of the spine and radicular in origin. A number of cases are attributable to trauma or pressure on the nerve in the aponeurotic canal through which it passes. Pregnancy is among the causes in women. It may be the result of irritation from the abdominal or pelvic organs and has followed the operation for appendicitis.

The *sensory* disturbances consist of various forms of paresthesia located over the outer side of the thigh, sometimes with diminished sensation or hyperesthesia. The symptoms may persist for years with such discomfort, exaggerated by walking or the touch of the clothing, that patients may be greatly incapacitated. Excision of the nerve as it passes under Poupart's ligament has given good results. Infiltration of the nerve with novocaine has been successful.

Sacral Plexus.—The sacral plexus is frequently involved in tumors and inflammations within the pelvis and may be injured during parturition. Neuritis is usually due to extension from the sciatic nerve.

Goldthwaite calls attention to the fact that the lumbosacral articulation varies very greatly in its stability, and displacement of the bones may result with separation of the posterior portion of the intervertebral disc. The cauda equina, or the nerve roots, may be compressed. With displacement on one side the spine is rotated and the articular process of the fifth is drawn into the spinal canal, with such narrowing that paraplegia may result, and he reports a remarkable case in which paralysis came on during the application of a plaster jacket. Weakness of the joints or displacements may cause irritation of the nerves inside and outside the canal with resulting sciatica.

Of the branches, the *sciatic nerve,* when injured at or near the notch, causes paralysis of the flexors of the legs and the muscles below the knee, but injury below the middle of the thigh involves only the latter muscles. There is also anesthesia of the outer half of the leg, the sole, and the greater portion of the dorsum of the foot. Wasting of the muscles and trophic disturbances may follow. In paralysis of one sciatic the leg is fixed at the knee by the action of the quadriceps extensor and the patient is able to walk.

Paralysis of the *small sciatic nerve* is rarely seen. The gluteus maximus is involved and there may be difficulty in rising from a seat. There is a strip of anesthesia along the back of the middle third of the thigh.

External Popliteal Nerve.—Paralysis involves the peronaei, the long extensor of the toes, tibialis anticus, and the extensor brevis digitorum. The ankle can not be flexed, resulting in foot drop, and as the toes can not be raised the leg must be lifted, producing the *steppage* gait seen in peripheral neuritis. In long-standing cases the foot is extended with wasting of the anterior tibial and peroneal muscles. The loss of sensation is in the outer half of the front of the leg and on the dorsum of the foot.

Internal Popliteal Nerve.—When paralyzed, plantar flexion of the foot and flexion of the toes are impossible. The foot can not be adducted, nor can the patient rise on tiptoe. In long-standing cases talipes calcaneus follows and the toes assume a claw-like position from secondary contracture, due to overextension of the proximal and flexion of the second and third phalanges.

SCIATICA

Definition.—The term sciatica is applied to any painful condition referred to the sciatic nerve. It may be defined as an interstitial inflammation of the sciatic nerve, a neurofibrositis, causing severe pain in the branches of distribution and, if long continued, atrophy of the muscles. Only rarely does marked motor paralysis or sensory loss result.

Etiology.—*Primary neuritis* of this nerve is very rare and is seen chiefly in diabetes and gout, sometimes being bilateral. In the vast majority the condition is *secondary* to a process elsewhere which affects the component cords or the trunk itself. Among the causal factors are: (1) *Arthritis* which may be of the lower spine, lumbosacral, sacro-iliac or hip joints. The arthritic lesion is often due to a focus of infection. (2) Anatomical *anomalies,* as an unusually long transverse process of the fifth lumbar vertebra. (3) Disease of the bones of the lower spine or pelvis, *e.g.,* tuberculosis. (4) *Strain,* which may be acute or chronic, especially of the sacro-iliac joint. Exposure to cold after heavy muscular exertion is said to be a cause. (5) *Pelvic* conditions, such as a solid ovarian or fibroid tumor in women and prostatic disease in men. Constipation and the pressure of the fetal head in labor are occasional causes. (6) *Syphilis* is responsible in a few cases. (7) It may be due to a focus of infection, which may cause fibrositis. (8) Among rare causes are an abnormal network of veins on the trunk and anomalies, such as the pyriform muscle passing through the nerve, spinal cord tumor and occupational strain.

Symptoms.—Pain is the most constant and troublesome symptom. The onset may be severe, with slight pyrexia, but, as a rule, it is gradual, and for a time there is only slight pain in the back of the thigh, particularly in certain positions or after exertion. Soon the pain becomes more intense and, instead of being limited to the upper portion of the nerve, extends down the nerve. The patient can often point out the most sensitive spots, usually at the notch or in the middle of the thigh; and on pressure these are extremely painful. The pain may occur particularly in the distribution of one of the branches, as the external popliteal. The pain is gnawing or burning, and is usually constant, but in some instances is paroxysmal, and often worse at night. On walking it may be very great; the knee is bent and the patient treads on the toes, so as to relieve the tension on the nerve. In protracted cases there may be wasting of the muscles, but the reaction of degeneration can seldom be obtained. In chronic cases cramp and fibrillary contractions may occur. Herpes may develop but this is unusual. The patient assumes the position in which there is least tension on the nerve and any position or movement which stretches the nerve increases the pain. The knee jerk is usually increased; the ankle jerk is decreased or lost. The ankle jerk may be absent for a long period afterwards. In rare instances the neuritis ascends and involves the spinal cord.

Duration and Course.—These are extremely variable and depend greatly on the cause. As a rule, it is an obstinate affection, lasting for months, or even, with slight remissions, for years. Relapses occur and the disease may be relieved in one nerve only to appear in the other. In the severer forms the patient is bedridden, and such cases prove among the most distressing and trying which we are called upon to treat.

Diagnosis.—It is important, in the first place, to determine whether the disease is primary, or secondary to some affection elsewhere. The diagnosis should determine the cause; lesions of the lower spine and sacro-iliac joints should be searched for especially. A careful rectal examination should be made, and, in women, pelvic tumor should be excluded. "Lumbago" may be confounded or associated with it. Affections of the hip joint are easily distinguished by the absence of tenderness in the course of the nerve and the pain on movement of the hip joint or on pressure in the region of the trochanter. Pressure on the nerve trunks of the cauda equina, as a rule, causes bilateral pain and disturbances of sensation, and, as double sciatica is rare, these suggest a lesion of the nerve roots. Pressure on the nerve roots by neoplasm must always be excluded. Between the lightning pains of tabes and sciatica the differences are usually well defined. In a certain number of cases the condition is a fibrositis. There is no tenderness along the course of the sciatic nerve, but there is pain in the gluteal region, with disability and Lasègue's sign, *i.e.*, inability to extend the leg completely when the thigh is flexed on the abdomen.

Treatment.—If the cause can be determined, treatment should be directed to correcting this as soon as possible. So many are due to bone conditions which themselves are secondary to disease elsewhere (such as foci of infection) that a very complete study is necessary. The removal of an infected tooth may cause a rapid improvement. In cases with diabetes or gout the usual treatment for these should be carried out. In all cases certain palliative measures are indicated and may be the only ones available in some cases. The most important is *rest* which should be absolute and in the position which gives the most relief. Fixation of the leg by a splint may be of aid. The patient should not be allowed up for any purpose. The application of heat in some form is helpful. An electric pad, a hot water bag or the cautery may be used. Counterirritation, especially by blisters, sometimes gives relief. Acupuncture is worth a trial in obstinate cases. Injections into the nerve have been frequently used and various solutions have been employed, *e.g.*, normal saline solution, sterile water or novocaine. Exposure of the nerve and incision of the sheath with stretching are indicated in severe cases. Electricity may give temporary relief but is often disappointing. X-ray exposures over the roots along the fourth and fifth lumbar and first four sacral vertebrae may be helpful. Diathermy is sometimes useful. In some cases time, usually months, seems necessary.

As to drugs, sedatives are usually necessary, the simple ones being preferred, and morphia avoided if possible. Salicylates *in full doses* (120 grains, 8 grams) are worth a trial and often give relief when combined with codeine. This may be given by rectum. The use of sedative suppositories is often helpful. If there is any suspicion of syphilis, active treatment should be given.

HERPES ZOSTER

(*Acute Posterior Ganglionitis*)

Definition.—An acute disease with localization in the cerebral ganglia and in the ganglia of the posterior nerve roots, associated with a vesicular inflammation of the skin of the corresponding cutaneous areas.

Distribution.—Herpes most frequently occurs in the region of the dorsal roots and extends in the form of a half girdle, on which account the names "zona" and "zoster" have been given. The trigeminal region may be involved, particularly the first branch.

Etiology.—It may occur with acute infections, particularly pneumonia, malaria and cerebrospinal fever. Epidemics have been described. In some cases, especially those in the lower part of the body, syphilis coexists and there may be repeated attacks. Even in nonsyphilitic cases the spinal fluid may show increase in the cells but the globulin is rarely much increased. Herpes zoster may occur with traumatic paraplegia or injury to the ganglia (fracture) or tumors may be responsible. It has followed the administration of arsenic. A curious association of occurrence with chicken-pox has been noted. A filterable virus is probably the cause in primary cases.

Pathology.—Bärensprung first showed that there was involvement of the spinal ganglia. There is an acute hemorrhagic inflammation of the ganglia of the posterior nerve roots and of the homologous cranial ganglia (Head and Campbell). There are inflammatory foci, hemorrhage in and destruction of certain of the ganglion cells leading to degeneration of the axis-cylinders. In herpes facialis in pneumonia W. T. Howard showed that similar lesions are found in the Gasserian ganglion, and Hunt found the same changes in the geniculate ganglion in herpes auricularis.

Symptoms.—There is often a slight prodromal period in which the patient feels ill, has moderate fever, and pain in the side, sometimes of such severity as to suggest pleurisy. On the third or fourth day the rash appears. The characteristic group of vesicles has a segmental distribution usually limited to one side of the body. One or more of the adjoining skin fields is usually affected. With involvement of the cervical, lumbar or sacral ganglia the zonal or girdle form of the vesicular crop is naturally lost owing to the distortion of the skin fields from the growth of the limbs. The typical zonal form is only seen in involvement of the thoracic ganglia. Groups of vesicles are regularly arranged on the hyperemic skin, at first filled with a clear or sometimes bloody serum, which later becomes purulent. The crop varies greatly, and the individual vesicles may be superficial, in which case they leave no scar, or they may be deep and leave superficial scars. The most serious form is that seen in the upper division of the fifth nerve. The fever may be high and the eruption very profuse with great swelling and much pain. Permanent disfigurement may follow the scarring.

It seems not improbable that there may be extension of the disease from the posterior ganglia to the neighboring meninges as there may be pains about the spine, the girdle sensation, exaggerated knee jerks, the Kernig sign, and lymphocytosis in the cerebrospinal fluid.

Herpes Zoster Oticus.—In this the vesicles may be very small and sometimes occur about the fauces, uvula or tongue. The pain may last for some time. There is sometimes an enlarged lymph node (pre-auricular). Facial paralysis may come on a few days later and with pain should suggest herpes zoster. Vertigo may occur. The application of cocaine to the sphenopalatine region is said to relieve the pain if there is swelling of the ganglion.

Complications.—The most serious of these is that occasionally seen in ophthalmic zoster, when there is intense inflammation of the conjunctiva and cornea with consecutive panophthalmitis and destruction of the eye. In some cases there may be scars on the cornea.

In a few cases the eruption becomes gangrenous. Swelling of the lymph nodes has ben noted, sometimes before the eruption. A bilateral distribution has occurred. A generalized herpes zoster is occasionally seen with a widespread vesicular rash on the face, neck, trunk and thighs. A facial paralysis may develop during or after ophthalmic or cervical herpes. Swelling of the parotid gland on the same side may occur. In rare cases paralysis of the extremities has occurred. A most distressing feature is *postzonal neuralgia.* After recovery from the herpes, hot burning sensations remain in the cutaneous distribution. In other instances, particularly in the aged, the pain persists and may be a terrible affliction. The victim may commit suicide.

Treatment.—Care should be taken to protect the vesicles; a one per cent cocaine ointment with lanolin applied on lint gives relief to the pain. Carbolized vaseline, stearate of zinc, menthol ointment or dusting powders may be used. Ultraviolet light therapy is often useful, given over the front, sides and back, for two minutes to each and repeating daily with an increase of two minutes each day. The salicylates or analgesic drugs aid in relieving pain. Benefit has been reported from the intramuscular injection of 1 cc. of pituitrin. With involvement of the ophthalmic division of the fifth nerve the greatest care should be taken to keep the conjunctiva clean. For the severe postherpetic neuralgia, alcohol injections into the posterior nerve roots have been tried, and in cases of great severity the posterior nerve roots may be cut.

SYMPATHETIC NERVOUS SYSTEM

This part of the nervous system is known also as the *Involuntary, Vegetative, Visceral* or *Autonomic* system and innervates the pupils, nonstriped muscles, glands, viscera, heart and blood vessels, and genital organs. It is outside the control of the will but can be influenced by the central nervous system, especially by emotional stimuli. The reverse may occur; disturbance in the realm of the sympathetic system may affect the general nervous system. Digestive disturbance may result from nervous anxiety or fatigue, and conversely disturbed function of the alimentary tract may cause marked nervous depression.

This involuntary or vegetative nervous system consists of two parts which are distinct anatomically and antagonistic physiologically.

(1) Sympathetic proper (thoracicolumbar).

(2) Parasympathetic (*a*) craniobulbar and (*b*) sacral.

There is some confusion in the use of the term "autonomic" which was applied by Langley to the whole vegetative system, but is also used by some to designate the parasympathetic alone. It would be well if the term were used as by Langley or not used at all.

The fibres of the sympathetic proper arise from cells in the intermedio-lateral region of the cord (preganglionic), pass by the anterior roots to end in ganglia which in turn send fibres (postganglionic) to the termination in smooth muscle, the heart, blood vessels, sweat glands, secreting glands, etc. The receptor (afferent) elements are concerned with visceral sensations and referred visceral pain. The excitor (efferent) elements form synapses in the ganglia and in this way one fibre may stimulate a number of cells. From these cells the postganglionic fibres pass directly to their destinations. The ganglia act as "distributing stations" and form a series in front of the vertebral column, one on each side. In the neck there are three ganglia in each chain, connected with the cord by the first and second thoracic roots. In the thoracic, lumbar and sacral regions there is a ganglion for each nerve root. It is suggested that there are centres in the hypothalamic area of the diencephalon which exercise some control over the sympathetic systems. The control of the sympathetic proper lies in the posterior hypothalamic region and that of the parasympathetic more anteriorly in the tuber cinereum at the base of the infundibulum. These "hypothalamic mechanisms" are of great importance and the explanation of many disturbances may lie in this important region.

The parasympathetic system (often termed autonomic or system of the "extended vagus") has the ganglia placed more peripherally. In the *craniobulbar* portion, fibres pass from the midbrain to the ciliary ganglion, constricting the pupil, from the medulla secretory fibres go to the submaxillary glands and by the vagus inhibitory fibres go to the heart, constrictor to the bronchi, motor to the esophagus, stomach and intestines, and secretory to the stomach and intestines. The vagus nerve is the most important constituent of the parasympathetic system. From the sacral portion by the pelvic nerve fibres go to the descending colon, rectum, anus, bladder and genital system. The vegetative system has three plexuses, cardiac, solar and hypogastric, which receive fibres from both systems. The sympathetic system has close relations to the endocrine glands. (1) The thyroid, adrenals and pituitary glands are in close relationship to the thoracicolumbar sympathetic and accelerate metabolism (*katabolic*). (2) The parasympathetic has close relations to the digestive tract and its glands and is engaged in storing energy (*anabolic*).

When the sympathetic and parasympathetic supply the same structure, their influences are antagonistic. Thus the sympathetic dilates the pupil, the other contracts it; the sympathetic increases the heart rate, the other slows it; the sympathetic inhibits the movements of the gastro-intestinal tract, the other increases them. In conditions of health there is a balance between the two systems. To describe the resulting condition when this balance is disturbed the terms sympathicotonia and vagotonia are employed, depending on which system is overactive. In the diagnosis of this the effects of certain drugs are important. Thus the sympathetic system proper is stimulated by epinephrine (1 cc. of 1-1000 solution) with resulting tremor, rigor, a sense of cold, glycosuria and a rise in blood pressure. The parasympathetic system is stimulated by pilocarpine (gr. 1/20-1/6, 0.003-0.01 gm.) with resulting salivation, nausea, sweating, flushing and a fall in blood pressure. Atropine (gr. 1/100-1/50, 0.00065-0.0013 gm.) paralyses the parasympathetic system with resulting dryness of the mouth and throat, palpitation and oppression.

Clinically among the features of *vagotonia* are small pupils, salivation, flushing, sweating, clammy hands and feet, dermographia, bradycardia, irregularity of respiration, hyperacidity, cardio- and pylorospasm, spastic constipation, and sphincter contraction. There may be increased sensitiveness to foreign proteins, as shown by urticaria, anaphylaxis; some include asthma. Among those of *sympathicotonia* are, dilated pupils, prominence of the eyes, dryness of the mouth and dry skin, tachycardia, decreased sugar tolerance and atony of the digestive tract. Actually it is found that many patients show features suggestive of disturbance in both systems. Some show vagotonia at one time and sympathicotonia later. The sympathetic system stands in close relation to the endocrine glands and its stimulation may cause increased activity of the adrenal and thyroid glands particularly.

GENERAL AND FUNCTIONAL DISEASES

PARALYSIS AGITANS

(*Parkinson's Disease; Shaking Palsy*)

Definition.—A chronic affection of the nervous system, characterized by disturbance of certain movements, tremors and rigidity. The efferent neurones of the corpus striatum are affected.

Etiology.—The disease affects men more than women. It rarely occurs under forty, but instances have been reported in which the disease began about the twentieth year. Direct heredity is rare, but the patients often belong to families in which there are other nervous affections. In some cases it may be caused by senile degeneration and arteriosclerotic changes. Among exciting causes are possibly worries and anxieties; in some instances the disease has followed severe mental shock or trauma especially cranial. Cases are described after the specific fevers.

Morbid Anatomy.—The changes are especially in the basal ganglia. In the juvenile type there are atrophy and decrease in number of the large motor cells of the globus pallidus system. These are regarded as a primary atrophy (abiotrophy). In the globus pallidus system the large cells are motor and the small ganglia cells are inhibitory and coordinating. If this destructive lesion involves both types of cells in the caudate nucleus and putamen, the *Vogt syndrome* results, that is, double athetosis with spastic contractures and pseudobulbar palsy. If the caudate nucleus and lenticular nucleus are the seat of this destructive lesion there results progressive lenticular degeneration—Wilson's disease—that is the paralysis agitans syndrome with rigidity, tremor, clonic and tonic spasms and perhaps choreic and athetoid movements (Gowers' tetanoid chorea).

Symptoms.—The disease begins gradually, usually in one or other hand, and the tremor may be constant or intermittent. With this may be associated weakness or stiffness. Rigidity may be the first manifestation. At first these symptoms may be present only after exertion. Although the onset is slow and gradual in nearly all cases, there are instances in which it sets in abruptly after fright or trauma. When well established the disease is very characteristic. The following are the prominent features.

The face—Parkinson's mask.—Even before the tremor begins the expressionless face, slow movement of the lips, the elevated eyebrows, and general facial immobility suggest the disease. When well developed it is the most characteristic—and pathetic—feature.

Tremor.—This may be in the four extremities or confined to hands or feet; the head is not so commonly affected. The tremor is usually marked in the hands, and the thumb and forefinger display the motion made in the act of rolling a pill. At the wrist there are movements of pronation and supination and though less marked, of flexion and extension. The upper arm muscles are rarely involved. In the legs the movement is most evident at the ankle joint, and less in the toes than in the fingers. Shaking of the head is less frequent and is usually vertical, not rotatory. The rate of oscillation is about five per second. Any emotion exaggerates the movement. The attempt at a voluntary movement may check the tremor (the patient may be able to thread a needle), but it returns with increased intensity. The tremors cease, as a rule, during sleep, but persist when the muscles are not in use. The writing is tremulous and zigzag. For months or years the chief tremor may be in one arm or one leg.

Weakness.—Loss of power is present in all cases, and may occur before the tremor, but is not very striking, until the late stages. The weakness is greatest where the tremor is most developed. The movements are remarkably slow. There is rarely complete loss of power.

Rigidity may early be expressed in a slowness and stiffness in the voluntary movements, which are performed with some effort and difficulty, and all the actions of the patient are deliberate. This rigidity is in all the muscles, and leads ultimately to the characteristic attitude.

Attitude and Gait.—The head is bent forward, the back bowed, and the arms held away from the body, somewhat flexed at the elbow joints. The fingers are flexed and in the position assumed when the hand is at rest; in the late stages they can not be extended. Occasionally there is overextension of the terminal phalanges. The hand is usually turned toward the ulnar side. In the late stages there are contractures at the elbows, knees and ankles. The movements of the patient are characterized by great deliberation. He rises from the chair slowly in the stooping attitude, with the head projecting forward. In attempting to walk the steps are short and hurried, and, as Trousseau remarked, he appears to be running after his centre of gravity. This is termed festination or propulsion, in contradistinction to a peculiar gait observed when the patient is pulled backward, when he makes a number of steps and would fall over if not prevented—retropulsion.

The *voice*, as pointed out by Buzzard, is at first shrill and piping, and there is often a hesitancy in beginning a sentence; then the words are uttered with rapidity, as if the patient was in a hurry.

The REFLEXES are normal in most cases but in a few they are exaggerated.

Of SENSORY disturbances Charcot noted alterations in the temperature sense. Some patients complain of subjective sensations of heat, general or local—which may be present on one side only and associated with an increase of the surface temperatures. In other instances, patients complain of cold. Localized sweating may be present. The skin, especially of the forehead, may be thickened. The mental condition rarely shows any change.

The disease is incurable. Periods of improvement may occur, but the tendency is for the affection to proceed progressively downward. It is a slow, degenerative process which lasts for years.

VARIATIONS IN THE SYMPTOMS.—The tremors may be absent, but the rigidity, weakness, and attitude are characteristic. The disease may be hemiplegic in character, involving only one side or even one limb. Usually these are but stages of the disease. Dull pain or discomfort may be present.

Diagnosis.—In well-developed cases the disease is recognized at a glance. The attitude, gait, stiffness, and mask-like expression are points of as much importance as the oscillations, and usually serve to separate the cases from senile and other forms of tremor. Disseminated sclerosis develops earlier and is characterized by the nystagmus and scanning speech, and does not present the *attitude* so constant in paralysis agitans. Yet Schultze and Sachs have reported cases in which the signs of multiple sclerosis have been associated with those of paralysis. The hemiplegic form might be confounded with posthemiplegic tremor, but the history, mode of onset and greatly increased reflexes distinguish the two. The Parkinsonian face and rigidity are of great importance in the diagnosis of the obscure forms. The history should distinguish the Parkinsonian sequel of epidemic encephalitis.

Treatment.—There is no satisfactory treatment. Fatigue should be avoided. Slowly performed muscular movements, with strong mental concentration, are sometimes useful in controlling the tremor. Hyoscine seems helpful in some cases (gr. $\frac{1}{200}$, 0.0003 gm. and gradually increased) alone or with small amounts of bromide. Stramonium may be used to relieve tremor. Hypnotics and sedatives should be used as indicated. Opium in some form may be required in late stages.

OTHER FORMS OF TREMOR

Simple Tremor.—This is occasionally found in persons in whom it is impossible to assign any cause. It may be transient or persist for an indefinite time. It is often extremely slight, and is aggravated by all causes which lower the vitality.

Hereditary Tremor.—C. L. Dana reported remarkable cases of hereditary tremor. It occurred in all the members of one family, and beginning in infancy continued without producing any serious changes.

Senile Tremor.—With advancing age tremulousness during muscular movements is extremely common, but is rarely seen under seventy. It is always a fine tremor, which begins in the hands and often extends to the muscles of the neck, causing slight movement of the head.

Toxic tremor is seen chiefly as an effect of tobacco, alcohol, lead or mercury; more rarely in arsenical or opium poisoning. In elderly men who smoke much it may be due to tobacco. A common form is the alcoholic tremor, which occurs only on movement and has considerable range. Lead tremor is an important symptom of lead poisoning.

Hysterical tremor, which usually occurs under circumstances which make the diagnosis easy, will be considered in the section on hysteria.

ACUTE CHOREA

(Sydenham's Chorea; St. Vitus's Dance)

Definition.—A disease, probably an acute infection, chiefly affecting children, characterized by irregular, involuntary contraction of the muscles, variable psychical disturbance, and a liability to acute endocarditis.

Etiology.—SEX.—Of 554 cases at the Philadelphia Infirmary for Nervous Diseases, 71 per cent were in females and 29 per cent in males (Osler). Of 808 Johns Hopkins Hospital cases, 71.2 per cent were females.

AGE.—The disease is most common between the ages of five and fifteen. Of 522 cases, 380 occurred in this period; 84.5 per cent in the Hopkins series. It is rare among the negroes and native races of America. Only 25 of the Johns Hopkins Hospital cases were in negroes.

RHEUMATIC FEVER.—Of the 554 cases, in 15.5 per cent there was a history of "rheumatism" in the family. In 88 cases, 15.8 per cent, there was a history of articular swelling, acute or subacute. In 33 cases there were pains, sometimes described as "rheumatic," in various parts, but not associated with joint trouble. Adding these to those with manifest articular trouble, the percentage is raised to nearly 21. It is rather remarkable that in the Baltimore series the percentage with a history of rheumatism was the same—21.6. It does not seem justified to regard chorea and rheumatic fever as one disease.

In one group the arthritis antedates by months or years the onset of the chorea, and does not recur before or during the attack. In the other the chorea sets in with or follows immediately upon the acute arthritis. It is difficult to differentiate the cases of irregular pains without definite arthritis. It is probable that many of them are rheumatic, but it is a mistake to regard as such all cases in children in which there are complaints of vague pains in the bones or muscles—so-called growing pains. It should never be forgotten that there may be no acute arthritis with rheumatic fever in a child.

HEART DISEASE.—Endocarditis is believed by some writers to be the cause of the disease. On this view chorea is the result of an embolic process occurring in the course of a rheumatic endocarditis.

INFECTIOUS DISEASES.—Scarlet fever with arthritic manifestations may be a direct antecedent. With the exception of rheumatic fever, there is no intimate relationship between chorea and the acute diseases incident to childhood. It may be noted in contrast to this that the so-called canine chorea is a common sequel of distemper. Chorea may follow gonorrhea, puerperal fever, and other forms of sepsis. The tonsils are frequently diseased.

SYPHILIS.—There is a small group, with features much like those of chorea, in which congenital syphilis is apparently the cause. Specific treatment results in rapid improvement.

ANEMIA is less often an antecedent than a sequence, and though cases occur in children who are anemic, this is by no means the rule.

PREGNANCY.—A choreic patient may become pregnant; more frequently the disease occurs during pregnancy; sometimes after delivery. Willson and Preece (1932) studied the records of 951 choreic pregnancies in 797 patients. More than half gave a history of previous chorea. Evidence of heart disease was found in about one third. In 690 cases, chorea preceded the pregnancy in 38, appeared in the first three months in 312, second three months in 219 and in the last three months in 101 cases. In 17 per cent the patient was single. Therapeutic abortion should not be done as a rule. The disease is often severe, and maniacal symptoms may occur.

A tendency to the disease is found in certain families. In 80 cases there was a history of chorea in other members. In one instance both mother and grandmother had been affected. High-strung, excitable, nervous children are especially liable. *Fright* is considered a frequent cause, but in a large majority of the cases no close connection exists between the fright and the onset of the disease. Occasionally the attack sets in at once. Mental worry, sudden grief or a scolding may apparently be the exciting cause. The strain of *education*, particularly in girls during the third hemidecade, appears to be an important factor. Bright, intelligent, active-minded girls, ambitious to do well at school, often stimulated by teachers and parents, form a large contingent of the cases—the so-called *school-made* chorea. *Imitation*, mentioned as an exciting cause, is extremely rare, and did not appear to have influenced the onset in a single case in the Infirmary records.

The disease may rapidly follow an injury or a slight surgical operation. Reflex irritation was believed to play an important rôle, particularly the presence of worms or genital irritation, but this is very doubtful. Ocular defects do not occur in greater proportion in choreic than in other children, and a majority of the cases in which operation has been followed by relief have been instances of *tic*, local or general.

The essential etiology is obscure. That it is an acute infection is suggested by (1) the association with rheumatic fever; (2) the acute febrile cases; (3) the frequency of involvement of the tonsils; (4) the seasonal relations; (5) the endocarditis; (6) the finding of micro-organisms—though no one organism is generally accepted as the cause; and (7) the occurrence of a chorea type in epidemic encephalitis in which the lesions are similar and in the same situation, basal ganglia, especially the red nucleus and corpus luysii.

Pathology.—Two anatomical changes are found: (1) *Endocarditis*, usually simple (and of the mitral valve), which was present in 62 of 73 fatal cases recorded.[1] In a few instances the lesion was ulcerative. (2) Foci of softening in the *basal ganglia*, in the situation and with the appearance of an *acute encephalitis*. Minute hemorrhages have been found elsewhere in the brain. Connected with the endocarditis there may be embolism of the central artery of the retina and cerebral embolism has occurred.

Symptoms.—Three groups of cases may be recognized—the mild, severe, and maniacal chorea.

[1] Osler, *Chorea and Choreiform Affections*, Philadelphia, 1894.

Mild Chorea.—In this the affection of the muscles is slight, the speech is not seriously disturbed, and the general health not impaired. Premonitory symptoms are shown in restlessness and inability to sit still, a condition well characterized by the term "fidgets." There are emotional disturbances, such as crying spells, or sometimes night terrors. There may be pains in the limbs and headache. Digestive disturbances and anemia may be present. A change in the temperament is frequently noticed, and a docile, quiet child may become cross and irritable. After these symptoms have persisted for a week or more the characteristic involuntary movements begin, and are often first noticed at the table, when the child spills a tumbler of water or upsets a plate. There may be only awkwardness or slight incoördination of voluntary movements, or constant irregular clonic spasms. The jerky, irregular character of the movements differentiates them from almost every other disorder of motion. In the mild cases only one hand, or the hand and face, are affected, and it may not spread to the other side.

In the *severe form* the movements become general and the patient may be unable to get about or to feed or undress herself, owing to the constant, irregular, clonic muscular contractions. The speech is affected, and for days the child may not be able to talk. Often with the onset of the severer symptoms there is loss of power on one side or in the limb most affected.

The third and most extreme form, maniacal chorea or *chorea insaniens,* is truly a terrible disease, and may arise out of the ordinary form. These cases are more common in adult women and may develop during pregnancy.

Chorea begins, as a rule, in the hands and arms, then involves the face, and subsequently the legs. The movements may be confined to one side—hemichorea. The attack begins oftenest on the right side, though occasionally it is general from the outset. One arm and the opposite leg may be involved. In a number of cases *speech* is affected; this may amount only to an embarrassment or hesitancy, but in other instances it becomes an incoherent jumble. In very severe cases the child will make no attempt to speak, perhaps for weeks. This is not marked by special choreic unrest of the muscles of speech; it is probably a motor weakness. Complete recovery follows. The tongue may be protruded and withdrawn with great rapidity. Paroxysms of panting and of hard expiration may occur, or odd sounds may be produced. As a rule the movements cease during sleep.

Weakness.—A prominent symptom is muscular weakness, usually no more than a condition of paresis. The loss of power is slight, but the weakness may be shown by an enfeebled grip or by a dragging of the leg or limping. In some cases there is flaccidity of the limbs (*limp chorea*). In his original account Sydenham refers to the "unsteady movements of one of the legs, which the patient drags." There may be extreme paresis with but few movements—the paralytic chorea of Todd. Occasionally a local paralysis or weakness remains after the attack. Hypotonia may be marked.

Cardiac.—As so many of the subjects of chorea are nervous girls, it is not surprising that a rapidly acting heart is common. Irregularity is not so special a feature. The patients seldom complain of pain about the heart.

Murmurs.—With anemia and debility, not uncommon with chorea in the third or fourth week, we find a corresponding cardiac condition. The impulse is diffuse, perhaps wavy in thin children. The carotids throb visibly, and in the recumbent posture there may be pulsation in the cervical veins. On auscultation a systolic murmur is heard at the base, perhaps, too, at the apex, soft and blowing in quality.

Endocarditis.—Acute valvulitis rarely gives symptoms. It must be sought, and usually shows murmurs at one or other of the cardiac orifices.

For the guidance of the practitioner these statements may be made:

(*a*) In thin, nervous children a systolic murmur of soft quality is extremely common at the base, with accentuation of the second sound, particularly at the second left costal cartilage, and is probably of no moment.

(*b*) A systolic murmur of maximum intensity at the apex, and heard also along the left sternal margin, is not uncommon in anemic, enfeebled states, and does not necessarily indicate either endocarditis or insufficiency.

(*c*) A murmur of maximum intensity at the apex, with rough quality, and transmitted to the axilla or angle of the scapula, indicates an organic lesion of the mitral valve, and is usually associated with enlargement of the heart.

(*d*) When in doubt it is much safer to trust to the evidence of eye and hand than to that of the ear. If the apex beat is in the normal position, and the area of dulness not increased vertically or to the right of the sternum, there is probably no serious valvular disease.

The *endocarditis* of chorea is almost invariably of the simple form, and in itself not dangerous; but it leads to those sclerotic changes in the valve which produce incompetency. Of 140 patients examined more than two years after the attack, the heart was normal in only 51; in 17 there was functional disturbance and 72 presented signs of organic heart disease. In an analysis of the Johns Hopkins Hospital cases, Thayer found evidence of involvement of the heart in 25 per cent of the out-patients and in more than 50 per cent of the ward patients. Cardiac involvement was more common in the cases with a history of rheumatic fever, and was much more frequent in the relapses. Pericarditis is an occasional complication. Aortic endocarditis is rare and in this it differs from rheumatic fever.

Sensory Disturbances.—Pain in the affected limbs is not common. Occasionally there is soreness on pressure. There are cases, usually of hemichorea, in which pain in the limbs is marked. Weir Mitchell spoke of these as *painful choreas.* Tender points along the lines of emergence of the spinal nerves or along the course of the nerves of the limbs are rare.

Psychical disturbances are common. Irritability of temper, marked wilfulness, and emotional outbreaks may indicate a complete change in the character. There is deficiency in the powers of concentration, the memory is enfeebled, and the aptitude for study is lost. The psychical element is apt to be neglected and it is always a good plan to tell the parents that it is not the muscles alone which are affected, but that the irritability and change of disposition really form part of the disease. Rarely there is progressive impairment of the intellect with termination in actual dementia. Acute melancholia has been described. Hallucinations of sight and hearing may occur. Patients may behave in an odd manner and do all sorts of meaningless acts. The most serious manifestation of this character is the maniacal delirium, occasionally associated with the very severe cases—*chorea insaniens.* Usually the motor disturbance in these cases is aggravated, but it has been overlooked and patients have been sent to an asylum.

The deep *reflexes* often show much variation, especially the knee jerk; the quadriceps contraction may be prolonged. Trophic lesions rarely occur.

FEVER, usually slight, was present in all but one of 110 cases (Thayer). Endocarditis may occur with little if any rise in temperature; but, on the other hand, with an acute arthritis, severe endocarditis or pericarditis, and in the maniacal cases the fever may range from 102° to 104°.

CUTANEOUS AFFECTIONS.—Pigmentation, which is not uncommon, is due to arsenic. Herpes zoster occasionally occurs. Erythema nodosum and purpuric urticaria have been described. There may be the condition of arthritis with purpura (Schönlein's disease), one of the varieties of anaphylactoid purpura. Subcutaneous nodules may be present.

Course.—From eight to ten weeks is the average duration of an attack of moderate severity. Cases described as chronic chorea following an acute attack are usually instances of cerebral sclerosis or Friedreich's ataxia, but occasionally an attack which has come on in the ordinary way persists for months or years and recovery ultimately takes place. A slight grade, particularly under excitement, may persist for months in nervous children. The tendency to *recur* is common; Sydenham first made the observation. Of 410 cases, 240 had one attack, 110 had two attacks, 35 three attacks, 10 four attacks, 12 five attacks, and 3 six attacks. The recurrence is apt to be in the spring.

Recovery is the rule. The statistics of outpatient departments are not favorable for determining the mortality. The Collective Investigation Committee of the British Medical Association found 9 deaths in 439 cases, about 2 per cent. There were 83 deaths in England and Wales in 1931.

The paralysis rarely persists. Mental dulness may be present for a time, but usually passes away; permanent impairment of the mind is exceptional.

Diagnosis.—In a majority of instances the diagnosis is made at a glance; but there are several affections which may be mistaken for it.

(*a*) *Multiple and Diffuse Cerebral Sclerosis.*—The cases may be mistaken for ordinary chorea, and have been described as *chorea spastica.* As a rule, the movements are readily distinguishable but the simulation is sometimes close; the onset in infancy, impaired intelligence, increased reflexes and in some instances rigidity with the chronic course separate them from true chorea.

(*b*) *Friedreich's Ataxia.*—Cases of this disease were formerly classed as chorea. The slow, irregular, incoördinate movements, the scoliosis, scanning speech, early talipes, nystagmus, and the family character give the diagnosis.

(*c*) In rare cases the paralytic form of chorea may be mistaken for *poliomyelitis* or, when both legs are affected, for paraplegia of spinal origin; but this can be the case only when the choreic movements are very slight.

(*d*) *Hysteria* may simulate chorea minor most closely, and unless there are other manifestations it may be impossible to make a diagnosis. Most commonly, however, the movements in the so-called hysterical chorea are rhythmic and differ entirely from those of ordinary chorea.

(*e*) The *mental symptoms* in maniacal chorea may mask the true nature of the disease especially if the choreic movements disappear.

(*f*) *Habit spasms* and *tics* should not be confused.

(*g*) *Epidemic encephalitis* with chorea-like movements is recognized by the other features of the disease.

Treatment.—Abnormally bright, active-minded children belonging to families with pronounced neurotic taint should be carefully watched and not allowed to overtax their mental powers. So frequently in children of this class does the attack of chorea date from the worry and stress incident to examinations that the competition for prizes should be emphatically forbidden.

The treatment of the attack consists largely in attention to hygienic measures, with which alone, in time, a majority of the cases recover. Parents should be told to scan gently the faults and waywardness of choreic children. The psychical element, strongly developed in so many cases, is best treated by quiet and seclusion. The child should be confined to bed in the recumbent posture, and mental as well as bodily quiet enjoined. In private practice this is often impossible, but with well-to-do patients the disease is always serious enough to demand the assistance of a skilled nurse. Toys and dolls should not be allowed at first, for the child should be kept amused without excitement. The rest allays the hyperexcitability and reduces to a minimum the possibility of damage to the valve segments should endocarditis exist.

The child should be kept apart from other children and, if possible, from other members of the family, and should see only those persons directly concerned with the care and nursing. The child should be protected against chilling. If the movements are violent care should be taken to prevent the child from falling out of bed or injuring herself. Especial care should be taken to prevent surface injury due to rubbing.

Diet.—Every effort should be made to give sufficient nourishment. Many patients do well on a diet principally of milk to which lactose may be added. Fruit juices, cooked fruits, ice cream and cocoa are allowed. Soft foods may be given if desired. The nasal tube should be used if necessary. After the fever is over a full varied diet should be given with abundance of vitamins.

Medicinal.—The salicylates may be used for fever; acetylsalicylic acid, (gr. 5-10, 0.3-0.6 gm.) is often the best. The use of arsenic is very general but it is a question if very large doses are indicated. It may be given as Fowler's solution in doses of 5 minims (0.3 cc.) three times a day. It should be stopped at once if there are any signs of overdosage. *Nirvanol* (a combination of urea and glycol) is given in amounts of 0.3 gm. per day until a marked morbilliform rash appears, usually with fever, fairly generally over the trunk and limbs. This occurs in from 8 to 14 days and is an indication to stop the drug. Drowsiness and stupor are common. The blood shows a leukopenia with eosinophilia. The reaction is termed "nirvanol disease" and must be produced if the drug is to be useful. Some give 90 grains (0.6 gm.) in 10 days. *Foreign protein therapy* (typhoid vaccine intravenously) has been used. Marked reactions are probably necessary if benefit is to result and this treatment should not be regarded as without danger. Fever therapy by diathermy is much safer and probably more efficient. The treatment is not without risk. *Sedatives* are usually necessary. Chloral hydrate is usually the best, the required dosage varying greatly. It may be begun in 10 grain (0.6 gm.) doses three or four times a day and increased if necessary. An equal amount of bromide may be added. Belladonna is useful in some cases. Hyoscine hydrobromide (gr. 1/100, 0.0006 gm.) sometimes is helpful. Barbital or phenobarbital in suitable dosage to the age is useful in securing sleep. In congenital syphilis active specific treatment should be given. Simple laxatives or enemata are used to keep the bowels regular. For anemia, iron and arsenic are indicated.

During convalescence carefully graduated exercises are beneficial. It is not well to send a choreic child to a school gymnasium, as the stimulus of other children and the excitement are very prejudicial.

In the severe cases with incessant movements, sleeplessness, dry tongue, and delirium, the important indication is to procure rest, for which purpose chloral may be freely given, and, if necessary, morphia. Chloroform may be necessary to control the paroxysms, but the high mortality in this form illustrates how often our endeavors are fruitless. A hot pack is sometimes soothing and should be tried.

There are cases which drag on from month to month without getting better or worse and resist all modes of treatment. In such cases a combination of suggestion and passive movements, followed by voluntary movements under control, and later simple exercises, may be useful. Change of air and scene is sometimes followed by rapid improvement, and in these cases the treatment by rest and seclusion should always be given a full trial.

Diseased tonsils and other foci of infection should be removed and nasal trouble treated. Ocular defects should be corrected. After the child has recovered, the parents should be warned that return is not infrequent, and liable to follow overwork at school or debilitating influences.

HABIT SPASMS AND TICS

Habit Spasm; Convulsive Tic.—Two groups of cases may be recognized under the designation of habit spasm—one in which there are simply localized spasmodic movements, and the other in which, in addition to this, there are explosive utterances and psychical symptoms, the French *tic convulsif.*

(*a*) Habit Spasm.—This is found chiefly in childhood, most frequently in girls from seven to fourteen years of age (Mitchell). There is usually a psychical basis; imitation is a factor in some cases. In its simplest form there is a sudden, quick contraction of certain of the facial muscles, such as rapid winking or drawing of the mouth to one side, or the neck muscles are involved and there are unilateral movements of the head. The head is given a sudden, quick shake, and at the same time the eyes wink. A not infrequent form is the shrugging of one shoulder. The movement is repeated at irregular intervals and is much aggravated by emotion. A short inspiratory sniff is not uncommon. Night terrors and enuresis may be associated. The cases are most frequent in children who are "out of sorts," who have been growing rapidly, or who have a tendency to neurotic disorders. Allied to or associated with this are some of the curious tricks of children. A boy was in the habit every few moments of putting the middle finger into the mouth, biting it, and at the same time pressing his nose with the forefinger. Hartley Coleridge is said to have had a somewhat similar trick, only he bit his arm. In all these cases the habits of the child should be studied, the nose and vault of the pharynx thoroughly inspected, and the eyes tested. As a rule the condition is transient, and after a few months gradually disappears. Occasionally a local spasm persists—twitching of the eyelids or the facial grimace.

Spasmus nutans, head nodding, is a coordinated tic in young infants usually of a harmless nature; it may be associated with nystagmus.

In *treatment,* comments on the condition and the mimicry of other children should be avoided. The child should lead a quiet open-air life with sufficient exercise and amusement. A tactful effort should be made to gain the child's confidence and learn his mental processes. The origin of the habit may be due to some curious idea or fear. In severe acute cases a period of rest and seclusion may be advisable. In older children and adults the effort should be made to learn to relax the muscles concerned. If there is much nervous excitement sedatives are useful.

(*b*) IMPULSIVE TIC (GILLES DE LA TOURETTE'S DISEASE).—This remarkable affection, often mistaken for chorea, more frequently for habit spasm, is really a psychosis allied to hysteria, psychical tic, though in some aspects it has the features of monomania. The disease begins, as a rule, in young children, as early as the sixth year, though it may occur after puberty. There is usually a neurotic family history. The special features are:

(1) Involuntary muscular movements, usually affecting the facial or brachial muscles, but in aggravated cases all the muscles of the body may be involved and the movements may be extremely irregular and violent.

(2) Explosive utterances, which may resemble a bark or an inarticulate cry. A word heard may be mimicked at once and repeated over and over again, usually with the involuntary movements. To this the term *echolalia* has been applied. A much more distressing disturbance in these cases is *coprolalia,* or the use of bad language. A small child may swear constantly when making the involuntary movements or utter all sorts of obscene words. Occasionally actions are mimicked—*echokinesis.*

(3) Some of these patients have curious mental disturbances; the patient has a form of obsession or a fixed idea. This may take the form of the impulse to touch objects, or a fixed idea about words—onomatomania—or he may feel compelled to count a number of times before doing certain actions—arithmomania. The disease is readily distinguished from ordinary chorea. The movements have a larger range and are explosive in character. Tourette regarded the coprolalia as the most distinctive feature. The prognosis is doubtful, but recovery may follow. In *treatment* every effort should be made to gain the patient's confidence and study his psychical processes, early in the course if possible. Psychical treatment is the most important. His life should be ordered in the most healthy fashion, physically and mentally. Complete separation from other members of the family may be advisable.

Saltatory Spasm (*Latah; Myriachit; Jumpers*).—Bamberger described a disease in which when the patient attempted to stand there were strong contractions in the leg muscles, which caused a jumping or springing motion. This occurs only when the patient attempts to stand. The affection has occurred in both men and women, more frequently in the former, and the subjects have usually shown marked neurotic tendencies. In many cases the condition has been transitory; in others it has persisted for years. Remarkable affections similar to this in certain points occur as a sort of epidemic neurosis. One of the most striking of these occurs among the "jumping Frenchmen" of Maine and Canada. The subjects are liable on any sudden emotion to jump violently and utter a loud cry or sound, and obey any command or imitate any action without regard to its nature. Echolalia is present in a marked degree. The "jumping" prevails in certain families.

A very similar disease prevails in parts of Russia and in Java and Borneo, where it is known by the names of myriachit and latah, the chief feature of which is mimicry by the patient of everything he sees or hears.

Rhythmic Chorea.—This is readily recognized by the rhythmical character of the movements. It may affect the muscles of the abdomen, producing the salaam convulsion, or involve the sternomastoid, producing a rhythmical movement of the head, or the psoas, or any group of muscles. In its orderly rhythm it resembles the canine chorea. It has to be distinguished from the myoclonic form of epidemic encephalitis.

INFANTILE CONVULSIONS

Convulsive seizures similar to those of epilepsy are not infrequent in children. The fit may be identical with epilepsy, from which the condition differs in that when the cause is removed there is no tendency for the fits to recur. Occasionally, however, the convulsions continue and pass into true epilepsy. It may be difficult for a time to decide which condition is present.

Etiology.—A convulsion may be due to many causes, all of which lead to an unstable condition of the nerve centres, permitting sudden, excessive, and temporary nervous discharges. The following are the most important:

(1) *Debility,* resulting usually from gastro-intestinal disturbance. Convulsions frequently supervene toward the close of an attack of enterocolitis and recur, sometimes proving fatal.

(2) *Irritation.*—Dentition alone is rarely a cause, but is often one of several factors in a feeble infant. The greatest mortality from convulsions is during the first six months, before the teeth have really cut through the gums. Another irritative cause is overloading the stomach with indigestible food. It has been suggested that some of these cases are toxic. Worms, to which convulsions are frequently attributed, probably have little influence. Among other possible sources are phimosis and otitis.

(3) *Rickets.*—Rickets and convulsions are often associated (Jenner). The spasms may be laryngeal, the so-called child-crowing, which, though convulsive in nature, can scarcely be reckoned under eclampsia. This condition is more apparent in Europe than in the United States. Spasms, local or general, in rickets are probably associated with the debility and malnutrition.

(4) *Infections.*—In young children the onset of the infectious diseases is frequently with convulsions, which may take the place of a chill in the adult. It is not known upon what they depend. Scarlet fever, measles and pneumonia are most often preceded by convulsions.

(5) *Congestion of the Brain.*—That extreme engorgement of the blood-vessels may produce convulsions is shown by their occasional occurrence in severe whooping cough, but their rarity in this disease really indicates how small a part mechanical congestion plays in the production of fits.

(6) *Severe convulsions* usher in or accompany many of the serious diseases of the nervous system in children. The acute encephalitis of children, which is followed by hemiplegia, usually has severe convulsions at the onset.

They less frequently precede a spinal paralysis. They occur with meningitis, tuberculous or simple, and with tumors and other lesions of the brain.

(7) Convulsions may occur after birth and persist for weeks or months, probably due to meningeal hemorrhage or injury to the cortex.

The relation of convulsions in children to true *epilepsy* is important. In Gowers' figures of 1,450 cases of epilepsy, the attacks began in 180 during the first three years of life. Of 460 cases of epilepsy in children, in 187 the fits began within the first three years and the greatest number, 74, was in the first year (Osler). In nearly all these instances there was no interruption in the convulsions. J. L. Morse regarded as the dangerous forms those in which the convulsions occur over a considerable period or in which there are repeated attacks suggesting *petit mal.*

Symptoms.—The attack may come on suddenly without any warning; more commonly it is preceded by restlessness, twitchings and perhaps grinding of the teeth. The convulsion is rarely so complete in its stages as true epilepsy. The spasm begins usually in the hands, most commonly in the right hand. The eyes are fixed and staring or are rolled up. The body becomes stiff and breathing is suspended for a moment or two by tonic spasm of the respiratory muscles, in consequence of which the face becomes congested. *Clonic* convulsions follows, the eyes are rolled about, the hands and arms twitch, or are fixed and extended in rhythmical movements, the face is contorted, and the head is retracted. The attack gradually subsides and the child sleeps or passes into a state of stupor. Following indigestion the attack may be single, but in rickets and intestinal disorders it is apt to be repeated. Sometimes the attacks follow each other with great rapidity, so that the child never rouses but dies in a deep coma. If the convulsion has been limited chiefly to one side there may be slight paresis after recovery, or if the convulsions usher in infantile hemiplegia, when the child arouses, one side is completely paralyzed. During the fit the temperature is often raised. Death rarely occurs from the convulsion itself, except in debilitated children or when the attacks recur with great frequency. In the co-called hydrocephaloid state in connection with protracted diarrhea convulsions may close the scene.

Diagnosis.—If the child is in full health, the attack is probably due to an overloaded stomach, to some peripheral irritation, or occasionally to trauma. Setting in with high fever and vomiting, it may indicate the onset of an exanthem, meningitis, encephalitis, or whatever the condition is which causes infantile hemiplegia. When associated with debility or rickets the diagnosis is easily made. The carpopedal spasms and pseudoparalytic rigidity often associated with rickets, laryngismus stridulus, and the hydrocephaloid state are usually confined to the hands and arms and are intermittent and usually tonic. The convulsions with tumor or which follow infantile hemiplegia are usually at first Jacksonian in character. After the second year convulsive seizures which come on irregularly without apparent cause and recur while the child is apparently in good health, are likely to prove true epilepsy.

Prognosis.—Convulsions play an important part in infantile mortality. In chronic diarrhea convulsions are usually of ill omen. Those ushering in fevers are rarely serious, and the same may be said of the fits associated with indigestion and peripheral irritation. However, there is frequently doubt as to the significance and therefore the prognosis of infantile convulsions.

Treatment.—Every source of irritation should be removed. If associated with indigestible food, an emetic should be given, followed by an enema. The teeth should be examined, and if the gum is swollen, hot, and tense, it may be lanced; but never if it looks normal. At first, if the paroxysm is severe, no time should be lost by giving a hot bath, but chloroform should be given at once, and repeated if necessary. A child is so readily put under chloroform and with such a small quantity that this procedure is quitc harmless and saves valuable time. The practice is almost universal of putting the child into a warm bath, and if there is a fever the head may be douched with cold water. The temperature of the bath should not be above 95°. The very hot bath is not suitable, particularly if the fits are due to indigestion. After the attack an ice-cap may be placed upon the head. If there is much irritability, particularly in rickets and severe diarrhea, small doses of opium will be found efficacious. When the convulsions recur after the child comes from under the influence of chloroform it is best to give morphia hypodermically, in doses of gr. 1/25 to 1/30 (0.0026 to 0.0022 gm.) for a child of one year. Other remedies are chloral by enema, in 5 grain (0.3 gm.) doses, and nitrite of amyl. After the attack has passed the bromides are useful, of which 5 to 8 grains (0.3 to 0.5 gm.) may be given in a day to a child a year old. Recurring convulsions, particularly if they come on without special cause, should receive careful treatment with bromides. When associated with rickets the treatment should be directed to this disease.

EPILEPSY

Definition.—An affection of the nervous system characterized by attacks of unconsciousness, with or without convulsions. The transient loss of consciousness without convulsive seizures is known as minor epilepsy (*petit mal*); the loss of consciousness with general convulsive seizures is known as major epilepsy (*grand mal*). Localized convulsions, occurring usually without loss of consciousness, are known as Jacksonian or cortical epilepsy.

Etiology.—Idiopathic or essential epilepsy, the form with an unknown or indefinite etiology, appears to depend upon a congenital tendency in the individual. Coarse anatomical changes in the brain are not present, but changes have been found, particularly a gliosis of the superficial layers of the cortex described by Alzheimer. Apart from this is the large group of *symptomatic* convulsive seizures due to toxemias, trauma, growths, chronic infections and arteriosclerosis, which should not be termed epilepsy. The loose use of the term leads to much confusion both in thought and treatment.

AGE.—In a large proportion the disease begins before puberty. Of 1,450 cases observed by Gowers, in 422 the disease began before the tenth year, and three-fourths of the cases began before the twentieth year. Of 427 cases of epilepsy in children, the age of onset was: First year, 74; second year, 62; third year, 51; fourth year, 24; fifth year, 17; sixth year, 18; seventh year, 19; eighth year, 23; ninth year, 17; tenth year, 27; eleventh year, 17; twelfth year, 18; thirteenth year, 15; fourteenth year, 21; fifteenth year, 34. Arranged in hemidecades the figures are as follows: From the first to fifth year, 229; from the fifth to the tenth year, 104; from the tenth to the fifteenth year, 95 (Osler). These figures show the early onset in a large proportion of cases.

It is well always to be suspicious of "epilepsy" beginning in adult life, for in a majority of such cases the disease is not epilepsy.

Sex.—No special influence is evident, certainly not in children. Of 435 cases, 232 were males and 203 were females. After puberty unquestionably, if a large number of cases are taken, the males are in excess.

Heredity.—Gowers remarks "there are few diseases in the production of which inheritance has a more marked influence." The study of the American Eugenics Bureau (Bulletin No. IV), analyzing data of 206 epileptics, shows how potent are inherited factors. Pierce Clark considered that there are more or less definite essential defects in epileptics which account in part for the predisposition. These are "egocentricity, supersensitiveness, an emotional poverty and an inherent lack of adaptability to normal social life." Stress and annoyance, and an intensive regression to day-dreaming, lethargy and somnolence are precipitating factors. "The attack occurs at the final break of a too severe tension."

Chronic alcoholism in the parents is regarded by many as a potent predisposing factor. Echeverria analyzed 572 cases and divided them into three classes, of which 257 cases could be traced directly to alcohol as a cause; 126 cases in which there were associated conditions, such as syphilis and traumatism; 189 cases in which the alcoholism was probably the result of the epilepsy. Figures equally strong are given by Martin, who in 150 insane epileptics found 83 with a marked history of parental intemperance. Spratling found 15 per cent with marked alcoholic history in the parents. Severe convulsive seizures may occur in steady drinkers.

Syphilis.—This in the parents is probably less a predisposing than an actual cause of epilepsy, which is the direct outcome of local cerebral manifestations. There is no reason for recognizing a special form of syphilitic epilepsy. Convulsive seizures due to acquired syphilitic disease of the brain are very common.

Of exciting causes fright is probably not important. Trauma is present in a certain number of instances. An important group depends upon a local disease of the brain existing from childhood, as seen in the posthemiplegic epilepsy. Occasionally cases follow the infectious fevers. Masturbation is stated to be a cause but its influence is overrated. Convulsive seizures like epilepsy are due to toxic agents, as in lead poisoning and uremia.

Reflex Causes.—Eye strain, dentition, worms, the irritation of a cicatrix, some local affection, such as adherent prepuce, or a foreign body in the ear or nose, are given as causes. In rare cases the fits cease after the removal of the irritating factor but usually the attacks persist. Genuine cases of reflex epilepsy are rare. A remarkable instance occurred in a man with a testis in the inguinal canal, pressure upon which caused a typical fit. Removal of the testis was followed by cure.

Cardiovascular "epilepsy" is usually a manifestation of advanced arteriosclerosis, and may be associated with a slow pulse (Stokes-Adams disease). The passage of a gallstone or the removal of pleuritic fluid may induce a fit. Digestive troubles are extremely common in epilepsy and the eating of indigestible articles seems often to precipitate an attack. Protein hypersensitiveness to certain foods is found in some patients. Convulsive seizures may occur in old people without obvious cause.

Symptoms.—(*a*) Major Epilepsy.—Preceding the fits there is usually a localized sensation, known as an *aura,* in some part of the body. This may be somatic, in which the feeling comes from some particular region in the periphery, as from the finger or hand, or is a sensation felt in the stomach or about the heart. The peripheral sensations are of great value, particularly those in which the aura always occurs in a definite region, as in one finger or toe. It is the equivalent of the signal symptom in a fit from a brain tumor. The varieties of these sensations are numerous. The epigastric sensations are most common. In these the patient complains of an uneasy sensation in the epigastrium or distress in the intestines, or the sensation may be not unlike that of heartburn and associated with palpitation. These groups are sometimes known as pneumogastric aurae or warnings.

Of *psychical* aurae one of the most common, as described by Hughlings Jackson, is a vague, dreamy state, a sensation of strangeness or sometimes of terror. The aurae may be associated with special senses; of these the most common are the visual, consisting of flashes of light or sensations of color; less commonly, distinct objects are seen. The auditory aurae consist of noises in the ear, odd sounds, musical tones or occasionally voices. Olfactory and gustatory aurae, unpleasant tastes and odors, are rare.

Occasionally the fit may be preceded not by an aura, but by certain movements; the patient may turn round rapidly or run with great speed for a few minutes, the so-called epilepsia procursiva. In an Elwyn case the lad stood on his toes and twirled with extraordinary rapidity, so that his features were scarcely recognizable. It is stated that the pulse sometimes stops just before the fit. The studies of Gibson and Good show that no alteration in the pulse occurred up to the point of clonic convulsions, and there was no lowering of the blood pressure suggesting anemia of the brain. At the onset of the attack the patient may give a loud scream or yell, the so-called *epileptic cry.* The patient drops as if shot, making no effort to guard the fall. In consequence, epileptics frequently injure themselves, cutting the face or head or burning themselves. In the attack, as described by Hippocrates, "the patient loses his speech and chokes, and foam issues from the mouth, the teeth are fixed, the hands are contracted, the eyes distorted, he becomes insensible, and in some cases the bowels are affected. And these symptoms occur sometimes on the left side, sometimes on the right, and sometimes on both." The fit may be described in three stages:

(1) *Tonic Spasm.*—The head is drawn back or to one side and the jaws are fixed. The hands are clinched and the legs extended. This tonic contraction affects the muscles of the chest, so that respiration is impeded and the initial pallor of the face changes to a dusky or livid hue. The muscles of the two sides are unequally affected, so that the head and neck are rotated or the spine is twisted. The arms are usually flexed at the elbows, the hand at the wrist, and the fingers are tightly clinched in the palm. This stage lasts only a few seconds, and then the clonic stage begins.

(2) *Clonic Stage.*—The muscular contractions become intermittent; at first tremulous or vibratory, they gradually become more rapid and the limbs are jerked and tossed about violently. The muscles of the face are in constant clonic spasm, the eyes roll, the eyelids are opened and closed convulsively. The movements of the muscles of the jaw are very forcible and strong, and

the tongue may be caught between the teeth and lacerated. The cyanosis, marked at the end of the tonic stage, gradually lessens. A frothy saliva, which may be blood stained, escapes from the mouth. The feces and urine may be discharged involuntarily. The duration of this stage is variable. It rarely lasts more than one or two minutes. The contractions become less violent and the patient passes into the condition of coma.

(3) *Coma.*—The breathing is noisy or even stertorous, the face congested, but no longer intensely cyanotic. The limbs are relaxed and the unconsciousness is profound. After a variable time the patient can be aroused, but if left alone he sleeps for some hours and then awakes, complaining only of slight headache or mental confusion. If the attack has been severe, petechial hemorrhages may occur over the neck and chest. In a young man in a severe convulsion both subconjunctival spaces were filled with blood, and blood oozed from them (James). Hemoptysis is a rare sequel.

After the attack the reflexes are often absent for a short time and later increased; ankle clonus can usually be obtained. The state of the urine is variable, particularly as regards the solids. The quantity is usually increased after the attack, and albumin or sugar may be present.

(4) *Status epilepticus.*—In this attacks occur in rapid succession, and the patient does not recover consciousness. The pulse, respiration, and temperature rise in the attack. It is serious and often proves fatal.

(5) *Postepileptic symptoms* are of great importance. The patient may be in a trance-like condition, in which he performs actions of which subsequently he has no recollection. More serious are the attacks of mania, in which the patient is often dangerous and sometimes homicidal. It is held by some that an outbreak of mania may be substituted for the fit. The mental condition of an epileptic patient is often seriously impaired.

(6) *Paralysis,* which rarely follows the epileptic fit, is usually hemiplegic and transient. Slight disturbances of speech may occur; in some instances, forms of sensory aphasia. Scripture draws attention to an inflexibility of speech of the epileptic which sounds "expressionless or wooden" and can be recognized by a trained ear. The absence of flexibility can be demonstrated by graphic records.

The attacks may occur at *night,* and a person may be epileptic for years without knowing it. As Trousseau remarks, when a person tells us that in the night he has incontinence of urine, awakes in the morning with headache and mental confusion, complains of difficulty in speech because he has bitten his tongue, and there are purpuric spots on the face and neck, the probability is very strong that he is subject to nocturnal epilepsy.

(*b*) Minor Epilepsy.—Epilepsy without convulsions consists of transient unconsciousness, which may come on at any time, with or without a feeling of faintness and vertigo. Suddenly, at the dinner table, the subject stops talking and eating, the eyes become fixed, and the face slightly pale. Anything which may have been in the hand is usually dropped. In a moment or two consciousness is regained and the patient resumes conversation as if nothing had happened. In other instances there is slight incoherency or the patient performs some almost automatic action. He may begin to undress and on returning to consciousness find that he has partially disrobed. He may rub his face, or spit about in a careless way. In other attacks the patient falls without convulsive seizures. A definite aura is rare. Though transient unconsciousness and giddiness are the most constant manifestations of *petit mal*, there are other equivalent manifestations, such as sudden jerkings in the limbs, sudden tremor, or a sudden visual sensation. Gowers gave no less than seventeen different manifestations. In occasional cases the patient has a sensation of losing his breath and may become red in the face. There may be myoclonic movements—"the jumps."

After the attack the patient may be dazed for a few seconds and perform automatic actions, which may seem to be volitional. Undressing is common, but many odd actions may be performed, some of which are awkward or serious. One patient after an attack was in the habit of tearing anything he could lay hands on, particularly books. Violent actions have been committed and assaults made, giving rise to medicolegal questions. This has been termed masked epilepsy or *epilepsia larvata*. In a majority of the cases of *petit mal* convulsions finally occur, at first slight, but ultimately major epilepsy is developed, and the attacks may then alternate.

(*c*) Jacksonian Epilepsy.—This is also known as cortical, symptomatic or partial epilepsy. It is distinguished from the ordinary epilepsy by the important fact that consciousness is retained or is lost late. The attacks are usually the result of irritative lesions in the motor zone, though there are probably also sensory equivalents of this motor form. Of 107 cases analyzed by Roland, there were 48 of tumor, 21 instances of inflammatory softening, 14 instances of acute and chronic meningitis, and 8 cases of trauma. The remaining cases were due to hemorrhage or abscess, or associated with sclerosis cerebri. A considerable number of the cases of Jacksonian epilepsy are found in children following hemiplegia, the so-called posthemiplegic epilepsy. The convulsions usually begin on the affected side, either in the arm or leg, and the fit may be unilateral and without loss of consciousness. Ultimately they become more severe and general.

In a typical attack the spasm begins in a limited muscle group of the face, arm or leg. The zygomatic muscles, for instance, or the limb may twitch, or the toes may first be moved. Prior to the twitching the patient may feel a sensation of numbness or tingling in the part affected. The spasm extends and may involve the muscles of one limb only or of the face. The patient is conscious throughout and watches, often with interest, the march of the spasm. The *onset* may be slow, and there may be time for the patient to place a pillow on the floor, so as to be as comfortable as possible during the attack. The spasm may be localized for years, but there is a great risk that the partial epilepsy may become general.

(*d*) Pyknolepsy.—This is a form of minor epilepsy occurring between four and twelve years of age and usually with an explosive onset. The attacks are slight, of short duration, without any distress and may be many in a day. The child rarely falls, although the limbs relax, and objects are rarely dropped from the hands. The head may turn, the eyes rotate up and the arms show a feeble tonic spasm. There are no clonic spasms. The child seems normal afterwards and the attacks are not harmful. Treatment seems to have no effect. The attacks stop spontaneously, usually by puberty.

Diagnosis.—In *major epilepsy* the suddenness of the attack, the abrupt loss of consciousness, the order of the tonic and clonic spasm, and the relaxation of the sphincters are distinctive features. The seizures due to uremia are usually readily recognized by the hypertension and the condition of the urine. In young adults hysteria causes the greatest difficulty and may closely simulate true epilepsy. Hysteroid attacks sometimes are postepileptic. A careful study and observation of an attack usually make the diagnosis clear. *Cysticercosis* should be considered if the attacks begin in adult life. It may cause epileptic-like seizures.

Recurring epileptic seizures in a person over thirty who has not had previous attacks is always suggestive of organic disease, usually syphilis.

Petit mal must be distinguished from attacks of syncope, and the vertigo of Ménière's disease, of a cardiac lesion, and of indigestion. Puzzling attacks occur especially about puberty, in which there is a slow and usually only partial loss of consciousness with dizziness, palpitation, slow pulse, low blood pressure and vasomotor disturbance. The subjects have often grown rapidly. Diagnosis may be difficult if an attack is not observed. The results from good hygiene, supervised activity, and long hours of sleep are an aid.

Jacksonian epilepsy has features so distinctive and peculiar that it is at once recognized. It is, however, by no means easy always to determine upon what the spasm depends. Irritation in the motor centres may be due to a great variety of causes, among which tumors and localized meningo-encephalitis are the most frequent; but in uremia localized attacks may occur. The most typical Jacksonian spasms may occur in general paresis.

Prognosis.—This may be given to-day in the words of Hippocrates: "The prognosis in epilepsy is unfavorable when the disease is congenital, and when it endures to manhood, and when it occurs in a grown person without any previous cause. . . . The cure may be attempted in young persons, but not in old." Of cases beginning under ten years few are arrested, whereas of those beginning at puberty the opposite is true (W. A. Turner).

Death during the fit rarely occurs, but it may happen if the patient falls into water or a fire, or if the fit comes on while he is eating. Occasionally the fits stop spontaneously. This is particularly the case in the epilepsy in children which has followed the convulsions of teething or the fevers. Frequency of the attacks and marked mental disturbances are unfavorable indications. The posthemiplegic epilepsy is rarely arrested.

Treatment.—General.—In the case of children the parents should be made to understand from the outset that epilepsy in the great majority of cases is incurable, so that the disease may interfere as little as possible with the education of the child. The subjects need firm but kind treatment. Indulgence and yielding to caprices and whims are followed by weakening of the moral control, which is so necessary in these cases. Sources of irritation should receive attention. The disease does not incapacitate a person for all occupation. It is much better for an epileptic to have some definite pursuit but he should not follow an occupation which involves climbing or working with machinery. He should not be allowed to drive a car or swim. The individual should take up an out-of-door occupation, or have manual training suited to his condition. This is best done in an institution where he is carefully watched and studied. Psychoanalysis, with reeducation, over a prolonged period is of value in some patients. There are instances in which epileptics have had extraordinary mental and bodily vigor, as, for example, Julius Cæsar and

Napoleon. One distressing feature is the mental impairment which follows in a certain number of cases. If such patients become extremely irritable or show signs of violence they should be placed in an institution. Epileptics should not marry.

During the *attack* a cork or bit of rubber should be placed between the teeth and the clothes should be loosened. The patient should be in the recumbent posture. If vomiting occurs he should be turned on the side and the mouth emptied of vomited material. As the attack usually passes off with rapidity, no special treatment is necessary, but in cases in which the convulsion is prolonged a few whiffs of chloroform or nitrite of amyl or a hypodermic of a quarter of a grain of morphia may be given.

DIETETIC.—The important points are to give the patient a light diet at fixed hours and on no account permit overloading of the stomach. Meat should not be given more than once a day. There are cases in which animal food seems injurious and a strict vegetable diet is sometimes useful. The possibility of protein sensitization should be considered and if found, these proteins should be excluded from the diet. The patient should not go to sleep until the completion of gastric digestion. The bowels should be kept freely open and colon irrigations are useful. A ketogenic diet, starvation and dehydration have not been proved to be of value.

MEDICINAL.—The *bromides* are extensively used. They act as a depressant and therefore should be used only after a careful study of each patient. Sodium bromide is probably less irritating than the potassium salt and is better borne for a long period. It may be given in milk, in which it is scarcely tasted. In all instances the dilution should be considerable. The dose for an adult should be from half a dram to a dram and a half (2 to 6 gm.) daily. It is often best to give but a single dose, daily, about four to six hours before the attacks are most likely to occur. For instance, in nocturnal epilepsy 30 to 60 grains (2 to 4 gm.) should be given in the evening. If the attack occurs in the morning, the patient should take a full dose when he awakes. When given three times a day it is less disturbing after meals. The diet should be salt-poor. Each patient should be carefully studied to determine how much bromide should be used. The individual susceptibility varies and some patients require more than others. Children take the drug well and stand proportionately larger doses than adults. Saturation is indicated by drowsiness, mental torpor, and gastric and cardiac distress. Loss of palate reflex is an early indication. Acne may appear but is diminished by giving the drug largely diluted in alkaline waters and administering arsenic from time to time. Written directions should be given to the mother or the friends of the patient, and he should not be held responsible for the administration of his medicine. The addition of belladonna to the bromide is recommended. *Phenobarbital* (luminal) is probably more useful than bromide, beginning with doses of one grain (0.065 gm.) one to three times a day and gradually increasing until the best dosage is found. Amounts over six grains a day should be given only for short periods. The drug may be given for four or five days a week and bromide given on the other days. If attacks occur at certain times, *e.g.*, with menstruation, the drugs should be given in larger doses for a few days before. In status epilepticus, hyoscine or morphine hypodermically may be useful. The use of sodium phenobarbital intravenously (gr. v-x, 0.3-0.6 gm.) has been successful.

Among other remedies are chloral, cannabis indica and nitroglycerin. Nitroglycerin is sometimes advantageous in *petit mal* in full doses, from 2 to 5 drops of the 1 per cent solution, until the physiological effects are produced. Calcium lactate in 20 grain (1.3 gm.) doses daily has been recommended. Counterirritation is rarely advisable. When the aura is very definite and constant in its onset, as from the hand or from the toe, a ligature tightly applied may stop the oncoming fit.

The subjects of a chronic and, in most cases, an incurable disease, epileptic patients form no small portion of the unfortunate victims of charlatans and quacks, who prescribe to-day, as in the time of the father of medicine, "purifications and spells and other illiberal practices of like kind."

SURGICAL.—In Jacksonian epilepsy the propriety of surgical interference is universally granted. It is questionable whether in the epilepsy following hemiplegia it is likely to be of any benefit. In idiopathic epilepsy, when the fit starts in a certain region—the thumb, for instance—and the signal symptom is invariable, the centre controlling this part may be removed. Operation, *per se*, appears in some cases to have a curative effect. The operation in the traumatic epilepsy, as after fracture, is much more hopeful. Operations have not been always on the skull, and White collected an interesting series in which various surgical procedures had been done, such as ligation of the carotid artery, castration, excision of the superior cervical ganglia, incision of the scalp, etc.

MIGRAINE

(*Hemicrania; Sick Headache*)

Definition.—A paroxysmal affection characterized by severe headache, usually unilateral, and often associated with vomiting or disorders of vision.

Etiology.—*Heredity* plays an important rôle in 90 per cent of cases according to Möbius. Women and members of neurotic families are most frequently attacked. Many distinguished men have been its victims, and the astronomer Airy gave a classical account of his case. The nature of the disease is in dispute, and many views have been entertained:

(*a*) That it is a *toxemia* from disorder of the intestinal digestion or from some self-manufactured poison. In some cases this may be added to another factor. Acetonuria is found in some cases.

(*b*) That it is a *vasomotor* affection with spasm of the arteries, in favor of which are the facts that in the attack the temporal arteries on the affected side may be felt to be small, the retinal arteries may sometimes be seen in spasm, and sclerosis of the arteries on the same side is found in a certain number of cases. There is also the temporary paralysis which may be associated with a monoplegic or hemiplegic attack. Mitchell Clarke reported recurring motor paralysis in eleven members in three generations of the same family. The characteristic visual phenomena preceded the unilateral headache, especially the hemianopia. In most of the attacks the hemiplegia was on the right side. It lasted from a few hours to a day and disappeared completely. It is difficult to explain such cases except on the view of a transient spasm of the arteries.

(*c*) Others regard the affection as of *reflex* origin arising from a refractive error in the eyes, or from trouble in the nose or sexual organs.

(*d*) A constitutional *anatomical defect* causing stenosis of the foramen of Monro, associated with hyperemia of the choroid plexus and increase of pressure in one or both lateral ventricles, is the view of Spitzner.

(*e*) Some regard it as a disturbance of the *sympathetic* nervous system, due to a number of conditions. The variety of suggested causal factors is striking; toxic states and psychosexual disturbances are among them.

(*f*) *Allergy*.—This may be the cause in some patients. Many patients are sensitive to a number of foods, perhaps markedly to one or two. In some there is associated hay fever or asthma. Others have curious abdominal attacks regarded as an equivalent of migraine (allergic?).

(*g*) *Hepatic dysfunction,* perhaps with subacute hepatitis and gallbladder disease (dyskinesia), is suggested in some patients.

(*h*) *Sella turcica*.—Abnormalities of this area have been suggested but the evidence is not convincing.

The majority of cases begin in young adults, but Sinclair refers to a case in a child of two years. Many circumstances bring on the attack: a powerful emotion, mental or bodily fatigue, digestive disturbances, or the eating of some particular food. The subjects often suffer from train- or seasickness. The paroxysmal character may be a striking feature of the attacks which may occur on the same day every week or every month. Headaches of the migraine type may occur for years with chronic nephritis and with tumors and other lesions of the base of the brain.

Symptoms.—Premonitory signs are present in many cases, and the patient can tell when an attack is coming on. There may be a sense of well-being or depression; some have marked hunger. Remarkable prodromata have been described, particularly in connection with vision. Apparitions may appear —visions of animals, such as mice, dogs, etc. Transient hemianopia or scotoma may be present. In other instances there is spasmodic action of the pupil on the affected side, which dilates and contracts alternately, the condition known as *hippus.* Frequently the disturbance of vision is only a blurring or there are balls of light, or zigzag lines, or the so-called fortification spectra (teichopsia), which may be illuminated with gorgeous colors. Disturbances of the other senses are rare. Numbness of the tongue and face and occasionally of the hand may occur with tingling. More rarely there are cramps or spasms in the muscles of the affected side. The blood sugar may be low at the onset. Transient *aphasia* may occur and be intermittent. The *paralysis* may be (1) of cerebral origin—hemiplegia or aphasia, or (2) due to lesions of cranial nerves—optic nerve and ophthalmoplegias, the oculomotor most often, abducens rarely, trochlearis very rarely. The supposed involvement of the facial in migraine is relapsing facial palsy (Ramsay Hunt). Some patients show marked *psychical* disturbance, either excitement or, more commonly, mental confusion or great depression. Dizziness occurs in some cases. The *headache* follows a short time after the prodromal symptoms or may be the feature of onset, especially on waking in the morning. It is cumulative and expansile in character, beginning as a localized small spot, which is generally constant on the temple, forehead or in the eyeball. It is usually described as of a penetrating, sharp, boring character. The pain gradually spreads and involves the entire side of the head, sometimes the neck, and may pass into the arm. In some cases both sides are affected. *Nausea* and *vomiting* are common and, if the attack comes on when the stomach is full, vomiting may give relief. *Vasomotor* symptoms may be present. The face may be pale, and there may be a marked difference between the two sides. Subsequently the face and ear on the affected side may become a burning red from vasodilator influences. The pulse may be slow. The temporal artery on the affected side may be firm and hard, and arteriosclerotic—confirmed anatomically by Thoma. Few affections are more prostrating and during the paroxysm the patient may scarcely be able to raise the head from the pillow. The slightest noise or light aggravates the condition.

The *duration* of the attack is variable. The severer forms usually incapacitate the patient for two or three days. In other instances the entire attack is over in a day. The disease recurs for years, and in patients with a marked hereditary tendency may persist throughout life. In women the attacks often cease after the menopause, and in men after the age of fifty.

Diagnosis.—In well-marked cases there is little difficulty, especially with a clear history, but nephritis and intracranial tumor should be considered in cases originating in later life. There are abortive attacks, with a variety of symptoms, not easily recognized until a typical attack appears.

Treatment.—The patient is usually aware of the causes which precipitate an attack. Avoidance of excitement, regularity in meals, and moderation in diet are important rules. Some patients suffer from too much protein and others from too much carbohydrate. It is well to try a low carbohydrate diet and if no benefit results cut out animal protein for a time. Some patients are helped by exclusion of eggs from the diet, others by a strict vegetarian diet. The intravenous injection of peptone has helped some patients. Treatment should be directed toward the removal of the conditions upon which the attacks depend. Much may be done by watchfulness and care in regulating the bowels and watching the diet. Errors of refraction should be adjusted. On no account should children with migraine be allowed to compete in school for prizes. A prolonged course of bromides sometimes proves successful. If anemia is present, iron and arsenic should be given. When the arterial tension is increased a course of nitroglycerin may be tried. Not too much, however, should be expected from preventive treatment as in a large proportion of cases the headaches recur in spite of all we (including the refractionists) can do. Lavage of the stomach with water at 105°, a brisk saline cathartic and irrigation of the colon with hot saline solution are sometimes of value at the onset. Alkaline water should be taken freely by mouth. During the paroxysm the patient should be kept in bed and absolutely quiet. If the patient feels faint and nauseated strong coffee may give relief. A prolonged course of cannabis indica may be tried. Antipyrine and phenacetine have been much used and given at the very outset are sometimes effective. Small, repeated doses are more satisfactory. Lauder Brunton advised sodium salicylate (gr. 15, 1 gm.) and potassium bromide (gr. 30, 2 gm.) at the onset. Combinations of acetylsalicylic acid, caffeine and phenacetine may be used. Phenobarbital (gr. ½ to 1½, 0.03 to 0.1 gm.) given daily for a considerable period is sometimes useful. Calcium lactate (gr. 30, 2 gm.) at the onset may avert an attack. Epinephrine hypodermically (10 minims, 0.6 cc., of a 1-1000 solution) may be useful if given at the onset (not if there is hypertension). Ergotamine tartrate has been used in doses of 0.25 mg. subcutaneously, and increased to 0.5 mg. sometimes every 2 or 3 hours. It should be given at the onset. Some give it both intravenously and subcutaneously at the same time. Caution should be used if there is vascular disease as it usually increases the systolic pressure. Pregnancy is a contra-indication. The drug stimulates the contraction of smooth muscle and depresses the activity of the sympathetic system. Intravenous injection of sodium thiosulphate (0.5-1 gram) twice a week for 12 doses has been of benefit. Right subtemporal decompression has given relief in severe cases. In women with menstrual attacks, theelin injections may be given for a week preceding menstruation or emmenin (ʒ ss-i, 2-4 cc.) twice a day.

Ophthalmoplegic Migraine.—This term was applied by Charcot to a special form in which there is weakness or paralysis of one or more eye muscles, with or after a migraine attack. The oculomotor nerve is usually involved. Ptosis, loss of certain movements, and double vision are the common features, which may persist for some days. Local causes, especially syphilis, should be excluded before the diagnosis is established.

NEURALGIA

Definition.—A painful affection of the nerves, due to functional disturbance of their central or peripheral extremities or to neuritis in their course.

Etiology.—Members of neuropathic families are most subject to the disease. It affects women more than men. Children are rarely attacked. The various forms of anemia are frequently associated with neuralgia. Inflammatory processes are often responsible, in the nerve roots, in a plexus or in the course of the nerves. In the last case fibrositis may be the cause by exudate or communicated inflammation. Exposure to cold is a cause in susceptible persons. Reflex irritation, particularly from carious teeth, and disease of the antrum and frontal sinuses are common causes of neuralgia of the fifth nerve. The disease occurs sometimes in gout, lead poisoning and diabetes. Persistent neuralgia may be a feature of latent nephritis.

Symptoms.—Before the onset of the pain there may be uneasy sensations, sometimes tingling, in the part to be affected. The pain is localized to a certain group of nerves, usually affecting one side. The pain is not constant, but paroxysmal, and is described as stabbing, burning or darting in character. The skin may be very tender in the affected region, particularly over certain points along the course of the nerve, the so-called tender points. Movements, as a rule, are painful. Trophic and vasomotor changes may accompany the paroxysm; the skin may be cool, and subsequently hot and burning; occasionally local edema or erythema occurs. More remarkable are the changes in the hair, which may become blanched (canities) or fall out. Fortunately, such alterations are rare. Twitchings of the muscles, or even spasms, may occur. After lasting a variable time—from a few minutes to many hours—the attack subsides. Recurrence may be at definite intervals—every day at the same hour, or at intervals of two, three, or even seven days. Occasionally the paroxysms develop only at the catamenia.

Cervico-occipital neuralgia involves the posterior branches of the first four cervical nerves, particularly the inferior occipital, at the emergence of which there is a painful point about half-way between the mastoid process and the first cervical vertebra. It may be caused by cold or be due to cervical caries or spondylitis.

Cervicobrachial neuralgia involves the sensory nerves of the brachial plexus, particularly in the cubital division. When the circumflex nerve is involved the pain is in the deltoid. The pain is most commonly about the shoulder and down the course of the ulnar nerve. There is usually a marked tender point upon this nerve at the elbow. This form frequently results from arthritis of the spine, fibrositis and trauma.

Neuralgia of the phrenic nerve is rare. It is sometimes found in pleurisy and in pericarditis. The pain is chiefly at the lower part of the thorax on a line with the insertion of the diaphragm, and there may be painful points on deep pressure. Full inspiration is painful, and there is great sensitiveness on coughing or any movement by which the diaphragm is suddenly depressed.

Intercostal Neuralgia.—Postzoster neuralgias may occur in this situation. The possibility of spinal disease, tumor, spondylitis, caries or aneurism must be borne in mind. The diagnosis of primary intercostal neuralgia should be made with hesitation. It is often a cover for ignorance and should not be made until other possibilities are excluded.

Lumbar Neuralgia.—The posterior fibres of the lumbar plexus, particularly the ilioscrotal branch, are affected. The pain is in the region of the iliac crest, along the inguinal canal, in the spermatic cord and the scrotum or labium. The affection known as irritable testis, probably a neuralgia of this nerve, may be accompanied by syncopal sensations.

Coccydynia.—This is regarded as a neuralgia of the coccygeal plexus. It is most common in women and aggravated by the sitting posture. It is very intractable, and may necessitate the removal of the coccyx, an operation, however, which is not always successful.

Neuralgias of the Nerves of the Feet.—Many of these cases accompany varying degrees of flatfoot. The condition is brought about by weakness or fatigue of the muscles supporting the arches of the foot, which consequently settle until the strain of the superimposed body-weight falls upon the ligamentous and aponeurotic attachments between the metatarsal and tarsal bones. Rest, massage, exercises and orthopedic measures are indicated.

PAINFUL HEEL.—There may be severe pains about the heel which interfere seriously with walking—the pododynia of S. D. Gross. There may be little or no swelling, no discoloration, and no arthritis. Some cases follow a gonococcus infection and are due to a bony spur.

PLANTAR NEURALGIA.—This is often associated with a definite neuritis, such as follows typhoid fever, and has been seen in caisson disease (Hughes). The pain may be limited to the tips of the toes or to the ball of the great toe. Numbness, tingling and hyperesthesia or sweating may occur.

METATARSALGIA.—Thomas G. Morton's "painful affection of the fourth metatarsophalangeal articulation" is a very trying disorder, most frequent in women, and usually in one foot. Morton regarded it as due to a pinching of the metatarsal nerve. In some cases there is a *metatarsophalangeal osteochondritis.* Trauma and infection are factors. There is pain referred to the head of the metatarsal bone, with swelling, due to exudate, and tenderness. The X-ray study is diagnostic. In treatment, weight should be taken entirely off the foot; operation may be required.

Causalgia (Thermalgia).—A form of neuralgia following gunshot wounds, most frequently of the median and sciatic branches, characteried by burning throbbing pains of the greatest intensity, glossy skin, vasomotor disturbances, and at last a condition of general hyperesthesia and nervousness that makes life unbearable. Nothing has been added to Weir Mitchell's classical description (1864), and later he gave the above name from the Greek words for burning and pain. Stopford suggested the name *thermalgia.* An explanation of causalgia is difficult. The median and posttibial nerves have a large number of vasomotor fibres, interference with which may cause the peculiar character of the pain; indeed, it has been suggested that the pain is caused by irritation of the peri-arterial sympathetic fibres and not by the wound of the nerve itself. Anatomically, partial division with perineural and intra-neural fibrosis is present, but these are found in many cases in which causalgia is not present.

Visceral Neuralgias.—The more important of these occur with cardiac and gastric neuroses. They are most frequent in women often with neurasthenia and hysteria. The referred pains represent a "viscerosensory reflex." With lesions in the viscera there may be alteration of sensation in the related skin areas. The distribution of the sensory nerves and their segmental relations are important in working out the source of the disturbance.

Treatment of Neuralgia.—The cause should be found and treated if possible. Causes of reflex irritation should be remedied and foci of infection removed. The neuralgia, as a rule, recurs unless the general health improves; so that tonic and hygienic measures should be employed. Often a change of air or surroundings relieves a severe neuralgia. A strict vegetable diet will sometimes relieve the neuralgia or headache of a gouty person. Of general remedies, iron is often a specific in cases associated with anemia. Arsenic is beneficial also and should be given in ascending doses. The value of quinine has been much overrated. It probably has no more influence than any other bitter tonic, except in the rare instances in which neuralgia is definitely associated with malaria. Strychnine, cod-liver oil and phosphorus are advantageous. Of remedies for the pain, phenacetine and acetylsalicylic acid are generally useful, and small doses of codeine may be added if necessary. Morphia should not be given. Gelsemium is highly recommended.

Of local applications, the cautery is invaluable, particularly in chronic forms. Acupuncture may be used. Counterirritation and the use of heat and various forms of light therapy are helpful. Chloroform liniment, camphor and chloral, and menthol, may be tried. Freezing over the tender point with ether spray is sometimes successful. The continuous current may be used. The sponges should be warm, and the positive pole placed near the seat of the pain. The current should cause a slight tingling or burning.

PROFESSIONAL SPASMS; OCCUPATION NEUROSES

The continuous and excessive use of the muscles in performing a certain movement may be followed by an irregular, involuntary spasm or cramp, which may completely check the performance of the action. The condition is found frequently in writers, hence the term writer's cramp or scrivener's palsy, and also occurs in typists, needle-workers, piano and violin players, telegraph operators, milkmaids, weavers, and cigar and cigarette rollers.

The most common form is *writer's cramp,* which is much more frequent in men than in women. Persons of a nervous temperament are more liable to the disease. Occasionally it follows slight injury. In a majority a faulty method of writing has been employed, using either the little finger or the wrist as the fixed point. Persons who write with the middle of the forearm or the elbow as the fixed point are rarely affected.

No anatomical changes have been found. A psychoneurosis is present in many patients, with anxiety states, obsessions or hysteria. It is "a combination of psychoneurotic symptoms and weak muscular coordination." There may be a deranged action of the centres presiding over the movements involved in the act of writing.

(*a*) Cramp or Spasm.—This is often an early symptom and most commonly affects the forefinger and thumb; or there may be a combined movement of flexion and adduction of the thumb, so that the pen may be twisted from the grasp and thrown to some distance. Weir Mitchell described a lock-spasm, in which the fingers become so firmly contracted upon the pen that it can not be removed.

(*b*) Paresis and Paralysis.—This may occur with the spasm or alone. The patient feels a sense of weakness and debility in the muscles of the hand and arm and holds the pen feebly. Yet the grasp of the hand may be strong and there may be no paralysis for ordinary acts.

(*c*) Tremor.—This is most commonly seen in the forefinger and may be a premonitory symptom of atrophy. It is not an important symptom and is rarely sufficient to produce disability.

(*d*) Pain.—Abnormal sensations, particularly a tired feeling in the muscles, are very constantly present. Actual pain is rare, but there may be irregular shooting pains in the arm. Numbness or soreness may exist. If, as sometimes happens, a subacute neuritis develops, there may be pain over the nerves and numbness or tingling in the fingers.

(*e*) Vasomotor Disturbances.—These may occur in severe cases. There may be hyperesthesia. Occasionally the skin becomes glossy, or there is a condition of local asphyxia resembling chilblains. In attempting to write, the hand and arm may become flushed and the veins increased in size. Early the electrical reactions are normal, but in advanced cases there may be diminution of faradic and sometimes increase in the galvanic irritability.

Diagnosis.—A well-marked case of writer's cramp or palsy could scarcely be mistaken. Care must be taken to exclude the existence of any cerebrospinal disease, such as progressive muscular atrophy or hemiplegia, or local affection, such as cervical rib. The physician is sometimes consulted by nervous persons who fancy they are becoming subject to the disease and complain of stiffness or weakness without displaying any characteristic features.

Prognosis.—The course is usually chronic. If taken in time and if the hand is allowed perfect rest, the condition may improve rapidly, but too often there is a strong tendency to recurrence. The patient may learn to write with the left hand, but this also may after a time be attacked.

Treatment.—Various prophylactic measures have been advised. It is important that a proper method of writing be adopted. Gowers suggested that if all persons wrote from the shoulder writer's cramp would practically not occur. Various devices have been invented for relieving the fatigue, but none of them are very satisfactory. The use of the typewriter has diminished the frequency of scrivener's palsy. Rest is essential and no measures are of value without it. Massage and manipulation, combined with systematic gymnastics, give the best results. The patient should systematically practise the opposite movements to those concerned in the cramp. This muscle training often gives good results. The psychical state should be carefully studied and an effort made to remedy any psychoneurotic condition. In very obstinate cases the condition remains incurable.

HYSTERIA

Definition.—A disorder of personality manifested by a heightened and perverted suggestibility, a change in character, together with certain mental and bodily states induced by suggestion—auto or hetero—and cured by persuasion. It is "an irrational answer to a conflict."

Etiology.—Persons with mobile emotional dispositions, especially women, are the chief subjects. In periods of great stress it becomes a widespread disorder. A community disease, often spreading widely in institutions, such as schools and convents, it may behave like an epidemic, as in the dancing mania. The essential element under the above definition is the first—*heightened suggestibility*. (*a*) With the chameleon we take the color of our surroundings. The company, physical conditions, weather, etc., send our spirits up and down like the mercury in a barometer. Suggestion, deliberate by speech, unconscious through imitation, is the most important part of education, and to free the mind as far as possible from the mastery of these external influences has been the goal from the days of the Greeks. Love, hate and fear, the three powerful emotions, control us individually or sway us in herds as the cattle on the plains. The dominant influence of *suggestion* is everywhere in the story of human progress; just as it is in the black chapters of superstition, folly and crime. Unconscious imitation, or an imitation against which the individual is powerless to fight, has been the important factor in outbreaks of hysteria as the dancing mania, epidemic chorea, and such tragedies as led to the persecutions for witchcraft.

(*b*) Right judgments are indispensable conditions to right action in mind or muscle and it is in this Stoic doctrine of the control of the will—the will to do and the will to avoid—that we find the key to many of the problems of hysteria. It may be a knee "locked" for months. An injury or pain induces the fixed belief that the joint can not be moved, loss of muscle judgment—there were many such war cases—but ten minutes at Seale-Hayne or a trip to Lourdes and the joint is flexible. After the shock of an explosion a man is blind (without a lesion), the condition persists—the judgment has been lost—to be restored months afterwards at a temple of Æsculapius or by some modern Galen. An emotional girl takes an aversion to her mistress. The moral judgment is lost and she plays pranks, sometimes harmless, but often serious as entailing great inconvenience and loss, as in the Norfolk case in which the walls of a house were so covered with paraffin, sandal oil and water that it had to be abandoned. Or craving sympathy, she will inflict injuries, even wound herself to such an extent as to necessitate amputation of a limb. Loss of right judgment in muscle action, sense action and conduct are essential factors. As the impulse—suggestion—is spontaneous we speak of it as autosuggestion—and in direct proportion to the feebleness of control by the will is the readiness with which muscles, sense and mind yield to impulses not prompted by right judgment.

Charcot and his followers regarded hysteria as a psychosis, in which morbid states are induced by ideas. The capability of responding to suggestion is the test of its existence. It is a disturbance in the sphere of personality, in which the emotions have an exaggerated influence on the sensory, motor and secretory functions. Babinski held that hysteria is a mental condition with certain primary phenomena and certain secondary accidental symptoms. The essence of the primary features is that they may be produced by suggestion, and may be made to disappear by persuasion (pithiatism). The primary symptoms include hemianesthesia, paralysis, contractures, etc.; secondary features, as muscular atrophy, are directly dependent upon the primary and can not themselves be induced by suggestion.

In the Breuer-Freud theory we return to the days of Aretæus, who originated (?) the views of sexual hysteria and believed the womb, "like an animal within an animal" and altogether erratic, caused all sorts of trouble in its wanderings. Freud's view is thus analyzed by Jelliffe in his article in our *System of Medicine*. "There develop usually on a constitutional basis, in the period before puberty, definite sexual activities which are mostly of a perverse nature. These activities do not, as a rule, lead to a definite neurosis up to the time of puberty, which in the psychic sphere appears much earlier than in the body, but sexual phantasy maintains a perverse constellated direction by reason of the infantile sexual activities. On constitutional (affect) grounds the increased fantasy of the hysteric leads to the formation of complexes which are not taken up by the personality and by reason of shame or disgust remain buried. There, therefore, results a conflict between the characteristic normal libido and the sexual repressions of these buried infantile perversions. These conflicts give rise to the hysterical symptoms. It is in his contributions to the sexual theory that Freud develops his later thoughts of the sexual origin of the hysterical reaction. By sexual it is important to remember that Freud is not speaking of sensual.

"Sexual experiences differ, however, from ordinary experiences—the latter have a tendency to fade out, while the idea of the former grows with increasing sexual maturity. There results a disproportionate capacity for increased reaction which takes place in the subconscious. This is the cause of the mischief.

"There must be, however, a connecting link between the infantile sexual traumata and the later manifestations. This connection Freud finds in the so-called 'hysterical fancies.' These are the day-dreams of erotic coloring, wish-gratifications, originating in privation and longing. These fancies hark back to the original traumatic moment, and, either originating in the subconscious or shortly becoming conscious, are transformed into hysterical symptoms. They constitute a defence of the ego against the revival, as reminiscences, of the repressed traumatic experiences of childhood" (White).

The affection is most common in females, and usually appears first about the time of puberty, but the manifestations may continue until the menopause, or even until old age. Men are by no means exempt, and hysteria in the male is not rare. It occurs in all races, but is much more prevalent, particularly in its severer forms, in members of the Latin race. In England and the United States the milder grades are common, but the graver forms are rare in comparison with the frequency with which they are seen in France.

Children under twelve years of age are not very often affected, but the disease may be well marked as early as the fifth or sixth year. One of the saddest chapters in the history of human deception, that of the Salem witches, might he headed *hysteria in children,* since the tragedy resulted directly from the hysterical pranks of girls under twelve years of age.

Of predisposing causes, two are important—*heredity* and *education.* The former acts by endowing the child with a mobile, abnormally sensitive nervous organization. We see cases most frequently in families with marked neuropathic tendencies, the members of which have suffered from neuroses of various sorts. Education at home too often fails to inculcate habits of self-control. A child grows to girlhood with an entirely erroneous idea of her relations to others, and accustomed to have every whim gratified and abundant sympathy lavished on every woe, however trifling; she reaches womanhood with a moral organization unfitted to withstand the cares and worries of everyday life. At school, between the ages of twelve and fifteen, when the vital energies are absorbed in the rapid development of the body, she is often cooped in close school rooms for six or eight hours daily. The result too frequently is an active, bright mind in an enfeebled body, ill adapted to subserve the functions for which it was framed, easily disordered, and prone to react abnormally to the ordinary stimuli of life. Among the more direct influences are emotions of various kinds, fright occasionally, more frequently love affairs, grief and domestic worries. Physical causes less often bring on hysterical outbreaks, but they may follow an injury or develop during the convalescence from an acute illness or be associated with disease of the generative organs.

"Chorea major": "Pandemic Chorea."—The common name, St. Vitus's dance, applied to chorea has come to us from the Middle Ages, when under the influence of religious fervor there were epidemics characterized by great excitement, gesticulations and dancing. For the relief of these symptoms, when excessive, pilgrimages were made, and, in the Rhenish provinces, particularly to the Chapel of St. Vitus in Zebern. Epidemics of this sort occurred also during the nineteenth century, and descriptions of them among the early settlers in Kentucky have been given by Robertson and Yandell. It was unfortunate that Sydenham applied the term chorea to an affection in children totally distinct from this chorea major, which is in reality a hysterical manifestation under the influence of religious excitement.

Symptoms.—A useful division is into convulsive and nonconvulsive forms.

Convulsive Hysteria.—(*a*) *Minor Forms.*—The attack, commonly following emotional disturbance, sets in suddenly or may be preceded by symptoms, called by the laity "hysterical," such as laughing and crying alternately, or a sensation of constriction in the neck, or of a ball rising in the throat—the *globus hystericus.* Sometimes, preceding the convulsive movements, there may be painful sensations arising from the pelvic, abdominal or thoracic regions. From the description these sensations resemble aurae. They become more intense with the rising sensation of choking in the neck and difficulty in getting breath, and the patient falls into a more or less violent convulsion. The fall is not sudden, as in epilepsy, but the subject goes down, as a rule, easily, often picking a soft spot, like a sofa or a chair, and in the movements apparently exercises care to do herself no injury. Yet at the same time she appears to be unconscious. The movements are clonic and disorderly, with the head and arms thrown about in an irregular manner. The paroxysm after a few minutes slowly subsides, then the patient becomes emotional, and gradually regains consciousness. When questioned the patient may confess to having some knowledge of the events which have taken place, but, as a rule, has no accurate recollection. During the attack the abdomen may be much distended with flatus, and subsequently a large amount of clear urine may be passed. These attacks vary greatly; there may be scarcely any movements of the limbs, but after a nerve storm the patient sinks into a torpid, semi-unconscious condition, from which she is roused with difficulty. In some cases the patient passes from this state into a condition of catalepsy.

(*b*) *Major Forms; Hystero-epilepsy.*—Typical instances are very rare in the United States and in England. The attack is initiated by certain prodromata, chiefly minor hysterical manifestations, either foolish or unseemly behavior, excitement, sometimes dyspeptic symptoms with tympanites, or frequent micturition. Areas of hyperesthesia may be marked, the so-called hysterogenic spots described by Richet. These are usually symmetrical and situated over the upper dorsal vertebra, and in front in a series of symmetrically placed areas on the chest and abdomen. Painful sensations or a feeling of oppression and a *globus* rising in the throat may be complained of prior to the onset of the convulsion, which, according to French writers, has four distinct stages: (1) Epileptoid condition, which closely simulates a true epileptic attack with tonic spasm (often leading to opisthotonos), grinding of the teeth, congestion of the face, followed by clonic convulsions, gradual relaxation, and coma. (2) Succeeding this is the period which Charcot has termed *clownism,* in which there is an emotional display and a remarkable series of contortions or of cataleptic poses. (3) Then in typical cases there is a stage in which the patient assumes certain attitudes expressive of ecstasy, fear, beatitude, or erotism. (4) Finally consciousness returns and the patient enters upon a stage in which she may display very varied symptoms, chiefly manifestations of a delirium with extraordinary hallucinations. Visions are seen, voices heard, and conversations held with imaginary persons. In this stage patients will relate imaginary events, and make extraordinary and serious charges against individuals. This sometimes gives a grave aspect to these seizures, for not only does the patient make and believe the statements, but when recovery is complete the hallucination sometimes persists. After an attack a patient may remain for days in a state of lethargy or trance.

NONCONVULSIVE FORMS.—So complex and varied is the picture that the manifestations are best considered according to the systems involved.

(*a*) *Disorders of Motion.*—(1) *Paralysis.*—These may be hemiplegic, paraplegic or monoplegic. Hysterical diplegia is extremely rare. The paralysis sets in abruptly or gradually, and may take weeks to attain its full development. *There is no type or form of organic paralysis which may not be simulated in hysteria.* Sensation is lessened or lost on the affected side. The hysterical paraplegia is more common than hemiplegia. The loss of power is not absolute; the legs can usually be moved, but do not support the patient. The reflexes may be increased, though the knee jerk is often normal. A spurious ankle clonus may be present. The feet are usually extended and turned inward in the equinovarus position. The muscles do not waste and the electrical reactions are normal. Other manifestations, as paralysis of the bladder or aphonia, are usually associated. Hysterical monoplegias may be facial, crural or brachial. A condition of ataxia sometimes occurs with paresis. Incoordination may be marked and there are usually sensory manifestations.

The following points are important in deciding between functional and organic hemiplegia. The absence of epigastric and cremasteric reflexes with Babinski's sign suggests organic disease. If the patient lies on a table, with the arms folded on the chest and the legs apart, and is asked to sit up without using the arms, in doing this the organically paralyzed leg is flexed at the hip and the heel raised from the table. The heel of the nonparalyzed leg is pressed against the table. In hysterical paralysis both heels remain pressed against the table. Another test is made with the patient lying on the back. When asked to raise the unaffected leg, the opposite leg, paralyzed for voluntary effort, is strongly pressed down (Hoover).

(2) *Contractures and Spasms.*—The hysterical contractures may attack almost any group of voluntary muscles and be of the hemiplegic, paraplegic or monoplegic type. They may come on suddenly or slowly, persist for months or years, and disappear rapidly. The contracture is most common in the arm, which is flexed at the elbow and wrist, while the fingers tightly grasp the thumb in the palm of the hand; more rarely the terminal phalanges are hyperextended. It may occur in one or in both legs, more commonly in one. Ankle clonus is present; the foot is inverted and the toes are strongly flexed. These cases may be mistaken for lateral sclerosis and the difficulty in diagnosis may be great. The spastic gait is typical, and with the exaggerated knee jerk and ankle clonus the picture may be characteristic. Other forms of contracture may be in the muscles of the hip, shoulder or neck; more rarely in those of the jaws—hysterical trismus—or in the tongue. There are remarkable local contractures in the diaphragm and abdominal muscles, producing a *phantom tumor,* in which just below and in the neighborhood of the umbilicus is a firm, apparently solid growth. According to Gowers, this is produced by relaxation of the recti and a spasmodic contraction of the diaphragm, together with inflation of the intestines with gas and an arching forward of the vertebral column. They are apt to occur in middle-aged women about the menopause, and are frequently associated with spurious pregnancy—*pseudocyesis.* The resemblance to a tumor may be striking. The only safeguard is in complete anesthesia, when the tumor disappears.

Rhythmic Hysterical Spasm.—The movements may be of the arm, either flexion and extension, or, more rarely, pronation and supination. Clonic contractions of the sternocleidomastoid or of the muscles of the jaws or of the rotatory muscles of the head may produce rhythmic movements of these parts. The spasm may be in one or both psoas muscles, lifting the leg in a rhythmic manner eight or ten times in a minute. In other instances the muscles of the trunk are affected, and every few moments there is a bowing movement—salaam convulsions—or the muscles of the back may contract, causing strong arching of the vertebral column and retraction of the head.

Tremor may be a purely hysterical manifestation, occurring either alone or with paralysis and contracture. It most commonly involves the hands and arms; more rarely the head and legs. The movements are small and quick. In the type described by Rendu the tremor may or may not persist during repose, but it is increased or provoked by volitional movements. Volitional or intention tremor may exist, simulating closely that of multiple sclerosis. Many instances of this disease are mistaken for hysteria.

(*b*) *Disorders of Sensation.*—Anesthesia is most common, and usually confined to one half of the body. It may not be noticed by the patient. Usually it is accurately limited by the middle line and involves the mucous surfaces and deeper parts. The conjunctiva, however, is often spared. There may be hemianopsia. This symptom may come on slowly or follow a convulsive attack. Sometimes the various sensations are dissociated and the anesthesia may be only to pain and to touch. The skin of the affected side is usually pale and cool, and a pin prick may not be followed by blood. With the loss of feeling there may be a loss of muscular power. Curious trophic changes may be present, such as unilateral swelling of the hemiplegic side.

By the application of certain metals, the anesthesia or analgesia can be transferred to the other side of the body. This may be caused by the electromagnet and by wood and other agents, and is an effect of suggestion.

Hyperesthesia.—Increased sensitiveness and pains occur in various parts. One of the most frequent complaints is of pain in the head, usually over the sagittal suture, less frequently in the occiput. This is described as agonizing, and is compared to the driving of a nail into the part; hence the name *clavus hystericus*. Neuralgias are common. Hyperesthetic areas exist on the thorax and abdomen, pressure upon which may cause minor manifestations or even a convulsive attack. Increased sensitiveness in the ovarian region is not peculiar to hysteria. Pain in the back is an almost constant complaint with sensitiveness limited to certain spinous processes or diffuse. In hysterical women the pains in the abdomen may simulate those of gastric ulcer, or the condition may be almost identical with that of peritonitis; more rarely the abdominal pains resemble those of appendix disease.

Special Senses.—Disturbances of taste and smell are not uncommon and may cause much distress. Of ocular symptoms, retinal hyperesthesia is common, and the patients prefer to be in a darkened room. Retraction of the field of vision is common and usually follows a convulsive seizure. It may persist for years. The color perception may be normal even with complete anesthesia. Hysterical deafness may be complete and alternate or come on with hysterical blindness. Hysterical amaurosis may occur in children. One must distinguish between functional loss of power and simulation.

(*c*) *Visceral Manifestations.*—*Respiratory Apparatus.*—Of disturbances in the respiratory rhythm, the most frequent, perhaps, is an exaggeration of the deeper breath, which is taken normally every fifth or sixth inspiration, or there may be a "catching" breathing, such as is seen when cold water is poured over a person. In hysterical *dyspnea* there is no special distress and the pulse is normal. In the syndrome of Briquet there are shortness of breath, suppression of the voice, and paralysis of the diaphragm. The anhelation is extreme. In rare instances there is bradypnea. *Aphonia* is frequent and may persist for months or years without other special symptoms. Spasm of the muscles may occur with violent inspiratory efforts and great distress, and lead to cyanosis. Hiccough, or sounds like it, may be present for weeks. Among the respiratory manifestations are the hysterical cries. These may mimic the sounds produced by animals, and epidemics of them have been observed. Attacks of gaping, yawning and sneezing may occur.

The hysterical *cough* is frequent, particularly in young girls. It may occur in paroxysms, but is often a dry, persistent, croaking cough, extremely monotonous and unpleasant. Sir Andrew Clark called attention to a loud, barking cough occurring about the time of puberty, chiefly in boys belonging to neurotic families. The attacks, which last about a minute, recur frequently. A form of hysterical *hemoptysis* may lead to a diagnosis of pulmonary disorder. The sputum is a pale-red fluid, not so bright in color as in ordinary hemoptysis, and probably comes from the mouth or pharynx.

Digestive System.—Disturbed or depraved appetite, dyspepsia and gastric pains are common. The patient may have difficulty in swallowing, apparently from spasm of the gullet. There are instances in which the food seems to be expelled before it reaches the stomach. In other cases there is incessant gagging. The *globus hystericus* is probably due to spasm of the esophagus. In the hysterical vomiting the food is regurgitated without much effort and without nausea. This may persist for years without great disturbance of nutrition. The most striking and remarkable digestive disturbance is the *anorexia nervosa* described by Sir William Gull. "To call it loss of appetite—anorexia—but feebly characterizes the symptom. It is rather an annihilation of appetite, so complete that it seems in some cases impossible ever to eat again. Out of it grows an antagonism to food which results at last and in its worst forms in spasm on the approach of food, and this in turn gives rise to some of those remarkable cases of survival for long periods without food" (Mitchell). There are three special features in anorexia nervosa: *First,* and most important, a psychical state, usually depressant, occasionally excited and restless. It is not always hysterical. *Secondly,* loss of appetite, regurgitation, vomiting, and the whole series of phenomena associated with nervous dyspepsia. *Thirdly,* emaciation, which reaches a grade seen only in cancer and dysentery. The patient finally takes to bed, and in extreme cases lies upon one side with the thighs and legs flexed, and contractures may occur. Food is either not taken at all or only upon urgent compulsion. The skin becomes wasted, dry, and covered with branlike scales. No food may be taken for several weeks, and attempts to feed may be followed by severe spasms. Although the condition looks so alarming, these patients, when removed from their home surroundings and treated by isolation, sometimes recover in a remarkable way. It may be months before improvement is noted. Death, however, may follow with extreme emaciation. In one fatal case the girl weighed only 49 pounds. No lesions were found postmortem.

Hysterical *tympanites* is common and may be associated with peristaltic unrest. Frequent movements may be due to disturbance in the small or large bowel. An obstinate diarrhea occurs in some hysterical patients, which proves very intractable and is associated especially with the taking of food. It seems an aggravated form of the looseness of bowels to which many nervous people are subject on emotion or of the tendency which some have to diarrhea immediately after eating. A different form is that produced by what Mitchell called the irritable rectum, in which scybala are passed frequently, sometimes with great force. Constipation is more frequent and may be due to lack of attention to the need for defecation or to spasm. In extreme cases the bowels may not move for two or three weeks. Other disturbances are anospasm or intense pain in the rectum apart from any fissure. Hysterical ileus and fecal vomiting are among the most remarkable hysterical phenomena. Following a shock there are constipation, tympanites, vomiting, sometimes hematemesis. The constipation grows worse, everything taken by mouth is rejected, the vomitus becomes fecal, even scybala are brought up, and suppositories and enemata are vomited. The symptoms may continue for weeks and then gradually subside. Laparotomy—even thrice in one patient—has shown a perfectly normal condition of the bowels (Parkes Weber).

Cardiovascular.—Rapid action of the heart on slight emotion, with or without the subjective sensation of palpitation, is often a source of great distress. A slow pulse is less frequent. Pains about the heart may simulate angina. Flushes in various parts are common. Sweating may occur, or the *seborrhoea nigricans,* causing a darkening of the skin of the eyelids.

Among the more remarkable vasomotor phenomena are the so-called *stigmata* or hemorrhages in the skin, such as were present in the celebrated case of Louise Lateau. In many cases these are undoubtedly fraudulent, but if, as appears credible, such bleeding may occur in the hypnotic trance, there seems no reason to doubt its possibility in the trance of religious ecstasy.

(*d*) *Joint Affections.*—To Sir Benjamin Brodie and Sir James Paget we owe the recognition of these extraordinary manifestations. Perhaps no single affection has brought more discredit upon the profession, for the cases are very refractory, and often fall into the hands of a charlatan or faith-healer, under whose touch the disease may disappear at once. Usually it affects the knee or the hip, and may follow a trifling injury. The joint is usually fixed, sensitive and swollen. The surface may be cool, but sometimes the local temperature is increased. To the touch it is very sensitive and movement causes great pain. In protracted cases the muscles are somewhat wasted, and in consequence the joint looks larger. The pains are often nocturnal, at which time the local temperature may be increased. While, as a rule, neuromimetic joints yield to proper management, there are instances in which organic change followed the functional disturbance. Intermittent hydrarthrosis may be a manifestation of hysteria, sometimes with transient paresis.

(*e*) *Mental Symptoms.*—Mental perversions of all kinds are common in hysterical patients and not much dependence can be placed on statements either about themselves or about others. A morbid craving for sympathy may lead to the commission of all sorts of bizarre and foolish acts.

Hallucinations and delirium may alternate with emotional outbursts of an aggravated character. There is a condition which may be spoken of as the *status hystericus.* For weeks or months they may be confined to bed, entirely oblivious to their surroundings, with a delirium sometimes associated with unpleasant objects. The nutrition may be maintained, but there is a heavy, foul breath. With care recovery usually takes place within a few months.

Of hysterical manifestations in the higher centres that of *trance* is the most remarkable. This may develop spontaneously without any convulsive seizure, but more frequently it follows hysteroid attacks. Catalepsy may be present, a condition in which the limbs are plastic and remain in any position in which they are placed.

(*f*) *Manifestations.*—(1) *Edema.* Puffiness of the face, even unilateral, and swelling of the hands are not uncommon and the features of Raynaud's disease may be met with. A white and a blue type of edema is recognized, and either may be associated with paralyses, motor and sensory. (2) *Stigmata.* Local bleedings have been described, sometimes, as in the so-called marks of the cross, on forehead, hands, feet and side, as in the famous case of Louise Lateau. Organic lesions of the skin (blisters) are claimed to have been produced by hypnotic suggestion (Hadfield) and the stigmata are probably produced by autosuggestion in the trance state. (3) *Pathomimia,* the self-inflicted injuries, usually of the skin, by caustics, etc. In a case seen at the Hôtel Dieu with Dieulafoy, the patient, supposed to be the subject of severe trophic disorders, submitted to amputation of the arm before a confession was obtained that the lesions were self-inflicted.

(*g*) *Hysterical Fever.*—In hysteria the temperature, as a rule, is normal. The cases with fever may be grouped as follows: (1) Instances in which the fever is the sole manifestation. These are rare, but there are cases in which the chronic course, the retention of nutrition, and the entirely negative condition of the organs leaves no other diagnosis possible. In one case the patient had for four or five years an afternoon rise of temperature, usually to 102° or 103°. She was well nourished and had no pronounced hysterical symptoms, beyond the interrupted sighing respiration so often seen.

(2) Cases of fever with spurious local manifestations. These are very troublesome and deceptive cases. The patient may be suddenly taken ill with pain in various regions and elevation of temperature. The case may simulate meningitis. There may be pain in the head, vomiting, contracted pupils, and retraction of the neck—which may persist for weeks—and some anomalous manifestation during convalescence may alone indicate to the physician that he has had to deal with hysteria, and has not, as he perhaps flattered himself, cured a case of meningitis. There is hysterical pseudophthisis with pain in the chest, slight fever, and the expectoration of blood-stained mucus. The cases of hysterical peritonitis may show fever.

(3) *Hyperpyrexia.*—It is a suggestive fact that the cases of paradoxical temperatures in which the thermometer has registered 112° to 120° have been in women. Fraud has been practised in nearly all these cases.

Astasia; Abasia.—These terms, indicating respectively inability to stand and to walk, were applied by Charcot and Blocq to conditions characterized by loss of the power of standing or of walking, with retention of muscular power, coordination and sensation. Blocq's definition is as follows: "A morbid state in which the impossibility of standing erect and walking normally is in contrast with the integrity of sensation, of muscular strength, and of the coordination of the other movements of the lower extremities." The condition forms a symptom group and is a functional neurosis. Knapp analyzed 50 cases; in 21, hysteria was present; in 3, chorea; in 2, epilepsy; and in 4, psychoses. As a rule, the patients, though able to move the feet and legs perfectly when in bed, are either unable to walk properly or can not stand at all. The disturbances are very varied and different forms have been recognized. The commonest, according to Knapp's analysis, is the paralytic, in which the legs give out as the patient attempts to walk and "bend under him as if made of cotton. There is no rigidity, no spasm, no incoordination. In bed, sitting, or even while suspended, the muscular strength is found to be good." Other cases are associated with spasm or ataxia; there may be movements which stiffen the legs and give to the gait a somewhat spastic character. In others there are sudden flexions of the legs, or of the arms, or a saltatory, spring-like spasm. The condition is a manifestation of hysteria.

Diagnosis.—Inquiry into the occurrence of previous manifestations and the mental conditions may give important information. These questions, as a rule, should not be asked the mother, who is least likely to give satisfactory information. The occurrence of the globus hystericus, of emotional attacks, of weeping and crying is always suggestive. The diagnosis between the convulsive attacks and true epilepsy may give difficulty at first. The hysterical paralyses are very variable and apt to be associated with anesthesia. The contractures may be deceptive, but areas of anesthesia, retraction of the visual field, and the development of minor hysterical manifestations give valuable indications. The contractures disappear under full anesthesia. A most careful study should be made to exclude the existence of organic disease; the presence of hysteria does not exclude this. Special care must be taken not to confound the spastic paraplegia of hysteria with lateral sclerosis.

The visceral manifestations are usually recognized without much difficulty.

The practitioner has constantly to bear in mind the strong tendency in hysterical patients to practise deception. The very elect have been fooled by these patients; their abilities in this regard are to be respected.

Treatment.—The prophylaxis may be gathered from the remarks on the relation of education to the disease. The successful treatment of hysteria demands qualities possessed by few physicians. The first element is a due appreciation of the nature of the disease on the part of the physician and friends. It is pitiable to think of the misery which has been inflicted on these unhappy victims by the harsh and unjust treatment which has resulted from false views of the nature of the trouble; on the other hand, worry and ill health, often the wrecking of mind, body, and estate, are entailed upon the near relatives in the nursing of a protracted case. The minor manifestations, attacks of the vapors, the crying and weeping spells, are not of much moment and rarely require treatment. The physical condition should be carefully looked into and the mode of life regulated so as to insure system and order in everything. A congenial occupation offers the best remedy for many of the manifestations. Any functional disturbance should be attended to and tonics prescribed. Special attention should be paid to the bowels.

PSYCHOTHERAPY, in which the important features are hypnosis, analysis, suggestion, and reeducation.

Hypnosis.—The majority of hysterical patients can be hypnotized, but the general opinion of those who know most on the subject is that by hypnosis alone hysteria is rarely cured. Sometimes a brilliant miracle is wrought but as a routine treatment it has fallen into disfavor even in France.

Suggestion.—Babinski defines suggestion as "the action by which one endeavors to make another accept or realize an idea which is manifestly unreasonable." On the other hand, persuasion is applied when the ideas are reasonable, or at least are not in opposition to good sense. Most writers, however, use the word "suggestion" as meaning the introduction of mental associations and modifications of the patient's mental state leading to betterment. In proper hands it is a powerful instrument, particularly when the patient has faith in the person who makes it. After a careful and sympathetic examination and testing the electrical reactions of the muscles of a paralyzed limb the suggestion, "Now you will be able to move it" may be all-sufficient. A strong, imperative command may have the same effect.

Reeducation.—In both hysteria and neurasthenia this should be the aim of all reasonable practice, but it is not always feasible: some of our patients would have to be rebuilt from the blastoderm. With patience and method much may be done, and the special merit of Weir Mitchell's work and of his system (which is not simply a rest cure, as many suppose) is that it is an elaborate plan of reeducation. The essentials are that the patient should be isolated and under the charge of an intelligent nurse. The physical condition is carefully studied and a rigid daily régime carried out: A milk diet of three to four quarts daily, varying the food as the patient improves, and as the weight increases. This may be followed by a rapid gain in weight and the disappearance of abdominal symptoms. Massage, hydrotherapy and electricity are adjuncts, but very much depends upon the tact, patience, and, above all, the personality of the physician; *the man counts more than the method.* The mental condition has to be carefully studied and the patient's attitude toward life influenced by specially selected literature, careful conversation, and suggestion.

The Analytical Method.—Introduced by Breuer and extended by Freud, it is partly the method of the confessional, in which the sinner poured out his soul in the sympathetic ear of the priest, but it also enables the patient to bring out into the open what he may not consciously know. It is a difficult procedure, not for all to attempt, exhausting alike to patient and doctor, and, when thoroughly carried out, time consuming. In the hands of those who have practised it skilfully, very good results have been obtained, particularly in young and carefully selected cases.

Hydrotherapy is of great value, especially wet packs, salt baths and various douches. General tonics, such as arsenic and iron, may be helpful, especially if the patients are nervous and anemic. Sedatives are rarely indicated. Occasionally they may be necessary, but for the relief of sleeplessness all possible measures should be resorted to before the employment of drugs. The wet pack given hot or cold at night will usually suffice.

NEURASTHENIA

(*Psychasthenia: Psychoneurosis*)

Definition.—A condition of weakness or exhaustion of the nervous system, giving rise to various forms of mental and bodily inefficiency.

The term, an old one, popularized by Beard, covers an ill-defined, motley group of symptoms, which may be either general and the expression of derangement of the entire system, or local and limited to certain organs.

Etiology.—The causes may be grouped as hereditary and acquired.

(*a*) Hereditary.—We do not all start in life with the same amount of nerve capital. Parents who have led irrational lives, indulging in excesses of various kinds, or who have been the subjects of nervous complaints or of mental trouble, may transmit to their children an organization which is defective in what, for want of a better term, we must call "nerve force." Such individuals start handicapped with a neuropathic predisposition, and furnish a considerable proportion of our neurasthenic patients. As Van Gieson, sonorously puts it, "the potential energies of the higher constellations of their association centres have been squandered by their ancestors." So long as these individuals are content to transact a moderate business with their life capital, all may go well, but there is no reserve, and in the exigencies of modern life these small capitalists go under and come to us as bankrupts. The influence of a nervous parent on the young child is also an important factor.

(*b*) Acquired.—The functions, though perverted most readily in persons who have inherited a feeble organization, may also be damaged in persons with no neuropathic predisposition by use which is excessive in proportion to the strength—*i.e.*, by strain. The cares and anxieties attendant upon the gaining of a livelihood may be borne without distress, but in many persons the strain becomes excessive and is first manifested as *worry*. The individual loses the distinction between essentials and nonessentials, trifles cause annoyance, and the entire organism reacts with unnecessary readiness to slight stimuli, and is in a state which the older writers called "irritable weakness." If such a condition be taken early and the patient given rest, the balance is quickly restored. In this group may be placed a large proportion of the neurasthenia which we see in professional and business men. Neurasthenia may follow the infectious diseases, particularly influenza, typhoid fever and syphilis. The abuse of alcohol or tobacco may predispose to neurasthenia.

(*c*) Sexual Causes.—Undoubtedly the part played in the production of neurosis by sex factors is of the first importance. As stated, Freud regards sexual trauma as the basis of hysteria, and he also regards neurasthenia as largely a product of disturbance in the sexual sphere. For him and his school the sex impulses furnish the basis of the psychoneuroses. Repressed as they have to be in so many in our modern civilization, without normal outlet, the thought formations, retained in the unconscious state, express themselves by means of somatic phenomena—the objective features of hysteria and neurasthenia. *Cherchez la femme* is a safe rule in investigating a neurotic male. Freud may have ridden his hobby too hard, particularly in the insistence upon the importance of infantile sexuality, but in recognizing the rôle of the younger Aphrodite in the lives of men and women he has but followed the great master, Plato, who saw, while he deplored, the havoc wrought by her universal dominance.

Symptoms.—These are extremely varied, and may be general or localized; more often a combination of both. The appearance of the patient is suggestive, sometimes characteristic, but difficult to describe. Important information can be gained by the physician if he observes the patient closely as he enters the room—the way he is clothed, his manner, his facial expression, and the humor which he is in. Loss of weight and slight anemia may be present. The debility may reach a high grade and the patient be confined to bed. Mentally the patients are usually low-spirited and despondent; women are frequently emotional. *Fatigue* is an important feature.

The *local* symptoms may dominate the situation, and there have accordingly been described a whole series of forms of the disease—cerebral, spinal, cardiovascular, gastric and sexual. In all there is a striking lack of accordance between the symptoms of which the patient complains and the objective changes discoverable by the physician. In nearly every form the predominant symptoms are referable to pathological sensations and the psychic effects of these. Disturbed sleep and distressing dreams are complained of by a majority of patients, or, if not complained of, are found to exist.

In the *cerebral* or psychic form the symptoms are chiefly connected with an inability to perform ordinary mental work. Thus, a row of figures can not be correctly added, the dictation or the writing of a few letters is a source of great worry, the transaction of petty details is a painful effort, and there is loss of power of fixed attention. With this condition there may be no headache, the appetite may be good, and the patient may sleep well. As a rule, however, there are sensations of fulness and weight or flushes, if not actual headache. Insomnia is frequent. Some patients are good-tempered and cheerful but a majority are moody, irritable and depressed.

Hyperesthesia, especially to sensations of pain, is one of the main characteristics of almost all neurasthenic individuals. The sensations are nearly always referred to some special region—the skin, eyes, joints, blood-vessels or viscera. It is frequently possible to localize a number of points painful to pressure (Valleix's points). In some patients there is marked vertigo, occasionally resembling that of Ménière's disease.

If such sensations continue for a time the mood and character of the patient gradually alter. Many obnoxiously egoistic individuals met with in daily life are in reality examples of psychic neurasthenia. Complaint is made of everything. The patient demands the greatest consideration for his condition; he feels that he has been insulted if his desires are not immediately granted, but at the same time he has but little consideration for others. Indeed, in the severer forms he may show a malicious pleasure in attempting to make people uncomfortable who seem happier than himself. Such patients complain frequently that they are "misunderstood."

In many cases the so-called "anxiety conditions" gradually come on; one scarcely ever sees a case of advanced neurasthenia without some form of anxiety or fear. In the simpler forms there may be a fear of impending insanity, of approaching death or of apoplexy. More frequently the anxious feeling is localized somewhere in the body—in the precordial region, the head, the abdomen, the thorax, or more rarely in the extremities. In some cases the anxiety becomes intense and the patients are restless, and declare that they do not know what to do with themselves. They may throw themselves upon a bed, crying and complaining, and making convulsive movements with the hands and feet. Suicidal tendencies may be present in such cases.

Involuntary mental activity may be very troublesome; the patient complains that when he is overtired thoughts which he can not stop or control run through his head with lightning-like rapidity. In other cases there is marked absence of ideas, the individual's mind being so filled up by latent memory pictures that he is unable to form the proper associations for ideas called up by external stimuli. Sometimes a patient complains that a definite word, a name, a number, or a song keeps running in his head in spite of all he can do to abolish it.

In the severer cases the *phobias* are common. A frequent form is *agoraphobia,* in which patients when they come into an open space are oppressed by a feeling of anxiety. They are frightened and commence to tremble; they complain of compression of the thorax and palpitation of the heart. They may break into profuse perspiration and assert that they feel as though chained to the ground or that they can not move a step. It is remarkable that in some such cases the open space can be crossed if the individual be accompanied by some one, even by a child, or if he carry a stick or an umbrella! Other people are afraid to be left alone (monophobia), especially in a closed compartment (claustrophobia).

The fear of people and of society is known as anthropophobia. A whole series of other phobias has been described—batophobia, or the fear that high things will fall; pathophobia, or fear of disease; siderodromophobia, or fear of a railway journey; siderophobia or astrophobia, fear of thunder and lightning. Occasionally we meet with individuals who are afraid of everything and every one—victims of pantophobia. By psycho-analysis it may be possible to explain the mechanism of these fears.

The *special senses* may be disturbed, particularly vision. An aching or weariness of the eyeballs after reading a few minutes or flashes of light are common symptoms. The "irritable eye," the so-called nervous or neurasthenic asthenopia, is familiar to every physician. There may be acoustic disturbances —hyperalgesia and even true hyperacusia.

A common symptom is *pressure in the head* which, variously described, may be diffuse, but is more frequently referred to some one part, especially the occipital region. When *spinal symptoms* predominate, in addition to many of the features mentioned, the patients complain of weariness on the least exertion, of weakness, pain in the back, intercostal neuralgiform pains, and of aching pains in the legs. There may be spots of local tenderness on the spine. The pain may be spontaneous, or noticed only on pressure or movement. Occasionally there may be disturbances of sensation, particularly numbness and tingling, and the reflexes may be increased. Visceral neuralgias, especially in the genital organs, are frequent. An aching pain in the back or in the back of the neck is a frequent complaint. In women it may be impossible to say whether the condition is neurasthenia or hysteria. It is in these cases that the disturbances of muscular activity are pronounced, and in the French writings *amyosthenia* plays an important rôle.

The symptoms may be irritative or paretic, or a combination of both. Disturbances of coordination are not uncommon in the severer forms. These particularly involve the associated movements of the eye muscles, leading to asthenopic lack of accommodation. Occasionally Romberg's sign is present, and the physician may fear a beginning tabes. More rarely there is disturbance of coordinated acts as writing and articulation, not unlike those at the onset of general paresis. Such symptoms are always alarming, and the greatest care must be taken in the diagnosis. That they may be the symptoms of pure neurasthenia can not be doubted.

The *reflexes* are usually increased, the deep reflexes especially never being absent. The condition of the superficial reflexes is less constant, though these, too, are usually increased. The pupils are often dilated and the reflexes are usually normal. There may be inequality of the pupils. Errors in refraction are common, the correction of which may give great relief.

In another form the weakness is extreme and thorough examination is necessary before deciding as to the nature of the affection, since serious mistakes may be made. Here belong *atremia, akinesia algera,* and the neurasthenic form of *astasia-abasia* described by Binswanger.

The *cardiovascular* symptoms may be the most distressing, and occur with only slight disturbance of the cerebrospinal functions, though the conditions are nearly always combined. Palpitation of the heart, irregular and very rapid action, and pains and oppressive feelings in the cardiac region are the most common. Some are due to the "dropped" heart which may be dilated. The slightest excitement may be followed by increased action of the heart, sometimes with sensations of dizziness and anxiety, and the patients fear that they have serious disease. Attacks of precordial pain may occur.

Vasomotor disturbances are marked in many cases. Flushes of heat, especially in the head, and transient hyperemia of the skin may be very distressing symptoms. Profuse sweating may occur, local or general, and sometimes nocturnal. The pulse may show interesting features, owing to the relaxation of the peripheral arterioles. The arterial throbbing may be almost as marked as in aortic insufficiency. The pulse may have a somewhat collapsing quality and the capillary pulse may be seen. Hypotension is common. A characteristic symptom in some cases is the *throbbing aorta.* This "preternatural pulsation in the epigastrium," as Allan Burns calls it, may be extremely forcible and suggest aneurism. The associated subjective sensations may be very unpleasant, particularly when the stomach is empty.

In women especially, and sometimes in men, the peripheral blood vessels are contracted, the extremities are cold, the nose is red or blue, and the face has a pinched expression. These patients feel much more comfortable when the cutaneous vessels are distended, and resort to various means to favor this (wearing of heavy clothing, use of diffusible stimulants).

The general features of *gastro-intestinal neurasthenia* have been dealt with under the section on nervous dyspepsia. The connection with dilatation of the stomach, floating kidney and *enteroptosis* has been mentioned.

In *sexual neurasthenia* there is an irritable weakness of the sexual organs manifested by nocturnal emissions, premature emission, depression after intercourse, and often a dread of impotence. The mental condition of these patients is pitiable and they fall an easy prey to quacks and charlatans. In males these symptoms are frequently due to diseased conditions in the deep urethra, especially of the verumontanum, and prostate. Spermatorrhea is the bugbear of many. They complain of losses especially with defecation or micturition. Psychical impotence is not uncommon. The "painful testicle" is a well-known neurasthenic phenomenon. In severer cases, there may be sexual perversion. In females it is common to find a tender ovary, and painful or irregular menstruation. There may be disturbances in the sex sphere with anxiety states.

Diagnosis.—*Psychasthenia.*—Under this term may be placed the cases characterized by mental, emotional, and psychical disturbances, imperative ideas, phobias of all sorts, doubts, enfeebled will, uncontrollable movements, and some of the borderland features of a psychosis. It is really an inherited psychoneurosis, while neurasthenia is usually acquired. Obessions of all sorts characterize it and there may be a feeling of unreality and even of loss of personality. How complicated the condition may be is shown from the varieties distinguished by Janet: (1) The *doubter,* in whom obsessive ideas are not very precise, more of the nature of a general indication than a specific idea, such as a craze for research, for explanation, for computing. (2) The *scrupulous,* whose obsessions are of a moral nature. Their manias are of literalness of statement, of exact truth, of conjuration, of reparation, of symbols, etc. (3) The *criminal,* whose obsessive ideas are of homicide, theft, and other overt acts. The impulsive idea is stronger in this than in the other varieties. (4) The *inebriates,* morphinomaniac, etc., in whom the impulse seems to be least resistible. (5) The *genesically perverted.* (6) *Delirious psychasthenia,* in which a delirious state occurs, connected with the obsession.

Neurasthenia, above all other diseases, has to be diagnosed from the subjective statements of the patient, and from a study of his general behavior rather than from the physical examination, which, however, is of the highest importance in excluding other diseases likely to be confounded with it. That somatic changes occur and that physical signs are often found is very true, but there is nothing typical or pathognomonic in the objective changes.

The *hypochondriac* differs from the neurasthenic in the excessive psychic distortion of the pathological sensations to which he is subject. He is the victim of actual delusions regarding his condition.

The confusion of neurasthenia with *hysteria* is frequent; in women especially a diagnosis of hysteria is often made when the condition is neurasthenia. In the absence of hysterical paroxysms, of crises, and of the marked emotional and intellectual characteristics of the hysterical individual the diagnosis of hysteria should not be made. If hysterical stigmata (paralyses, convulsions, contractures, anesthesias, alterations in the visual field, etc.) are present, the diagnosis is not difficult.

Epilepsy is not likely to be confounded with neurasthenia if there be definite epileptic attacks, but cases of *petit mal* may be puzzling.

The onset of *exophthalmic goitre* may be mistaken for neurasthenia, especially if there be no exophthalmos at the beginning. The emotional disturbances and the irritability of the heart may mislead the physician. *Tuberculosis* should always be excluded and careful search made for signs of any *internal secretion* disturbance. In pronounced cases of neurasthenia the differential diagnosis from various psychoses may be extremely difficult.

The two forms of *organic disease* of the nervous system with which neurasthenia is most likely to be confounded are tabes and general paresis. The symptoms of the spinal form of neurasthenia may resemble those of tabes, while the symptoms of the psychic form of neurasthenia may be very similar to those of general paresis. The diagnosis, as a rule, presents no difficulty if the physician makes a thorough routine examination. It is only a superficial study that is likely to lead one astray. In tabes a consideration of the sensory disturbances, the deep reflexes, and the pupillary findings will establish the diagnosis. In general paresis there is sometimes more difficulty. The onset is often characterized by symptoms quite like those of neurasthenia, and the physician may overlook the real malady. The mistake in the other direction is perhaps just as common. A physician who has seen a case of general paresis arise out of what appeared to be neurasthenia is too prone afterward to suspect every neurasthenic to be developing the malign affection. The most marked symptoms of psychic exhaustion do not justify a diagnosis of general paresis even when the history is suspicious, unless along with it there is a definite paresis of the pupils, of the facial muscles, or of the muscles of articulation. The physician should be sharply on the lookout for intellectual defects, paraphasia, facial paresis and sluggishness of the pupils. The examination of the spinal fluid will remove any doubt.

Treatment.—PROPHYLAXIS.—Many patients come under our care a generation too late for satisfactory treatment, and it may be impossible to restore the exhausted capital. The greatest care should be taken in the rearing of children of neuropathic predisposition. From a very early age they should be submitted to a process of "psychic hardening," every effort being made to strengthen the bodily and mental condition. Even in infancy the child should not be pampered. Later on the greatest care should be exercised with regard to food, sleep and school work. Complaints of children should not be too seriously considered. Much depends upon the example set by the parents. An emotional, constantly complaining mother will rack the nervous system of a child. In some instances, for the welfare of a developing boy or girl, the physician may find it necessary to advise removal from home.

Neurotic children are especially liable during development to fits of temper and of emotional disturbance. These should not be too lightly considered. Above all, violent chastisement in such cases is to be avoided, and loss of temper on the part of the parent or teacher is particularly pernicious for the nervous system of the child. Where possible, in such instances, the best treatment is to put the obstreperous child immediately to bed, and if the excitement and temper continue a warm bath followed by a cool douche may be effective. If he be put to bed after the bath sleep soon follows.

Special attention is necessary at puberty in both boys and girls. If there be at this period any marked tendency to emotional disturbance or to intellectual weakness the child should be removed from school and every care taken to avoid unfavorable influences.

PERSONAL HYGIENE.—Throughout life individuals of neuropathic predisposition should obey scrupulously certain hygienic and prophylactic rules. Intellectual work especially should be judiciously limited and alternate frequently with periods of repose. Excitement of all kinds should be avoided, and such individuals do well to be abstemious in the use of tobacco, tea, coffee and alcohol, if, indeed, they be permitted to use them at all. The habit of taking at least once a year a prolonged holiday should be urgently enjoined upon every neuropathic individual. In many instances it gives great relief and rest if the patient can take his holiday away from his relatives.

During ordinary life nervous people should, during some portion of each day, pay rational attention to the body. Cold baths, swimming, exercises in the gymnasium, gardening, golf, lawn tennis, cricket, hunting, shooting, rowing and bicycling are of value in maintaining the general health. Such exercises are to be recommended only to individuals physically equal to them. If neurasthenia is well established the greatest care must be observed in the ordering of exercise. Many nervous girls have been completely broken down by following injudicious advice with regard to exercise.

Treatment.—The treatment of neurasthenia when once established presents a varied problem to the thoughtful physician. Every case must be handled upon its own merits, no two, as a rule, requiring exactly the same methods. In general it will be the aim to remove the patient as far as possible from the influences which have led to his downfall, and to restore to normal the nervous mechanisms which have been weakened by injurious influences. The general character of the individual, his physical and social status, must be considered and the therapeutic measures carefully adjusted to these.

Certain things are essential—time, patience, understanding of the weakness of human nature, sympathy (as a motive, not emotional) and the desire to help. The patient must be allowed to tell his story, however long it takes, and then the physician has to reconstruct the background and development of the patient and his disease. The physical examination must be thorough so that organic disease is not overlooked and the patient convinced that this does not exist. When the proper time comes explanations are given but placeboes such as "It is only nervousness" or "Forget it" should never be given.

The diagnosis having been settled, the physician may assure the patient that with prolonged treatment, during which his cooperation is absolutely essential, he may expect to get well. He must be told that much depends upon himself and that he must make a vigorous effort to overcome certain of his tendencies, and that all his strength of will will be needed to further the progress of the cure. In business or professional men, in whom the condition develops as a result of strain and worry, it may be sufficient to enjoin absolute rest with change of scene. A trip abroad or, if there is nervous dyspepsia, a residence at one of the spas will usually prove sufficient. The excitement of large cities should be avoided. The longer the disease has lasted and the more intense the symptoms, the longer the time necessary for the restoration of health. In cases of any severity the patient must be told that at least six months' complete absence from business, under strict medical guidance, will be necessary. Shorter periods may be of benefit, which, however, as a rule, is only temporary.

It is often advisable to make out a daily programme, which shall occupy almost the whole time of the patient. At first he need know nothing about this, the care being given over entirely to the nurse. With improvement, moderate physical and intellectual exercises, alternating frequently with rest and the administration of food, may be undertaken. Part of the day may be left free for reading, correspondence, conversation and games. In some instances the writing of letters is particularly harmful and must be prohibited or limited. Cultured individuals may find benefit from drawing, painting, modelling, translating, the making of abstracts, etc., for short periods.

In some cases, including a large proportion of neurasthenic women, a systematic rest treatment rigidly carried out should be tried. The patient must be isolated and all regulations must be strictly adhered to, the consent of the patient and the family having first been gained. The treatment of the gastric and intestinal symptoms has been considered. For the irregular pains, particularly in the back and neck, the cautery is invaluable.

Hydrotherapy is indicated in nearly every case if it can be properly applied.

Much can be done at home or in a hospital, but for systematic hydrotherapeutic treatment residence in a suitable sanitarium is better. The wet pack is of especial value and, particularly at night, is perhaps the best remedy against insomnia. Salt baths are helpful to some patients. The various forms of douches, partial packs, etc., may be valuable in individual cases. Electrotherapy is of some value, though only in combination with psychic treatment and hydrotherapy.

Special care should be given to the recognition of local disease and proper measures instituted. Attention to the eyes is important. Infection of the nasopharynx, teeth or tonsils, sinus disease, visceroptosis or anemia should be corrected. In women the pelvic organs and in men the deep urethra and prostate may require treatment.

Treatment by drugs should be avoided as much as possible. They are of benefit chiefly in the combating of single symptoms. Alcohol, morphia, opium or cocaine should never be given. General tonics may be helpful, especially with anemia, when arsenic and iron are indicated. For the severer pains and nervous attacks some sedative may be necessary, especially at the beginning of the treatment. The bromides may be given or an occasional dose of phenacetine or acetylsalicylic acid but the less of these we use the better. Phenobarbital may be useful. For the relief of insomnia all possible measures should be resorted to before the use of drugs. The wet pack will usually suffice. If necessary to give a drug, chloral hydrate, sulphonal, barbital, or other hypnotics may be employed.

Psychotherapy.—Hypnotism is rarely indicated. Carefully practised suggestion is most helpful and psycho-analysis is of value.

The use of religious ideas and practices has come into vogue in various forms, as Christian Science, Mental Healing, etc. It is an old story. In all ages, and in all lands, the prayer of faith, to use the words of St. James, has healed the sick; and we must remember that amid the Æsculapian cults, the most elaborate and beautiful system of faith healing the world has seen, scientific medicine took its rise. As a profession, consciously or unconsciously, more often the latter, *faith* has been one of our most valuable assets and Galen expressed a great truth when he said, "He cures most successfully in whom the people have the greatest confidence." It is in neurasthenia and psychasthenia, with the weak brothers and the weaker sisters, that the personal character of the physican comes into play, and once let him gain the confidence of the patient, he can work the same miracles as Our Lady of Lourdes or Ste. Anne de Beaupré. Three elements are necessary: first, a strong personality in whom the individual has faith—Christ, Buddha, Æsculapius (in the days of Greece), one of the saints, or, what has served the turn of common humanity very well, a physician. Secondly, certain accessories—a shrine, a sanctuary, the services of a temple, or for us a hospital or its equivalent, with a skillful nurse. Thirdly, suggestion, either of the "only believe," "feel it," "will it" attitude of mind, which is the essence of every cult and creed, or of the active belief in the assurance of the physician that health is within reach.

THE TRAUMATIC NEUROSES

Definition.—A morbid condition following shock which presents the symptoms of neurasthenia or hysteria or both.

Erichsen regarded the condition as the result of inflammation of the meninges and cord, and gave it the name "railway spine." Walton and J. J. Putnam, of Boston, were the first to recognize the hysterical nature of many of the cases, and to Westphal's pupils we owe the name traumatic neurosis.

Etiology.—The condition follows an accident, often in a railway train, in which injury has been sustained, or succeeds a shock or concussion, from which the patient may apparently not have suffered in his body. A man may appear well for several days, or even a week or more, and then the symptoms appear. Bodily shock or concussion is not necessary. The affection may follow a profound mental impression; thus, an engine-driver ran over a child, and received a very severe shock, subsequent to which the most pronounced symptoms of neurasthenia developed. Severe mental strain with bodily exposure may cause it, as in a naval officer who was wrecked in a violent storm and exposed for more than a day in the rigging before he was rescued. A slight blow, a fall on a pavement or on the stairs may suffice. The possibility of actual injury of the spine should always be considered and in the determination of this the X-ray study is important.

Symptoms.—The cases may be divided into three groups: simple neurasthenia, cases with marked hysterical manifestations, and cases with severe symptoms indicating or simulating organic disease.

(1) Simple Traumatic Neurasthenia.—The first symptoms usually develop a few weeks after the accident, which may or may not have been associated with actual trauma. The patient complains of headache and fatigue. He is sleepless and finds himself unable to concentrate his attention upon his work. A condition of nervous irritability develops, which may have a host of trivial manifestations, and the entire mental attitude of the person may be changed. He dwells constantly upon his condition, becomes despondent and in extreme cases melancholia may develop. He may complain of numbness and tingling in the extremities, and in some cases of much pain in the back. The bodily functions may be well performed, though such patients usually have, for a time at least, disturbed digestion and loss in weight. The physical examination may be entirely negative. The reflexes are slightly increased, as in ordinary neurasthenia. Cardiovascular symptoms may be marked.

(2) Cases with Marked Hysterical Features.—Following an injury of any sort, neurasthenic symptoms, like those described above, may develop, and in addition symptoms regarded as characteristic of hysteria. The emotional element is prominent and there is but slight control over the feelings. The patients have headache, backache and vertigo. A violent tremor may be present and constitute the most striking feature. In an engineer who developed subsequent to an accident a series of nervous phenomena the most marked feature was an excessive tremor of the entire body, specially manifest during emotional excitement. The most pronounced hysterical features are the sensory disturbances. Hemianesthesia may occur as a consequence of trauma, more common in France than in England and the United States. Achro-

matopsia may exist on the anesthetic side. A second, more common, manifestation is limitation of the field of vision, similar to that in hysteria.

(3) Cases in which the Symptoms Suggest Organic Disease.—As a result of spinal concussion, without fracture or external injury, symptoms may subsequently develop suggestive of organic disease, which may come on rapidly or at a late date. In a case reported by Leyden the symptoms following the concussion were at first slight and the patient was regarded as a simulator, but finally the condition became aggravated and death resulted. The postmortem showed a chronic pachymeningitis, doubtless from the accident. The cases in this group about which there is so much discussion are those which display marked sensory and motor changes. Following an accident in which the patient has not received external injury a condition of excitement may develop within a week or ten days; he complains of headache and backache, and sensory disturbances are found, either hemianesthesia or areas in which the sensation is much benumbed; or painful and tactile impressions may be felt in certain regions; and the temperature sense is absent. The distribution may be bilateral and symmetrical in limited regions or hemiplegic in type. Limitation of the field of vision is usually marked, and there may be disturbance of taste and smell. The superficial reflexes may be diminished; usually the deep reflexes are exaggerated. The pupils may be unequal; the motor disturbances are variable. The French writers describe cases of monoplegia with or without contracture, symptoms upon which Charcot laid great stress as a manifestation of profound hysteria. The combination of sensory disturbances with paralysis, particularly if monoplegic, and the occurrence of contractures without atrophy and with normal electrical reactions, may be regarded as distinctive of hysteria.

In rare cases following trauma and symptoms regarded as neurasthenic or hysterical there are organic changes which may prove fatal. That this occurs has been demonstrated by autopsies. The features upon which the greatest reliance can be placed as indicating organic change are optic atrophy, bladder symptoms, particularly with tremor, paresis and exaggerated reflexes.

The anatomical changes are not very definite. When death follows spinal concussion within a few days there may be no apparent lesion, but in some instances the brain or cord showed punctiform hemorrhages. Edes reported 4 cases in which degeneration in the pyramidal tracts followed concussion or injury of the spine; but in all these cases there was marked tremor and the spinal symptoms developed early, or followed immediately upon the accident.

Diagnosis.—A condition of fright and excitement following an accident may persist for days or even weeks, and then gradually pass away. The symptoms of neurasthenia or of hysteria which subsequently develop present nothing peculiar and are identical with those which occur under other circumstances. Care must be taken to recognize simulation, and, as in these cases the condition is largely subjective, this is sometimes extremely difficult. In a careful examination a simulator will often reveal himself by exaggeration of certain symptoms, particularly sensitiveness of the spine, and by increasing voluntarily the reflexes. Mannkopff suggests as a good test to take the pulse rate before, during, and after pressure upon an area said to be painful. If the rate is quickened, it is held to be proof that the pain is real but this is not always the case. It may require careful study to determine whether the individual is honestly suffering from the symptoms of which he complains. A still more important question is, Has the patient organic disease? The symptoms given under the first two groups of cases may exist in a marked degree and persist for several years without the slightest evidence of organic change. Hemianesthesia, limitation of the field of vision, monoplegia with contracture, may all be present as hysterical manifestations, from which recovery may be complete. The diagnosis of an organic lesion should be limited to those cases in which optic atrophy, bladder troubles, and signs of sclerosis of the cord are well marked—indications either of degeneration of the lateral columns or of multiple sclerosis. Examination by the X-rays is an important aid and has showed in some cases definite injury to the spine.

Prognosis.—A majority of patients with traumatic hysteria recover. In railway cases, so long as litigation is pending and the patient is in the hands of lawyers, the symptoms usually persist. Settlement is often the starting-point of a speedy and perfect recovery. On the other hand, there are a few cases in which the symptoms persist even after the litigation has been closed; the patient goes from bad to worse and psychoses develop, such as melancholia, dementia, or occasionally progressive paresis. And, lastly, in extremely rare cases organic lesions may result as a sequence.

The function of the physician acting as medical expert in these cases consists in determining (*a*) the existence of actual disease, and (*b*) its character, whether simple neurasthenia, severe hysteria, or an organic lesion. The outlook for ultimate recovery is good except in patients who present the more serious symptoms above mentioned. Nevertheless traumatic hysteria is one of the most intractable affections which we are called upon to treat. In the treatment of the traumatic neuroses the practitioner may be guided by the principles laid down for the treatment of hysteria and neurasthenia.

NARCOLEPSY

There are two forms. In one, perhaps after a feeling of severe fatigue, the patient suddenly falls into what appears to be normal sleep which lasts a short time. He can be waked and appears normal. In the other form are curious attacks usually produced by emotion, especially laughter, in which the patient falls to the floor (cataplexy). He is unable to move or speak but does not lose consciousness. There may be convulsive movements suggesting epilepsy. The *etiology* is obscure; disturbance of the pituitary gland and adjoining structures has been suggested. It appears to have followed epidemic encephalitis in a few cases. Males are affected more often than females. In *treatment* ephedrine should be tried, gr. 3/8 (0.37 gm.) two or three times a day. The malady is chronic and persists through life.

VASOMOTOR AND TROPHIC DISEASES

RAYNAUD'S DISEASE

Definition.—A vascular change, without organic disease of the vessels, chiefly seen in the extremities, but occurring also in the internal parts, in which a persistent ischemia or a passive hyperemia leads to disturbance of function or to loss of vitality with necrosis.

Etiology.—It is a comparatively rare disease. There were only 19 cases in about 20,000 medical patients admitted to the Johns Hopkins Hospital. Women are much more frequently attacked than men. Sixty per cent of the cases occur in the second and third decades, but no age is exempt. It has occurred in a six-month-old child and in a woman of 77 years.

Several members of a family may be affected. Neurotic and hysterical patients are more prone to the disease. Damp and cold weather appears to favor its occurrence. Severe chilblain leading to superficial necrosis represents a type of the malady. In the infectious diseases areas of multiple necrosis occur, but such should not be included under Raynaud's disease, nor the local gangrene associated with arteritis. Syphilis is suggested in some cases.

Pathology.—According to the definition, cases are excluded in which organic disease of the vessels is present. In advanced cases sclerosis of the blood vessels has been found; and neuritis has been described, but neither is an essential factor. Changes in the spinal cord have been reported, but in a majority of cases the examination has been negative. The *local ischemia* is an expression of a constrictor influence causing spasms of the arteries and arterioles, so that no blood enters a part. This may be followed in an hour or two, or less, by active *hyperemia;* the arteries and arterioles dilate widely and the white finger becomes a bright pink. While hyperemia may follow the ischemia directly, more commonly there is an intervening period of *asphyxia* in which the finger becomes blue. In frost-bite, active hyperemia, cyanosis, and ischemia is the order. In Raynaud's disease the order is usually ischemia, asphyxia, and hyperemia. In frost-bite it seems that the asphyxia is due to a backward flow from the veins, to which the ischemia yields as the part thaws, before the arteries passing to the part can be felt to pulsate. In moderate grades of asphyxia some little blood trickles through the sluice gates, but in the deep purple skin of a typical example of Raynaud's disease the circulation has ceased and death of the part is imminent. The necrosis is a simple matter, as simple as if a string is tied tightly about the finger.

The disease is probably the result of some instability of the vasomotor system rather than disease of the vessels. The *capillaries* are contracted in the syncopal stage. In the cyanotic state they are dilated but there is no movement of the blood. There is loss of coordination between the arterioles and capillaries. Even in the stage of hyperemia many of the capillaries show stagnation of the blood stream.

Symptoms.—There are various grades of the disease, of which mild, moderate, and severe types may be recognized. In the *mild* forms the disease never gets beyond the stage of such vascular disturbance as is frequently seen in chilblains. The hands alone may be affected. In the winter, on the slightest exposure, there is acrocyanosis, which gives place in the warmth to active hyperemia, sometimes with swelling, throbbing and aching. The so-called "beefsteak" hand is often a great annoyance to women. It is a vasomotor disturbance representing a potential case of Raynaud's disease. In these mild attacks one finger may be white and others red and blue.

The condition may persist for years and never pass on to necrosis. In a case of *moderate* severity a woman, aged say twenty or twenty-five, after a period of worry or ill health, has pains in the fingers, or a numbness or tingling; then she notices that they are white and cold, and in an hour or so they become red and hot. Within a day or two a change occurs; they remain permanently blue perhaps as far as the second joint or to the knuckles. There is pain, sometimes severe enough to require morphia. The cyanosis persists and the tip of one finger or the terminal joint of another gets darker and a few blebs form. The other fingers show signs of restored circulation, but necrosis has occurred in the pad of one finger and perhaps the terminal inch of another. The necrotic parts gradually separate, and the patient may never have another attack, or in a year or two there is a recurrence.

The *severe* form is a terrible malady, and may affect fingers and toes at once and sometimes the tip of the nose and the ears. The pain is of great severity. Both feet may be swollen to the ankle with the toes black. It may look as if both feet would become gangrenous, but as a rule the process subsides, and in a case of great severity only the tips of the toes are lost. A severe attack may last for months, when the patient recovers with the loss of two or three fingers or toes, a snip off the edge of both ears and a scar on the tip of the nose. Such attacks may occur year by year, and there are terrible instances in which the patients have lost both hands and feet.

Of the parts affected Monro states that in 43 per cent one or both of the arms is involved. Parts other than the extremities may be attacked, as the chin, lips, nates and eyelids.

Complications.—Temporary amblyopia due to spasm of the retinal vessels, transient aphasia and transient hemiplegia have been met with. In one case there were three attacks of aphasia with hemiplegia and complete recovery. Associated with these were the features of Raynaud's disease. The patient died in a severe attack with pain in the right hand, gangrene to the elbow, and coma. Epilepsy occurs with some cases, and in one case the attacks occurred only in the winter when he had Raynaud's disease.

Albuminuria may occur during the attacks. Hemoglobinuria occurs in some cases, and was studied by the well-known surgeon, Druitt, in his own case. It is of the same nature as the paroxysmal hemoglobinuria.

Scleroderma of the fingers may follow recurring attacks. Occasionally true generalized scleroderma begins with the features of Raynaud's disease. Arthritis has been present in certain cases.

Diagnosis.—Gangrene or trophic changes limited largely to the skin, symmetrical or bilateral involvement, absence of occlusive lesions in the arteries and intermittent attacks of change in color which precede the trophic changes are important points. One condition may simulate it, namely, local gangrene of the toes with obliterative arteritis; but this occurs most frequently in older persons, in diabetic subjects or with well-marked arteriosclerosis. As a rule, the pulse in such cases is not to be felt in the dorsal artery. Thrombo-angiitis obliterans has constant features; it is not paroxysmal. In acute infections, particularly typhus fever, occasionally in typhoid fever and malaria, areas of multiple gangrene occur. The distribution is usually different, and there is rarely any difficulty in distinguishing this form.

There are cases of multiple neurotic skin gangrene in hysterical and nervous patients, in the majority of which the lesions are self-inflicted. In military recruits local gangrene of the toes has been caused by phenol and many of these lesions are simulated.

Treatment.—Every effort should be made to improve the general health. Residence in a warm climate is an advantage. Placing the hands or feet alternately in hot and cold water is useful. In the forms of local asphyxia in the feet, the patient should be kept in bed with the legs elevated. The toes should be wrapped in cotton wool. The pain is often intense and may require morphia. Carefully applied, systematic massage of the extremities is sometimes of benefit. Galvanism may be tried. Nitroglycerin has been warmly recommended. Calcium lactate in 15 grain (1 gm.) doses, three or four times a day, is sometimes effectual. It often relieves chilblains. Small doses of thyroid extract or anterior lobe pituitary gland substance (gr. ii, 0.12 gm.) sometimes are useful. Cushing used a treatment which proved successful in several cases. An elastic bandage or a pneumatic tourniquet is applied to the extremity tight enough to shut off the arterial circulation and left for some minutes. On releasing the constriction the member flushes brightly, owing to vasomotor relaxation. This may have to be repeated at intervals. Peri-arterial sympathectomy has been useful in some cases. Operation on the sympathetic nervous system has been of great value. Removal of the related ganglia is done.

ERYTHROMELALGIA (*Red Neuralgia*)

Definition.—"A chronic disease in which a part or parts—usually one or more extremities—suffer with pain, flushing and local fever, made far worse if the parts hang down" (Weir Mitchell). The name signifies a painful red extremity. There are attacks of bilateral symmetrical burning pain in the hands and feet, made worse by standing, exercise or heat, and relieved by elevation and cold. In attacks the temperature of the affected parts is increased.

Mitchell speaks of it as a "painful nerve-end neuritis." Excision of the nerves to the parts has been followed by relief. In one of Mitchell's patients gangrene of the foot followed excision of four inches of the musculocutaneous nerve and stretching of the posterior tibial. Sclerosis of the arteries was found. In 9 cases in which the local conditions were studied, the only constant change was a chronic endarteritis (Batty Shaw).

Symptoms.—In 1872 (*Phila. Med. Times*, November 23d), Weir Mitchell described the case of a sailor, aged forty, who after an African fever began to have "dull, heavy pains, at first in the left and soon after in the right foot. There was no swelling at first. When at rest he was comfortable and the feet were not painful. After walking the feet were swollen. They scarcely pitted on pressure, but were purple with congestion; the veins were everywhere singularly enlarged, and the arteries were throbbing visibly. The whole foot was said to be aching and burning, but above the ankle there was neither swelling, pain, nor flushing." As the weather grew cool he got relief but no treatment seemed to benefit him.

The disease is rare. The feet are much more often affected than the hands. The pain may be of the most atrocious character. It is usually, but not always, relieved by cool weather; in one case winter aggravated the trouble. Cold applications, faradism, massage and radium have been employed in treatment. Excision of nerves and amputation have been done.

ANGIONEUROTIC EDEMA

(*Quincke's Disease*)

Definition.—An affection characterized by the occurrence of local edematous swellings, more or less limited in extent, and of transient duration. Severe colic is sometimes associated.

Etiology.—There is a marked hereditary predisposition, sometimes through many generations, transmitted by males and females. In one family in five generations 22 members were affected (Osler). The sexes are affected equally and the disease occurs most often in the second, third and fourth decades. It often occurs with urticaria. *Allergy* is probably responsible and there may be many causes, foods and drugs perhaps being most frequent. Foci of infection are sometimes important.

Symptoms.—The edema appears suddenly and is usually circumscribed. It may appear in the face; the eyelid is a common situation, or it may involve the lips or cheek. The backs of the hands, the legs, or the throat may be attacked. Usually it is transient, associated perhaps with slight gastro-intestinal distress, and the affection is of little moment. There may be a remarkable periodicity in the attacks. In Matas' case this was very striking; the attack came on every day at eleven or twelve o'clock. The swellings appear in various parts; only rarely are they constant in one locality. The hands, face, pharynx, glottis and genitalia are most frequently affected. Itching, heat, redness, or in some instances urticaria, may precede the outbreak. Sudden edema of the larynx may prove fatal. Two members of one family died of this complication. The lower lip may be so swollen that the mouth can not be opened. The hands enlarge suddenly, so that the fingers can not be bent. There may be gastro-intestinal attacks with severe colic, pain, nausea, and sometimes vomiting, suggesting involvement of the gastro-intestinal mucous membrane. It is possible that some of the cases of intermittent vomiting belong to this group. The colic is of great intensity and usually requires morphia. Arthritis apparently does not occur. Periodic attacks of cardialgia may also occur with the edema. Hemoglobinuria has occurred in several cases. There is a hysterical variety in which the edema affects geometrical areas, has abrupt edges and may be accompanied by sensory disturbances but not by gastro-intestinal attacks.

The disease has affinities with urticaria, the giant form of which is probably the same disease, and with Henoch's purpura. The prognosis is good in the nonhereditary forms; the duration varies from one to three years. A large proportion of deaths occurs from edema of the larynx.

The **treatment** is unsatisfactory. In cases with anemia and general nervousness, iron and large doses of strychnia do good. Improvement may follow the prolonged use of nitroglycerin; calcium lactate may be tried, in doses of 15 grains (1 gm.) thrice daily. A spray of epinephrine or ephedrine may be used if the throat is involved. Epinephrine, 1-1000 solution, (♏ vii, 0.5 cc.) given hypodermically and repeated in fifteen minutes has been helpful. In the search for a causal factor, skin tests are rarely helpful. A study of possibilities with withdrawal of suspicious objects is more useful. Attempts to desensitize are rarely successful. In cases due to food susceptibility, the causal food should be avoided. In one case in which there was susceptibility to any albumin, the administration of peptone was successful.

ERYTHREDEMA

(*Acrodynia: "Pink Disease"*)

To this disease other names have been given, *e.g.*, epidemic erythema, erythredema polyneuritis, and dermatopolyneuritis. The term acrodynia has been used in France for a condition of infective polyneuritis. The chance of confusion should be noted. It is difficult to know where to place it. Swift, of Adelaide, Australia, drew attention to it in 1914. Since then cases have been reported from many countries, with some difference in the main features. The disease occurs at ages from four months to four years. There is a change in disposition with irritability and discomfort; the child is fretful and miserable. Photophobia, anorexia, weakness, slight fever occasionally, and increased pulse rate occur. The *rash* is important and is variable in character, sometimes like "prickly heat." It may fade and reappear. Erythema and eczema-like are used by some to describe it. The exact color varies from pink to a dark red. There are marked itching and excessive perspiration. The hands and feet are red, swollen and cold, are compared to raw beef, and show desquamation. Stomatitis and gingivitis with loss of the teeth may be present. There may be loss of hair and the nails may fall off. Disturbance of sensation is common and there is a varying degree of hypotonia and pseudoparesis. Peripheral neuritis and changes in the spinal cord and nerve roots have been found. The children are subject to respiratory disorders. A leukocytosis is common. The usual course is 5 to 6 months. The mortality is about 5 or 6 per cent. The *diagnosis* should be made from the peculiar features. The *treatment* is symptomatic. Artificial light treatment and the use of atropine are advised. Some emphasize the importance of removing infected tonsils and adenoids, and treating sinusitis if present.

CHRONIC HEREDITARY EDEMA OF THE LEGS

(*Milroy's Disease*)

This condition, described by Milroy of Omaha, is characterized by persistent edema of the legs, without any traceable cause or constitutional features. It affects males and females equally. In Milroy's series 22 persons were affected among 97 in six generations; in Hope and French's series 13 of 42 persons in five generations. The edema is limited to the legs and varies very slightly. In some instances there are acute attacks, with chill, fever and increase of swelling. Except mechanically the condition does not seriously interfere with health. Constant support by bandages is advisable.

There is a familial affection described by Edgeworth of Bristol (1911), with a general subcutaneous edema. Of six infants, five died within the first few months, with general edema, following diarrhea. The cases differ essentially from those of edema neonatorum.

FACIAL HEMIATROPHY

A rare affection characterized by progressive wasting of the bones and soft tissues of one side of the face. The atrophy starts in childhood, but in a few cases has not come on until adult life. Perhaps after a trifling injury or disease it begins, either diffusely or more commonly at one spot on the skin. It gradually spreads, involving the fat, then the bones, more particularly the upper jaw and last and least the muscles. The wasting is sharply limited at the middle line, and the appearance is remarkable, the face looking as if made up of two halves from different persons. There is usually change in the color of the skin and the hair falls. Owing to the wasting of the alveolar processes the teeth become loose and drop out. The eye on the affected side is sunken, owing to loss of orbital fat. There is usually hemiatrophy of the tongue on the same side. Disturbance of sensation and muscle twitching may precede or accompany the atrophy. In a majority of cases the atrophy is confined to one side of the face, but there are instances in which the disease was bilateral, and a few cases with areas of atrophy on the back and arm of the same side.

In Mendel's case an interstitial neuritis was found in all the branches of the trigeminus, most marked in the superior maxillary branch. Changes may be found in the Gasserian ganglion.

The disease is recognized at a glance. The facial asymmetry with congenital wryneck must not be confounded with facial hemiatrophy. Other conditions to be distinguished are: Facial atrophy in poliomyelitis and in the hemiplegia of infants and adults; the atrophy following nuclear lesions and sympathetic nerve paralysis; acquired facial hemihypertrophy, which may by contrast give an atrophic appearance to the other side and scleroderma, if confined to one side of the face. The precise nature of the disease is doubtful, but it is suggestive that in many cases the atrophy followed an acute infection. It is incurable.

SCLERODERMA

Definition.—A condition of localized or diffused induration of the skin.

Varieties.—Two forms are recognized; the circumscribed, which corresponds to the keloid of Addison and to morphea; and the diffuse, in which large areas are involved.

Etiology.—The disease affects females more frequently than males and occurs most commonly at the middle period of life. *Sclerema neonatorum* is a different affection. The disease is more common in the United States than statistics indicate. The senior author saw 20 cases in sixteen years. It is regarded as a trophoneurosis, as due to changes in the arteries of the skin, and to endocrine disturbance, especially of the thyroid, adrenal and pituitary glands. The thyroid has been found atrophied.

Pathology.—There is pigment deposit in the epidermis with an increased amount of connective tissue in the corium and subcutaneous tissues. The superficial vessels are contracted and the deeper vessels are surrounded by leukocytes. Calcinosis of the skin and subcutaneous tissues may occur.

Symptoms.—In the *circumscribed form* there are patches, from a few centimetres in diameter to the size of the hand or larger, in which the skin has a waxy or dead-white appearance, and to the touch is brawny, hard and inelastic. Sometimes there is a preliminary hyperemia and subsequently there are changes in color, either areas of pigmentation or of complete atrophy of the pigment—leukoderma. The sensory changes are rarely marked. The secretion of sweat is diminished or entirely abolished. The areas are situated most frequently about the breasts and neck, sometimes in the course of the nerves. The patches may develop with great rapidity and persist for months or years; sometimes they disappear in a few weeks.

The *diffuse form,* though less common, is more serious. It begins in the extremities or in the face, and the patient notices that the skin is unusually hard and firm, or that there is a sense of stiffness or tension in making movements. Gradually the skin becomes firm and hard, and so united to the subcutaneous tissues that it cannot be picked up or pinched. It may look natural, but more commonly is glossy, drier than normal, and unusually smooth. With reference to the localization, in Lewin and Heller's statistics, in 66 cases the disease was universal; in 203, regions of the trunk were affected; in 193, parts of the head or face; in 287, portions of one or other of the upper arms; and in 122, portions of the legs. In 80 cases there were disturbances of sensation. The disease may gradually extend and involve an entire limb. When universal, the face is expressionless, the lips can not be moved, mastication is hindered, and it may become extremely difficult to feed the patient. The hands become fixed and the fingers immobile, on account of the extreme induration of the skin. Remarkable vasomotor disturbances are common, as extreme cyanosis of the hands and legs. Tachycardia may be present. The disease is chronic, lasting for months or years; there are instances of more than twenty years. Recovery may occur or the disease be arrested. One patient, with extensive involvement of the face, ears and hands, improved very much. The patients are apt to succumb to pulmonary complaints or nephritis. Arthritis has been noted in some instances; in others, endocarditis. Raynaud's disease may be associated with it. The *pigmentation* of the skin may be as deep as in Addison's disease, for which it has been mistaken; scleroderma may occur with exophthalmic goitre.

In the dystrophy known as *sclerodactylia* there is symmetrical involvement of the fingers, which become deformed, shortened and atrophied; the skin is thickened, of a waxy color, and sometimes pigmented. Multiple subcutaneous nodules, not unlike tophi, but not uratic, occur about the fingers. Bullae and ulcerations have occurred and great deformity of the nails. The disease has usually followed exposure; the patients are worse during the winter and curiously sensitive to cold. There may be changes in the skin of the feet, but deformity similar to that in the hand has not been noted. Some patients present diffuse sclerodermatous changes of the skin of other parts. In Lewin and Heller's monograph there are 35 cases of isolated sclerodactylism, and 106 cases in which it occurred with scleroderma.

Poikiloderma is a condition which shows marked pigmentation of the skin in some areas while other areas are pale and atrophic. It may begin as a dermatomyositis. There are ulcerated lesions and telangiectasis. It may accompany sclerodactylism, fibrous myositis and calcinosis. In some cases calcification has occurred in the pleura.

Treatment.—The patients require to be warmly clad and to be guarded against exposure, as they are particularly sensitive to cold. Warm baths followed by frictions with oil should be systematically used. Thyroid gland extract should be tried thoroughly in the diffuse form. In one case the disease appeared to be arrested; the patient took the extract for seven years. In a second case, after a year the face became softer, and there was permanent improvement. In a case of extensive localized scleroderma the patches became softer and the pigmentation much less intense. The views as to the value of X-ray treatment are conflicting. In morphea, injections of fibrolysin have been useful.

Scleredema adultorum has progressive induration of the deeper structures of the skin. It may follow an acute infection. The onset may be with malaise and fever of short duration. The skin is hard and board-like and does not pit on pressure. The surface is smooth and shiny. The back of the neck is first affected with progress to the face and trunk. The hands and feet usually escape. The face is mask-like and it may be difficult to open the mouth. The duration varies from a few weeks to years but it usually clears within a year. Myxedema may be suggested. From scleroderma, the freedom of the epidermis and the hands and feet, with absence of pigmentation are helpful in diagnosis. Massage and hot baths are useful in treatment. A trial of thyroid gland extract should be carried out.

AINHUM

This is a disease of the fifth, rarely of the fourth and other toes, in which a groove forms at the digitoplantar fold and deepens until the toe drops off. Described first by Da Silva Lima in 1852, it occurs in many tropical regions, in the southern states of America, and very rarely in temperate regions. Nothing is determined as to the *etiology*. It may occur in families, and is more common in males. There is endarteritis, with proliferation of the epidermis. Parasites have not been found. It is a local disease without symptoms and in the affected toe there is no disability and rarely pain, except when the skin of the groove ulcerates. The toe drops off in about two years. It is said that it may occur in the fingers. A longitudinal section across the groove may stop the progress, otherwise the toe should be removed.

LIPODYSTROPHIA PROGRESSIVA

A rare affection, more common in females, in which the subcutaneous fat gradually disappears from the face, arms and trunk. The cause is unknown (a trophic neurosis?). The midbrain may be the site of the causal lesion. Beginning usually before the eighth year, the wasting is progressive, but limited to the parts mentioned. The buttocks and legs remain normal and by contrast look abnormally plump. The breasts are spared. In rare cases the legs and pelvic girdle only are affected. In the early stages it resembles the "bilateral atrophy of the face." There is no treatment.

ERYTHROCYANOSIS CRURUM PUELLARUM FRIGIDA

This elaborate designation is applied to a condition which occurs most often in the legs of young women. There is a cyanotic swelling of the back of the leg and ankle, and the foot and leg are cold, especially the former. Chilblains are often present. There is a painful swelling over the insertion of the tendo Achilles. Ulcers may form on the back of the lower part of the leg where the coldness and swelling are most marked. In *treatment* an elastic stocking may be helpful. Elevation of the heel in the shoe may give relief. Slices of fat have been removed from the leg. In some cases a bilateral lumbar sympathectomy has given good results, suggesting a vasomotor origin for the condition.

SECTION XIII

DISEASES OF THE LOCOMOTOR SYSTEM

DISEASES OF THE MUSCLES

MYOSITIS

Definition.—Inflammation of the voluntary muscles.

A primary myositis occurs as an acute, subacute, or chronic affection. It is seen in two chief forms—the suppurative and non-suppurative.

I. Suppurative myositis (infectious myositis) is especially frequent in Japan, where Miyake took cultures from 32 cases; in 27 a pure culture of *Staphylococcus aureus* was obtained, while in another a streptococcus and in 2 the *albus* with the *aureus* was grown. The malady may involve one or many muscles, and is usually sudden in its onset with high fever and marked prostration. Subsequently abscesses occur in the indurated muscles, and pyemia may ensue if the implicated areas are not thoroughly evacuated.

II. Dermatomyositis.—An acute or subacute inflammation of the muscles of unknown origin associated with edema and dermatitis. Steiner collected 28 cases from the literature and reported two cases from the Hopkins clinic. The nature of the disease is unknown. The muscle inflammation is multiple and associated with edema and dermatitis. The muscles are stiff and firm, but fragile, with serous infiltration, great proliferation of the interstitial tissue, and fatty degeneration. The *onset* is usually gradual, the muscles of the extremities being first involved and later those of the trunk. There is moderate fever with sweating and enlargement of the spleen. The skin over the affected muscles is edematous and the dermatitis takes various forms, erythematous, urticarial or erysipelatoid. Pain is present, worse on movement or pressure, and sensory changes may occur. The *course* is usually progressive and after some months death may result from involvement of the muscles of deglutition and respiration, perhaps with bronchopneumonia. The duration is usually one to three months. Of Steiner's 28 cases, 17 died. If recovery results there is atrophy of the muscles. The features suggest trichiniasis which may be distinguished by examination of a portion of muscle. The *treatment* is symptomatic.

III. Polymyositis hemorrhagica.—This form resembles the dermatomyositis in general features, but differs in the presence of hemorrhages into and between the muscles. Of the ten cases analyzed by Thayer four recovered. Purpura and hemorrhages from the mucous membranes may occur.

IV. Secondary Myositis.—This may occur in some infections, as septicemia and typhoid fever, and is constant in trichiniasis. It is very rare in tuberculosis. In scurvy a chronic myositis may occur, sometimes with hemorrhages. In chronic alcoholism, myositis may occur with neuritis. In some cases of fibrositis there is an associated myositis, difficult to distinguish. Syphilis may cause myositis.

MYOSITIS OSSIFICANS PROGRESSIVA

This is a progressive inflammatory affection of the locomotor system of unknown origin, characterized by the gradual formation of bony masses in the fasciae, muscles, aponeuroses, tendons, ligaments and bones, with resulting ankylosis of most of the articulations (Steiner). The process begins in the neck or back, usually with swelling of the affected muscles, redness of the skin, and slight fever, or with small nodules in the muscles which appear and disappear. After subsiding an induration remains, which becomes progressively harder as the transformation into bone takes place. The disease may ultimately involve a majority of the skeletal muscles. Microdactylism of the thumbs and big toes is present in 75 per cent of the cases.

Local myositis ossificans may occur after repeated injuries or a single severe one. There are also nontraumatic and neurotic forms. It may follow an abdominal incision. The diagnosis has to be made from hematoma, new growth and exostoses. The history and X-ray study are important. This form usually reaches its maximum size rapidly, to remain stationary or diminish, usually the latter.

FIBROSITIS

Definition.—An inflammation of fibrous tissue which may occur in many parts of the body, involving ligaments, tendons, muscle sheaths, fasciae, aponeuroses, periosteum, nerve sheaths, or any part where fibrous tissue is found. It is associated with arthritis in many cases and to designate the involvement of special parts certain terms are employed, as synovitis, tenosynovitis, bursitis and perineuritis. Fibrositis is very common and causes many painful conditions often termed myalgia, "muscular rheumatism," neuritis, etc.

Etiology.—The essential cause is infection in the great majority of cases and usually from a local focus. Trauma, muscular strain and exposure to cold and wet are determining factors, especially in acute attacks. Prolonged strain on tendons or ligaments may be responsible for a chronic fibrositis, but infection is often added. It may follow exposure to a draught of air, as from an open window in a carriage or sudden chilling after heavy exertion may bring on an attack. Gouty persons seem prone to it. One attack renders an individual more liable to another. It is usually acute at first, but may become subacute or chronic, the last being more common in later life.

Pathology.—The changes are usually in the white fibrous tissue and are of an inflammatory nature. In acute cases there is a serous exudation in the affected parts and following this there may be proliferation of the fibrous tissue. This may extend between the muscle fibres and cause stiffness and pain. Disability with muscular atrophy may result. Nodules sometimes form which may be painful.

Symptoms.—In the acute forms the affection is usually local. The constitutional disturbance is slight, and, even in severe cases, there may be no fever. *Pain* is a prominent feature and may be constant or occur only when the structures are in certain positions or moved. It may be a dull ache, like the pain of a bruise, or sharp, severe, and cramp-like. It is often sufficiently intense to cause the patient to cry out. Pressure on the affected part usually gives relief. As a rule, the pain lasts from a few hours to a few days, although occasionally it is prolonged for weeks. It is very apt to recur.

There is a form occurring chiefly in the muscles of the head and neck, causing at first swelling and puffiness, later indurations. They are found particularly in the muscles at the back of the neck, but they are occasionally present in the muscles of the abdomen and limbs. The affection of the muscles of the head and neck may be associated with headache, the so-called *indurative headache.* Some are very similar to migraine. In the abdominal muscles these limited swellings may cause pain and suggest appendicitis.

The following are the principal varieties:

(1) "*Lumbago,*" a term which means nothing more than pain in the lower back, is due to many causes. (*a*) *Fibrositis,* in the muscles or fibrous tissue about the spine, is a common cause and may recur at short intervals. It comes on suddenly and may incapacitate the patient, any movement, particularly stooping or turning, causing severe pain. (*b*) *Ischemic lumbago,* described as a form of intermittent claudication, may be bilateral or unilateral and is excited by movement. The pain is between the twelfth rib and the crest of the ilium and may radiate forward. The area is not tender and the pain is dependent on muscular exertion. (*c*) *Static* conditions, due to faulty posture, which may be lateral (one leg shorter) or anteroposterior, flat feet, stooping, occupation, etc. (*d*) *Anatomical variations* of the fifth lumbar vertebra. (*e*) *Arthritis of the spine.* (*f*) *Sacro-iliac* joint strain or relaxation. (*g*) *Lumbosacral strain.* (*h*) *Neuritis* of the posterior nerve roots. (*i*) Pain due to *pelvic disease* in males (prostate, etc.) or females. (*j*) *Trauma,* especially with lifting in a stooped position. The diagnosis of "backache" as being due to fibrositis should only be made after other possibilities are excluded. In every case the effort should be made to arrive at an etiological diagnosis as only then is proper treatment possible. For the cases due to spondylitis or sacro-iliac joint disease some form of fixation is useful; faulty posture should be corrected and flat feet receive attention.

(2) Stiff neck or *torticollis* affects the muscles of the anterolateral or back region of the neck. It is very common, often unilateral, and occurs most frequently in the young. The patient holds the head in a peculiar manner turned to one side, and rotates the whole body in attempting to turn it.

(3) *Pleurodynia* involves the intercostal muscles on one side, and in some instances the pectorals and serratus magnus. This is, perhaps, the most painful form of the disease, as the chest can not be at rest. A deep breath or coughing causes pain, sometimes over a very limited area. It may be difficult to distinguish from intercostal neuralgia, in which the pain is usually more circumscribed and paroxysmal, and there are tender points along the course of the nerves. It is sometimes mistaken for pleurisy, but careful examination readily distinguishes between the affections.

(4) Among other forms are cephalodynia, affecting the muscles of the

head; scapulodynia, omodynia, and dorsodynia, affecting the muscles about the shoulder and upper part of the back. Fibrositis also occurs in the abdominal muscles, in the muscles of the extremities, in the tendons and about the joints. Bursitis (especially subdeltoid) may be due to it. In the legs it causes tenderness and pain, increased by use. Areas of thickening or infiltration may be palpated. Nodules are sometimes felt in the sole of the foot and in the hands. The chronic forms have soreness or pain associated with varying degrees of disability. There may be marked stiffness of the muscles, which are sometimes painful on pressure and may show definite tender areas of induration. Periosteal involvement gives pain and tenderness on pressure.

Panniculitis designates chronic inflammation of the panniculus adiposus. It occurs more often in women. The skin has a hard brawny feel over many areas and on the inner surfaces of the arms and thighs, over the abdomen and upper thorax there are small masses about the size of a pea, subcutaneous and tender. There may be tender lipomata also. Christian described a *relapsing febrile nodular panniculitis* with recurring attacks of fever and nodular inflammation of the subcutaneous tissue. There may be necrosis (gangrene?) of the fatty tissue with resulting atrophy and depression of the skin.

Diagnosis.—If a careful examination is made there should be little difficulty in recognizing the surface lesions but deeper ones give difficulty. Disease of the nerve roots or viscera should be excluded.

Treatment.—As a focus of infection is often responsible careful search should be made for any such and proper treatment given. If done early the chronic conditions are not likely to result. *Rest* of the affected parts is of the first importance, and it is well to protect them from cold by a covering of flannel. Fixation by strapping should be done wherever possible. No belief is more widespread among the public than in the efficacy of porous plasters for pains of all sorts. If the pain is severe and agonizing, a hypodermic of morphia gives relief. For lumbago acupuncture is, in acute cases, an efficient treatment. Needles of from three to four inches in length (ordinary bonnet-needles, sterilized, will do) are thrust into the lumbar muscles at the seat of pain, and withdrawn after five or ten minutes. In many cases the cautery gives relief and in obstinate cases blisters may be tried. *Heat* or counter-irritation in any form is useful and at the outset a Turkish bath may cut short an acute attack. Infra-red and ultraviolet light treatment may give relief. The bowels should be freely opened and large amounts of water taken. The salicylates are usually effectual; sodium salicylate (gr. x to xv, 0.6 to 1 gm.), acetylsalicylic acid (gr. x, 0.6 gm.), or salol (gr. v, 0.3 gm.) may be given. Some patients respond well to colchicum (♏ xv, 1 cc. of the wine). In chronic cases iodide may be used. Persons subject to this affection should be warmly clothed, and avoid, if possible, exposure to cold and damp. Massage usually is helpful; it should be given gently at first and more vigorously later. Use of the affected parts is advisable after the acute features are over. For the lumbar form, fixation is most useful by strapping or some form of support.

MYOTONIA CONGENITA (*Thomsen's Disease*)

Definition.—An affection characterized by tonic cramp of the muscles on attempting voluntary movements. The disease received its name from the physician who first described it, in whose family it existed for five generations.

While the disease is in a majority of cases hereditary, there are other forms of spasm very similar which may be acquired, and others still which are quite transitory. The nature of the affection is unknown. Dejerine and Sottas found hypertrophy of the primitive fibres with multiplication of the nuclei of all the muscles but not the heart. The spinal cord and nerves were intact. From Jacoby's studies it is doubtful whether these changes in the muscles are characteristic or peculiar to the disease. J. Koch found, with the muscle hypertrophy, degenerative and regenerative changes.

Etiology.—All the typical cases have occurred in family groups; a few isolated instances have been described in which similar features were present. Males are much more frequently affected; in 102 recorded cases, 91 were males and only 11 females (Hans Koch). The disease is rare in America and England; it seems more common in Germany and Scandinavia.

Symptoms.—The onset is in childhood. It is noticed that on account of the stiffness the children are not able to take part in ordinary games. The peculiarity is noticed only during voluntary movements. The contraction which the patient wills is slowly accomplished; the relaxation which the patient wills is also slow. The contraction often persists for a little time after he has dropped an object which he has picked up. In walking, the start is difficult; one leg is put forward slowly, it halts from stiffness for a second or two, and then after a few steps the legs become limber and he walks without any difficulty. The muscles of the arms and legs are those usually implicated; rarely the facial, ocular or laryngeal muscles. Emotion and cold aggravate the condition. In some instances there is mental weakness. The sensation and reflexes are normal. G. M. Hammond reported three cases in one family, in which the disease began at the eighth year and was confined to the arms. It was accompanied with slight mental feebleness. The condition of the muscles is interesting. The patients appear and are muscular, and there is sometimes definite muscular hypertrophy. The force is scarcely proportionate to the size. Erb described a characteristic reaction—the so-called *myotonic* reaction, the chief feature of which is that the contractions caused by either current attain their maximum slowly and relax slowly, and vermicular, wave-like contractions pass from the cathode to the anode. The disease is incurable but may be arrested temporarily. No treatment is known.

MYOTONIA ATROPHICA (*Dystrophia Myotonica*)

This is a slowly progressive form of muscular atrophy affecting special muscles, with delayed relaxation of muscular contractions. It was formerly regarded as an atypical form of Thomsen's disease. The disease is hereditary and familial in many cases but not in all. Males are affected more often; the onset is usually between the ages of 20 and 30. There is an overgrowth of connective tissue with degeneration of the muscle fibres.

Symptoms.—The onset is insidious, usually with the myotonia preceding the atrophy but the reverse may occur. The myotonia is usually most evident in the hands. The atrophy appears in one of several groups of muscles: (1) The head and neck group, especially the muscles of the eyelids and the sternomastoids, (2) the muscles of the forearms, and (3) the anterior and lateral muscles of the legs, especially the quadriceps extensor and vasti. The inability to close the eyes, the hanging lower lip and the curious facial expression, if myotonia is present, give a characteristic appearance. There are many associated conditions. *Cataract* develops in one-third of the cases, usually matures rapidly and may occur in otherwise healthy members of the family. Loss of hair, changes in the teeth and skin, emaciation, loss of tendon reflexes and sensory disturbances may follow. The *diagnosis* from Thomsen's disease is made by the muscular atrophy and by the dystrophic features. The *course* is prolonged and in some the progress stops. The treatment is directed to the general health and to the relief of symptoms.

PARAMYOCLONUS MULTIPLEX (*Essential Myoclonia*)

Definition.—An affection described by Friedreich, characterized by irregular clonic contractions, chiefly of the muscles of the extremities, occurring either constantly or in paroxysms.

Etiology.—Hysteria, emotion, fright, trauma and parathyroid disease have been suggested as possible causes but the etiology is unknown. The disease may occur in several generations.

Pathology.—The nature of the disease is unknown. Pierce Clark suggested that it is an abiotrophy of the *corpus striatum.*

Symptoms.—The characteristic features are the short, sudden and lightning-like contractions, not rhythmic and of equal intensity, and without the synergic quality of a purposive movement. The two sides may be unequally involved and single muscles may be affected. The face and fingers are not often affected. Sensation is not involved; the reflexes are increased. The movements are usually absent during sleep.

Diagnosis.—The disease may be confounded with the various symptomatic myoclonias seen in the tics, chronic chorea and the rhythmic movements associated with midbrain lesions. The myoclonia with epilepsy (Unverricht) is described elsewhere.

Treatment.—Various forms of suggestion may be tried, but the disease may prove very resistant. The movements may cease spontaneously.

MYASTHENIA GRAVIS

Definition.—A disease with fatigue symptoms in the muscular system, due to failure of innervation without definite changes in muscles or nerves.

Etiology.—Of 180 cases collected by McCarthy, 83 were males and 96 females. In women the disease usually occurs before the age of twenty-five, in males in middle life. Of 56 autopsies, 17 showed hyperplasia or persistence of the thymus and 10 a thymic tumor, one of which was malignant. Degenerative lesions are found in the adrenal glands. Examination of the nervous system has revealed no constant abnormality. There may be degenerative lesions such as chromatolysis, hemorrhages and pigment formation. Lymphorrages are found in the skeletal muscles and occasionally in the myocardium.

The excretion of creatinine is decreased. The difficulty may be at the myoneural junction and acetylcholine seems to be concerned in the transmission of the stimulus from the nerve endings to the muscle fibres. There may be disturbance of the liberation of acetylcholine or it may be too rapidly destroyed.

Symptoms.—The striking feature is weakness of the voluntary muscles, rapidly produced by exertion and disappearing with rest. Ptosis is the first manifestation in many cases. The muscles innervated by the bulb are first affected—those of the eyes, face, of mastication and of the neck. After effort the muscles show fatigue, and if persisted in they fail to act and paresis or complete paralysis follows. All the voluntary muscles may become involved. After rest the power is recovered. In severe cases paralysis may persist. The *myasthenic reaction* of Jolly is the rapid exhaustion of the muscles by faradism, not by galvanism. There are marked remissions and fluctuations in the symptoms. Very acute cases occur. Probably there are many unrecognized mild cases.

The *diagnosis* is made from the ptosis, the facial expression, the nasal speech, the rapid fatigue of the muscles, the myasthenic reaction, the absence of atrophy, tremors, etc., and the remarkable variations in the intensity of the symptoms. Of 180 collected cases 72 proved fatal; sudden death may occur, sometimes from respiratory paralysis. The patient may live for many years and recovery take place. In *treatment,* absolute rest, both general and local, is important. Muscular fatigue should be avoided. Strychnine may be given in large doses hypodermically. Alternate courses of iodide and mercury may be tried. X-ray treatment of the thymus gland seems worthy of a trial. The use of glycocoll (glycine—*not glycin*) and ephedrine as in muscular dystrophies seems worth a trial. They should be given for a period of months, the glycocoll in doses of 10 to 20 grams a day and ephedrine gr. 1/8 to 3/8 three times a day. The use of physostigmine (eserine) or prostigmin (an analogue of physostigmine) results in improvement in a short time which lasts for five to eight hours. Physostigmine salicylate is given hypodermically (gr. 1/60-1/50) or by mouth (gr. 1/30 but larger amounts have been used apparently safely). Prostigmin is given hypodermically in doses of 2-5 cc. of the preparation. Belladonna or atropine in the usual dosage is given before or with the other drugs to lessen unpleasant effects.

AMYOTONIA CONGENITA (*Oppenheim's Disease*)

A congenital affection characterized by general or local hypotonus of the voluntary muscles. Oppenheim gave the name *myatonia,* but this is so similar to *myotonia* (Thomsen's disease) that the name *amyotonia* of English writers is preferable. Collier and Wilson give the following definition: "A condition of extreme flaccidity of the muscles, associated with an entire loss of the deep reflexes, most marked at the time of birth and always showing a tendency to slow and progressive amelioration. There is great weakness, but no absolute paralysis of any of the muscles. The limbs are most affected; the face is almost always exempt. The muscles are small and soft, but there is no local wasting. Contractures are prone to occur in the course of time. The faradic excitability in the muscles is lowered and strong faradic stimuli are borne without complaint. No other symptoms indicative of lesions of the nervous system occur." The changes are variable—increase in the muscle nuclei, many very small muscle fibres, a few large fibres, marked increase in connective tissue and fat, defective myelination of the nerves, and reduction in the number of ventral horn cells of the cord. The disease seems to come in the group of abiotrophies—a failure in the proper development of the lower motor neurone. Complete recovery is rare but considerable improvement may occur.

DISEASES OF THE JOINTS

ARTHRITIS DEFORMANS

Definition.—A disease of the joints, often the result of infection, characterized by changes in the synovial membranes, cartilage, and peri-articular structures, and in some cases by atrophic and hypertrophic changes in the bones. A tendency to a chronic course is the rule.

Long believed to be associated with gout and rheumatic fever, this relationship is disproved. There is a difference of opinion as to whether there are two distinct diseases or varying forms of the same disease included under this heading. Those who hold the former view consider that in one disease the synovial membranes and peri-articular tissues are particularly affected (rheumatoid arthritis) and in the other disease the cartilage and bone (osteo-arthritis). There are general differences in the age of the patients and character of the lesions. One is more inflammatory and the other more degenerative, but rheumatoid arthritis may attack an elderly person and osteo-arthritis a young individual. Certain patients show lesions of both forms. Many seem to have an infective process at first and later degenerative changes. The disease is common and to it belong many of the cases termed "chronic rheumatism."

Etiology.—AGE.—A majority of the cases are between the ages of twenty and fifty. In A. E. Garrod's analysis of 500 cases there were only 25 under twenty years of age. In 40 per cent of our series of 500 cases, the onset was before the age of thirty years. In the group with rheumatoid changes predominating the age of onset is usually lower than in the group with osteo-arthritic changes.

SEX.—Among Garrod's cases there were 411 in women. Practically half of our series were males. The incidence as to sex is influenced by the inclusion of the cases of spondylitis, of which a large majority is in males. In women an association with the menopause has been noted.

In America the incidence in the negro is relatively much less than in the white. Occupation and the station in life do not seem to have any special influence. Exposure to cold, wet and damp, errors in diet, worry and care, and local injuries are spoken of as causes, but play only a predisposing part.

INFECTION.—This is the most important single factor and the evidence suggests varieties of streptococci as responsible. This seems more probable than that the disease is due to a specific organism. The divergent results of bacteriological studies are striking. The significance of the presence of agglutinins is not clear. The possible sources of infection are many but infection of the mouth and throat probably takes first place. Abscesses about the teeth should always be searched for (X-ray study) and the tonsils carefully examined. Other sources are: infection of the nose or sinuses, pyorrhea alveolaris, otitis media, chronic bronchitis, infection of the biliary or urinary tract, pelvic disease in women, and infection of the prostate and seminal vesicles in men. The possibility of streptococcal infection from the intestinal tract must be considered although this is difficult to prove.

The acute onset, with fever in many cases, the polyarthritis, the presence of enlarged glands, the frequent enlargement of the spleen, the occurrence of pleurisy, endocarditis and pericarditis in some cases, are all suggestive of an infection. The likeness of the lesions to those in arthritis from a specific cause, such as the gonococcus, is suggestive and also the association of the arthritis with definite foci of infection in many cases.

METABOLIC.—While the nutrition suffers in many cases there does not seem evidence that the disease is due to disturbance of metabolism. Pemberton has emphasized the lowered carbohydrate tolerance in some cases.

Thyroid Gland.—There are forms of joint disturbance with hypothyroidism, usually degenerative, which may belong here.

Heredity.—A striking incidence of the disease is found in certain families but beyond this little can be said.

Morbid Anatomy.—The usual descriptions are of the late stages when extensive damage has occurred, for opportunities to study the early changes are few, although operations and skiagrams have aided much. There are three main forms of change: (1) Lesions principally in the synovial membranes and peri-articular tissues (rheumatoid arthritis), (2) with atrophic changes in the cartilage and bones predominating, and (3) with hypertrophy and overgrowth of bone (osteo-arthritis). The first and second are most frequent in the joints of the extremities, the third in the spine. In some cases all forms of change are found, which speaks against the view that there are two distinct diseases. The changes in general are: (1) *Effusion,* which is not constant and shows no special features. (2) Changes in the *synovial membrane.* These are inflammatory and often hemorrhagic at the onset. There may be marked thickening and proliferation of the synovial fringes with the formation of villi—*villous arthritis.* (3) The *capsule* and surrounding tissues may be infiltrated and swollen. The peri-articular tissues show infiltration and swelling, and the enlargement of the joint is often due to swelling about it. (4) *Cartilage.* This may show erosion, ulceration, atrophy or proliferation. It may disappear entirely, but the changes are often irregular and uneven and the cartilage may be replaced by fibrous tissue or by bone, the latter being most common at the edge of the cartilage. The cartilages may be soft and gradually absorbed or thinned (this often begins opposite the point of greatest involvement of the synovial membrane). (5) *Bone.* This may show atrophy of varying grade. If the cartilage is completely absorbed the surface of the bone may become hard and eburnated. In the *hypertrophic* form there is new bone formation which is most common at the edge of the articular surfaces. In the hip joint this may form an irregular ring of bone about the joint cavity. The commonest example of overgrowth of bone is seen in the "Heberden's nodes," bony outgrowths at the terminal interphalangeal joints. There may be deposit of new bone in the ligaments, particularly in the spine, which may be converted into a rigid bony column. Proliferation of bone usually occurs at the margins of the joints in the form of irregular nodules—osteophytes. Bony ankylosis is rare in the peripheral joints but common in the spine.

There may be extensive *secondary* changes. Muscular atrophy is common and may appear with great rapidity. Subluxation may occur, especially in the knee and finger joints. The hands often show great deformity, particularly ulnar deflection. Contractures may follow and the joints become fixed in a flexed position. Neuritis and trophic disturbances may be associated; the neuritis is sometimes due to direct extension of the inflammatory process. Subcutaneous nodules occasionally occur. Local changes in the circulation are marked.

The skiagrams show the changes very well. Erosion of the cartilage is easily seen. In the type with predominant peri-articular changes the cartilage and bone may show little alteration. The occurrence of various changes in different joints or even in the same joint is common and bony change may occur with marked involvement of the peri-articular tissues.

Symptoms.—The *onset* may be acute or gradual. In the acute form a number of joints may be involved with high fever and the picture suggests rheumatic fever. In other cases the onset is acute in one joint and others are involved a few days later. With the gradual onset one joint is attacked and others follow. Some cases are between and may be termed subacute. In cases with an acute onset the attack may not persist very long; with the chronic onset the duration is usually prolonged. The acute onset occurs more frequently in the rheumatoid form.

ARTHRITIS.—In the acute form the joints are swollen, tender, and hot to the touch, but do not often show marked redness. There may be effusion in the larger joints. *Pain* is severe and increased by movement, the patient usually taking the position of greatest ease. When a joint is once attacked, the process does not subside quickly, and when the arthritis lessens some change remains in the joint which, however, may be very slight. The joints of the spine, especially in the cervical region, may be involved in the more acute forms, and in these there is rarely any permanent change. The temporomaxillary joint is often involved, and arthritis here is always suggestive of this disease. The hands, when involved, show very characteristic changes. The knuckle joints are red, swollen, tender and show limitation of motion. The fingers are often involved; swelling of the interphalangeal joints is common with a resulting thickening which gives a fusiform appearance. Partial dislocation, particularly at the terminal joint, is common. The knee joints are often affected, with pain, effusion, limitation of motion and later villous arthritis or subluxation. Thickening of the capsule usually occurs early.

In the *hypertrophic* (osteo-arthritic) form the process is rarely as acute as in rheumatoid arthritis but is usually polyarticular. The terminal finger joints, the hip joint and the spine are especially affected. Pain is usually severe and the local features not so marked. This form is likely to be chronic. However, it may not be very disabling.

HEBERDEN'S NODES.—These are small bony outgrowths ("little hard knobs" —Heberden) at the terminal phalangeal joints. They are much more common in women than in men. Heberden says "they have no connection with gout," yet they are often regarded as gouty. In the early stage the joints may be swollen, tender, and slightly red, particularly when injured. The attacks of pain and swelling may come on at long intervals or follow injury. Sometimes they are the first manifestation of a general arthritis. Their distribution is not always regular and they are often largest on the fingers most used. They may be found in patients in whose larger joints the arthritis is of the other form. The condition is not curable; but the subjects whose arthritis begins in this way rarely have severe involvement of the larger joints.

The MONARTICULAR FORM affects chiefly old persons, particularly in the hip and shoulder. It is identical with the general disease. The muscles show wasting early and in the hip the condition is that described as *mobus coxae senilis*. These cases not infrequently follow injury. They differ from the polyarticular form in occurring chiefly in men and in later life.

THE VERTEBRAL FORM (*Spondylitis*).—This may occur alone or with involvement of the peripheral joints. With an acute polyarthritis of the peripheral joints the spine may be involved, but there is usually no permanent change. With the *hypertrophic* form there is often bony proliferation and some spinal rigidity results which may involve the whole spine or only a part; in the latter case the lower dorsal and lumbar regions suffer most frequently. It may not involve more than a few vertebrae. The features are as variable as in the peripheral joints and there may be repeated acute attacks or a steady progressive process. In the general involvement the ribs may be fixed, the thorax immobile, and the breathing abdominal. There are two varieties of general involvement which are sometimes regarded as special diseases. In one (von Bechterew) the spine alone is involved, and there are pronounced nerve root symptoms—pain, anesthesia, atrophy of the muscles, and ascending degeneration of the cord. In the other—Strümpell-Marie type—the hip and shoulder joints may be involved (spondylose rhizomélique), and the nervous symptoms are less prominent. Both are forms of arthritis deformans, and should neither be regarded nor described as separate diseases. Spondylitis deformans is more frequent in males, and trauma plays a part in its etiology. Local involvement is particularly common in the lumbar region and may cause sciatica and a great variety of referred pains (radicular syndrome). Pressure on the nerve roots causes pain, paresthesia and muscle atrophy. These nerve root pains may be mistaken for evidence of thoracic or abdominal disease. Movement of the spine is usually restricted.

ARTHRITIS DEFORMANS IN CHILDREN.—Some cases are like the disease in adults, in others there are striking differences. In a variety described by Still, the arthritis is associated with enlargement of the lymph nodes and the spleen. The onset is usually before the second dentition and girls are more frequently affected than boys. At first there is slight stiffness in one or two joints; others are gradually involved. The onset may be acute with fever or chills. The enlargement of the joints is due rather to peri-articular thickening than to bony change. The limitation of movement may be extreme and there may be much muscular wasting. The enlargement of the lymph nodes is striking, increases with fever, and may be general; the epitrochlear glands may be very large. The spleen can usually be felt. Sweating is often profuse and there may be anemia, but heart complications are rare. The children look puny and generally show arrest of development.

GENERAL FEATURES.—*Fever*.—In acute attacks this may be 102° or 103° F., but is frequently lower and often persists for weeks with a maximum about 100° F. The *pulse* is rapid in proportion to the fever, a frequent range being from 90 to 110. Cardiac changes are found in a small proportion of cases. *Glandular enlargement* is common and may be general or especially marked in the glands related to the affected joints. The *spleen* is enlarged in some cases, the frequency being greater in the younger patients. *Subcutaneous nodules* occur and are sometimes tender. The *blood* often shows a slight anemia, not as marked as might be expected from the appearance of the patients. There is rarely much increase in the leukocytes and the differential count shows no peculiarity. The *sedimentation rate* may show acceleration, more in the rheumatoid group. The *urine* does not show any change of moment. The *skin* sometimes shows irregular areas of yellow pigmentation, especially on the face and arms. It may have a glossy appearance over the affected joints. Profuse sweating of the hands and feet is common. The *reflexes* are usually increased in acute cases and a return to normal is of good significance. They are sometimes absent. Muscular *atrophy* is common and sometimes advances rapidly. It is most marked in the hands. Muscular twitching is not uncommon.

In some patients the bony atrophy is very marked. This is most common in females. In these disorganization of the joints occurs and the cartilage rapidly disappears. These cases usually progress rapidly downward. This atrophy is to be distinguished from that due to disuse.

COURSE.—*General Progressive Form.*—This occurs in two varieties, acute and chronic. The *acute* form may resemble, at its outset, rheumatic fever. There is involvement of many joints; swelling, particularly of the synovial sheaths but not often redness; there is fever which is often persistent and may be from 99° to 100° F. for weeks. This pulse rate is usually high in proportion to the fever. There may be repeated acute attacks, perhaps at intervals of years, or there may be repeated attacks in various joints. These usually leave definite changes, which may be slight at first, but tend to increase with subsequent attacks. Some cases progress very rapidly with loss of weight and strength; atrophy and arthritic deformity are marked.

The *chronic* form is more common, although many have an acute attack at some time, especially at the onset. The first symptoms are pain on movement and slight swelling, which may be in the joint itself or peri-articular. In some cases the effusion is marked, in others slight. The local conditions vary greatly, and periods of improvement alternate with remissions. At first only one or two joints are affected, gradually others are involved, and in extreme cases every joint is affected. Pain is variable; some proceed to the most extreme deformity without severe pain; in others the suffering is very great, particularly at night and during exacerbations. There are cases in which pain of an agonizing character is almost constant, quite apart from acute disturbances. Pain has an important influence in the production of deformity, as it hinders movement and the joints are kept in the position of greatest ease. An onset about the *menopause* is not rare and usually in women who are overweight. The features are rarely acute with pain and stiffness predominating. The course tends to be chronic. The possibility of hypothyroidism, which may have arthritic features, should be remembered.

Gradually the shape of the joints is altered, partly by thickening of the capsule and surrounding tissues, perhaps by osteophytes, and by muscular contraction. Crepitus may be felt in the affected joint. Ultimately the joints may become immobile, not by a true bony ankylosis, although it may be by the osteophytes which form around the articular surfaces, but more often from adhesions and peri-articular thickening. There is often an acute atrophy of the muscles and atrophy from disuse supervenes, so that contractures tend to flex the thigh upon the abdomen and the leg upon the thigh. Numbness, tingling, pigmentation, or glossiness of the skin, and onychia may be present. In extreme cases the patient is helpless, and lies with the legs drawn up and the arms fixed. Fortunately, in these severe cases the joints of the hand may not be much affected, and the patient can knit or write, though unable to walk. In many cases, after involving two or three joints, the disease becomes arrested. A majority of the patients finally reach a quiescent stage, in which they enjoy fair health, suffering from the inconvenience and crippling. Coincident affections are not uncommon. A small number show cardiac lesions and the pulse rate is usually higher than normal. In the *Felty syndrome* there is chronic arthritis, splenomegaly and leukopenia in adults.

Diagnosis.—The cases with an acute onset may be difficult to distinguish from *rheumatic fever*. The affected joints are rarely as tender as in rheumatic fever, and the smaller joints are more often involved. The presence of thickening in a joint, rapid muscular atrophy, a relatively high pulse rate in relation to the fever (in the absence of endocarditis), and the absence of response to salicylate medication speak against rheumatic fever. The diagnosis from *gonorrheal arthritis* may be difficult, but in this the small joints are usually not attacked so often, and after an onset with polyarthritis the majority of the affected joints clear, leaving one joint particularly involved. This rarely occurs in arthritis deformans. A careful search for gonococci is an aid. In the chronic stage there may be difficulty in distinguishing this disease from *gout*. This is particularly marked in either disease without marked joint changes. The study of the skiagrams is helpful and marked peri-articular changes speak for arthritis deformans. The finding of tophi or the estimation of the uric acid content of the blood may give the diagnosis of gout. Changes in joints due to "wear and tear" are much like those of arthritis deformans. It is important to distinguish *subdeltoid bursitis* from the monarticular form in the shoulder; the X-ray study is a great aid, as also in the recognition of disease of the *sacro-iliac* joint, *tuberculosis* of the *hip joint* and spondylitis. Special importance attaches to the diagnosis of the spinal forms. There is no difficulty in the case of general involvement, but with local changes in the lower spine it is not so easy. Pain on and restriction of movement are important; the patient is careful to limit any motion of the spine. The root pains may be mistaken for evidence of visceral disease. Tuberculosis of the spine rarely offers any difficulty, especially with skiagrams.

Prognosis.—The age, general circumstances, character of the patient, the extent of arthritis, and the variety are all important. The outlook is not as dark as is usually described. If the source of infection can be found *early* and properly treated the prognosis is encouraging. In many patients the disease runs a certain course, and, if they can be brought through it with a minimum of damage, the ultimate outlook is good. In the rheumatoid form, early diagnosis, treatment of the source of infection, the preservation of good nutrition, and a patient who is willing to fight are encouraging factors. The outlook in the cases with the acute attacks is usually better than in those with a more chronic progressive course. Rapid muscular atrophy is of grave import. Cases in women beginning about the menopause are usually obstinate. Rapid advancement in the joint changes is serious. In children the outlook is not good but some recover entirely. The group with osteoarthritis usually do well. Heberden's nodes are permanent, but in the larger joints it is rare for the condition to advance to absolute crippling, although there may be considerable interference with function. Spondylitis rarely advances to complete immobility of the whole spine. The outlook is good in the local cases, but depends somewhat on the occupation and possibility of trauma. The general condition is of importance and in those with marked nervous features the prognosis is not good.

Treatment.—Much depends on proper management and the pessimistic attitude is not justified. Too much stress can not be placed on the need of early diagnosis; the disease is often regarded as "rheumatic" and the treatment directed to this (especially restriction of diet and the giving of salicylates for long periods) is usually harmful. The patient should be studied as a whole; he needs treatment as much as his joints.

Source of Infection.—Every effort should be made to find any such and prompt treatment carried out. Infection of the teeth and tonsils has always to be excluded. The possible sources of infection are many.

General Measures.—The patient should be kept out of doors as much as possible and every effort made to improve the general health. The *diet* should be the most nourishing possible. The mistake of cutting down the proteins is often made. Regard must be had to the digestion and it is more often the carbohydrates which should be reduced. Water should be freely given, as elimination is important. The bowels should be kept open, and for this the salines are useful. It is important to see that the patients are warmly clad in cold weather and guarded against chilling. *Hydrotherapy* is useful locally in the form of compresses. The hot bath treatment, so often given, often does harm, particularly in acute cases. Baths, when taken, should be of short duration. In more chronic cases bathing is sometimes of value. *Massage* is especially useful in the rheumatoid form and in it passive motion should be used early. *Climate* is of value in so far as the patient is able to be out of doors and avoids rapid changes of temperature. In obese women about the menopause, a low diet, iodide, thyroid gland extract sometimes, and physiotherapy are useful.

Medicinal.—There is no drug which essentially influences the disease. The salicylates may aid in relieving pain, but should not be given for long periods. Iron, arsenic, and iodine are often useful. Iodine may be given as the tincture in doses of five to ten drops. Thyroid and thymus gland extracts given persistently are sometimes beneficial. For the *pain* it is necessary to give drugs, although local measures should be used as much as possible. There are many which are available. Acetylsalicylic acid (gr. v, 0.6 gm.), guaiacol carbonate (gr. v, 0.3 gm.), antipyrine (gr. iii, 0.2 gm.), and sometimes codeine (gr. ½, 0.03 gm.), are useful. Morphia should not be given on account of the danger of a habit.

Local.—(*a*) Use of the joints must be governed by the condition. When the cartilage and bones are not involved, passive motion and massage are useful, followed later by active motion. The patient should be taught simple exercises. When the cartilage and bones are involved, *rest* is usually advisable for a time. Every effort should be made to avoid contracture and displacement, and in this the use of splints during the night is often valuable. Caution should be exercised in advising complete fixation. This is sometimes useful for short periods but may result in fixation and is usually not advisable. (*b*) *Counterirritation.* This is usually an aid, and the cautery, blisters, mustard and iodine may be used. It is usually better to use light counterirritation frequently than severe at longer intervals. (*c*) *Hyperemia.* This may be active. Various forms of light therapy may be used. (*d*) *Hydrotherapy.* The persistent use of compresses is often of value. (*e*) With diminished circulation in and about the joints measures to improve this are indicated, such as histamine subcutaneously in doses of 0.1-0.5 mg., two or three times a week. The reaction varies greatly. It may be used with ionization. *Vaccines* and *filtrates.* These may be of definite value. The dose should be small and reactions avoided.

Surgical Measures.—These are useful for the correction of deformities. In villous arthritis operation is usually indicated. In the group with marked hypertrophy of bone removal of the outgrowths may be helpful.

Special Forms.—(*a*) *Heberden's nodes.* Avoidance of irritation and injury is important, and in the case of pain the use of compresses is helpful. (*b*) *Spondylitis.* During the acute stages rest is essential and should be secured by a plaster jacket or simple apparatus. In the milder forms firm strapping may give relief. Trauma should be avoided. (*c*) *Knee joint.* An elastic support is useful and may save the joint from injury.

Foreign Protein.—This has proved useful, given intravenously as proteose (1-2 cc. of a 4 per cent solution) or as typhoid vaccine (75-150 millions). A sharp reaction is necessary if benefit is to result.

Arthritis Secondary to Acute Infection.—While the majority of cases of arthritis are secondary to some infection, it is important to recognize various forms. (1) Those with a definite bacterial cause, such as gonorrheal or tuberculous arthritis. These usually have fairly well defined features. (2) Those secondary to infections of doubtful etiology, such as typhus fever or measles. In some of these the arthritis is due to a secondary infection but in others it appears to be due to the specific cause of the disease. (3) Arthritis secondary to infections with no evidence of any organism in the joint. These are comparatively common and are difficult to designate. For example, arthritis, which is not of long duration, may occur with tonsillitis. These have been termed "toxic" or "toxemic" arthritis. The term "infectious" arthritis, sometimes applied, is not a satisfactory one. The cases in this group usually clear without permanent damage, but if long continued they may result in the changes included under arthritis deformans.

"Chronic Rheumatism."—This term deserves mention because it is so commonly used, but its retention is not justified. There is no uniformity in its usage and it is applied without discrimination to all kinds of arthritis and frequently to conditions which have nothing to do with the joints. Painful conditions of the joints, muscles, faciae, bones, and nerves are all termed "rheumatism." There is no disease entity to which the term can be applied, and it would be an advantage to give it up entirely.

INTERMITTENT HYDRARTHROSIS

The condition was described by Perrin in 1845. It is characterized by a remarkable periodic swelling of one or several joints without fever. The knee is usually involved, sometimes the hip, elbow or wrist joints. The intervals between attacks vary from 2 to 20 days with an average of 12 days. The swelling may take place with great rapidity, and there may be a sensation of water rushing into the joint. There are usually pain and stiffness. The periods may be from ten to twelve days, a month or even three months. Many of the cases are in women and sometimes with marked nervous symptoms. While some cases are secondary and represent a phase in the evolution of various articular lesions, there is a primary form characterized by periodic swelling and nothing else. It is sometimes the joint equivalent to Quincke's edema and may be associated with erythema or angioneurotic edema. Some cases are due to allergy and treatment of this may be useful. The prognosis is not good; the attacks are apt to occur in spite of all treatment. Miller and Lewis obtained good results from the use of foreign protein (dead typhoid bacilli).

DISEASES OF THE BONES

HYPERTROPHIC PULMONARY OSTEO-ARTHROPATHY

Definition.—A symmetrical enlargement of the bones of the hands and feet, and of the distal ends of the long bones, occurring in association with certain chronic diseases, particularly affections of the lungs.

Bamberger in 1889 described abnormal thickening of the long bones in bronchiectasis, and in 1890 Marie described cases and gave the name.

Etiology.—*Clubbing* of the fingers, or the Hippocratic fingers, represent a minor manifestation of this condition. Many varieties occur; there is a monograph with sketches of some thirty forms. It is met with perhaps most constantly in congenital disease of the heart, in tuberculosis and in other affections of the lungs, particularly bronchiectasis, in chronic jaundice, and in other chronic affections. In thoracic aneurism it may involve only one hand. It usually comes on very slowly, but cases have been described of an acute appearance within a week or two. It may disappear. There is no bony alteration, but a fibrous thickening of the connective tissues with turgescence of the vessels. The condition is not easy to explain. The mechanical effect of congestion, the usual feature, explains the heart and lung cases, but not those of congenital syphilis and diseases of the liver. Some attribute it to a toxin.

Marie's syndrome is met with: (1) In diseases of the lungs and pleura, as in 43 of 55 cases collected by Thayer and in 68 of Wynn's 100 cases. Bronchiectasis is the most common, then pulmonary tuberculosis and empyema. (2) Other affections, such as chronic diarrhea, chronic jaundice, nephritis, and congenital syphilis. Marie regards the process as resulting from the absorption of toxins causing a periostitis; others have regarded it as a low form of tuberculous infection. The bones most frequently involved are the lower ends of the radius and ulna and the metacarpals, more rarely the lower end of the humerus, and the lower ends of the tibia and fibula.

Symptoms.—The affection comes on gradually, unnoticed by the patient. In other cases there is great sensitiveness of the ends of the long bones and of the fingers and toes. The fully developed condition is easily recognized. The hands are large, the terminal phalanges swollen, the nails large and much curved. Similar changes occur in the toes, and the feet look large, especially the toes and the malleoli. The bones of the forearms are diffusely thickened, particularly near the wrist, and the tibiae and the fibulae are greatly enlarged. Sometimes in advanced cases both ankles and knee joints stand out prominently. The hypertrophy rarely affects the other long bones, though occasionally the extremities of the humerus and femur may be involved. The bones of the head are not attacked. Kyphosis may occur.

Diagnosis.—There is rarely any difficulty, as the picture presented by the hands and feet differs from that in acromegaly, and in practically all cases it is a secondary condition. *Treatment* should be directed to the primary disease; otherwise it is symptomatic.

OSTEITIS DEFORMANS (*Paget's Disease*)

Definition.—A chronic affection of the bones characterized by enlargement and deformity, affecting the skull, tibiae, femora, pelvis, spine, clavicle, ribs and radii. These are especially dorsocervical kyphosis, enlargement of the clavicles, spreading of the lower thorax and forward bowing of the legs.

The affection was described first by Sir James Paget, in 1877.

Etiology.—The generalized form is a rare disease. The etiology is unknown. Some have regarded it as luetic, others as due to arteriosclerosis, which is a constant lesion. Internal secretion disturbance is not proved.

Pathology.—The skull, spine, and long bones are chiefly affected; those of the face, hands and feet are less involved. The skull may be three quarters of an inch in thickness and its circumference is increased. In one of Paget's cases it measured 71 cm. The shafts of the long bones are greatly thickened and they may weigh twice as much as a normal bone. The femur is bent, the convexity forward, the tibae may be huge and very much bowed anteriorly. The bones of the arms are less often involved; the spine shows marked kyphosis, sometimes partial ankylosis; the pelvis is broadened.

The process is a rarefying osteitis involving the centre of the bones with new bone formation, especially subperiosteal. The calcium and phosphorus content of the blood are normal but the blood phosphatase is high.

Symptoms.—The disease begins, as a rule, in the sixth decade, sometimes with indefinite pains, but more frequently the patient notices first that the head begins to enlarge, so that he has to buy a larger hat. Then his friends notice that he is growing shorter, and that the legs are getting more and more bowed. There is a painful variety with great soreness of the arms and legs, which may be much worse at night. Headache, bronchitis and pigmentation of the skin have been noted. The reduction in stature is very remarkable; one patient lost 13 inches in height.

Diagnosis.—The disease is readily recognized. The face differs from acromegaly, in which it is ovoid or egg-shaped with the large end down, while in Paget's disease the face is triangular with the base upward. In a few cases the disease may be limited to one or a few bones. There is a variety involving the tibiae and fibulae alone, and in some the femurs to a slight extent. These bones gradually enlarge, are bowed anteriorly and laterally, so that the only obvious features are a reduction in height with bowing of the legs. There is also a variety, sometimes known as tumor-forming osteitis deformans, in which the bones are much deformed with multiple hyperostosis and new growths. The X-ray findings in Paget's disease are characteristic and it is recognized first, not infrequently, by the X-ray study.

Treatment.—With evidence of syphilis active treatment should be given. Sedatives may be required to relieve the pain. Calcium and vitamin D should be given freely. Ultraviolet light and X-ray therapy may be tried.

LEONTIASIS OSSEA

In this disease there is hyperostosis of the bones of the cranium, and sometimes those of the face. The disease usually begins in early life. The *symptoms* are due to encroachment on the cranial contents and contraction of the orbits and nasal fossae with pressure on the vessels and nerves. Headache may be an early symptom. The bony tumors may compress the brain and cause cerebral symptoms which may suggest tumor. The enlargement of the head is usually marked and the X-ray study is important in diagnosis especially of the tumors of the inner table of the skull. Surgery may be required to relieve pressure.

OSTEOGENESIS IMPERFECTA

(*Fragilitas Ossium, Osteopsathyrosis, Lobstein's Disease*)

Definition.—A prenatal and postnatal defective activity of the osteoblasts, rendering the bones abnormally brittle. It is often hereditary and is sometimes associated with a peculiar shape of the head and blue sclerotics.

History.—Lobstein described the disease as osteopsathyrosis in 1833, while Vrolik in 1849 described the prenatal form as *osteogenesis imperfecta.* Some thought the conditions were not identical but the general opinion is that they are the same, and that *idiopathic fragilitas ossium,* whether prenatal or postnatal, is due to a deficient activity of the osteoblasts, whether in subperiosteal or chondral ossification (Bronson). The terms *osteogenesis imperfecta congenita* and *tarda* describe the two conditions.

Etiology.—Nothing is known except the single factor of heredity which occurs in a variable number of cases. Davenport and Conrad state that the heredity is typically direct and that the factor is a dominant one. The younger half of the family of an osteopsathyrotic parent will be affected, "but if neither parent, though of affected stock, has shown the tendency, then the expectation is that none of the children will have brittle bones." Biotypes occur, in some families the femur only, in some the humerus only is affected. The utilization of calcium, phosphorus and magnesium seems to be low.

Symptoms.—In the prenatal cases the child is often premature and stillborn, the extremities short and thick with many fractures in all stages of healing. The head may feel like a crepitant bag of bones. The head may show a bitemporal enlargement. In the postnatal cases the onset is usually after infancy. While the liability to fracture, as a rule, decreases with years, it may persist until the age of fifty. Slight blows may cause a fracture, of which a child may have a score or more before puberty. As a rule, they are painless and heal readily.

Treatment.—Care should be taken to avoid fractures and, if they occur, every effort made to prevent deformity. Calcium, phosphorus and vitamin D should be given. Thymus gland appears to have been useful.

Blue Sclerotics.—Eddowes first described this remarkable condition which is more common in the inherited form. It may occur in individuals of the family who have never had fractures. It is not due to any color in the sclera itself but to increased transparency, possibly depending upon the absence of lime salts in the connective tissue. Some patients have otosclerosis also.

OSTEOMALACIA (*Mollities Ossium*)

This disease is characterized by pain, muscular weakness, and softness of the bones, due to decalcification, resulting in fractures and deformity. The great majority of the cases are in women; repeated pregnancies may play a part. Deficiency in vitamin D may be a factor. A relationship to rickets is doubtful. Infection may have an influence. Disturbance of internal secretion, perhaps of the ovary, may be responsible. The onset is usually between the age of twenty and thirty. The bones are soft and show decalcification and new formation of uncalcified tissue. The earliest *symptom* is pain, especially in the back and sacral regions, increased by movement. Weakness is marked and there may be stiffness with contractures. The gait may be uncertain, sometimes spastic. The bony deformity is usually first in the spine or pelvis. Later there is marked deformity with fractures, callus formation and muscular wasting. The course is usually over some years and death may result from exhaustion or a terminal infection. The early *diagnosis* is difficult and may only be made when deformities appear. The blood calcium is not increased. The X-rays are of value. In *treatment*, phosphorus in oil should be given (gr. 1/20, 0.003 gm.). Calcium should be given as the lactate. Vitamins A and D are given freely and a varied diet with abundance of milk. The removal of the ovaries has been useful. Heliotherapy may be helpful. Proper treatment for the symptoms should be given.

ACHONDROPLASIA (*Chondrodystrophia Fetalis*)

Definition.—A dystrophy of the epiphyseal cartilages due to connective tissue invasion from the periosteum, in consequence of which the epiphyses and diaphyses are prematurely united and there is failure of the normal growth of the long bones. In consequence the subjects become dwarfs with normal heads and trunks, but short, stumpy extremities.

Description.—Achondroplasic dwarfs are easily recognized. They are well nourished and strong, and of average intelligence. Their height varies from 3 to 4 feet; the head and trunk are of about normal size, but the extremities are very short, the fingers, when the arms are at the sides, reaching little below the crest of the ilium. The important point is that in the shortness of the limbs it is the proximal segments which are specially involved, the humerus and femur being even shorter than the ulna and tibia (rhizomelia). The limbs are considerably bent, but this is more an exaggeration of normal curves and abnormalities in the joints than pathological curves. The features of rickets are absent. The hand is short, and has a trident shape, since the fingers, which are of almost equal length, often diverge somewhat. The root of the nose is depressed, the back flat, and the lumbar lordosis abnormally deep, owing to a tilting forward of the sacrum. The scapulae are short, the fibulae longer than the tibiae, and the pelvis is contracted; hence, the number of these cases reported by obstetricians. Heredity plays some part.

Pathology.—Virchow described the disease as fetal cretinism, others as fetal rickets. Of late it has been associated with disturbance of the pituitary function or of its hormonic relations. Jansen suggested that it results from a disturbance of the amniotic pressure, and brings it into relationship with other fetal malformations. An argument in favor of some endocrine disturbance is that achondroplasics often show precocious sexual development.

HEREDITARY DEFORMING CHONDRODYSPLASIA

Given also the designation *multiple cartilaginous exostoses*, the disease is characterized by multiple, usually symmetrical, cartilaginous or osteocartilaginous growths, generally benign, which result from proliferation and ossification of bone-forming cartilage, and cause bony deformities. The disease is hereditary in many instances; in one family there were 26 cases in four generations. The American cases were collected by Ehrenfried, who found that males were more often affected (3 to 1). The changes begin in infancy or early childhood, increase with skeletal growth and cease about the age of 22 years. The height is often less than normal. There are "irregular juxta-epiphyseal hyperostoses" most marked at the hips, knees, ankles, shoulders and wrists. There is often knock-knee and pes valgus, and the ulna may be relatively shortened. There may be symptoms due to pressure of the exostoses on nerves or vessels. Removal of the exostoses is indicated if they cause troublesome symptoms.

OXYCEPHALY

Definition.—A cranial deformity associated with exophthalmos and impairment of vision.

Description.—The condition, known as *tower* or *steeplehead,* is characterized by great height of the forehead, sloping to a pointed vertex, with feebly marked supra-orbital ridges, and the hairy scalp may be raised above the normal level, looking as if perched on the top of a comb. The intelligence is unimpaired. The condition is usually present at birth, though in some instances it develops from the second to the sixth year. As this curious growth of the head proceeds, headache may be present, exophthalmos develops, and the vision becomes impaired, due to progressive *optic atrophy*. Smell is often completely lost. The deformity appears to be due to premature synostosis of certain sutures, notably the sagittal and coronal, so that the growth of the vault of the skull is restricted in both its anteroposterior and transverse diameters. To accommodate the increasing bulk of the brain a compensatory increase in height takes place. Eventually the anterior fontanelle closes, but there is reason to think that this occurs at a later date than normal, and its former site is marked by a slight protuberance with thinning of the bone.

The optic neuritis and atrophy result from pressure exerted by the growing brain and may be compared to that of cerebral tumor. The cause of this premature synostosis is not known. Rickets and syphilis are not responsible. The condition is one for which a decompression operation with ventricular puncture is indicated.

HEREDITARY CLEIDOCRANIAL DYSOSTOSIS

This is a familial and hereditary disease in which the skull is large and the fontanelles and sutures close late. There may be enlargement of the large fontanelle. There are prominent cranial bosses. The clavicles are defective, the acromial end usually being absent. There may be pseudo-arthrosis or absence of a part or the whole of the clavicles. The mobility of the shoulders is increased and they can be made to meet under the chin. Many patients show genu valgum, hereditary and familial, transferred through either parent.

MISCELLANEOUS AFFECTIONS

Albers-Schönberg Disease (*Marble Bones*).—This is characterized by extremely dense changes in the bones. Associated features are a marked anemia (perhaps due to diminution of the medullary spaces), enlargement of the liver and spleen, pressure on the cranial nerves with optic atrophy, nystagmus, hydrocephalus and necrosis of the jaw.

Spondylolisthesis.—In this there is a forward subluxation of the fifth, occasionally the fourth, lumbar vertebra. Congenital defects, a long sacralized transverse process and sacro-iliac disease may contribute but trauma is usually the determining factor. There is backache, usually relieved by rest, and some stiffness on movement. The trunk is shortened, the upper posterior border of the sacrum is prominent, one side of the pelvis is usually higher and there is lumbar lordosis. There may be restriction of bending movements. With caudal involvement there are pain and disturbed sensations in the sciatic distribution of one or both sides and occasionally sensory changes and alteration of the deep reflexes. The X-ray study is important in diagnosis. In *treatment* some stabilizing operation may be indicated.

Compression Fractures of the Spine.—These comprise nearly half the spinal fractures and are caused by forced hyperflexion of the spine. Usually the body of the vertebra only is concerned and the majority are in the lower thoracic or lumbar regions. The picture varies in early and late stages. (1) *Early stage.* There is pain and limitation of movement in the region of the lesion with tenderness over the spine of the injured vertebra, which may be prominent. Neurological signs are few and paralysis is rare. (2) *Late stage* (Kummell's Disease). After the initial injury there may be a period with no symptoms followed, perhaps months later, by pain and an angular kyphosis. In *diagnosis,* the X-ray study is important but demands care in interpreting the films. In *treatment* fixation may be sufficient or operation may be required.

Morquio's disease is a familial osseous dystrophy with some characteristics of achondroplasia. The bones show deformity, rarefaction and delay in development. In the cases reported by Davis and Currier (1934) there were extensive changes in the skull with optic atrophy and cerebral disturbance but these are unusual. The children are healthy at birth and for the first year. The trunk is symmetrical but the extremities are deformed.

Hereditary Arthrodysplasia and Dystrophy of the Nails.—In a study of two families, Turner (1933) found 35 of 79 members affected. There are changes in bones and joints, especially the apparent absence of the patella, which may be rudimentary and displaced, and congenital dislocation of the head of the radius. The nails may be almost completely absent or be very thin. The dystrophy of the nails may be present in members of these families without any joint abnormality.

Arachnodactyly.—This was described by Marfan in 1896 as "pieds d'araigne" or spider feet and named by Achard in 1902. There is an abnormal increase in the length of the bones, especially of the hands and feet, with laxity of the joint ligaments and general dystrophy of the muscles without paralysis. The bones appear normal in the X-ray studies. The cause is not known.

Hypertelorism.—Described and named by Grieg in 1924, this is a developmental congenital anomaly of the lesser wings of the sphenoid bone. There is a familial tendency. Due to excessive growth the orbits are widely separated, giving a "fetal facies." Mental deficiency may be associated.

INDEX

A

B

C

D

E

G

I

J

K

M

N

O

P

Q

R

S

T

U

X

Y

Z